Occupational Therapy in Mental Health

A Vision for Participation

Occupational Therapy in Mental Health

A Vision for Participation

Editors:

Catana Brown, PhD, OTR, FAOTA
Associate Professor
School of Occupational Therapy
Touro University–Nevada
Las Vegas, Nevada

Virginia C. Stoffel, PhD, OT, BCMH, FAOTA
Chair, Associate Professor
University of Wisconsin–Milwaukee
College of Health Sciences
Department of Occupational Therapy
Milwaukee, Wisconsin

Associate Editor:

Jaime Phillip Muñoz, PhD, OTR/L, FAOTA
Associate Professor
Department of Occupational Therapy
Duquesne University
Pittsburgh, Pennsylvania

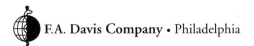 F.A. Davis Company • Philadelphia

F. A. Davis Company
1915 Arch Street
Philadelphia, PA 19103
www.fadavis.com

Printed in the United States of America

Last digit indicates print number: 10 9 8 7

Senior Acquisitions Editor: Christa A. Fratantoro
Manager of Content Development: George W. Lang
Developmental Editor: Nancy Peterson
Art and Design Manager: Carolyn O'Brien

As new scientific information becomes available through basic and clinical research, recommended treatments and drug therapies undergo changes. The author(s) and publisher have done everything possible to make this book accurate, up to date, and in accord with accepted standards at the time of publication. The author(s), editors, and publisher are not responsible for errors or omissions or for consequences from application of the book, and make no warranty, expressed or implied, in regard to the contents of the book. Any practice described in this book should be applied by the reader in accordance with professional standards of care used in regard to the unique circumstances that may apply in each situation. The reader is advised always to check product information (package inserts) for changes and new information regarding dose and contraindications before administering any drug. Caution is especially urged when using new or infrequently ordered drugs.

Library of Congress Cataloging-in-Publication Data

Occupational therapy in mental health: a vision for participation/editors, Catana Brown, Virginia C. Stoffel; associate editor, Jaime Phillip Munoz.
   p. ; cm.
   Includes bibliographical references and index.
   ISBN-13: 978-0-8036-1704-9
   ISBN-10: 0-8036-1704-6
  1. Occupational therapy. 2. Mentally ill—Rehabilitation. I. Brown, Catana. II. Stoffel, Virginia C. III. Munoz, Jaime Phillip.
   [DNLM: 1. Mental Disorders—therapy. 2. Occupational Therapy—methods. 3. Patient Participation.   WM 450.5.02 0148 2011]
   RC487.0252 2011
   616.89'165—dc22
                                                                                          2010008001

To Alan

—TB

To Bob

—GS

Foreword

This is a text we have all been waiting for—a contemporary occupational performance, client-centered, and evidence-based approach to occupational therapy in mental health. People, regardless of their diagnosis, are individuals with roles, goals, hopes, and aspirations to live life to the fullest. Mental illness touches each of us. It is so prevalent today, with problems ranging from developmental disabilities and autism to eating and substance-related disorders, from personality and mood disorders to schizophrenia. People we know and love have these conditions, and they require the knowledge and skills that occupational therapists and occupational therapy assistants can provide to help them manage their condition in home, family, work, and community activities. The overall objective of occupational therapy is to enable participation, and that is the focus of this book.

The editors and chapter contributors have employed a contemporary approach to their effort by organizing the text with a person-environment-occupation approach; such an approach situates the book in most contemporary models being developed in occupational therapy today. They want the learner to understand the lived experience of people with mental illness and have used a very personal and innovative approach called PhotoVoice, using narratives of persons with mental illness to give the reader lived experiences. They also use first-person narratives written by people with mental illness or their family members or service providers. They use Evidence-Based Practice boxes to support the practice of occupational therapy. These approaches support a very personal level of learning and are actually a gift to the profession, as we are being called upon to support the health and participation of all our citizens and to do it using evidence that will direct resources to approaches known to be effective.

This book advances the practice of occupational therapy, reframing much of practice from group skill training to a life skill and occupational approach that fosters participation. It also integrates knowledge from the behavioral, environmental, and occupational sciences.

I can't finish this foreword without saying a few words about the editors. Tana Brown and Ginny Stoffel have dedicated their careers to a vision of occupational therapy as a far-reaching helping science that, within its practice guidelines, can be shaped and applied to benefit people in new ways and in broader areas of need. This textbook is a result of their vision. They are both passionate about their profession and about the people who will benefit from the knowledge they have compiled. I can't help but think that our earlier leaders in mental health—Dr. Adolph Meyer, Dr. William Dutton, and Eleanor Clark Slagle, to name a few—who knew the power of occupation and stressed the importance of engagement in an enabling environment, would be pleased to see this work come to a format that would guide clinicians to make a difference in the everyday lives of people with mental challenges who require the skills of an occupational therapist. This book should be required reading for all occupational therapists who work with people experiencing vulnerabilities due to health and situational circumstances.

Carolyn Baum, PhD, OTR/L, FAOTA
Professor of Occupational Therapy
and Neurology
Washington University School of Medicine
St. Louis, Missouri

Preface

Occupational therapy has its roots in mental health practice, with its founders including individuals who worked in psychiatry at the prestigious Johns Hopkins Hospital and Sheppard and Enoch Pratt Hospitals. However, the role of occupational therapy as a health care and service profession is broad in scope. Occupational therapists work with individuals and populations with both physical and psychiatric disabilities, as well as individuals without disabilities who struggle with occupational performance problems. All age groups, from newborns to older adults, and a variety of settings, including medical, educational, community, and industry, are served by occupational therapists.

Mental health occupational therapy is one important area of specialized practice, and occupational therapists who work primarily as mental health practitioners must acquire specific knowledge and abilities. Yet an appreciation for the *whole* person, which includes mental health issues, is so integral to our practice that it is essential for occupational therapists in all practice areas to develop competencies associated with mental health practice. It is safe to assume that all people deal with mental health issues at some point in their lives and that individuals who have challenges related to occupational performance will almost certainly experience mental health concerns, be it anxiety, depression, ineffective coping, or some other challenge.

Participation is the primary goal of occupational therapy; that is, occupational therapists work to support individuals in their efforts to engage in all aspects of everyday life. This textbook strives to be visionary in providing established as well as newly emerging practices for occupational therapists working in mental health, hence the title *Occupational Therapy in Mental Health: A Vision for Participation.*

This comprehensive textbook provides both a breadth and depth of information related to mental health practices. There is content presented in this text that is essential for all occupational therapists regardless of practice area, as well as more specific information relevant to occupational therapists who specialize in mental health practice. This text is primarily intended for entry-level occupational therapy students, but it is also a useful reference book for practicing therapists. As occupational therapy curricula vary greatly, the comprehensive nature of the text and its intuitive organizational structure make it applicable across multiple occupational therapy courses, including courses with a focus on mental health and those organized around specific client factors, areas of occupation, and environments.

As an edited text, *Occupational Therapy in Mental Health: A Vision for Participation* utilizes experts within the field to author chapters on their particular area of expertise. The numerous contributors and the breadth of the text resulted in several areas in which significant and relevant content for occupational therapy is published for the first time. In addition, the contributors come from six different countries, including the United States, Canada, Australia, China, England, and Sweden. The international authorship offers a broader point of view of occupational therapy in mental health.

Guiding Principles

Several philosophical principles guide the tone and content of the book:

- The person-environment-occupation model is used as the organizing structure for the text. Each is examined in a comprehensive manner to ensure that the learner will have a strong grounding in client-centered, occupation-based practices that promote full participation in the everyday lives of persons with mental illness and others struggling with psychosocial issues.
- The lived experience of mental illness and recovery is highlighted so that the learner develops a full appreciation for the real people who will be future recipients of occupational therapy services. Recognition of the whole person—the individual's state of physical, emotional, spiritual, and mental health—and the need to address co-occurring conditions are emphasized.
- Occupational therapy interventions are grounded theoretically and in the evidence based on occupational therapy and mental health literature.
- Active learning strategies are incorporated into the text to emphasize self-reflection and the experiential application of learning. The reflective nature of these activities is useful for promoting the development of therapeutic engagement as a skill.
- The text utilizes a client-centered, optimistic, recovery-oriented perspective that empowers clients to be in control of their own lives and therapists to recognize their unique contribution in promoting full participation in daily life.

Organization Using the Person-Environment-Occupation Framework

Occupational Therapy in Mental Health: A Vision for Participation is organized around the person-environment-occupation (PEO) model. There are several conceptual models in occupational therapy that we could have selected, but the PEO model was chosen for its simple but all encompassing structure. This does not mean that PEO is the only model used in this textbook; many other models are described and referenced throughout the text when relevant. The model works well as a framework for the text because it addresses the full practice domain of occupational therapy in mental health and gives equal attention to person, occupation, and environment factors. The text is divided into four parts:

Part 1 Foundations
Part 2 The Person
Part 3 Environment
Part 4 Occupation

Part 1: Foundations

The introductory section provides information on overarching issues in mental health occupational therapy. The first chapter, on recovery, sets the tone for the text by acknowledging the expertise and point of view of the individual with mental illness. In addition, the recovery model promotes optimism and hope that individuals with psychiatric disabilities can achieve their occupational wants and needs. Other chapters in Part 1 provide further perspective and background for mental health occupational therapy practice that is (1) person centered, (2) occupation based, (3) grounded in theory, (4) supported by evidence, and (5) cognizant of the historical roots of occupational therapy in mental health.

Part 2: The Person

Part 2 is further divided into "Diagnosis" and "Client Factors" sections. It is important for occupational therapists to thoroughly understand the conditions of the individuals with whom they work. Therefore, major psychiatric diagnoses are presented with a focus on symptoms, etiology, medications, and impact on occupational performance. Although occupational therapy practice is not driven by symptomatology, practitioners can better understand the experience of the individual with a mental illness if they are aware of symptoms the person may be experiencing. In addition, a working knowledge of psychiatric diagnoses is useful when participating on a multidisciplinary treatment team.

Because occupational therapy assessment and intervention are not based on diagnosis, the chapters in Part 2 include minimal information on assessment and intervention. More thorough explanations are included in other chapters of the text, with equal attention given to assessment and intervention targeting client factors, environments, and occupations. For easy reference, see the Index of Assessments and Index of Interventions.

The "Client Factors" section addresses skills and abilities that are important for occupational performance. These chapters provide detailed content about the skills addressed, theories related to those skills, and specific information on particular diagnoses associated with impairments in those skill areas.

Part 3: Environment

Part 3 is also divided into two sections: "Lived Environment" and "Practice Settings." Although recognized as important by occupational therapists, the environmental component of the PEO model has received the least attention. The "Lived Environment" section of the text aims to correct this neglect by providing the mental health practitioner with (1) an explicit understanding of the environment and its impact on occupational performance, (2) specific environmental

assessments, and (3) interventions aimed at creating a supportive environment.

The "Practice Setting" section is devoted to the places that occupational therapists work, including settings with either a primary or secondary focus on mental health practice. Some of these settings are emerging areas of practice that have received little attention in previous texts. Each chapter includes a general description of the setting with information on the needs of the population served. The role of occupational therapy is discussed, including assessments and interventions common to those settings.

Part 4: Occupation

Few occupational therapy texts attempt to comprehensively address areas of occupational performance. This part of the text covers the more familiar occupations of work, self-care, and leisure, along with some areas of occupation that have been neglected, such as sleep and spirituality. Attention is paid to the character or purpose of different occupations across the lifespan. Many of these chapters include descriptions of specific assessments and intervention models and techniques.

Special Features

Educators and students alike find special features to be useful in helping the learner comprehend and retain new information as well as envision how it will apply to practice. *Occupational Therapy in Mental Health: A Vision for Participation* includes several unique features:

PhotoVoice

This feature includes photographs with accompanying narratives that utilize the PhotoVoice methodology. PhotoVoice was developed by Caroline C. Wang and Mary Ann Burris as a means for marginalized people to have their voices heard. Its goal is social action and influence. PhotoVoice follows a particular structure in which the group involved in the project identifies a particular mission or message to convey, brainstorms about images, takes photographs, and discusses the significance of the photos. Then, the person who took the photo writes a narrative that describes its meaning.

The PhotoVoice methodology typically involves identifying a target audience. In this case, the audience is the reader of this textbook. Each of the editors of the text held separate PhotoVoice groups with individuals with mental illness. The purpose was to collect photos and narratives that convey the content of the text from the perspective of the individuals with the lived experience of mental illness. This was a powerful experience that goes far beyond the confines of this text; however, we hope readers will find the PhotoVoice features particularly useful to illustrate the rich information we can accumulate when we listen to the people we serve as occupational therapists.

The Lived Experience

First-person narratives reflect the chapters' major concepts and allow the reader to gain an understanding of the lived experience. We have taken care to maintain each writer's unique voice. Most of these narratives are written by individuals with a psychiatric disability, but a few are written by family members or service providers. In some cases, an interview was conducted to help the individual tell his or her story. The Lived Experience and PhotoVoice features reinforce the importance of the person-first, client-centered philosophy of the book.

Evidence-Based Practice

Although research evidence is an important component of each chapter, evidence is also highlighted in Evidence-Based Practice boxes. A primary purpose of this feature is to distill important research in a particular content area with specific applications to occupational therapy practice. Each box uses a standard format in which the evidence is cited, followed by a bulleted list of implications for practice, and then the full reference. The research is drawn from the occupational therapy literature as well as the larger interdisciplinary mental health literature.

Active Learning Strategies and Reflective Journal Prompts

When using this textbook within a course, students are encouraged to start a Reflective Journal. The Reflective Journal is a separate notebook used to record individual impressions, reactions, and insights gained from the learning experience. Each chapter includes one or more experiential activities that promote active learning of concepts within the chapter. In many cases, the activity involves developing an appreciation for the lived experiences of people with mental illness. In others, the reader has the opportunity to engage in an assessment or intervention experience. Many activities are followed by a set of reflective questions, which is where the Reflective Journal comes in. The student can use these questions or others developed by the instructor to help personalize and process the experience. The questions are intended to enhance the reader's understanding of the chapter and facilitate the synthesis of applicable person, environment, and occupation concepts. The journals also provide a means of preparation by which the students can more meaningfully engage in a discussion around the content of the chapter.

Resources

Most chapters includes information on resources that the student and instructor can use to augment the text and utilize in practice. Examples of resources include books, assessment or intervention manuals, videos, and websites.

A Note About the Cover

The image chosen for the cover is significant as well as beautiful: During an art group meeting at Spectrum, a community meeting place of consumers, Cherie Bledsoe did a finger painting. She was about to throw it in the trash, but Jan Kobe, the art teacher, saw its potential and the images emerging from it. Jan claimed it for the Art Coalition to salvage and complete, using a Monet-like impressionist theme. The Art Coalition finished the painting, adding a pond, flowers, and swans. Due to the quality of the work, it was chosen for the "Sunshine from Darkness" exhibit in 2008. The painting reflects reclaiming quality of life after the losses of mental illness and the rebirth of regained skills and recovery. Contributors: Cherie Bledsoe, Ella Devosha, Jan Kobe, and the Art Coalition of Painters.

Closing Thoughts

Many experts in the field, both occupational therapists and people with mental illness, have come together to create this work. In doing so, these individuals have created the most comprehensive occupational therapy in mental health textbook available. It is our desire that the reader finds the information accessible and useful for occupational therapy practice, but perhaps more important, that the vision of the book is realized. Our hope is that this text contributes to the revitalization of occupational therapy practice in mental health and that the profession plays a significant role in supporting participation in everyday life for those people with psychiatric disabilities.

Contributors

Katie C. Alexander, MS, OTR
Program Development Consultant
The Model Asperger Program
The Ivymount School, Inc.
Rockville, Maryland

Cherie Bledsoe
Executive Director
S.I.D.E. Inc.
Kansas City, KS

Charles Christiansen, EdD, OTR, OT(C), FAOTA
Executive Director
American Occupational Therapy Foundation
Bethesda, Maryland

Patricia Crist, PhD, OTR, FAOTA
Chairperson and Professor
Department of Occupational Therapy
John G. Rangos Sr. School of Health Sciences
Duquesne University
Pittsburgh, Pennsylvania

Jeanenne Dallas, MA, OTR/L, CPRP
Instructor and Academic Fieldwork Coordinator
Program in Occupational Therapy
Washington University
St. Louis, Missouri

Noralyn Davel Pickens, PhD, OT
Assistant Professor
School of Occupational Therapy
Texas Woman's University
Dallas, Texas

Janis Davis, PhD, OTR/L
Associate Professor
Department of Occupational Therapy
Dominican University of California
San Rafael, California

Frank P. Deane, PhD, BS., MSc, Clinical Psychology Diploma
School of Psychology and Illawarra Institute for Mental Health
University of Wollongong
Australia

Mary Egan, PhD, OT Reg. (Ont.), FCAOT
Associate Professor
School of Rehabilitation Sciences
University of Ottawa
Ottawa, Ontario, Canada

Mona Eklund, PhD, Reg OT
Professor
Department of Health Sciences
Division of Occupational Therapy and Gerontology
Lund University
Lund, Sweden

Joyce M. Engel, PhD, OTR, FAOTA
Professor and Program Director
University of Wisconsin–Milwaukee
College of Health Sciences
Department of Occupational Therapy
Milwaukee, Wisconsin

Pamela Erdman, MS, OTR
Quality Assurance Director
Wraparound Milwaukee Program
Milwaukee, Wisconsin

S. Megan Exley, MOT, OTR/L
Occupational Therapist
Landmark Home Health Care
Pittsburgh, Pennsylvania

Judith Gonyea, OTD, MSEd, OTR/L
Assistant Professor
Occupational Therapy Department
Ithaca College
Ithaca, New York

Sharon A. Gutman, PhD, OTR, FAOTA
Associate Professor
Programs in Occupational Therapy
Columbia University
New York, New York

Kristine Haertl, PhD, OTR/L
Associate Professor
Department of Occupational Science and Occupational Therapy
St. Catherine University
St. Paul, Minnesota

Carol Haertlein Sells, PhD, OTR, FAOTA
Professor, Occupational Therapy
University of Wisconsin–Milwaukee
College of Health Sciences
Department of Occupational Therapy
Milwaukee, Wisconsin

Carole Hays, MA, OTR/L, FAOTA
Director of Rehabilitation Services
Springfield Hospital Center
Sykesville, Maryland

Christine A. Helfrich, PhD, OTR/L, FAOTA
Assistant Professor
Department of Occupational Therapy
Boston University
Boston, Massachusetts

Alexis D. Henry, ScD, OTR/L, FAOTA
Senior Research Scientist
Center for Health Policy and Research
University of Massachusetts Medical School
Shrewsbury, Massachusetts

Brian Holmquist, MOT, OTR
Lead Occupational Therapist
Child and Adolescent Psychiatry Program
Madison, Wisconsin

Valerie Howells, PhD, OTR
Professor
School of Health Sciences, Occupational Therapy
    Program
Eastern Michigan University
Ypsilanti, Michigan

Barbara Jacobs, MS, OT
Clinical Associate Professor, Retired
University of Wisconsin–Milwaukee
Milwaukee, Wisconsin

Vaune Kopeck, OTR/L
Senior Occupational Therapist
Mann Residential Treatment Center
Sheppard Pratt Health System
Baltimore, Maryland

Terry Krupa, PhD, MEd, OT Reg. (Ont.)
Associate Professor
School of Rehabilitation Therapy
Queen's University
Kingston, Ontario, Canada

Chris Lloyd, PhD
Senior Occupational Therapist
Homeless Health Outreach Team
Ashmore City, Queensland
Australia

Laura C. Lock, Dip. COT, SROT
Head Occupational Therapist
St. George's Eating Disorders Service and Chair
    of the College of Occupational Therapists Specialist
    Section–Mental Health
Special Interest Group in Eating Disorders
London, United Kingdom

Lisa Mahaffey, MS, OTR/L
Assistant Professor
Occupational Therapy-Downers Grove
Midwestern University
Downers Grove, Illinois

Deane B. McCraith, MS, OT/L, LMFT
Clinical Associate Professor, Retired
Department of Occupational Therapy
Boston University College of Health and Rehabilitation
    Sciences: Sargent College
Boston, Massachusetts

Ann E. McDonald, PhD, OTR/L, SWC
Pediatric Occupational Therapist
Private Practice: (EI/MH/SS)
Sierra Madre, California

M. Beth Merryman, PhD, OTR/L
Associate Professor
Department of Occupational Therapy
    and Occupational Science
Towson University
Towson, Maryland

Penelope A. Moyers, EdD, OTR/L, BCMH,
FAOTA
Professor and Chair
Department of Occupational Therapy
University of Alabama at Birmingham
Birmingham, Alabama

Jaime Phillip Muñoz, PhD, OTR/L, FAOTA
Associate Professor
Department of Occupational Therapy
Duquesne University
Pittsburgh, Pennsylvania

Rebecca S. Baker Nicholson, MS Ed, OTR/L
Clinical Assistant Professor
Occupational Therapy Education
University of Kansas Medical Center
Kansas City, Kansas

Geneviève Pépin, PhD
Senior Lecturer
Occupational Science and Therapy
School of Health and Social Development
Deakin University
Victoria, Australia

Christine Peters, PhD, OTR/L
Chairperson and Clinical Associate Professor
Occupational Therapy Program
Stony Brook University
Stony Brook, New York

Suzette Phillips, PhD, OT
Mental Health Therapist
Alberta Health Services
Camrose Mental Health Clinic
Camrose, Alberta, Canada and Lecturer
Saint Paul University
Ottawa, Ontario, Canada
Newman Theological College
Edmonton, Alberta, Canada
University of Alberta
Edmonton & Camrose, Alberta, Canada

Doris Pierce, PhD, OTR/L, FAOTA
Endowed Chair in Occupational Therapy
Eastern Kentucky University
Richmond, Kentucky

Deborah B. Pitts, PhD (cand.), MBA, OTR/L,
BCMH, CPRP
Clinical Faculty
Division of Occupational Science and Occupational
Therapy
University of Southern California
Los Angeles, California

Kris Pizur-Barnekow, PhD, OTR/L
Assistant Professor
University of Illinois at Chicago
College of Applied Health Science
Department of Occupational Therapy
Chicago, Illinois

Heidi Plach, MS, OTR
Clinical Instructor
University of Wisconsin–Milwaukee
College of Health Sciences
Department of Occupational Therapy
Milwaukee, Wisconsin

Karen L. Rebeiro Gruhl, MScOT, OT Reg (Ont)
PhD Candidate, School of Rural and Northern Health
Laurentian University,
Sudbury, Ontario
Canada

Patricia Schaber, PhD, OTR/L
Assistant Professor
Program in Occupational Therapy
University of Minnesota
Minneapolis, Minnesota

Marian K. Scheinholtz, MS, OT/L
Public Health Advisor
Substance Abuse and Mental Health Services
Administration (SAMHSA)
Rockville, Maryland

Victoria P. Schindler, PhD, OTR, BCMH, FAOTA
Associate Professor of Occupational Therapy
Master of Science in Occupational Therapy Program
Richard Stockton College of New Jersey
Pomona, New Jersey

Emily Schulz, PhD, OTR, CFLE
Associate Professor
Arizona School of Health Sciences
Occupational Therapy Program
Mesa, Arizona

Andrew M. H. Siu, PhD
Assistant Professor
Department of Rehabilitation Sciences
Hong Kong Polytechnic University
Hunghom, Kowloon,
Hong Kong Sar, China

Nancy Spangler, MS, OTR/L
President, Spangler Associates, Inc.
Leawood, Kansas
Consultant to the Partnership for Workplace Mental Health
Arlington, Virginia

Susan Strong, MSc (DME), BSc, OT Reg (Ont)
Coordinator of Program Evaluation
Schizophrenia & Community Integration Service
St Joseph's Healthcare and Associate Clinical Professor
(PT), School of Rehabilitation Science
McMaster University
Hamilton, Ontario, Canada

Karen Summers, MS, OTR/L
Doctoral Student in Rehabilitation Sciences
University of Kentucky
Lexington, Kentucky and Occupational Therapist for
Model Laboratory School
Eastern Kentucky University
Richmond, Kentucky

Margaret (Peggy) Swarbrick, PhD, OTR,
CPRP
Assistant Professor
University of Medicine and Dentistry of New Jersey
School of Health Related Professions
Department of Psychiatric Rehabilitation and Counseling
Professions and Director of the Institute for Wellness
and Recovery Initiatives
Collaborative Support Programs of New Jersey
Clifton, New Jersey

C. Annette Thompson, MS, OTR/L
Director of Rehabilitation Services
Springfield Hospital Center
Sykesville, Maryland

Jeffrey Tomlinson, OTR, MSW, FAOTA
Washington Heights Community Service
New York, New York

Hector W.H. Tsang, PhD, TOR
Associate Professor and Occupational Therapy Program
Director
Department of Rehabilitation Sciences
Hong Kong Polytechnic University
Hong Kong

Christine Urish, PhD, OTR/L, BCMH, FAOTA
Occupational Therapist, Board Certified in Mental
Health
Professor of Occupational Therapy
St. Ambrose University
Davenport, Iowa

Reviewers

Nancy E. Carson, MHS, OTR/L
Assistant Professor
Occupational Therapy
Medical University of South Carolina
Charleston, South Carolina

Mariana D'Amico, EdD, OTR/L, BCP
Assistant Professor
Occupational Therapy
Medical College of Georgia
Augusta, Georgia

Priscilla Ennals, MOT, BAppSci OT, BCouns
Lecturer
Occupational Therapy
La Trobe University
Brunswick, Australia

Ellie Fossey, MSc, DipCOT, AccOT
Lecturer and MOT Course Coordinator
School of Occupational Therapy
La Trobe University
Brunswick, Australia

Robert W. Gibson, PhD, MS, OTR/L
Associate Professor
Occupational Therapy
Medical College of Georgia
Augusta, Georgia

Liane Hewitt, PhD, OTR/L
Associate Professor
Occupational Therapy
Loma Linda University
Loma Linda, California

Joanne T. Jeffcoat, OTR/L, MEd
Professor, Fieldwork Coordinator
Occupational Therapy Assistant
Community College of Allegheny County
Monroeville, Pennsylvania

Kathryn M. Loukas, MS, OTR/L, FAOTA
Associate Clinical Professor
Occupational Therapy
University of New England
Portland, Maine

MaryBeth Merryman, PhD, OTR/L
Associate Professor
Occupational Therapy & Occupational Science
Towson University
Towson, Maryland

Jaime P. Muñoz, PhD, OTR/L, FAOTA
Assistant Professor
Occupational Therapy
Duquesne University
Pittsburgh, Pennsylvania

Ann H. Nolen, PsyD, OTR
Chair, Associate Professor
Occupational Therapy
University of Tennessee Health Science Center
Memphis, Tennessee

Jane O'Brien, PhD, OTR/L
Associate Professor
Occupational Therapy
University of New England
Portland, Maine

Christine Peters, PhD, OTR/L
Associate Professor
Occupational Therapy
Pacific University
Hillsboro, Oregon

Regi Robnett, PhD, OTR/L
Director, Associate Professor
Occupational Therapy
University of New England
Portland, Maine

Janeene C. Sibla, OTD, MS, OTR/L
Program Director and Associate Professor
Occupational Therapy
University of Mary
Bismarck, North Dakota

Margaret Swarbrick, PhD, OTR, CPRP
Director
Institute for Wellness and Recovery Initiatives
Collaborative Support Programs of New Jersey
Freehold, New Jersey

Mary P. Taugher, PhD, OT, FAOTA
Assistant Professor (Retired), Ad Hoc Instructor
Occupational Therapy
University of Wisconsin–Milwaukee
Milwaukee, Wisconsin

Janet H. Watts, PhD, OTR
Emeritus Associate Professor
Occupational Therapy
Virginia Commonwealth University
Richmond, Virginia

Marla J. Wonser, MS, OT, OTR/L
Program Director
Occupational Therapy Assistant
Casper College
Casper, Wyoming

Acknowledgments

When we embarked on the journey to create this text, little did we know how many people would contribute to and shape this book. We had a vision about what we wanted to create, and we were open and willing to learn from each step of the process. We first want to thank our publisher, F.A. Davis, for giving us the support and guidance to create a product that required time, careful review and development, and the inclusion of many voices to convey the vibrant opportunities that support occupational therapy mental health practice.

Christa Fratantoro, the acquisitions editor who kept us afloat and upbeat as we engaged one author after another, chapter by chapter; Elizabeth Y. Stepchin, who worked behind the scenes to set up conference calls, send chapters out for review, convey documents to and from the many authors and reviewers; and Nancy Peterson, our developmental editor, who truly joined with us in our aspirations for this text and was instrumental in the marathon of getting chapters analyzed, edited, and fully developed while gently checking in around deadlines—their professionalism and commitment to the quality of this project never wavered, and we are grateful to them for their legacy of quality publishing practices.

We particularly want to acknowledge the contributions of Jaime Muñoz, who authored several chapters and joined us as an associate editor in the final phase of the editing process. Jaime's deep understanding of occupational therapy mental health practice, his cultural insights and experiences, and his expertise as an educator were invaluable in providing finishing touches to a significant number of chapters. We are also grateful that he was willing to author the instructor resources, which we hope will provide best practices in occupational therapy education.

We acknowledge the authors who shared their professional knowledge, resources, and stories and who invited the first-person narrative writers so that each chapter would speak to the reader with the clear perspective of the lived experience of mental illness and recovery. We appreciate our team of PhotoVoice participants, whose visual images and narratives in the text provide another way of understanding and celebrating their personal wisdom and insights. PhotoVoice participants include Cindy-Sue, Caroline, Marty, Barbara, Henry, Willard, Doug, Judith, Brian, Neil, Marsha, and Bruce from Transitional Living Services and the Grand Avenue Club in Milwaukee and Willetta, Jan, Jill, Bobby, Betty, Dennis, Viola, Mary, Glen, Janet, Barbara, Sterling, Grady, Helen, and Marca from the Wyandot Center in Kansas City, Kansas.

Additional photographs that help to capture real people in real life were submitted from a number of sources. We thank the individuals who submitted photographs as well as those who are pictured. In particular, we thank the Northern Initiative for Social Action, a consumer-driven, occupationally oriented program in Sudbury, Ontario, Canada; S.I.D.E., a consumer-run organization in Kansas City, Kansas; Jeannine Dallas, Virginia Leeson, Jaime Muñoz, Kristi Haertl, Art Hsieh, and Al Chernov.

We are grateful that we were able to engage authors from across the United States as well as our occupational therapy colleagues from around the world. We know that the practice of mental health occupational therapy globally reflects the varied health and social service systems of their respective countries and hope that we continue to share and enrich our global and cultural understanding.

We acknowledge the support of our colleagues at Kansas University Medical Center, the University of Wisconsin–Milwaukee, and Touro University–Nevada. We acknowledge the contributions of several graduate students who contributed to this project, especially Yeojin Choi, who assembled the glossary from all 55 chapters; Rebecca Barbosa, Hannah Miller, and Heidi Plach, who all assisted in facilitating PhotoVoice Workshops at Transitional Living Services and Mental Health America of Wisconsin; and Teresa Vente, who helped assemble the assessment and intervention indices. We acknowledge the training in PhotoVoice that we received from Sasha Bowers at the very start of the process, in September 2005, and Jan Kobe, who helped lead the PhotoVoice project at the Wyandot Center.

We acknowledge the occupational therapy educators and clinicians who carefully reviewed each chapter and whose comments helped improve and enrich the focus and content of each chapter. They were integral to the development of the text over time, and we appreciate their enthusiastic response to many of the features in the text.

We acknowledge the support and understanding we received from family and friends. We missed many a meal and stole many evenings and weekends to get the volume of work done in order to complete this project. Alan and Lauren, Bob, Brian, Eric, and Adam were closest to us as we carried out these activities, and we know they celebrate having this project published. And to Owen Brown, you won't have to ask me again, "When do you think THAT book is going to be published?"

We close with acknowledging the people who, across time, have shared their journey of mental illness and recovery with us. We hope that the lessons we have learned from and with you are reflected in the different aspects of this book. And we look forward to learning even more so that future versions of this kind of text will be shaped by and will shape mental health practice in occupational therapy. Our hope is that the "Vision of Participation" becomes a reality for all!

Tana Brown
Ginny Stoffel

Contents in Brief

Contents

Foundations

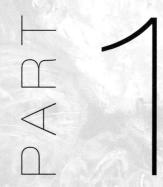

Part I provides information on overarching issues in mental health occupational therapy. The first chapter on recovery sets the tone for the text, which acknowledges the expertise and point of view of the individual with mental illness. In addition, the recovery model promotes optimism and hope that individuals with psychiatric disabilities can achieve their occupational wants and needs. The other chapters in this part of the text provide further perspective and background for mental health occupational therapy practice that is (1) person centered, (2) occupation based, (3) grounded in theory, (4) supported by evidence, and (5) cognizant of the historical roots of occupational therapy in mental health.

Recovery

Virginia Carroll Stoffel

> "As recovery belongs to people with psychiatric disabilities, and as it is up to them to define what it is and what it entails, it is key that people in recovery lead the way.
> —Davidson et al, 2007

Introduction

This chapter on **recovery** is a collection, a tapestry of perspectives from many sources, with careful attention being paid to those shared by persons who have the lived experience of recovery. True to the principles of **client-centered practice** in occupational therapy (Law, 1998), the emphasis is placed on what is important to the person. As such, recovery planning is guided by the individual's goals and dreams in the context of his or her personal gifts, strengths, and skills while pursuing occupations in his or her lived environments.

Occupational therapy practitioners who are surrounded by people working on their recovery from mental illness and/or substance abuse and dependence can find ways of joining with, listening, and reflecting sensitively in order to gain a view of each person's individually held picture of recovery. The journey of recovery that each mental health practitioner is privy to when invited, involves an assumption of a collaborative partnership

Occupational therapy has as its primary domain (American Occupational Therapy Association [AOTA], 2002, 2008) an emphasis on "supporting health and participation in life through engagement in occupation" (p. 626), which takes place within a context, including the social and physical environments. This perspective is compatible with and linked to the concept of recovery. In fact, recovery is a major theme of this text. A "vision for participation," part of the textbook title, supports the view that, through participating in everyday activities that are needed and desired, persons with mental illness and/or substance use disorders will achieve a state of health, well-being, and recovery.

Definitions of Recovery

As reflected in this chapter's opening quote (Davidson et al, 2007), recovery is best defined by those individuals who have the lived experience of disability and recovery. In the United States, the Substance Abuse and Mental Health Services Administration (SAMHSA) engaged groups from across the country that represented people who live with mental illness, their families and supporters, mental health advocates, and mental health professionals to arrive at a definition of recovery.

In April 2006, this definition was released by SAMHSA as a consensus statement (Box 1-1): "Mental health recovery is a journey of healing and transformation enabling a person with a mental health problem to live a meaningful life in a community of his or her choice while striving to achieve his or her full potential" (p. 5).

In addition, 10 components of recovery that are fundamental to understanding this journey were identified:

- Self-direction
- Individualized and person centered
- Empowerment
- Holistic
- Nonlinear
- Strengths based
- Peer support
- Respect
- Responsibility
- Hope

Gagne, White, and Anthony (2007) suggest that a common recovery vision for both psychiatric and/or addiction disorders includes a desire to live with or a lessening of symptoms, an emphasis on participation in valued roles, and a sense of life purpose and meaning (p. 33). Crowley (2000) coined the term **procovery** to emphasize the process of "attaining a productive and fulfilling life regardless of the level of health assumed attainable" (p. 4). In her book, *The Power of Procovery in Healing Mental Illness,* Crowley offers tips for simple everyday living that allow a person living with mental illness to move forward at his or her own pace and grounded in hope. This book is a tool for persons who live with mental illness and their staff and family, with strategies for typical challenges such as partnering with health-care practitioners, managing medication, uncovering hope, creating change, dissolving stigma, using feelings constructively, gathering support, providing self-care, and living intentionally through work and activities.

Occupational therapy practitioners can facilitate recovery and procovery by teaching symptom management and coping strategies to structure one's routines in a manner that supports well-being, promotes occupational role function, and facilitates engagement in occupations that are purposeful and meaningful to the individual.

BOX 1-1 ▧ National Consensus Statement on Mental Health Recovery and the 10 Fundamental Components of Recovery

Mental health recovery is a journey of healing and transformation enabling a person with a mental health problem to live a meaningful life in a community of his or her choice while striving to achieve his or her full potential.

- *Self-Direction:* Consumers lead, control, exercise choice over, and determine their own path of recovery by optimizing autonomy, independence, and control of resources to achieve a self-determined life. By definition, the recovery process must be self-directed by the individual, who defines his or her own life goals and designs a unique path toward those goals.

- *Individualized and Person Centered:* There are multiple pathways to recovery based on an individual's unique strengths and resiliencies, and his or her needs, preferences, experiences (including past trauma), and cultural background in all its diverse representations. Individuals also identify recovery as being an ongoing journey and an end result, as well as an overall paradigm for achieving wellness and optimal mental health.

- *Empowerment:* Consumers have the authority to choose from a range of options and to participate in all decisions—including the allocation of resources—that will affect their lives, and are educated and supported in doing so. They have the ability to join with other consumers to collectively and effectively speak for themselves about their needs, wants, desires, and aspirations. Through empowerment, an individual gains control of his or her own destiny and influences the organizational and societal structures in his or her life.

- *Holistic:* Recovery encompasses an individual's whole life, including mind, body, spirit, and community. Recovery embraces all aspects of life, including housing, employment, education, mental health, and health-care treatment and services, complementary and naturalistic services, addictions treatment, spirituality, creativity, social networks, community participation, and family supports, as determined by the person. Families, providers, organizations, systems, communities, and society play crucial roles in creating and maintaining meaningful opportunities for consumer access to these supports.

- *Nonlinear:* Recovery is not a step-by-step process, but one based on continual growth, occasional setbacks, and learning from experience.

Recovery begins with an initial stage of awareness in which a person recognizes that positive change is possible. This awareness enables the consumer to move on to fully engage in the work of recovery.

- *Strengths Based:* Recovery focuses on valuing and building on the multiple capacities, resiliencies, talents, coping abilities, and inherent worth of individuals. By building on these strengths, consumers leave stymied life roles behind and engage in new life roles (e.g., partner, caregiver, friend, student, employee). The process of recovery moves forward through interaction with others in supportive, trust-based relationships.

- *Peer Support:* Mutual support—including the sharing of experiential knowledge and skills and social learning—plays an invaluable role in recovery. Consumers encourage and engage other consumers in recovery and provide each other with a sense of belonging, supportive relationships, valued roles, and community.

- *Respect:* Community, systems, and societal acceptance and appreciation of consumers—including protecting their rights and eliminating discrimination and stigma—are crucial in achieving recovery. Self-acceptance and regaining belief in one's self are particularly vital. Respect ensures the inclusion and full participation of consumers in all aspects of their lives.

- *Responsibility:* Consumers have a personal responsibility for their own self-care and journeys of recovery. Taking steps toward their goals may require great courage. Consumers must strive to understand and give meaning to their experiences, and identify coping strategies and healing processes to promote their own wellness.

- *Hope:* Recovery provides the essential and motivating message of a better future—that people can and do overcome the barriers and obstacles that confront them. Hope is internalized, but can be fostered by peers, families, friends, providers, and others. Hope is the catalyst of the recovery process. Mental health recovery not only benefits individuals with mental health disabilities by focusing on their abilities to live, work, learn, and fully participate in our society, but also enriches the texture of American community life. America reaps the benefits of the contributions individuals with mental disabilities can make, ultimately becoming a stronger and healthier nation.

Source: Substance Abuse and Mental Health Services Administration (SAMHSA). (n.d.). "National Consensus Statement on Mental Health Recovery." Brochure. Available at: http://download.ncadi.samhsa.gov/ken/pdf/SMA05-4129/trifold.pdf (accessed October 16, 2009).

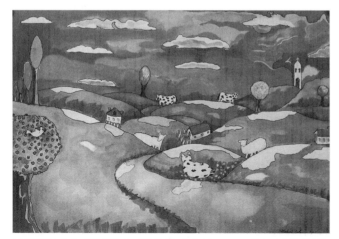

FIGURE 1-1. "Earth" by Michelle Cohen, a member of Fountain House. Painting courtesy of the Fountain Gallery.

Based on a comprehensive analysis of recovery definitions and elements in the literature, Onken, Craig, Ridgway, Ralph, and Cook (2007) offer a dimensional perspective that considers the individual and his or her environment in a dynamic interaction—from an ecological framework. Similar to Gagne et al (2007), they suggest that recovery involves first order change in which the person reestablishes mental health through symptom reduction/amelioration, and second order change by mitigating oppressive community barriers so that full social integration and community inclusion are achieved.

These are also concepts embraced by occupational therapists, who focus their interventions at the individual, family, and community levels to help transform home, school, community, and work environments to be open and accessible to all persons, embracing their talents and gifts while offering needed supports. Rebeiro Gruhl (2005) asserts that "core occupational therapy beliefs and assumptions are strikingly similar to those purported to be important to fostering recovery" (p. 96), citing such shared assumptions as self-determination, social support, strengths based, uniqueness, and client centeredness.

Occupational therapists who use a Person-Environment-Occupation (PEO) model (Law et al, 1996) and the Ecology of Human Performance model (Dunn, Brown, & Youngstrom, 2003) further add to the understanding of the ecological framework by considering not only the individual and his or her environment, but also his or her occupation, which is often imbued with meaning, purpose, and identity. This book is organized to embrace a recovery philosophy based on a deep understanding of people; the varied environments in which they live, work, learn, worship, and play; and their chosen and needed occupations.

The vision of recovery, hope, inclusion, community integration, and full participation contrasts with earlier paradigms of mental illness, which were almost exclusively focused on pathology, negative consequences, and hopelessness. Onken, Dumont, Ridgway, Dornan, and Ralph (2002) conducted a series of focus groups with 115 participants to identify factors that help and hinder recovery in a manner that contrasts the recovery paradigm (what helps recovery) with the pathology paradigm (what hinders recovery). Onken et al (2002), in their publication "Mental Health Recovery: What Helps and What Hinders?" suggest that

Recovery is a product of dynamic interaction among characteristics of the individual (the self/whole person, hope/sense of meaning and purpose), characteristics of the environment (basic material resources, social relationships, meaningful activities, peer support, formal services, formal service staff), and the characteristics of the exchange (hope, choice/empowerment, independence/ interdependence). (p. vii)

This complex description of recovery focuses on what the individual is experiencing within the environment, as well as the dynamic interaction of the person with their environment. "This emerging paradigm is integrative and holistic (i.e., focusing on the whole person functioning in his or her environment), while acknowledging the interrelations, multiple dimensions, individuality and the complexity of the recovery phenomenon" (Onken et al., 2002, pp. 68–69). Table 1-1 shows examples of the factors reported by Onken et al that help and hinder recovery. These factors can be used as a checklist by occupational therapy and mental health practitioners to self-evaluate their practices and incorporate more factors that facilitate recovery. Being mindful of those practices that may be working against a recovery philosophy is critical to transforming the mental health system. Throughout this chapter, the reader is encouraged to find ways that recovery concepts link with the domain of occupational therapy.

Insights Into Recovery—The Lived Experience

The **lived experience** of mental illness and recovery provides important insights into the nature of recovery. The following narratives are selected from a qualitative study

Table 1-1 ● Factors That Help and Hinder Mental Health Recovery

Factors Impacting Mental Health Recovery	What Helps	What Hinders
Self/whole person	• Positive traits and attitudes • Self-reliance, personal resourcefulness	• Negative beliefs and attitudes • Not taking personal responsibility
Basic material resources	• Livable income • Safe and affordable housing • Transportation	• Poverty • Unsafe and unaffordable housing • Lack of transportation
Hope, sense of meaning, and purpose	• Developing a sense of meaning/purpose • Staff hopeful with realistic optimism • Positive personal attitudes • Spirituality acknowledged	• Dreams, goals, and desires demeaned • Staff pessimistic • Sense of hopelessness and negativity • Spirituality discounted or ignored
Choice	• Freedom of whether and how to participate • Self-determination • Individualized services and planning • More job choices	• Forced treatment and coercion • Family and professional control • Limited treatment options • Unemployment and underemployment
Independence	• Voice in the system/make own choices • Self-determination and advanced directives	• Paternalistic system/lack of respect • Involuntary/long-term hospitalization
Social relationships	• Extended networks, friendships • Supportive and accepting kin • Personal ties and intimate relationships	• Inadequate social network and isolation • Controlling family members • Emotional withdrawal and isolation
Meaningful activities	• Choice among meaningful jobs • Educational advancement • Meaningful volunteer work • Advocacy participation	• Unemployment, role loss, limited options • Lack of educational opportunities • Exploitation of volunteer work • Prejudice, stigma, discrimination limit
Peer support	• Diverse peer support options (e.g., support groups, warm lines, case managers) • Support resources run by consumers • Consumers employed in mental health services	• Limited participation opportunities • Lack of independent peer support resources • Professional mistrust of peer support

Continued

Table 1-1 ● Factors That Help and Hinder Mental Health Recovery—cont'd

Factors Impacting Mental Health Recovery	What Helps	What Hinders
Formal services	• Vision of recovery and consumer driven • Partnership and tailored to person	• Pathology-focused organization • Expert centered, few choices
Formal service system staff	• Hopeful, positive expectations, belief in recovery as possible • Continuity, available, partnership in therapeutic relationship • Listened to; believed in; staff as authentic, responsive, humble	• Low expectations and negative messages • Discontinuity, burnout, overworked • Paternalism; no understanding of caring, consumer's experiences; disrespectful

Note: Examples drawn from Onken, S. J., Dumont, J. M., Ridgway, P., Dornan, D. H., & Ralph, R. O. (2002, October). "Mental Health Recovery: What Helps and What Hinders? A National Research Project for the Development of Recovery Facilitating System Performance Indicators." Phase One Research Report: A National Study Of Consumer Perspectives on What Helps and Hinders Mental Health Recovery. Alexandria: VA: National Technical Assistance Center for State Mental Health Planning; pp. 25–60.

of mental health recovery and how engagement in a psychosocial clubhouse impacts recovery (Stoffel, 2008). One member commented that

Recovery is not a destination, not a fixed place . . . I think it is part of a journey, our life long journey . . . a process of recovering. I'll always be taking my medications. I'll always visit a psychiatrist a few times a year for check-ins. I'll have a therapist for a period of time while I work on closure for some of the major wounds in my life. But recovery is about becoming and for me, especially, it's about becoming more whole as a person. (p. 114)

This statement resonates with the work of Anne Wilcock, an occupational therapist and occupational scientist, whose work on being and becoming as it relates to health highlights a link between recovery and occupational therapy. In Wilcock's (2006) book, *An Occupational Perspective of Health,* the concepts of being, doing, and becoming are explored as determinants of health. Wilcock suggests that, for individuals for whom meaning, purpose, and belonging are associated with being through doing, an absence from illness and a state of physical, mental, and social well-being are more likely.

Becoming implies a lifelong process of growth and fulfilling one's human potential (Wilcock, 2006). The participant quoted previously described recovery as a process that will occur across his lifetime, during which he will do a number of health-related self-care activities, such as take medication, see his psychiatrist, and work through issues with a therapist. These activities then open the door to many other possibilities that will make him become "more whole as a person," linking to many other life activities that offer opportunities for him to explore his human potential.

The journey of recovery has many ups and downs, as noted in the following narrative:

There's many a thing I could be doing right now but trying to motivate myself more by being in a recovery program for alcohol and drug abuse really helps me to learn what things I need to be around. So I chose the clubhouse and it works for me . . . with my schizophrenia and anxiety, there's lots of things that can trigger me back . . . so I need to be in a safe place like this. (Stoffel, 2008, p. 115)

Occupational therapy practitioners who embrace the PEO model (Law et al, 1996) will recognize how this person carefully chooses places that support his goal of recovery and spends time around people who support his avoidance of alcohol and drug use. The PEO model supports the availability

of a variety of opportunities to engage in occupations that hold meaning for individuals. This meaningfulness was confirmed by the following participant in a comment he made about discovering what was available to do at the clubhouse:

I just went to the library to see all the books and computers . . . I thought that was great. I could pick up a book and sit back, reading something with help because I'm slow a little bit, you know. My schizophrenia triggers me every now and then . . . but everyone appreciated me for being there, doing a good job. I could name a whole bunch of things I got credit for. I was working really hard just to be me, the new me, actually. (Stoffel, 2008, p. 96)

Strong and Rebeiro Gruhl (Chapter 3, this volume) suggest that therapists who apply the PEO model consider the "fit (or lack of fit) between the person's abilities and skills, the demands of the occupation, and the environmental conditions in which the occupation takes place" (p. 37). Congruence across the three aspects of person, environment, and occupation guides the therapist's interventions to facilitate the optimal occupational performance.

The complexity and multiple layers of recovery are exemplified in the following narrative:

Recovery from mental illness, from addictions, from my eating disorder . . . recovery is overwhelming because it is very painful dealing with issues from the past and the present . . . they pile up and then I get overwhelmed and then I get suicidal and end up back at the hospital. (Stoffel, 2008, p. 115–116)

The fact that the recovery experience evolves slowly and gradually, with individuals making gains as well as experiencing setbacks interspersed with plateau periods, was also reflected on by the participants. One participant who developed a resilient approach stated

In mental illness, we don't fix it, we either accept it and learn to live with it, or we make it our focus . . . it's the pebble, the rock in our shoe, it's something that in dealing with it, we become better. We become better because calluses build up around the pebble and we become stronger. It hurt in the beginning, but it hurts less and less. I don't feel ill, even though I know I have it—sometimes I feel paranoid or I feel a little suspicious . . . but I'm actually stronger in some ways than others who don't have mental illness are because I've had to overcome this and in overcoming it, makes me stronger. (Stoffel, 2008, pp. 115–116)

A Recovery Poem

by: Marie DiMenna (2007)

People recover
from illness
from sorrow
from addiction
from acts of violence.

People recover—
our voices joined together
in harmonic song.

People recover
from death
from persecution
from divorce
from prejudice.

People recover
with courage
and strength of character.

We hope
we dream
we dare to live again.

People recover
from abuse
from injury
from injustice
from natural disaster.

People recover.
We triumph—
creating networks of support
finding one another
in the fabric of community.

People recover
from poverty
from trauma
from abandonment
from homelessness.

People recover
in time with hope
the strength to continue
lies within the core of our beings.

We recover
from mental disturbances
from loneliness
from low self-esteem
from feeling violated.

We recover
with the love and commitment
of our sisters and brothers.

We recover
from fear
from isolation
from imprisonment
from acts of terrorism.

We recover.
The limitations of yesterday
shall not prevent us
from seeing and believing
in the promise of a beautiful tomorrow.

We recover
from anger
from war
from slavery
from the Holocaust.

We recover—
The desire to be well
shall make us whole again.

We recover
from hatred
from doubt
from despair
from dishonesty.

We are liberated.
We are healed.
We find mercy.
We seek love.
We find grace.

We sow seeds of compassion.
We acknowledge truth.
We witness reconciliation.
We devote ourselves
to loving one another.
We affirm the goodness
we see in humanity.

Learning to grow and adjust to the challenges of living with a mental illness or substance use disorder, and finding ways to strengthen oneself through what can be painful struggles, are also consistent with Wilcock's (2006) perspective on being through doing and becoming. The previous narrative highlights being through doing and becoming; that is, experiencing oneself authentically (being) through learning from coping with symptoms and struggles (doing) builds resiliencies and strengths (becoming).

Another interviewee talked about what recovery might look like:

I want to have a balanced, whole life. I don't have that yet, but I'm trying to achieve that. I need to nurture my friendships, including twelve step friends. I need to have fun at some points and be serious at other points.

I have a hard time getting it all to work in conjunction with each other. I really need a sense of humor—I don't know how to, but I'd like to be able to laugh at myself; it's very hard to do. I tend to focus more on my problems and that's not always good . . . when I was young I was laughed at and teased and bullied by a lot of people growing up. So I have a hard time just looking at myself and seeing the humor in what I do and how I do things. Other people see it and they laugh at me sometimes and I get offended by it. So then I get defensive, I feel like it's malicious and it's not always. (Stoffel, 2008, p. 116)

Recovery seems to involve continual self-discovery, overcoming past issues and struggles with oneself and others, and building solid relationships that are supportive of recovery. The previous narrative, which speaks to the challenge of developing one's sense of humor when one has past negative experiences resulting in vulnerabilities, also speaks to the role that emotional regulation skills play in regard to engaging in occupations with others (AOTA, 2008).

Each participant's story captured the challenges of recovery and the ups and downs of the journey, providing a perspective on the nature of recovery as a process that encompasses the person, environment, and occupation as important factors in one's recovery. Recovery as a process of becoming whole and more than simply a person struggling with mental illness was an important lesson learned from these psychosocial clubhouse colleagues.

Recovery as a Process and Journey

The journey of recovery is highlighted in the narratives and definitions of recovery presented here. Rather than focusing only on problems associated with mental illness, Ridgway (2001) suggests that constructing recovery narratives focused on strengths, hopefulness, active coping, and a positive sense of self with meaning and purpose in life involving support and partnership can facilitate the journey of recovery. Occupational therapists can ask their clients to reflect on their recovery stories as a means of tracking where they are on the journey, where they have come, and where they hope to go. Given that stories can be written, read out loud, developed over time, and shared with others, using narrative as a means to help clients construct their recovery stories also facilitates peer interaction and self-understanding. Throughout this book, you will find first person accounts of the lived experience, as well as **PhotoVoice** images and stories that serve as examples of recovery-oriented narratives.

Roe, Rudnick, and Gill (2007) considered what is meant by "being in recovery" and suggest that, rather than considering all persons with mental illness to be in recovery, it might be more helpful to think of recovery on a continuum, with a number of stages that characterize its process. They also note that "the process of recovery can be a goal in itself as well as a possible predictor of what are considered to be traditionally good outcomes" (p. 172). Occupational therapists trained in a recovery orientation can facilitate engagement in the process of recovery by promoting a hopeful perspective for the future, while helping the person build external supports such as housing, employment, pursuit of academic goals, and engagement in meaningful service to strengthen social connections.

Anthony, Cohen, Farkas, and Gagne (2002) framed the 21st century as a time when mental health systems of care are guided by a vision of recovery. They defined recovery as

a deeply personal, unique process of changing one's attitudes, values, feelings, goals, skills, and/or roles. It is a way of living a satisfying, hopeful, and contributing life, with or without limitations caused by the illness. Recovery involves the development of new meaning and purpose in one's life as one grows beyond the catastrophic effects of a mental illness. (p. 31)

This definition offers another way to understand the complex process of recovery—a process that occurs within an individual, shaping cognitive beliefs and motivations, tapping into emotions, and impacting coping responses. This text explores these and many other client factors that contribute to recovery. Important aspects of recovery include

- Importance of hope
- Coping and adaptation
- Empowerment and self-determination
- Social and community integration

Importance of Hope

The importance of **hope**, or a sense that recovery is possible (Jacobson & Greenley, 2001), and the possibility of a life with meaning and purpose, self-determination, and engagement in valued occupational roles that are important to the person have been reflected in the writings of Patricia Deegan (1988, 1996, 2001). Deegan (2001) and Graham et al (2001) also note barriers to recovery that are imposed by professionals who practice in a manner that conveys a lack of hope, an overemphasis on symptoms, diagnosis, and deficits, and engenders overdependence on mental health experts. Shared decision-making about using psychiatric medications (Deegan, 2007) and broader mental health care (Schauer, Everett, del Vecchio, & Anderson, 2007) reinforces the importance of collaboration and mutual respect as practitioners travel with people on their recovery journey. The role that the environment plays in promoting hope is conveyed in Deegan's (1996) message, "we are learning that the environment around people must change if we are to be expected to grow into the fullness of the person who, like a small seed, is waiting to emerge from within each of us" (p. 2).

When mental health practitioners engage in shared decision-making with their clients in a manner that conveys their respect, hope is reinforced. The implicit message to the client is "You are worth it. You have capacity to shape your future in a positive manner. What you know counts." Onken et al (2007) speak of hope as being a catalyst for the recovery process. Sheyett, Kim, Swanson, and Swartz (2007) note that, by developing psychiatric advance directives, hope is supported from the perspective that pain and past crises offer learning opportunities for creating a more positive future.

Occupational therapists need to carefully consider their message of hope in all that they reflect on and convey to the people with whom they work. Helping clients find their own answers and exercise their own judgment, with the therapist offering information or advice only when given permission (techniques used by practitioners trained in motivational interviewing) (Miller & Rollnick, 2002), are techniques that are consistent with an implicit message of hope. Both verbal and nonverbal exchanges are important in conveying a realistic optimism associated with a sense of hopefulness.

The following PhotoVoice feature offers one person's perspective on how she gains hope from her environment and symbolic items that offer meaning to her.

PhotoVoice

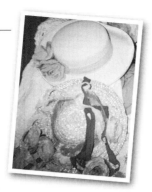

This is a picture of beautiful Easter bonnets, which are a symbol of spring, new beginnings, and new life. Being surrounded by beautiful things creates hope for my future.

Coping and Adaptation

The journey of recovery involves cycles of **coping and adaptation** as a nonlinear, complicated process that includes setbacks that result in greater coping responses over time (Strauss, 1989). Hatfield and Lefley (1993) frame mental health recovery as a "process of adaptation at increasingly higher levels of personal satisfaction and interpersonal functioning" (p. 141). Profiles of recovery identified in an analysis of qualitative interviews (Provencher, Grigg, Mead, & Mueser, 2002) reflect that, at different points in time during the journey, some individuals view their recovery as uncertain, others view it as a self-experience of reconstructing self and reconnecting with others, and others view recovery as a reachable challenge, including feeling empowered, being involved in satisfying social relationships, and looking forward to a promising future.

This characterization of adaptation and coping is consistent with perspectives held by occupational therapy practitioners. As individuals build on their strengths, overcome challenges, and begin to move toward personal goal achievement, a sense of personal self-efficacy develops. In turn, engagement in occupations is enhanced by self-efficacy and actively pursuing meaningful occupations, which further strengthens the journey to recovery.

Empowerment and Self-Determination

Empowerment has been identified as an important factor in the recovery process. Cohen (2005) identify the elements of empowerment as including

- Decision-making power
- Access to information and resources
- Variety of options from which to choose
- Assertive communication
- Hopeful future
- Constructive means of expressing anger
- Promoting change within oneself and the community
- Image of self as improving and overcoming stigma

Consistent with empowerment, **self-determination** has been described by Cook (n.d.) as ". . . having the freedom to be in charge of your own life, choosing where you live, who you're with, and what you do. It means having the resources you need to create a good life and to make responsible decisions that are best for you and others around you. It also means choosing where, when, and how you will get support and assistance for mental health problems when needed" (p. 2).

Occupational therapists who work with people recovering from substance abuse and/or psychiatric disabilities are in key positions to facilitate empowerment, self-determination, and constructive decision-making about everyday routines, occupational roles that are important to the person, and choosing people and places (social and physical environments) that support the person's optimum performance. For example, empowering a mother in recovery from cocaine addiction might include providing her with information about self-help groups that meet during the same times her children are in school so that she can balance her personal self-care with her cherished parenting role. Helping a person explore how he or she might alternatively cope with hearing voices to reduce the side effects of certain medications, such as getting engaged in activities that are calming (e.g., deep breathing or focusing on tensing and relaxing muscle groups to mindfully distract oneself, listening to music, folding laundry) can be empowering to an individual with a psychiatric disability.

Another example from the occupational therapy literature (Le Granse, Kinebanian, & Josephsson, 2006) is as follows: "The occupational therapist is not the person who determines the content of the client's daily life, but is the one who creates the conditions that enable the client to determine the content of his or her own daily life" (p. 153). Creating conditions by helping position the person in the best environment for carrying out their chosen goals and exploring resources that might make a difference are among those strategies that can facilitate empowerment and self-determination.

Social and Community Integration

Social connection has been studied as an important aspect of recovery (Davidson, 2007; Spaniol, Bellingham, Cohen, & Spaniol, 2003), as well as being connected to familiar and welcoming places that hold a larger purpose or meaning. Erdner, Magnusson, Nystrom, and Lutzen (2005) found that social connectedness versus being socially alienated and seeing oneself as an outsider was important to recovery. Boydell, Gladstone, and Crawford (2002) highlight the importance of having friends with and without psychiatric disabilities. Occupational therapists who work in community support programs can facilitate exploration of new people and places by first accompanying the person to various events and gatherings. In that way, as personal competence and resilience increase over time, an occupational therapy intervention might be simply pointing out opportunities that the individual can choose to pursue. Such opportunities can include education, employment, volunteer, leisure/recreation, spiritual, and citizenship options available to all community members.

Baron (2007) invited consumers, family members, and mental health providers to generate recommendations as to how **community integration** might be promoted in the areas of civic engagement, competitive employment, educational advancement, social participation, housing supports, and religious/spiritual connection. Encouraging civic reciprocity (i.e., the concept that people give to others as well as take); working with businesses to increase employment opportunities and supports; and enhancing educational paths toward GED completion, technical, baccalaureate, and graduate options with educational funding were among the 20 strategies generated. Employing strategies to enhance access to free or low-cost community events for social participation, providing resources for safe and affordable housing, and stimulating religious and spiritual congregations to be more open and welcoming rounded out their recommendations (Baron, 2007).

Occupational therapy practitioners need to focus their attention not only on the individual and family levels, but also on the community advocacy level to create new avenues for inclusion and participation. Building on the individual's own natural communities (church, school, social, and recreational), occupational therapists can promote outreach to all persons in the community.

Occupational Therapy and Recovery

Throughout this chapter and the text overall, the reader will note many links between the emphasis of occupational therapy and its fit with recovery and recovery-related concepts. In this section, specific contributions from the occupational therapy literature are reviewed that add to the overall understanding of recovery.

Rebeiro Gruhl (2005) asserts that occupational therapists should attend to the construct of recovery and lead research and practice in promoting recovery, given the strong fit between core occupational therapy beliefs and assumptions and what the literature indicates is important to fostering recovery. Occupational therapists contribute to the complexity and meaning of the recovery vision and integrate recovery with occupational therapy practice (Krupa & Clark, 2004).

Krupa (2004) suggests that, at any point in recovery, work participation can occur. Contributions made by occupational

---

Evidence-Based Practice

Work participation can occur at any point in recovery. The optimum work environment is one that supports the individual's confident engagement.

➤ Occupational therapists can promote engagement in work based on client interest and goals, not on specific mental health recovery status.

➤ Careful attention to a work environment that best matches the individual's interests, talents, and competent involvement may help promote recovery.

Krupa, T. (2004). Employment, recovery, and schizophrenia: Integrating health and disorder at work. *Psychiatric Rehabilitation Journal, 28,* 8–14.

Strong, S. (1998). Meaningful work in supportive environments: Experiences with the recovery process. *American Journal of Occupational Therapy, 52,* 31–38.

Woodside, H., Schell, L., & Allison-Hedges, J. (2006). Listening for recovery: The vocational success of people living with mental illness. *Canadian Journal of Occupational Therapy, 73,* 36–43.

---

therapists in the recovery literature include helping people find those environments that best support their confident engagement in meaningful occupations such as work (Woodside, Schell, & Allison-Hedges, 2006), where the match of values in the workplace with values of the person impacts vocational success (Kirsch, 2000), and where meaningful work in a supportive environment leads to a sense of self as competent and capable (Strong, 1998).

At the 2007 conference hosted by the American Occupational Therapy Foundation entitled "Habit and Rehabilitation: Promoting Participation," Davidson (2007) posited that action theory be applied to rethinking psychiatric research and practice. This theory states that actions precede and generate insight; that is, humans are viewed as active beings who create and are simultaneously shaped by their environment. Based on an understanding of persons with psychiatric disability as having habits of living that are limited because of the institutional environments created for persons with psychosis, a newer understanding emphasizing habit formation as supporting recovery is considered. Helping persons with psychiatric disabilities form habits of daily living that permit them to more fully participate in everyday life in communities brings a different understanding of what is needed. Davidson promotes the development of two habits that are critical to recovery: developing caring relationships and being grounded in the present. These habits could form the basis for living more successfully in the community as a person in recovery. The text by Crowley (2000) referenced previously in this chapter offers a multitude of strategies that would be consistent with being grounded in the present and dealing with everyday life.

To summarize, recovery is the personal journey of an individual with serious mental illness or substance use disorder that involves living beyond the diagnosis and symptoms and achieving purpose, meaning, and life satisfaction. Personal growth resulting from managing and adapting to everyday challenges is part of that journey. Hope is an essential ingredient in initiating one's recovery, which is further fostered by a sense of empowerment, being connected with others, having access to resources, practicing self-determination, and having a clear sense of one's values and life goals.

Evidence-Based Practice

Social connectedness and developing caring relationships is important to recovery, as is having friends with and without psychiatric disability. Having someone who is trustworthy and loyal through positive and challenging times plays a role in supporting mental health recovery.

➤ Occupational therapists can use skillful group facilitation to promote social connectedness.

➤ Occupational therapy practitioners should encourage seeking and providing social support as a means to develop competence in reciprocal relationships that are important to recovery.

Boydell, K. M., Gladstone, B. M., & Crawford, E. S. (2002). The dialectic of friendship for people with psychiatric disabilities. *Psychiatric Rehabilitation Journal, 26,* 123–131.

Davidson, L. (2007). Habits and other anchors of everyday life that people with psychiatric disabilities may not take for granted. *OTJR: Occupation, Participation and Health, 27*(Suppl), 60S–68S.

Davidson, L., Tondora, J., O'Connell, M. J., Kirk, T., Rockholz, P., & Evans, A. C. (2007). Creating a recovery-oriented system of behavioral health care: Moving from concept to reality. *Psychiatric Rehabilitation Journal, 31,* 23–31.

Erdner, A., Magnusson, A., Nystrom, M., & Lutzen, K. (2005). Social and existential alienation experienced by people with long-term mental illness. *Scandinavian Journal of Caring Sciences, 19,* 373–380.

The following PhotoVoice highlights how, despite the challenges faced when living with mental illness, when on the journey of mental health recovery, strength and hope can result.

Measurement of Recovery

Given the increasing interest in recovery as an outcome for persons with psychiatric disabilities, researchers and practitioners have generated evidence and tools to measure recovery and aspects of recovery, such as hope, empowerment, and self-determination. In addition, a number of instruments have been designed to evaluate the degree to which mental health programs, services, and systems have embraced various concepts and best practices associated with recovery.

Ralph, Kidder, and Phillips (2000) produced a compendium of such measures entitled *Can We Measure Recovery? A Compendium of Recovery and Recovery-Related Instruments, Volume I.* In 2005, Campbell-Orde, Chamberlin, Carpenter, and Leff produced *Measuring the Promise: A Compendium of Recovery Measures, Volume II*, which provided updates on two of the instruments published in Volume I, additional measures of individual recovery and service, and program- and system-level tools for measuring recovery in the respective environments.

Several of the measurement tools are described here to encourage occupational therapists to consider their utility in program evaluation and individual assessment.

Recovery Enhancing Environment Scale

The importance of a person's movement toward positive recovery and an awareness of the recovery facilitating/inhibiting aspects of the person's environment deserve careful analysis.

PhotoVoice

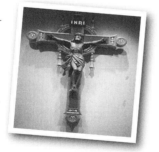

She accompanies me everywhere, yet I have never seen her. She attended many of my birthday parties—uninvited. At my 24th birthday, I said, "No presents, only presence," but her presence was no gift, she sent me to the hospital. She has been a boss, a tormenter, my constant companion—my worst enemy. She crashed my wedding and ruined my marriage. My children have never seen her, but they know her m.o. Like a spouse, I have learned to live with her, till death do us part.

I can see her presence in my life now as a gift that I accept with gratitude. For if we had not met, I would be bereft of the travel, experiences, friends, maturity, wisdom, and grace I have received. She is not my partner, best friend, lover, or roommate. She is not even a person, place, or thing. She is a cross, not made of wood, that I have carried all my life....She is mental illness.

One tool, the Recovery Enhancing Environment (REE) scale (Ridgway, 2005; Ridgway, Press, Anderson, & Deegan, 2004), includes both individual and systems measures. The REE assesses individual recovery (stage of recovery, service utilization, recovery markers) and factors in the service environment that are considered to be resilience- and recovery-enhancing from the perspective of the service user's ratings (recovery practice elements and resilience-promoting factors in the organizational climate).

The consumer perspective, when considering one's recovery and how the environment affects the recovery journey, is a central concern (Ridgway & Press, 2004). The questionnaire can be completed by the individual (average time, 25 minutes) or as an interview (average time, 30–45 minutes). The REE has been used for program evaluation and assessment of change over time in adolescent programs, state hospital programs, and internationally. Table 1-2 provides a sample item for each of the parts of the REE.

Recovery Self-Assessment

The Recovery Self-Assessment (RSA; O'Connell, 2005; O'Connell, Tondora, Evans, Croog, & Davidson, 2005) was developed in conjunction with the Connecticut Department of Mental Health and Addiction Services to assess the degree to which its recovery-supporting practices were evident to service users. This 36-item tool was developed based on the following nine principles (O'Connell et al, 2005):

- Renewing hope and commitment
- Redefining self
- Incorporating illness
- Being involved in meaningful activities
- Overcoming stigma
- Assuming control
- Becoming empowered and exercising citizenship
- Managing symptoms
- Being supported by others

Table 1-2 ● **Sample Items in Ridgway Recovery-Enhancing Environment Measure**

Section of Tool (No. of Elements)	Sample Item
Stage of recovery (9)	I've been thinking about recovery, but haven't decided to move on it yet.
Elements of recovery and recovery-enhancing programs (24)	Having a positive sense of personal identity beyond my psychiatric disorder is important to my recovery.
Special needs (5)	Healing trauma, including sexual abuse and/or physical abuse, is important to my recovery.
Organizational climate (14)	The program provides opportunities for meaningful participation and contribution.
Recovery markers (27)	I have more good days than bad.
Final questions (4)	What are one or two of the most important things you have learned so far on your journey of recovery?

Source: Ridgway, P. (2005). Recovery enhancing environment measure. In T. Campbell-Orde, J. Chamberlin, J. Carpenter, & H.S. Leff (Eds.), Measuring the Promise: A Compendium of Recovery Measures, Volume II (pp. 213–228). Cambridge, MA: The Evaluation Center @ HSRI.

These principles were derived from an extensive literature review and input from persons in recovery, family members, service providers, and administrators. There are four versions of the tool: Persons in Recovery Version, Family/Significant Others/Advocates Version, Provider Version, and CEO/Agency Director Version. Administration time is less than 10 minutes, and the tool has been tested in inpatient and outpatient settings as well as in peer-run residential and social programs. The five domains (life goals, involvement, diversity of treatment options, choice, and individually tailored services) showed internal consistency, with Cronbach's alpha ranging from 0.76 to 0.90 for each domain. The RSA has been used by the state of Connecticut and has been selected for use by the Veterans Administration as it conducts system-level analysis of its recovery-oriented practices (O'Connell, 2005). Salyers, Tsai, and Stultz (2007) studied the Provider Version of the RSA in a sample of hospital workers and reported internal consistency and test–retest reliability as good to excellent, with adequate convergent and discriminant validity.

The REE and RSA are two examples of recent tools that are in various phases of development. Occupational therapy practitioners practicing in mental health settings might find them to be useful in examining the recovery orientation of their own programs and practices. Given the paradigm shift from a pathological and medical model of care to a recovery model, knowing how aligned staff and programs are with principles of recovery is an important process to monitor across time as a continuous quality improvement activity.

Making Decisions Empowerment Scale

The Making Decisions Empowerment scale (Rogers, Chamberlin, Ellison, & Crean, 1997), a 28-item scale, measures the personal construct of empowerment. Tested on 271 members of six self-help programs across six states and administered to 56 state hospital inpatients and 200 college students, it discriminates among respondent groups.

Factor analyses revealed five factors: self-efficacy—self-esteem, power—powerlessness, community activism, righteous anger, and optimism—control over the future, which accounted for 54% of the variance. Statistical significance was found for relationships between empowerment and community activities, total monthly income, quality of life, social support, self-esteem, and satisfaction with self-help programs. An inverse correlation between empowerment and traditional use of mental health services ($p = 0.02$) was reported, and empowerment was not related to such demographic variables as gender, race, marital status, education level, or previous psychiatric hospitalizations. Cronbach's alpha was reported to be 0.86, showing high internal consistency. Occupational therapists working in recovery-oriented mental health programs that emphasize empowerment may find this scale helpful in tracking changes in personal empowerment.

Hope Scale

Although the Hope scale (Snyder et al, 1991) is a generic tool for studying hopefulness that was not specifically developed for a population of adults with serious mental illness, it was recommended for use in mental health settings by its inclusion in *Measuring the Promise: A Compendium of Recovery Measures, Volume II* (Campbell-Orde et al, 2005).

The Hope scale is a self-report measure with 12 items, 8 of which are aspects of hope and 4 of which are fillers, answered using a 4-point Likert-type scale (definitely false, mostly false, mostly true, definitely true). It has a Cronbach's alpha of 0.74 to 0.84, and a test–retest reliability of 0.85 over a 3-week period. Convergent and discriminant validity are well documented (Snyder et al, 1991).

Given that hope is a construct considered important to understanding recovery, this scale can be useful for occupational therapists who are interested in tracking program impact on sense of hope in the people they serve.

Measurement of Community Integration

Salzer and Baron (2006) offer a conceptual framework for measuring participation and community integration that considers opportunities for involvement in "community integration domains: Housing, Employment, Education, Health, Leisure/Recreation, Spirituality, Citizenship, Social Roles, Peer Support, and Self Determination" (p. 2). Their framework incorporates objective and subjective measures of opportunity, participation in varied activities across domains, presence in the community, well-being and quality of life, and recovery as "living a satisfying, fulfilling, and hopeful life" (p. 2).

Considerations regarding the level of segregated activity within institutions/agencies versus integrated participation in the community; involvement with others who do not have a psychiatric disability; the degree of individual choice; and important benchmarks associated with recovery, such as employment status, level of income, educational status, and housing conditions as compared to people with similar sociodemographic profiles, are all monitored to determine overall level of community integration. Their model views increased participation of any kind as positive "regardless of where it falls on the varied dimensions" (Salzer & Baron, 2006, p. 3).

To summarize, measures associated with recovery at the program and system levels can determine to what degree the paradigm of recovery has been embraced based on input from mental health consumers, families, staff, and administrators. Individual measures of recovery, empowerment, hope, and community integration all hold promise for tracking change at the individual, group, and community levels.

Recovery as Public Policy Leading Mental Health System Transformation

Recovery concepts and outcomes have been the focus of mental health systems at a global level. In New Zealand, recovery principles were identified in The Mental Health Commission's (1998) "Blueprint for Mental Health Services in New Zealand," and "Recovery Competencies for New Zealand Mental Health Workers" was published in 2001 to provide educators from the varied disciplines with broad guidelines for preparing the mental health workforce.

In the United States, the New Freedom Commission on Mental Health (2003) and the SAMHSA Consensus Conference in 2006 promoted mental health recovery as the desired outcome of mental health services. The vision of recovery included full participation in communities, living a productive life, working and learning (New Freedom Commission on Mental Health, 2003), and the importance of hope. Mental health recovery has emerged as an important concept that validates the lived experience of mental illness and recovery; provides insights to mental health service providers and families as to how they can be involved in supporting recovery; and serves as the focus of public policy, programs, and services. In April 2006, the U.S. Department of Health and Human Services released its "National Consensus Statement on Mental Health Recovery," citing recovery as "the single most important goal for the mental health service delivery system" (SAMHSA, n.d., p. 5).

In addition to the initiatives led by the federal government, as of January 2006, the Joint Commission on Accreditation of Healthcare Organizations' (JCAHO's) Behavioral Health Care Standards required programs to support a recovery-oriented philosophy and approach to care, treatment, and services (JCAHO, 2005). Focusing on strengths, facilitating people's ability to successfully cope with life's challenges (not just on managing distressing symptoms of one's mental illness), and offering services that are consumer- and family-driven are consistent with such a philosophy.

Occupational therapy practitioners worldwide have also joined with the recovery movement and apply the recovery principles to facilitate full participation in everyday community life (Krupa, 2004; Rebeiro Gruhl, 2005; Strong, 1998). The final section of this chapter provides an overview of the recovery principles that govern recovery-oriented mental health systems.

Recovery Principles

Principles governing recovery are consistent with the PEO perspective that is built into the design of this text. These principles have been incorporated into state and federal policies in the United States and internationally.

Anthony et al (2002) suggest a number of assumptions to consider regarding the recovery process:

- Recovery occurs at an individual level and can be facilitated by families, friends, self-help groups, and professionals.
- An array of activities—which may or may not include formal mental health services, such as sports, clubs, adult education, and church activities—can facilitate recovery.
- Essential to recovery are people who can be trusted to "be there" in times of need and who convey their belief in and support of the person's recovery.
- Diagnoses and medical interventions are not part of the recovery vision.
- Recovery can occur despite symptoms of the illness.
- Symptoms play a lesser role as a person recovers.

- Like life, recovery has growth and setbacks; yet, when viewed over time, it has a gradual upward trend.
- The consequences of mental illness—such as loss of rights and equal opportunities related to employment, housing, and parenting, and other discrimination related to stigma, even if the person is recovered—may be more challenging than the illness itself.
- Recovery for a person means that he or she has much to offer others in recovery, not that he or she was not ill in the first place.

These principles direct psychiatric rehabilitation professionals, including occupational therapy practitioners, to pay attention to the recovery process and facilitate favorable outcomes associated with mental health recovery, as well as guide public policy and programs with a paradigm of recovery.

In the United States, Connecticut has been involved in mental health recovery as a statewide system of care since 2000. Their definition of recovery was based on the perspectives of those in recovery: "a process of restoring a meaningful sense of belonging to one's community and positive sense of identity apart from one's condition while rebuilding a life despite or within the limitations imposed by that condition" (Davidson et al, 2007, p. 25). As opposed to the medical model, which emphasizes compliance with treatment, the disability/civil rights model of recovery encourages consumers to pursue their hopes and dreams based on their assets and strengths.

Operationalization of the recovery components (e.g., being supported by others, renewing hope and commitment, engaging in meaningful activities, redefining self, incorporating illness, overcoming stigma, assuming control, managing symptoms, becoming empowered and exercising citizenship) on the part of persons in recovery, direct support providers, and manager/administrators was carefully planned. The Recovery Self-Assessment (O'Connell et al, 2005) was adopted as the outcome measure to determine the extent to which their recovery system transformation was successful. The most significant need and the most significant facilitator of recovery was found to be "having someone I can trust who will stick with me over time, through the good times and the bad, to support me in my recovery" (Davidson et al, 2007, p. 28).

New York State adopted eight basic principles of recovery-centered service planning (Felton, Barr, Clark, & Tsemberis, 2006) and conducted statewide training with all mental health workers. The principles include the following:

1. At every stage of service delivery and support, the individual's *own stated needs, wants, and goals* in his or her *own language* drive the nature and the development of the service plan.
2. We must very *patiently* develop an honest, trustworthy *partnership-based relationship* that is marked by *"true mutuality"* and *"shared humanity,"* which fosters *recovery, respect, and responsibility.*
3. Our charge is to foster and *"form a community of hope"* surrounding each individual we serve.
4. Individuals must be afforded the ability to learn from their own mistakes in a supportive atmosphere (*the dignity of risk and the right to failure.*)
5. For each self-defined goal, relying on and/or helping develop each individual's own skills and capacities

should be the first approach (e.g., wellness self-management techniques, self-advocacy).

6. Crisis planning and relapse prevention strategies that draw on the individual's preferences and accounts of what has worked in the past should be developed as early as the relationship allows.

7. Determining long-term goals at the outset of the relationship will assist both parties in deciding when *discharge planning* should occur.

8. We should always seek to *favor the use of natural supports* that are available or can be developed in natural community settings. These should include sources of self-help and mutual support. (p. 114)

After completing a statewide training initiative promoting these principles, Felton et al (2006) conducted a study to determine which aspects of recovery-oriented practices were most easily adopted and identify stumbling blocks to adoption. They found that these principles could be applied to persons living with serious mental illness and substance use disorders, but not when the person did not recognize that he or she had a mental illness. In addition, when a person was in a crisis situation, the use of a recovery orientation was considered to be less applicable. Working collaboratively and reflecting goals important to the individual were accomplished when the therapists learned about the individual as a whole person. A wellness orientation using Copeland's

(1997) Wellness Recovery Action Plan (also referred to as WRAP) was endorsed by participants who stated "Wellness works!" (Felton et al, 2006). WRAP is a manual approach to holistic self-management in which the individual analyzes the resources available to him or her (internal and external) to use in support of recovery (Copeland, 1997). Creating a personal toolbox for being successful in everyday life is built into a person's WRAP, from planning diet, exercise, and rest and filling treasured life roles to planning for crisis situations and returning to recovery post-crisis.

Summary

The recovery orientation toward living a full and meaningful life is supported by the occupational therapy domain: "Supporting health and participation in life through engagement in occupation" (AOTA, 2008, p. 626). This chapter provides the reader with definitions of recovery guided by persons with the lived experience of mental illness and recovery. Occupational therapy practitioners and other mental health providers who promote hope, resilience, coping, adaptation, empowerment, self-determination, and community integration, while supporting the individual's goals and personal vision of recovery in community of his or her choice, help make recovery possible.

Active Learning Strategies

1. Helps and Hinders

Review the content presented in Table 1-1 and the first person narratives in the "Insights Into Recovery—The Lived Experience" section. Make notes as to whether each person described what helped or hindered his or her recovery, and compare them with Table 1-1.

 In your **Reflective Journal**, describe any insights gained from this reflection. How would you approach a person in a manner that would facilitate the recovery process?

2. Recovery Orientation

Spend a day in a mental health setting (e.g., clubhouse, consumer-operated center, drop-in center, day treatment program) and observe staff–consumer interactions to determine

to what extent they have integrated recovery-oriented practices. Use Table 1-1 as a checklist to collect evidence based on the practices you observe that support or hinder recovery. Download one of the recovery assessment tools available at www.tecathsri.org, and interview either a therapist or a person served at the site.

 Describe the experience in your **Reflective Journal**.

3. Exploring Narratives

Read first person narratives at any of the sites listed in the "Resources" section. Listen carefully for the description of practices that supported or hindered the person's recovery. Describe how you would treat the person differently if you were to make a positive difference in his or her recovery.

Resources

- Examples of how participation might be measured and a copy of the full report entitled "Community Integration and Measuring Participation" can be accessed at the UPenn Collaborative on Community Integration website: www.upennrrtc.org
- Self-determination resources can be accessed at the University of Illinois at Chicago website: www.psych.uic.edu/uicnrtc

- The Evaluation Center, supported by the Center for Mental Health Services, SAMHSA, maintains a website where people can access documents online and find updates to reports and recovery measurement tools: www.tecathsri.org
- Mental Health America website: www.nmha.org
- National Mental Health Consumers' Self-Help Clearinghouse website: www.mhselfhelp.org
- National Empowerment Center website: www.power2u.org
- Mental Health Recovery website: www.mhrecovery.com

References

American Occupational Therapy Association (AOTA). (2002). Occupational therapy practice framework: Domain and process. *American Journal of Occupational Therapy, 56,* 609–639.

American Occupational Therapy Association (AOTA). (2008). Occupational therapy practice framework: Domain and process, 2nd ed. (Framework). *American Journal of Occupational Therapy, 62,* 625–683.

Anthony, W., Cohen, M., Farkas, M., & Gagne, C. (2002). *Psychiatric Rehabilitation* (2nd ed.). Boston: Center for Psychiatric Rehabilitation.

Baron, R. C. (2007, August). "Promoting Community Integration for People With Serious Mental Illnesses: A Compendium of Local Implementation Strategies." Philadelphia: University of Pennsylvania Collaborative on Community Integration. Available at: http://www.upennrrtc.org/var/tool/file/139-BH%20Unite.pdf (accessed October 15, 2009).

Boydell, K. M., Gladstone, B. M., & Crawford, E. S. (2002). The dialectic of friendship for people with psychiatric disabilities. *Psychiatric Rehabilitation Journal, 26,* 123–131.

Campbell-Orde, T., Chamberlin, J., Carpenter, J., & Leff, H. S. (2005, September). *Measuring the Promise: A Compendium of Recovery Measures, Volume II.* Cambridge, MA: The Evaluation Center @ HSRI. Available at: http://www.power2u.org/downloads/pn-55.pdf (accessed October 15, 2009).

Cohen, O. (2005). How do we recover? An analysis of psychiatric survivor oral histories. *Journal of Humanistic Psychology, 45*(3), 333–354.

Cook, J. A. (n.d.) "Web-Survey on Self-Determination and Technology." Interview protocol. Chicago: University of Illinois at Chicago National Research and Training Center (UIC NRTC) on Psychiatric Disability. Available at: http://www.cmhsrp.uic.edu/download/websurvey.pdf (accessed October 15, 2009).

Copeland, M. E. (1997). *Wellness Recovery Action Plan.* W. Dummerston, VT: Peach Press.

Crowley, K. (2000). *The Power of Procovery in Healing Mental Illness: Just Start Anywhere.* San Francisco: Kennedy Carlisle.

Davidson, L. (2007). Habits and other anchors of everyday life that people with psychiatric disabilities may not take for granted. *OTJR: Occupation, Participation and Health, 27*(Suppl), 60S–68S.

Davidson, L., Kirk, T., Rockholz, P., Tondora, J., O'Connell, M. J., & Evans, A. C. (2007). Creating a recovery-oriented system of behavioral health care: Moving from concept to reality. *Psychiatric Rehabilitation Journal, 31,* 23–31.

Deegan, P. E. (1988). Recovery: The lived experience of rehabilitation. *Psychosocial Rehabilitation Journal, 11*(4), 11–19.

Deegan, P. E. (1996). "Recovery and the Conspiracy of Hope." Presented at the sixth annual Mental Health Services Conference of Australia and New Zealand, Brisbane, Australia. Available at: http://www.bu.edu/resilience/examples/deegan-recovery-hope.pdf (accessed October 15, 2009).

Deegan, P. E. (2001). "Recovery as a Self-Directed Process of Healing and Transformation." Available at: http://intentionalcare.org/articles/articles_trans.pdf (accessed October 15, 2009).

Deegan, P. E. (2007). The lived experience of using psychiatric medication in the recovery process and a shared decision-making program to support it. *Psychiatric Rehabilitation Journal, 31,* 62–69.

Dunn, W., Brown, C., & Youngstrom, M. J. (2003). Ecological model of occupation. In P. Kramer, J. Hinojosa, & C. B. Royeen (Eds.), *Perspectives in Human Occupation: Participation in Life* (pp. 222–263). Baltimore: Lippincott William & Wilkins.

Erdner, A., Magnusson, A., Nystrom, M., & Lutzen, K. (2005). Social and existential alienation experienced by people with long-term mental illness. *Scandinavian Journal of Caring Sciences, 19,* 373–380.

Felton, B. J., Barr, A., Clark, G., & Tsemberis, S. J. (2006). ACT team members' responses to training in recovery-oriented practices. *Psychiatric Rehabilitation, 30,* 112–119.

Gagne, C., White, W., & Anthony, W. A. (2007). Recovery: A common vision for the fields of mental health and addictions. *Psychiatric Rehabilitation, 31,* 32–37.

Graham, C., Coombs, T., Buckingham, B., Eager, K., Trauer, T., & Callaly, T. (2001). "The Victorian Mental Health Outcomes Measurement Strategy: Consumer Perspectives on Future Directions for Outcome Self-Assessment. Report of the Consumer Consultation Project." Victoria: Department of Human Services. Available at: http://www.health.vic.gov.au/mentalhealth/outcomes/consumer-consult-report.pdf (accessed October 15, 2009).

Hatfield, A. B., & Lefley, H. P. (1993). *Surviving Mental Illness: Stress, Coping and Adaptation.* New York: Guilford Press.

Jacobson, N., & Greenley, D. (2001). What is recovery? A conceptual model and explication. *Psychiatric Services, 52,* 482–485.

Joint Commission on Accreditation of Healthcare Organizations (JCAHO). (2005). Behavioral health care standards supporting recovery and resilience. *Joint Commission Perspective, 25,* 6-6(1).

Kirsch, B. (2000). Factors associated with employment for mental health consumers. *Psychiatric Rehabilitation Journal, 24,* 13–21.

Krupa, T. (2004). Employment, recovery, and schizophrenia: Integrating health and disorder at work. *Psychiatric Rehabilitation Journal, 28,* 8–14.

Krupa, T., & Clark, C. (2004). Occupational therapy in the field of mental health: Promoting occupational perspectives on health and well-being. *Canadian Journal of Occupational Therapy, 71,* 69–74.

Law, M. (1998). *Client-Centered Practice in Occupational Therapy.* Thorofare, NJ: Slack.

Law, M., Cooper, B., Strong, S., Stewart, D., Rigby, P., & Letts, L. (1996). The Person-Environment-Occupation model: A transactive approach to occupational performance. *Canadian Journal of Occupational Therapy, 63,* 9–23.

Le Granse, M., Kinebanian, A., & Josephsson, S. (2006). Promoting autonomy of the client with persistent mental illness: A challenge for occupational therapists from The Netherlands, Germany and Belgium. *Occupational Therapy International, 13*(3), 142–159.

The Mental Health Commission. (1998, December). "Blueprint for Mental Health Services in New Zealand: How Things Need To Be." Wellington, NZ: Author. Available at: http://www.mhc.govt.nz/users/Image/Resources/1998%20Publications/BLUEPRINT1998.PDF (accessed October 15, 2009).

The Mental Health Commission. (2001, March). "Recovery Competencies for New Zealand Mental Health Workers." Wellington, NZ: Author. Available at: http://www.mhc.govt.nz/users/Image/Resources/2001%20Publications/RECOVERY_COMPETENCIES.PDF (accessed October 15, 2009).

Miller, W. R., & Rollnick, S. (2002). *Motivational Interviewing* (2nd ed.). New York: Guilford Press.

New Freedom Commission on Mental Health. (2003). *Achieving the Promise: Transforming Mental Health Care in America.* Final Report. DHHS Publ. No. SMA-03-3832. Rockville, MD: Author.

O'Connell, M. (2005). Recovery Self-Assessment (RSA). In T. Campbell-Orde, J. Chamberlin, J. Carpenter, & H. S. Leff (Eds.), *Measuring the Promise: A Compendium of Recovery Measures, Volume II* (pp. 91–96). Cambridge, MA: The Evaluation Center @ HSRI.

O'Connell, M., Tondora, J., Evans, A. C., Croog, G., & Davidson, L. (2005). From rhetoric to routine: Assessing recovery-oriented practices for recovery-oriented practices in a state mental health and addiction system. *Psychiatric Rehabilitation Journal, 28,* 378–386.

Onken, S. J., Craig, C. M., Ridgway, P., Ralph, R. O., & Cook, J. A. (2007). An analysis of the definitions and elements of recovery: A review of the literature. *Psychiatric Rehabilitation Journal, 31,* 9–22.

Onken, S. J., Dumont, J. M., Ridgway, P., Dornan, D. H., & Ralph, R. O. (2002, October). "Mental Health Recovery: What Helps and What Hinders?" A National Research Project for the Development of Recovery Facilitating System Performance Indicators. Phase One Research Report: A National Study of Consumer Perspectives on What Helps and Hinders Mental Health Recovery. Alexandria: VA: National Technical Assistance Center for State Mental Health Planning.

Provencher, H. I., Grigg, R., Mead, S., & Mueser, K. (2002). The role of work in the recovery of persons with psychiatric disabilities. *Psychiatric Rehabilitation Journal, 26,* 132–144.

Ralph, R. O., Kidder, K., & Phillips, D. (2000). *Can We Measure Recovery? A Compendium of Recovery and Recovery-Related Instruments, Volume I.* Cambridge, MA: The Evaluation Center @ HSRI.

Rebeiro Gruhl, K. L. (2005). Reflections on...The recovery paradigm: Should occupational therapists be interested? *Canadian Journal of Occupational Therapy, 75,* 96.

Ridgway, P. (2005). Recovery enhancing environment measure. In T. Campbell-Orde, J. Chamberlin, J. Carpenter, & H. S. Leff (Eds.), *Measuring the Promise: A Compendium of Recovery Measures, Volume II* (pp. 213–228). Cambridge, MA: The Evaluation Center @ HSRI.

Ridgway, P. A. (2001). Re-storying psychiatric disability: Learning from first person recovery narratives. *Psychiatric Rehabilitation Journal, 24,* 335–343.

Ridgway, P. A., & Press, A. N. (2004, June 3). "An Instrument to Assess the Recovery and Resiliency Orientation of Community Mental Health Programs: The Recovery Enhancing Environment Scale (REE), Version 1." Lawrence: University of Kansas, School of Social Welfare, Office of Mental Health Training and Research.

Ridgway, P. N., Press, A. N., Anderson, D., & Deegan, P. E. (2004). *Field Testing the Recovery Enhancing Environment Measure: The Massachusetts Experience.* Byfield, MA: Pat Deegan & Associates.

Roe, D., Rudnick, A., & Gill, K. J. (2007). The concept of "being in recovery". *Psychiatric Rehabilitation Journal, 30,* 171–173.

Rogers, E. S., Chamberlin, J., Ellison, M. L., & Crean, T. (1997). A consumer-constructed scale to measure empowerment among users of mental health services. *Psychiatric Services, 48,* 1042–1047.

Salyers, M. P., Tsai, J., & Stultz, T. A. (2007). Measuring recovery orientation in a hospital setting. *Psychiatric Rehabilitation Journal, 31,* 131–137.

Salzer, M.S., & Baron, R.C. (2006, November). "Promoting Community Integration: Increasing the Presence and Participation of People With Psychiatric and Developmental Disabilities in Community Life." Philadelphia: University of Pennsylvania Collaborative on Community Integration. Available at: http://www.upennrrtc.org/var/tool/file/32-Promotingcommunityintegration%20-%20Salzer,Baron.pdf (accessed October 15, 2009).

Schauer, C., Everett, A., del Vecchio, P., & Anderson, L. (2007). Promoting by value and practice of shared decision-making in mental health care. *Psychiatric Rehabilitation Journal, 31,* 54–61.

Sheyett, A. M., Kim, M. M., Swanson, J. W., & Swartz, M. S. (2007). Psychiatric advance directives: A tool for consumer empowerment and recovery. *Psychiatric Rehabilitation Journal, 31,* 70–75.

Snyder, C. R., Harris, C., Anderson, J. R., Holleran, S. A., Irving, L. M., Sigmon, S. T.,Yoshinobu, L., Gibb, J., Langelle, C., & Harney, P. (1991). The will and the ways: Development and validation of an individual-difference measure of hope. *Journal of Personality and Social Psychology, 60,* 570–585.

Spaniol, L., Bellingham, R., Cohen, B., & Spaniol, S. (2003). *The Recovery Workbook II: Connectedness.* Boston: Center for Psychiatric Rehabilitation, Boston University.

Stoffel, V. C. (2008). Perception of the clubhouse experience and its impact on mental health recovery. *Dissertation Abstracts International Section A: Humanities and Social Sciences, 68*(8-A), 3300.

Strauss, J. S. (1989). Mediating processes in schizophrenia. *British Journal of Psychiatry, 155,* 22–28.

Strong, S. (1998). Meaningful work in supportive environments: Experiences with the recovery process. *American Journal of Occupational Therapy, 52,* 31–38.

Substance Abuse and Mental Health Services Administration (SAMHSA). (n.d.) "National Consensus Statement on Mental Health Recovery." Brochure. Available at: http://download.ncadi.samhsa.gov/ken/pdf/SMA05-4129/trifold.pdf (accessed October 16, 2009).

Wilcock, A. A. (2006). *An Occupational Perspective of Health* (2nd ed.). Thorofare, NJ: Slack.

Woodside, H., Schell, L., & Allison-Hedges, J. (2006). Listening for recovery: The vocational success of people living with mental illness. *Canadian Journal of Occupational Therapy, 73,* 36–43.

History of Mental Health: Perspectives of Consumers and Practitioners

Christine Peters

> "We as a Nation have long neglected the mentally ill. . . . This neglect must end if our nation is to live up to its own standards of compassion and dignity and achieve the maximum use of its manpower. I am convinced that . . . the mentally ill can eventually achieve a wholesome and constructive social adjustment.
>
> —John F. Kennedy, Message from the president to the U.S. Congress, February 5, 1963

Introduction

President John F. Kennedy delivered the previous message of hope and dignity about mental illness to the U.S. Congress in 1963. Kennedy's concern for people with mental illness led to changes in mental health policy, some of which are regarded as advances and others as failures. The message remains relevant today. Achieving dignity and empowerment for individuals with mental illness has been a difficult struggle and, for the most part, a hidden chapter when compared with other civil rights movements in American history.

When reading mental health history, it is important to understand that history is not simply a chronology of events in time, nor should it be considered a whole truth. There are several sides to any event, depending on the point of view of the individual telling the story. This author views history as making connections or weaving threads. Memorizing names and dates, although a commendable effort, results in knowledge of linear and somewhat static information. What is missing is a reconstruction of *who* these people were, both occupational therapists and consumers, in the context of their times, and *why* their decisions and contributions worked or did not work.

This chapter presents history from multiple perspectives; unlike many works of occupational therapy history, it includes a strong voice from consumers who have lived the history. Various historical social movements are explored to demonstrate how changes in thinking in the United States influenced society's views of people with mental illness and the provision of mental health services. As with all historical accounts, the reader should recognize that this chapter presents only part of the story, with the goal of stimulating further interest in the topic.

History of Mental Health Practice in America

Occupational therapy as a profession was established in 1917, with strong roots in mental health settings (Schwartz, 2003). However, to understand the beginnings of occupational therapy, it is necessary to put those beginnings in context. Therefore, this section provides a more general overview of the evolution of practices and policies, the way the mental illness was understood, and the experiences of people with mental illness during these times.

Mental Illness in Colonial America

Misunderstood and mislabeled as "cursed souls," people with mental illness were banished from society in 17th-century America (McKown, 1961; Rosen, 1968). Keeping people with mental and physical illnesses secluded at home was a norm in Colonial America. Tending to the sick at home had both positive and negative consequences. On the one hand, it promoted health through maintaining daily rhythms in familiar environments. On the other hand, the isolation created a barrier for those in society who saw mental illness as taboo and did not want to acknowledge the ill in their communities. It is plausible that in Colonial America, like today, those individuals coping with mental illness and their families desired the best care available. However, in reality, the care for people with mental illness was frequently inferior or misguided.

Homeless individuals, who were viewed as "deranged," wandered the country and were auctioned off to work for minimal or no wages. The middle-class and wealthier people who were labeled as mentally ill wasted away at home. Not adequately cared for and lacking adequate food and clean clothes, these individuals were sometimes chained in unheated attics and occasionally tended to by physicians who used bleeding or purging methods (Dain, 1964). The prevailing belief was that mental illness was God's punishment for evil.

In agrarian Colonial America, where people commonly lived long distances from each other, responsibility for care of people with mental illnesses rested on the family, and it is likely that these families dealt with their own struggles. In moralistic and puritanical America, there existed the practical belief that every adult in the newly developing country had an obligation to contribute to society. Individuals with various mental illnesses were viewed as a drain on society because they were unable to enter the workforce and financially contribute to their communities. As a result, people with mental illness were grouped with destitute widows, orphans, the disabled, aged, and sick (Grob, 1994).

To remedy some of these shortcomings, Massachusetts created the first legal code in 1641, which assumed the financial burden for the "distracted and idiots." Other similarly populated states, including Connecticut, Rhode Island, New York, Vermont, and Virginia, followed suit in 1694. Although financial support was a practical solution, these legislative acts fell short because they did not address treatment needs (Grob, 1983; Starr, 1982).

Urbanization and the Rise and Fall of Asylums

Urbanization at the time of the Industrial Revolution gave rise to hospitalization, with the first hospitals established in Philadelphia in the mid-18th century. As poor immigrant populations flooded into America, overpopulation and disease spread quickly (Tomes, 1998). New solutions were sought for the mentally ill, including building large psychiatric hospitals or asylums. Literally translated from the Greek "without seizure," **asylums** were conceptualized as safe havens. These refuges were often built with acres of open space for walks and gardening activities. Staff cottages and other living quarters were built on the grounds.

Described by Dr. T. Romeyn Beck of New York City in 1811, in his address about moral treatment: "Moral management consists of removing patients from their residence to some proper asylum; and for this purpose, a calm retreat in the country is preferred" (Dain, 1964, p. 12). The Pennsylvania Hospital, the first general hospital in the United States to admit patients with mental illness, began an institutional transformation in the late 18th century under the leadership of American psychiatrist Benjamin Rush (Dain, 1964). Modeling British merchant William Tuke's York Retreat, large asylums in this country built before 1835 promoted humane treatment. The Quakers, or the Enlightened Friends, a progressive religious order that had a strong foothold in Pennsylvania, became influential as lay people promoting humanitarian values and care. The Quakers' beliefs in humane treatment of mentally ill individuals influenced the **mental hygiene movement** that came into spotlight at the turn of the 20th century.

Psychiatrist Benjamin Rush, drawing from the **moral treatment** momentum in the 1800s, became an influential figure in American medicine. He helped change the view that mental illness was due to possession or some other religious cause. Rush proposed various ideas about the etiology of mental illness, including the existence of predisposing psychological causes such as imaginative "occupations," damaging political and economic environments, and heredity (Dain, 1964). Adopting the belief that a biological and environmental balance was needed in mental diagnosis and treatment, the psychiatry profession began to develop (Starr, 1982).

A respected physician, Rush aligned himself with influential friends, such as Thomas Jefferson, John Adams, and Benjamin Franklin, who could politically promote his humane ideas. On a personal level, Rush coped with his own son John's lifelong commitment to the Pennsylvania Hospital, after John killed a close friend in a duel in 1810 (Dain, 1964). Consoling Rush at the time, Jefferson wrote a letter stating, ". . . he knew many persons who recovered from insanity and that he had always believed it was one of those diseases with a cure . . ." (p. 33). Rush understood mental illness not only as a physician, but also as a father who hospitalized his son in the very institution he founded.

Ultimately, these havens, which were intended to protect and treat people with mental illness, failed for several reasons, including training of the providers, questionable practices allowed in the asylums, and major issues of overcrowding. Still a developing profession in the 1800s, psychiatrists continued to prescribe purges and few visited "inmates." In Rush's day, less than 10% of all practitioners held degrees; therefore, there was a lack of licensing laws to enforce standards of care and education to promote moral treatment perspectives (Dain, 1964; Ludmerer, 1999). Clearly, there was a lack of qualified physicians in large hospital settings, thus contributing to the poor care for individuals with mental illness (Flexner, 1910). In the 1900s, dubious practices such as indiscriminant electroshock, lobotomies, cold sheet packs, and insulin shock therapy were prevalent.

The number of individuals needing care increased, which resulted in increased asylum commitments and the eugenics movement, or the sterilization process of individuals with mental illnesses (Whitaker, 2002). Adolph Meyer, who is often identified as the philosophical founder of occupational therapy, was a prominent psychologist in the early 1900s. Meyer presented a paper at the Conference on Mental Hygiene in 1913 in Raleigh, North Carolina. He spoke about common misunderstandings regarding state hospitals: "At present the (state) hospital is stamped as a receptacle for cases with whom nobody likes to be associated. Most states have not enough beds and provisions . . . and resent taking in cases of alcoholism and senile dementia, which they would rather leave to authorities . . ." (p. 186). In a more hopeful tone, Meyer continued, "The time will come when states and communities will be judged according to the way they are able to work for mental health, and when our people will have as much pride in their hospitals for mental cases as they are now justly proud of their schools and churches and public health boards" (p. 189). Idealistically, the state hospital system continued to face challenges.

Decaying, overpopulated American asylums built in the last quarter of the 19th century became structurally unsafe in the early to mid-20th century. Simultaneously, much needed federal funding required to upgrade these large hospitals was diverted away from mental health care concerns due to World Wars I and II and the Great Depression. Increasingly, the asylums became warehouses rather than treatment centers. Prior to the 1880s, psychiatric hospitalization typically lasted less than a year (Grob, 1994). After 1923, more than half of these patients remained hospitalized for 5 or more years.

It was in 1917 that occupational therapy was established as a profession. Occupational therapy was part of the humanistic movement, with its focus on the needs of people with mental illness. Although occupational therapists were working in many of the asylums, they held roles of lesser authority in these institutions (Grob, 1994). The patients were the group with the lowest rank, yet ironically it was their voice that needed to be heard the most. However, as conditions declined, the need for reform took precedence, leading to the mental hygiene movement.

Mental Hygiene Movement

One former patient who was heard, Clifford Whittingham Beers (1876–1943), spearheaded the mental hygiene movement. Beers (1912) wrote about his experience as a hospitalized patient in *A Mind That Found Itself*:

This story is derived from as human a document as ever existed . . . for in telling the story of my life, I must relate the history of another self. My history of a mental civil war, which I fought single-handed on a battlefield. . . . An Army of Unreason, composed of the cunning and treacherous thoughts of an unfair foe, attacked my bewildered consciousness with cruel persistency. Reason finally interposed a superior strategy that saved me from my unnatural self. (p. 1)

Born into a middle-class family from New Haven, Connecticut, Beers was one of five sons who showed early "chronic restlessness" in grammar school. Graduating from high school with no great desire to seek a job, he chose entrance into the Sheffield Scientific School, which offered a business course requiring 3 years of study rather than the more rigorous Yale College, which required 4 years. He was popular and involved in extracurricular activities. However, Beers began feeling mood fluctuations during his last 2 years of college, and by 1900, he experienced acute depression followed by nervousness. He also experienced difficulties at work. While visiting his family at home in August 1900, Beers attempted suicide and required hospitalization. It was his personal account of conditions at the Hartford Retreat that put an identified voice to the patient's movement.

"Few if any prison in this country contains worse holes than this cell proved to be. It was one of five about six feet wide by ten feet. A heavily screened and barred window admitted light and a negligible air quality" (Beers, 1912, p. 151). Seeing support for his book, Beers forwarded his manuscript to philosopher and psychologist William James. Although he was able to garner support from psychologists, psychiatrists such as Adolf Meyer were more guarded, seeing Beers' work as hypercritical of colleagues in his profession (Grob, 1983).

Gaining support, in 1909, Beers became a founding member of the National Committee for Mental Hygiene (NCMH), which was later renamed the National Mental Health Association (NMHA). Without the support of leading psychiatrists like Adolph Meyer, Beers held fast, and was successful in seeking funding sources and alliances, including the Rockefeller Foundation.

With Rockefeller's seed money, the NCMH was founded February 19, 1909, with the following goals:

- Protect the public's mental health.
- Promote research pertaining to etiology and prevention of mental disease.
- Seek government aid.
- Establish state societies.

In 1911, Beers was appointed secretary to NCMH. He was thereafter affiliated with the organization for 15 years, during which time he witnessed much growth, including the creation of an International Congress representing 41 nations. Beers struggled with his mental health from 1939 until his death in 1943, at the age of 67. In 1933, at the 25-year anniversary of the NCMH, various leaders in mental health reflected on their memories and involvement with the movement, including occupational therapy supporters Adolph Meyers, Richard Dunton, and Eleanor Clark Slagle. Dunton wrote that Beers showed that "mental illness is no more a shameful subject than . . . physical disease. I always wondered why Beers was not awarded a Nobel Prize . . ." (Letter to Welch from Dunton, February 13, 1933). In 1952, acknowledging Beers' contribution to mental health care, an hour-long dramatization of *A Mind That Found Itself* was made into a play entitled "My Name is Legion." The play opened on Broadway in 1952, and toured throughout the United States in 1953 for the purposes of education, fund raising, and supporting the mental hygiene movement.

Mental Health Policy

In the 1900s, several policies were established that promoted better services for people with mental illness. The Rehabilitation Act of 1920 addressed the needs of individuals with physical disabilities. In 1943, the Barden La Follette Amendment (PL 113) broadened the Rehabilitation Act to include individuals diagnosed with mental illness. This affected community transition, particularly for returning soldiers. Vocational counselors began to function as liaisons among hospitals, schools, and the work environment for individuals who experienced psychiatric problems. Because of the inherent problems of a stressful community reentry, various transitional community supports were established, including sheltered workshops, day hospitals, and outpatient clinics (Greenblatt, York, & Brown, 1955).

The National Institute of Mental Health (NIMH) was established in 1949 (Ridenour, 1961). The NIMH supported research relating to cause, diagnosis, and treatment of mental illness; provided fellowships and institutional grants to train personnel; and established clinics and treatment centers to deal with prevention, diagnosis, and treatment. Robert Felix, the director of NIMH from 1949 to 1964, created an optimism for community mental health that led to the adoption of important legislation.

The Community Mental Health Services Act of 1954, a New York State law supported by Governor Thomas E. Dewey, stated that any county or city with 50,000 or more residents could create a local mental health board with a psychiatrist director. Perhaps still medically authoritative, rather than consumer based, this law gave precedence to the idea that persistent mental illnesses could be prevented by early intervention in the community (Grob, 1994).

The National Mental Health Act, sponsored by Senator Lister Hill in 1955, addressed mental illness at the national level. This act supported the study of mental illness, the development of treatment methods, the evaluation and training of personnel, and the conduction of a national survey by the newly formed Joint Commission on Mental Illness Health (JCMIH). Given this new cash flow for treatment gains, new therapies evolved, including psychotropic drugs, milieu therapies (therapeutic communities, typically established on a hospital ward), electroshock, psychosurgery, and psychodynamic approaches.

A landmark act, the Community Mental Health Act of 1963, is criticized as being one of the most unsuccessful pieces of legislation (Torrey, 1977). The hope was that this legislation would reshape policy, creating more direct links with local communities to effectively and autonomously address their unique community mental health needs. Instead, it was the beginning of a poorly executed deinstitutionalization movement in which doors to large state hospitals opened with inadequate or scant community care available to individuals with serious mental illness. Deinstitutionalization and inflation in real estate led to high rates of homelessness among people with serious mental illness, a significant problem that continues today.

The Americans with Disabilities Act (ADA) of 1990 set a tone for the 1990s. The act spotlighted and described the isolation and segregation of individuals with disabilities. In 1999, the ADA was cited in the U.S. Supreme Court case of *Olmstead, Commissioner, Georgia Department of Human Resources, et al. v. L.C. and E.W.* As stated in the legal brief, the respondents L.C. and E.W. are mentally retarded women. In addition, L.C. was diagnosed with schizophrenia, and E.W. with personality disorder. When both women were admitted voluntarily to Georgia Regional Hospital in Atlanta, they were confined to a psychiatric unit. Although the treatment team concluded that they could be cared for appropriately in the community, they remained hospitalized. In a mixed opinion ruling (five supporting and three opposing), Justice Ginsberg announced that these women had the right to reasonable accommodations in the community. Identifying that parallel support existed for individuals with medical rather than mental disabilities, institutionalization was not justified.

For decades, mental health advocates have been working to establish better health care coverage for mental illness. The Mental Health Parity Act of 2007 (S. 558) and the Paul Wellstone Mental Health and Addiction Equity Act of 2007 are not only seen as progress, but also as a compromise. Although mental health coverage is not mandated, when mental health coverage is included, the coverage (including addiction) should be on par with physical illnesses. Seeing this as a step in the right direction and understanding that health insurance and business lobbyists were successful in their efforts to move against mandating mental health coverage, the American Occupational Therapy Association (AOTA) joined the National Alliance on Mental Illness in viewing this as a positive compromise (AOTA, 2007).

The Consumer Movement

The consumer or survivor's movement is akin to other equal rights movements. The purpose of any social movement is to change policy and culture, and gain jurisdiction (Abbott, 1988). Linked to counterculture ideology, the Insane Liberation Front, founded in 1969 in Oregon, is identified as the first consumer-run rights group (Tomes, 2006). Anchored by Judi Chamberlin's (1977) work, *On Our Own*, the consumer/survivor movement challenged an antiquated mental health belief system. In questioning labeling, Chamberlin states: "We can see this judgmental process at work when we look at the effect that a diagnosis of mental illness has on an individual's life. Unlike physical illnesses . . . once it has been decided that a person has a sick mind, enormous social consequences ensue . . . frequently loss of liberty" (p. 3).

Owning their identity and right not to be second-class citizens who need to hide an illness, some survivors are choosing to share their stories. Russell Pierce (2004), a consumer of mental health services, compared historical racial

struggles in the United States to the stigmatization of mental illness. The following passage shows how this former history student believes that a "sense of the past" promotes one's own recovery from the challenge of mental illness: "I believe . . . those of us who are already marginalized by history have a remarkable capacity to fight back. I gather strength from the struggles of black Americans, that . . . was just another label that had to be disproved, dealt with or more compassionately understood and appreciated in context" (p. 407). Although racial discrimination and mental illness can be challenged as dissimilar, the perils of discrimination and the challenges of various types of social injustice are shared experiences.

Thus far, this chapter has reviewed mental health history in the United States from Colonial America to current legislative and social policy. Moving from ineffective care to a more humane approach that ultimately brought with it empowerment and activism, consumers of mental health services have experienced many shifts in the "tides." Most recently, "prosumers," or mental health professionals who are consumers, have joined colleagues to show the effectiveness of peer-operated services (see Chapter 35) in forming mental health partnerships, research, and practice shifts in the community.

The next section reviews specific occupational therapy developments that occurred in the context of larger historical events in the United States. The reader is introduced to therapists who played prominent roles in occupational therapy mental health practice, policy, education, and research. These outstanding leaders and scholars shaped occupational therapy practice while responding to social change. When information is available, first person accounts are drawn on to show the meaning of occupational therapy to consumers.

Occupational Therapy Mental Health History

There is consensus that the roots of occupational therapy are in mental health practice and the moral treatment movement (Bing, 1981; Peloquin, 2005; Quiroga, 1995; Schwartz, 1992). The history of occupational therapy in mental health is presented first from the perspective of the consumer, using literature in which the individual receiving occupational therapy services describes his or her experiences. This is followed by the perspective of the mental health practitioner, primarily a leader in mental health occupational therapy. These two sections highlight the different focus on history when told from differing viewpoints.

Consumers' Perspectives

Historically, first person accounts about occupational therapy treatment were not always complimentary. Barbara Field Benziger (1969) writes about her 1960s hospitalization in *The Prison of My Mind*. She remembered her encounter with an occupational therapist with mixed reviews: "The first person I met who made any real sense . . . was the occupational therapist—a term I've always hated. She was kind, interested, enthusiastic . . . and intelligent. She had hit a gold mine in me, who all my life I have loved doing work with my hands—knitting, designs, painting. I told her that they (hospital staff) had taken away my knitting and tapestry needles . . . and my little scissors" (p. 47).

Mrs. Benziger's personal interests and willingness to embrace occupational therapy could have led to a therapeutic alliance; however, the author presents a different view. After the therapist returned with some sewing supplies and scissors, she asked, "Do you think I can trust you with these?" and suggested leaving the door open. The end result was a sense of powerlessness in Mrs. Benziger.

Other 1960s writings are published about Hillside Hospital and Creedmore Psychiatric Center (known as Creedmore State Hospital until 1974) in New York. Susan Sheehan (1983) received a Pulitzer Prize for her nonfiction book *Is There No Place on Earth for Me?* Beginning in June 1977, the author spent 1 year shadowing Sylvia Frumkin, a 28-year-old white middle-class woman of Jewish descent, who was hospitalized at Creedmore Psychiatric Center. Creedmoor opened in 1926, and consisted of 70 buildings sitting on 300 acres in Queens, New York, a borough of New York City. The center was riddled with overcrowding problems; in 1956, there were 6018 patients in a hospital that had a maximum capacity of 4188 (Sheehan, 1983). Frumkin's first Creedmore admission was in 1964, at the age of 15. With a total of nine hospitalizations through her mid-30s, during which she received electroshock therapy and insulin-coma therapy. Significant to occupational therapy is Sheehan's portrayal of Hermine Plotnick, who was the Clearview Unit Chief. Although Plotnick was identified as an able administrator, she was also an occupational therapist (AOTA, 1980). Through her years of hospitalizations, discharges, and rehospitalizations, Frumkin continued her relationship with Plotnick. During her 1977 hospitalization, Plotnick saw Frumkin's potential, suspecting that "Frumkin could have had a glamorous career if she hadn't spent so much of her life as a mental patient."

Occupational therapist Mary Donohue was then Supervisor of the After Care Activity Program at Long Island Jewish-Hillside Medical Center in the 1970s (M. Donahue, personal communication, May 3, 2007). Frumkin attended the woman's group that Donohue developed at Hillside. However, she dropped out because things said in the group were "very offensive" to her deep Christian beliefs (Sheehan, 1983, p. 286). Donohue (1982) developed and facilitated the women's group using an occupational therapy framework and life stimulation activities, readings, "rap" sessions, and exercise for body image building.

During the late 1970s and early 1980s, Donohue's (1982) woman's groups paralleled the consciousness-raising groups that many women involved in the feminist movement attended in their neighborhoods (Friedan, 1963). Thus, it provided a model for community transition and reintegration if newly discharged patients wanted to continue their activism and self-exploration. Although these women's consciousness-raising groups were framed in the feminist movement, what is innovative about the advocacy work is that it echoes the same issues that were discussed in the turn-of-the-century mental hygiene movement and current consumer's movement. Common to the mental hygiene movement, ex-patients were gaining a political voice of equality while owning their right to empowerment.

Another first person account is Irene Turner (1989) writing about her various hospitalizations while experiencing depression. At times feeling punished and humiliated in the most restrictive settings, she recalled the occupational therapist empowering her to decide which activities she believed were important to her own treatment. Turner also expressed difficulties and feelings of rejection when participating in interpersonal skills groups led by the occupational therapist, stating that the treatment approach did not meet her needs at the time. Hers is another mixed picture of occupational therapy intervention.

Moving into the "decade of the brain," the 1990s, occupational therapists attending the AOTA's annual conference in March 1992 in Houston, Texas, heard psychologist Frederick Frese and his wife, Penny Frese, talk about the personal experience of living with a psychiatric disability. Frese told the audience about his diagnosis of schizophrenia. He suggested that "OTs should encourage clients to participate in activities that are part of 'this world,' but that allow them to work through their trauma" (Egan, Joe, & Tapper, 1992, p. 33). Presenting the importance of a meaningful and dignified life with hope, the Freses advocated for occupational therapy's involvement in the consumer's movement.

These client's or patient's perspectives paralleled the time when individuals diagnosed with mental illness became more open in disclosing their stories. This was in part related to the feminist/equal rights movement, the independent living moving, and the consumers' movement.

More recently, occupational therapists have shared their personal life experiences as consumers or family members of individuals diagnosed with a mental illness (Mack, 2001; McGruder, 2001). Occupational therapist Suzette Mack (2001), rather than using the phrase "recovery from mental illness," sees her path as a "road to discovery." Occupational therapist Juli McGruder (2001) wrote about a family member's hospitalization and the formation of her interest in mental health practice: "I was attracted, as an adolescent, to consider occupational therapy as a career when I saw intriguing paintings at a mental hospital. None of these experiences compares with last year, when a beloved family member went missing . . ." (pp. 5–6). McGruder also writes about the mixed dilemma health-care professionals experience when they know both sides of the situation.

Health Providers' Perspectives

Until the 1950s, psychiatrists were the most prevalent spokespeople for occupational therapy in mental health. Early occupational therapy supporters included physicians William Rush Dunton, Jr., and Adolph Meyer. An unidentified psychiatrist stated the following: "As a psychiatrist, I point with considerable pride to the fact that it was in work with mental and nervous patients that the occupational therapist first made her official bow to the medical profession and to the public" (Slagle & Robeson, 1933, p. 18).

The idea of curative workshops became prominent in the 1930s. Curative occupations are "an essential treatment of persons suffering with mental disorder, of the feeble minded or of delinquents and criminal" (Ellis, 1930, p. 213). In April 1930, the Honorable William J. Ellis, Commissioner of the Department of Institutions and Agencies in Trenton, New Jersey, delivered a paper entitled "The Growing Need and Value of

The Lived Experience

Timeline of Recovery Through Mental Illness

Cherie Bledsoe

The comprehensiveness of this narrative reflects the importance that this chapter places on understanding history from multiple perspectives. For this reason, it includes quotes from multiple people.

> *We envision a future when everyone with a mental illness will recover, a future when mental illness can be prevented or cured, a future when mental illnesses are detected early, and a future when everyone with a mental illness at any stage of life has access to effective treatment and supports—essentials for living, working, learning, and participating fully in the community.*
>
> —THE PRESIDENT'S NEW FREEDOM ON COMMISSION ON MENTAL HEALTH, ACHIEVING THE PROMISE: TRANSFORMING MENTAL HEALTH CARE IN AMERICA, JULY 2003

I was born in the mid-1950s—an era of a restless but hopeful time of evolution for African Americans. For me, these times were about growing up in inner-city Kansas City, Kansas. My family and community village lived under the umbrella of poverty, oppression, and societal racism. We, however, found ways to create our own adventures and favorable memories. My father, who struggled with raising a family of 10 children, would often talk about having "bad nerves" as he spun into conflicting episodes of kindness and battles of rage. I now realize that he was doing his best to combat his own symptoms of mental illness. In my culture, topics such as mental illness were silenced and hushed, and thought of as private family matters.

Many consumers/clients/survivors of mental health services conclude that the mental health service delivery system has not remarkably changed since the 1950s. The history of the consumer movement revealed people on a journey of challenging, rebelling, and pushing for reform of our mental health service delivery system. This revolution was also the struggle of people who by the very nature of having an illness became marked as societal outsiders, labeled dangerous and given life sentences as hopeless cases. In my earlier childhood years, I remember community members joking about how they would pay you money to take people down to the "crazy house" and using phrases like "that person is as nutty as a fruitcake." I shuddered at the idea of being outcast from my community, committed to living in "the nut house." Life was hard enough living the black experience. To be further discriminated against because of the onset of mental illness was scary to think about.

As a person with mental illness, I have often felt the sting of stigma. Initially, I tried to find my way in understanding this illness. I did not feel the same sense of care and concern from people as those who were challenged with other physical sicknesses. No one really talked much to me about it. My world became silent.

Of note, in the 1950s, antipsychotic medications such as lithium to control symptoms of bipolar disorder were introduced to the mental health community. The 1960s marked the peak of the civil rights movement, to fight against inequality and social injustice. It was also the beginning of the introduction of television. I had a chance to see history being made. I can remember my grandmother, a strong and spiritual woman, intensely watching the news reports of black people challenging our nation's conscientious on our black-and-white television set. She would say, "Pray for Dr. King. You (girls) gotta be strong to live in times like these." These images depicted on television and their commentary by news reporters greatly influenced opinions, attitudes, and interpretation of this cause, but little did I realize that this same technology would play such a critical role later in my life because it would cast a negative light on people with mental illness.

> *In the very beginning, there was darkness. Persons experiencing mental illness were called "mental patients," "mental," "clients," and "chronic mental patients" or "chronics." All aspects of a patient's life were considered a "treatment modality." Therefore, there was no privacy in the patient's life and professionals exerted total control.*
>
> —SU BUDD, KANSAS CONSUMER ADVISORY COUNCIL LEADERSHIP COORDINATOR, PERSONAL COMMUNICATION, 2008

I listened to pioneer consumer leaders and advocates tell stories of the mental health system in the 1960s and was brought to an awareness—just like the struggles of the civil rights movement for African Americans, individuals with mental illness were also involved in their own civil rights reform. I am appreciative of these unwavering pioneers that led this cause for people with mental illness to be seen as human beings with dignity. The consumer movement was advanced in 1960, when the first mental health consumer-run organization in the nation was established. Consumer-run organizations and consumer-operated services create communities where consumers have ready access to peers who provide a circle of support. Consumers have hope that they can not only recover themselves, but also that they can play a role contributing to the recovery of others.

In 1961, the Report of the Joint Commission on Mental Illness and Health recommended upgrading hospitals and establishing community-based treatment centers. President John F. Kennedy in 1963 signed legislation for the creation of community mental health centers. President Kennedy defined mental illness as a real medical disability similar to heart disease and diabetes. Mental illness began to be viewed as a physical illness. President Kennedy set up a program to fight negative stigma.

> *I got ill in 1975, after a car wreck. From that time to 1980, I was having extreme feelings of paranoia and was challenged with delusional thinking; examples—like the FBI had bugged me and were listening and following me. In 1979, I was hospitalized and given a diagnosis of paranoid schizophrenia. I remember Reagan and Carter were presidents in the 70s. I can recall a world event where American hostages were taken in Iran. I remember trying to get to Iran to save the hostages. I had a belief that I could save them.*
>
> —DONALD C., A MENTAL HEALTH CONSUMER, PERSONAL COMMUNICATION, 2008

The Lived Experience—cont'd

The 1970s brought about the emergence of the women's liberation, gay rights, and disabilities rights movements. This was also the time of the first mental health ex-patients survivor's conference. The 1970s also brings to mind the era of empowerment for people of color. "Black Power" and "Black Is Beautiful" flourished pride and dignity, especially in young African Americans, and challenged the generally accepted standards of beauty. My self-esteem was at an all-time high as I picked my hair into afro and begged my mom to sew me a dashiki.

I started getting depressed after I graduated high school, lying in bed all day. It was hard to find jobs—unemployment was high for blacks. I went for treatment at our local community mental health center in 1984/1985, after being hospitalized in a state psychiatric facility. I received a case manager and attended the day program most of the time. Clients would sometimes receive certificates for perfect attendance, time out of the hospital, and being a kitchen volunteer. Smoking, sitting around, stuff to keep us busy was the agenda for the day. I remember President Ronald Reagan's campaign, "Say No to Drugs." For me, street drugs became my coping tool and alternative medication to deal with the changes within me and how the world responded to me.

—LESLIE W., A CONSUMER LEADER, PERSONAL COMMUNICATION, 2008

The foundation of the recovery movement took root through the consumer empowerment movement. It was energized with the disability rights movement, which started having a major impact around the 1970s and changed the way we view people with disabilities. The disability rights movement made it clear that the opportunities and supports that people with disabilities have are more important to their active participation in life than is their personal condition. The disability right movement has shown us that people with disabilities can live positive contributing lives if they have the right resources and supports.

As the consumer movement picked up momentum, consumers called for increased involvement in policy-setting and decision-making and increased attention to human rights. One of the major slogans of the disability rights movement is "Nothing about us without us." In fact, consumer control of services has increasingly been stressed in the disability field.

Another movement taking place around the 1970s was the emergence of self-help groups with a growing emphasis on the self-management of many long-term health challenges. Some of these models are in the fields of substance abuse such as AA's 12 steps. Other models were deaf/hearing impaired, HIV disease, cancer awareness, obesity, heart disease, and diabetes. Self-care and self-management of psychiatric problems began to follow this trend. In 1989, the National Association of State Mental Health Program Directors took the position that mental health consumers "have a unique contribution to make to the improvement of quality mental health care services . . . and

their contribution should be valued and sought . . . in provision of direct services. All of this greatly impacted the mental health consumer movement as consumer/clients/survivors themselves began to document their recovery journeys and started to share their stories.

In the mid-1970s, I graduated high school and had plans on becoming a special education teacher. I had compassion for special needs children. During this time, I managed to get through college, marry, and was raising three children. I carried hope for a promising future. The way I saw and knew life changed for me in the mid-1980s. During the summer of 1987, I can recall experiencing an intense overwhelming sadness, coupled with a lack of energy and motivation. Slowly, I could no longer keep up the pace of my work duties and taking care of my children. I thought this state of being was due to the numerous losses I had experienced that year, including my grandmother, mother-in-law, and brother-in-law.

With the support and intervention of coworkers, I was hospitalized for a psychiatric illness. The doctors at that time called it major depression and schizoaffective disorder. I had periods of dissociation, panic attacks, and delusions. I experienced symptoms of paranoia and anxiety, and was plagued by hallucinations. I was also confused and depressed, and an even deeper emotional depression set in because I was depressed. I felt caught up in what I simply referred to as hell. This was the beginning of my journey through recovery from mental illness. According to my faith community, the state of depression and "depressed people" were people separated from God. My community considered going to a mental health treatment center a taboo.

I moved into the social security system and the confines of poverty. I enrolled in the mental health center's partial hospital program, where the treatment focus was about stabilization of symptoms. I saw faces that looked like mine. These faces reflected my own feelings and emotions. They included some of my old childhood friends, neighbors, and church members, as well as many who were unknown to me. Some faces were of college students, parents, single moms, and grandmothers. I met a woman there, my age, with small children. I knew her as the daughter of a prominent minister in our community. Her face, like many of the others, was real, like mine. They mirrored back my fear, confusion, anxiety, and embarrassment. They reflected my hopelessness, but they also became my comfort. They became my friends and comrades as I became more detached from my family and community. They also reassured me that I wasn't alone.

Being part of the day program provided me the realization that there were others just like me—people I knew, and some I didn't, with their own unique story of how they came through the same door I had. This was the beginning of my awareness of what it is like to live with a mental illness. I came to understand that mental illness was no respecter of person—it happens to people regardless of who they are, what they look like, or where they come from.

The 1980s brought us the amazing shrinking hospitals and the explosion of community support programs. In 1980,

Continued

The Lived Experience—cont'd

Compeer, a project that brought together community people and people with mental illness as mentors and pals, was established. I received a case manager and therapist. At this time, mental health centers used the medical model of treatment, which was illness focused with the goal to stabilize symptoms. My treatment goals designed by my treatment team became my life focus—get out of the house, socialize with friends, stay out of the hospital, and learn to relax. I can remember being told, don't think about work, just take your medications and don't worry. My life became a merry-go-round of hospitals, pill medicines, therapy, day programs, and extensive stays in inpatient psychiatric hospitals and mental health treatment facilities.

In 1982, the Strengths Model of Case Management was being explored and introduced to mental health community supportive services. This transforming model of treatment focused on the mental health client's abilities versus illness, dreams versus past histories, and possibilities versus mistakes.

The 1990s ushered in the decade of "power to the mental health consumer." "Nothing about us without us" was echoed throughout the consumer movement. "Empowerment" was embraced as a pathway to finding your social voice and raising the consciousness of our world that individuals with mental illness are people, citizens with guaranteed universal rights. Consumers were encouraged by peers to see themselves as being more than a diagnosis of mental illness. More consumers started to share their stories of recovery. Consumer leadership, peer-driven services, and peer support were now being examined as emerging best practices in promoting recovery and wellness. The consumer movement held on to a hope that people with mental illness would be looked on with new lenses.

In 1990, the Americans with Disabilities Act (ADA), landmark legislation, provided protections against discrimination of people with disabilities. In 1997, Mary Ellen Copeland, mental health consumer, launched the "Wellness Recovery Action Plan" to assist consumers in developing a personalized plan to stay well. And, in 1999, the Olmstead v. L.C. U.S. Supreme Court decision affirmed the right of individuals with disabilities to live in community settings. A National Recovery Summit was held in Portland, Oregon, in 1999. At this summit, I recall discussions from peers on how they defined recovery in their own lives.

Recovery and resiliency are not new concepts to people adjusting to mental illness. People with mental illness understand that our survival depends on this spirit. The philosophy of recovery helps consumers through painful experiences of everything attached to a diagnosis of mental illness.

In 1999, the Surgeon General reported that the mental health system was in shambles and declared that stigma was a major barrier to why people shun mental health care. Community mental health centers began embracing recovery ideas and empowering consumers to build meaningful lives above and beyond symptom control and stability.

The road to recovery for me is a journey of hope, discovery, and change. My life is acceptance of the fact that I am a person with mental illness, but mental illness does not define all that I am. My change is constant, up and down, backward and forward—but my eyes stay on the prize of living a good life.

In 2003, The President's New Freedom Commission on Mental Health's "Achieving the Promise: Transforming Mental Health Care in America," stated, "Services and treatments must be consumer and family centered, geared to give consumers real and meaningful choices about treatment options and providers . . . care must focus on increasing consumers' ability to successfully cope with life's challenges, on facilitating recovery, and on building resilience, not just on managing symptoms" (p. 7).

This reform called for the transformation of an entire mental health service delivery system where consumers drive and participate in the decisions that affect their lives. The core values provide opportunities for consumers to lead, direct their treatment goals, and have genuine alliances with mental health providers who facilitate the consumer's recovery, and the community is there ready to support it.

Survivors/clients/consumers talked about visions of transformation of mental health services where consumers are engaged, visible, and participating in every area of policy-making and planning. We desire to have peer supporters, peer extenders, consumer providers, consumer advisory officers, and/or consumer advisory councils. Mental health consumers talk about the need to feel comfortable and welcome to express opinions about mental health services that are received without reservation of negative consequences.

Consumers are also beginning to talk to each other about raising the standards and expectations for their lives. We challenge ourselves to think about those perceived entitlements of care and learned helplessness behaviors that have been pasted on from the old school of treatment to moving toward self-responsibility, self-ownership, and pride in our own accomplishments. We look more to testing uncharted waters, understanding the dignity of risk to fail and learn from our experiences and discoveries. We are coming to the place where we no longer have to look at ourselves through the lens of the illness, but can see all the facades that make us human beings.

Currently, there are promising grassroots to federal initiatives to improve mental health care in America, that is, national and state recovery conferences, the development of a national toolkit for consumer-operated services, antistigma campaigns aimed at reducing stigma and discrimination associated with mental illness, and exploring shared decision aids to engage mental health consumers and providers in genuine alliances that support the recovery philosophy.

I believe recovery from mental illness and "having a life in the community" takes a community effort. Consumers ask our community of helpers and providers to accord us with equality, dignity, and respect. We want to be seen as human beings with all the rights and privileges that infers. We desire that our stories be told. We ask to be seen as unique people with various personalities, diverse life experiences, beliefs, skills,

The Lived Experience — cont'd

talents, and abilities. We ask that we have opportunities to contribute and participate in our communities. We ask that we not be seen as an illness, diagnosis, or label. We ask that you know we could be your family member, sister or brother, neighbor, coworker, or community member, not a person to be feared. We ask that we be full partners in our treatment and our recovery. We ask for a chance to live a quality life with you. We are all worthy.

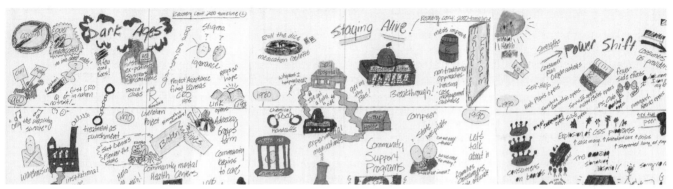

Timeline of mental health treatment from the perspective of consumers in Kansas attending the annual Recovery Conference in Wichita, Kansas, 2000. *Timeline courtesy of Cherie Bledsoe.*

PhotoVoice

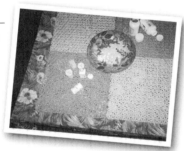

A little of this, a little of that . . . so many pretty pellets.

My experience with medication has, far too often, ended in an increase of misery— being more bane than benefit. That history has made the trial-and-error process of psychiatric treatment difficult to tolerate, and it's increasingly difficult to hold onto hope during periods of regression. My current prescription is successful in lessening my symptoms without creating a plethora of stressful side effects, and I am grateful. Still I wonder about the effects of long-term use. We bring the best of our knowledge and intentions to practicing the art of medicine and yet it seems that there are always trade-offs to be made. There are no easy answers.

—Willetta

Curative Occupations in All Types of Institutions for Mental Cases and in the Penal and Correctional Institutions," at the annual Institute and Conference of Chief Occupational Therapists of the State of New York's Department of Mental Hygiene. Ellis presented an exemplary system at the time. Physician McMurray, as chief director of occupational therapy at Greystone Park, reported a therapeutic program that included men's and women's arts and crafts, printing and bookbinding, concrete block making, and physical education (Fig. 2-1). However, of the 1126 patients, only 32% of the population was engaged in occupational therapy work (p. 214). It is not clear if this minority percentile was due to patient disinterest, illness acuity, or availability of services to all wards. For those involved in rehabilitation in the state prisons, training in occupations included manufacturing shoes, kitchen utensils, sheet metal work, and concrete road building through the cooperation of the State Highway Commission (p. 218). In his paper, Ellis presents a progressive program of rehabilitation; however, some of these programs were criticized and eventually eliminated because it was believed that patients were being exploited to supply part of the workforce of the institution.

Gail Fidler, an occupational therapy leader in mental health practice, spoke about early experiences that shaped her thinking about occupational therapy's place in community practice. While a student at the Philadelphia School of Occupational Therapy, studying with mentor Willard from 1938 until 1940, she remembered the following: "I got a job in the settlement house in south Philadelphia located in an area called Devil's Pocket. There were fights constantly between Italians and the Shanty Irish. And the front steps would be covered with drunk men (sic). Everybody said you can't take a job there, that dangerous. It was the safest post, because those men took care of me, would watch out for me . . ." (Fidler/Peters oral history, March 6, 2003, pp. 2917–2933). Fidler, who was known for her ability to see no barriers, carried this perspective into her occupational therapy work, forging new paths in the profession and challenging therapists to go beyond conservative paths.

Maintaining momentum while expanding the profession's presence, occupational therapy grew in the 1940s. This was influenced by the rehabilitation movement when returning World War II soldiers coped with physical and psychological

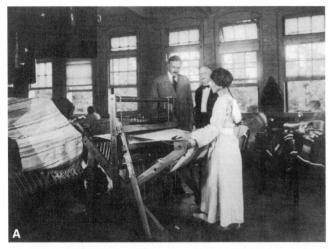 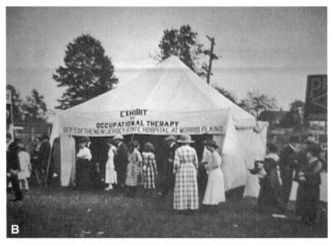

FIGURE 2-1. Occupational therapy was an integral component of treatment in the state hospitals during the 1920s. Both photos were taken by the Greystone Park Hospital's photographer, Fredrick Wainwright. **A:** Occupational Therapy Loom at Greystone Park Hospital, 1928. **B:** The Occupational Therapy Exhibit from Greystone Park Hospital at the Trenton State Fair, October 1926. *Photos courtesy of Greystone Park Hospital.*

war trauma. Occupational therapists shared their views about the effectiveness of their treatment anecdotally. For example, two unknown therapists on staff at the Bedford Veterans Administrative (VA) Hospital in Massachusetts shared their perception about the therapeutic environment in working at the hospital in 1945. The Bedford VA Hospital, typical of other hospitals of its kind, opened in 1928 as an outgrowth of the Rehabilitation Act for veterans of World War I. By the 1940s, following World War II, the staff expanded to include physicians, nurses, clinical psychologists, social workers, occupational therapists, manual arts therapists, education specialists, recreation therapists, and psychiatric technicians.

The rehabilitation department, including occupational therapy, helped patients transition to the community by focusing on problems of daily living. Two occupational therapists presented their account of occupational therapy intervention and outcome (Greenblatt et al, 1955, pp. 342–343):

> **First Therapist:** *"We went from painting the chairs to painting colored checker tables. Having made the things themselves, the men were more interested in playing with them later."*
> **Chief Nurse:** *"I'm interested to know if anyone has observed changes in the patients' socialization or communication?"*
> **Second Therapist:** *"The way they used to be lined up against the wall was awful to see. That has changed, and they seem proud of what they're doing and tell you about it."*

Underscored in this dialogue are two interpretations. The first therapist described how simple activities helped the men transcend their bleak surroundings, while they were able to stimulate new interests, such as simple craft construction and eventual games of checkers. The second therapist more clearly stated the reality of such environments and presented how potentially debilitating an illness can be in a less than supportive environment.

Similarly, at Boston Psychopathic Hospital, occupational therapist Marion Plotnick wrote in her journal about the ward environment for people with dementia: "The radio didn't work and there were no books or magazines available.

I felt that not so many baths (for incontinence) would have to be given and not so many disciplinary measures taken if there was something interesting for the patients to do" (Greenblatt et al, 1955, p. 119). Another journal entry reflects similar conditions on the children and adolescent unit: "The children were ill, but they had no materials for them to play with. The younger children who were psychotic were huddled together in a back room . . ." (p. 120). Plotnick was able to impact these environments by training aides and developing therapeutic programs.

The 1950s occupational therapy community mental health programs were led by physicians. For example, Maurice E. Linden, MD, director of the Division of Mental Health at the Department of Public Health in Philadelphia, mapped out a plan for community and social development in a paper he delivered at the Mid-Atlantic Regional Occupational Therapy Conference in Atlantic City in 1955. Linden (1956) urged occupational therapists to prepare for community-based practice, stating that rehabilitation does not stop at an institutional level, but "must be woven into a complete pattern of social reintegration" (p. 46).

Linden identified the occupational therapy skills that were most needed in community mental health practice. For example, guidance and habilitation of individuals with psychiatric disabilities requires the learning of "doing" skills, that is, arts and crafts that develop self-esteem through productivity. Community health priorities included "the mentally well who desire benefits from preventive services, those emotionally disturbed requiring readjustment to community living, and antisocial individuals requiring guidance" (Linden, 1956, p. 44). Although this was written more than 40 years ago, the ideas of emerging practice, prevention, and nontraditional occupational therapy settings were introduced.

Another shift in mental health practice was the emphasis on the theoretical support for practice. Theoretical underpinnings to practice surfaced between the 1950s and 1970s, with mental health occupational therapists Fidler and Fidler (1954), King (1974), Llorens (1960), Mosey (1968), and Reilly (1965), writing about psychoanalytic, developmental, behavioral, group development and adaptation, and sensory integration frameworks, respectively. Weighing how different frames of reference can better serve individuals, occupational therapists working in mental health began to understand the unique demands of shifting practice from hospital to community-based practice. Illustrating this, Patricia Ostrow (1960) discussed the "care and feeding" of theories, stating that theories evolve, change, and can become obsolete; "surely as a violet would become stunted and cease to flower if treated as a cactus, so will a theory become useless and cease to grow . . . " (p. 54). Mary Reilly (1965) believed in the importance of a theoretical foundation for practice, particularly in mental health, and also argued for the importance of research in occupational therapy. Theory development remained a topic of discussion from the 1960s to the 1980s.

Expanding the importance of theory development, the AOTA invited therapists to regional institutes that were financially sponsored by the Vocational Rehabilitation Administration to support field training and consultancy programs in psychiatric rehabilitation (Fig. 2-2). In these 5-day regional institutes, topics included group processes, object relationships, evaluation, the meaning of work, and human relationships (Mazer, 1964). When the American Psychiatric Association (APA) met in San Francisco in 1965, a coalition of mental health occupational therapists representing the AOTA and the California Occupational Therapy Association met. It was chaired by occupational therapist Dale Houston, and several occupational therapists presented papers on community-based occupational therapy. Describing how mental health services were undergoing rapid change, Lucy D. Ozarin (1965), of the NIMH, identified occupational therapy's place as part of the new mental health program and acknowledged the need for a partnership with the medical profession. Concluding the importance of transitioning to the community, this APA/AOTA workshop summarized the important shift to community practice.

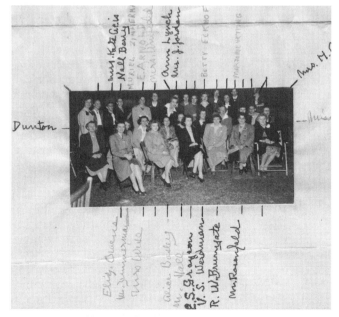

FIGURE 2-2. Maryland Occupational Therapy Association meeting in Maryland during the 1960s. This photograph belonged to Dr. William Dunton, whose handwriting identifies the therapists. Ruth Brunyate was the president of the American Occupational Therapy Association at the time. *Photo courtesy of William Dunton Furst, MD.*

Occupational therapy's involvement in community mental health projects expanded, thanks to occupational therapy leader Wilma L. West's position as consultant of the Occupational Therapy Maternal and Child Health (MCH) Service of the Health Services and Mental Health Administration, in which she promoted cutting-edge practice. In that role, she recruited occupational therapist Lela A. Llorens, who at the time was involved in child mental health research, for the "Mount Zion" project. Llorens accepted the MCH Service–funded position as occupational therapy consultant of the Comprehensive Child Care Project at Mount Zion Hospital in San Francisco, where she worked from 1968 to 1971. Working with at-risk families living in San Francisco's Western Addition housing projects, she demonstrated a new direction for community mental health prevention and occupational therapy practice. Based on this work, Llorens was invited to participate in a White House Conference on Children and Youth, highlighting occupational therapy's role in community practice with children (Peters, 2006).

Another significant community mental health symposium was sponsored in Philadelphia in 1970, under the support of the Psychiatric Special Interest Group, Council on Practice, AOTA. West (1970) proposed an occupational therapy trajectory, stating that "tomorrow's health care will be designed for the community as well as for the individual. For ours is a day of consumer involvement, of confrontation with demands for participation. . . . It is no longer satisfactory to people that we simply do things to and for them" (pp. 3, 5). West saw occupational therapy provision in new environments that provided a bridge between hospitals and community, such as in-home service and halfway houses.

Moving through the 1970s and 1980s, AOTA presidents Florence Cromwell, Jerry Johnson, and Robert K. Bing looked at emerging practice. Cromwell remembers Johnson, a strong proponent of preventive mental health services: "Johnson was very strong on moving into the community and not many had done that yet" (Cromwell/Peters oral history, April 28–29, 2003, p. 7013). In 1973, Johnson also chaired a social issues task force that looked at community mental health needs, including at-risk populations. Bing, a mental health practitioner, moved into the rank of dean at the University of Texas. While there, he developed multidisciplinary pilot programs along the border of Texas and Mexico for at-risk youth in the public school system. Once again, occupational therapy addressed mental health concerns in community settings.

Earlier issues in occupational therapy have been repeated from the 1980s to the present. Collaboration between disciplines is not new to occupational therapy, particularly when discussing community mental health services. However, while occupational therapists have been building new roads in community services, other professionals in social work, psychology, and medicine have also promoted psychosocial or psychiatric rehabilitation intervention. These individuals, based in various community mental health settings, have worked toward community reentry and supported employment and education, social skills training, jail diversion programs, homeless shelters, and clubhouse models (Anthony, 1977; Anthony, Cohen, & Farkas, 1983; Anthony & Liberman, 1992; Chamberlin, 1977; Deegan, 1994; Rutman, 1994).

Currently, occupational therapy is addressing the need for collaborative relationships with other disciplines, while also identifying the role and place of occupational therapy in the mental health system and establishing core competencies for mental health practitioners. Some examples of how the AOTA is addressing these issues is through the creation of Board Certification in Mental Health in 2006, and current efforts at the state level to add occupational therapy to the list of "Qualified Mental Health Practitioners."

At this time, occupational therapists are also managing issues related to evidence-based practice both for mental health occupational therapy and the profession as a whole. There are two separate concerns: (1) training practitioners to include research evidence as part of the clinical reasoning process, and (2) generating evidence to support occupational therapy practices in mental health. One AOTA initiative to address this need was the formation of the 2007 Ad Hoc Mental Health Evidenced-Based Literature Review Resource Advisory Group (M. Scheinholt, personal correspondence, May 18, 2007). This group is working to create literature reviews that can be used to guide occupational therapy practice in mental health.

Recovery

Occupational therapists are taking note of the recovery movement and its implications for mental health practice. Several historical events have marked the paradigm shift toward a widespread adoption of recovery-oriented principles. The President's New Freedom Commission on Mental Health (2003), *Achieving the Promise: Transforming Mental Health Care in America,* and An Action Plan for Behavioral Health Workforce Development, which was prepared for the Substance Abuse and Mental Health Services Administration (SAMHSA) by The Annapolis Coalition on the Behavioral Health Workforce (2007), are interdisciplinary task force projects that have generated reports stating that people with a mental illness can recover. In his vision statement, President Bush (President's New Freedom Commission on Mental Health, 2003) identified "a future when everyone with a mental illness will recover . . . and has access to effective treatment and supports essential for living, working, learning and participating fully in the community" (p. 1). In 2001, Bush cited the ADA and the *Olmstead v. L.C.* decision, adding that there are problems remaining: "the stigma that surrounds mental illnesses; unfair treatment limitations and financial requirements placed on mental health benefits in private health insurance; and a fragmented mental health service delivery system" (President's New Freedom Commission on Mental Health, Executive Summary, 2003, p. 1).

Targeting workforce needs, The Annapolis Coalition (Hoge, 2007), which is a not-for-profit organization focused on improving workforce development, concluded a 2-year strategic planning process that involved more than 5000 leaders in mental health across the United States. Strategic plans that evolved from the coalition focus on meeting workforce shortages, understanding recovery, and promoting community wellness. The report suggests that mental health providers can "learn from persons in recovery, youth and their families; become community mentors, and convey hope" (p. 24). Occupational therapy was involved in these meetings and is working to identify ways in which the profession can address the workforce shortages and promote recovery-oriented practices.

For example, following the Representative Assembly's recommendation, AOTA President Baum created ad hoc committees to address the need for occupational therapy to position itself in the mental health system (Brown et al, 2006; Pitts et al, 2005). Two AOTA ad hoc committee reports presented to the AOTA Board of Directors in 2005 and 2006 addressed potential action plans. For example, committee members suggested an exploration of the readiness of practitioners to participate in the mental health system, while additionally influencing public policy and payment streams (Pitts et al, 2005). A second AOTA report recommended exploring core competencies, payment reimbursement, and evidence to support occupational therapy practicing in mental health (Brown et al, 2006).

Occupational therapy is working to position itself as a discipline that embraces recovery-oriented principles. In occupational therapy, there is a slow but growing literature base specifically focused on occupational therapy and recovery (Brown, 2001; Inman, McGurk, & Chadwick, 2007; Lloyd, Wong, & Petchkovsky, 2007). In addition, there is a need to inform other disciplines about occupational therapy. In 2008, a special issue of the *Psychiatric Rehabilitation Journal* was devoted to occupational therapy's role in a recovery-oriented system of mental health care. Occupational therapy's continuing challenge includes educating occupational therapists about recovery and promoting the inclusion of occupational therapy within recovery-oriented service systems.

Summary

This chapter reviews occupational therapy's history in community mental health from the vantage point of individuals who received services. Autobiographical accounts showed how occupational therapy treatment was considered effective and noneffective, particularly in the 1960s through 1980, when the equal rights movement, combined with the seedlings of the consumers' movement came together in American history. It also reviewed occupational therapy history from the perspective of the profession, identifying its leaders in the mental health and mental hygiene movement from the 1920s to the present. This overview shows how social and historical events converged to bring about change, build bridges, and promote professional partnerships. The evolution of the mental health practice was fueled by changes in public policy and attitudes toward people labeled as mentally disabled. Learning from those who directly experienced mental disabilities, occupational therapy also changed practice directions. New frames of references better supported mental health practice. Transitions from hospital-based therapy to community-based therapies also changed the direction of occupational therapy practice. Most notable, founders such as Slagle, Dunton, and Meyer, to some degree, were supportive of the mental hygiene movement, which was closely linked to today's consumer-driven voice. Finally, history informs current practice in the area of recovery and evidence-based practice. Responding to government initiatives, the AOTA is evaluating the work ahead to better understand its role in today's mental health system, including having a better grasp of recovery and wellness, as well as training and education. Thus, occupational therapy, with its legacy of mental health advocacy, is moving forward in finding its unique contribution to all aspects of mental health care.

Active Learning Strategies

1. Interview

Interview a person with mental illness regarding his or her own experience with the history of mental health services. Has this individual's own perspective on mental illness changed? Has he or she seen a change in services? A change in health-care professionals? A change in stigma and acceptance? More or fewer opportunities? Did he or she receive occupational therapy services? Did these services play a role in his or her recovery? What are the most important changes he or she has seen? What changes are still needed?

 Describe the experience in your **Reflective Journal**.

Reflective Questions

- What did you learn from this interview? What insights did you gain about the experience of mental illness, mental health services, and the providers of those services?
- Did the individual experience discrimination? If so, what factors do you believe contributed to the discrimination? Did the person express any feelings of self-stigmatization (seeing the self in a negative light because of mental illness)?
- Based on the interview, what changes do you believe need to be made in terms of mental health services, society's view of mental illness, and occupational therapy's role?

Resources

Books

- Beers, C. W. (1912). *A Mind That Found Itself: An Autobiography.* New York: Longmans.
- Benziger, B. F. (1969). *The Prison of My Mind.* New York: Walker.
- Chamberlin, J. (1977). *On Our Own: Patient Controlled Alternatives to the Mental Health System.* Lawrence, MA: National Empowerment Center.
- Foucault, M. (1988). *Madness and Civilization: A History of Insanity in the Age of Reason.* New York: Vintage.
- Goffman, E. (1961). *Asylums: Essays on the Social Situation of Mental Patients and Other Inmates.* New York: Doubleday.
- Goldman, H. H., & Grob, G. N. (2006). Defining mental illness in mental health policy. *Health Affairs, 25*(3), 737–749.
- Jamison, K. R. (1995). *An Unquiet Mind: A Memoir of Moods and Madness.* New York: Random House.
- Sheehan, S. (1983). *Is There No Place on Earth for Me?* New York: Vintage/Random House.

Museums

- American Visionary Art Museum
  800 Key Highway
  Baltimore, MD 21230
  (410) 244-1900
  www.avam.org
  Includes many works by people with mental illness. According to the museum's website, "The AVAM refers to art produced by self-taught individuals, usually without formal training, whose works arise from an innate personal vision that revels foremost in the creative act itself."
- Glore Psychiatric Museum
  3408 Frederick Avenue
  Saint Joseph, MO 64506
  Chronicles 130 years of history of the "State Lunatic Asylum No. 2."
- Walter Anderson Museum of Art
  510 Washington Avenue
  Ocean Springs, MS 39546
  (228) 872-3164
  www.walterandersonmuseum.org
  Highlights the art of Walter Anderson, a prominent American artist that lived with serious mental illness.

Websites

- History of the American Occupational Therapy Association: http://www.aota.org/About/39983.aspx
- Patricia Deegan—includes information on several history projects: http://www.patdeegan.com/cp_socialjustice.html#state
- The Willard Suitcase Exhibit—an online exhibit of suitcases left behind by former patients of a New York State Hospital: http://suitcaseexhibit.org/indexhasflash.html

References

Abbott, A. (1988). *The System of Professions: An Essay on Division of Expert Labor.* Chicago: The University of Chicago Press.

American Occupational Therapy Association (AOTA). (1980). *1980 Yearbook.* New York: Author.

American Occupational Therapy Association (AOTA). (2007). "AOTA Supports Mental Health and Substance Abuse Parity." Available at: http://www.aota.org/Archive/FedReimbA/Issues/MentalHealth/40333.aspx (accessed January 7, 2010).

The Annapolis Coalition on the Behavioral Health Workforce (2007). "An Action Plan on Behavioral Health Workforce Development." Report for the U.S. Department of Health and Human Service (DHHS), Substance Abuse and Mental Health Service Administration (SAMHSA). Contract No. 280-02-0302.

Anthony, W. A. (1977). Psychological rehabilitation: A concept in need of a method. *American Psychologist, 32,* 658–662.

Anthony, W. A., Cohen, M., & Farkas, M. (1983). Philosophy, treatment process and principles of psychiatric rehabilitation approach. In I. Bahrach (Ed.), *New Directions for Mental Health Services: Deinstitutionalization* (pp. 67–79). San Francisco: Jossey-Bass.

Anthony, W. A., & Liberman, R. P. (1992). Principles and practice of psychiatric rehabilitation. In R. P. Liberman (Ed.), *Handbook of Psychiatric Rehabilitation* (pp. 95–126). New York: Macmillan.

Beers, C. W. (1912). *A Mind That Found Itself: An Autobiography.* New York: Longmans.

Benziger, B. F. (1969). *The Prison of My Mind.* New York: Walker.

Bing, R. H. (1981). Occupational therapy revisited: A paraphrastic journey. *American Journal of Occupational Therapy, 35,* 499–518.

Brown, C. (2001). *Recovery and Wellness: Models of Hope and Empowerment for People With Mental Illness.* New York: Haworth Press, Inc.

Brown, C., Moyers, P., Haerlein Sells, C., Learnard, L., Mahaffey, L., Pitts, D., Ramsay, D., Bonder, B., Hudkins, A., Giles, G., Nanoff, T., Scheinholtz, M., & Willmarth, C. (2006). "Report of Ad Hoc Committee on Mental Health Practice in Occupational Therapy to the AOTA Board of Directors, December 18, 2006." Unpublished paper, American Occupational Therapy Association.

Chamberlin, J. (1977). *On Our Own: Patient Controlled Alternatives to The Mental Health System.* Lawrence, MA: National Empowerment Center.

Chamberlin, J. (1994). An ex-patient's view of people who are homeless and mentally ill. In L. Spaniol (Ed.) *An Introduction to Psychiatric*

Rehabilitation (pp. 135–138). Columbia, MD: International Association of Psychosocial Rehabilitation Services.

Dain, N. (1964). *Concepts of Insanity in the United States 1789–1865*. New Brunswick, NJ: Rutgers University Press.

Deegan, P. E. (1994). The independent living movement and people with psychiatric disabilities: Taking back control over our own lives. In *An Introduction to Psychiatric Rehabilitation* (pp. 121–134). Columbia, MD: International Association of Psychosocial Rehabilitation Services.

Donohue, M. V. (1982). Designing activities to develop a women's identification group. *Occupational Therapy in Mental Health, 2*(1), 1–19.

Dunton, W. R. (1928/1945). *Prescribing Occupational Therapy*. Springfield: Thomas.

Egan, M., Joe, B. E., & Tapper, B. E. (1992). Consumer thrust evident at general plenary sessions. *OT Week, April 16*, 32–33.

Ellis, W. J. (1930). The growing need and value of curative occupations in all types of institutions for mental cases and in penal and correctional institutions. *Occupational Therapy and Rehabilitation, IX*(4), 213–220.

Fidler, G. S., & Fidler, J. W. (1954). *Introduction to Psychiatric Occupational Therapy*. New York: Macmillan.

Flexner, A. (1910). *Medical Education in the United States and Canada*. Boston: Merrymount Press.

Freidan, B. (1963). *The Feminine Mystique*. New York: Dell.

Goffman, E. (1961). *Asylums: Essays on the Social Situation of Mental Patients and Other Inmates*. New York: Doubleday.

Greenblatt, M., York, R. H., & Brown, E. L. (1955). *From Custodial to Therapeutic Patient Care in Mental Hospitals*. New York: Russell Sage Foundation.

Grob, G. N. (1983). *Mental Illness and American Society 1875–1940*. Princeton, NJ: Princeton University Press.

Grob, G. N. (1994). *The Mad Among Us: A History of the Care of America's Mentally Ill*. Cambridge, MA: Harvard University Press.

Inman, J., McGurk, E., & Chadwick, J. (2007). Is vocational rehabilitation a transition to recovery? *British Journal of Occupational Therapy, 70*(2), 60–66.

King, L. J. (1974). A sensory integrative approach to schizophrenia. *American Journal of Occupational Therapy, 28*(9), 529–536.

Linden, M. E. (1956). A community organizes for mental health programming. *American Journal of Occupational Therapy, 10*(2 pt 1), 43–46, 74.

Llorens, L. A. (1960). Psychological tests in planning therapy goals. *American Journal of Occupational Therapy, 14*, 243–246.

Lloyd, C., Wong, S. R., & Petchkovsky, L. (2007). Art and recovery in mental health: A qualitative investigation. *British Journal of Occupational Therapy, 70*(5), 207–214.

Ludmerer, K. M. (1999). *Time to Heal: American Medical Education from the Turn of the Century to the Era of Managed Care*. New York: Oxford University Press.

Mack, J. (2001). Where the rainbow speaks and catches the sun: An occupational therapist discovers her true colors. *Occupational Therapy in Mental Health, 17*(3), 43–58.

Mazer, J. L. (1964). "Summary of the New Psychiatric Consultancy Grant." Proceeding of the special programs of the Psychiatric Subcommittee at the American Occupational Therapy Association annual conference, October 27, Denver.

McGruder, J. (2001). Life experience is not a disease or why medicalizing madness is counterproductive to recovery. *Occupational Therapy in Mental Health, 17*(3), 59–80.

McKown, R. (1961). *Pioneers in Mental Health*. New York: Dodd, Mead & Company.

Mosey, A. C. (1968). "Occupational Therapy Theory and Practice." Training program supported in part by Training Grant No. 543-T-65 from the Rehabilitation Services Administration, Department of Health, Education and Welfare, Washington, DC, to the Medical Foundation, Inc., in collaboration with Massachusetts Department of Mental Health. Medford, MA: Pothier Brothers Printers.

Olmstead, Commissioner, Georgia Department of Human Resources, et al. v. L.C. and E.W. 98-536 (U.S. Supreme Court, 1999).

Ostrow, P. C. (1960). "The Care and Feeding of Theories." Proceedings from 1960 AOTA Conference, 55–57.

Ozarin, L. D. (1965). "Mental Health Services in Transition: Implications of Community Health Programs for Occupational Therapy." Paper presented at the Patterns for Progress in Psychiatric Occupation Therapy meeting for psychiatric occupational therapists, 17th Mental Hospital Institute of the American Psychiatric Association, September 26, San Francisco.

Peloquin, S. M. (2005). Embracing our ethos, reclaiming our heart. *American Journal of Occupational Therapy, 59*(6), 611–625.

Peters, C. (2005). "Powering Professionalization of Occupational Therapy: 1950–1980." Unpublished doctoral dissertation. New York University.

Peters, C. O. (2006). "Power and Professionalization: Occupational Therapy 1950 to 1980." PhD dissertation, New York University.

Pierce, R. D. (2004). A narrative of hope. *Psychiatric Rehabilitation Journal and Innovations Research, 27*(4), 403–409.

Pitts, D., Lamb, A., Ramsay, D., Learnard, L., Clark, F., Scheinholtz, M., Metzler, C., & Nanoff, T. (2005). "OT in Mental Health Systems." Report to the American Occupational Therapy Association Board of Directors, October 12, 2003.

President's New Freedom Commission on Mental Health. (2003). *Achieving the Promise: Transforming Mental Health Care in America, Final Report*. Publ. No. SMA-03-3832. Rockville, MD: U.S. Department of Health and Human Services.

Quiroga, V. (1995). *Occupational Therapy: The First 30 Years*. Bethesda, MD: American Occupational Therapy Association.

Reilly, M. (1965). "A Psychiatric Occupational Therapy Program as a Teaching Model." Paper presented at the meeting for psychiatric occupational therapists, held in conjunction with the 17th Mental Hospital Institute of the American Psychiatric Association, September 26, San Francisco.

Reverby, S. M. (1987). *Ordered to Care: The Dilemma of American Nursing, 1850–1945*. New York: Cambridge University Press.

Ridenour, N. (1961). *Mental Health in the United States: A 50 Year History*. Cambridge, MA: Harvard University Press.

Rosen, G. (1968). *Madness in Society: Chapters in the Historical Sociology of Mental Illness*. New York: Harper & Row.

Rutman, I. D. (1994). What is psychiatric rehabilitation? In *An Introduction to Psychiatric Rehabilitation* (pp. 4–8). Columbia, MD: International Association of Psychosocial Rehabilitation Services.

Schwartz, K. B. (1992). Examining the profession's legacy. *American Journal of Occupational Therapy, 46*, 9–10.

Schwartz, K. B. (2003). History of occupation. In P. Kramer, J. Hinojosa, & C. B. Royeen (Eds.), *Perspective in Human Occupation: Participation in Life* (pp. 18–31). Philadelphia: Lippincott Williams & Wilkins.

Sheehan, S. (1983). *Is There No Place on Earth for Me?* New York: Vintage/Random House.

Slagle, E. C., & Robeson, H. (1933). *Syllabus for Training Nurses in Occupational Therapy*. Utica, NY: State Hospitals Press.

Starr, D. (1982). *The Social Transformation of American Medicine*. New York: Basic Books.

Tomes, N. (1998). *The Gospel of Germs: Men, Women and the Microbe in American Life*. Cambridge, MA: Harvard University Press.

Tomes, N. (2006). The patient as a policy factor: A historical case study of the consumer/survivor movement in mental health. *Health Affairs, 25*(3), 720–729.

Torrey, E. F. (1997). *Out of the Shadows: Confronting America's Mental Illness Crisis*. New York: Wiley.

Turner, I. M. (1989). The healing power of respect: A personal journey. *Occupational Therapy in Mental Health, 9*(1), 17–22.

West, W. L. (1970). "Occupational Therapy in Community Health Care." Paper presented at Our Changing Partnership symposium, Psychiatric Special Interest Group, Council on Practice, American Occupational Therapy Association, September 21, Philadelphia.

Whitaker, R. (2002). *Mad in America: Bad Science, Bad Medicine and the Enduring Mistreatment of the Mentally Ill*. Cambridge, MA: Perseus Publishing.

Person-Environment-Occupation Model

Susan Strong and Karen Rebeiro Gruhl

> "Far and away the best prize that life offers is the chance to work hard at work worth doing.
>
> —Theodore Roosevelt, 1903

Introduction

Amidst their efforts to enable clients' satisfying participation in meaningful occupations of their choosing, occupational therapists must make sense of occupational performance issues. To begin, they use clinical reasoning skills to determine what is interfering with occupational performance. For example, there are many reasons why a child may have difficulty completing homework, such as attentional problems that interfere with focusing on the homework. In this case, the barrier relates to the child's cognitive abilities. However, there could be family issues that make working at home difficult, which is an environmental issue. Finally, the occupation itself may present the problem; the homework may be too difficult, or the child does not find it interesting.

Occupational therapists work under the assumption that successful engagement in meaningful occupations is central to an individual's well-being and health (Wilcock, 2006). Although success is personally defined by the client, the elements that contribute to that success can be understood by the interplay of factors concerning the person, environment, and occupation. The **Person-Environment-Occupation (PEO) model** is a conceptual framework that was developed by a group of Canadian occupational therapy clinicians and researchers to provide a systematic way to analyze complex occupational performance issues within the context of occupational therapy practice (Law et al, 1996). In fact, the PEO model is the organizing construct for this textbook; each aspect is examined in a comprehensive way to ensure that learners have a strong grounding in client-centered, occupation-based practices that occur in natural environments in order to promote individuals' full participation in their everyday lives in communities.

There are several broad theoretical frameworks in occupational therapy that provide direction for considering the relationships of the person, environment, and occupation in occupational performance. Other prominent frameworks include the Person, Environment, Occupational Performance model (Christiansen, Baum, & Haugen, 2005), the Ecology of Human Performance (Dunn, Brown, & Youngstrom, 2003), and the Model of Human Occupation (Kielhofner, 2008). These frameworks are useful and provide slightly different perspectives on the constructs. One reason for using the PEO model to organize this text is its parsimony. Although each individual construct of person, environment, and occupation is complex and deep, these three central constructs provide a straightforward system for organizing the material in the text.

Development of the PEO Model

In the 1990s, several Canadian occupational therapists came together to develop the PEO model in an effort to more comprehensively describe the constructs that affect occupational performance (Law et al, 1996). The PEO model was built on the work of many environmental-behavioral theorists who studied the relationships between people and environments. For example, Lewin (1933) and Murray (1938) wrote about the concept of **environmental press**, in which forces in the environment, together with individual need, evoke a response. For example, the environmental press of a large sporting event encourages, or presses, the individual in attendance to root for the team. However, the environment and needs of the student in a classroom testing situation promotes quiet and concentration.

The concept of **adaptation** was identified by Lewin (1933) and Murray (1938) as the achievement of a good fit between a person and his or her environment. Baker and Intagliata (1982) looked at an individual's perception of the environment and concluded that people actively engage in efforts to achieve a level of satisfaction, or fit, between themselves and their perceived environment.

Lawton's (1986) Model of Competency described adaptive and maladaptive behaviors as the result of the environmental press and an individual's competence to meet the demands of that press. Therefore, what Lawton termed "maladaptive behavior" with negative effect was conceptualized as resulting from someone with too low skills being met with too high challenges or, conversely, someone with too high skills being met with weak or limited challenges. As an individual's personal competence decreases, vulnerability to environmental influences increases. For example, people are more vulnerable to getting into a car accident when under the influence of alcohol or drugs. And individuals who are stressed or anxious may find it more challenging to deal with the demands of young children.

These theories were primarily developed with an interactive framework that simplified the realities of human behavior as consisting of cause-and-effect relationships. What was needed, however, was a transactive model that supported the diversity of therapists' observations. In a transactive model, the relationships are bidirectional. For example, the environment can influence the person and vice versa; in the process, this interaction creates a change in the occupation. For example, a parent who is preparing a meal for the family creates changes in the food during the cooking process. In addition, the parent is creating a social context for eating together. The reaction of the family then impacts the food preparer. If the family likes the meal and compliments the cook, then the parent will feel affirmed and appreciated, and he or she is likely to repeat the experience. However, if a family member complains about the food or misses dinner to attend an event with friends, a different social context is created, which affects the parent who prepared the meal and, potentially, subsequent meals together. The experience is laden with personal meaning for everyone involved, and any one change in the people, environment, or occupation of the situation can result in a much different experience.

Another reason for the need for a new model for occupational therapists was that, in the 1990s, therapists were expanding their practice and were working with individuals, groups, organizations, and communities in a variety of roles and settings. Also, the environmental-behavioral theorists did not inform therapists about occupation, which is the core of occupational therapy.

Another influence of the PEO model was Csikszentmihalyi and Csikszentmihalyi's (1988) Theory of Optimal Experience, which described people engaging in occupations. In this theory, adaptation is viewed as the congruence between challenges present within an activity and the environment and a person's skills. They coined the term "**flow**" to describe the experience of losing oneself in an inherently satisfying activity; this can occur when an individual is engaged in an activity in a given environment with the just right challenge (i.e., when the perceived challenge matches the individual level of skill for that particular activity in that given environment).

A few other theorists looked at individuals beyond their immediate environment. Bronfenbrenner's (1977) Ecological Systems model assumed the interdependence of "nested" social systems, with the individual's microsystem in the center, surrounded by a mesosytem of families and work/school, which was surrounded by an exosystem of formal and informal social structures, which in turn was enveloped by a macrosystem of institutions in society (e.g., government).

The Healthy Communities Conceptual model (Trainor, Pomeroy, & Pape, 1983) introduced the influence of community, culture, and social policy on the mind, body, and spirit of an individual. This model expanded conceptually what was considered the environment and introduced the need to change environments rather than changing people to fit the environment.

The creation of the PEO model was influenced by these and the following factors:

- Rise in the use of the environment as a treatment modality for occupational therapy
- Publication of the *Occupational Therapy Guidelines for Client-Centered Practice* (Canadian Association of Occupational Therapists [CAOT], 1991)

- Occupational therapists reclaiming occupation as a central focus of practice
- Health care's shift to a health and wellness focus with health linked to people having autonomy over their environments (National Health and Welfare Canada, 1988)
- Recognition that professional intervention services are not to be assumed to be the best or only intervention, with government policies making self-help and supportive, caring communities a new focus
- Societal changes of a growing consumer movement and legislation such as the American With Disabilities Act (1990)

For a more detailed explanation of its early development, the reader is directed to Law et al's (1996) article in the *Canadian Journal of Occupational Therapy*. At this time, occupational therapy was redefining itself within a changing global community and new understandings of health. The PEO model was used, and continues to be used, to explain and define the occupational therapy field and practices, and to communicate what it is all about to others.

The PEO model has become even more relevant as the concept of disabling environments has come to be understood. Jongbloed and Crichton (1990) encouraged therapists to consider the handicapping effects of the environment and target efforts on the social circumstances that sustain disability, rather than focusing on fixing the individual with a disability. Fougeyrollas et al's (1998) Quebec Committee of the International Classification of Impairment, Disability and Handicap (ICIDH) published a conceptual model of the handicap creation process, in which handicap is viewed as the interaction between the person's organic systems (impairments), abilities (disabilities), environmental factors (obstacles), and life habits (handicap situations). Environments came to be classified according to their enabling and disabling effects (Law, 1991).

Writing about the outcry of "not in my back yard" to the creation of transitional housing for persons with mental illness, Kearns and Taylor (1989) were some of the first researchers to draw the public's attention to how mental disability is reinforced and compounded by poverty, unemployment, limited social networks, and negative public attitudes. Social and health service systems have been described as a labyrinth of bureaucratic barriers that compromises clients' pursuit and participation in meaningful community occupations (Rebeiro, 1999).

Patricia Deegan (1992) eloquently wrote about a series of environmental barriers faced by individuals with psychiatric disabilities that create helplessness and dependency. Her Cycle of Disempowerment and Despair (p. 12) identified professionals' and other service providers' attitudes and beliefs about people with psychiatric disabilities as the central driving force for transferring control over consumers' lives to the health-care system. Occupational therapists came to understand how they could be an enabling or disabling element in a client's environment.

The now considerable writings about client-centered practice in occupational therapy are in essence about therapists creating enabling environments. An occupational therapist, Deborah Corring (1996), studied clients' perceptions of client-centered practice and found that some service providers have added to the stigma that already exists in their clients' lives. For example, therapists may suggest that the individual with a mental illness "settle" for a limited life due to the disability. Corring's study participants suggested that therapists can foster a client-centered practice by creating a supportive social environment that demonstrates valuing the client, believing in the client's potential, taking time to arrive at a common ground, and actively supporting choice- and decision-making by the client.

Description of the PEO Model

The PEO model describes the transactive, dynamic relationships that occur when people engage in occupations within given environments over time. Environments, occupations, and people have both enabling and constraining effects on one another; they shape each other, change over time, and ascribe meaning in the process. Change within one part affects the other parts on many levels. Students can consider the transactive relationship involved in working on group projects for school. Differences in the individuals who comprise the group, along with the particular assignment, can create different enabling and constraining effects. In addition, the experience will undoubtedly affect each student involved, but each student's experience will be unique. Furthermore, the transaction creates a whole that is greater than any of the individual parts. This does not necessarily mean that it is a positive experience, but one that is dynamic and complex.

The transactive relationships are interwoven and interdependent, with the result being greater than the sum of individual elements. The product of these relationships is the quality of a person's experience with regard to being able to satisfactorily perform meaningful occupations (i.e., occupational performance). The person's experiences shape performance and vice versa, ascribing ever-changing meanings. The PEO model enables the therapist to conceptualize, analyze, and communicate these dynamic, transactive relationships.

The definitions of the model's main components—person, environment, occupation/occupational performance—are synonymous with the definitions used by the Canadian Model of Occupational Performance (CMOP; CAOT, 1997).

Person

The person is viewed as "an integrated whole who incorporates spirituality, social and cultural experiences, and observable occupational performance components" (CAOT, 1997, p. 41). The performance components refer to what the person is feeling (affective), thinking (cognitive), and doing (physical), which "contribute to successful engagement in occupation" (p. 43).

Spirituality is considered to be at the core of all PEO interactions. "Spirituality resides in the person, is shaped by the environment, and gives meaning to occupations" (CAOT, 1997, p. 33). A person's spirituality is imbued with his or her individual beliefs, values, and goals, all of which guide choices and provide a source of self-determination and personal control. In client-centered practice, the client can be an individual person, a group of individuals, or an organization.

The person as a component of the PEO model is further described in Chapter 6.

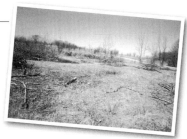

PhotoVoice

What I see here is the contrast between the sky, which is bright and stands for hope, and the ground, which is dismal. I see this as a comparison of mental health and mental illness.

Environment

The environment is "the context within which occupational performance takes place" (CAOT, 1997, p. 44). The environment encompasses local situations, such as families and neighborhoods, and broader influences involving community, provincial/state, and national and international factors, such as health insurance, transportation systems, and industry or employment opportunities. Elements of the environment are classified as cultural, institutional, physical, and social. The cultural environment involves beliefs, customs, and traditions. The institutional environment is made up of organized systems, such as legislative bodies, health-care systems, and educational institutions. The physical environment is made up of things that can be seen and includes objects such as furniture and cookware, buildings, and the natural environment. The social environment includes friends, family, and larger social networks that interact with the individual.

The environment as a component of the PEO model is further described in Chapter 26.

Occupation

Occupations are "clusters of activities and tasks in which people engage while carrying out various roles in multiple" locations (Strong et al, 1999, p. 125). Canadian occupational therapists use three classifications of purpose, which are culturally defined: self-care, productivity, and leisure (CAOT, 1997, p. 37). American occupational therapists use the classifications of activities of daily living (ADLs), instrumental activities of daily living (IADLs), education, work, play, leisure, and social participation (AOTA, 2002). Canadian "productivity" occupations are viewed differently than American "work." Both classifications include volunteering, but in Canada productivity includes home maintenance and parenting, and, for children, productivity includes play and school work. Occupations place affective, cognitive, and physical demands on the individual performing the occupation.

Occupation as a component of the PEO model is further described in Chapter 45.

Occupational Performance

Occupational performance is "the result of a dynamic relationship between persons, environment and occupation over a person's lifespan . . . refers to the ability to choose, organize, and satisfactorily perform meaningful occupations that are culturally defined and age appropriate for looking

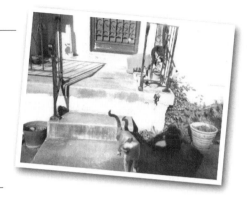

after one's self, enjoying life, and contributing to the social and economic fabric of a community" (CAOT, 1997, p. 30). Occupational performance refers to both the subjective experience of engaging in an occupation in a given environment and the observable performance.

In Figure 3-1, the person, environment, and occupation components are represented by three interrelated spheres (Venn diagrams) that move with respect to one another to illustrate the components that dynamically transact over a person's life span. The congruence, or fit, among these components is illustrated by the extent of the overlap of the person, environment, and occupation spheres. The overlap in the center of the spheres represents occupational performance, or the dynamic experience of a person engaged in an occupation within an environment over time.

To illustrate the continuity of these elements transacting throughout life, the three-dimensional components extend into a cylindrical form that reflects the temporal and spatial dimensions. Theoretically, one could examine the dynamic interactions and forces at play for a slice in time by making a cross-section of the cylinder. The slice enables an analysis of the P × O, O × E, P × E relationships by examining the fit between each set of components within the meanings ascribed at that particular point of time and space. Therefore, discrete moments in a person's life can be captured by a series of cross-sections at different points in time; each will have a different composition of P-E-O interplay and a different expression of occupational performance as the person proceeds through time and space. Figure 3-1 includes three cross-sections, each with different expressions of occupational performance depicted by different combinations of overlapping spheres.

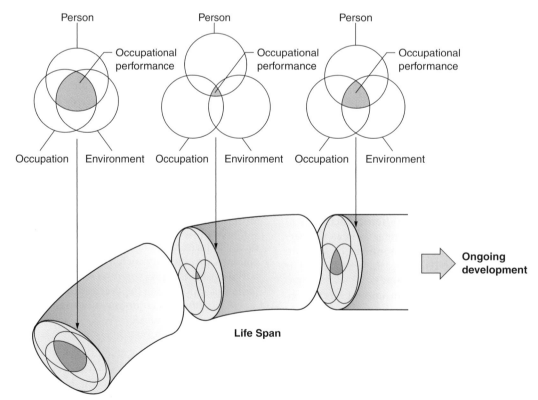

FIGURE 3-1. Depiction of the Person-Environment-Occupation (PEO) model across the life span. The PEO components are represented by three interrelated spheres (Venn diagrams) that illustrate hypothetical changes in occupational performance at three different points in time. *(Adapted with permission from Law, M., Cooper, B., Strong, S., Stewart, D., Rigby, P., & Letts, L., 1996). The Person-Environment model: A transactive approach to occupational performance. Canadian Journal of Occupational Therapy, 63(1), 9–23.*

For example, at one point in time, a student may experience satisfaction with his or her schoolwork, and successful performance demonstrates a fit among his or her abilities, interests, and values, and schoolwork's demands (P × O); a fit between the schoolwork's requirements and the school environment's expectations (O × E); and a fit between the student's needs and support given in his or her environment (P × E). This is illustrated in the first cross-section in Figure 3-1. However, at another point in time, the same student may have a negative experience and is unable to perform when presented with a new assignment or task that invokes anxiety and expectations of failure (P × O). At that time, the student's environmental supports and resources are not engaged or not helpful for this particular assignment (P × E). The result is poor occupational performance, which is illustrated by limited overlap in the spheres (the second cross-section). At a later point in time, the student has asked for help, and useful environmental supports and resources are engaged (P × E). The assignment's instructions are clarified, there is flexibility in the assignment being presented orally or written, and the time requirements are altered (P × O). Also, the different manner in which the assignment is to be completed is viewed as acceptable by the school (O × E). At this point, occupational performance is improved, which is illustrated by increased overlap in the spheres (third cross-section). Therefore, discrete moments in a person's life can be captured by a series of cross-sections at different points in time; each will have a different composition of P-E-O interplay and a different expression of occupational performance as the person proceeds through time and space.

Dimension of Time

The PEO reflects how individuals grow and change over the course of their lives. For example, when a young adult leaves home, he or she assumes new roles and responsibilities by engaging in additional occupations, thus expanding the number of spheres that transact. There may be added time pressures with less environmental supports (i.e., reduced fit between occupation and environment) and, initially, inadequate skills to satisfactorily cook meals (i.e., reduced fit between person and occupation). As cooking skills increase and time becomes better managed, there is greater P-E-O overlap, or congruence, and the experience of occupational performance improves, which is depicted by enlarged center overlap. Over a person's life span, their roles, occupations, and meanings change. For example, being a member of a faith community will likely have very different meanings as an adolescent in a youth group, the same person as the parent of a young child, and still another meaning as an older adult facing end-of-life issues. Occupations and/or roles may be discontinued, which reduces the number of occupation spheres and any dependent environment spheres, or occupations may be restored, which increases occupation spheres and the corresponding environments.

Time is also an experienced dimension. That is, individuals experience the present while remembering the past and holding ideas of their future. This ability to experience time in three facets shapes individuals' perceptions of themselves (e.g., beliefs of what they can and cannot perform well), the choices they make, and their evaluation of their own occupational performance. This makes it important for therapists to obtain information about changes and perceived changes in self, occupations, and environments.

Dimension of Space

One aspect of space is location. People can engage in an occupation in multiple locations. For example, the space in which students choose to study can vary widely. Within the PEO model, this is represented by multiple layers of the environment sphere transacting with the occupation and person spheres (Fig. 3-2). When engaged in occupations, each person has a personally defined use of space and unique standards of what physical space is required to engage comfortably; the extent of fit or congruence can be shown in the PEO model by the extent of O-E overlap. The use of space can be further restrained by functional limitations due to illness or aging, which is reflected in the model by adding the consideration of the person component or examining the relationships for P-E-O congruence.

Another aspect of space is emotional space. Particularly when working with others, people refer to whether they have sufficient emotional space to meet their personal emotional privacy/protection requirement; the extent of fit can be illustrated by the extent of P-E overlap.

Emotional spaces are socially constructed and given meanings by ourselves and others. An individual who is going through a divorce will have emotional needs that may or may not be met by others, and the way in which the divorce is interpreted (e.g., who is at fault or whether it is an acceptable option) will assume meaning from the individual going through the experience as well as others.

O'Brien, Dyck, Caron, and Mortenson (2002) wrote about how the meanings of places and spaces are related to the enabling and constraining features of the environment and whether a person is labeled or inscribed by others as being different. A person's inscription with a diagnosis (e.g., mental illness) and his or her own ascription of what that diagnosis means, in addition to functional limitations, mediate a person's use of space. For example, the stigma of mental illness can prevent an individual from obtaining or even interviewing for a particular job. The same individual may be reluctant to interact with new people or, after meeting someone new, may be rejected once a diagnosis of mental illness is revealed. The meanings of places are dynamic and ever changing, as in the progression of a disease.

Rowles (2003) expands on the dynamic concept of meaning-making of place, such as the meaning of home and how people can strive to make a space into a personally meaningful place. Individuals who are homeless or are living in substandard housing may lack a place that fulfills the emotional needs of a home.

In a study of the Northern Initiative for Social Action (NISA) (Rebeiro, Day, Semeniuk, O'Brien, & Wilson, 2001), an occupation-based, mental health program, space was found to be an important aspect of clients' sense of belonging. Belonging is important to social inclusion, which is why many mental health consumers choose to remain in programs where the social environment is inclusive instead of venturing into a community where they may not feel included and may be stigmatized. Often, study participants would not engage fully in occupations until they had secured a sense of belonging to the organization. This sense of belonging also reinforced one's sense of being, or of self, which is important to the individuals' capacity to fully engage in occupations.

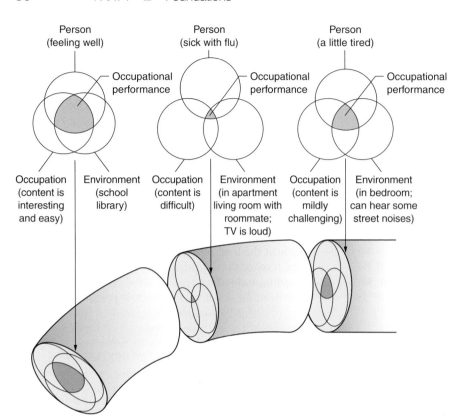

Person
(feeling well)

Occupational
performance

Occupation
(content is
interesting
and easy)

Environment
(school
library)

Person
(sick with flu)

Occupational
performance

Occupation
(content is
difficult)

Environment
(in apartment
living room with
roommate;
TV is loud)

Person
(a little tired)

Occupational
performance

Occupation
(content is
mildly
challenging)

Environment
(in bedroom;
can hear some
street noises)

FIGURE 3-2. Person-Environment-Occupation model in three different situations across time for a person studying (occupation) who prefers a quiet space (environment). *(Adapted with permission from Law, M., Cooper, B., Strong, S., Stewart, D., Rigby, P., & Letts, L. (1996). The Person-Environment model: A transactive approach to occupational performance. Canadian Journal of Occupational Therapy, 63(1), 9–23.)*

As an element of the environment and in relation to geographic location, place is a very important consideration for occupational therapists in rural and remote areas. Often, opportunities in small or remote communities are less available than in larger urban centers, and this fact influences the degree of community support for individuals with mental illness. If, for example, an individual with schizophrenia were interested in seeking work in a rural community, the small community may mean that he or she is more likely to experience social exclusion and marginalization, and not be able to secure a job interview. It is also likely that the individual will have fewer options for employment and less services available to provide employment supports.

The focus of occupational therapy is to improve the PEO fit to improve occupational performance. The PEO model enables therapists to understand how maximizing fit can optimize occupational performance (Fig. 3-3). In the case of supporting employment for people with psychiatric disabilities, there are interventions that can target the person, the environment, or the occupation. For example, the person can receive training in social skills to enhance the development of positive relationships with coworkers and supervisors. At the environment level, the individual may be offered a quiet place to retreat when feeling overwhelmed and a job coach to assist with on-the-job training. The occupation is targeted when specific job duties are adapted or modified to increase successful performance. These approaches may be fruitless if the PEO fit is compromised by a high-expectation, fast-paced work environment and an individual who is experiencing high job anxiety.

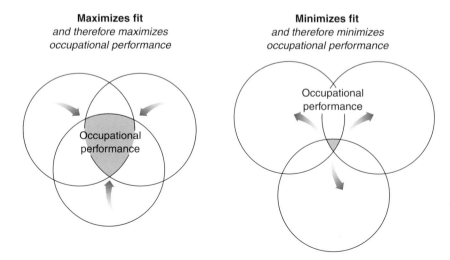

Maximizes fit
*and therefore maximizes
occupational performance*

Occupational
performance

Minimizes fit
*and therefore minimizes
occupational performance*

Occupational
performance

FIGURE 3-3. Changes to occupational performance as a consequence of variations in person, environment, and occupation fit. *(Adapted with permission from Law, M., Cooper, B., Strong, S., Stewart, D., Rigby, P., & Letts, L. (1996). The Person-Environment model: A transactive approach to occupational performance. Canadian Journal of Occupational Therapy, 63(1), 9–23.)*

Using the PEO model, a therapist can analyze and explain how different PEO relationships can influence occupational performance. The therapist can reflect on the fit (or lack of fit) between a person's abilities and skills, the demands of the occupation, and the environmental conditions in which the occupation takes place. In this way, the model can illustrate the current PEO relationships surrounding a particular occupational performance issue and how changes to components will enable improvements in occupational performance. For example, as shown in Figure 3-4, if changes were made to a person's environment (e.g., eliminated time pressures) that improved the P × E congruence and the O × E congruence, these changes could be depicted by moving the environment sphere inward to increase its overlap with the person and occupation spheres, resulting in the increased overlap in the center, which depicts improved occupational performance. If the intervention only influenced the P × E transaction and not the O × E transaction, the E sphere would not be moved uniformly toward the center; rather, it would move toward the P sphere to increase the P-E overlap and not the P-O overlap in spheres. Similarly, interventions could be focused on the person component or on the occupation component to improve the congruence with one or all components of the model.

The PEO Model in Mental Health Practice

The PEO model is effective in mental health practice because it promotes clients' full participation in their everyday lives in several ways:

- Embodies principles of client-centered practice—Therapists will be most effective when their practice is grounded in the daily realities of their clients' lives and experiences. The PEO model facilitates understanding occupational performance issues from the lived experiences of clients, and supports clients' participation in the intervention planning process. A shared understanding of issues and priorities enables a strong therapeutic alliance and effective working partnership. Because the PEO model considers human growth, development across the life span, and changes over the course of one's life and life circumstances, therapists can use an individualized approach for each client.

- Supports reflective evidence-based practice—The PEO model offers a systematic approach to the analysis of occupational performance issues. It promotes the gathering of evidence, reflection, and the use of clinical reasoning.
- Enables therapists to see both the forest and the trees—Using the PEO model as a conceptual framework, therapists can reach a clear, comprehensive understanding of the complexities of human performance and experience, while considering influential relationships at the micro and macro levels.
- Expands options for intervention—The PEO model broadens the focus of analysis and offers guidance regarding potential areas for intervention that involve the environment and occupation, in addition to the person. Also, therapists can consider interventions not only at the level of the individual or group, but also at the level of the organization, local environment, community, and system.
- Identifies focused interventions with relevant outcomes—Successful occupational performance is dependent on the transaction of the person, environment, and occupation. Therefore, it becomes important for the occupational therapist to measure all three components in the assessment process so that the relevant barrier can be targeted in the intervention.
- Frames the scope of practice—The PEO model helps occupational therapists place their activities into a framework that defines the scope of occupation-based practice. Therapists have been able to use this model in a variety of roles (e.g., direct service provider, consultant, change agent, manager, advocate) and settings (e.g., community, hospitals, businesses, schools).
- Facilitates communication of practice within and outside occupational therapy practice—The PEO model is easily understood by other health-care professionals, consumers, and family members. Its broad application in multiple contexts has illustrated the fact that the model can be used with other theories and combined with other perspectives. Constructive teamwork is facilitated by focusing discussions on the shared PEO fit issues rather than placing responsibility on any one person or organization, thus reducing potential feelings of defensiveness.
- Supports advances in the occupational therapy profession—By clearly articulating its theory and practical application, the PEO model enables therapists to discuss, reflect on, and systematically evaluate practice. The model provides a tool with which to build on what is known and move the profession forward.

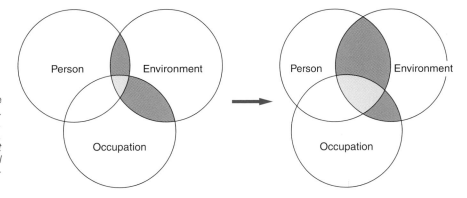

FIGURE 3-4. Effect of intervention to change the environment on occupational performance. *(Adapted with permission from Law, M., Cooper, B., Strong, S., Stewart, D., Rigby, P., & Letts, L. (1996). The Person-Environment model: A transactive approach to occupational performance. Canadian Journal of Occupational Therapy, 63(1), 9–23.)*

Analyzing Occupational Performance

The relationships among the PEO components are examined systematically by reflecting on the elements that influence the fit and the lack of fit between the models' main components ($P \times O$, $O \times E$, $P \times E$) individually and as a whole, within the ascribed meanings, in the context of the particular occupational performance issue. This analysis can be described as looking at different layers of relationships and then synthesizing the understandings into a formulation as a whole to identify options for improving the PEO fit. The relationships are examined systematically in the context of the identified occupational performance issue by

1. Assessing important elements that influence the client's identified occupational performance with respect to each of the three main components: person, environment, and occupation.
2. Assessing the PEO transactions by reflecting on the $P \times O$, $O \times E$, and $P \times E$ relationships.
3. Recognizing the meanings ascribed.
4. Considering all three components and the transactional relationships, identify strategies to improve occupational performance by removing barriers/constraints and developing supports to improve the quality of the PEO fit.

It is important to examine relationships from the client's perspective in order to properly recognize the ascribed meanings. For example, Bejerholm and Eklund's (2006) study of people with schizophrenia found that engagement in occupations provided rhythm and meaning to their days. Even quiet activities that would be easy to dismiss as "just passing time" were ascribed different meanings to these individuals within the enabling or constraining home environments. Another example is Strong's (1998) ethnographic study of individuals with schizophrenia who worked at an affirmative business, which found that meaningful occupation is uniquely individual and changes over time. The study illustrated how meaning ascribed to work changes with the person's relationship to his or her own illness and recovery. For example, when illness was the main focus in their lives, work was a bolster against the daily battle with illness and a buffer for dealing with society's negative attitudes. When workers viewed themselves as becoming capable people with a future, work took on the meaning of providing concrete evidence that they were more than just an illness and may have a future. When workers were engaged in recovery and getting on with their lives, work became the modality to practice and develop the interests, skills, and habits necessary for being a worker and friend. When finding a place in the world was considered important, work was a means to feel valued and a place to belong.

Figure 3-5 illustrates the use of the PEO model to systematically analyze an occupational performance issue for a client. Shelly is a 20-year-old woman whose university studies were interrupted with a second admission to a hospital for anorexia nervosa. She intends to reapply to attend university in 10 months. In the meantime, she has returned home to live with her parents and has been attending a day hospital eating disorders program. With Shelly's consent, the occupational therapist arranged for Shelly to help a counselor run a photography interest group at a program for inner-city children. After two photography interest groups, Shelly told her occupational therapist that she is very nervous volunteering and expressed doubts that she has anything to offer the children ("I'm sure they see right through me. Who am I anyway? A fake, a fraud. . . . I don't know what I am doing there.").

By examining the problem using the PEO model, the therapist was able to conceptualize the issue in terms of a complex set of transactions that constrained Shelly's satisfaction and restricted her occupational performance. The therapist drew the PEO's intersecting Venn diagram circles to explain what strategies might be helpful to improve the PEO fit. The diagrams helped Shelly reframe her experience, take control, and participate in planning strategies to remove or reduce barriers and add supports. Shelly was able to frame her volunteering experience as a repeat of negative cognitive attribution patterns in the past. She was determined to challenge her avoidant coping pattern and thoughts of herself as not being good enough. She affirmed her belief that photography can help people deal with emotions and experiences, as it has helped her deal with her own life. She views volunteering as a way to help others, get away from a focus on herself and food, and begin to get to know herself better.

In an article by Strong and colleagues (1999), the PEO model is described as a practical analytical tool for the analysis of occupational performance problems, intervention planning and evaluation, and communication of practice to others. In this article, three scenarios illustrate the application of the model to common situations encountered in different occupational therapy practice settings: an elderly man wanting to return home from a hospital after a hip fracture, a child with cerebral palsy feeling frustrated with written work at school, and a man with schizophrenia expressing that he cannot return to a transitional work placement.

Applying PEO to the Occupational Therapy Process

Understanding and incorporating the constructs of the PEO model is useful throughout the occupational therapy process. It begins with the initial evaluation and is carried out through the intervention. The following scenario illustrates the steps involved in applying the PEO framework in the occupational therapy treatment process. The person described in the scenario has experienced a cerebrovascular incident. A physical disability was intentionally chosen to illustrate the mental health considerations that are inherent in all aspects of occupational therapy practice.

Identifying a Priority Occupational Performance Issue

Daryl Fox, a 61-year-old retired physical education teacher, has been referred to occupational therapy 1 month after having a right cerebrovascular accident. After spending

Shelly's Occupational Performance Issue

❑ Feeling of discomfort when volunteering at a photography interest group

Assessment of Main Components

Person (affective, cognitive, physical, spirituality)	**Environmental Conditions (cultural, institutional, physical, social)**	**Occupational Demands (affective, cognitive, physical)**
❑ Emotionally immature, impulsive ❑ Intellectually bright ❑ Rigid thinking when stressed ❑ Limited coping strategies ❑ Talented photographer ❑ Values photography for dealing with life experiences and healing	❑ Shelly is viewed as an adult by the children and as an expert photographer. ❑ Shelly reports the E as unpredictable regarding what questions are asked and how children respond to her. ❑ Group counselor is confident, easy going, and appears to really enjoy working with the children.	❑ Shelly is not able to identify any of the "do's" and "don'ts" of the job. ❑ The pace is hectic for short periods. ❑ No impeding physical factors

Assessment of PEO Transactions

Person-Occupation (P × O)	**Occupation-Environment (O × E)**	**Person-Environment (P × E)**
❑ Values the work ❑ Low self-efficacy ❑ Skills/abilities match work activities ❑ Unrealistic expectations ❑ Lack of structure and connection of being in place	❑ Organization of work activities by counselor ❑ Shelly has not received any feedback about her contributions ❑ The children have been responding with interest to the photography activities	❑ Unclear communication regarding Shelly's and counselor's roles, responsibilities, and expectations ❑ Her relationships with children are strained ❑ Match of organization's goals and activities with her goal's and needs

Interventions/Strategies to Improve Occupational Performance

❑ Shelly will meet with photography group counselor to discuss a set of questions she will have prepared on paper regarding roles, responsibilities, and expectations.

❑ Shelly will request a regular, informal, post-group debriefing session to check out perceptions, learn from experiences, plan the next session, improve the program for the children, and develop a supportive working alliance with the counselor.

❑ Explore things Shelly can do to feel better prepared, determine aspects of the occupation that she can take over and feel some aspect of control, and identify the choices she can make.

❑ Identify with her OT potential environmental stressors, and triggers for returning to negative self-talk and destructive behaviors, and practice cognitive-behavioral techniques.

FIGURE 3-5. Example of a systematic analysis of an occupational performance issue using the Person-Environment-Occupation model.

2 weeks in the hospital, he is now living at home with his wife. During an interview using the Canadian Occupational Performance Measure, the therapist learns that Daryl's most important occupational performance issue is not being able to drive. Daryl expresses feelings of depression and frustration related to these limitations.

Exploring Factors That Influence PEO

As the interview continues, the therapist and client together explore the strengths and challenges of the person, environment, and occupation related to the selected priority occupational performance issue (Table 3-1). Daryl tells the therapist about himself, including his interests, values, self-concept, what he is able to do and not do, and his thoughts and feelings surrounding driving.

Examining Relationships Among the PEO Components

Next, the relationships among the P-E-O components are examined by reflecting on the congruence, or fit, and lack of fit among the transactions (P × O, O × E, and P × E).

Table 3-1 ● **Strengths and Challenges of P-E-O Components Related to Driving**

	Person Component
Physical	• Able to walk unassisted for short distances with a left leg limp • Left hand cannot grip or hold things; fingers are curled into a fist that hurts when he tries to open the fingers with his other hand; and left hand does not feel the same as the right hand when he touches it • Left feels tight on flexion and external rotation • He has not been sleeping well and wakes early in the morning
Affective	• Frustrated with difficulties performing routine two-handed tasks (e.g., buttons, cutting food) • Worried about relationship with wife, which has been strained since he retired 1 year ago • Frightened he will not get back to living a "good" life • Feels like doing nothing all day, and spends long periods in bed
Cognitive	• Tires easily • He reports no difficulties with memory, planning, or decision-making
Spiritual	• Believes he is not able to drive today but will be able to do so soon • Values his independence and views driving as essential for independence • Previously prided himself on his fitness, strength, and ability to help others as a teacher; now feels lost
	Environment Component
Cultural	• Prior to stroke, Daryl and wife assumed relatively traditional gender roles in terms of roles and responsibilities at home and on the farm • Wife currently drives him to the bank and medical appointments • Since his stroke, his wife now does all the shopping, cooking, maintenance of home, and taking care of farm animals
Physical	• Lives on a rural 50-acre hobby farm • His home is 30 minutes drive from town, with no public transit and variable road conditions
Institutional	• They receive financial support from Daryl's pension from teaching
Social	• Wife is frequently angry • Wife works part time at a nursing home • Prior to the stroke, they followed a routine they had begun many years before; both preferring to work on tasks alone and getting together for socializing • Their grown children live some distance away • Daryl has many friends; a few have visited, but most live some distance away
	Occupation Component
	• Daryl explains the type of driving he would like to be able to do (e.g., distances, time of day, type of traffic) • Therapist examines Daryl's vehicle to determine physical requirement for driving • Organizational, decision-making, problem-solving requirements of driving are discussed • Stress and coping with stressors related to driving

Person-Occupation

- Daryl values and sees himself being able to drive in the future.
- There is a mismatch between his current abilities and the physical, affective, and cognitive demands of driving.

Occupation-Environment

- Driving would be on challenging rural roads under varied weather conditions for lengthy distances.
- Community resources for driver rehabilitation and adaptive driving equipment are available and affordable.

Person-Environment

- Daryl's relationship with his wife is strained, although his wife continues to perform the necessary supporting tasks.
- His wife is available to drive Daryl to the driver rehabilitation center.
- He has a supportive social network, but physical distances and the inability to drive reduce the opportunity to be with friends.

Formulating a Plan

After examining the relationships among the PEO components, the therapist presents this information to Daryl and his wife to discuss potential barriers and supports. The formulation is communicated to the client to confirm, elaborate, disconfirm, refine, or refocus. Together with the client, an intervention plan is developed to improve the PEO fit. The plan involves using strategies to eliminate or reduce the effects of barriers and increase supports to improve occupational performance. Given that occupational performance is influenced by complex transactional processes among the person and his or her environment and occupation, therapists need to direct their interventions at all three components.

Daryl confirmed the therapist's formulation that he experienced a loss of role when he retired, and his sense of self was further undermined with losses accompanying his stroke. Driving was important to him, not only to allow him to return to engaging in productivity and social occupations, but it was fundamental to Daryl's sense of self and the support of their marriage. The main barriers to participation in driving were not only the physical setup of the vehicle's controls, but also Daryl's mental and physical endurance. The extent to which mood, lethargy, and poor sleeping might be contributing to Daryl's cognitive impairment was unknown.

Completion of the Beck Depression Inventory, a screen for psychiatric services, indicated that Daryl should be referred for a psychiatric evaluation and possible treatment. The therapist planned to assist Daryl in reengaging in healthy self-care routines (e.g., regularly eating nutritious meals, regular sleep, exercise). Cognitive-behavioral therapy techniques would be used to assist Daryl to reframe his self-talk and cognitive responses, and consider alternative interpretations and behavioral responses to daily encounters with occupational challenges.

The extent to which the stroke influenced Daryl's cognitive abilities to meet the demands of driving was unknown. Cognitive abilities could be evaluated and strategies put into place at a driver rehabilitation center, including adapted vehicle controls, once the potential depression was resolved. His overall endurance could be improved, which would assist his driving endurance, by engaging in a graduated return to productivity roles and use of energy conservation strategies.

The therapist recommended that Daryl and his wife discuss the importance of social experiences, and identify strategies to maintain social contacts. Also, the therapist suggested they seek short-term marital counseling.

Evaluating Intervention Plans

Intervention plans are evaluated by the client and therapist by examining changes in the occupational performance of the priority occupational performance issue. For Daryl, the plans were evaluated with respect to whether they helped him drive safely.

Initially, interventions focused on the steps to achieve his driving goal. Each intervention in turn is evaluated with the client to examine progress and potential readjustment of plans. The PEO model provides the framework for analysis and joint communication. For Daryl, the initial focus was to reengage in healthy routines concerning meals, exercise, and sleep routines. The therapist drew circle diagrams to explain the lack of PEO fit and the intentions of interventions relating to the PEO relationships.

Daryl chose to begin by getting up regularly at a time chosen by him, limiting himself to one nap a day with unlimited rest periods, and reinstituting a bedtime routine coupled with daily walks of progressively longer durations. He maintained a daily log to track his own progress. His wife was asked to support him in his plans. After 2 weeks, he complained of still being very tired and of being disappointed in his performance. His log reported walking each day and limited nap times, but he often continued to stay in bed in the morning.

The situation was reviewed to recognize accomplishments and potential opportunities for changing the plans using the PEO. Although changes had been made in the environment (wake-up alarm, wife's encouragement), tasks surrounding bedtime routine (bath, reading), physical activity, and expectations of himself, he had not been taking medication for depression for a sufficient length of time for effect (person), and no changes had been made surrounding the tasks of his morning routine (occupation). Daryl noted that nothing is expected of him, and there is nothing scheduled to do in the morning (i.e., no meaningful morning occupation). Daryl

chose to walk the length of their lane to pick up the newspaper, and to make coffee for his wife and himself each morning. The PEO model was useful to facilitate Daryl to move away from blaming himself for what he viewed as a lack of progress and focus on aspects of occupation and environment, areas over which he had some control while waiting for the medications to take effect.

Application of the PEO Model

The PEO model has been applied in numerous settings in which therapists provide direct service and consultation to individuals, groups, or organizations, and engage in teaching, research, and advocacy in countries around the world. A review of 36 publications that cited the PEO model from 1998 to 2007 reveals how the model has permeated occupational therapy practice. Those works that merely quoted the PEO as background literature or to substantiate a viewpoint were not included in this review.

Collectively, these citations illustrate the diversity of PEO use. The citations involve descriptions of interventions, the development of theory or practice principles, and research that examines practice and theory across the breadth of occupational therapy. The PEO model is taught in occupational therapy academic programs as a tool for therapists to use in the systematic analysis of occupational performance issues, and it is included in the CAOT Certification Examination. Two publications reported using the PEO model for occupational therapy curriculum development in Russia (Patterson, Krupa, & Packer, 2000) and Thailand (Pongsaksri, 2004).

The PEO is cited as a framework for planning, evaluating, and making recommendations for individual client interventions (4 publications) and for OT services (4 papers). In research, the PEO is cited as a framework for developing data collection measures/questions to capture occupational performance (7 papers), a framework for research design (3 papers), and a framework for data analysis and interpretation of findings or formulation of recommendations (13 publications).

In the seven theory citations, the PEO model is used to

- Advance a discussion about evidence-based practice (Bennett & Bennett, 2000; Egan, Dubouloz, von Zweck, & Vallerand, 1998).
- Articulate what therapists can offer in forming partnerships with other sectors to address clients' needs (Baum, 2002).
- Place concepts from sociology and geography concerning the meaning of "place" and use of spaces into an understanding of disability experiences over a life span (O'Brien et al, 2002; Rowles, 2003).
- Explore the concept of boredom and reflect on the delivery of occupational therapy mental health inpatient services (Molineux, 2004).
- Study the transactional nature of the P-E-O relationships (Schult, 2002).

Throughout these citations, the PEO is used to communicate occupational therapy practice principles, as well as the role and scope of the profession within and outside the profession, and advocate for occupational performance issues

The Lived Experience

Lisa

Lisa is a 37-year-old mother of one who has had extensive experience with mental health services and programs, including several hospital admissions over a 2-year period. Lisa was diagnosed with bipolar affective disorder and, during the time of her involvement with occupational therapy, rapidly cycled between depression and varying levels of mania, accompanied by delusional ideas.

For many years, Lisa identified seeking purpose, a job, and, specifically, a career as being important to her. Despite the unrelenting nature of her illness, she somehow always persevered with her education and obtained a degree in social work and a diploma in marketing. Lisa held the belief that she would successfully work at some point in the future. She experimented with a variety of occupations, but had difficulty concentrating and was left dissatisfied with many of the jobs. Her career orientation was the reason that Lisa initially sought out involvement in the Northern Initiative for Social Action (NISA), an occupation-based, mental health program, and with occupational therapy. The following PEO issues were found to interfere with her occupational performance and, subsequently, her occupational goal attainment.

Person-Occupation

Lisa views herself as both a professional and a social worker. She is personally sensitive to many of the issues dealt with by her profession, such as abuse, alcoholism, and dysfunctional relationships. Lisa has attempted other careers, including marketing, but found that they were not stimulating to her, nor did this kind of work provide her with a sufficient sense of satisfaction with her work. In addition, Lisa has used both art and writing as ways to express her experiences of health and illness, and Lisa recognized that these occupations were primarily therapeutic. Lisa understood that in order to participate as a helping professional, she would need to better manage her own illness/health issues.

Occupation-Environment: Working at NISA among other consumers of mental health services, Lisa was able to experiment with a variety of occupations without fear of failure or social rejection. Mistakes were handled in a low-key, matter-of-fact manner, and she was given the opportunity to make corrections. Lisa was able to make real, often concrete and meaningful, contributions to something that was bigger than her. Her occupations met the needs of others and the organization.

Environment-Person: Lisa grew up in an abusive family environment, punctuated by alcohol use and abuse. For her recovery, at the beginning, she needed a place that not only felt safe, but also offered the flexibility for her to make choices. NISA seemed to be a good fit for Lisa. An environment in which Lisa felt she belonged and that offered her choices (and subsequent responsibility for the consequences of these choices) assisted her in gaining a different perspective of herself as a person with her own skills and capabilities. Her peers and therapist expressed their belief in her and held the hope for a better life for her when she could not do so for herself. They supported her and reminded her of the instrumental things she needed to do to manage her illness in order to work.

Person-Environment-Occupation: An environment that was neither competitive nor punitive allowed Lisa the flexibility to experiment with different roles and occupations, which helped her feel more capable as a person and, ultimately, more competent. Her experiences and performances shaped each other, ascribing new meanings to who she was as a worker and imbuing her performances with new purpose and meaning (in the words of Roosevelt, "a work worth doing"). In this environment, while participating in helping occupations, Lisa realized that helping others was the type of career that she needed to pursue.

Lisa's Own Story

One morning, I was parked in the slowly creeping line-up at Tim Horton's waiting for my morning coffee before work. It occurred to me that most people would probably be irritated with the line-up. I, however, was thinking to myself how grateful I was to be "part of" this world. It hasn't always been this way. I remember a time not so long ago (5 years) when I wasn't feeling part of anything. I was standing on a chair, noose around my neck, wishing for the will to push the chair and let myself fall to my death and end the pain that was my daily existence. I had been labeled bipolar affective disorder, suffered from the delusions of mania and the crashing lows of depression ever since I was 13 years old. I was 31 when I started to turn things around for myself.

How does one come back from the depths of such despair to work as a counselor in a nationally recognized program? I believe that several factors came together to bring about this change. A change in medication and quitting drugs and alcohol were two important factors. I became involved in an organization called Northern Initiative for Social Action, the brain child of a local occupational therapist. NISA is an occupation-based program predicated on three essential components of recovery: Being, Belonging, and Becoming needs.

It was at NISA that I began to feel that I belonged to society again. And, importantly, that I had something worthwhile to contribute to society. I contributed a painting to an art show, designed ads, and wrote poetry and articles for the *Open Minds Quarterly Journal,* which was produced by NISA. Actually, I did so much more. In short, I was encouraged to become involved, to participate in occupations of choice, and I felt I was contributing. I felt empowered. It was like I was evolving again as a person instead of sitting at a standstill, wasting my life away. I again belonged in this world. I learned from the occupational therapist that I had to eat and sleep regularly to be well, and slowly I began to learn how to go about doing that. What needed to happen for my recovery all seems so obvious now that I have 20/20 hindsight. It wasn't so obvious to me at that time.

After reaping the benefits of my newfound sense of worth for almost a year, I became pregnant with my first child. I gave birth to my son and, subsequently, to another purpose for my life. Routine, such an important factor in my recovery, became paramount. I stayed with my father and stepmother for 1.5 months after my son was born. I was blessed with a child who slept through the night at 2 months and had a regular feeding schedule. We both returned home very content. I slipped into the role of mother like a glove. Now, I was not only staying well for myself, but for my son.

The Lived Experience—cont'd

I felt I no longer had a choice to break down, decompensate, or become hospitalized because someone was depending on me for stimulation, affection, love, basic needs . . . for everything. I needed to stay well to take care of these things. At this point, I was still on a Canada Pension and the Ontario Disability Support program, the criteria for which is "a severe and prolonged disability." When the application for disability was made, my prognosis was placed as "guarded," but I knew that others believed I would never work again. I am thankful that they were all wrong!

With the confidence given me by my occupational therapist and peers, and with more than 2 years of psychiatric stability behind me, I began to think that I could work again and started to consider my options. I was educated and had received my bachelor's degree in social work. Dare I think I could return to my field? At the recommendation of my doctor, I applied for a part-time job as a social worker to work with troubled youth.

Since then, and with an additional 2 years of continued stability, I have recently applied for and secured a full-time position. I am now happily a part of the workforce, Tim Horton's line-ups and all!

Since becoming employed, I have required slight adjustments to my medication and short periods of time off to deal with the medication adjustments for which my boss has been kind and accommodating. My family, friends, and coworkers never let me stray too far from the things that have kept me well for the past 5 years. I have meaning, purpose, and a wonderful life. I am so grateful to everyone who was and is part of my recovery from mental illness. It cannot be underestimated the importance of occupation even for those who seemingly are beyond hope. I was . . . but now am no longer . . . beyond hope.

Read more about Lisa's perspectives on client-centered occupational therapy in Bibyk et al (1999).

---

from the client's perspective. This clear articulation enables reflection, discussion, and further development of occupational therapy theory and practice.

Five of the 36 PEO citations focused on individuals with established mental illness. Using a mixed methods design, Bejerholm and Eklund (2006) examined the engagement and experience of daily occupations within context over time for a Swedish group of men and women with schizophrenia to reveal how this group could have meaningful lives, experience pleasure, and enjoy life. Molineux (2004) wrote a discussion paper and used the PEO model to substantiate the position that occupational therapists working in inpatient psychiatry would better use their time determining how clients experience boredom to enable people to develop more adaptive time use and coping skills.

In New Zealand, McWha, Pachana and Alpass (2003) compared the perceptions of a group of women in late life with depression to the health-care team's perceptions concerning the impact of a group activity and the environment on rehabilitation. Rebeiro (2001) reported a secondary analysis of qualitative data from three studies exploring the meaning and experience of occupational engagement for persons with mental illness at a clubhouse program in Canada. The study highlighted key elements of social environments that occupational therapists need to address to avoid a handicapping environment.

In Strong's (1998) ethnographic study examining the meaning of work and the role of work in recovery, the PEO model was used to answer why the experience at an affirmative business was satisfying and successful for some clients, but not for others with persistent mental illness.

These 36 citations also offer implications for the PEO model. Several cited papers demonstrate the cultural neutrality of the PEO model by illustrating how the PEO concepts are being used in diverse settings, with individuals who are not imbued by the occupational therapy culture, in sectors other than hospital health care, and in societies other than the Canadian society, where the model was developed (e.g., Netherlands, Australia, Slovenia, India). However, for relevant use, the person, occupation, and environment constructs may

need to be labeled with locally meaningful phrase(s). For example, in Jarus and Ratzon's (2005) use of the PEO model in planning musculoskeletal disorder prevention programs at workplaces, they fit the PEO concepts into ergonomics and neurobehavioral sciences culture by explicitly labeling PEO terms with locally recognizable terms (e.g., labeling "occupation" as "task" or "work," labeling "person" as "learner" or "worker," labeling "environment" as "structure of practice" or "analysis of worksite").

Pongsaksri's (2004) study identified how therapists in Thailand perceived the PEO model as not matching their culture's emphasis on collectivism, viewing the PEO model as a Western tool focusing on the individual. This view is similar

Evidence-Based Practice

What is significant in reflecting on the 36 publications discussed previously is how the evidence serves to uphold the assumptions underpinning the PEO model.

➤ Occupational performance is the product of the person, occupation, environment (PEO) component areas.

➤ Occupational performance involves both the subjective experience and the performance of the occupation within a given environment, and is experienced uniquely for each person.

➤ Occupational performance will be affected by changes in any of the PEO component areas.

➤ The fit, or congruence, of the PEO components determines the quality of the outcome (i.e., occupational performance). The greater the congruence, the better the occupational performance, and vice versa.

➤ The relationship of the components is dynamic (i.e., PEO relationships enable and constrain participation and are ever changing) and transactive (i.e., experience and performance shape each other, ascribing of meaning, multiple layers of influence).

to Iwama's (1999) discourse on client-centered practice in Japan. Perhaps if the PEO model were reinterpreted within a client-centered framework in which the "client" is not an individual, but rather a family or societal group, the PEO would become more relevant to occupational therapists beyond our Western world.

Vrkljan (2006) interpreted the "person" as both the driver and copilot when she applied the PEO to analysis of case studies of the use of in-vehicle navigation technology among older drivers.

Summary

This chapter introduces the PEO model, which serves as the organizing framework for the textbook. The book is separated into sections of person, environment, and occupation, but as this chapter points out, the core principles of the model stress the transaction among the concepts. It is the overlap of person, environment, and occupation that determines occupational performance. Therefore, when reading each chapter, remember that nothing occurs in isolation. For example, cognition or thinking (a person factor) is always occurring within a particular environment and while a person is engaged in an occupation. Each act of thinking will be unique and dependent on the environment and occupation. One way that this book consistently explores the multifaceted nature of life experience is through the inclusion of first person narratives. The first person narratives tell a real life story and, in doing so, exemplify the complexities and distinctiveness of each individual.

Active Learning Strategies

1. Personal Assessment

Choose an activity that you really enjoy. Reflect on what makes it a successful experience for you. Identify how the P-E-O transactions are congruent at this time.

Reflective Questions
- Has this activity always been a positive experience for you?
- Think about a negative experience with an activity. What was different at that time? Was there a fit with your skills, abilities, values, demands of the occupation, and environmental conditions?

2. Teaching

Explain to a friend the PEO model using your own language and Venn diagrams. When describing the model, use as an example someone who experiences a mental health problem. What happens to their ability to choose, organize, and satisfactorily perform culturally and personally meaningful occupations?

Reflective Questions
- What examples did you include in your description?
- Was it easier to describe the person, environment, or occupation constructs?
- How did you explain the transactional nature of the model?
- Do you think your friend understood the model after your explanation?

3. Case Study: Shelly

Examine Figure 3-5. Looking at only the information in the first row of the table (i.e., the person, occupation, and environment elements), isolating it from the other information, what picture do you form in your mind of this person and her circumstance? Next, looking at the second row of information (i.e., the P × O, O × E, and P × E relationships), in what way does this information provide a new understanding of this person and her occupational performance issue?

Reflective Questions
- What personal meanings do you now understand?
- What can this information tell you about time and space?

4. Revisiting the Lived Experience

Revisit the client in the chapter's Lived Experience narrative, and complete a Systemic Analysis of Occupational Performance Issue Form (similar to Fig. 3-5) to further examine Lisa's experiences both with the mental health system and with NISA.

Reflective Questions
- What is noteworthy from an occupational therapist's perspective with respect to the environment? The occupation?
- Did anything really change with the person? For example, was the person the focus of the intervention, or was the environment? The occupation?
- In your opinion, what were the salient qualities of the client-centered relationship for Lisa?

Resources

Books
- Law, M., Baum, C. M., & Baptiste, S. (2002). *Occupation Based Practice: Fostering Performance and Participation*. Thorofare, NJ: Slack.
- Law, M., Cooper, B., Strong, S., Stewart, D., Rigby, P., & Letts, L. (1996). The Person-Environment model: A transactive approach to occupational performance. *Canadian Journal of Occupational Therapy, 63*(1), 9–23.
- Letts, L., & Rigby, P. (2003). *Using Environments to Enable Occupational Performance*. Thorofare, NJ: Slack.
- Strong, S., & Rebeiron, K. (2003). Creating supportive work environments for people with mental illness. In L. Letts, P. Rigby, & D. Stewart (Eds.), *Using Environment to Enable Occupational Performance* (pp. 137–154). Thorofare, NJ: Slack.

- Strong, S., Rigby, P., Stewart, D., Law, M., Cooper, B., & Letts, L. (1999). The Person-Environment-Occupation model: A practical intervention tool. *Canadian Journal of Occupational Therapy, 66,* 122–133.
- Strong, S., & Shaw, L. (1999). A client-centred framework for therapists in ergonomics. In K. Jacobs & C. M. Bettencourt (Eds.), *Ergonomics for Therapists* (2nd ed., pp. 22–46). Woburn, MA: Butterworth-Heinemann.

Measures
- Canadian Occupational Performance Measure (COPM): www .caot.ca/copm
- CHORES: Dunn, L. (2004). Validation of the CHORES: A measure of school-aged children's participation in household tasks. *Scandinavian Journal of Occupational Therapy, 11,* 179–190.
- Test of Playfulness: Muys, V., Rodger, S., & Bundy, A. (2006). Playfulness in children with autistic disorder: A comparison of the Child's Playfulness Scale and the Test of Playfulness. *OTJR: Occupation, Participation and Health, 26,* 159–170.

References

American Occupational Therapy Association (AOTA). (2002). Occupational therapy practice framework: Domain and process. *American Journal of Occupational Therapy, 56,* 609–639.

Baker, F., & Intagliata, J. (1982). Quality of life in the evaluation of community support systems. *Evaluation and Program Planning, 5,* 69–79.

Baum, C. (2002). Creating partnerships: Constructing our future. *Australian Occupational Therapy Journal, 49,* 58–62.

Bejerholm, U., & Eklund, M. (2006). Engagement in occupations among men and women with schizophrenia. *Occupational Therapy International, 13*(2), 100–121.

Bennett, S., & Bennett, J.W. (2000). The process of evidence-based practice in occupational therapy: Informing clinical decisions. *Australian Journal of Occupational Therapy, 47,* 171–180.

Bibyk, B., Day, D. G., Morris, L., O'Brien, M. C., Rebeiro, K. L., Seguin, P., Semeniuk, B., Wilson, B., & Wilson, J. (1999). Who's in charge here? The client's perspective on client-centred care. *Occupational Therapy Now, Sept/Oct,* 11–12.

Bronfenbrenner, U. (1977). Toward an experimental ecology of human development. *American Psychologist, 32,* 513–531.

Canadian Association of Occupational Therapy (1991). *Occupational therapy guidelines for client-centred practice.* Ottawa: CAOT Publications ACE.

Canadian Assocation of Occupational Therapy (1997). *Enabling occupation: An occupational therapy perspective.* Ottawa: CAOT Publications ACE.

Christiansen, C. H., Baum, C. M., & Haugen, J. B. (2005). *Occupational Therapy: Performance, Participation and Well-Being.* Thorofare, NJ: Slack.

Corring, D. (1996). "Client-Centred Care Means That I Am a Valued Human Being." Unpublished master's thesis, The University of Western Ontario, London, Ontario, Canada.

Csikszentmihalyi, M., & Csikszentmihalyi, I. S. (1988). *Optimal Experience: Psychological Studies in Flow in Consciousness.* Cambridge, MA: Cambridge University Press.

Deegan, P. (1992). The Independent Living Movement and people with psychiatric disabilities: Taking back control over our own lives. *Psychosocial Rehabilitation Journal, 15,* 3-19.

Dunn, W., Brown, C., & Youngstrom, M. J. (2003). Ecological model of occupation. In P. Kramer, J. Hinojosa, & C. B. Royeen (Eds.), *Perspectives in Human Occupation: Participation in Life* (pp. 222–263). Baltimore: Lippincott William & Wilkins.

Egan, M., Dubouloz, C., von Zweck, C., & Vallerand, J. (1998). The client-centred evidence-based practice of occupational therapy.

Canadian Journal of Occupational Therapy: Revue Canadienne d'Ergotherapie, 65(3), 136–143.

Fougeyrollas, P., Noreau, L., Bergeron, H., Cloutier, R., Dion, S. A., & St-Michel, G. (1998). Social consequences of long term impairments and disabilities: Conceptual approach and assessment of handicap. *International Journal of Rehabilitation Research, 21,* 127–141.

Iwama, M. (1999). Are you listening? Cross-cultural perspectives on client-centred occupational therapy practice: A view from Japan. *Occupational Therapy Now, 1*(6), 4–6.

Jarus, T., & Ratzon, N. Z. (2005). The implementation of motor learning principles in designing prevention programs at work. *Work, 24,* 171–182.

Jongbloed, L., & Crighton, A. (1990). A new definition of disability: Implications for rehabilitation practice and social policy. *Canadian Journal of Occupational Therapy, 57,* 32–38.

Kearns, R. A., & Taylor, S. M. (1989). Daily life experiences of people with chronic mental disabilities in Hamilton, Ontario. *Canada's Mental Health, 37*(4), 1–4.

Kielhofner, G. (2008). *Model of Human Occupation: Theory and Application* (4th ed.). Baltimore: Lippincott William & Wilkins.

Law, M. (1991). The environment: A focus for occupational therapy. *Canadian Journal of Occupational Therapy, 58,* 171–179.

Law, M., Cooper, B., Strong, S., Stewart, D., Rigby, P., & Letts, L. (1996). The Person-Environment-Occupation model: A transactive approach to occupational performance. *Canadian Journal of Occupational Therapy, 63*(1), 9–23.

Lawton, M. P. (1986). *Environment and Aging* (2nd ed.). Albany, NY: The Center for the Study of Aging.

Lewin, K. (1933). *Dynamic Theory of Personality.* New York: McGraw-Hill.

McWha, J. L., Pachana, N. A., & Alpass, F. M. (2003). Exploring the therapeutic environment for older women with late life depression: An examination of the benefits of an activity group for older people suffering from depression. *Australian Occupational Therapy Journal, 50,* 158–169.

Molineux, M. (2004). Occupation in occupational therapy: A labour in vain? In M. Molineux (Ed.), *Occupation for Occupational Therapists* (pp. 79–88). Ames, IA: Blackwell.

Murray, H. (1938). *Explorations in Personality.* New York: Oxford.

National Health and Welfare Canada. (1988). *Mental Health for Canadians: Striking a Balance.* Ottawa: Minister of Supplies and Services Canada (ISMN 0-662-16347-8 Cat.#H39-128).

O'Brien, P., Dyck, I., Caron, S., & Mortenson, P. (2002). Environmental analysis: Insights from sociological and geographical perspectives. *Canadian Journal of Occupational Therapy, 69*(4), 229–238.

Patterson, M., Krupa, T., & Packer, T. (2000). Canada Russia Education Project. *Occupational Therapy Now, 2*(3), 10–12.

Pongsaksri, A. (2004). *A Trans-Cultural Study of Practice of Occupational Therapists in Thailand and Australia: Reframing Theories of Practice.* Doctoral dissertation, Curtin University of Technology, Thailand. Available at: http://espace.library.curtin.edu.au/R/?func=dbin-jump-full&object_id=15810&local_base=GEN01-ERA02 (accessed January 15, 2010).

Rebeiro, K. L. (1999). The labyrinth of community mental health: In search of meaningful occupation. *Psychiatric Rehabilitation Services, 23,* 143–152.

Rebeiro, K. L. (2001). Enabling occupation: The importance of an affirming environment. *Canadian Journal of Occupational Therapy: Revue Canadienne d'Ergotherapie, 68*(2), 80–89.

Rebeiro, K. L., Day, D. G., Semeniuk, B., O'Brien, M. C., & Wilson, B. (2001). NISA: An occupation-based, mental health program. *American Journal of Occupational Therapy, 55,* 493–500.

Rowles, G. D. (2003). The meaning of place as a component of self. In E. B. Crepeau, E. S. Cohn, & B. A. B. Schell (Eds.), *Willard and Spackman's Occupational Therapy* (10th ed., pp. 111–119). Philadelphia: Lippincott Williams & Wilkins.

Schult, M. (2002). *Multidimensional assessment of people with chronic pain: A critical appraisal of the Person, Environment, Occupation model.* Doctoral thesis, Uppsala University, Faculty of Medicine, Department of Public Health and Caring Services, Uppsala, Sweden. Available at: http://urn.kb.se/resolve?urn=urn:nbn:se:uu:diva-2555 (accessed October 19, 2009).

Strong, S. (1998). Meaningful work in supportive environments: Experiences with the recovery process. *American Journal of Occupational Therapy, 52,* 31–38.

Strong, S., Rigby, P., Stewart, D., Law, M., Cooper, B., & Letts, L. (1999). The Person-Environment-Occupation model: A practical intervention tool. *Canadian Journal of Occupational Therapy, 66,* 122–133.

Trainor, J., Pomeroy, E., & Pape, B. (1983). *A New Framework for Support for People With Serious Mental Health Problems.* Toronto: Canadian Mental Health Association.

Vrkljan, B. H. (2006). *In-Vehicle Navigation Systems and Driving Safety: The Occupational Performance of Older Drivers and Passengers—A Mixed Methods Approach.* Doctoral dissertation, Rehabilitation Science, University of Western Ontario, Ontario, Canada.

Wilcock, A. A. (Ed.). (2006). *An Occupational Perspective of Health* (2nd ed.). Thorofare, NJ: Slack.

Psychosocial Concerns With Disability

Patricia Crist

> "Having a disability shapes a person's life, but it is not their total destiny.
>
> —Senator Robert Dole, 1999

Introduction

At the heart of holistic practice in occupational therapy is integration of the psychosocial and physical aspects of productive and meaningful living that contribute to one's state of health and well-being. To put this concept into practice, the practitioner must consider not only the performance and participation issues associated with mental health conditions, but also the **psychosocial issues** related to the broader perspective of **disability**, whether a mental, physical, or developmental condition. Consider, for example, the loss of confidence that is exacerbated by the stigma of mental illness for a person with depression, the anxiety and overwhelming feelings for new parents after the birth of a child with severe developmental disorders, or the anger and despair that comes with a spinal cord injury in the life of a young adult athlete. Add to that issues of external environmental stress, such as financial or legal problems, discrimination, and prejudice.

Because occupation is the active process by which a person engages in everyday life with a disability, the person–environment–occupation interactions are framed by these broad sociopolitical influences. Considerations regarding the psychosocial aspects of disability and chronic illness must also reflect the context, or environment, in which the individual lives to fully appreciate one's potential for quality of life.

Although many occupational therapy practitioners advocate that they "treat the whole individual," service delivery systems may drive care to be less than holistic. For example, school-based practice exclusively emphasizes educationally related services and may not allow other natural occupations and contexts that are a part of a typically developing child to be considered unless educationally related. As evidence of the discipline's commitment to holism, the Accreditation Council for Occupational Therapy Education (ACOTE) included in its 2006 educational standards a specific fieldwork requirement to encourage consideration of the importance of the psychosocial aspects of care, regardless of area of practice (ACOTE, 2006a, 2006b, 2006c). All entry-level occupational therapy practitioners, as a result, are expected to address the psychosocial concerns presented by any population in any practice setting.

Standard B.10.15. Provide Level II fieldwork in traditional and/or emerging settings, consistent with the curriculum design. In all settings, psychosocial factors influencing engagement in occupation must be understood and integrated for the development of client-centered, meaningful, occupation-based outcomes. (ACOTE, 2006a, 2006b, 2006c, p. 12)

The occupational therapy profession is particularly well positioned to address the contingent influences between psychosocial issues and disabilities. In mental health settings, occupational therapists can offer effective intervention strategies that can lead to participation in daily life activities for individuals with both physical and mental or behavioral health conditions. Individuals receiving physical rehabilitation services who struggle with mental health and self-esteem issues of depression, poor body image, low self-efficacy, stressed interpersonal relationships, and/or loneliness or isolation can be challenging for other mental health professionals to address because few have formal preparation in the interaction between mental and physical health problems. For example, consider complex clinical cases such as an elderly man with aphasia who does not want to leave his home, even though he reports feeling lonely and isolated, because he fears being moved into a nursing home if he gets lost repeatedly. Or, consider a woman with a traumatic disability who is abandoned by her husband, even though he vowed to be true "for better or worse." Occupational therapy practitioners work to rebuild lives toward recovery that involves addressing the whole person in his or her environment and around his or her chosen and needed occupations.

For some clients, independence is an aspiration that is likely unachievable. For them, independence is the ability to have self-control of their destiny with as little assistance from others as possible, while being able to usefully navigate environmental resources, otherwise understood as **self-determination**. This chapter contributes to the understanding that healthy **interdependence** is the result of an individually chosen balance among personal abilities and aspirations and environmental resources that support occupational functioning.

The chapter begins with an understanding of response to disability and chronic illness followed by perspectives on addressing psychosocial aspects of disability as they emerge across time. Psychosocial issues that impact an individual's ability to be self-determining, participate, and advocate for oneself are explored, closing with a suggested protocol for teaching self-advocacy to support adaptation to disability. Critical review of evidence regarding psychosocial aspects of disability is emphasized throughout the chapter.

Disability Versus Chronic Illness

It is important to remember that the individual person-environment response to disability and chronic illness are not the same. Researchers have questioned over the years whether "having a disability" is different from "having a chronic illness." Buck and Hohmann (1983) stated:

> *A person with a stabilized disability can assume his/her physical health is intact and thus devote time and energy to pursuing personal, social and vocational goals. The ill person may attend more to the course and prognosis of the illness and emotionally invest time and interest in life-sustaining activities to the relative exclusion of other aspects of his/her life. (p. 212)*

Many chronic illnesses are frequently accompanied by not only continuous adaptation, but also physical disabilities.

Although disability and chronic illness have essentially different related processes and issues from each other, these two are combined in this chapter. However, in intervention, the occupational therapy practitioner should reflect the different trajectory or prognosis presented by the individual's performance challenges resulting from their experience with their disability or their chronic illness, cognizant that, in many cases, a combination of living with both simultaneously occurs.

Addressing Psychosocial Aspects of Disabilities

The ways in which an individual adapts to having a disability reflect the interactions among his or her personal psychological characteristics (e.g., life experience, needs, values, hope) and socioenvironmental factors (e.g., support, resources, objects), as well as the nature and level of severity of the condition or disability (Livneh, 2001; Livneh & Antonak, 1997). The prognosis or trajectory of a given condition or diagnosis also presents challenges to adapting to the course of the illness. For example, a person with an amputation secondary to trauma will experience a different life course than a child born with a physical disability. An adult who has a stroke will have a different lifestyle than a person who is continually adjusting to multiple sclerosis, a condition in which the course of illness might become more challenging over time.

The psychosocial aspects of living with a disability or chronic illness have been known for many years, but many times they were considered secondary to addressing the physical or medical aspects of conditions. Beatrice Wright (1959) wrote the first edition of the landmark textbook *Psychology and Rehabilitation*. This significant work advocated for all rehabilitation specialists to attend to the psychosocial issues that occur with physical disabilities. In a 1983 edition (titled *Physical Disability: A Psychological Approach*), she provided a

set of 20 value-laden beliefs and principles (modified from her earlier 1972 work) that still resonates today as a guide for understanding the psychosocial aspects of the disability experience.

Although Wright (1983) wrote these beliefs and principles based on her experience with people living with physical disabilities, they speak to all persons who live with disabilities, including persons with psychiatric disabilities. These primary principles provide a foundation for occupational therapy traditions and warrant current reaffirmation in daily practice (despite dated use of language such as "handicap" and less consistent person first language). They include

1. Every individual needs respect and encouragement; the presence of a disability, no matter how severe, does not alter these fundamental rights.
2. The severity of handicap can be increased or diminished by environmental conditions.
3. Issues of coping and adjusting to a disability cannot be validly considered without examining real problems that exist as barriers in the social and physical environment.
4. The assets of the person must receive considerable attention in the rehabilitation effort.
5. The significance of a disability is affected by the person's feelings about the self and his or her situation.
6. The active participation of the client in the planning and execution of the rehabilitation program is to be sought as fully possible.
7. Because each person has unique characteristics and each situation its own properties, variability is required in rehabilitation.
8. Interdisciplinary and interagency collaboration and coordination of services are essential.
9. In addition to the special problems of particular groups, rehabilitation clients commonly share certain problems by virtue of their disadvantaged and devalued position.
10. Society as a whole must continuously and persistently strive to provide the basic means toward fulfillment of the lives of all its inhabitants, including those with disabilities.
11. People with disabilities, like all citizens, are entitled to participate and contribute to the general life of the community. (pp. x–xvii)

These statements are helpful in understanding the individual psychosocial response to disability, as well as illuminating the core of the disability rights movement. Occupational therapy practitioners, other health-related professionals, and all citizens can view these principles as a call for action representing ideals for an inclusive society.

Despite these well-articulated principles, inclusion of people with disabilities in all aspects of everyday community life is far from being achieved. The gap between the ideal and reality is wide. In addition, despite efforts for more than 40 years to actively improve the employability and employment environments for individuals with disabilities, unemployment and underemployment continue to be problematic for those who live with a disability. According to the 2000 U.S. Census data (U.S. Census Bureau, 2003), although 24.4% of people between the ages of 5 and

64 have a disability, 38% of working age adults with disabilities live in households with annual incomes under $15,000, and 30% do not have either checking or savings accounts. In addition, Census 2000 showed that disability status impacts employment status among people ages 16 to 64, where almost 80% of people without disabilities were employed versus 60% of those with disabilities (U.S. Census Bureau, 2003).

In its early years, occupational therapists adopted a psychodynamic approach to understanding disability, which was viewed as a loss. The object relations approach hypothesized that the response to any form of loss was uniform. However, the impact of the loss for an individual was directly proportional to the degree of psychic energy tied to the lost object (Ogden, 2002). Applied to occupational therapy, a disability was equated to the loss of a specific, self-rewarding function or ability. The reaction to the loss was tempered by how important the lost or altered function was to the individual.

The fundamental components of response to loss according to object relations theory remain in the foundations of most models today that address adaptation to disability. Early in the quest for understanding individual reaction to disability, Kübler-Ross's (1973, 2005) stages of dying were considered relevant to understanding an individual's response to having a disability as a sense of loss, particularly a new one:

- Denial that one has lost function or has a disability
- Anger that one will no longer be able to perform certain activities because of the disability
- Bargaining as one attempts to do, give, or purchase something in exchange for having the lost function returned
- Depression over the frustration that bargaining is not working as desired
- Acceptance of one's disability includes integrating the disability into one's daily life activities.

However, referencing the Kübler-Ross stages fell into disfavor by disability rights advocates whose intent was not to equate the highly emotional, negative passage of death and dying with experiencing a disability. Further, words such as *coping, adjustment, adaptation,* and *acceptance* were believed to "pathologize" the experience of disability, meaning a disability was automatically assumed to be an undesirable state (Smart, 2001, p. 229).

Instead, the use of the word *response* is considered to be more accurate and less stigmatizing. Smart (2001) advocates for the use of "response to a disability" because it communicates the meaning that the individual attaches to his or her disability as more important than just having a disability. Further, once a person has a disability or chronic illness, he or she experiences challenges in responding to activities and occupations for the duration of life. Thus, in reality, words such as *acceptance* and *adaptation* are inaccurate in describing living with a disability.

To summarize, consideration of the individual with a disability or chronic illness might best be addressed by following Wright's (1983) principles, in which the disability is considered an experience in which the person responds to the challenges associated with their disability, while pursuing his or her valued occupations based on personal and social strengths and supports.

Evidence Regarding Response to Disability

A review of the evidence regarding response to disability is significantly limited. First, there is a paucity of research on this dimension. Second, as we value and understand that each disability may have its own unique pattern of response, the application of methods or assessments used in one study of disability to another may not be appropriate.

For example, a simple historical review conducted by this author indicates that 10 years ago, one or two major instruments were used to measure quality of life. Now, nearly every major disability or chronic illness has at least one specific quality-of-life measure related to unique disability-specific variables considered or found to be important. Third, studies of acquired disabilities, which affect the largest percentage of the population, seldom look at the influence of premorbid psychosocial or personality variables or lifestyle considerations in regard to the current response to disability.

Finally, the influence of culture or ethnic traditions in understanding the response to disability is seldom isolated or recognized. For example, Sobralske (2006) found that Mexican American men who hold cultural beliefs associated with machismo waited to access health care until their pain or disability reached a level at which they could no longer work or carry out their personal activities of daily living. Littlewood (2006) notes that the dominant culture identifies disabilities such as mental illness and intellectual disabilities at higher rates among those groups over which they dominate. Family religious beliefs may impact how a family affected by disability participates in the rehabilitation process (Callicott, 2003).

Smart (2001) points out that the primary evidence for response to disability has been based on the medical model, which creates limitations about information on individual experience with a disability. Most published information focuses on intervention outcomes and little on social and environmental issues. Smart cautions readers of evidence regarding living with a disability or chronic illness with the following:

1. Response to disability is multidimensional. However, most studies are unidimensional.
2. Stigma associated with disability is a well-known social issue, but it is seldom accounted for as a variable contributing to findings from studies.
3. Response to disability is best understood across time, yet very little longitudinal research is available.
4. Knowledge about response to disability primarily centers on men with physical disabilities, which limits generalizability to others such as women, and those from varied age and ethnic groups.
5. Erroneously, symptoms associated with a disability become labeled as response when in fact they are not.
6. Lack of accepted psychometric procedures, such as using a psychosocial instrument focusing on adjustment or quality of life that has not been standardized on a sample of individuals with a disability, may result in biased and unfounded outcomes.
7. Although qualitative studies of response to disability are emerging to present rich, enlightening descriptions of the individual response to the disability experience, accepting this type of research as evidence is very slow to be accepted by traditional researchers who are bound to quantitative methodologies. (pp. 235–240)

The number of military personnel returning from war with traumatic brain injuries (TBIs), posttraumatic stress disorder (PTSD), and depression related to physical trauma are addressed in this evidence:

➤ In a study of 613 U.S. soldiers hospitalized following serious combat injury, early severity of physical problems was strongly predictive of PTSD (12%) or depression (9.3%) 7 months later (Grieger et al, 2006). Other mental health problems also increased substantially between the two screenings.

➤ A more recent study of the general military population, including 56,350 active and 31,885 National Guard and Reserve soldiers, reported PTSD (active soldiers, 11.8%–16.7%; reservists, 12.7%–24.5%), depression (active, 4.7%–10.3%; reserve, 3.8%–13.0%), and overall mental health risk (active, 17.0%–27.1%; reserve, 17.5%–35.5%) (Milliken, Auchterlonie, & Hoge, 2007). Many had a higher rate of general physical health concerns as well.

➤ At minimum, returning to the individual's community on completion of a deployment requires learning how to reintegrate with a society that is not in combat and probably does not understand the daily influence from one's prior combat experience (Association of the United States Army, 2008). If the person is returning with a new physical disability, support for changes in lifestyle are essential.

➤ Battle fatigue is viewed as a response to the overwhelming psychosocial stressors associated with combat. Along with attending to physiological needs, providing structured occupations and support of occupational roles has been effective in creating high return-to-duty rates in soldiers by providing occupational therapy rooted in the model of human occupation (Geraldi, 1996).

➤ A randomized clinical trial to rehabilitate 67 active duty military service members with TBI who have the potential to return to duty demonstrated success. The intervention included an 8-week rehabilitation program combining group therapies (fitness, planning and organization, cognitive skills, work skills, medication and milieu groups, and community reentry outings) and individual therapy (neuropsychology, work therapy, occupational therapy, and speech and language pathology). The results were that 96% returned to work, and 66% (n = 44) returned to duty (Braverman et al, 1999).

➤ The implications of this evidence indicate the challenges and opportunities for occupational therapy with our wounded warriors regarding community reentry; response to ongoing psychosocial issues related to PTSD, depression, and/or suicidal ideation, TBI, and what might be the late effects of battle fatigue, not to mention the stress of multiple return deployments.

Association of the United States Army (AUSA). (2008). "Mental Health Care—Before, During and After Deployment." Available at: http://www.ausa.org/webpub/DeptHome.nsf/byid/RBOH-7D9N9V (accessed October 19, 2009).

Braverman, S. E., Spector, J .S., Warden, D. L., Wilson, B. C., Ellis, T. E., Bamdad, M. J., & Salazar, A. M. (1999). A multidisciplinary TBI inpatient rehabilitation programme for active duty service members as a part of a randomized clinical trial. *Brain Injury, 13,* 405–415.

Geraldi, S. S. (1996). The management of battle-fatigued soldiers: An occupational therapy model. *Military Medicine, 161,* 483–488.

Grieger, T. A., Cozza, S. J., Ursano, R. J., Hoge, C., Martinez, P. E., Engel, C. C., & Wain, H. J. (2006). Posttraumatic stress disorder and depression in battle injured soldiers. *American Journal of Psychiatry, 163,* 1777–1783.

Milliken, C. S., Auchterlonie, J. L., & Hoge, C. W. (2007). Longitudinal assessment of mental health problems among active and reserve component soldiers returning from the Iraq War. *Journal of the American Medical Association, 298,* 2141–2148.

Response to Disability

As stated previously, the response to disability has primarily been studied among acquired disabilities using the historical stage-specific model, mainly on disabling conditions. This has limited application to congenital disabilities, the aging population, and disabilities such as chronic illnesses in which the individual gradually declines naturally.

Research literature focusing on the major chronic illness patterns is now emerging. Livneh (2001) identifies the psychosocial reactions to disability as being short term (including the shock, anxiety, and denial that might rise immediately after being diagnosed with a disabling condition), intermediate (including affective reactions to the life change such as depression, grief, anger, and aggressiveness), and long term (those that occur down the road and show evidence of adaptation such as "passive and active acceptance, environmental mastery, behavioral adaptation, affective equilibrium, and disability integration") (p. 153). Adaptive responses occur when the person integrates the disability into a reconstructed self, whereas maladaptive responses might move an individual toward hopelessness and helplessness. The reader may compare the stages of Kübler-Ross (1973, 2005) with Livneh's model and see a similar understanding of the reaction to living with a disabling condition.

Shock

Shock is the reaction to the initial impact of realizing that one has acquired a new disability. This occurs both with acknowledgment of either a recent trauma or a new condition associated with an existing diagnosis. The person may be frightened, overwhelmed, and disorganized in his or her behavior while attempting to integrate this new experience (Livneh & Antonak, 2005). Information flow is fast paced, and it is often difficult to understand what is being said. Shock may recur when a major new step occurs in rehabilitation, such as being sent to a new supported living situation, getting a wheelchair, or acquiring some new ability, such as with cochlear implants. During this early phase, the occupational therapist might offer support and empathy, and encourage the person to vent their feelings and vulnerabilities (Livneh & Antonak, 1997) by using therapeutic use of self.

Defensive Retreat or Denial

Defensive retreat, or **denial**, is considered to be a healthy, typical response to the disability. Denial can take three basic forms: denial of the presence of the disability, denial of the implications of the disability, or denial of the permanence of the disability (Langer, 1994; Smart, 2001; Stewart, 1994). Denial might be considered a healthy response because it lessens anxiety and might allow a person to hope for the best possible outcome; however, it might also result in a lack of engagement in the full rehabilitative program based on unrealistic expectations (Livneh & Antonak, 2005). Consistent with **motivational interviewing**, strategies addressing **precontemplation** (similar to the concept of denial but based on little to no awareness of how their condition might have serious disabling consequences), offering information and reflection on performance issues observed, and giving clear feedback would be consistent with a motivational approach (Miller & Rollnick, 2002; Stoffel & Moyers, 2004).

The Lived Experience

John Jones

Can you look back and pick a single day that changed your life? Think about it.

The day you got married? Maybe the day your kids were born? Perhaps the day you graduated from school? For me, picking the day that changed my life is easy. June 11, 2006. The day I nearly died . . .

Before that Sunday morning, I was living a dream, the dream I'd worked 20 years in the National Football League to achieve. I was the 10th president in the history of the Green Bay Packers, the team I'd loved since I was a teenager growing up in New Orleans. Everything about my life was on track. I was doing all the right things personally and professionally. My sights were set on leading the Packers franchise to continued success. Then, on a Sunday morning in June a few years back, my dreams slipped away. Literally, in a heartbeat. Everything changed.

If it weren't for my friends—doctors Pat McKenzie and John Gray—and my doctors at Bellin Health in Green Bay—cardiologist Matt Fuchs and cardiothoracic surgeon Tom Cain—I wouldn't be here telling this story.

On that Sunday morning in June 2006, my aorta dissected, and I suffered a stroke during surgery. Everything changed. Since that day, I have never stopped fighting to return to the life I once knew.

Not the Packers part. The stroke took care of that.

I've spent the past year and a half fighting to reclaim as much of myself as I can, always supported by loving family and friends.

I continue to seek a way to make sense of how to use a post-stroke brain.

It became a painful truth that the stroke's damage to my brain looks like it truly is permanent. I still haven't fully come to terms with that. I keep praying for a miracle.

Some of the doctors told me that I needed to learn to live with it.

That was never an option, the way I looked at it. One thing the stroke didn't take from me was my determination to do things the best that I can, to keep fighting in hopes my condition will somehow improve.

I never quit. Not when the docs weren't sure my kidneys would come back on line after surgery.

Not when the docs weren't sure the paralysis in my left leg would subside.

Truth is, I am doing this the only way I know how.

Never surrender.

I choose to believe that someday, some way I will find my way back to who I was. I pray that my brain will shake off the pallor of the stroke, that my neurons will start popping like they used to. No more forgetfulness. No more messing up dates and time sequences. No more asking the same question 5 minutes after I last asked it. No more forgetting—as Crosby, Stills, and Nash once harmonized: "Where you have to be at noon."

Until that day comes, if ever, I am setting my sights on new goals, goals that I can attain as I am.

My new goal on my mission is to get out regionally, even nationally, to speak about men's health. I want to speak to businesses, civic groups, churches, and professional and business organizations.

I measure my successes in the personal stories I hear from men or wives and other loved ones who tell me their guy got his checkup after hearing me speak.

My biggest joy comes when I get word that a guy who heard my message got his checkup. A few of those guys have undergone same-day heart surgery to save their lives. They wouldn't have been in the doc's office in the first place if they hadn't heard me speak or been pushed by loved ones, who happened to be armed with my story.

At moments like that, the bad things that happened to me seem very small. At times like that, I say a prayer of thanks. It's not about me. It's about finding a way to make sure that my story doesn't become some other guy's story.

The truth is that men need to take care of themselves like their lives depend on it.

Because they do.

Nobody is bulletproof.

Used with permission of John Jones, former president of the Green Bay Packers. For more information, go to www.bulletproofmyth.com.

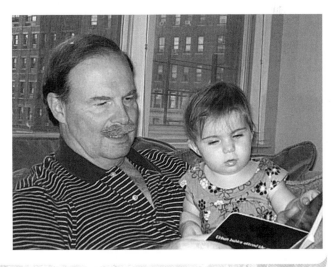

Depression or Mourning

Whereas denial is focused on losing past functions and abilities, **depression** or **mourning** is related to considering the future (Kübler-Ross, 1973). The person is grieving for dreams that no longer seem possible, coupled with fear or anxiety about what lies ahead. As with depression of any kind, the individual will have very limited energy and ability to focus on participation in intervention programs, and may view the world as "better off without them." The individual may express guilt, self-blame, loss of hope, apathy, and depression. The occupational therapist might not only encourage the person to vent these feelings, but would also want to move the individual toward social engagement, finding and seeking out support and activities with others that emphasize self-assertiveness and determination, and reengagement in everyday life activities that hold meaning for the person (Livneh & Antonak, 2005). Being aware that depression and grief reactions may also increase the likelihood of other more serious issues, such as coping with feeling down by drinking or using other mood-altering substances (Grant et al, 2006), might also be explored with the person as a preventive measure.

In addition, another area that deserves attention of the occupational therapist relates to suicidal ideation or gestures. The suicidal thoughts may not only be related to depression, but could also be understood as an attempt to exercise control over one's existence (Shontz, 1993). Ensuring safety, referring for more intense psychological services, and helping the individual work with close social supports would all be consistent with handling protracted depression (Livneh & Antonak, 2005).

This is also the time when family and friends may drop away as they grieve for their own reasons or become weary of engaging with the person who is depressed. Anyone who has sat next to the bed of someone seriously ill for great lengths of time knows this feeling of helplessness, hopelessness, and even the desire to be able to absorb pain for the individual (Gorman, 1993). At this point, contact with other individuals who are living with the disability is beneficial for the individual and significant others as they consider how to create the new story of living with a disability. Support groups for family members are also helpful contexts in which to express shared feelings safely and learn about ways in which they can productively help their loved ones and consider their own new future.

The practitioner can help the individual with the disability and his or her significant others understand that adapting to a disability happens in cycles; it is not linear. Past issues that the individual dealt with may resurface as new issues, for example, choosing to begin a family may look quite different when one has a disability that also has a genetic basis. New knowledge may lead to a downward spiral to an earlier stage, which medical experts label "**regression**," as the individual idealized images of what he or she used to be and cannot be anymore. This is a natural response (Livneh & Antonak, 1997). For instance, a person dealing with a chronic illness is doing relatively well, but suddenly learns about a new diagnosis, related or unrelated, that will permanently change his or her functional ability again. Cancer survivors are frequently unprepared for the late effects of earlier interventions that put their cancer in remission. For instance, the late onset of life-altering cardiopathies, neuropathies, and cognitive changes can cause them to revisit their history and question their future with these new disabilities. As the grief subsides, energy returns to participate.

Personal Questioning and/or Anger

Personal questioning and/or **anger** are related to feeling of helplessness, fear, frustration, anxiety, and irritability. Often, two questions are trying to be answered: "Why me (hopelessness and abandonment)?" and "How did I let myself get into this condition (self-blame and guilt)?" (Livneh & Antonak, 1997).

The goal of occupational therapy at this time is to help the person work toward creating new meaning and purpose in life activities. Therapists can focus on helping individuals reestablish independent daily life routines at this time. Individuals

with disabilities can learn their capabilities, identify who to ask for support when needed, and begin to create their own story about living with a disability through experience with everyday life. The individual with the disability and even family members begin to clarify beliefs about the purpose and meaning of the disability experience.

Occupational therapy provides an excellent channel and expression for dealing with anger. Engaging in heavy, repetitive work; physical exercise; or, if possible, sports activities offers an excellent tool for anger management or redirection, as well as expressive media and movement in which feelings can be put on paper or into artistic creations for outside release and reflection (Livneh & Antonak, 2005).

Integration and Growth

Integration and **growth** occur when the individual sees the disability as an opportunity for personal growth and new learning. Carolyn Vash (1981) called this "transcendence of the disability." Typically, individuals in this stage become interested in leading change in the person–environment interaction through service, advocacy, and/or political action. Seeing their experience with responding to disability as a personal strength, they look for activities that give meaning and purpose to their disability experience.

Smart (2001) encourages practitioners to educate individuals with disabilities and their families about these response stages because it "normalizes" or "universalizes" their response to disability as a common, rather than lonely, experience. Occupational therapy practitioners can use this response model to validate the concerns of clients, establish intervention goals, and show clients what may lie ahead.

This information serves as a general guide for individuals with disabilities; however, no two persons go through these stages in the same way. In fact, earlier stages may recur when new challenges in living are confronted. Some individuals may never experience one or more of the stages. Learning to respond to one's disability is a complex process that involves drawing on the resources within and outside the individual, integrated with the personal meaning attributed to the disability. The complexity in individual response to disability reflects the following considerations related to the type of disability experienced, including the time of onset (congenital or acquired, as well as related developmental issues) (Smart, 2001, pp. 261–331):

- Type of onset (insidious or acute and phases)
- Functions impaired
- Severity of disability
- Visibility of the disability
- Degree, if any, of disfigurement
- Degree of stigma
- Course of the disability (stable, progressive, episodic, including predictability, acute, chronic, exacerbation, degenerative, remission)
- Prognosis of the disability
- Treatment required
- Resources available

These factors, coupled with the environmental issues, which are discussed briefly in the next section, combine to create quality of life for persons with disabilities.

Disability Conditions and the Environment

In the 1970s, groups of people with and without disabilities joined forces to create **disability communities** in order to eradicate stigma and advocate for inclusion and participation, which impacted the quality of life for persons with disabilities. The University of California–Berkeley led the way in moving the sociopolitical interests of individuals into the mainstream (DeJong, 1979). Popular press publications, such as the *Disability Rag* and *Accent on Living*, pointed to the atrocities in the environment, including discrimination, exclusion, and inaccessible environments, and identified the person-environment changes needed to provide opportunities and eliminate barriers to full engagement of individuals with disabilities.

Major legislation changed the context that frames disability in the United States, that is, the **disability rights movement**, which is transforming the years of stigma, social prejudice, and discrimination surrounding disabilities into a healthier environment for all citizens. A series of landmark court decisions, along with sustained advocacy by people with disabilities for legislation such as the Rehabilitation Act of 1973 (PL 93-112), the Individuals With Disabilities Education Act of 1975 (PL 99-457), and, most notably, the Americans With Disabilities Act of 1990 (PL 101-336), were major leaps forward for inclusionary employment, environments, and education.

Also, additional resources were created to comprehensively eliminate barriers and create opportunities for individuals with disabilities based on these laws and associated regulations. The reader is encouraged to review Chapters 2, 17, and 28, which provide a deeper understanding of the sociopolitical influences on mental health and disability-related issues.

Supporting the deinstitutionalization movement that began in the late 1960s, with the goal to move individuals out of long-term care institutions into the community (now known as the "least restrictive environment"), the **independent living (IL) movement** has been a major contributor to the broader issue of self-determination for persons with physical and psychiatric disabilities (The National Council on Independent Living, 2006). The IL movement advocates that people with even the most severe disabilities should have a choice regarding their living situation in the community. It focuses on personal assistance services and the removal of architectural and transportation barriers to allow individuals with disabilities to manage their daily life activities and fully participate in the life of the community.

The IL movement has resulted in the establishment of hundreds of **independent living centers (ILCs)** around the globe, more than 500 in the United States alone (www.ilusa.com). The goal of ILCs is to assist individuals with disabilities achieve their maximum potential within their families and communities. Most ILCs are typically nonresidential, nonprofit, consumer-controlled, community-based organizations that provide services and advocacy by and for persons with all types of disabilities.

In 1978, the National Institute for Disability Research and Rehabilitation (NIDRR) was founded as a branch of the National Institutes of Health in Washington, DC, with the mission to generate research to improve the ability of people with disabilities to perform self-selected activities in the community, and enhance society's capacity to provide full opportunities and accommodations for its citizens with disabilities. Full inclusion, social integration, employment, independent living, and community integration of individuals of all ages with disabilities are the focus of NIDRR activities.

Although multiple legal and government acts and bills are now in place for individuals with disabilities, a significant law related to this text is the 1985 Mental Illness Bill of Rights Act, which resulted in the Protection and Advocacy for Individuals With Mental Illness Act of 1986 (PAIMI Act). This act (updated most recently in 2002) requires protection and advocacy services for people with mental illness and serious emotional disturbance. The primary objectives of this law are to

- Protect and advocate the rights of individuals with mental illness
- Investigate incidents of abuse and neglect among individuals with mental illness
- Investigate incidents of serious injury and deaths in public and private care and treatment facilities and nonmedical community-based facilities for children and youth
- Receive reports of all serious injuries and deaths related to incidents of seclusion and restraint in public and private care and treatment facilities in the states and territories

The sociopolitical influences presented here provide a strong and convincing case for occupational therapy practitioners to work with and among all service recipients (persons with disabilities, their families, friends, employers, and neighbors) to create change across the spectrum (personal to societal) by being advocates and facilitating self-advocacy.

Occupational Therapy Role in Advocacy

Occupational therapy practitioners, through advocacy at the societal level, can support the passage and implementation of regulations that modify the environment to prevent exclusion and promote full community engagement. Some practitioners make careers of providing environmental modification recommendations as consultants. With the growing number of empowered individuals with disabilities, frail elderly, and the desire of baby boomers to age in place, there are numerous possibilities to practice, consult, and educate about accessible environments for independent living.

Although occupational therapy practitioners can promote environmental accessibility for full community participation, it is also important to prepare our clients to advocate for their own full participation. One individual may need the skills to be able to disclose his or her mental illness to an employer, and a parent with a child who has a physical disability may need help securing supports for educational activities. A person using a wheelchair may be frustrated by the community places that cannot be accessed, and a frail elderly person may be afraid to ask a physician important questions or admit to symptoms that might change their options regarding driving or housing. Preparing individuals with disabilities to be self-advocates and to be self-empowered is central to productive living.

Self-advocacy in the health-care arena can begin by focusing on core concepts from the patient bills of rights (U.S. Office of Personnel Management, n.d.):

1. Information Disclosure—the right to receive accurate, easily understood information, including health plans and making health decisions
2. Choice of Providers and Plans—the right to a choice of health-care providers
3. Access to Emergency Services—the right to access emergency health-care services when and where the need arises
4. Participation in Treatment Decisions—the right and responsibility to fully participate or be represented by a designated individual in all decisions related to health care
5. Respect and Nondiscrimination—the right to considerate, respectful care from all members of the health-care system at all times and under all circumstances
6. Confidentiality of Health Information—the right to confidentially communicate with health-care providers and to have the confidentiality of individually identifiable health-care information protected
7. Access to Health Information—the right to review and copy your own medical records as well as request amendments to the records
8. Complaints and Appeals—the right to a fair and efficient process for resolving differences with health-care providers, including a systematic internal review and an independent external review, if requested
9. Consumer Responsibilities—the right to be actively involved in decisions and processes of getting health care for oneself to achieve the best outcomes in terms of quality and cost efficiencies

All intervention should address some form of advocacy or empowerment. Two types of self-advocacy preparation are requisite:

- Education regarding laws and regulations that support the access and rights of individuals with disabilities, and how individuals can engage these resources in their daily lives
- Individual skill development in being a self-advocate

Education can occur through providing community resource or fact sheets that outline what can be expected or accessed to support oneself. Alerting individuals with disabilities to ombudsman services, employee assistance programs, and legal aid societies can also be useful. An **ombudsman** is an official who is typically appointed by an agency, government, employer, or school and charged to investigate and address complaints reported by individuals. **Employee assistance programs** are confidential resources to assist employees with life issues that impact their ability to focus on or meet employment expectations. **Legal aid societies** are nonprofit entities that provide civil legal assistance for individuals who cannot afford their own legal counsel.

As part of helping an individual adapt to his or her disability, providing skills or resources to prepare for self-advocacy, or to be empowered, is essential. Tips regarding the basics of teaching self-advocacy are included in Box 4-1.

BOX 4-1 ■ Information for Occupational Therapists Addressing Self-Advocacy

Teaching Self-Advocacy to Support Adaptation to Disability

The process of taking control of one's life when living with a disability is essential—that is, being able to self-advocate for needs, interests, and rights, and to promote self-efficacy and autonomy. Every person with a disability needs self-advocacy in their tool kit for life. Occupational therapists can address the primary facets of self-advocacy to assist individuals with disabilities in gaining these skills.

1. **Admit and accept your disability.** Focus on abilities or accommodations you need to participate. Avoid using disability as an excuse.
2. **Know your rights and responsibilities.** Educate yourself on these expectations.
3. **Know what you need or want.** Consider alternatives and prioritize them.
4. **Negotiate regarding issues that interfere with your ability to self-advocate and be willing to compromise.** Look for the "win-win" in decisions. Be flexible and accept appropriate shared responsibilities to enact a desired change.
5. **Know where to go for support or resources.** Know what is available in the community and on the Internet. Research supports, risks, and benefits of what you find.
6. **Plan for the future.** Be able to state your goals and then articulate what you are doing now or what you believe needs to occur next for you to be successful.

Cues for Successful Self-Advocacy

- Negotiating health care and one's rights can be complicated. Before you make contacts, make a checklist of the questions or concerns you want to address.
- Consider keeping a log of contacts or copies of written communication that includes:
  1. What you wanted
  2. Who you contacted: name, title, address, phone number, e-mail
  3. When: date and time of contact
  4. What they said
  5. What needs to happen next or what you expect to happen (and by when)
- Be respectful.
- Become informed about your disability and related issues. Consider retaining
  1. Copies of medical records, medication lists, lab tests, and self-care instructions
  2. Literature on disability and other major health conditions
  3. List of beneficial websites
- Gain an understanding of the perspective or the concerns of the other party.
- Rehearse your request or dialogue in the various ways you believe it might go.

BOX 4-1 ■ Information for Occupational Therapists Addressing Self-Advocacy—cont'd

- Practice a convincing, clear voice and good eye contact while minimizing negative emotions (anger, screaming, walking out, slamming objects down, whining, saying "yes, but . . .").
- Establish or set a good time for discussion to be unhurried and completed.
- Take time to say what you want, and ask for time to think about something before you answer.
- Be willing to compromise, but also know your threshold below which a decision is not acceptable.

- If you meet resistance, do not push; instead, ask for another time to meet and consider bringing someone along for support or to request additional information.
- Be willing to actively contribute to the desired change.
- Pushing for a decision quickly may lead to the wrong one. Also, if decision is clearly not going to be acceptable, avoid having the decision stated. Buy time for more thought and discussion by stopping discussion and requesting a future meeting.

Disability rights advocates initiated the concept of self-advocacy to assist individuals with confronting the limitations, stigma, and injustices experienced during the medical response to their disability. This included promoting treatment as humans versus objects and the ability to self-direct versus being asked to comply. Self-advocacy, or empowerment, is now generalized to mean self-pursuit of all aspects leading to healthy, self-directed participation in all aspects of living to ensure the best quality of life possible.

The basics of self-advocacy and empowerment are universal. Self-advocacy is more individual and person centered, whereas empowerment is more person-environment centered and moves groups of people toward collective action or outcomes, such as bettering communities or systems. Regardless, the outcome of both is to transform choices into desired outcomes or actions for more fully engaged living and quality of life for persons with disabilities.

Summary

Adaptation to disability or illness is a process, and occupational therapy practitioners are skilled at engaging both person characteristics and environmental resources to enhance quality of life. This chapter extends understanding of the individual response to disability and psychosocial practice with individuals who experience disability of all types, given the influence of the sociopolitical environment. Because of occupational therapy's philosophy to be holistic practitioners who use occupational engagement to interface personal abilities with context, this chapter provides a broad insight of influences that impact response to disability among the individuals we serve. Occupational therapy practitioners are called to use this broader understanding to challenge all aspects of living with a disability in order to help our clients reach their full potential and desired quality of life.

Active Learning Strategies

1. Reflection on Wright's 11 Foundational Beliefs

Consider contact you have had with a close family member or friend with a disability whom you know well. Review each of the 11 beliefs described in this chapter. Apply each belief to that individual, and reflect on how these beliefs impact how you might ethically work with this person. How can you ensure that these traditions are carried out in your everyday practice?

2. Promotional Brochure

Imagine that you work for a nonprofit organization and are expected to work with your facility's marketing and development units on a brochure that will reflect the benefits of occupational therapy. It will be used to raise funds to purchase beneficial equipment and cover costs for treating individuals who do not have funding sources for care. What visual images and narratives would you include about your program? Share a draft of your brochure with another student in your class. Compare your images with one another, and critique one another's brochure as to content that might be considered as prejudicial, discriminating, or dehumanizing.

3. Disability Experience and Reflection

Simulate a disability by attempting three typical daily tasks (e.g., mobility impairment: wheelchair- or crutch-assisted gait problems; hearing impairment: ear plugs; visual impairment: scotch tape over lenses, remove eyeglasses or contacts or patch). What challenges or loss of function did you experience? How did you feel about this loss? How did people react to you differently because of your disability? What happened that you did not expect? Did you have experiences that came from being or others seeing you as disadvantaged or devalued? What would be the difference between your experience and living with this disability daily? What has this experience taught you about your future practice?

 Describe the experience in your **Reflective Journal**.

Caution: Some do not advocate simulations because they believe that they present false pictures of reality. Simulating a disability does not totally parallel the lived experience. An alternative is to shadow a person with a disability or accompany the person simulating the same disability to obtain a better perspective. To experience others' reactions, minimize visual cues and behaviors that you are not "really disabled."

4. Acquired Versus Congenital Disability Reflection

Some consider the experience with an acquired disability occurring later in life as different from what an individual with a congenital disability experiences. What are the comparative opportunities created by having either type of disability? What are the comparative challenges or negatives by having either? Is acquiring a disability or chronic illness experienced differently at each of the major developmental life stages? How does this impact your response to disability or chronic illness during practice?

Resources

- Independent Living Centers: www.ilusa.com
- Disability Rag: http://www.ragged-edge-mag.com/
- disABILITY Magazines: http://www.netreach.net/~abrejcha/magazine.htm

References

Accreditation Council for Occupational Therapy Education (ACOTE). (2006a). *Accreditation Standards for a Doctoral-Degree-Level Education Program for the Occupational Therapist.* Rockville, MD: Author.

Accreditation Council for Occupational Therapy Education (ACOTE). (2006b). *Accreditation Standards for a Master's-Degree-Level Education Program for the Occupational Therapist.* Rockville, MD: Author.

Accreditation Council for Occupational Therapy Education (ACOTE). (2006c). *Accreditation Standards for the Occupational Therapy Assistant.* Rockville, MD: Author.

Americans With Disabilities Act of 1990 (PL 101-336), 42 U.S.C. § 12101.

Association of the United States Army (AUSA). (2008). "Mental Health Care—Before, During and After Deployment." Available at: http://www.ausa.org/webpub/DeptHome.nsf/byid/RBOH-7D9N9V (accessed October 20, 2009).

Braverman, S. E., Spector, J., Warden, D. L., Wilson, B. C., Ellis, T. E., Bamdad, M. J., & Salazar, A. M. (1999). A multidisciplinary TBI inpatient rehabilitation programme for active duty service members as part of a randomized clinical trial. *Brain Injury, 13,* 405–415.

Buck, F. M., & Hohmann, G. W. (1983). Parental disability and children's adjustment. In E. L. Pan, T. E. Backer, & C. L. Vash (Eds.), *Annual Review of Rehabilitation* (Vol. 3; pp. 203–241). New York: Springer.

Callicott, K. J. (2003). Culturally sensitive collaboration within person-centered planning. *Focus on Autism and Other Developmental Disabilities, 18,* 60–68.

DeJong, G. (1979). Independent living: From social movement to analytic paradigm. *Archives of Physical Medicine and Rehabilitation, 60*(10), 435–446.

Geraldi, S. S. (1996). The management of battle-fatigued soldiers: An occupational therapy model. *Military Medicine, 161,* 483–488.

Gorman, K. K. (1993). Addicted and disabled: One man's journey from helplessness to hope. In A. W. Heinemann (Ed.), *Substance Abuse and Physical Disability* (pp. 11–20). New York: Haworth Press.

Grant, B.F., Stinson, F.S., Dawson, D.A., Chou, P., Dufour, M.C., Compton, W., Pickering, R.P., & Kaplan, K. (2006). Prevalence and co-occurrence of substance use disorders and independent mood and anxiety disorders. *Alcohol Research & Health, 29,* 107–120.

Grieger, T. A., Cozza, S. J., Ursano, R. J., Hoge, C., Martinez, P. E., Engel, C. C., & Wain, H. J. (2006). Posttraumatic stress disorder and depression in battle injured soldiers. *American Journal of Psychiatry, 163,* 1777–1783.

Individuals With Disabilities Education Act of 1975 (PL 99-457), 20 U.S.C. § 1400.

Kübler-Ross, E. (1973). *On Death and Dying.* New York: Routledge.

Kübler-Ross, E. (2005). *On Grief and Grieving: Finding the Meaning of Grief Through the Five Stages of Loss.* New York: Simon & Schuster.

Langer, K. G. (1994). Depression and denial in psychotherapy of persons with disabilities. *American Journal of Psychotherapy, 48,* 181–194.

Littlewood, R. (2006). Mental health and intellectual disability: Culture and diversity. *Journal of Intellectual Disability Research, 50,* 555–560.

Livneh, H. (2001). Psychosocial adaptation to chronic illness and disability: A conceptual framework. *Rehabilitation Counseling Bulletin, 44,* 151–160.

Livneh, H., & Antonak, R. F. (1997). *Psychosocial Adaptation to Chronic Illness and Disability.* Gaithersburg, MD: Aspen.

Livneh, H., & Antonak, R. F. (2005). Psychosocial adaptation to chronic illness and disability: A primer for counselors. *Journal of Counseling & Development, 83,* 12–20.

Miller, W. R., & Rollnick, S. (2002). *Motivational Interviewing: Preparing People to Change Addictive Behavior* (2nd ed.). New York: Guilford Press.

Milliken, C. S., Auchterlonie, J. L., & Hoge, C. W. (2007). Longitudinal assessment of mental health problems among active and reserve component soldiers. *Journal of the American Medical Association, 298*(18), 2141–2148.

The National Council on Independent Living (NCIL). (2006). "The Disability Rights and Independent Living Movements." Available at: http://www.ncil.org/about/WhatIsIndependentLiving.html (accessed October 20, 2009).

Ogden, T. H. (2002). A new reading of the origins of object-relations theory. *The International Journal of Psychoanalysis, 83,* 767–782.

Rehabilitation Act of 1973 (PL 93-112), 29 U.S.C. § 791.

Shontz, F. C. (1993). A personological integration of chemical dependence and physical disability. In A. W. Heinemann (Ed.), *Substance Abuse and Physical Disability* (pp. 21–39). New York: Haworth Press.

Smart, J. (2001). *Disability, Society, and the Individual.* Austin, TX: PRO-ED.

Sobralske, M. (2006). Machismo sustains health and illness beliefs of Mexican American men. *Journal of the American Academy of Nurse Practitioners, 18,* 348–350.

Stewart, J. R. (1994). Denial of disabling conditions and specific interventions in the rehabilitation counseling setting. *Journal of Applied Rehabilitation Counseling, 25*(3), 7–15.

Stoffel, V. C., & Moyers, P. A. (2004). An evidence-based and occupational perspective of interventions for persons with substance-use disorders. *American Journal of Occupational Therapy, 58,* 570–586.

U.S. Census Bureau. (2003, March). *Census 2000 Briefs.* Washington, DC: U.S. Department of Commerce.

U.S. Office of Personnel Management. (n.d.). "Patients' Bill of Rights and the Federal Employees Health Benefits Program." Available at: http://www.cancer.org/docroot/MIT/content/MIT_3_2_Patients_Bill_Of_Rights.asp (accessed October 19, 2009).

Vash, C. L. (1981). *The Psychology of Disability.* New York: Springer.

Wright, B. A. (1959). *Psychology and Rehabilitation.* Washington, DC: American Psychological Association.

Wright, B. A. (1983). *Physical Disability: A Psychological Approach.* New York: Harper & Row.

Evidence-Based Practice in Mental Health

Hector W.H. Tsang, Andrew M.H. Siu, and Chris Lloyd

> *The deepest sin against the human mind is to believe things without evidence.*
>
> —Thomas H. Huxley, 1893

Introduction

Imagine that you are a new occupational therapist working in a community-based mental health setting. Your primary job responsibilities involve working with individual consumers to successfully manage their independent living. Some consumers are living in their own apartments for the first time. You are also in charge of running groups at the mental health center with a focus on developing supportive relationships among friends and family. You have several ideas in mind as to how you might approach these responsibilities based on your occupational therapy education and fieldwork experiences. However, you are wondering how to make a decision about which approach to take. Along with considering the wants and needs of your clients, the philosophy of the setting, and the available resources, an essential component of this decision should include an appraisal of the available research evidence. By selecting intervention approaches with sound research evidence, you will increase the likelihood that the services you provide will result in positive outcomes.

This chapter reviews the historical roots and development of evidence-based practice for people with psychiatric disabilities. It reviews research involving or conducted by occupational therapists and discusses how the field of occupational therapy can strengthen its base of evidence-based practice. The chapter also reviews established evidence-based practices in the field of mental health so that occupational therapists can become familiar with these practices and consider adopting them in their practice settings.

Development of Evidence-Based Practice

"What exactly is **evidence-based practice?**" There is a tremendous amount of literature that attempts to address this simple question. Evidence-based practice is defined as the conscientious and judicious use of current best evidence in making decisions about the care of our clients (Sackett, Rosenberg, Gray, Haynes, & Richardson, 1996). A simpler and yet specific definition was suggested by Torrey, Rapp, van Tosh, McNabb, and Ralph (2005): "Evidence-based practice (EBP) refers to health services that are bolstered by a strong scientific base, preferably accumulated through a plethora of randomized clinical trials performed by different research teams in multiple research sites and even in different places of the world. (p. 94)" Going further, a meta-analysis would be even better, providing a statistical summary of multiple studies that allows for an objective judgment about the magnitude of the effect of a particular intervention.

Although evidence-based practice has had a sweeping effect on the current provision of health and rehabilitation services, it does not have a long history. The history, according to Tanenbaum (2006), can be dated back to the astonishing findings of small area variation studies conducted by a physician, John Wennberg, in the 1980s. Dr. Wennberg found that physicians treated the same medical condition differently, depending not on scientific evidence, but largely on their demographic similarity. His conclusion was that physicians were uncertain about how to treat their patients and that the treatment decision was heavily dependent on factors such as tradition and norm. Wennberg and others therefore suggested the shift of paradigm that is now known as **evidence-based medicine**.

In the 2000 Eleanor Clarke Slagle Lecture, Holm (2000) remarked that the *Occupational Therapy Code of Ethics* has affirmed the importance of and need for evidence based-practice. In fact, Principle 4.E of the *Code of Ethics* states, "Critically examine evidence so they may perform their duties on the basis of current information" (American Occupational Therapy Association, 2005, p. 641). Occupational therapists need to be able to identify and select the best evidence for their practice.

A hierarchy has been suggested with which to classify evidence based on its strengths at five levels, as shown in Table 5-1 (Moore, McQuary, & Gary, 1995).

To further elucidate the levels of evidence hierarchy, we use anger management interventions for youth as an example. Level I evidence is the strongest because it is not based on a single study, but recognizes the importance of replication of positive findings before a practice can truly be evidence based. Blake and Hamrin (2007) conducted a systematic review of psychosocial approaches to anger management for youth ages 5 to 17 years. This means that they reviewed all studies that met their criteria. They found that the techniques

Table 5-1 ● **Classification of Strength of Evidence**

Level	Description
I	Level I evidence is the strongest. It is generated through meta-analytic or systematic reviews on multiple, well-designed, randomized controlled trials.
II	Level II evidence is originated from sound randomized controlled trials with appropriate sample size.
III	In Level III evidence, there is a control group, but the design lacks randomization to group assignment.
IV	Level IV evidence is generated from desirable nonexperimental studies such as single-subject and pre- and post-test studies.
V	Level V qualitative research and evidence is generated from the opinions of respected authorities.

used most commonly were based on cognitive behavioral or skills training approaches, and included affective education, relaxation training, cognitive restructuring, problem-solving skills, social skills, and conflict resolution. The greatest number of studies, which also produced the strongest effect sizes (i.e., the largest improvements) were interventions using cognitive behavioral approaches.

Level II evidence is randomized controlled trials (RCTs) of adequate sample size. At this point, the levels of evidence hierarchy are focused on a single study. An RCT provides the strongest evidence for a single efficacy study because the design itself controls for many other factors that might account for a difference among groups. In other words, with an RCT, the results are more likely to be attributable to the intervention itself and not some other factor (e.g., natural recovery or placebo effect).

Greene et al (2004) studied the efficacy of the collaborative problem-solving (CPS) approach for managing disruptive behavior in children with oppositional defiant disorder. In this RCT, children were assigned to either the CPS intervention or parent management training. Both interventions resulted in improvements, but the CPS intervention resulted in greater effects, particularly related to limit setting and communication.

In level III evidence, a control or comparison group exists to be compared with the intervention group; however, participants are not randomly assigned to the group. Lack of randomization causes some threats to the validity of the study because the method of group assignment could influence the results. For example, if initial volunteers are placed in the intervention group, then these individuals may be more motivated and eager to change. In some studies, one setting will receive an intervention, and the other setting the control. In this case, the setting itself could affect the outcomes.

Botvin, Griffin, and Nichols (2006) studied a life skills training program administered to sixth-grade students in a school setting. Children were not randomly assigned to the intervention or control groups; instead, schools were randomly selected for participation. Results indicated that the intervention participants had less verbal and physical aggression, fighting, and delinquency. Although these results are promising, the potential effects of setting (e.g., the selected intervention schools may have been more motivated to work toward change) should be taken into account.

Level IV evidence is based on nonexperimental studies. This could be a study that uses a pre-post or a single-subject design. With these designs, there is a lack of information regarding what would occur for individuals who do not receive the intervention. Gaines and Barry (2008) used a single-subject design to examine relaxation training for aggressive adolescents. Only two of the six participants improved on targeted behaviors.

Level V evidence is drawn from expert opinion or qualitative studies. An example is a program description that does not include a research component. Qualitative studies typically do not provide efficacy evidence, but can provide information that is useful to the topic that may not be obtained through quantitative methods. For example, in a qualitative study of adolescent perceptions of violence, adolescents in focus groups discussed what constitutes a fight and a weapon (Marsh, McGee, Nada-Raja, & Currey, 2007). The participants believed that adults did not always distinguish between play fights and real fights, and that there was a difference between fighting that occurred at school and outside school. This information could be useful in both assessing and providing interventions for youth violence.

The previous example illustrates that an analysis of the literature can be useful in identifying evidence-based practices. Overall, there is research support for anger management programs. An occupational therapist interested in using anger management approaches would need to do further investigation into the research to identify the most effective programs, the best match for a particular setting, and the logistics of implementing a particular approach (e.g., training, time).

Issues of Evidence-Based Practice— Beyond Efficacy Studies

The concept of levels of evidence is applicable to efficacy studies in which the research question is focused on whether a particular intervention works. In this case, RCTs, by design, are best at answering causal questions and provide the strongest type of evidence. However, occupational therapists and other practitioners are frequently interested in other types of research questions that can be better answered with other designs.

Tickle-Degnen and Bedell (2003) argue that there is more to choosing and communicating about an intervention than simply understanding its probability of causing a beneficial outcome in a population. They suggest that practitioners are concerned not only with causality and probability, but also with patterns and possibility when it comes to selecting an intervention. This information is drawn from quantitative descriptive, observational, and correlational designs, as well as qualitative narrative analysis, ethnographic, and phenomenological designs. Tickle-Degnen and Bedell recommend that evidence-based practice must build models that help practitioners to evaluate and synthesize research evidence from multiple studies, and then integrate it with information coming from other sources in a manner that is useful and practical for clinical decision-making.

For example, questions about patterns are typically answered using correlation or regression designs (which would fall under level IV evidence). An example of a predictive question that an occupational therapist might pose is the relationship between self-efficacy and engagement in health-promoting behaviors.

Qualitative research ranks low on the levels of evidence hierarchy, but answers essential questions that cannot be answered using quantitative methods (Fossey, Harvey, McDermott, & Davidson, 2002). In qualitative research, the methods focus on subjective methods of gathering information, such as interviews, focus groups, and observations. Qualitative research provides information about the lived experience and meaning. It values the individual and recognizes the limitations associated with aggregating data. For example, in a weight loss study, the average weight loss data for the group does not tell the story of the individual who gained weight or the person who lost much more than the average. In addition, qualitative research is useful in theory development. A qualitative study can help uncover concepts and theories that would have been left unknown using other methods.

The important point is that the research design should match the research question. Although the levels of evidence hierarchy establishes the importance of RCTs for efficacy questions, other designs are better for answering questions of meaning, relationship, and description.

There are other limitations to the notion of evidence-based practice. Current research tends to focus on medically oriented outcomes, such as hospitalization and symptoms, and is typically less focused on occupational performance and constructs associated with recovery (e.g., empowerment, quality of life) (Solomon & Stanhope, 2004). Another limitation is the fact that evidence cannot keep up with practice. The research process is a lengthy one, as is the time period from when a study is completed until when it is published. Therefore, there will always be a lag between when a practice is initiated and when there is a significant body of research that either supports or rejects a particular practice.

In addition, many of the controls applied to increase the internal validity of a study may actually limit the generalizability of the findings. In other words, the strict protocol of the study (e.g., criteria for participants, training of leaders, or intensity of the intervention) may be so different from traditional practice that the usefulness of the study may be limited for real life occupational therapy (Fig. 5-1).

All that being said, there is a body of research that already exists (and is growing substantially as this chapter is written) and can inform practitioners about best practices in mental health occupational therapy. Consequently, it is important that occupational therapists become informed about evidence-based practice and use that information to make decisions about their own practice. Competent and ethical occupational therapy practice requires that evidence is considered in the clinical reasoning process.

Evidence-Based Practice and Occupational Therapy

Cusick and McClusky (2000) urged occupational therapists to incorporate evidence-based practice into their professional role in order to remain competent, relevant, and clinically

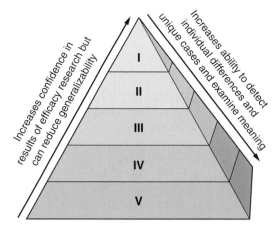

FIGURE 5-1. The levels of evidence construct is most relevant for evaluating studies examining the efficacy of interventions for groups of people. Randomized controlled trials and systematic reviews are generally not useful for studying individual experiences and unique or rare situations.

effective. Has this happened in mental health? The literature shows that occupational therapists are active in conducting mental health research. Currently, there is a lack of RCTs and meta-analyses reported by occupational therapists, and typical studies are small and often report pilot work. However, the increase in doctorally prepared occupational therapists and emphasis on evidence-based practice is leading to higher-quality research.

Tse, Lloyd, Penman, King, and Bassett (2004) discussed the importance of evidence-based practice and the necessity for occupational therapists to become evidence-based practitioners. They highlighted the importance of therapists and academic researchers being involved in clinical research. Table 5-2 provides a sampling of research since 2000 that has been conducted by mental health occupational therapists and/or provides evidence about occupational therapy interventions in mental health.

Clearly, mental health occupational therapists have been active in conducting research and contributing to the evidence base for practice in mental health. Occupational therapy can continue to improve its status as a health profession for people with psychiatric disabilities by contributing to the research literature. An area of improvement that is needed is more occupational therapy research using RCTs in efficacy studies. However, occupational therapy research is providing valuable information related to functional assessment, understanding occupational performance, intervention planning and development, and efficacy of interventions.

Recommendations for Increasing Occupational Therapy Research

Although growing, the research evidence originating from occupational therapy in mental health is limited. The following recommendations are made for increasing the contribution of occupational therapy to mental health research:

1. Occupational therapists need to be more involved in intervention research that supports the core occupational therapy approaches of therapeutic activities and activity groups.

Table 5-2 ● **Occupational Therapy Research**

Author/Date	Design	Purpose	Results
Employment			
O'Brien (2007)	Quantitative and qualitative	Prevocational program to build motivation for people with mental illness	Participants increased confidence and motivation in vocational activity
Basset, Lloyd, & Bassett (2001)	Qualitative	Identify issues of young people with psychosis seeking employment	Themes identified included loss, low self-confidence, treatment issues, need for support, and difficulty achieving goals
Lee, Tan, Ma, Tsai, & Liu (2006)	Randomized crossover	Efficacy of a work-related stress management program for people with schizophrenia	Large but short-term positive effect on work-related stress
Eklund, Hansson, & Alquist (2004)	Descriptive	Compared work with other forms of occupation for people with mental illness	People who worked were more satisfied with daily activities and rated as better functioning
Kin Wong et al (2008)	RCT	Efficacy of supported employment in Hong Kong	Supported employment was more effective than conventional vocational rehabilitation for finding and sustaining employment
Henry, Lucca, Banks, Simon, & Page (2004)	Controlled trial	Effect of individual placement and support (IPS) vocational models on mental health hospitalizations	Individuals receiving IPS who also regularly used mental health services were more likely to have fewer hospitalizations and emergency visits
Tsang & Pearson (2001)	RCT	Efficacy of a work-related social skills training (WSST) program for people with schizophrenia	Participants in the WSST program had better social competence and greater employment outcomes
Leisure			
Lloyd, King, McCarthy, & Scanlan (2007)	Correlational	Examine relationship between motivation to engage in leisure and perception of recovery	Significant positive relationship exists between leisure motivation and recovery
Lloyd, Wong, & Petchkovsky (2007)	Qualitative	Ways that an arts program contributes to recovery	Themes included art as a medium of expression and self-discovery and the promotion of spirituality, empowerment, and self-validation
Health Promotion			
Lloyd, Williams, & King (2004)	Pre- and post-test	Efficacy of a sexual health education program for people with mental illness	Participants increased knowledge related to sexual health
Almomani, Brown, & Williams (2006)	RCT	Efficacy of a toothbrushing intervention for people with mental illness	Intervention resulted in significant improvements in oral hygiene
Brown, Goetz, Van Sciver, & Sullivan (2006)	Controlled trial	Efficacy of a weight loss intervention for people with mental illness	Individuals in the intervention had significant weight loss, whereas individuals in control group gained weight
Family/Caregivers			
Reid, Lloyd, & de Groot (2005)	Qualitative	Experiences of parents of adults with mental illness	Themes included usefulness of psychoeducation, barriers to accessing information and support, unmet caregiver needs, and negotiating the best care for family members
Bassett, Lloyd, & King (2003)	Pre- and post-test	Efficacy of nutrition program for mothers with mental illness	Mothers reported a change in how the family shopped and cooked, and less money spent on foods identified in the "eat least" group
Gitlin, Hauck, Dennis, & Winter (2005)	RCT	Efficacy of REACH intervention—six-session OT for caregivers of people with Alzheimer's disease to modify environment to support daily functioning	Caregivers in the intervention group reported improved skills, fewer behavioral occurrences, less need for help, and a long-term improvement in affect
Self-Awareness			
Chan, Lee, & Chan (2007)	RCT	Efficacy of the TRIP program to increase self-awareness and treatment adherence for people with schizophrenia	Intervention participants had increased awareness of health and lower readmission rate than controls
Assertive Community Treatment (ACT)			
Krupa et al (2005)	Qualitative	Experience of individuals receiving ACT	Participants were primarily positive about ACT, but also reported tension regarding conflicts with providers, stigma, and lack of autonomy
Krupa, McLean, Eastabrook, Bonham, & Baksh (2003)	Descriptive	Time use of individuals receiving ACT	Individuals in ACT have imbalance of time use, primarily spending time in leisure activities and sleeping

Table 5-2 ● Occupational Therapy Research—cont'd

Author/Date	Design	Purpose	Results
Life Skills Training			
Helfrich & Fogg (2007)	Pre- and post-test	Efficacy of life skills training for individuals who are homeless	Improvements in self-care and community safety
Duncombe (2004)	RCT	Compared life skills training (cooking) in home and clinic for people with schizophrenia	Training in home was no more effective than training in clinic
Brown, Rempfer, & Hamera (2002)	Controlled trial	Efficacy of grocery shopping intervention for people with schizophrenia	Individuals in the intervention improved in grocery shopping accuracy and efficiency when compared to controls
Substance Abuse			
White (2007)	Pre- and post-test	Efficacy of time management and organization program for people with mental illness and substance abuse disorders	Participants increased knowledge of time management, improved punctuality, and ability to maintain appointment books
Stoffel & Moyers (2004)	Systematic review	Reviewed effective interventions for substance abuse	Identified four effective intervention approaches: brief interventions, cognitive behavioral therapy, motivational interviewing, and 12-step programs
Peer Interaction in Children			
Tanta, Deitz, White, & Billingsley (2005)	Single subject	Children with delayed play skills were matched with one child with higher skills and one child with lower skills	Children with delayed play skills had more initiation and response when playing with higher-skilled peers
Marr, Mika, Miraglia, Roerig, & Sinnott (2007)	Single subject	Efficacy of sensory stories for improving target behaviors in children with autism	Sensory stories were effective in making changes in individualized target behaviors
Measurement Development			
Bassett, King, & Lloyd (2006)	Psychometric	Development of a parent–child assessment for parents with mental illness	Evidence for reliability, discriminative and concurrent validity
Katz, Golstand, Bar-Ilan, & Parush (2007)	Psychometric	Usefulness of the dynamic cognitive assessment for children	Useful for discriminating children with ADHD, good interrater reliability and internal consistency
Quake-Rapp, Miller, Ananthan, & Chiu (2008)	Psychometric	Usefulness of direct observation as a means of observing problem behaviors in youth unwilling to answer questions	Proved to be an effective method for identifying behaviors that interfere with group participation
Pan, Chung, & Hsin-Hwei (2003)	Psychometric	Reliability and validity of the Canadian Occupational Performance Measure for clients with psychiatric disorders	Identified occupational performance issues not collected with others measures (particularly leisure), good test–retest reliability
Hamera & Brown (2000)	Psychometric	Reliability and validity of the Test of Grocery Shopping Skills	Good test–retest reliability and alternate forms, support for construct validity
Brown, Cromwell, Filion, Dunn, & Tollefson (2002)	Psychometric	Discriminant validity of the Adult Sensory Profile for individuals with schizophrenia and bipolar disorder	Identified distinct patterns of sensory processing for people with schizophrenia and bipolar disorder when compared with individuals without mental illness

RCT, randomized controlled trial; ACT, assertive community treatment; ADHD, attention deficit-hyperactivity disorder.

2. Psychosocial occupational therapists around the world have developed a wide spectrum of mental health services. Occupational therapy programs and intervention protocols that are standardized with protocols or manuals are ready candidates for evaluation research. Occupational therapists can incorporate pre- and post-measures to collect outcome data that would support the efficacy of the intervention. The unique and innovative programs could be brought to the attention of other professions via presentations at international conferences and publications in peer-reviewed multidisciplinary journals.

3. Lloyd, King, and Bassett (2005) reported the benefits of forming a collaborative partnership between occupational therapy clinicians and a university in order to conduct research within a clinical setting. They demonstrated that collaboration has the potential to overcome the low level of involvement in clinical research, and outlined the steps involved in developing a collaboration between clinicians and academic researchers. Clinicians can provide access to the population and the therapists to carry out the intervention, whereas academic researchers can design the study, select outcome measures, and analyze the data.

4. Although there are a number of barriers to the implementation of experimental research, quasi-experimental and observational studies also provide important quantitative evidence, and qualitative research helps us answer "how" and "why" occupational therapy interventions works. When experimental studies are not feasible, occupational therapists can consider these other research designs.

5. Case studies in journals and textbooks should attempt to knit theory, practice, and research together by demonstrating how evidence-based practice can be implemented within a coherent theoretical framework. Occupational therapists can submit case studies to journals that describe the approach to an individual case in terms of a theoretical perspective, the clinical reasoning and intervention provided, and the outcomes collected.

Evidence-based practice includes the assimilation of empirical evidence for clinical decisions. Therapists and the profession should conduct regular reviews to synthesize empirical evidence from occupational therapy and other fields to support clinical reasoning. An excellent example of this is the review conducted by Stoffel and Moyers (2004) on substance abuse treatments. In this review, they identified four evidence-based practices: brief intervention, cognitive behavioral therapy, motivational interviewing, and 12-step programs. Especially helpful in this review was an analysis of the role of occupational therapy within each of these practices.

Evidence-Based Psychosocial Interventions

Medication is a standard treatment for people with psychiatric disabilities. However, medications rarely provide total relief from psychiatric symptoms and disability. For example, 30% to 50% of individuals with psychotic illnesses do not respond adequately to traditional antipsychotic medication (Lacro, Dunn, Dolder, Leckband, & Jeste, 2002). Furthermore, many individuals taking psychiatric medications (just like those who take medications for other illnesses) do not adhere to the recommended medication regimes (Cramer & Rosenback, 1998; Lacro et al, 2002). The main reasons for poor compliance are the side effects associated with the medication (Corrigan, Liberman, & Engel, 1990) and internalized stigma (Tsang, Fung, & Corrigan, 2006). Due to the limitations of medication, the current emphasis on recovery, and the availability of psychiatric rehabilitation, psychosocial intervention is widely accepted for people with psychiatric disabilities.

Psychosocial interventions refer to those modalities that are designed to help clients attain independence, recovery, employment, meaningful interpersonal relationships, and an improved quality of life (Antai-Otong, 2003). These interventions address person factors, such as symptom management, social skills, and cognitive performance; target occupational performances, such as work, parenting, and independent living; and consider environmental barriers that interfere with successful and satisfying community living. For the past three decades, a wide range of psychosocial interventions have been developed and used with individuals with mental illness.

However, not all psychosocial interventions are evidence based. A common way of identifying evidence-based practices is through established **guidelines for best practice**. In the past few years, a number of indicators for determining whether a particular psychosocial intervention may be regarded as evidence based have been put forward.

The Substance Abuse and Mental Health Service Administration (SAMHSA) has released the three foundation guidelines to promote the implementation of evidence-based practice (Center for Substance Abuse Prevention, 2007):

- Guideline 1 suggests that the intervention should be formed with solid and validated theoretical framework.
- Guideline 2 asserts that its effectiveness should be supported by empirical evidence.
- Guideline 3 suggests that the intervention should be judged by a group of informed experts to be effective in terms of its underlying theoretical framework, research outcomes, and practice experience.

The SAMHSA has established a Web-based searchable database, the National Registry of Evidence-based Programs and Practices, to provide information about evidence-based programs for individuals with co-occurring disorders.

The next section describes several intervention approaches that fall within occupational therapy's domain and that meet SAMHSA's criteria for evidence-based practices. A brief description of the practice, along with supporting evidence, is presented. Each intervention is discussed in fuller detail in other chapters of the book, and the corresponding chapter is identified in each section. The strong research support for these practices increases the likelihood of positive outcomes for consumers. Therefore, it is important that occupational therapists are familiar with these practices and, when applicable, consider adopting them.

Assertive Community Treatment

One goal of mental health services and occupational therapy is to enable community functioning among people with psychiatric disabilities (Bustillo, Lauriello, Horan, & Keith, 2001). The coordination and thoughtful allocation of mental health services are promoted by proper case management systems (Antai-Ontog, 2003). **Assertive community treatment (ACT)** is a community-oriented intensive case management approach (Dhillon & Dollieslager, 2000; Lehman et al, 2003; Mueser, Bond, Drake, & Resnick, 1998; Philips et al, 2001) that originated from the Mendota Mental Health Institute in Madison in the late 1970s (Stein & Santos, 1998; Stein & Test, 1980). ACT was developed in response to the deinstitutionalization movement of psychiatric rehabilitation (Marshall & Lockwood, 1998).

The key objectives of ACT are to reduce the hospital admission rate among individuals with the most serious disabilities, develop skills for community living, and promote proper utilization of mental health services (Antai-Otong, 2003; Marshall & Lockwood, 1998). The unique principles of ACT enable it to be distinguished from traditional case management models.

One such principle is the importance of multidisciplinary teamwork (Bustillo et al, 2001; Lehman et al, 2003; Mueser et al, 1998; Philips et al, 2001). The team draws on the expertise of its members to provide targeted services to clients. The composition of each team may vary, but a team typically consists of 10 to 12 mental health professionals, such as an occupational therapist, nurse, psychiatrist, social worker, psychologist, employment specialist, substance abuse specialist, peer specialist, or other related experts. All team members are able to serve as case managers (Stein & Santos, 1998). The caseload of staff members is generally low, with approximately 1 staff member for every 10 clients. This ensures that staff members have the capacity to cope with the intensive needs of service recipients (Philips et al, 2001). The service provided is tailor-made to meet the individualized needs of participants and is delivered on a 24-hour basis with no arbitrary time limit (Mueser et al, 1998; Philips et al, 2001). In other words, clients receive services for as long as needed, whenever they are needed.

Numerous studies of ACT provide empirical support regarding its effectiveness in reducing the number of hospital admissions, reducing the total length of stay in psychiatric hospitals, and improving housing stability among people with psychotic disorders (Bustillo et al, 2001; Holloway & Carson, 1998; Marshall & Lockwood, 1998; Mueser et al, 1998; Nelson, Aubry, & Lafrance, 2007; Salyers & Tsemberis, 2007). Studies indicate a range of 10% to 85% reduction in hospitalization rates among participants who had engaged in ACT programs (Latimer, 1999). The best outcomes were demonstrated for individuals with serious symptoms and functional impairments (Philips et al, 2001).

In addition to reducing hospitalization rates, the effectiveness of ACT on improving other clinical outcomes is less conclusive (Clark & Samnaliev, 2005), and consensus regarding its effectiveness in promoting competitive employment, social functioning, and symptom management has not been demonstrated (Marshall & Lockwood, 1998; Mueser et al, 1998). (Assertive community treatment is described in more detail in Chapter 40.)

Social Skills Training

Social skills are the basis of effective social performance (Bellack & Mueser, 1993), enabling individuals to succeed in daily life (Kopelowicz, Liberman, & Zarate, 2006). **Social skills training (SST)** is founded on social learning theory (Bandura, 1969) and the principles of operant conditioning (Liberman, 1972). The objectives of SST are to promote the social functioning of individuals and enhance specific skills, such as identifying and mending problems in social relationships, daily life, work, and leisure (Lauriello, Bustillo, & Keith, 1999). SST works to optimize the social functioning of people with psychiatric disabilities (Antai-Otong, 2003) and improve their repertoire of skills for community functioning (Corrigan, Schade, & Liberman, 1993).

The key elements of SST include warm-up activities, behaviorally based instructions, demonstration, corrective feedback, and homework assignments (Lehman et al, 2003; Wallace et al, 1980). Behavioral techniques such as prompting, shaping, reinforcing, and modeling are used to help individuals acquire and maintain social skills (Glynn, 2003).

There are three models of SST (Bellack & Mueser, 1993; Bustillo et al, 2001): basic, social problem-solving, and cognitive remediation. The basic model focuses on corrective learning, in which complex social repertoires have been broken down into simple steps for practice. The social problem-solving model works on the hypothesis that social skill deficits are caused by impairments in information processing. The skill deficit of corresponding daily life domains is thus targeted and corrected in terms of reception, processing,

and transmission. The cognitive remediation model assumes that learning and generalization of social skills can be achieved by reducing the level of cognitive deficits, and thus fundamental cognitive skills are trained with this model.

The effectiveness of SST for skill acquisition of people with psychiatric disabilities has been widely demonstrated (Benton & Schroeder, 1990; Bustillo et al, 2001; Corrigan, 1991; Heinssen, Liberman, & Kopelowicz, 2000; Lehman et al, 2003); that is, the SST evidence finds that people with psychiatric disabilities are able to acquire and maintain new skills. A meta-analysis conducted by Mojtabai, Nicholson, and Carpenter (1998) found a moderate effect size for SST. In view of the importance of social skills for success in employment, Tsang and Pearson (1996; 2001) developed a structural work-related social skills training (WSST) program for people with psychotic disorders. In addition to practicing basic social skills and basic social survival skills, participants were required to learn the social skills necessary for handling general and specific work-related situations (Tsang & Pearson, 1996).

Tsang and Pearson (2001) conducted an RCT to test the effectiveness of the WSST program. The findings suggest that the participants had better social competence than those who received standard treatment without WSST. The competitive employment rate of participants of the WSST program reached 46.7%. The WSST program is currently being used as a part of psychiatric rehabilitation programs in Hong Kong, Australia, and Germany (Tsang & Cheung, 2005).

Skills training programs should be tailored to the required skills of a particular job (Becker et al, 1998). In view of the importance of job-specific social skills for success in the workplace, Cheung, Tsang, and Tsui (2006) continued earlier efforts along this line of study and developed a Job-specific Social Skills Training (JSST) program with a specific focus on the job of a salesperson because this job was found to be common for people with psychotic disorders (Tsang, Ng, & Chiu, 2002). Tsang and colleagues (2005) conducted a study of 106 salespeople to identify the required specific social skills and used these findings to develop the JSST program.

A systematic literature review (Tsang & Cheung, 2005) on the effectiveness of SST for people with psychiatric disabilities suggests a consistently strong and positive impact on social skills acquisition among participants. However, inconsistent findings include symptom and relapse reduction, rehospitalization prevention, and short-term maintenance of skills. In addition, the long-term outcomes of SST and generalization of behaviors remain unclear. (Also see Chapter 47.)

Supported Employment

Work is an important domain of life that promotes positive mental health and community participation. Unfortunately, people with psychotic disorders have poor outcomes related to employment, with only 15% to 30% able to obtain competitive employment (Equal Opportunities Commission, 1997; Massel et al, 1990). Among those individuals with psychiatric disabilities who are employed, problems with job adjustment and tenure are prevalent (Marwaha & Johnson, 2004; Tsang, Ng, & Chiu, 2002).

Vocational rehabilitation aims to help people with psychotic disorders succeed in employment (Mueser & Bond, 2000) and facilitate their recovery process (Antai-Otong, 2003). Traditionally, the "train and then place" approach was the essential philosophy of vocational rehabilitation. Under this approach, people were expected to develop the necessary skills *before* seeking employment through sheltered workshops or prevocational training programs. However, this approach was associated with unfavorable outcomes (Clark & Samnaliev, 2005; Glynn, 2003); Tsang, Chan, and Bond (2004) found that only 2.5% of individuals who received this type of intervention went on to obtain competitive employment.

In view of the limitations of the traditional vocational rehabilitation model, the Individual Placement and Support (IPS) model was developed to enhance treatment outcomes (Becker & Drake, 1993; Drake & Becker, 1996). IPS is a specific model of **supported employment** (SE) that aims to help people with psychiatric disabilities obtain competitive employment (Drake & Becker, 1996). According to Bond et al (2001; Bond, 2004), instead of a "train and then place" approach, the IPS model adopts a "place and then train" approach. The seven key principles of this SE model are

- Seeking competitive employment
- Conducting a rapid job search
- Integrating mental health services
- Emphasizing individuals' preferences
- Implementing continuous and comprehensive assessment
- Providing time-unlimited support
- Conducting benefits counseling

Empirical evidence indicates that the IPS model improves short-term employment of people with psychotic disorders (Drake et al, 1999; Lehman et al, 2002). Bond (2004) reviewed nine RCTs investigating the effectiveness of IPS and found, on average, that 56% of the participants were able to achieve competitive employment. Overall, supported employment is superior to traditional methods of vocational rehabilitation (e.g., prevocational training, sheltered workshops), as demonstrated by multiple RCTs (Bond, Drake, & Becker, 2008; Cook et al, 2008). Still, nearly one-half of the individuals in SE do not obtain sustained employment, and the effectiveness of the IPS model in enhancing job satisfaction, job tenure, and other nonvocational outcomes has not been demonstrated (Drake et al, 1999).

Vocational researchers have integrated skills training elements into the IPS model in order to augment its treatment outcomes (Cook et al, 2005; McGurk, Mueser, & Pascaris, 2005; Tsang, Chan, Wong, & Liberman (2009). For example, individuals tended to work more hours and earn more after they had engaged in the IPS program with cognitive training (McGurk et al, 2005). Tsang, Fung, Leung, Li, & Cheung (2010) incorporated SST in their program and found that the competitive employment rate was raised to 78.8%, and the participants tended to work longer (23.84 weeks) within the 15 months of service. Current research is exploring various versions of enhanced SE. (Also see Chapter 50.)

Cognitive Behavioral Therapy

Cognitive behavioral therapy (CBT) is a problem-oriented approach that works to improve emotional states by changing distorted thinking (Reinecke, Ryan, & Dubois, 1998). CBT was first developed to treat depression and anxiety (Beck, 1976; Haddock et al, 1998). It has subsequently been used as a supplement to pharmacotherapy for people with schizophrenia and bipolar disorders (Gould, Mueser, Bolton, Mays, & Goff, 2001) to diminish hallucinations and delusions, and reduce the level of social disability and risk of relapse (Bustillo et al, 2001; Glynn, 2003).

CBT assumes the symptom or problem is manifested and maintained by the mediation of cognitive and environmental processes, and modification of those processes can be accomplished by teaching individuals more adaptive cognitive and behavioral skills (Haddock et al, 1998). Kingdon, Turkington, and Beck (1993) described the two-pronged approach of CBT; testing the validity of potential irrational beliefs by logical reasoning is the first step, followed by management strategies such as problem-solving and distraction if the targeted concern could not be eliminated via logical reasoning. Modalities such as psychoeducation, cognitive reconstruction, and skills trainings are integrated in CBT programs (Kingdon & Turkington, 1994).

CBT was initially developed for individuals with depression, with the focus on changing negative thinking. There is strong support for the efficacy of CBT for reducing depressive symptoms and that it is equally effective when compared to medication (Feldman, 2007). There is also evidence that CBT may be more beneficial than medication for preventing relapse (Butler, Chapman, Forman, & Beck, 2006). There is similar evidence for the efficacy of cognitive therapy in reducing symptoms associated with anxiety disorders (Hendriks, Oude Voshaar, Keijsers, Hoogdwin, & van Balkom, 2008). CBT can be run in individual or group formats; the efficacy of groups suggest this may be an efficient method for offering this intervention (Oie & Dingle, 2008).

Several clinical trials demonstrate the effectiveness of CBT in reducing psychotic symptoms such as delusions and auditory hallucinations (Clark & Samnaliev, 2005; Gould et al, 2001; Lehman et al, 2003). A meta-analysis conducted by Tarrier and Wykes (2004) investigated 19 controlled trials of CBT that suggested that CBT programs offered moderate effect size reduction for positive symptoms (mean effect size = 0.37; SD = 0.39). Another meta-analysis included 14 controlled studies of CBT, which showed a mean effect size of 0.37 in eliminating positive symptoms (Zimmermann, Favrod, Trieu, & Pomini, 2005). However, its beneficial effects on prevention of relapse, reduction in hospital admissions, and promotion of social functioning for people with schizophrenia have been limited (Dickerson & Lehman, 2006). (Also see Chapter 19.)

Family Intervention

Research suggests that outcomes for people with psychiatric disabilities are associated with the family environment (Glynn, 2003). **Expressed emotion** is a concept used to indicate the level of family stress due to factors such as criticism, overinvolvement, and hostility (Antai-Otong, 2003). At the same time, it is important to understand that taking care of mentally ill family members does increase the stress and burden of the family (Tsang, Tam, Chan, & Cheung, 2003). The purpose of **family intervention** (**FI**) is to reduce relapse rates, enhance the social adjustment of people with psychotic disorders, and reduce caregiver stress and burden (Glynn, 2003).

Effective FIs consist of psychoeducation, problem-solving, crisis management, and crisis intervention (Dixon & Lehman, 1995; Lehman et al, 2003). FI can be conducted with an individual family or in multiple family groups. Research suggests that the multiple family groups method is more effective due to the additional benefit of increased social support among members (Glynn, 2003; McFarlane, Dushay, Stastny, Deakins, & Link, 1996).

The effectiveness of FIs in the reduction of symptoms, improvement in functioning, reduction of family burdens, and promotion of family subjective well-being are well verified by RCTs (Dixon, Adams, & Lucksted, 2000; Klingberg, Buckremer, Holle, Monking, & Hormung, 1999; Lehman et al, 2003; Pharoah, Mari, Rathbone, & Wong, 2006). Mueser and Glynn (1998) reported that the relapse rate of individuals who had participated in FI was 24%, compared to 64% for those without FI. Moreover, FIs can also enhance medication compliance and improve the coping skills and knowledge of family members to take care of their mentally ill relatives (McFarlane et al, 1996; Pharoah et al, 2006). Empirical evidence supports the durable effect of long-term FI (Mueser & Glynn, 1998; Tarrier, Barrowclough, Porceddu, & Fitzpatrick, 1994), and the beneficial effects of FIs are sustained after the termination of services (Tarrier et al, 1994). (Also see Chapter 29.)

Motivational Interviewing

Motivational interviewing was originally developed to address problems associated with making behavioral changes for people with substance abuse disorders (Miller et al, 2006); however, it has since been applied to many other interventions for behavioral change (e.g., smoking cessation, weight loss, exercise). One of the primary differences between motivational interviewing and earlier approaches to substance abuse treatment is the style of interaction. Traditionally, substance abuse treatment used a confrontational approach and was based on the belief that people could not change until they "hit rock bottom" or were ready to change. In contrast, motivational interviewing uses a collaborative approach that seeks to engage the client to want to change.

The four general principles of motivational interviewing (Miller & Rollnick, 2002) include

1. Express empathy (let the client know that the change process is difficult)
2. Develop discrepancy (identify differences between current behavior and personal goals and values)
3. Roll with resistance (avoid confrontation)
4. Support self-efficacy (indicate that you believe the client is capable of making a change)

There is strong evidence supporting the efficacy of motivational interviewing for substance abuse treatment. A meta-analysis found that motivational interviewing was more effective than no treatment, and was particularly useful for establishing a therapeutic relationship and increasing engagement in treatment (Burke, Arkowitz, & Mencholam, 2004). Another review found that motivational interviewing was equal to or more effective than other substance abuse interventions (Babor & DelBoca, 2003). Motivational interviewing is typically offered in a very brief format (sometimes as brief as one session). Empirical evidence provides additional support for these short-term approaches (Vasilaki, Hosier, & Cox, 2006). (Also see Chapter 23.)

Dialectical Behavior Therapy

Dialectical behavior therapy is based on both cognitive and behavioral approaches (Linehan, 1993). It combines both individual psychotherapy and group skills training. Dialectical behavior therapy was originally developed for individuals with borderline personality disorder and focuses on emotion regulation, impulse control, and reducing self-harm and suicidal behaviors. In dialectical behavior therapy, the primary dialectic (the coming together of opposites) is acceptance and change. In terms of acceptance, there is a validation of the person's experience of emotions and interventions that involve tolerating unpleasant emotions. However, the change component of dialectical behavior therapy emphasizes the development of healthy coping skills. The group skills training component of dialectical behavior therapy is best suited for occupational therapy. The four modules include mindfulness, interpersonal effectiveness, emotion modulation, and distress tolerance.

Multiple RCTs demonstrate the efficacy of dialectical behavior therapy (Linehan, Armstrong, Suarez, Allmon, & Heard, 1993; Linehan et al, 1999, 2006). These studies indicate that individuals with borderline personality disorder that participate in dialectical behavior therapy are less likely to drop out of therapy, and have reduced hospitalizations, fewer parasuicidal and suicidal behaviors, and better social adjustment. (Also see Chapter 24.)

Summary

Occupational therapists are involved in demonstrating evidence for practice; however, occupational therapy as a profession may lag behind some other health-care disciplines in terms of their contributions. Evidence-based practices in mental health include assertive community treatment, social skills training, supported employment, cognitive behavioral therapy, family interventions, motivational interviewing, and dialectical behavior therapy. Unfortunately, none of these interventions is unique to occupational therapy. However, although occupational therapists have developed an array of innovative programs for people with mental illness, these treatments are generally not known outside the occupational therapy community. The previous recommendations serve to guide occupational therapists to cross the bridge and contribute in a more effective way to the development of evidence-based practice in our profession.

Active Learning Strategies

1. Applying Research

Read a research study about a mental health intervention that is of interest to you. Consider one of the interventions discussed in this chapter or another chapter in this book. After reading the study, identify the following information:

- Describe the population, intervention (including how it was implemented, frequency, and leaders/therapists), and outcomes measured.
- Summarize the findings.
- Identify any study limitations.

Reflective Questions

Now that you've gathered this information, what are your impressions of the intervention?

- Would you recommend it for occupational therapy practice? Why or why not?
- What is the risk of making judgments based on a single study? What other information should you gather before making a decision about this intervention?

2. Journal Club

Start a journal club. The purpose of a journal club is to discuss research with a group of individuals with similar interests. With a group of students or fellow practitioners, decide on a regular meeting time and place. You might organize the journal club so that each member is responsible for identifying a research study or so that you might decide which studies to consider as a group. When together, some possible discussion questions could include

- What did you learn from this study?
- What are the study's strengths and weaknesses?
- How is the population, intervention, setting, etc., similar to your knowledge or experiences of real life practice?
- What are the clinical implications of this study? What does it teach you about your own practice?

Resources

- **American Occupational Therapy Association (AOTA):** AOTA's resources for evidence-based practice include evidence briefs on particular conditions and focused literature reviews called Critically Appraised Topics on a particular research question. http://www.aota.org/Educate/Research.aspx
- **National Guideline Clearinghouse:** Website for evidence-based practice guidelines that can be searched by condition or intervention. www.guidelines.gov
- **OTSeeker:** Provides summaries and evaluations of systematic reviews and randomized controlled trials that are relevant to occupational therapy. www.otseeker.com
- **Substance Abuse and Mental Health Services Administration (SAMHSA):** Provides a guide to evidence-based practice and searchable links for information on evidence-based practices in mental health. http://www.samhsa.gov/ebpwebguide/index.asp

References

Almomani, F., Brown, C., & Williams, K. B. (2006). The effect of an oral health promotion program for people with psychiatric disabilities. *Psychiatric Rehabilitation Journal, 29,* 274–281.

American Occupational Therapy Association. (2005). Occupational Therapy Code of Ethics. *American Journal of Occupational Therapy, 59,* 639–642.

Antai-Otong, D. (2003). Psychosocial rehabilitation. *Nursing Clinics of North America, 38*(1), 151–160.

Babor, T. F., & DelBoca, F. K. (2003). *Treatment Matching in Alcoholism.* New York: Cambridge University Press.

Bandura, A. (1969). *Principles of Behavior Modification.* New York: Holt, Rinehart and Winston.

Bassett, H., King, R., & Lloyd, C. (2006). The development of an observation tool for use with parents with psychiatric disability and their preschool children. *Psychiatric Rehabilitation Journal, 30,* 31–37.

Bassett, H., Lloyd, C., & King, R. (2003). Food Cent: Educating mothers with a mental illness about nutrition. *British Journal of Occupational Therapy, 66,* 369–375.

Bassett, J., Lloyd, C., & Bassett, H. (2001). Work issues for young people with psychosis: Barriers to employment. *British Journal of Occupational Therapy, 64,* 66–72.

Beck, A. T. (1976). *Cognitive Therapy and the Emotional Disorders.* New York: International Universities Press.

Becker, D. R., & Drake, R. E. (1993). *A Working Life: The Individual Placement and Support (IPS) Program.* Concord: New Hampshire-Dartmouth Psychiatric Research Center.

Becker, D. R., Drake, R. E., Bond, G. R., Xie, H., Dain, B. J., & Harrison, K. (1998). Job terminations among persons with severe mental illness participating in supported employment. *Community Mental Health Journal, 34,* 71–82.

Bellack, A. S., & Mueser, K. T. (1993). Psychosocial treatment for schizophrenia. *Schizophrenia Bulletin, 19*(2), 317–336.

Benton, M. K., & Schroeder, H. E. (1990). Social skills training with schizophrenics: A meta-analytical evaluation. *Journal of Consulting and Clinical Psychology, 58,* 741–747.

Blake, C. S., & Hamrin, V. (2007). Current approaches to the assessment and management of anger and aggression in youth: A review. *Journal of Child and Adolescent Psychiatric Nursing, 20,* 209–221.

Bond, G. R. (2004). Supported employment: Evidence for an evidence-based practice. *Psychiatric Rehabilitation Journal, 27*(4), 345–359.

Bond, G. R., Becker, D. R., Drake, R. E., Rapp, C. A., Meisler, N., Lehman, A. F., & Bell, M. D. (2001). Implementing supported employment as an evidence-based practice. *Psychiatric Services, 52*(3), 313–322.

Bond, G. R., Drake, R. E., & Becker, D. R. (2008). An update on randomized controlled trials of evidence-based supported employment. *Psychiatric Rehabilitation Journal, 31,* 280–290.

Botvin, G. J., Griffin, K. W., & Nichols, T. R. (2006). Preventing youth violence through a universal school-based prevention approach. *Prevention Science, 7,* 403–408.

Brown, C., Cromwell, R. L., Filion, D., Dunn, W., & Tollefson, N. (2002). Sensory processing in schizophrenia: Missing and avoiding information. *Schizophrenia Research, 55,* 187–195.

Brown, C., Goetz, J., Van Sciver, A., & Sullivan, D. (2006). A psychiatric rehabilitation approach to weight loss. *Psychiatric Rehabilitation Journal, 29,* 267–273.

Brown, C., Rempfer, M., & Hamera, E. (2002). Teaching grocery shopping skills to people with schizophrenia. *Occupational Therapy Journal of Research, 22*(suppl 1), 90S–91S.

Burke, B. L., Arkowitz, H., & Mencholam, M. (2004). The emerging evidence for motivational interviewing: A meta-analytic and qualitative review. *Journal of Cognitive Psychotherapy, 18,* 309–322.

Bustillo, J. R., Lauriello, J., Horan, W. P., & Keith, S. J. (2001). The psychosocial treatment of schizophrenia: An update. *The American Journal of Psychiatry, 158*(2), 163–175.

Butler, A. C., Chapman, J. E., Forman, E. M., & Beck, A. T. (2006). The empirical status of cognitive-behavioral therapy: A review of meta-analyses. *Clinical Psychology Review, 26,* 17–31.

Center for Substance Abuse Prevention. (2007). *Identifying and Selecting Evidence-Based Interventions: Guidance Document for the Strategic Prevention Framework State Incentive Grant Program.* Washington, DC: Substance Abuse and Mental Health Services Administration.

Chan, S. H., Lee, S. W., & Chan, I. W. (2007). TRIP: A psychoeducational programme in Hong Kong for people with schizophrenia. *Occupational Therapy International, 14,* 86–98.

Cheung, L. C. C., Tsang, H. W. H., & Tsui, C. U. (2006). Job-specific Social Skills Training (JSST) for people with severe mental illness in Hong Kong. *Journal of Rehabilitation, 72*(4), 14–23.

Clark, R. E., & Samnaliev, M. (2005). Psychosocial treatment in the 21st century. *International Journal of Law and Psychiatry, 28,* 532–544.

Cook, J. A., Blyler, C. R., Leff, H. S., McFarlane, W. R., Goldberg, R. W., Gold, P. B., Mueser, K. T., Shafer, M. S., Onken, S. J., Donegan, K., Carey, M. A., Kaufmann, C., & Razzano, L. A. (2008). The employment intervention demonstration program: Major findings and policy implications. *Psychiatric Rehabilitation Journal, 31,* 291–295.

Cook, J. A., Lehman, A. F., Drake, R., McFarlane, W. R., Gold, P. B., Leff, H. S., Blyler, C., Toprac, M. C., Razzano, L. A., Burke-Miller, J. K., Blankertz, L., Shafer, M., Pickett-Schenk, S. A., & Grey, D. D. (2005). Integration of psychiatric and vocational services: A multisite randomized, controlled trial of supported employment. *American Journal of Psychiatry, 162*(10), 1948–1956.

Corrigan, P. W. (1991). Social skills training in adult psychiatric populations: A meta-analysis. *Journal of Behavior Therapy and Experimental Psychiatry, 22,* 203–210.

Corrigan, P. W., Liberman, R. P., & Engel, J. D. (1990). From noncompliance to collaboration in the treatment of schizophrenia. *Hospital and Community Psychiatry, 41*(11), 1203–1211.

Corrigan, P. W., Schade, M. L., & Liberman, R. P. (1993). Social skills training. In R. P. Liberman (Ed.), *Handbook of Psychiatric Rehabilitation* (pp. 95–126). Boston: Allyn & Bacon.

Cramer, J. A., & Rosenbeck, R. (1998). Compliance with medication regimens for psychiatric and medical disorders. *Psychiatric Services, 49,* 196–210.

Cusick, A., & McClusky, A. (2000). Becoming an evidence-based practitioner through professional development. *Australian Occupational Therapy Journal, 47,* 159–170.

Dhillon, A. S., & Dollieslager, L. P. (2000). Overcoming barriers to individualized psychosocial rehabilitation in an acute treatment unit of a state hospital. *Psychiatric Services, 51*(3), 313–317.

Dickerson, F. B., & Lehman, A. F. (2006). Evidence-based psychotherapy for schizophrenia. *Journal of Nervous and Mental Disease, 194*(1), 3–9.

Dixon, L., Adams, C., & Lucksted, A. (2000). Update on family psychoeducation for schizophrenia. *Schizophrenia Bulletin, 26*(1), 5–20.

Dixon, L. B., & Lehman, A. F. (1995). Family interventions for schizophrenia. *Schizophrenia Bulletin, 21*(4), 631–643.

Drake, R. E., & Becker, D. R. (1996). The individual placement and support model of supported employment. *Psychiatric Services, 47*(5), 473–475.

Drake, R. E., McHugo, G. J., Bebout, R. R., Becker, D. R., Harris, M., Bond, G. R., & Quimby, E. (1999). A randomized clinical trial of supported employment for inner-city patients with severe mental disorders. *Archives of General Psychiatry, 56,* 627–633.

Duncombe, L. W. (2004). Comparing learning of cooking in home and clinic for people with schizophrenia. *American Journal of Occupational Therapy, 58,* 272–278.

Eklund, M., Hansson, L., & Alquist, C. (2004). The importance of work as compared to other forms of daily occupations for well being and functioning among persons with long term mental illness. *Community Mental Health Journal, 40,* 465–477.

Equal Opportunities Commission. (1997). *Full Report: A Baseline Survey on Employment Situation of Persons With a Disability in Hong Kong.* Hong Kong: Author.

Feldman, G. (2007). Cognitive and behavioral therapies for depression: Overview, new directions and practice recommendations for dissemination. *Psychiatric Clinics of North America, 30,* 39–50.

Fossey, E., Harvey, C., McDermott, F., & Davidson, L. (2002). Understanding and evaluating qualitative research. *Australian and New Zealand Journal of Psychiatry, 36,* 717–732.

Gaines, T., & Barry, L. M. (2008). The effect of a self-monitored relaxation breathing exercise on male adolescent aggressive behavior. *Adolescence, 43,* 291–302.

Gitlin, L. N., Hauck, W. W., Dennis, M. P., & Winter, L. (2005). Maintenance of effects of the home environmental skill-building program for family caregivers and individuals with Alzheimer's disease and related disorders. *Journal of Gerontology, Biological Science and Medical Science, 60,* 368–374.

Glynn, S. M. (2003). Psychiatric rehabilitation in schizophrenia: Advances and challenges. *Clinical Neuroscience Research, 3*(1–2), 23–33.

Gould, R. A., Mueser, K. T., Bolton, E., Mays, V., & Goff, D. (2001). Cognitive therapy for psychosis in schizophrenia: An effect size analysis. *Schizophrenia Research, 48*(2–3), 335–342.

Haddock, G., Tarrier, N., Spaulding, W., Yusupoff, L, Kinney, C., & McCarthy, E. (1998). Individual cognitive-behavior therapy in the treatment of hallucinations and delusions: A review. *Clinical Psychology Review, 18*(7), 821–838.

Hamera, E., & Brown, C. (2000). Developing context-based performance measures: Grocery shopping skills in individuals with schizophrenia. *American Journal of Occupational Therapy, 54,* 20–25.

Heinssen, R. K., Liberman, R. P., & Kopelowicz, A. (2000). Psychosocial skills training for schizophrenia: Lessons from the laboratory. *Schizophrenia Bulletin, 26,* 21–46.

Helfrich, C. A., & Fogg, L. F. (2007). Outcomes of a life skills intervention for homeless adults with mental illness. *Journal of Primary Prevention, 28,* 313–326.

Hendriks, G. J., Oude Voshaar, V. C., Keijsers, G. P., Hoogdwin, C. A., & van Balkom, A. J. (2008). Cognitive behavioural therapy for late life anxiety disorders: A systematic review and meta-analysis. *Acta Psychiatrica Scandinavica, 117,* 403–411.

Henry, A. D., Lucca, A. M., Banks, S., Simon, L., & Page, S. (2004). Inpatient hospitalization and emergency service visits among participants in an Individual Placement and Support model program. *Mental Health Services Research, 6,* 222–237.

Holloway, F., & Carson, J. (1998). Intensive case management for the severely mentally ill: Controlled trial. *British Journal of Psychiatry, 172,* 19–22.

Holm, M. B. (2000). Our mandate for the new millennium: Evidence-based practice, 2000 Eleanor Clarke Slagle lecture. *American Journal of Occupational Therapy, 54,* 575–585.

Huxley, T. H. (1893). *Evolution and Ethics.* New York: Harper.

Katz, N., Golstand, S., Bar-Ilan, R. T., & Parush, S. (2007). The Dynamic Occupational Therapy Cognitive Assessment for Children (DOTCA-CH): A new instrument for assessing learning potential. *American Journal of Occupational Therapy, 61,* 41–52.

Kin Wong, K., Chiu, R., Tang, B., Mah, D., Liu, J., & Chiu, S. N. (2008). A randomized controlled trial of a supported employment program for persons with long term mental illness. *Psychiatric Services, 59,* 84–90.

Kingdon, D. G., & Turkington, D. (1994). *Cognitive-Behavioral Therapy of Schizophrenia.* New York: Guilford Press.

Klingberg, S., Buckremer, G., Holle, R., Monking, H. S., & Hormung, W. P. (1999). Differential therapy effects of psychoeducational psychotherapy for schizophrenic patients: Results of a two-year follow-up. *European Archives of Psychiatry and Clinical Neuroscience, 249*(2), 66–72.

Kopelowicz, A., Liberman, R. P., & Zarate, R. (2006). Recent advance in social skills training for schizophrenia. *Schizophrenia Bulletin, 32,* S12–S23.

Krupa, T., Eastabrook, S., Hern, L., Lee, D., North, R., Percy, K., Von Briesen, B., & Wing, G. (2005). How do people who receive assertive community treatment experience this service. *Psychiatric Rehabilitation Journal, 29,* 18–24.

Krupa, T., McLean, H., Eastabrook, S., Bonham, A., & Baksh, L. (2003). Daily time use as a measure of community adjustment for persons served by assertive community treatment teams. *American Journal of Occupational Therapy, 57,* 558–565.

Lacro, J. P., Dunn, L. B., Dolder, C. R., Leckband, S. G., & Jeste, D. V. (2002). Prevalence of and risk factors for medication nonadherence in patients with schizophrenia: A comprehensive review of recent literature. *Journal of Clinical Psychiatry, 63*(10), 892–909.

Latimer, E. (1999). Economic impact of assertive community treatment: A review of the literature. *Canadian Journal of Psychiatry, 45*(5), 443–454.

Lauriello, J., Bustillo, J., & Keith, S. J. (1999). A critical review of research on psychosocial treatment of schizophrenia. *Biological Psychiatry, 46*(10), 1409–1417.

Lee, H. L., Tan, H. K., Ma, H. I., Tsai, C. Y., & Liu, Y. K. (2006). Effectiveness of a work-related stress management program in patients with chronic schizophrenia. *American Journal of Occupational Therapy, 60,* 435–441.

Lehman, A., Goldberg, R., Dixon, L., McNary, S., Postrado, L., Hackman, A., & McDonnell, K. (2002). Improving employment outcomes for persons with severe mental illnesses. *Archives of General Psychiatry, 59,* 165–172.

Lehman, A. F., Buchanan, R. W., Dickerson, F. B., Dixon, L. B., Goldberg, R., Green-Paden, & Kreyenbuhl, J. (2003). Evidence-based treatment for schizophrenia. *Nursing Clinics of North America, 26,* 939–954.

Lehman, A. F., Kreyenbuhl, J., Buchanan, R. W., Dickerson, F. B., Dixon, L. B., Goldberg, R., Green-Paden, C. D., Tenhula, W. N., Boerescu, D., Tech, C., Sandson, N., & Steinwachs, D. M. (2004). The schizophrenia Patient Outcomes Research Team (PORT): Updated treatment recommendations 2003. *Schizophrenia Bulletin, 30*(2), 193–217.

Liberman, R. P. (1972). *A Guide to Behavioral Analysis and Therapy.* New York: Pergamon.

Linehan, M. M. (1993). *Cognitive Behavioral Treatment for Borderline Personality Disorder.* New York: Guilford Press.

Linehan, M. M., Armstrong, H. E., Suarez, A., Allmon, D., & Heard, H. L. (1993). Cognitive behavioral treatment of chronically parasuicidal borderline patients. *Archives of General Psychiatry, 50,* 157–158.

Linehan, M. M., Comtois, K. A., Murray, A. M., Brown, M. Z., Gallop, R. J., Heard, H. L., Korslund, K. E., Tutek, D. A., Reynolds, S. K., & Lindenboim, N. (2006). Two-year randomized controlled trial and follow-up of dialectical behavior therapy vs therapy by experts for suicidal behaviors and borderline personality disorder. *Archives of General Psychiatry, 63*(7), 757–766.

Linehan, M. M., Schmidt, H., Dimeff, L. A., Kanter, J. W., Craft, J. C., Comtois, K. A., & Recknor, K. L. (1999). Dialectical behavior therapy for patients with borderline personality disorder and drug-dependence. *American Journal on Addiction, 8,* 279–292.

Lloyd, C., King, R., & Bassett, H. (2005). Occupational therapy and clinical research in mental health rehabilitation. *British Journal of Occupational Therapy, 68,* 172–176.

Lloyd, C., King, R., McCarthy, M., & Scanlan, M. (2007). The association between leisure motivation and recovery: A pilot study. *Australian Occupational Therapy Journal, 54,* 33–41.

Lloyd, C., Williams, P. L., & King, R. (2004). A sexual healing programme implemented in a psychiatric inpatient unit. *New Zealand Journal of Occupational Therapy, 52,* 26–32.

Lloyd, C., Wong, S. R., & Petchkovsky, L. (2007). Art and recovery in mental health: A qualitative investigation. *British Journal of Occupational Therapy, 70,* 207–214.

Marr, D., Mika, H., Miraglia, J., Roerig, M., & Sinnott, R. (2007). The effect of sensory stories on targeted behaviors in preschool children with autism. *Physical and Occupational Therapy in Pediatrics, 27,* 63–79.

Marsh, L., McGee, R., Nada-Raja, S., & Currey, N. (2007). Adolescents' perceptions of violence and its prevention. *Australian and New Zealand Journal of Public Health, 31,* 224–229.

Marshall, M., & Lockwood, A. (1998). Assertive community treatment for people with severe mental disorders. *Cochrane Review, 4.*

Marwaha, S., & Johnson, S. (2004). Schizophrenia and employment—A review. *Social Psychiatry and Psychiatric Epidemiology, 39,* 337–349.

Massel, H. K., Liberman, R. P., Mintz, J., Jacobs, H. E., Rush, T. V., Giannini, C. A., & Zarate, R. (1990). Evaluating the capacity to work of the mentally ill. *Psychiatry, 53,* 31–43.

McFarlane, W. R., Dushay, R. A., Stastny, P., Deakins, S. M., & Link, B. (1996). A comparison of two levels of family-aided assertive community treatment. *Psychiatric Services, 47,* 744–750.

McGurk, S. R., Mueser, K. T., & Pascaris, A. (2005). Cognitive training and supported employment for persons with severe mental illness: One-year results from a randomized controlled trial. *Schizophrenia Bulletin, 31*(4), 898–909.

Miller, W. R., Baca, C., Compton, W. M., Ernst, D., Manuel, J. K., Pringle, B., Schermer, C. R., Weiss, R. D., Willenbring, M. L., & Zweben, A. (2006). Addressing substance abuse in health care settings. *Alcohol Clinical and Experimental Research, 30,* 292–302.

Miller, W. R., & Rollnick, S. (2002). *Motivational Interviewing: Preparing People for Change* (2nd ed.). New York: Guilford Press.

Mojtabai, R., Nicholson, R. A., & Carpenter, B. N. (1998). Role of psychosocial treatments in management of schizophrenia: A meta-analytic review of controlled outcome studies. *Schizophrenia Bulletin, 24*(4), 569–587.

Moore, A., McQuary, H., & Gary, J. A. M. (1995). Evidence-based everything. *Bandolier, 1*(12), 1.

Mueser, K. T., & Bond, G. R. (2000). Psychosocial treatment approaches for schizophrenia. *Current Opinion in Psychiatry, 13,* 27–35.

Mueser, K. T., Bond, G. R., Drake, R. E., & Resnick, S. G. (1998). Models of community care for severe mental illness: A review of research on case management. *Schizophrenia Bulletin, 24*(1), 37–74.

Mueser, K. T., & Glynn, S. M. (1998). Family intervention for schizophrenia. In K. S. Doboson & K. D. Craig (Eds.), *Developing and Promoting Empirically Supported Interventions* (pp. 157–186). Newbury Park, CA: Sage.

Nelson, G., Aubry, T., & Lafrance, A. (2007). A review of the literature on the effectiveness of housing and support, assertive community treatment, and intensive case management interventions for persons with mental illness who have been homeless. *American Journal of Orthopsychiatry, 77,* 350–361.

O'Brien, L. (2007). Pre-vocational group intervention program for building motivation in mature aged unemployed people with a disability. *Journal of Rehabilitation, 73,* 22–28.

Oie, T. P., & Dingle, G. (2008). The effectiveness of group cognitive behavioural therapy for unipolar depressive disorders. *Journal of Affective Disorders, 107,* 5–21.

Pan, A. W., Chung, L., & Hsin-Hwei, G. (2003). Reliability and validity of the Canadian Occupational Performance Measure for clients with psychiatric disorders in Taiwan. *Occupational Therapy International, 20,* 269–277.

Pharoah, F., Mari, J., Rathbone, J., & Wong, W. (2006). Family intervention for schizophrenia. *Cochrane Database of Systematic Reviews, 4.*

Philips, S. D., Burns, B. J., Edgar, E. R., Mueser, K. T., Linkins, K. W., Rosenheck, R. A., Drake, R. E., & McDonell Herr, E. C. (2001). Moving assertive community treatment into standard practice. *Psychiatric Services, 52*(6), 771–779.

Quake-Rapp, C., Miller, B., Ananthan, G., & Chiu, E. C. (2008). Direct observation as a means of assessing frequency of maladaptive behavior in youths with severe emotional and behavioral disorders. *American Journal of Occupational Therapy, 62,* 206–211.

Reid, J., Lloyd, C., & de Groot, L. (2005). The psychoeducation needs of parents who have an adult son or daughter with a mental illness. *Australian e-Journal for the Advancement of Mental Health, 4*(2).

Reinecke, M., Ryan, N., & Dubois, D. (1998). Cognitive-behavioral therapy of depression and depressive symptoms during adolescence: A review and meta-analysis. *Journal of the American Academy of Child and Adolescent Psychiatry, 37*(1), 26–34.

Sackett, D. L., Rosenberg, W. M., Gray, J. A., Haynes, R. B., & Richardson, W. S. (1996). Evidence-based medicine: What it is and what it isn't. *British Medical Journal, 312,* 71–72.

Salyers, M. P., & Tsemberis, S. (2007). ACT and recovery: Integrating evidence-based practice and recovery orientation on assertive community treatment teams. *Community Mental Health Journal, 43,* 619–641.

Scottish Intercollegiate Guidelines Network (SIGN). (1999). *An Introduction to Sign Methodology for the Development of Evidence-Based Clinical Guidelines.* Edinburgh, Scotland: Author.

Solomon, P., & Stanhope, V. (2004). Recovery: Expanding the vision of evidence based practice. *Brief Treatment and Crisis Intervention, 4,* 311–321.

Stein, L. I., & Santos, A. B. (1998). *Assertive Community Treatment of Persons With Severe Mental Illness.* New York: Norton.

Stein, L. I., & Test, M. A. (1980). Alternative to mental-hospital treatment. 1. Conceptual model, treatment program, and clinical-evaluation. *Archives of General Psychiatry, 37*(4), 392–397.

Stoffel, V. A., & Moyers, P. A. (2004). An evidence based and occupational perspective of interventions for persons with substance-use disorders. *American Journal of Occupational Therapy, 58,* 570–586.

Tanenbaum, S. J. (2006). The role of "evidence" in recovery from mental illness. *Health Care Analysis, 14,* 195–201.

Tanta, K. J., Deitz, J. C., White, O., & Billingsley, F. (2005). The effects of peer-play level on initiations and responses of preschool children with delayed play skills. *American Journal of Occupational Therapy, 59,* 437–445.

Tarrier, N., Barrowclough, C., Porceddu, K., & Fitzpatrick, E. (1994). The Salford Family Intervention Project: Relapse rates of schizophrenia at 5 and 8 years. *British Journal of Psychiatry, 165,* 829–832.

Tarrier, N., & Wykes, T. (2004). Is there evidence that cognitive behaviour therapy is an effective treatment for schizophrenia? A cautious or cautionary tale? *Behaviour Research and Therapy, 42*(12), 1377–1401.

Tickle-Degnen, L. (1998). Communicating with patients about treatment outcomes: The use of meta-analytic evidence in collaborative treatment planning. *American Journal of Occupational Therapy, 52,* 526–530.

Tickle-Degnen, L., & Bedell, G. (2003). Evidence-based practice forum—Heterarchy and hierarchy: A critical appraisal of "levels of evidence" as a tool for clinical decision-making. *American Journal of Occupational Therapy, 57,* 234–237.

Torrey, W. C., Rapp, C. A., van Tosh, L., McNabb, C. R. A., & Ralph, R. O. (2005). Recovery principles and evidence-based practice: Essential ingredient of service improvement. *Community Mental Health Journal, 41*(1), 91–100.

Tsang, H. W. H. (2001). Applying social skills training in the context of vocational rehabilitation for people with schizophrenia. *Journal of Nervous and Mental Disease, 189,* 90–98.

Tsang, H. W. H., Chan, A., Wong, A., & Liberman, R. P. (2009). Vocational outcomes of an integrated supported employment program for individuals with persistent and serious mental illness. *Journal of Behavioral and Therapeutic Experimental Psychiatry, 40,* 292–305.

Tsang, H. W. H., Chan, F., & Bond, G. R. (2004). Cultural considerations for adapting psychiatric rehabilitation models in Hong Kong. *American Journal of Psychiatric Rehabilitation, 7,* 35–51.

Tsang, H. W. H., & Cheung, L. C. C. (2005). Social skills training for people with schizophrenia: Theory, practice and evidence. In J. E. Pletson (Ed.), *Progress in Schizophrenia Research* (pp. 181–207). New York: Nova Science.

Tsang, H. W. H., Fung, K. M. T., & Corrigan, P. W. (2006). The Psychosocial Treatment Compliance Scale (PTCS) for people with psychotic disorders. *Australian and New Zealand Journal of Psychiatry, 40,* 561–569.

Tsang, H. W., Fung, K. M., Leung, A. Y., Li, S. M., & Cheung, W. M. (2010). Three year follow-up study of integrated supported employment for individuals with serious mental illness. *Australian and New Zealand Journal of Psychiatry, 44,* 49–58.

Tsang, H. W. H., Ng, B. F. L., & Chiu, F. P. F. (2002). Job profiles of people with severe mental illness: Implications for rehabilitation. *International Journal of Rehabilitation Research, 25,* 189–196.

Tsang, H. W. H., & Pearson, V. (1996). A conceptual framework for work-related social skills in psychiatric rehabilitation. *Journal of Rehabilitation, 62,* 61–67.

Tsang, H. W. H., & Pearson, V. (2001). Work-related social skills training for people with schizophrenia in Hong Kong. *Schizophrenia Bulletin, 27,* 139–148.

Tsang, H. W. H., Tam, P., Chan, F., & Cheung, W. M. (2003). Sources of burdens on families of individuals with mental illness. *International Journal of Rehabilitation Research, 26*(2), 123–130.

Tse, S., Lloyd, C., Penman, M., King, R., & Bassett, H. (2004). Evidence-based practice and rehabilitation: Occupational therapy in Australia and New Zealand experiences. *International Journal of Rehabilitation Research, 27,* 269–274.

Vasilaki, E. I., Hosier, S. G., & Cox, W. M. (2006). The effectiveness of motivational interviewing as a brief intervention for excessive drinking: A meta-analytic review. *Alcohol and Alcoholism, 41,* 328–335.

Wallace, C. J., Nelson, C. J., Liberman, R. P., Aitchison, L. D., Elder, J. P., & Ferris, U. (1980). A review and critique of social skills training with schizophrenic patients. *Schizophrenia Bulletin, 6,* 42–63.

White, S. (2007). Let's get organized: An intervention program for persons with co-occuring disorders. *Psychiatric Services, 58,* 713.

Zimmermann, G., Favrod, J., Trieu, V. H., & Pomini, V. (2005). The effect of cognitive behavioral treatment on the positive symptoms of schizophrenia spectrum disorders: A meta-analysis. *Schizophrenia Research, 77*(1), 1–9.

The Person

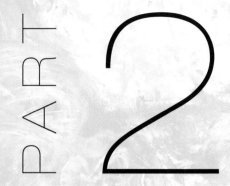

Part 2 is divided into diagnosis and client factors sections. It is important that occupational therapists have a thorough understanding of the conditions of the individuals with whom they work. For this reason, major psychiatric diagnoses are presented with a focus on symptoms, etiology, impact on occupational performance, and, when appropriate, medications used to treat the condition. Although occupational therapy practice is not driven by symptomatology, practitioners can better understand the experience of the individual with a mental illness if the occupational therapist is aware of symptoms the person may be experiencing. In addition, a working knowledge of psychiatric diagnoses is useful when participating on a multidisciplinary treatment team.

Because occupational therapy assessment and intervention are not based on diagnosis, these chapters only provide minimal information on the topics. However, assessment and intervention are covered in other chapters, with equal attention given to assessment and intervention targeting client factors, environments, and occupations.

The client factors section addresses skills and abilities that are important for occupational performance. In addition to the information on assessment and intervention, these chapters provide detailed content about the skills addressed, theories related to those skills, and specific information on particular diagnoses that are associated with impairments in those skill areas.

CHAPTER

6

Introduction to the Person

Catana Brown

> "The goal of the recovery process is not to become normal. The goal is to embrace our human vocation of becoming more deeply, more fully human. The goal is not normalization. The goal is to become the unique, awesome, never to be repeated human being that we are called to be.
> —Pat Deegan (1996)—a person who has recovered from mental illness

Introduction

The **Person-Environment-Occupation (PEO)** model provides the organizing framework for this book; that is, the chapters are categorized and focused on one aspect of the model, with the understanding that the three components are inextricably interlinked (Law et al, 1996). Section 1 addresses content that is most strongly associated with the person. In the PEO model, the person is viewed holistically with spiritual, social, and cultural experiences that shape the individual's unique identity. In addition, the person has abilities, known as occupational performance components, that include affective, cognitive, and physical skills. This part of the text includes chapters on psychiatric diagnoses, and client factors. This introductory chapter provides information on rethinking the person with a psychiatric disability from a recovery perspective, acknowledging the importance of the person's expertise and narrative, and an orientation to the subsequent chapters in this section.

Recovery-Oriented Practice: Rethinking the Person

The emphasis in mental health practice is often placed on what is "wrong" with a person. Symptoms and impairments are assessed and then identified as limitations. The professional as expert then prescribes what is best for the person, whether it be medications or a rehabilitation program; if the person does not follow the prescribed plan, he or she is labeled noncompliant. However, the **recovery movement** (see Chapter 1) is creating a paradigm shift in mental health practice (Davidson, Flanagan, Roe, & Styron, 2006; Deegan & Drake, 2006).

People with psychiatric disabilities are speaking out, and their message is both shocking and compelling (Davidson, 2006; Dunn, Wewiorski, & Rogers, 2008; Nelson, Clarke, Febbraro, & Hatzipantelis, 2005). What are they saying? The mental health system can be more harmful than helpful. People with serious mental illness can live full, productive lives. All individuals are due the same civil rights. The expertise of the individual living with mental illness should be respected. People with psychiatric disabilities have the same opportunities to access housing and employment of their choice and to make the same mistakes as everyone else in society. Frequently, when people with psychiatric disabilities express feelings of anger, sadness, and disappointment, these feelings are labeled as symptoms. Instead, people with psychiatric disabilities should be expected to experience and express these feelings as part of the natural experience of being human.

Some mental health professionals can be uncomfortable with adopting recovery-oriented principles. Practitioners may believe that their expertise is not valued, may be reluctant to acknowledge dehumanizing practices that have taken place in mental health service delivery, or may simply be unskilled at working within this new paradigm. Furthermore, recovery is typically described as a unique process for each individual (Jacobson, 2001). If each individual experiences recovery differently, practitioners can no longer rely on diagnosis, deficit-based protocols, and/or practices that are applied uniformly to all people within a diagnostic category.

Davidson and colleagues (2006) contend that moving from a deficit model to one that focuses on enhancing participation and real world supports will require a significant transformation of the current mental health system. They state that ". . . the challenge posed by transformation therefore is whether we choose to continue to confine adults with serious mental illnesses to the second- or third-class status of mental patient, or do we view and treat them as full, contributing citizens capable of self-determination and worthy of being included fully in community life" (p. 1145). Central to this transformation is asking people with mental illness what they want and need.

Acknowledging the Person

The recovery paradigm is consistent with **client-centered practice** in occupational therapy (Law, 1998). Many practitioners, including occupational therapists, are beginning to embrace recovery-oriented approaches and, as a result, find that their practice is more effective and rewarding (Gruhl, 2005). Thinking about a person from a recovery-oriented perspective includes

- Hearing the person's unique story
- Respecting the person's expertise of lived experience
- Relating to the person as an equal member of society

Recovery-oriented practices are also consistent with occupational therapy models such as Person-Environment-Occupation (Stewart et al, 2003; also see Chapter 3) and the Ecology of Human Performance (Dunn, Brown, & Youngstrom, 2003), which recognize that the person cannot be understood outside his or her context and valued occupations. In her Eleanor Clark Slagle Lecture, Suzanne Peloquin (2005) discusses the ethos of occupational therapy. She states, "When in spite of constraints, practitioners make their interventions meaningful, lively and even fun, they infuse therapy's purposive aims with its capacity to encourage and inspire. Acting on the belief that occupation fosters dignity, competence and health, we embrace the spirit of the profession. As we enable healing occupations, we reclaim our heart" (p. 623).

When occupational therapists employ client-centered, recovery-oriented, occupation-based practices, they move beyond merely providing a predetermined number of sessions that follow a prescribed protocol to inspire individuals to reclaim their hope and success.

Person First Language

Language is powerful, and this is particularly true with the language used to describe disability (Blaska, 1993). Words such as "crazy," "deranged," and "insane" are laden with strong negative images that contribute to the stigma associated with having a mental illness. In addition, referring to people by their diagnoses, such as "manic depressives," "anorexics," or "schizophrenics" is demeaning and disrespectful. When the diagnosis becomes the label, the person is lost and becomes known as the mental illness. The focus is on the schizophrenia or depression and not on the unique qualities of the individual. Using **person first language** is one step toward valuing the individual and seeing the person first. Therefore, in client-centered practice, it is crucial that occupational therapists avoid labels and only use them when necessary. When it is necessary to refer to a diagnosis, the person should always come first. For example, instead of "the schizophrenic," it is more respectful to refer to a "person with schizophrenia."

Addressing Symptoms and Diagnosis

Some occupational therapists may argue that diagnoses and symptoms are associated with the medical model and therefore irrelevant to occupational therapy practice. Although a medical model approach can overemphasize symptoms at the expense of the person, the symptoms and diagnoses are still important in the provision of recovery-oriented services. Occupational therapists need to recognize and understand the symptoms associated with mental disorders and psychiatric disabilities. However, in a recovery-oriented system, the occupational therapist does not consider the illness and associated symptoms to be a "life sentence of disablement." Instead, the occupational therapist uses the information to better understand the experiences of the individual, including how the diagnosis and symptoms impact his or her occupational performance. For example, what role might severe depression play in a person's desire to engage in self-care activities? Does an individual's anxiety interfere with him or her using public transportation? Could auditory hallucinations make test-taking challenging for a college student?

Occupational therapists are primarily concerned with occupational performance, and psychiatric symptoms can interfere with successful or satisfying engagement in meaningful occupations. Therefore, it is essential to take symptoms into account in the assessment and intervention processes, along with the other person, environment, and occupational factors that combine to determine the individual's performance.

One example of a recovery-oriented intervention that addresses symptoms along with overall health is the Wellness Recovery Action Plan (WRAP). Mary Ellen Copeland (2000) developed this plan when providers of mental health services failed to assist her in creating an individualized self-management program. Frustrated with the mental health system, Copeland assembled a group that included other people with psychiatric disabilities, which identified the ways in which people implemented wellness and recovery strategies into daily life. Consequently, WRAPs have addressed a much neglected need and have experienced widespread adoption among people with psychiatric disabilities (Buckley et al, 2007). There is also a role for occupational therapists in helping individuals create and follow WRAPs. In addition, the occupational therapist's interest in task analysis, habits, and routines can be useful in supporting individuals as they implement their plans.

Identifying Client Factors

Occupational therapists use different taxonomies to describe skills that are inherent to the person. Part II, Section 3 of this text includes chapters on the following client factors:

- Cognition (skills and beliefs)
- Sensation
- Communication
- Coping
- Motivation
- Emotion
- Pain

The Lived Experience

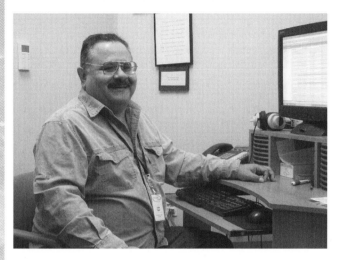

Recovery from mental illness has been a long, hard, exhaustive road to travel. Being African American, however, has made the trek more excruciatingly perilous.

I grew up in a household of "nerves." There was my mother, my grandmother, and two uncles. I guess you could say they were all a bit dysfunctional. Through no fault of their own, each displayed some form of mental illness.

My grandmother's mother died in childbirth, and she was raised by her father, a relatively wealthy African American in late 1800s Arkansas. My grandmother taught school, married, and moved north to Kansas City, Kansas—part of the great migration of the 1930s, when blacks sought better jobs and social conditions. My grandmother and grandfather raised seven children. There was, however, a breakdown. Grandmother went to some "rest home," leaving her family. When she finally came back, I was told that some of her children didn't recognize her.

My mother gave birth to me in 1954. About 3 years later, she had some mental disturbances. She was gone for 9 months. Because grandmother was older and my two uncles knew nothing about raising kids, I stayed with some family friends. I remember from that experience only that I used to destroy the toys they gave me and cry a lot. I guess I was angry. When my mother returned it was, "Oh, happy day." I didn't want her to leave my sight.

It wasn't that bad growing up in a segregated neighborhood in the '60s. Each of us went to segregated schools, churches, and movie theatres. I saw the world in our living room on glorious black-and-white TV. There was the civil rights movement, Viet Nam, assassinations, and "The Ed Sullivan Show." I also observed my grandmother and mother taking different colored pills. One of my uncles would work hard at the Missouri Pacific Railroad, while the other worked construction. Then on the weekend, they'd disappear to get drunk and entertain the ladies.

I had my first breakdown in college, where I experienced anxiety, depression, and suicidal thoughts. It passed when I dropped out of school. I took a blue-collar job, where I experienced racism and panic attacks. I lasted for 3 years, then quit and landed in a mental facility for the first time. I was also prescribed medication that was available at that time of the early '80s. The doctors and therapist also told me to get a job (any kind of job). I didn't bring up the racism factor, fearing they would believe or conclude that I was bringing it on myself. So I got another job, and racism reared its ugly head with racist jokes and comments and the threat of bodily harm. This went on for 6 years 'til finally I had my first psychotic break.

I ended up in another facility, drugged and restrained. I was verbally and mentally abused by staff because of conflicts at home and the fact that I quit my job. I was referred to as a deadbeat and accused of laziness. I dared not bring up the subject of racism, for I knew I would be mocked and declared delusional. On release, I would look for work, but would become ill again and would end up back in the hospital. This went on for about 4 years until I received a new diagnosis and new medications, and for the first time got a social worker.

I started going to a community mental health support center, where I felt extremely comfortable with both staff and clients. There was no hint of discrimination of any kind. I was encouraged, now that I was more stable, to go back to school. I decided I would major in human services, where I felt I could help others like me and provide a guiding hand. Presently, I am a social worker, a certified "peer specialist" giving counsel to other peers snared in the web of mental illness. On my job I see different kinds of people, different races, gender, religion, ages, sexual orientation, etc.

Before, I had my own prejudice, that blacks were treated more harshly under the mental health system. I had preconceived notions that went all the way back to slavery. The cruel psychological aspects of enslavement, lynchings, segregation, and the modern-day subtle racism has haunted me for a long time. However, after all the devastating blows to the psyche, I realize that one can still survive, perhaps become stronger, and continue to carry on. It is a blueprint for us all. I've heard different stories from a lot of different people; everyone has had it rough. The message I try to convey to my peers, however, is that life is a struggle by itself, but having a mental illness adds an extra burden. That burden can be overcome with love, understanding, and forgiveness.

These factors were selected because they are important in mental health practice. Occupational therapists use task analysis to identify the client factors that are necessary for successful and satisfying engagement in particular occupations. Client factor strengths and difficulties are then considered when designing interventions to support occupational performance. Each client factor is briefly introduced here, but their corresponding chapters provide detailed descriptions of the factor, its relationship to occupational performance, and specific assessments and intervention approaches that target the client factor.

Cognitive Skills

In this text, cognitive skills refer to underlying cognitive functions, such as attention, memory, and executive functions (see Chapter 18). Cognitive impairments are central to some diagnoses, such as memory loss in Alzheimer's disease and attentional impairments in attention deficit-hyperactivity disorder. In other diagnoses, cognitive impairments may not form the core symptoms, but difficulties in cognition are associated with the particular psychiatric disability. For example, difficulties across several cognitive domains are common in schizophrenia. In fact, cognitive impairments in schizophrenia are much more limiting in terms of community functioning than are the actual symptoms of the illness (Bowie & Harvey, 2005).

Individuals with autism spectrum disorders typically experience executive dysfunctions, particularly problems with working memory and refocusing attention from one topic to another (Russo et al, 2007). These impairments contribute to the perseveration that is prevalent in autism. In depression, the mood disturbance is the core symptom, but another common symptom is difficulty concentrating (American Psychiatric Association [APA], 2000).

Generally speaking, the primary interventions that target cognitive skills include cognitive rehabilitation, which works to ameliorate a particular cognitive difficulty, and environmental or task modification, which compensates for cognitive impairments.

Cognitive Beliefs

Cognitive beliefs concern how people think about themselves and the world (see Chapter 19). Distorted cognitive beliefs can lead to occupational performance problems. For example, a client's belief that he is incompetent may prevent him from applying for a job. A client who believes that she is undesirable might avoid social interaction. Cognitive behavioral therapy, which originated as an intervention for depression, is based on the underlying theory that distorted thoughts cause depressed mood and other maladaptive behavior; interventions are aimed at altering cognitive distortions (Garrett, Ingram, Rand, & Sawalani, 2007). Cognitive behavioral therapy is now applied to many psychiatric disabilities, both to understand and provide interventions for the particular thought distortion. For example, in eating disorders, the cognitive approach recognizes the overemphasis that body image plays in the evaluation of self-worth (Wilson, 2005). In schizophrenia, delusions (actually defined as a false belief) are challenged by providing evidence to the contrary (Beck & Rector, 2005).

Sensory Processing

In occupational therapy, sensory integration and other related models are well-established specialties within pediatric practice. Chapter 20 describes child-based practice and addresses emerging practices that apply sensory models to adults with psychiatric disabilities. There is evidence suggesting that people with psychiatric disabilities have particular sensory processing preferences. For example, individuals with schizophrenia tend to simultaneously avoid and miss sensory information (Brown, Cromwell, Filion, Dunn, & Tollefson, 2002), and mental health occupational therapists who work with adults are beginning to use sensory interventions in their work to promote occupational performance.

Understanding sensory processing and the sensory features of the environment can be particularly helpful in vocational rehabilitation, where person/environment "fit" is a core intervention approach. Furthermore, occupational therapists are using sensory approaches to reduce the use of restraints and seclusion in psychiatric hospitals (Champagne & Stromberg, 2004). Occupational therapists are teaching nurses and other staff how to prevent and/or reduce agitation and aggression by meeting sensory needs with strategies such as reducing noise levels, creating calming environments, and using weighted jackets.

Communication

Occupational performance is often conducted in the presence of, or in collaboration with, other individuals. Much of the enjoyment that is experienced in certain play and leisure activities comes from the interaction with others. There are few jobs that do not involve some level of interpersonal communication. Instrumental activities of daily living can also require communication, such as when using public transportation, shopping, and attending medical appointments.

People with psychiatric disabilities can experience challenges with communication (see Chapter 21). In fact, a core component of autism is difficulty with communication (APA, 2000), which can profoundly affect play, social development, and success in school. Anxiety disorders can cause people to avoid social situations because they are uncomfortable or fearful of embarrassment or shame, and people with depression often isolate themselves during periods of sorrow. Individuals with schizophrenia frequently have difficulty interpreting social cues (Couture, Penn, & Roberts, 2006) and may be perceived as "odd" by others because of their thought-disordered speech.

Intervention approaches to address communication depend on the particular concern. Social skills training may be useful for teaching communication to individuals with schizophrenia (Penn, Roberts, Combs, & Sterne, 2007), whereas cognitive behavioral approaches may be useful for addressing social anxiety (Hoffman, 2007). For children with autism, modeling and reinforcement are often applied in school settings (Matson, Matson, & Rivet, 2007).

Coping

Everyone uses coping mechanisms to manage difficult life experiences (see Chapter 22). There are two overarching classification systems that are commonly used to categorize coping strategies (Nes & Segerstrom, 2006):

- Emotion focused or problem focused—With emotion-focused strategies, the person seeks to reduce the negative emotional consequences of a negative life event. Problem-focused coping involves changing or confronting the stress.
- Approach or avoidance oriented—Approach-oriented strategies involve dealing with the issue, whereas avoidance strategies involve escaping from the situation by distraction, denial, or some other method of avoidance.

Although certain mechanisms are typically identified as more adaptive than others, it can depend on the circumstance. For example, emotional coping is important when grieving the loss of a loved one, and problem-focused strategies are likely more effective when it comes to dealing with poor performance in school. Recently, acceptance has been acknowledged as a useful strategy for particular situations and conditions (Hayes, Luoma, Bond, Masudo, & Lillis, 2006). More specifically, distress tolerance, a skill taught in dialectical behavior therapy, recognizes that distress and uncomfortable experiences are part of being human (Linehan, 1993). Therefore, it is important that people learn to tolerate distressful feelings.

People with psychiatric disabilities may be more likely to overuse particular coping mechanisms or apply the wrong strategy to a particular situation. Occupational therapists can help individuals learn alternative coping strategies, as well as how and when to apply appropriate strategies to the certain situations. For example, the occupational therapist can teach problem-solving skills to an individual who is easily overwhelmed when facing a problem.

Motivation

One distinction sometimes made between people with physical and psychiatric disabilities is that a person with a psychiatric disability may have the physical and cognitive capacity to engage in a particular occupation, but may still be unsuccessful in initiating, performing, or completing the activity because he or she lacks motivation. Clearly, this belief contributes to the stigma of mental illness. Still, impaired motivation, or avolition, is one client factor that interferes with performance (see Chapter 23). Therapists and other healthcare providers sometimes label an individual as unmotivated and consequently undeserving of therapy, such that the individual is discharged from services after refusing a specified number of sessions. However, if motivation is conceptualized differently—that is, as a client factor that occupational therapists address and one that is frequently disrupted due to psychiatric mental illness—then the concern is approached in a completely different way.

In occupational therapy, the Model of Human Occupation (Kielhofner, 2004) identifies motivation for occupation as part of the volition subsystem. The volitional system drives the person to action. Regardless of whether an individual engages in an occupation is greatly influenced by volition. The individual's belief that he or she has the capacity to be successful, along with the person's interests and values, plays an important role in motivation for occupation. Through understanding the person's interests and values, and by promoting self-efficacy, occupational therapists can enhance motivation.

Emotion Regulation

The experience of emotions is primary to our understanding of who we are as humans. Every moment of every day is colored by our emotional state. In addition, everyone experiences intense emotions from time to time—from the exuberance that follows a major accomplishment to the sorrow associated with the loss of a loved one. Although our emotions are affected by what we experience at the time, people are also constantly working to regulate their emotions (see Chapter 24). For example, before speaking in front of an audience, an individual may need to get his or her anxiety under control in order to successfully deliver the message. On other occasions, crying or expressing anger may not be appropriate to the situation.

Some individuals with psychiatric disabilities find it more challenging to regulate their emotions. Yet, the ability to regulate emotions is essential to health (Cooney, Joormann, Atlas, Eugene, & Gotlib, 2007) and successful occupational engagement. In addition, individuals with psychiatric disabilities are more likely to experience unpleasant emotions for longer periods of time, and the intensity of the emotional experience may be more severe, so that emotional regulation is more difficult (Schore, 2003).

The development of emotion regulation strategies is associated with temperament and early childhood experiences (Feng et al, 2008). However, individuals with ineffective emotion regulation can learn better strategies. Emotion regulation is a core component of dialectical behavior therapy (Linehan, 1993), whereas other approaches, such as social rhythm therapy and relaxation techniques, can also help individuals feel more in control of their emotions.

Pain

There is a reciprocal relationship between pain and psychiatric disabilities. Pain, particularly chronic pain, can contribute to the development or exacerbation of psychiatric disabilities; likewise, psychiatric disabilities can contribute to the development of pain (see Chapter 25). For example, pain is common among people with major depression (Husein, Rush, & Trivedi, 2007). The experience of negative emotions intensifies pain, whereas pleasant emotions diminish it (Zelman, Howland, Nichols, & Cleeland, 1991). In addition, the experience of pain can significantly affect an individual's engagement in daily activities and, in extreme cases, makes engagement in even the most basic activities impossible. One study of older adults who experience pain indicated that the presence of pain was a primary barrier to engagement in health-promoting behaviors aimed at reducing pain (Patil, Johnson, & Lichtenberg, 2008). Clearly, pain and mental health are strongly related, and their relationship is complicated.

It is generally recognized that the treatment of chronic pain benefits from an interdisciplinary approach, and occupational therapists can play an important role in pain management (Stanos & Houle, 2006). The relationship of pain and mental illness necessitates that occupational therapists use holistic practices that consider both physical and psychosocial aspects of the person. For example, an individual who has taken a leave of absence from work due to back pain may be able to return to work through occupational therapy that includes teaching body mechanics and joint protection techniques, along with cognitive behavioral approaches and relaxation.

Recognizing Individual Nature of Client Factors

It is important to emphasize that each person is unique, as is each situation. There is great heterogeneity among people with psychiatric disabilities, even those who have similar diagnoses. Therefore, occupational therapists must resist making assumptions that a person with a particular diagnosis also has an impairment in a particular client factor. Furthermore, an impairment in a client factor does not directly translate to impaired occupational performance. For example, although cognition is associated with community functioning in schizophrenia, only a small percentage of problems in community functioning for people with schizophrenia can be attributed to impairments in cognition (Green, Kern, & Braff, 2000). In children with attention deficit-hyperactivity disorder, it appears that attentional problems are only partially associated with scholastic achievement and that classroom behavior and other unknown factors play a larger role in school success (Rapport, Scanlan, & Denne, 1999).

The Person-Environment-Occupation model (Stewart et al, 2003) implores occupational therapists to consider the occupation itself, along with the environment, in determining barriers and supports for occupational performance. For people with psychiatric disabilities, lack of transportation, poverty, stigma, limited social networks, and the complexity of the occupation are just a few of the factors that can contribute to successful community functioning. Occupational therapists should always use a holistic approach and be careful not to overemphasize person factors when evaluating occupational performance.

Appreciating the Lived Experience

The recovery-oriented model of providing mental health services offers two different ways to understand the person. When describing recovery, several authors identify an objective, or outsider, view, whereas other authors describe recovery from a subjective, or insider, perspective (Brown, Rempfer, & Hamera, 2008; Jacobson, 2001). The outsider perspective of recovery is based on objective assessments of outcomes, such as symptom reduction, hospitalization, and employment. This method is useful for measuring the effectiveness of services. However, if recovery is a unique, nonlinear process, these outcomes fall short of truly understanding the recovery process. Consequently, the insider view becomes essential to appreciating the lived experience of psychiatric disability.

Using Narrative for Assessment

A person's **narrative** can provide the occupational therapist with insights into the uniqueness of that individual. Schell (2003) includes narrative as a component of clinical reasoning, which involves taking the perspective of the client and understanding the meaning of the disability from his or her point of view. Occupational therapists are often interested in how disability disrupts an individual's life story and how individuals re-create stories to once again become full occupational beings. They may or may not be involved in the process of re-creation; however, by listening to life stories, the occupational therapist demonstrates that he or she values the expertise of the individual's lived experience. Furthermore, this process promotes the establishment of a therapeutic alliance that goes beyond treating symptoms and impairments.

One method of gathering narrative information is through structured interviews. The Occupational Performance History Interview is one tool that allows occupational therapists to gather such information (Kielhofner et al, 2004). This extensive list of questions (with possible variations and probes) addresses the client's occupational life history and a life history narrative. The measure includes a quantitative scoring system and a qualitative description of the life history. The Child Occupational Self Assessment (Keller, Kafkes, & Kielhofner, 2005) provides a method for children and youth to describe their own perceptions regarding occupational competence and values. Designed for children ages 7 and older, the measure fosters client-centered care and self-determination. It can be administered through an interview with a checklist or by using a card sort technique for children who are less verbal.

Evidence-Based Practice

A process called recovery preference exploration provides a framework for facilitating storytelling among consumers and providers. The process can result in improved communication, a deepening of the consumer–therapist relationship, and increased empowerment for the consumer.

➤ The use of recovery preference exploration is one narrative tool that occupational therapists can use to enhance the therapeutic relationship and promote recovery.

Kurz, A. E., Saint-Louis, N., Burke, J. P., & Stineman, M. G. (2008). Exploring the personal reality of disability and recovery: A tool for empowering the rehabilitation process. *Qualitative Health Research, 18,* 90–105.

PhotoVoice

Dolls and toys bring beauty, comfort, and security. Together, they all form their own little community. I think they give a sense of connectedness and fulfillment, completeness and joy. They make life more beautiful and secure. They show the importance of beauty in daily life. If I had more room, I would have more. Toys and dolls also can symbolize unity and fulfillment. Toys and dolls give strength, routine, and order to my life. They bring a fresh perspective to daily life. Some of the dolls in the picture are wearing pearls because they like to dress up. It's symbolic of the individual personalities they have. Each doll has its own personality, but at the same time they all belong together.

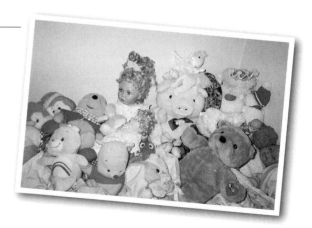

Occupational therapists can also use less formal methods, such as the narrative interview, which can offer the advantage of opening up lines of communication. This method also helps foster the therapeutic relationship because the person feels listened to and appreciated. Broad, open-ended questions can provide good starting points for the narrative interview (Box 6-1).

With children who are too young and adults with some disabilities (e.g., late-stage Alzheimer's disease), it may not be possible for occupational therapists to gather narrative information using verbal means. Creative media can often be useful, such as engaging children in play or having children or adults use art media to express their stories. In some cases, narrative may need to be gathered from family members or caregivers. In such cases, it is important to acknowledge the secondhand nature of these narratives because an individual can never truly tell the story of another person.

Using Narrative for Intervention

Although narrative is often identified in the occupational therapy literature as a qualitative research method and a component of clinical reasoning (Schell, 2003), the creation of narratives is less often identified as an intervention approach. Yet, telling one's story can have powerful therapeutic benefits. First, creating a narrative encourages self-discovery and promotes cognitive and psychological processing of the experience. Telling one's story causes the person to reflect on life experiences and integrate the experience into his or her sense of self. In addition, narratives allow the person to connect with others. Individuals who share their stories, particularly about topics that are often avoided (e.g., mental illness), often explain that they want to share their story so that others will feel more comfortable speaking out about their own experiences (DeSalvo, 1999). People also find that sharing their stories connects them to others with similar experiences.

Pennebaker and Chung (2007) studied the benefits of writing about difficult life events. Interestingly, Pennebaker and Chung's method does not include the sharing of the story; their approach emphasizes the processing and self-discovery benefits of expressive writing. They argue that, when the individual writes knowing that he or she will not share the story, the individual is less likely to spend time trying to craft a well-written story and more time actually capturing the experience. In fact, Pennebaker and Chung encourage people to burn, throw away, or destroy the writing as part of the therapeutic process.

However, the sharing of personal experience by people with disabilities can result in many positive outcomes. When stories are shared with students, they develop a more personal and empathic view of individuals with disabilities (Smith & Sparkes, 2008). Narratives benefit practitioners by enhancing collaboration and understanding (Simmons, Crepeau, & White, 2000). Frantis (2005) suggests that narratives provide the medium by which occupational therapists can understand disability from an insider perspective. A profound example of the power of narrative sharing is the recovery movement. People with psychiatric disabilities are telling their stories, and the revelation of the life experiences of people with psychiatric disabilities has altered our understanding of mental illness and impacted the way in which mental health services are delivered (Davidson, Sells, & Songster, 2005; Ridgway, 2001).

Writing and verbal expression are not the only ways in which narratives can be shared. Other creative media can be useful tools for sharing narratives. Photography, art, drama, music, and dance provide a variety of options for self-expression. The importance of narrative is recognized in this text with the inclusion of written narratives and the PhotoVoice feature to capture the lived experience of the person with mental illness.

BOX 6-1 ■ Sample Questions for Gathering Narrative Information

- Tell me a little bit about yourself.
- What's something I don't know about you?
- Tell me about a very difficult time in your life. Tell me about a very happy time in your life.
- What are your hopes and dreams for the future?
- What has it been like living with a psychiatric disability?
- What do you like most about yourself? What do you like least about yourself?
- What has been your greatest accomplishment?

Evidence-Based Practice

Occupational therapy practice should incorporate narrative in both assessment and intervention processes. Narrative data can provide information that is not available through other assessments methods. For example, the inclusion of narrative data allows occupational therapists to be more accurate in predicting occupational therapy outcomes.

➤ Occupational therapists should always include narrative as a component of clinical reasoning.

➤ Occupational therapists should consider methods for eliciting narrative during the assessment process.

Simmons, D. C., Crepeau, E. B., & White, B. P. (2000). The predictive power of narrative data in occupational therapy evaluation. *American Journal of Occupational Therapy, 54,* 471–476.

Evidence-Based Practice

Writing about difficult experiences can promote better mental and physical health.

➤ Occupational therapists should consider writing as an occupation that can address mental and physical health issues, particularly when the person is dealing with difficult experiences.

Pennebaker, J. W., & Chung, C. K. (2007). Expressive writing, emotional upheavals, and health. In H. S. Friedman & R. C. Silver (Eds.), *Foundations of Health Psychology* (pp. 263–284). New York: Oxford University Press.
Pennebaker, J. W., & Seagal, J. D. (1999). Forming a story: The health benefits of narrative. *Journal of Clinical Psychology, 55,* 1243–1254.

Summary

In understanding the person, occupational therapists consider underlying client factors or skills, as well as diagnoses and symptoms. In addition, occupational therapists who operate from a recovery-oriented perspective recognize that the person's lived experience, or narrative, can guide the occupational therapy process. This collaboration enriches the therapeutic relationship and increases the potential for positive outcomes to occur.

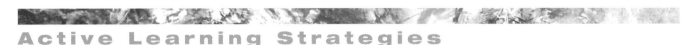

Active Learning Strategies

1. Writing a Narrative

Write a story about yourself. Think of something that's been troubling you. Maybe it is something that you have been avoiding thinking about, or it could be something you cannot stop thinking about. Decide ahead of time whether you plan to keep the story to yourself or share it with others. This will influence how you write. Find a time when you can devote at least 30 minutes to writing without interruption. Locate a quiet, comfortable place. When you write, do not just describe the event, but express your reactions to the experience and what you were thinking and feeling at the time.

 Describe the experience in your **Reflective Journal.**

Reflective Questions

- How did you decide what to write about?
- How would you describe the process? Was it easy or difficult? Was it emotional? Cathartic? Unpleasant?
- When you look back on the writing, are there things that surprised you about what you wrote?
- If you plan to share what you wrote, who will you share it with? Why?
- If you do not plan to share it, what might you do with it?
- Reflect on this experience and consider doing more writing, either about the same topic or other events.

2. Eliciting the Narrative of a Person With a Psychiatric Disability

Ask an individual with a psychiatric disability to tell you his or her story. You may not have a connection to a mental health center, but most people know someone, such as a family member or friend, who has experienced or is experiencing a mental illness. Approach the topic with sensitivity, acknowledging that some people may not want to share their experiences. However, you will find that people with psychiatric disabilities are often pleased when someone asks them to talk about the topic that everyone else seems to avoid. Explain that you are trying to learn more about psychiatric disability and that this learning includes the knowledge that comes from the lived experience. You may leave it open ended (e.g., "Tell me about your experience as a person with . . ."), or, if you know the individual, you may ask him or her about particular events or experiences (e.g., "What was it like when . . . ?").

 Describe the experience in your **Reflective Journal.**

Reflective Questions

- Were you uncomfortable approaching this experience? Having gone through it once, will it be easier to ask others to share their stories?
- What did you learn from this experience?
- Do you have insights into the person that you did not have before?
- What did you learn that you will take with you as an occupational therapist?

3. Person First Language

"Mayra is a mental patient. She was recently discharged from a psychiatric hospitalization, which was precipitated by a serious suicide attempt. As a borderline, she has been hospitalized three times previously. Mayra recently returned to school to complete her college degree. The recent brief hospitalization has set her back in her schoolwork and she would like assistance in advocating for herself to receive accommodations as a student."

Reflective Questions

- What picture is created by this presentation of Mayra? What seems most important?
- How could you rewrite the story so that it avoids labeling and incorporates person first language?
- Once the scenario is rewritten, what is different?

Resources

Narrative Assessment

- Kielhofner, G., Mallinson, T., Crawford, C., Nowak, M., Rigby, M., Henry, A., & Walens, A. (2004). *A User's Manual for the Occupational Performance History Interview (Version 2.1) (OPHI-II)*. Chicago: Model of Human Occupation (MOHO) Clearinghouse, Department of Occupational Therapy, College of Applied Health Sciences, University of Illinois at Chicago.

Child Occupational Self Assessment (COSA)

- Keller, J., Kafkes, A., Basu, S., Federico, J., & Kielhofner, G. (2005). *Child Occupational Self Assessment (COSA)*. Chicago: Model of Human Occupation (MOHO) Clearinghouse, Department of Occupational Therapy, College of Applied Health Sciences, University of Illinois at Chicago.

Narratives and Writing for Therapy

- DeSalvo, L. (1999). *Writing as a Way of Healing: How Telling Our Stories Transforms Our Lives*. Boston: Beacon Press.

- Pennebaker, J. W. (2004). *Writing to Heal: A Guided Journal for Recovering From Trauma and Emotional Upheaval.* Oakland, CA: New Harbinger Press.
- James Pennebaker, PhD, home page with instructions on writing for health: http://homepage.psy.utexas.edu/HomePage/Faculty/Pennebaker/Home2000/JWPhome.htm
- Precin, P. (2002). *Client-Centered Reasoning: Narratives of People With Mental Illness.* Boston: Butterworth Heinemann.

Wellness Recovery Action Plan
- Copeland, M. E. (2000). *Wellness Recovery Action Plan.* West Dummerston, VT: Peach Press.
- Mary Ellen Copeland's Mental Health Recovery and WRAP web site: http://www.mentalhealthrecovery.com/

References

American Psychiatric Association (APA). (2000). *Diagnostic and Statistical Manual of Mental Disorders* (4th ed., text revision). Washington, DC: American Psychiatric Association.

Beck, A. T., & Rector, N. A. (2005). Cognitive approaches to schizophrenia: Theory and therapy. *Annual Review of Clinical Psychology, 1,* 577–606.

Blaska, J. (1993). The power of language: Speak and write using "person first." In M. Nagler (Ed.), *Perspectives on Disability.* (pp. 25–32). Palo Alto, CA: Health Markets Research.

Bowie, C. R., & Harvey, P. D. (2005). Cognition in schizophrenia: Impairments, determinants and functional importance. *Psychiatric Clinics of North America, 28,* 613–626.

Brown, C., Cromwell, R. L., Filion, D., Dunn, W., & Tollefson, N. (2002). Sensory processing in schizophrenia: Missing and avoiding information. *Schizophrenia Research, 55,* 187–195.

Brown, C., Rempfer, M., & Hamera, E. (2008). Correlates of insider and outsider perspectives of recovery. *Psychiatric Rehabilitation Journal, 32,* 23–31.

Buckley, P., Bahmiller, D., Kenna, C. A., Shevitz, S., Powell, I., & Fricks, L. (2007). Resident education and perceptions of recovery in serious mental illness: Observations and commentary. *Academic Psychiatry, 31,* 435–438.

Champagne, T., & Stromberg, N. (2004). Sensory approaches in inpatient psychiatric settings: Innovative alternatives to seclusion and restraint. *Journal of Psychosocial Nursing and Mental Health Service, 42*(9), 34–44.

Cooney, R. E., Joormann, J., Atlas, L. Y., Eugene, F., & Gotlib, I. H. (2007). Remembering the good times: Neural correlates of affect regulation. *Neuroreport, 18,* 1771–1774.

Copeland, M. E. (2000). *Wellness Recovery Action Plan.* West Dummerston, VT: Peach Press.

Couture, S. M., Penn, D. L., & Roberts, D. L. (2006). The functional significance of social cognition in schizophrenia: A review. *Schizophrenia Bulletin, 32*(suppl 1):S44–S63.

Davidson, L. (2006). What happened to civil rights? *Psychiatric Rehabilitation Journal, 30,* 11–14.

Davidson, L., Flanagan, E., Roe, D., & Styron, T. (2006). Leading a horse to water: An action perspective on mental health policy. *Journal of Clinical Psychology, 62,* 1141–1155.

Davidson, L., Sells, D., & Songster, S. (2005). Qualitative studies of recovery: What can we learn from the person? In R. O. Ralph & P. W. Corrigan (Eds.), *Recovery in Mental Illness: Broadening Our Understanding of Wellness* (pp. 147–170). Washington, DC: American Psychological Association.

Deegan, P. E. (1996). Recovery as a journey of the heart. *Psychiatric Rehabilitation Journal, 19*(3), 91–97.

Deegan, P. E., & Drake, R. E. (2006). Shared decision making and medication management in the recovery process. *Psychiatric Services, 57,* 1636–1639.

DeSalvo, L. (1999). *Writing as a Way of Healing: How Telling Our Stories Transforms Our Lives.* Boston: Beacon Press.

Dunn, E. C., Wewiorski, N. J., & Rogers, E. S. (2008). The meaning and importance of employment to people in recovery from serious mental illness: Results of a qualitative study. *Psychiatric Rehabilitation Journal, 32,* 59–62.

Dunn, W., Brown, C., & Youngstrom, M. J. (2003). Ecological model of occupation. In P. Kramer, J. Hinojosa, & C. B. Royeen (Eds.), *Perspectives in Human Occupation: Participation in Life* (pp. 222–263). Baltimore: Lippincott William & Wilkins.

Feng, X., Shaw, D. S., Kovacs, M., Lane, T., O'Rourke, F. E., & Alarcon, J. H. (2008). Emotion regulation in preschoolers: The roles of behavioral inhibition, maternal affective behavior, and maternal depression. *Journal of Child Psychology and Psychiatry, 49,* 132–141.

Frantis, L. (2005). The issue is—Nothing about us without us: Searching for the narrative of disability. *American Journal of Occupational Therapy, 59,* 577–579.

Garrett, G., Ingram, R. E., Rand, K. L., & Sawalani, G. (2007). Cognitive processes in cognitive therapy: Evaluation of mechanisms of change in the treatment of depression. *Clinical Psychology: Science and Practice, 14,* 224–239.

Green, M. F., Kern, R. S., & Braff, D. L. (2000). Neurocognitive deficits and functional outcome in schizophrenia: Are we measuring the "right stuff"? *Schizophrenia Bulletin, 26,* 119–136.

Greene, R. W., Ablon, J. S., Goring, J. C., Raezer-Blakely, L., Markey, J., Monuteaux, M. C., Henin, A., Edwards, G., & Rabbitt, S. (2004). Effects of collaborative problem solving in affectively dysregulated children with oppositional defiant disorder: Initial findings. *Journal of Consulting and Clinical Psychology, 72,* 1157–1164.

Gruhl, K. L. (2005). Reflections on . . . the recovery paradigm: Should occupational therapists be interested? *Canadian Journal of Occupational Therapy, 72,* 96–102.

Hayes, S. C., Luoma, J. B., Bond, F. W., Masudo, A., & Lillis, J. (2006). Acceptance and commitment therapy: Model, processes and outcomes. *Behavioural Research and Therapy, 44,* 1–25.

Hoffman, S. G. (2007). Cognitive factors that maintain social anxiety disorder: A comprehensive model and its treatment implications. *Cognitive Behavior Therapy, 36,* 193–209.

Husain, M. M., Rush, A. J., & Trivedi, M. H. (2007). Pain in depression: STAR*D study findings. *Journal of Psychosocial Research, 63,* 113–122.

Jacobson, N. (2001). Experiencing recovery: A dimensional analysis of recovery narratives. *Psychiatric Rehabilitation Journal, 24,* 248–256.

Keller, J., Kafkes, A., & Kielhofner, G. (2005). Psychometric characteristics of the Child Occupational Self Assessment (COSA), part one: An initial examination of psychometric properties. *Scandinavian Journal of Occupational Therapy, 12,* 118–127.

Kielhofner, G. (2004). *Conceptual Foundations of Occupational Therapy* (3rd ed.). Philadelphia: FA Davis.

Kielhofner, G., Mallinson, T., Crawford, C., Nowak, M., Rigby, M., Henry, A., & Walens, A. (2004). *A User's Manual for the Occupational Performance History Interview (Version 2.1) (OPHI-II).* Chicago: Model of Human Occupation (MOHO) Clearinghouse, Department of Occupational Therapy, College of Applied Health Sciences, University of Illinois at Chicago.

Kingdon, D. G., & Turkington, D. (1993). *Cognitive Behavioral Therapy of Schizophrenia.* New York: Guilford.

Law, M. (1998). *Client-Centered Occupational Therapy.* Thorofare, NJ: Slack.

Law, M., Cooper, B., Strong, S., Stewart, D., Rigby, P., & Letts, L. (1996). The Person-Environment-Occupation model: A transactive approach to occupational performance. *Canadian Journal of Occupational Therapy, 63*(1), 9–23.

Linehan, M. M. (1993). *Skills Training Manual for Treating Borderline Personality Disorder.* New York: Guilford Press.

Matson, J. L., Matson, M. L., & Rivet, T. T. (2007). Social-skills treatments for children with autism spectrum disorders: An overview. *Behavior Modification, 31,* 682–707.

Nelson, G., Clarke, J., Febbraro, A., & Hatzipantelis, M. (2005). A narrative approach to the evaluation of supported housing: Stories of homeless people who have experienced serious mental illness. *Psychiatric Rehabilitation Journal, 29,* 98–104.

Nes, L. S., & Segerstrom, S. C. (2006). Dispositional optimism and coping: A meta-analytic review. *Personality and Social Psychology Review, 10,* 235–251.

Patil, S. K., Johnson, A. S., & Lichtenberg, P. A. (2008). The relation of pain and depression with various health-promoting behaviors in African American elders. *Rehabilitation Psychology, 53,* 85–92.

Peloquin, S. M. (2005). The 2005 Eleanor Clark Slagle Lecture: Embracing our ethos, reclaiming our heart. *American Journal of Occupational Therapy, 59,* 611–625.

Penn, D. L., Roberts, D. L., Combs, D., & Sterne, A. (2007). Best practices: The development of the Social Cognition and Interaction Training program for schizophrenia spectrum disorders. *Psychiatric Services, 58,* 449–451.

Pennebaker, J. W., & Chung, C. K. (2007). Expressive writing, emotional upheavals, and health. In H. S. Friedman & R. C. Silver (Eds.), *Foundations of Health Psychology* (pp. 263–284). New York: Oxford University Press.

Rapport, M. D., Scanlan, S. W., & Denne, C. B. (1999). Attention deficit/hyperactivity disorder and scholastic achievement: A model of dual developmental pathways. *Journal of Child Psychology and Psychiatry, 40,* 1169–1183.

Ridgway, P. (2001). ReStorying psychiatric disability: Learning from first person recovery narratives. *Psychiatric Rehabilitation Journal, 24,* 335–343.

Russo, N., Floanagan, T., Iavocci, G., Berringer, D., Zelazo, P. D., & Burak, J. A. (2007). Deconstructing executive deficits among people with autism: Implications for cognitive neuroscience. *Brain and Cognition, 65,* 77–86.

Schell, B. A. B. (2003). Clinical reasoning: The basis of practice. In E. B. Crepeau, E. S. Cohn, & B. A. B. Schell (Eds.), *Willard and Spackman's Occupational Therapy* (pp. 131–139). Philadelphia: Lippincott William & Wilkins.

Schore, A. (2003). *Affect Dysregulation and Disorders of the Self.* New York: Norton.

Simmons, D. C., Crepeau, E., & White, B. P. (2000). The predictive power of narrative data in occupational therapy evaluation. *American Journal of Occupational Therapy, 54,* 471–476.

Smith, B., & Sparkes, A. C. (2008). Narrative and its potential contribution to disability studies. *Disability and Society, 23*(1), 17–28.

Stanos, S., & Houle, T. T. (2006). Multidisciplinary and interdisciplinary management of chronic pain. *Physical Medicine and Rehabilitation Clinics of North America, 17,* 435–450.

Stewart, D., Letts, L., Law, M., Cooper, B. A., Strong, S., & Rigby, P. J. (2003). The Person-Environment-Occupation model. In E. B. Crepeau, E. S. Cohn, & B. A. B. Schell (Eds.), *Willard and Spackman's Occupational Therapy* (pp. 227–233). Philadelphia: Lippincott William & Wilkins.

Wilson, G. T. (2005). Psychological treatment of eating disorders. *Annual Review of Clinical Psychology, 1,* 439–465.

Zelman, D. C., Howland, E. W., Nichols, S. N., & Cleeland, C. S. (1991). The effects of induced mood on laboratory pain. *Pain, 46,* 105–111.

CHAPTER

7

Pervasive Developmental Disorders

Katie Alexander

> "*If you've met one person with autism, you've met one person with autism.*
>
> —Stephen Shore, EdD, an author and international leader in the field
> of autism who lives with an autism spectrum disorder

Introduction

For individuals who live with intact social abilities, it is difficult to imagine the profound impact that a social skill impairment can present. The way that a typically developing brain can make sense of the complex and obscure social world is remarkable, and when there is a breakdown, it affects every domain of human participation and engagement. At their core, pervasive developmental disorders (PDDs) are disorders of social participation; it is this social skills impairment that binds the various disorders together, despite their marked distinctions. Individuals who live with a PDD can offer the world their different perspectives and unique talents.

Occupational therapists are concerned with social participation, and those who work in schools, early intervention programs, and other child-based settings will often have a caseload that includes many children with PDDs. Adults with PDDs also continue to have occupational performance needs; however, occupational therapy services for adults with PDD are less available. Unlike the commonly used approach of discrete trial training in which small skills (e.g., saying the word "apple" when presented with the fruit) are taught in a time-intensive program, occupational therapists are more likely to focus on enhancing engagement in occupational performance within natural environments (e.g., mealtime at home, on the playground at school) (Case-Smith & Arbesman, 2008). Approaches commonly used by occupational therapists include structuring the environment to support performance, meeting sensory needs, enhancing socialization through engagement with typically developing children, and parent training. In addition, occupational therapists use the individual's strengths and interests to enhance the efficacy of the intervention. For example, individuals with autism often have strengths in visual perceptions; therefore, visual cues and pictures are integrated into the intervention (Panerai, Farrante, & Zingale, 2002).

This chapter introduces the PDDs, including information on etiology, prevalence, course, and gender and cultural influences, and explains the impact of PDDs on occupational performance. Although the chapters in Section 2 do not focus on intervention, this chapter provides information o n medication and a general discussion of interventions used by occupational therapists. For more information on assessment and intervention in PDDs, refer to Chapters 18, 20, 21, 48, and 52.

Description of the Disorder

Pervasive developmental disorder (PDD) is a set of childhood onset disorders that includes the following diagnoses:

- Autism spectrum disorder (including autistic disorder, Asperger's disorder, and pervasive developmental disorder not otherwise specified [PDD-NOS])
- Rett's disorder
- Childhood disintegrative disorder

Together, these disorders share a triad of impairments in social skills, communication, and behavior (American Psychiatric Association [APA], 2000). Although each PDD includes these traits, there is also vast heterogeneity among the separate disorders and within each disorder. This significant variability exists with regard to cognitive ability, social reciprocity, speech, language, course, and outcome. This heterogeneity has given rise to the term "spectrum disorders." The term **autism spectrum disorder (ASD)** commonly includes autistic disorder, Asperger's disorder, and PDD-NOS.

Each individual with a PDD presents with a different constellation of areas of strength and need. By definition, the impairment encompasses many areas of functioning and is sustained across the life span; however, its impact on occupational performance is highly variable. In some cases, individuals make significant progress, and independent participation in the community, at home, and at work is possible. This degree of participation is more likely with the diagnoses of Asperger's disorder and PDD-NOS. In other cases, such as with Rett's disorder, childhood disintegrative disorder, and some cases of autistic disorder, significant progress is less likely, and substantial support is usually required for participation in the community.

Autism Spectrum Disorders

The autism spectrum is complex, and each person on the spectrum is unique in his or her abilities and impairments. It can be helpful to think of autism spectrum disorders (ASDs) as a spectrum within a spectrum. For example, consider a spectrum of cognitive abilities. Individuals with an ASD can have cognitive abilities that range from below average to above average. There is also a spectrum of language ability, and individuals with an ASD can have no verbal language to verbal language that far exceeds his or her chronological age and typical developmental expectations. The spectrum of social skills is equally varied, but distinguished from the aforementioned areas in that it is always an area of impairment in ASDs. Even so, the ways in which and the degree to which it manifests itself vary from individual to individual. For example, an individual with autistic disorder may initiate social interaction with extremely limited frequency, whereas an individual with **Asperger's disorder** may frequently initiate social interaction, but the attempts often fail in producing the desired results due to deficient skills.

Finally, there is a spectrum of behavioral manifestations of ASDs. An individual may demonstrate frequent stereotypical behavior, such as moving his fingers every time he walks past a window, hand flapping when excited, or rocking. On the other end of the spectrum, an individual may not demonstrate any stereotypical behavior, but his or her range of interests is extremely limited. For example, an individual with Asperger's disorder may become preoccupied with trains to the exclusion of other themes of play or topics of conversation.

The *Diagnostic and Statistical Manual of Mental Disorders, Fourth Edition, Text Revision* (DSM-IV-TR) provides specific criteria for the diagnosis of autism, Asperger disorder, and autistic disorder not otherwise specified (APA, 2000). A diagnosis of autistic disorder requires the presence of three core features, including impaired social skills development; impaired communication; and marked restricted, stereotyped, and/or repetitive activities and interests (APA, 2000). Furthermore, these impairments are gross and sustained, and can present with varying topography and intensity. The detailed DSM-IV-TR diagnostic criteria for autistic disorder are listed in Box 7-1.

Asperger's Disorder

A diagnosis of Asperger's disorder requires that three of the core criteria identified previously in the autism diagnosis are met (APA, 2000):

- Significant, qualitative impairment in social interaction
- Presence of stereotyped, restricted, or repetitive behaviors, activities, and/or interests
- Impairments must interfere significantly with participation in daily life

---

BOX 7-1 ▒ DSM-IV-TR Diagnostic Criteria for Autistic Disorder

A. Criteria must be met from a total of at least six of areas 1, 2, and 3, with at least two criteria from area 1 and at least one criteria from 2 and 3:

1. Qualitative impairment in social interaction
   a. Impairment in nonverbal social behaviors
   b. Failure to develop developmentally appropriate peer relationships
   c. Lack of spontaneous seeking to share enjoyment, interests, or achievements
   d. Lack of social and/or emotional reciprocity

2. Qualitative impairment in communication
   a. Impaired spoken language, including possible absence of spoken language
   b. Impairment in ability to initiate and sustain conversation
   c. Stereotyped or repetitive use of language or idiosyncratic language
   d. Impairment in development of play appropriate to developmental level

3. Stereotyped, restricted, or repetitive activities, interests, and/or behaviors
   a. Encompassing preoccupation, abnormal in either intensity and/or focus, with one or more stereotyped or restricted areas of interest
   b. Rigid adherence to specific, nonfunctional routines or rituals
   c. Stereotyped and repetitive motor mannerisms
   d. Persistent preoccupation with parts of objects

B. With an onset prior to 3 years of age, impaired development in at least one of the following areas: social interaction, language as used in social conversation, and symbolic or imaginative play

From American Psychiatric Association. (2000). *Diagnostic and Statistical Manual of Mental Disorders* (4th ed., Text Revision). Washington, DC: Author.

Unlike autistic disorder, there need not be impairment in early language development in order to assign a *Diagnostic and Statistical Manual of Mental Disorders, Fourth Edition, Text Revision* (DSM-IV-TR) diagnosis of Asperger's disorder. In addition, the development of early cognitive, self-help, and adaptive behavior skills are age appropriate.

Pervasive Developmental Disorder Not Otherwise Specified

PDD-NOS is a diagnostic category reserved for patterns of behavior and development that are typical for a PDD (e.g., significant impairment in social interaction; communication; and/or repetitive, restricted, and stereotyped areas of interests and/or activities), but that do not satisfy the diagnostic criteria for autistic disorder or Asperger's disorder (APA, 2000). This category includes **atypical autism,** which means either that there were no characteristics of autism before age 3 or that the child does not meet the criteria for one of the areas of impairment as identified in the DSM-IV-TR diagnosis of autism.

Rett's Disorder

The course and gender distribution of **Rett's disorder (RD)** distinguish it from its PDD counterparts. This neurodevelopmental disorder occurs almost exclusively in females and is characterized by typical early development followed by stagnation and ultimate developmental regression (APA, 2000; Hagberg, Hanefeld, Percy, & Skjeldal, 2002).

RD is a complex disorder that features physical, psychomotor, and behavioral areas of impairment. Head circumference decelerates between 5 and 48 months of age. It is also possible that the child will experience overall growth retardation (Hagberg et al, 2002). RD results in a loss of acquired purposeful hand skills. In addition, the child develops stereotyped movements involving the hands and hands to mouth, both at midline and laterally (Temudo et al, 2007). These movements most frequently include hand wringing/squeezing, clapping, hand tapping, hand "washing," and hand rubbing.

RD can affect other aspects of motor development, such as gait ataxia, truncal apraxia/ataxia, and ataxia. During this period of skill loss, severely impaired expressive/receptive language and communication skills typically accompany the development of mental retardation (Hagberg, 2002). RD leads to the development of autistic-like social withdrawal and poor social and emotional reciprocity. However, eye contact is typically preserved (Hagberg, 2002). The detailed DSM-IV-TR diagnostic criteria for RD are listed in Box 7-2.

Childhood Disintegrative Disorder

Although individuals with **childhood disintegrative disorder (CDD)** present with the same heterogeneity found with other PDDs, CDD is distinguished by a later age of onset (at least 2 years of age), and the course associated with CDD is consistent across individuals. Once the initial, regressive course of CDD is complete, it is indistinguishable from autistic disorder, and individuals with the disorder demonstrate marked social, language, and communication impairments, in addition to the presence of stereotyped behavior (Malhotra & Gupta, 1999). However, individuals with CDD are more likely to be nonverbal than individuals with autism (Kurita, Osada, & Miyake, 2004). The detailed DSM-IV-TR diagnostic criteria for CDD are listed in Box 7-3.

Etiology

It is generally accepted that the behaviors associated with the PDDs are due to underlying genetic and neurobiological mechanisms (Buxbaum et al, 2001; Temudo et al, 2007). As such, the perplexing etiology of these disorders is likely the result of a combination of many factors and, to a great extent, yet unknown. Current research indicates that genetics, neurobiology, and environment play interrelated roles in the development and expression of PDDs (Armstrong, 2002; Fred, Volkmar, Klin, & Cohen, 2005). In addition, research investigating the etiology of these disorders has only begun to provide important answers while new questions continually surface. As science unveils the etiology of PDDs, new hope for effective methods of prevention and intervention emerges.

Autism Spectrum Disorders

A great deal of research is currently focused on understanding the cause of the ASDs. The multiple factors presented here illustrate the complexity of these disorders and why individuals living with an ASD present with such varying behaviors, skills, and abilities. For occupational therapists, this

---

BOX 7-2 ■ DSM-IV-TR Diagnostic Criteria for Rett's Disorder

A. All of the following:
   1. Apparently normal prenatal and perinatal development
   2. Apparently normal psychomotor development through the first 5 months after birth
   3. Normal head circumference at birth
B. Onset of all of the following after the period of normal development:
   1. Deceleration of head growth between ages 5 and 48 months
   2. Loss of previously acquired purposeful hand skills between ages 5 and 30 months with subsequent development of stereotyped movements (e.g., handwringing or hand washing)
   3. Loss of social engagement early in the course
   4. Appearance of poorly coordinated gait or trunk movements
   5. Severely impaired expressive and receptive language development with severe psychomotor retardation

From American Psychiatric Association. (2000). *Diagnostic and Statistical Manual of Mental Disorders* (4th ed., Text Revision). Washington, DC: Author.

BOX 7-3 ■ DSM-IV-TR Diagnostic Criteria for Childhood Disintegrative Disorder

A. Apparently normal development for at least the first 2 years after birth as manifested by the presence of age-appropriate verbal and nonverbal communication, social relationships, play, and adaptive behaviors
B. Clinically significant loss of previously acquired skills (before age 10 years) in at least two of the following areas:
   1. Expressive or receptive language
   2. Social skills or adaptive behavior
   3. Bowel or bladder control
   4. Play
   5. Motor skills
C. Abnormalities of functioning in at least two of the following areas:
   1. Qualitative impairment in social interaction
   2. Qualitative impairments in communication
   3. Restricted, repetitive, and stereotyped patterns of behavior, interests, and activities, including motor stereotypies and mannerisms

From American Psychiatric Association. (2000). *Diagnostic and Statistical Manual of Mental Disorders* (4th ed., Text Revision). Washington, DC: Author.

variability highlights the importance of appreciating the uniqueness of each individual in the assessment and intervention process.

Genetic Factors

Substantial evidence indicates ASDs are highly genetic (Bailey et al, 1995; Folstein & Rutter, 1977) and that multiple genes are involved (Pickles et al, 1995). The exact manner in which the genes are related to symptoms or severity of autism is relatively unknown and a continued subject of research. For example, one study found that in monozygotic twins (identical twins that share the same genetic material), if one twin has autism, the other twin has a 60% chance of also having the disorder (Bailey et al, 1995). However, when the criteria are broadened to include lower-level autistic symptoms (e.g., PDD-NOS), 92% of monozygotic twins fall somewhere on the autistic spectrum. Furthermore, 3% to 8% of siblings of individuals with ASDs have inherited the disorder (Bolton et al, 1994; Chudley, Gutierrez, Jocelyn, & Chodirker, 1998). Even when monozygotic twins have an autistic disorder, the two individuals can present with highly different patterns and severity of symptoms (Le Couteur et al, 1996), suggesting that the expression of ASDs is not purely the product of genetics.

Neuroanatomical Factors

The neuropathology of autism involves the structure of specific brain regions and connectivity between brain regions (Stanfield et al, 2007). In individuals with ASDs, total brain volume is increased, as are both the cerebral hemispheres and the cerebellum (Stanfield et al, 2007). In addition, the caudate nucleus is larger, whereas the corpus callosum and midbrain are smaller. The cortical language areas appear to have unusual asymmetry, which reflects atypical brain development (Rojas, Bawn, Benkers, Reite, & Rogers, 2002). The net result of these brain differences coincide with the behavioral manifestations of ASDs, meaning that the neurological abnormalities are consistent with the pervasive impairment in the higher-order skills of language and social participation. It can be helpful for parents, professionals, and the general public to understand that the behaviors exhibited in autism are related to neurological abnormalities and not poor parenting or intentional bad behavior from the individual with autism.

Functional Neuroimaging

In autism, social participation is affected by breakdowns in the connections between the frontal, limbic, and temporal lobes. With regard to social perception (e.g., finding salience in facial affect, reading facial expressions and body language), recent studies have established underactivation of three critical brain structures during social tasks: the fusiform gyrus (in particular, an area known as the fusiform face area [FFA]), the superior temporal sulcus (STS), and the amygdala (amy) (Schultz et al, 2003). The FFA allows an individual to perceive faces, and the STS plays an important role in interpreting dynamic social signals (e.g., eye gaze patterns, facial affect, body language) (Pelphrey, Morris, McCarthy, & Labar, 2007; Schultz et al, 2003). Although each of these brain regions operates differently under social conditions when compared with controls, ASDs appear to be a product of a disruption to the networking among these regions and other areas of the brain (Pelphrey et al, 2007; Schultz et al, 2003).

With regard to social cognition (i.e., the ability to think about and interpret another's thoughts, beliefs, and expectations), areas of the temporal and frontal lobes are primarily liable for breakdowns in social cognition. Specifically, areas of the prefrontal cortex (PFC), fusiform gyrus, and amygdala operate differently in individuals with ASDs when compared with controls (Pinkham, Hopfinger, Pelphrey, Piven, & Penn, 2007; Schultz & Robins, 2005)

Immunizations

Vaccinations, specifically the measles, mumps, and rubella vaccine (MMR), have been implicated in the etiology of ASDs. Although many individuals have strongly held beliefs about the relationship of vaccinations and the onset of autism, to date, the research conducted in this area has found no causative relationship between immunizations and ASDs (Fombonne, Zakarian, Bennett, Meng, & McLean-Heywood, 2006).

Rett's Disorder

RD is associated with a specific genetic mutation that results in particular neurological disturbances.

Genetic Factors

Through a benchmark Amir and colleagues (2005) identified the genetic cause for most cases of RD. Approximately 80% to 85% of individuals with this disorder have mutations or deletions of methyl-CpG binding protein 2 (*MECP2*); the cause of the remaining RD is yet unknown (Amir et al, 2005; Van den Veyver & Zoghbi, 2001). The *MECP2* mutation is de novo (i.e., a genetic mutation exists that neither parent possessed or transmitted; it is a new, spontaneous mutation) in most cases (Dragich, Houwink-Manville, & Schanen, 2000). *MECP2* is a protein that is critical to typical central nervous system (CNS) development. In the case of the RD-specific mutations, this dysregulation results in the arrest of CNS development and the expression of RD (Lombroso, 2000; Van Acker, Loncola, & Van Acker, 2005).

Neuroanatomical Factors

The brain of the individual with RD is small in both size and weight given the height and weight of the individual, which is apparently due to an arrest of cortical maturation during infancy, as opposed to cortical atrophy (Armstrong, 2002; Kaufmann, Naidu, & Budden, 1995). In addition, there is a significant reduction in grey matter throughout the cortex, which is predominantly distributed in the prefrontal, posterior frontal, and anterior temporal regions. Although gray matter sustains the greatest impact by RD, research has also indicated reductions in white matter, predominately in the caudate, putamen, and thalamus (Naidu et al, 2001; Subramaniam, Naidu, & Reiss, 1997).

The gross brain differences associated with RD are accompanied by significant deviations in the maturation, distribution, size, and density of projection neurons located in the frontal, motor, inferior temporal, hippocampus, and visual cortex (Armstrong, Dunn, Antalffy, & Trivedi, 1995). Neuroimaging and use of the rapid Golgi technique reveals a paucity of dendrites in these locations, and in those dendrites that exist, a simplified branching pattern is present. Therefore, information is not transmitted or is transmitted less efficiently and effectively.

Neurochemical Factors

Current literature suggests that there is a reduction in the overall number of neurotransmitters in RD. Furthermore, serotonin, dopamine, and norepinephrine have been implicated by different studies, although their precise contribution to RD is still unclear (Guideri et al, 2004; Viemari et al, 2005; Zoghbi, Percy, Glaze, Butler, & Riccardi, 1985). Studies have also found neurochemical impairments present in the brainstem, including the autonomic nervous system (Deguchi et al, 2000).

Childhood Disintegrative Disorder

There is less research on CDD when compared to the other PDDs; that, coupled with the rarity of the disorder, yields limited information regarding its causes. The precise etiology of CDD is unknown. The symptomology and associated medical conditions suggest that neurobiological factors contribute to etiology of the disorder.

Genetic Factors

CDD commonly occurs in families in which there is no other individuals with the disorder, and concordance among siblings has not been reported. This sporadic occurrence of CDD does suggest a complex pattern or lack of genetic etiology (Malhotra & Gupta, 2002). Although no specific genetic loci or chromosomal abnormalities have been identified, these possibilities have not been ruled out (Volkmar, Koenig, & State, 2005).

Neurobiological Factors

There is extremely limited evidence regarding the neurobiology or neurophysiology of CDD, and there are no consistent findings that indicate the neuropathology of the disorder (Malhotra & Gupta, 2002). However, electroencephalogram abnormalities and frequent comorbidity of seizure disorder in combination with the course of the disorder suggest that neurobiological factors are fundamental contributors to the development of this disorder.

Environmental Factors

Current literature reports the possible role of life stressors, both psychological and physical, as a precipitating factor in the development of CDD (Malhotra & Gupta, 2002; Volkmar et al, 2005). Seizures are one such stressor cited by families, and research indicates a high rate of seizures with CDD (Malhotra & Gupta, 2002). However, the possible causative role of seizures or other stressors has not been determined and is suspect because of their relatively common occurrence in early childhood (Volkmar et al, 2005). It has been hypothesized that CDD develops due to an interplay between complex genetic mechanisms and environmental events, but substantially more research is required to determine the exact cause of the disorder (Volkmar et al, 2005).

Prevalence

In the most rigorous and expansive epidemiologic study of ASDs to date, the Centers for Disease Control and Prevention (CDC; 2007) have found that the prevalence of ASDs among children is increasing and currently estimate the prevalence of ASDs at 1 in 110 children. The remaining two PDDs, RD and CDD, are considered rare, and each disorder has been estimated at a prevalence rate of approximately 0.6 per 10,000 individuals (Chakrabarti & Fombonne, 2001). Figure 7-1 shows an increase in the cases of autism between school years 1992 and 2007.

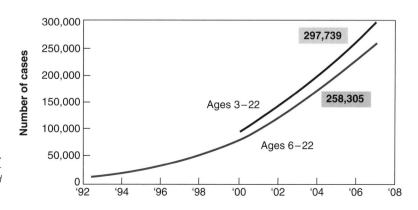

FIGURE 7-1. Increase in number of cases of autism. *Data from the Data Accountability Center (www.idea-data.org) and the Centers for Disease Control and Prevention.*

Course

The course of all PDDs is chronic. However, individuals with ASD can and often do progress in terms of their abilities to engage in occupational performance. In contrast, RD and CDD are conditions that result in a loss of or inability to develop skills, and in RD, there is a shortened life span.

Autism Spectrum Disorders

An ASD presents as a lifelong, continuous impairment. Across the autism spectrum, there are variations with regard to age of diagnosis and long-term outcomes. Autistic disorder is typically detected earlier in life than Asperger's disorder due to the early presentation of the disorder, resulting in more subtle and qualitative developmental differences (Fombonne & Tidmarsh, 2003). ASDs begin early in life, typically first diagnosed between 49 and 66 months of age (CDC, 2007). The most frequently reported developmental concern is language followed by social skills. In addition, parents may report limited eye contact, social smiling, social referencing, and/or different responses to physical touch in infancy and early childhood. Although the course of autism most often begins at birth, there are some reports of a loss of skills. The CDC reports a median percentage of children with autism who have a documented regression of skills as ranging from 13.8% to 31.6%, and the median age of regression onset ranges from 18 to 33 months.

As children with autism disorders get older, the deficits in activities of daily living and communication become more apparent (Mazfesky, Williams, & Minshew, 2008). This is partially due to the increased expectations associated with school and peer relationships. Children with autism may have problematic behaviors that interfere with participation in school, such as temper tantrums, aggressiveness with other children, or difficulties transitioning from the classroom to the cafeteria or playground (Hartley, Sikora, & McCoy, 2008). Particularly difficult for children with ASD is reciprocal play, so the development of friendships is challenging. Approximately one-half of children with ASD have an average or better than average IQ (Chakrabarti & Fambonne, 2005), but comorbid mental retardation can have a significant impact on school performance and the development of adaptive skills. Overall, in children with ASD, the acquisition of adaptive skills (e.g., communication, activities of daily living [ADLs], instrumental activities of daily living [IADLs]) is lower than would be expected given the child's IQ (Bolte & Poutska, 2002).

However, the course of ASD can be positively impacted with early intervention. Evidence indicates that behavioral interventions can result in significant improvements in language, daily living skills, and social behavior (Remington et al, 2007; Rogers & Vismara, 2008). Although controversial, there is some belief that the prevention of autism is plausible if infants receive treatment very early to alter the course of behavioral and brain development (Dawson, 2008). Still, a comprehensive review of the evidence suggests that, although early intervention is highly successful, there is little evidence to indicate whether these changes lead to increased

independence in vocational and social function in adulthood (Rogers & Vismara, 2008).

Although children with ASD grow to be adults, this is an understudied area. However, the evidence that does exist suggests that the concerns in childhood persist into adulthood. A qualitative study found that adults with ASD reported a strong sense of isolation, difficulty communicating with others, and a longing for intimacy (Muller, Schuler & Yates, 2008). The higher-order cognitive impairments such as executive dysfunction, which is prevalent in children with ASD, is also present in adults with ASD (Barnard, Muldoon, Hasan, O'Brien, & Stewart, 2008). There is a lack of services for adults with ASD, although occupational therapists have the skills to assist with transitioning these individuals into adulthood. For some, this could include supports for independent living, college, and work, whereas others may need more basic assistance, such as supported employment or assisted living environments.

Rett's Disorder

RD is not degenerative; it is a neurodevelopmental disorder with a course that shifts over time. Hagberg and Witt-Engerstrom (1986) proposed a staging system to describe and categorize the course of RD in four clinical phases. This system is generally accepted, and the stages are most commonly referenced by number as opposed to name (Van Acker et al, 2005):

1. **Early onset stagnation** begins at 5 months of age and continues from weeks to months.
2. **Developmental regression** begins from 2 to 4 years of age, and its duration can range from weeks up to 1 year. This stage includes the loss of skills characteristic for the developmental stage.
3. The **pseudostationary period** begins once the second phase subsides and continues for years or decades. It has also been termed the "wake-up" period, and marks a time during which regression slows so that it is unapparent, and some communication skills may return.
4. **Late motor deterioration** begins when the third stage and ambulation ceases, and this stage can continue for decades. The fourth stage also has subgroups for individuals who once walked and for those who never walked, and is characterized by severe disability, wheelchair dependency, and distortion and wasting of the extremities (Hagberg, 2002; Hagberg & Witt-Engerstrom, 1986).

Childhood Disintegrative Disorder

The course of CDD is a critical defining feature of the disorder, and central to its course is age of onset. The mean age of onset for CDD is approximately 3.76 years, but it can range from 2 to 7 years, following at least 2 years of typical development (Malhotra & Gupta, 2002). The initial course of the disorder has been described as insidious (lasting weeks to months) or acute (lasting days to weeks) (Volkmar et al, 2005). Following the initial period of regression, the course of the disorder is typically static, and individuals with CDD demonstrate features that are indistinguishable from autism

The Lived Experience

Sabrina

Sabrina, a mother of a child with an autism spectrum disorder, shares her journey to illustrate the unique challenge of raising a child with an "invisible" disability.

A friend visited our family for a few hours during a particularly difficult period. At the time, episodes of dangerous physical aggression were occurring frequently, and irritability was nearly constant. The sweet, funny, engaging child we adored and who loved us back seemed unreachable, lost to us and to himself. The friend phoned that night to express concern. "I felt like I was watching one of those drownings," she said, "where the child goes under and then one by one the people who go in after him drown trying to save him. He's pulling you all under."

It felt that way, too: like we were struggling to breathe air. Other days, the metaphor is different: it's like walking through a minefield. Or it's as if he sucks all the air out of the room, leaving nothing for anyone else to breathe.

Those are the worst times, of course, and it isn't always like that, not at all. Our life with our son is rich and warm and deeply rewarding; he is often funny and brilliant and generous, and all of us truly are better and stronger people for having lived with his struggles and triumphs. But my point is that when one person has this sort of disability, the whole family is affected, and you cannot cross our threshold, even on a good day, without feeling it. Even on a good day, everyone is taking care. Everyone is stressed to some extent. Everyone's energy and patience is depleted as we try to avoid the pitfalls we can anticipate and attempt to think 2 or 5 or 10 steps ahead so that

we can anticipate even more. Nothing is simple and straightforward, and always each of us is thinking: how will it affect *him*? What can I preview for him? What can I help him prepare for? What will he encounter? Will there be too many people? Will it be noisy? Will someone say something that bothers him? Will he say something inappropriate that people will perceive as rude? Will he refuse to do what he's supposed to do in this situation? And what will happen if he does?

My child's disability is invisible to people. He is handsome, big for his age, and strong. He's quite verbal, has a remarkable vocabulary, and a very sharp wit. Although they are wonderful strengths, these delightful attributes are also liabilities. They suggest to the world that he is a healthy, fully responsible individual, which he isn't. Life is very, very hard for my child, and making it through a day is enormously taxing. He has frequent "meltdowns," and his interactions with others often result in conflict. But unlike a child whose hair is visibly thinning under a baseball cap, or one who rides gamely in a wheelchair, or one with the distinctive facial features of a genetic syndrome, my son doesn't get the benefit of the doubt. He gets no credit for the extent of his disability, or even for its existence. Because the stigmata of disability are not physically apparent, and because he uses sophisticated language when he speaks, people don't recognize my child's inappropriate conduct as reflecting his brain-based disorder. Consequently, I am very quick to explain to people we encounter that he has an autism spectrum disorder, hoping this will result in a more sympathetic and accurate interpretation of his social missteps and difficult behavior.

(Malhotra & Gupta, 1999). Generally, the outcome for individuals with CDD is poorer than that for individuals with autistic disorder (Mouridsen, Rich, & Isager, 1998).

CDD is identified more frequently among males, who outnumber females at a ratio of approximately 5:1 (Malhotra & Gupta, 2002).

Gender Differences

Consistently, males outnumber females across all ASDs. Due in part to differences in study methodology, the gender ratio for all ASDs varies depending on the region of study. The CDC reports a male:female ratio of 3.4–6.5:1 (CDC, 2007). There are also gender differences with regard to cognitive impairments in that females (58.2%) are more likely than males (41.8%) to have a cognitive impairment (CDC, 2007). In addition, as the severity of the cognitive impairment increases from mild to profound, the male-to-female gender ratio shifts from 4:4 to 1:3 (Yeargin-Allsopp et al, 2003).

RD is almost exclusively identified among females. Because *MECP2* is located on the X chromosome, females have an additional, nonmutated chromosome that is able to produce sufficient protein to preserve early development and support life (Lombroso, 2000). With only one X chromosome, males have insufficient genetic material to sustain life. With rare exceptions, this results in fetal death of males carrying the *MECP2* genetic mutation (Lombroso, 2000).

Culture-Specific Information

There is inadequate research regarding the cultural factors relevant to PDDs. Current research indicates that rates of autism in the United States are similar across ethnic groups (Yeargin-Allsopp et al, 2003). However, there is initial evidence to indicate some diagnostic and intervention differences among different socioeconomic classes, but these differences appear to be a product of case ascertainment (i.e., children of families in higher socioeconomic status [SES] are more likely to be diagnosed by sources other than educational sources, such as a private psychologist) (Bhasin & Schendel, 2007). In addition, African American children are more likely to be identified by educational sources only (i.e., school) (Yeargin-Allsopp et al, 2003). These findings are important because they indicate that children who are African American or from families of lower SES are less likely to be identified early in life and, consequently, less likely to access early intervention services. Occupational therapists involved in early intervention services can assist with outreach and other public health initiatives to identify PDD in neglected populations.

Impact on Occupational Performance

Because the PDDs are social disorders, the impact on relationships is substantial. Because social skills are important for most other areas of occupational performance (e.g., school, work, many IADLs), these areas are affected as well.

Autism Spectrum Disorders

Most of the research that attempts to explain the social impairments in ASD focuses on cognitive impairments. In addition, adaptive skills and sensory processing differences contribute to difficulties with occupational performance.

Intellectual Impairments

The CDC (2007) estimated that 40% to 62% of children diagnosed with an ASD also have an intellectual impairment (IQ ≤70). Conversely, a more recent study indicated that the mean IQ score for individuals with Asperger's syndrome was 103 (Cederlund, Hagberg, Billstedt, Gillberg, & Gillberg, 2008).

Executive Function

Individuals with ASDs demonstrate impairments in **executive function,** which is the mental control required for the brain to maintain goal-directed behavior. Specifically, individuals with ASDs demonstrate impairments in organization, cognitive flexibility, visual working memory, planning, verbal fluency, inhibition, and interference control (Kenworthy et al, 2005; Verte, Geurts, Roeyers, Oosterlaan, & Sergeant, 2006). The following are examples of the role of executive function in participation:

- Frequently, students with Asperger's disorder obtain lower grades in school due to missing assignments, and adults may have difficulty prioritizing work tasks (organization).
- Individuals interacting with people with ASDs may be offended or avoid future interactions when the individual with ASD makes comments the instant they come to mind (inhibition).
- Cognitive flexibility allows a person to smoothly shift from one activity to another or quickly cope with and manage a change in routine. It is common for an individual with an ASD to experience profound anxiety if he or she arrives at school or work and finds that the schedule has changed. Intact cognitive flexibility would make this transition easier to bear.

Occupational therapists are often involved in adapting activities to reduce the executive function requirements of a particular task. For example, occupational therapists may create organizational systems such as picture schedules to help the individual with ASD complete schoolwork or manage job tasks in the workplace. In addition, the occupational therapist may work with teachers, families, and employers to reduce unexpected changes and maintain routines. Strategies can also be implemented to prepare the individual with ASD for altered routines. This might include giving the individual adequate notice to adjust to the change, allowing for self-soothing behaviors, or making small adjustments along the way to a larger change.

Theory of Mind

The Theory of Mind (ToM) deficit is one type of social cognition impairment that is present in ASDs (Baron-Cohen, 1989; Rutherford, Baron-Cohen, & Wheelwright, 2002). There are two ToM levels: first order and second order. First-order ToM is the ability to infer another person's mental state, including his or her beliefs, values, feelings, and perceptions. Second-order ToM is the ability to consider what another person may be thinking about a third person's mental state. For example, when Susan presents the findings of a report to her board, she scans the body language and facial expressions of her audience to ensure the desired effect (first order). Following the report, the executive officer challenges one of the other board members, and Susan watches both the executive officer and the other board member to gauge what each might be thinking about the other (second order). If Susan has an ASD, she might miss the board members' reactions to her and how the board members are responding to one another.

Interventions that focus on socialization, such as social stories, may address ToM impairments in children with autism (Reynout & Carter, 2006). Social stories are individualized scenarios that provide information to the individual with ASD about how to understand and respond to a social situation. Figure 7-2 is a drawing made by an individual with Asperger's disorder, depicting how he struggles with socialization and showing factors that have been helpful, including occupational therapy.

Central Coherence

Central coherence has emerged as a way of understanding the cognitive style of individuals with ASD (Jolliffe & Baron-Cohen, 2001). Central coherence is the ability to take in data and assess the gestalt or big picture meaning, at the risk of compromising memory for the details. This is a useful strategy because it prevents individuals from becoming focused on irrelevant details as opposed to the important meaning of the larger situation. An individual with weak central coherence is better able to secure an understanding of the details without assessing the gestalt meaning. Therefore, the cognitive style of individuals with ASD would be described as weak central coherence. For example, a child with Asperger's disorder (with weak central coherence) is led into a new room and asked to describe it. On leaving the area, he is able to report that there was a small plastic slide, a toy box with dinosaurs in it, cars next

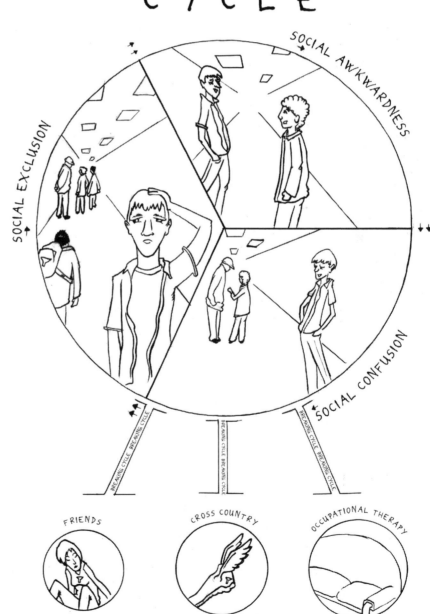

FIGURE 7-2. Nathan is a person with an autism spectrum disorder who is studying graphic design. Here, he depicts struggles with socialization and identifies factors that have been helpful, including occupational therapy.

to a window, and a small table with Legos on it. A child without a disability (with strong central coherence) is brought into the same room and, on leaving, reports that he was in a playroom. When entering a new situation, it can be helpful to identify the bigger picture for the child. The occupational therapist could provide a verbal explanation to the individual who can process it, or use pictures or single words to provide cues as to the most important information. For high school or college students, the individual may need assistance with highlighting or distilling a lecture for the main message.

Adaptive Skills

Adaptive skills include those abilities that are necessary to translate cognitive endowments into an ability to participate in the world, including engagement in social, communication, and daily living skills (Sparrow & Cicchetti, 1985). Consistently, individuals with ASDs demonstrate significantly impaired adaptive skills, which are most notably present in the social and communication domains, with relative strengths in self-care skills (Carter et al, 1998; Volkmar, Carter, Sparrow, & Cicchetti, 1993).

Children and adults with ASD are less likely to have close friendships and to assume roles that involve significant interaction. For example, individuals with ASD who are capable of working are more likely to assume jobs in which they can work in relative isolation and may have difficulties if required to work collaboratively with others. A high schooler who enjoys sports may be challenged with interacting as a team member.

Although individuals with ASDs and lower cognitive ability demonstrate the greatest difficulty with adaptive skills, individuals with average to above average cognitive ability also experience adaptive skill impairments, particularly in the area of socialization (Klin et al, 2007). Consequently, occupational therapists are involved in providing interventions to help children with ASDs acquire adaptive skills, particularly in relation to social interaction. This might include social skills training in which the individual role-plays particular situations and then practices those skills in real life interactions with others. The therapist can provide feedback along the way to strengthen the skills.

Sensory Processing

In her book *Thinking in Pictures*, Temple Grandin (1995) describes her experiences of touch:

> *From as far back as I can remember, I always hated to be hugged. I wanted to experience the good feeling of being hugged, but it was just too overwhelming. It was like a great, all-engulfing tidal wave of stimulation. . . . I was overloaded and would have to escape, often by jerking away suddenly. (p. 58)*

This is one example of the type of sensory processing differences experienced by individuals with ASDs. Sensory processing differences are present across sensations (e.g., oral, auditory, touch, proprioception) and can exist in patterns of low and/or high thresholds (e.g., sensitive to sound and/or does not detect the presence of food on one's face) (Kern et al, 2006). One study of children with ASD found that 95% of children demonstrated some

degree of sensory processing difficulties (Tomcheck & Dunn, 2007).These sensory processing differences vary in modality, threshold, and intensity across individuals (Kientz & Dunn, 1997). In many cases, individuals with ASDs report this as a significant barrier to participating in the world. Specific evidence indicates that problems with auditory processing and underresponsiveness are associated with poorer academic performance (Ashburner, Ziviani, & Rodger, 2008), and tactile defensiveness is associated with community use and social skills (Pfeiffer, Kinnealey, Reed, & Herzberg, 2005).

In a systematic review of interventions for ASD, Case-Smith and Arbesman (2008) found evidence for improved modulation of arousal, which led to better social interactions. The same review found that therapeutic touch may decrease self-stimulation. However, thus far, the research is limited, and the designs are weak. Still, the prevalence of sensory processing concerns suggests a need for occupational therapy intervention. Occupational therapists can intervene by providing a sensory diet to meet the sensory needs of the individual with autism, which might include activities that provide tactile, vestibular, or proprioceptive input. Playground activities, weighted vests, and balls for seating are some examples. Occupational therapists may also modify the environment so that it is more consistent with sensory processing preferences. For example, visual cues in the form of action pictures may be used to augment the verbal requests (e.g., get in line, time for lunch) that are challenging for individuals with ASD to process.

Figure 7-3, a drawing made by an individual with Asperger's disorder, poignantly illustrates the intensity of the experience of sensory overload.

Rett's Disorder

Individuals with RD typically function within the severe to profound range of mental retardation and are particularly vulnerable to significant communication, language, and fine motor delays (Perry, Sarlo-McGarvey, & Haddad, 1991; Van Acker et al, 2005). However, some children can learn to meet their needs through interaction within their environment using situation-specific skills, and these skills can be missed by typical assessments (Demeter, 2000). For example, parents can identify certain actions or vocalizations as meaningful, such as recognition of a familiar face or place.

Individuals with RD experience significant motor and feeding impairments in addition to impaired cognition (Perry et al, 1991; Reilly & Cass, 2001). Some individuals may benefit from referrals to feeding and nutrition specialists because feeding impairments can include swallowing difficulties, aspiration, limited self-feeding, low texture tolerance, and poor appetite (Isaacs, Murdock, Lane, & Percy, 2003; Reilly & Cass, 2001).

One focus of occupational therapy assessment and intervention is strategies for motor skills, paying particular attention to fine motor skills, especially purposeful hand use (Van Acker et al, 2005). Occupational therapists assess participation in context through strategies that include interviews with parents and/or caregivers. Topics include

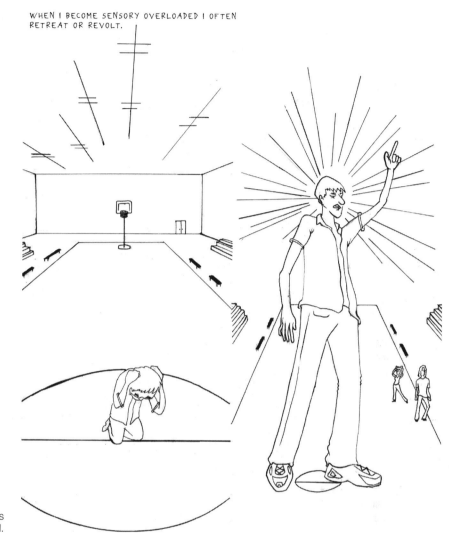

FIGURE 7-3. In this drawing, Nathan illustrates the intensity of the experience of sensory overload.

what an individual appears to have learned (e.g., daily routines, meeting needs), stimuli that has acquired meaning (e.g., photos, objects, activities), and behavior changes that appear to result from the learning process (e.g., eye pointing, producing sounds).

Childhood Disintegrative Disorder

Individuals with CDD typically function within the mild to profound range of mental retardation, and individuals evaluated in a recent study obtained a mean IQ score of 34 (Malhotra & Gupta, 2002). These cognitive impairments interfere significantly with an individual's ability to acquire the daily living and social skills required to navigate the world. Instead of focusing on skill acquisition, occupational therapists can provide parent training to make daily routines such as dressing, feeding, and bathing more efficient and effective. This could include adaptations to objects, such as Velcro fasteners on clothing, or task simplification. Occupational therapists should also consider the social support needs of the parents and provide interventions or referrals for this support.

Evidence-Based Practice

Current literature indicates a poorer prognosis for individuals with CDD as opposed to individuals with ASDs (Mouridsen et al, 1998). It has been hypothesized that the higher rates of institutionalization found among individuals with CDD may contribute to this finding (Kurita et al, 2004).

➤ Occupational therapists can work with families to maintain an individual's participation in the community.

➤ Whether in a community or an institutionalized setting, individuals may profit from environments rich with stimulation, language, and opportunities for activity.

Kurita, H., Osada, H., & Miyake, Y. (2004). External validity of childhood disintegrative disorder in comparison with autistic disorder. *Journal of Autism and Developmental Disorders, 34*(3), 355–362.

Mouridsen, S. E., Rich, B., & Isager, T. (1998). Validity of childhood disintegrative psychosis: General findings of a long-term follow-up study. *British Journal of Psychiatry, 172,* 263–267.

Medications

There are no pharmacological cures that exist for PDDs. To date, studies that explore medication management of both core and peripheral symptoms are limited, and those that incorporate randomized controlled trials are more limited still. However, there are medications that result in documented improvements for individuals with PDDs.

Autism Spectrum Disorders

Empirical support for the pharmacological management of core and peripheral symptoms of ASDs is limited and has been primarily restricted to the investigation of atypical antipsychotic, selective serotonin reuptake inhibitor, and stimulant agents. Of these, atypical antipsychotic medications currently offer the greatest potential for managing symptoms of ASDs.

Atypical Antipsychotics

Atypical antipsychotic medications are used to target the symptoms of aggression, self-injury, severe tantrums, impulsivity, language skills, and social impairments (Scahill, 2005). For individuals across the life span with aggression, self-injury, and severe tantrums, risperidone (Risperdal) has emerged as the standard treatment (Miral et al, 2008; Scahill, 2005). Some other atypical antipsychotics, including clozapine (Clozaril), olanzapine (Zyprexa), and ziprasidone (Geodon), have potential as effective medications, but require more research.

Selective Serotonin Reuptake Inhibitors

Selective serotonin reuptake inhibitors have been the subject of limited research. This class of medications has the potential for some therapeutic benefit for individuals with ASDs, reduction of repetitive thoughts, repetitive behaviors, and anxiety (Kolevzon, Mathewson, & Hollander, 2006). However, individuals with ASDs are at a higher risk for medication-induced agitation, which is a significant complication (Kolevzon et al, 2006).

Stimulants

Preliminary research indicates that stimulants, specifically methylphenidate (Ritalin), can work effectively to manage hyperactivity, impulsivity, and inattention in individuals with ASD that co-occurs with attention deficit-hyperactivity disorder (Santosh, Baird, Pityaratstian, Tavare, & Gringras, 2006). The individuals in this study reported only mild side effects.

Rett's Disorder

Trials of medications that target the fundamental underlying mechanisms of RD have failed to demonstrate lasting or significant improvements (Van Acker et al, 2005). Difficulties associated with RD are treated symptomatically (e.g., medication to treat coexisting epilepsy). Since the discovery of the role of *MECP2* in RD, researchers have begun to use mouse models to explore the mechanisms of the disorder and interventions (e.g., Roux, Dura, Moncla, Mancini, & Villard, 2007). Most recently, researchers have used a mouse model to demonstrate the reversibility of RD neurological impairments, which raises the possibility that the impairment associated with this and related disorders is not irrevocable (Guy, Gan, Selfridge, Cobb, & Bird, 2007).

Childhood Disintegrative Disorder

There are no fixed guidelines for the pharmacological treatment of CDD. The behavior, attention, and other difficulties associated with this disorder are treated symptomatically. Antipsychotics, benzodiazepines, antidepressants, and lithium have been tried with minimal effectiveness (Malhotra & Gupta, 1999). Seizures are treated with antiepileptics, most commonly with carbamazepine (Tegretol) (Malhotra & Gupta, 1999).

Summary

Throughout this chapter, the variability among individuals with PDDs was highlighted. Although all individuals share some level of impairment in social interaction, the severity of this impairment differs widely across individuals. Other concerns, such as stereotypical behavior, cognitive or intellectual impairments, and tactile defensiveness may or may not be present in any one individual. Another theme of this chapter was the strong support for genetic and neurological causes for PDDs. Knowing this information is important so that occupational therapists recognize the uniqueness of each individual and appreciate the neurological contributions of perceived maladaptive behaviors. In doing so, more effective assessment and intervention procedures can be implemented.

Active Learning Strategies

1. Observation

The best way to understand what it means to live with an ASD is to observe an individual with autism across settings. Contact a local chapter of the Autism Society of America to locate an individual or the family of an individual with an ASD who would be interested in sharing their life with you. Ask if you can spend some time observing and talking with them. Using what you have learned from this chapter, develop questions that will promote your understanding of living with an ASD. If possible, observe the individual across settings. For example, if you are in contact with a family of a child, schedule an observation of the child both at school and at home. Many families are eager to promote understanding of ASDs and will welcome you into their lives, but please remember the vulnerability that a family or an individual experiences when opening their lives to another person.

Reflective Questions
- In what ways did the individual encounter success in his or her day? In what ways did he or she encounter difficulty?
- What were the discrepancies between the individual/family's desired roles and activities, and what was actually possible for them?

- Imagine this individual participating in the different contexts of your life. What would be his or her difficulties? What would need to be done to support his or her participation?

Describe the experience in your Reflective Journal.

2. Theory of Mind

Read the section on ToM. Observe an interaction between two individuals with good social skills that involves both verbal and nonverbal communication. You could observe an interaction in real life or watch a video clip from a movie or television show. Identify examples of first-order ToM (the ability to infer another person's mental state) and second-order ToM (consider what another person may be thinking about a third person's mental state). Now consider how the interaction would differ if one of the individuals communicating was lacking in the ability to take another's perspective.

In your Reflective Journal, respond to the following questions.

Reflective Questions

- How observable was ToM perspective-taking in action?
- Describe behaviors that you observed that reflected inferences about another person's mental state?
- How did these behaviors affect the communication?
- What might have occurred if these behaviors were absent? How might it affect communication? How might it affect the feelings that the two individuals have about one another?

Resources

Books

- Grandin, T. (1995). *Thinking in Pictures*. New York: Random House.
- Myles, B. S., & Southwick, J. (2005). *Asperger Syndrome and Difficult Moments: Practical Solutions for Tantrums, Rage, and Meltdowns—Revised and Expanded Edition*. Shawnee Mission, KS: Autism Asperger.
- Robison, J. E. (2007). *Look Me in the Eye: My Life With Asperger's*. New York: Crown.

Organizations

- Autism Society of America: www.autism-society.org
- Autism Speaks: www.autismspeaks.org
- International Rett Syndrome Foundation: www.rettsyndrome.org
- National Institute of Mental Health: www.nimh.nih.gov
- Online Asperger Syndrome Information and Support: www.aspergersyndrome.org
- Organization for Autism Research: www.researchautism.org
- Wrong Planet (an online community for individuals on the spectrum): www.wrongplanet.net

References

American Psychiatric Association (APA). (2000). *Diagnostic and Statistical Manual of Mental Disorders* (4th ed., Text Revision). Washington, DC: Author.

Amir, R. E., Fang, P., Yu, Z., Glaze, D. G., Percy, A. K., Zoghbi, H. Y., Roa, B. B., & Van den Veyver, I. B. (2005). Mutations in exon 1 of *MECP2* are a rare cause of Rett syndrome. *Journal of Medical Genetics, 42*(2), e15.

Armstrong, D., Dunn, J. K., Antalffy, B., & Trivedi, R. (1995). Selective dendritic alterations in the cortex of Rett syndrome. *Journal of Neuropathology and Experimental Neurology, 54*(2), 195–201.

Armstrong, D. D. (2002). Neuropathology of Rett syndrome. *Mental Retardation and Developmental Disability Research Review, 8*(2), 72–76.

Ashburner, J., Ziviani, J., & Rodger, S. (2008). Sensory processing and classroom emotional, behavioral, and educational outcomes in children with autism spectrum disorder. *American Journal of Occupational Therapy, 62*(5), 564–573.

Bailey, A., Le Couteur, A., Gottesman, I., Bolton, P., Simonoff, E., Yuzda, E., & Rutter, M. (1995). Autism as a strongly genetic disorder: Evidence from a British twin study. *Psychological Medicine, 25*(1), 63–77.

Barnard, L., Muldoon, K., Hasan, R., O'Brien, G., & Stewart, M. (2008). Prevalence of executive dysfunction in adults with autism and comorbid learning disability. *Autism, 12,* 125–141.

Baron-Cohen, S. (1989). The autistic child's theory of mind: A case of specific developmental delay. *Journal of Child Psychology and Psychiatry, 30*(2), 285–297.

Bhasin, T. K., & Schendel, D. (2007). Sociodemographic risk factors for autism in a US metropolitan area. *Journal of Autism and Developmental Disorders, 37*(4), 667–677.

Bolte, S., & Poutska, F. (2002). The relation between genetics, cognitive level and adaptive behavior domains in individuals with autism with and without comorbid mental retardation. *Child Psychiatry and Human Development, 33,* 165–172.

Bolton, P., Macdonald, H., Pickles, A., Rios, P., Goode, S., Crowson, M., Bailey, A., & Rutter, M. (1994). A case-control family history study of autism. *Journal of Child Psychology and Psychiatry, 35*(5), 877–900.

Buxbaum, J. D., Silverman, J. M., Smith, C. J., Kilifarski, M., Reichert, J., Hollander, E., Lawlor, B. A., Fitzgerald, M., Greenberg, D. A., & Davis, K. L. (2001). Evidence for a susceptibility gene for autism on chromosome 2 and for genetic heterogeneity. *American Journal of Human Genetics, 68*(6), 1514–1520.

Carter, A. S., Volkmar, F. R., Sparrow, S. S., Wang, J. J., Lord, C., Dawson, G., Fombonne, E., Mesibov, G., & Schopler, E.. (1998). The Vineland Adaptive Behavior Scales: Supplementary norms for individuals with autism. *Journal of Autism and Developmental Disorders, 28*(4), 287–302.

Case-Smith, J., & Arbesman, M. (2008). Evidence based review of interventions for autism used in or relevant to occupational therapy. *American Journal of Occupational Therapy, 62,* 416–429.

Cederlund, M., Hagberg, B., Billstedt, E., Gillberg, I. C., & Gillberg, C. (2008). Asperger syndrome and autism: A comparative longitudinal follow-up study more than 5 years after original diagnosis. *Journal of Autism and Developmental Disorders, 38*(1), 72–85.

Centers for Disease Control and Prevention (CDC). (2007). *Prevalence of Autism Spectrum Disorders—Autism and Developmental Disabilities Monitoring Network, 14 Sites, United States, 2002.* http://www.cdc.gov/mmwr/preview/mmwrhtml/ss5601a2.htm. Retrieved January 18, 2010.

Chakrabarti, S., & Fombonne, E. (2001). Pervasive developmental disorders in preschool children. *JAMA, 285*(24), 3093–3099.

Chakrabarti, S., & Fombonne, E. (2005). Pervasive developmental disabilities in preschool children: Confirmation of high prevalence. *American Journal of Psychiatry, 162,* 1133–1141.

Chudley, A. E., Gutierrez, E., Jocelyn, L. J., & Chodirker, B. N. (1998). Outcomes of genetic evaluation in children with pervasive developmental disorder. *Journal of Developmental and Behavioral Pediatrics, 19*(5), 321–325.

Dawson, G. (2008). Early behavioral intervention, brain plasticity and prevention of autism spectrum disorders. *Developmental Psychopathology, 20,* 775–803.

Deguchi, K., Antalffy, B. A., Twohill, L. J., Chakraborty, S., Glaze, D. G., & Armstrong, D. D. (2000). Substance P immunoreactivity in Rett syndrome. *Pediatric Neurology, 22*(4), 259–266.

Demeter, K. (2000). Assessing the developmental level in Rett syndrome: An alternative approach? *European Child and Adolescent Psychiatry, 9*(3), 227–233.

Dragich, J., Houwink-Manville, I., & Schanen, C. (2000). Rett syndrome: A surprising result of mutation in *MECP2. Human and Molecular Genetics, 9*(16), 2365–2375.

Folstein, S., & Rutter, M. (1977). Infantile autism: A genetic study of 21 twin pairs. *Journal of Child Psychology and Psychiatry, 18*(4), 297–321.

Fombonne, E., & Tidmarsh, L. (2003). Epidemiologic data on Asperger disorder. *Child and Adolescent Psychiatry Clinics of North America, 12*(1), 15–21, v–vi.

Fombonne, E., Zakarian, R., Bennett, A., Meng, L., & McLean-Heywood, D. (2006). Pervasive developmental disorders in Montreal, Quebec, Canada: Prevalence and links with immunizations. *Pediatrics, 118*(1), e139–e150.

Fred R. P., Volkmar, R., Klin, A., & Cohen, D. (2005). *Handbook of Autism and Pervasive Developmental Disorders.* Hoboken, NJ: John Wiley & Sons.

Grandin, T. (1995). *Thinking in Pictures.* New York: Random House.

Guideri, F., Acampa, M., Blardi, P., de Lalla, A., Zappella, M., & Hayek, Y. (2004). Cardiac dysautonomia and serotonin plasma levels in Rett syndrome. *Neuropediatrics, 35*(1), 36–38.

Guy, J., Gan, J., Selfridge, J., Cobb, S., & Bird, A. (2007). Reversal of neurological defects in a mouse model of Rett syndrome. *Science, 315*(5815), 1143–1147.

Hagberg, B. (2002). Clinical manifestations and stages of Rett syndrome. *Mental Retardation and Developmental Disability Research and Review, 8*(2), 61–65.

Hagberg, B., Hanefeld, F., Percy, A., & Skjeldal, O. (2002). An update on clinically applicable diagnostic criteria in Rett syndrome. Comments to Rett Syndrome Clinical Criteria Consensus Panel Satellite to European Paediatric Neurology Society Meeting, Baden Baden, Germany, 11 September 2001. *European Journal Paediatric Neurology, 6*(5), 293–297.

Hagberg, B., & Witt-Engerstrom, I. (1986). Rett syndrome: A suggested staging system for describing impairment profile with increasing age towards adolescence. *American Journal Medical Genetics, 1*(suppl), 47–59.

Hartley, S. C., Sikora, D. M., & McCoy, R. (2008). Prevalence and increased risk factors of maladaptive behavior in young children with autistic disorder. *Journal of Intellectual Disability Research, 52,* 819–829.

Isaacs, J. S., Murdock, M., Lane, J., & Percy, A. K. (2003). Eating difficulties in girls with Rett syndrome compared with other developmental disabilities. *Journal of the American Dietetic Association, 103*(2), 224–230.

Jolliffe, T., & Baron-Cohen, S. (2001). A test of central coherence theory: Can adults with high-functioning autism or Asperger syndrome integrate fragments of an object? *Cognitive Neuropsychiatry, 6*(3), 193–216.

Kaufmann, W. E., Naidu, S., & Budden, S. (1995). Abnormal expression of microtubule-associated protein 2 (MAP-2) in neocortex in Rett syndrome. *Neuropediatrics, 26*(2), 109–113.

Kenworthy, L. E., Black, D. O., Wallace, G. L., Ahluvalia, T., Wagner, A. E., & Sirian, L. M. (2005). Disorganization: The forgotten executive dysfunction in high-functioning autism (HFA) spectrum disorders. *Developmental Neuropsychology, 28*(3), 809–827.

Kern, J. K., Trivedi, M. H., Garver, C. R., Grannemann, B. D., Andrews, A. A., Savla, J. S., Johnson, D.J., Mehta, J. A., & Schroeder, J. L. (2006). The pattern of sensory processing abnormalities in autism. *Autism, 10*(5), 480–494.

Kientz, M. A., & Dunn, W. (1997). A comparison of the performance of children with and without autism on the Sensory Profile. *American Journal of Occupational Therapy, 51*(7), 530–537.

Klin, A., Saulnier, C. A., Sparrow, S. S., Cicchetti, D. V., Volkmar, F. R., & Lord, C. (2007). Social and communication abilities and disabilities in higher functioning individuals with autism spectrum disorders: The Vineland and the ADOS. *Journal of Autism and Developmental Disorders, 37*(4), 748–759.

Kolevzon, A., Mathewson, K. A., & Hollander, E. (2006). Selective serotonin reuptake inhibitors in autism: A review of efficacy and tolerability. *Journal of Clinical Psychiatry, 67*(3), 407–414.

Kurita, H., Osada, H., & Miyake, Y. (2004). External validity of childhood disintegrative disorder in comparison with autistic disorder. *Journal of Autism and Developmental Disorders, 34*(3), 355–362.

Le Couteur, A., Bailey, A., Goode, S., Pickles, A., Robertson, S., Gottesman, I., & Rutter, M. (1996). A broader phenotype of autism: The clinical spectrum in twins. *Journal of Child Psychology and Psychiatry, 37*(7), 785–801.

Lombroso, P. J. (2000). Genetics of childhood disorders: XIV. A gene for Rett syndrome: News flash. *Journal of the American Academy of Child and Adolescent Psychiatry, 39*(5), 671–674.

Malhotra, S., & Gupta, N. (1999). Childhood disintegrative disorder. *Journal of Autism and Developmental Disorders, 29*(6), 491–498.

Malhotra, S., & Gupta, N. (2002). Childhood disintegrative disorder: Re-examination of the current concept. *European Child and Adolescent Psychiatry, 11*(3), 108–114.

Mazfesky, C. A., Williams, D. L., & Minshew, N. J. (2008). Variability in adaptive behavior in autism: Evidence for the importance of family history. *Journal of Abnormal Child Psychology, 36,* 591–599.

Miral, S., Gencer, O., Inal-Emiroglu, F. N., Baykara, B., Baykara, A., & Dirik, E. (2008). Risperidone versus haloperidol in children and adolescents with AD: A randomized, controlled, double-blind trial. *European Child and Adolescent Psychiatry, 17*(1), 1–8.

Mouridsen, S. E., Rich, B., & Isager, T. (1998). Validity of childhood disintegrative psychosis: General findings of a long-term follow-up study. *British Journal of Psychiatry, 172,* 263–267.

Muller, E., Schuler A., & Yates, G. B. (2008). Social challenges and supports from the perspective of individuals with Asperger's disorder and other autism spectrum disorders. *Autism, 12,* 173–196.

Naidu, S., Kaufmann, W. E., Abrams, M. T., Pearlson, G. D., Lanham, D. C., Fredericksen, K. A., et al. (2001). Neuroimaging studies in Rett syndrome. *Brain Development, 23*(suppl 1), S62–S71.

Panerai, S., Ferrante, L., & Zingale, M. (2002). Benefits of the Treatment and Education of Autistic and Communication Handicapped Children (TEACCH) program compared to a non-specific approach. *Journal of Intellectual Disability Research, 46,* 318–327.

Pelphrey, K. A., Morris, J. P., McCarthy, G., & Labar, K. S. (2007). Perception of dynamic changes in facial affect and identity in autism. *Social, Cognitive and Affect Neuroscience, 2*(2), 140–149.

Perry, A., Sarlo-McGarvey, N., & Haddad, C. (1991). Brief report: Cognitive and adaptive functioning in 28 girls with Rett syndrome. *Journal of Autism and Developmental Disorders, 21*(4), 551–556.

Pfeiffer, B., Kinnealey, M., Reed, C., & Herzberg, G. (2005). Sensory modulation and affective disorders in children and adolescents with autism spectrum disorders. *American Journal of Occupational Therapy, 59,* 335–345.

Pickles, A., Bolton, P., Macdonald, H., Bailey, A., Le Couteur, A., Sim, C. H., Rutter, M. (1995). Latent-class analysis of recurrence risks for complex phenotypes with selection and measurement error: A twin and family history study of autism. *American Journal Human Genetics, 57*(3), 717–726.

Pinkham, A. E., Hopfinger, J. B., Pelphrey, K. A., Piven, J., & Penn, D. L. (2007). Neural bases for impaired social cognition in schizophrenia and autism spectrum disorders. *Schizophrenia Research, 99,* 164–175.

Reilly, S., & Cass, H. (2001). Growth and nutrition in Rett syndrome. *Disability Rehabilitation, 23*(3–4), 118–128.

Remington, B., Hastings, R. P., Kovshoff, H., Espinosa, F., Jahr, E., Brown, T., Alsford, P., Lemaic, M., & Ward, N. (2007). Early intensive behavioral intervention: Outcomes for children with autism and their parents after two years. *American Journal of Mental Retardation, 112,* 418–438.

Reynout, G., & Carter, M. (2006). Social stories for children with disabilities. *Journal of Autism and Developmental Disabilities, 36,* 445–469.

Rogers, S. J., & Vismara, C. A. (2008). Evidence-based comprehensive treatments for early autism. *Journal of Clinical Child and Adolescent Psychology, 37*(1), 8–38.

Rojas, D. C., Bawn, S. D., Benkers, T. L., Reite, M. L., & Rogers, S. J. (2002). Smaller left hemisphere planum temporale in adults with autistic disorder. *Neuroscience Letters, 328*(3), 237–240.

Roux, J. C., Dura, E., Moncla, A., Mancini, J., & Villard, L. (2007). Treatment with desipramine improves breathing and survival in a mouse model for Rett syndrome. *European Journal of Neuroscience, 25*(7), 1915–1922.

Rutherford, M. D., Baron-Cohen, S., & Wheelwright, S. (2002). Reading the mind in the voice: A study with normal adults and adults with Asperger syndrome and high functioning autism. *Journal of Autism and Developmental Disorders, 32*(3), 189–194.

Santosh, P. J., Baird, G., Pityaratstian, N., Tavare, E., & Gringras, P. (2006). Impact of comorbid autism spectrum disorders on stimulant response in children with attention deficit hyperactivity disorder: A retrospective and prospective effectiveness study. *Child Care Health Development, 32*(5), 575–583.

Scahill, L. A. M. (2005). Psychopharmacology. In F. R. Volkmar, R. Paul, A. Klin, & D. Cohen (Eds.), *Handbook of Autism and Pervasive Developmental Disorders* (3rd ed., Vol. 2, pp. 1102–1117). Hoboken, NJ: John Wiley & Sons.

Schultz, R. T., Grelotti, D. J., Klin, A., Kleinman, J., Van der Gaag, C., Marois, R., Skudlarski, P. (2003). The role of the fusiform face area in social cognition: Implications for the pathobiology of autism. *Philosophical Transactions of the Royal Society B: Biological Sciences, 358*(1430), 415–427.

Schultz, R. T., & Robins, D. L. (2005). Functional neuroimaging studies of autism spectrum disorders. In F. R. Volkmar, R. Paul, A. Klin, & D. J. Cohen (Eds.), *Handbook of Autism and Pervasive Developmental Disorders* (3rd ed., Vol. 1, pp. 515–533). Hoboken, NJ: John Wiley & Sons.

Sparrow, S. S., & Cicchetti, D. V. (1985). Diagnostic uses of the Vineland Adaptive Behavior Scales. *Journal of Pediatric Psychology, 10*(2), 215–225.

Stanfield, A. C., McIntosh, A. M., Spencer, M. D., Philip, R., Gaur, S., & Lawrie, S. M. (2007). Towards a neuroanatomy of autism: A systematic review and meta-analysis of structural magnetic resonance imaging studies. *European Psychiatry, 24,* 1–16.

Subramaniam, B., Naidu, S., & Reiss, A. L. (1997). Neuroanatomy in Rett syndrome: Cerebral cortex and posterior fossa. *Neurology, 48*(2), 399–407.

Temudo, T., Oliveira, P., Santos, M., Dias, K., Vieira, J., Moreira, A., Calado, E., Carrilho, I., Oliveira, A., Levy, C., Barbot, M., Fonseca, A., Cabral, A., Dias, P., Cabral, J., Monteiro, L., Borges, R., Gomes, C., Barbosa, G., Mira, G., Eusebio, F., Santos, M., Sequeiro, J., & Maciel, P. (2007). Stereotypies in Rett syndrome: Analysis of 83 patients with and without detected *MECP2* mutations. *Neurology, 68*(15), 1183–1187.

Tomcheck, S. D., & Dunn, W. (2007). Sensory processing in children with and without autism: A comparative study using the Short Sensory Profile. *American Journal of Occupational Therapy, 61,* 190–200.

Van Acker, R., Loncola, J. A., & Van Acker, E. Y. (2005). Rett syndrome: A pervasive developmental disorder. In R. P. F. R. Volkmar, A. Klin, & D. Cohen (Eds.), *Handbook of Autism and Pervasive Developmental Disorders* (3rd ed., Vol. 1).(pp. 60–93). Hoboken, NJ: John Wiley & Sons.

Van den Veyver, I. B., & Zoghbi, H. Y. (2001). Mutations in the gene encoding methyl-CpG-binding protein 2 cause Rett syndrome. *Brain Development, 23*(suppl 1), S147–S151.

Verte, S., Geurts, H. M., Roeyers, H., Oosterlaan, J., & Sergeant, J. A. (2006). Executive functioning in children with an autism spectrum disorder: Can we differentiate within the spectrum? *Journal of Autism and Developmental Disorders, 36*(3), 351–372.

Viemari, J. C., Roux, J. C., Tryba, A. K., Saywell, V., Burnet, H., Pena, F., Zanella, S., Bevengut, M., Barthelemy-Requin, M., Herzing, L.B.K., Moncla, A., Mancini, J., Ramirez, J. M., Villard, L. & Hilaire, G. (2005). *Mecp2* deficiency disrupts norepinephrine and respiratory systems in mice. *Journal of Neuroscience, 25*(50), 11521–11530.

Volkmar, F. R., Carter, A., Sparrow, S. S., & Cicchetti, D. V. (1993). Quantifying social development in autism. *Journal of American Academy of Child and Adolescent Psychiatry, 32*(3), 627–632.

Volkmar, F. R., Koenig, K., & State, M. (2005). Childhood disintegrative disorder. In F. R. Volkmar, R. Paul, A. Klin, & D. J. Cohen (Eds.), *Handbook of Autism and Pervasive Developmental Disorders* (3rd ed., Vol. 1, pp. 70–87). Hoboken, NJ: John Wiley & Sons.

Yeargin-Allsopp, M., Rice, C., Karapurkar, T., Doernberg, N., Boyle, C., & Murphy, C. (2003). Prevalence of autism in a US metropolitan area. *JAMA, 289*(1), 49–55.

Zoghbi, H. Y., Percy, A. K., Glaze, D. G., Butler, I. J., & Riccardi, V. M. (1985). Reduction of biogenic amine levels in the Rett syndrome. *New England Journal of Medicine, 313*(15), 921–924.

Attention and Disruptive Behavior Disorders

Judith S. Gonyea and Vaune Kopeck

> Pooh needs intervention. We feel drugs are in order. We cannot but wonder how much richer Pooh's life might be were he to have a trial of low-dose stimulant medication. With the right supports, including methylphenidate, Pooh might be fitter and more functional and perhaps produce (and remember) more poems.
> I take a PILL-tiddley pom It keeps me STILL-tiddley pom, It keeps me STILL-tiddley pom Not fiddling . . .
> We acknowledge that Tigger is gregarious and affectionate, but he has a recurrent pattern of risk-taking behaviours. Look, for example, at his impulsive sampling of unknown substances when he first comes to the Hundred Acre Wood. With the mildest of provocation he tries honey, haycorns and even thistles. Tigger has no knowledge of the potential outcome of his experimentation. Later we find him climbing tall trees and acting in a way that can only be described as socially intrusive. He leads Roo into danger.
>
> —Shea, Gordon, Hawkins, Kawchuk, and Smith, 2000

Introduction

From the moment we are born, the world provides each of us with a wide array of interesting and not-so-interesting information to gather, sort, and recall. Most individuals will, in time, learn to manage this complex task with enough efficiency to engage in a lifetime of occupations. Others are not so fortunate and find the task of attending to each day's events difficult, if not impossible. Those individuals who are challenged by attention-based disorders struggle to maintain the threads of each process and filter or sort the barrage of incoming information. Other individuals with conduct disorders miss the cues that provide the parameters of expected social engagement.

The clinical review of Pooh and friends from the Hundred Acre Wood (Shea, Gordon, Hawkins, Kawchuk, & Smith, 2000) aroused some controversy because these familiar characters were identified as being like countless children and adults who are challenged with attention and disruptive behavior disorders. It is significant that, despite the unique challenges of each of A.A. Milne characters in the Pooh series, each was beloved by many. Individuals with similar disorders deserve the same fond regard.

Occupational therapists can play a key role in influencing an individual's or family's decisions regarding attention deficit and disruptive behavior disorders. Occupational therapists' knowledge of the components of function and the environment can help individuals and families create options to manage sensory and organizational challenges, giving each individual the opportunities to succeed in his or her own way. This can make the difference between an individual's exclusion from or avoidance of daily activities and the ability to fully participate in a functional daily routine.

Description of the Disorders

Children are typically curious and often adventurous, which makes the diagnosis of attention and disruptive disorders challenging. Knowing when, despite his or her best attempts, a child cannot sustain attention to complete his or her most interesting tasks, is a critical factor in helping determine the potential presence of attention deficit or disruptive disorders. A complex process of ruling out a multitude of potential alternative disorders with careful attention to patterns or frequency of behaviors is required. Parents, teachers, therapists, and others who frequently observe the individual within his or her daily contexts may be engaged in this process.

Generally, attention-based and disruptive disorders are diagnosed "when problems with attention, hyperactivity, and impulsiveness develop in childhood and persist, in some cases into adulthood" (American Psychiatric Association, 2000, p. 85). Diagnoses within this category include

- Attention deficit-hyperactivity disorder and its variations
- Conduct disorder
- Oppositional defiant disorder
- Disruptive behavior disorder, not otherwise specified

Individuals with these disorders are now increasingly recognized within the adult population, and research into the characteristics of attention and disruptive behavior disorders in this life stage continues to emerge (Volkmar, 2005). Further research is exploring the association between these disorders and development of personality, as well as personality disorders in adults (Anckarsater et al, 2006).

DSM-IV-TR Criteria

A review of the criteria indicates that varying degrees of inattention, disorganization, excess activity, and impulsivity interplay to determine each specific diagnosis. The hallmark of this diagnostic category is that the inability to focus and control movement and behavior results in maladaptive skills, including impaired social engagement.

Scheres et al (2004) support theories of response inhibition (in prefrontal cortical areas) and executive function deficits in childhood **attention deficit-hyperactivity disorder (ADHD).** These neurological descriptions help identify the difficulty many children with attention deficit demonstrate in social situations, for example, saying or doing something that is inconsistent with the social demands at the time.

Although many individuals with ADHD present with symptoms of both inattention and hyperactivity-impulsivity, there are individuals in whom one or the other pattern is predominant. The appropriate subtype for a current diagnosis is based on the predominant symptom pattern for the past 6 months. Subtypes of ADHD include

- Attention deficit-hyperactivity disorder, combined type
- Attention deficit-hyperactivity disorder, predominantly inattentive type
- Attention deficit-hyperactivity disorder, predominantly hyperactive-impulsive type

The **attention deficit-hyperactivity disorder, combined type** subtype is used if six (or more) symptoms of hyperactivity-impulsivity have persisted for at least 6 months. Most children and adolescents with the disorder have the combined type. It is not known whether the same is true of adults with the disorder.

The **attention deficit-hyperactivity disorder, predominantly inattentive type** is used if six (or more) symptoms of inattention (but less than six symptoms of hyperactivity-impulsivity) have persisted for at least 6 months. Hyperactivity may still be a significant clinical feature in many such cases, whereas other cases are more purely inattentive.

The **attention deficit-hyperactivity disorder, predominantly hyperactive-impulsive type** is used if six (or more) symptoms of hyperactivity-impulsivity (but less than six symptoms of inattention) have persisted for at least 6 months. Inattention may often still be a significant clinical feature in such cases.

The detailed *Diagnostic and Statistical Manual of Mental Disorders, Fourth Edition, Text Revision* (DSM-IV-TR) criteria for ADHD are outlined in Box 8-1.

Conduct disorder has far more significant social elements than ADHD and is noted when the individual also engages in high-risk or harmful activity. Searlight, Rottnek, and Abby (2001) note that this disorder "increases the risk of several public health problems including violence, weapon use, teenage pregnancy, substance abuse, and dropping out of school" (p. 1579). Age of onset plays a factor in the selection of this diagnosis, and criteria have been revised as more specific data about age groups have emerged. Behaviors that are elements of social- or peer-influenced adolescent defiance may also suggest other diagnoses such as **antisocial personality disorder**. The detailed DSM-IV-TR criteria for conduct disorder are outlined in Box 8-2.

BOX 8-1 ■ DSM-IV-TR Diagnostic Criteria for ADHD

A. Either (1) or (2):

1. Six (or more) of the following symptoms of **inattention** have persisted for at least 6 months to a degree that is maladaptive and inconsistent with developmental level:

Inattention

a. Often fails to give close attention to details or makes careless mistakes in schoolwork, work, or other activities
b. Often has difficulty sustaining attention in tasks or play activities
c. Often does not seem to listen when spoken to directly
d. Often does not follow through on instructions and fails to finish schoolwork, chores, or duties in the workplace (not due to oppositional behavior or failure to understand instructions)
e. Often has difficulty organizing tasks and activities
f. Often avoids, dislikes, or is reluctant to engage in tasks that require sustained mental effort (e.g., schoolwork, homework)
g. Often loses things necessary for tasks or activities (e.g., toys, school assignments, pencils, books, tools)
h. Is often easily distracted by extraneous stimuli
i. Is often forgetful in daily activities

2. Six (or more) of the following symptoms of **hyperactivity-impulsivity** have persisted for at least 6 months to a degree that is maladaptive and inconsistent with developmental level:

Hyperactivity

a. Often fidgets with hands or feet or squirms in seat
b. Often leaves seat in classroom or in other situations in which remaining seated is expected
c. Often runs about or climbs excessively in situations in which it is inappropriate (in adolescents or adults, may be limited to subjective feelings of restlessness)
d. Often has difficulty playing or engaging in leisure activities quietly
e. Is often "on the go" or acts as if "driven by a motor"
f. Often talks excessively

Impulsivity

g. Often blurts out answers before questions have been completed
h. Often has difficulty waiting turn
i. Often interrupts or intrudes on others (e.g., butts into conversations or games)

B. Some hyperactive-impulsive or inattentive symptoms that caused impairment were present before age 7 years.

C. Some impairment from the symptoms is present in two or more settings (e.g., at school [or work] and at home).

D. There must be clear evidence of clinically significant impairment in social, academic, or occupational functioning.

E. The symptoms do not occur exclusively during the course of a pervasive developmental disorder, schizophrenia, or other psychotic disorder and are not better accounted for by another mental disorder (e.g., mood disorder, anxiety disorder, dissociative disorder, or personality disorder).

From American Psychiatric Association. (2000). *Diagnostic and Statistical Manual of Mental Disorders* (4th ed.). Washington, DC: Author.

BOX 8-2 ■ DSM-IV-TR Diagnostic Criteria for Conduct Disorder

A. A repetitive and persistent pattern of behavior in which the basic rights of others or major age-appropriate societal norms or rules are violated, as manifested by the presence of three (or more) of the following criteria in the past 12 months, with at least one criterion present in the past 6 months:

Aggression to people and animals

1. Often bullies, threatens, or intimidates others
2. Often initiates physical fights
3. Has used a weapon that can cause serious physical harm to others (e.g., a bat, brick, broken bottle, knife, gun)
4. Has been physically cruel to people
5. Has been physically cruel to animals
6. Has stolen while confronting a victim (e.g., mugging, purse snatching, extortion, armed robbery)
7. Has forced someone into sexual activity

Destruction of property

8. Has deliberately engaged in fire-setting with the intention of causing serious damage
9. Has deliberately destroyed others' property (other than by fire-setting)

Deceitfulness or theft

10. Has broken into someone else's house, building, or car

11. Often lies to obtain goods or favors or to avoid obligations (i.e., "cons" others)
12. Has stolen items of nontrivial value without confronting a victim (e.g., shoplifting, but without breaking and entering; forgery)

Serious violations of rules

13. Often stays out at night despite parental prohibitions, beginning before age 13 years
14. Has run away from home overnight at least twice while living in parental or parental surrogate home (or once without returning for a lengthy period)
15. Is often truant from school, beginning before age 13 years

B. The disturbance in behavior causes clinically significant impairment in social, academic, or occupational functioning.

C. If the individual is age 18 years or older, criteria are not met for antisocial personality disorder.

Specify type based on age at onset:

■ *Childhood-Onset Type:* onset of at least one criterion characteristic of conduct disorder prior to age 10 years
■ *Adolescent-Onset Type:* absence of any criteria characteristic of conduct disorder prior to age 10 years
■ *Unspecified Onset:*

From American Psychiatric Association. (2000). *Diagnostic and Statistical Manual of Mental Disorders* (4th ed.). Washington, DC: Author.

Oppositional defiant disorder (ODD), usually diagnosed in childhood, is a psychiatric disorder characterized by two separate behavioral categories. These behaviors include aggression and the tendency to be purposefully bothersome, annoying, and/or irritating to others. These behaviors are often the reason that caregivers, clinicians, and teachers seek treatment (Chandler, 2008). The detailed DSM-IV-TR criteria for ODD are outlined in Box 8-3.

Disruptive behavior disorder, not otherwise specified, provides a more general category for diagnosis, and this designation is used when an individual presents with many of the same signs and symptoms that are noted in the attention deficit, conduct disorder, and ODD categories, but may not fit neatly into a diagnostic criteria as noted. Use of this category may enable initial intervention toward management of the disorder until further evaluation can be performed. In some cases, this diagnosis may remain throughout the course of treatment.

For each diagnostic category, it is important to note that much research continues across many disciplines. As Andres Martin (2005) notes in his editorial review of emerging studies, "For now, optimism and enthusiasm in the context of these studies, and awareness about the risky business of complacency, should together spur us to do more for the many with ADHD" (p. 1577).

Etiology

No specific cause (or causes) is cited for these disorders at this time, although neural regulatory processes are specific areas of concern. Research continues into the many variants of

---

BOX 8-3 ■ DSM-IV-TR Diagnostic Criteria for Oppositional Defiant Disorder

A. A pattern of negativistic, hostile, and defiant behavior lasting at least 6 months, during which four (or more) of the following are present:

1. Often loses temper
2. Often argues with adults
3. Often actively defies or refuses to comply with adults' requests or rules
4. Often deliberately annoys people
5. Often blames others for his or her mistakes or misbehavior
6. Is often touchy or easily annoyed by others
7. Is often angry and resentful
8. Is often spiteful or vindictive

Note: Consider a criterion met only if the behavior occurs more frequently than is typically observed in individuals of comparable age and developmental level.

B. The disturbance in behavior causes clinically significant impairment in social, academic, or occupational functioning.

C. The behaviors do not occur exclusively during the course of a psychotic or mood disorder.

D. Criteria are not met for conduct disorder, and, if the individual is age 18 years or older, criteria are not met for antisocial personality disorder

From American Psychiatric Association. (2000). *Diagnostic and Statistical Manual of Mental Disorders* (4th ed.). Washington, DC: Author.

attention and disruptive behavior disorders (Pliszka, Carlson, & Swanson, 1999). Genetic patterns across families and into adulthood have been considered (Martin, 2005), as well as a variety of neurobiological processing patterns of unknown etiology (Volkmar, 2005). Neuroimaging is leading to information about potential deficits in inhibitory control areas of the brain in individuals with ADHD (Pliszka et al, 2006) and the effects of medication on these regions. The complex process of differential diagnosis and information gathering through family history, neuroimaging, blood chemistry studies, and medication trials continue to build this body of knowledge.

Prevalence

In a review of data from 2003 by the Centers for Disease Control and Prevention, Visser and Lesesne (2005) estimate that, based on parent-reported data, 4.4 million children ages 4 to 17 years, or approximately 7.8%, were diagnosed with ADHD in the year 2003. Of those reported, they also noted that 56% were identified as receiving medication. It should be noted that diagnosis of these disorders often begins under a primary care physician's care (Searlight et al, 2001); thus, data regarding diagnosis and treatment may be difficult to gather because the primary care provider may not be coding or reporting data that are identified with aggregate samples for these diagnoses.

Although prevalence of conduct disorders is also subject to coding difficulties, the U.S. Department of Health and Human Services (1999) reported that conduct disorders were more likely to be found in boys than girls and more likely in urban areas than rural areas. Overall, conduct disorders affect 1% to 4% of youth ages 9 to 17 years, depending on exactly how each disorder is defined.

In addition, the growing body of knowledge and research regarding medications and their indications and contraindications (Pliszka et al, 2006) makes decisions regarding diagnosis and treatment even more complex. Several categories of medication may be used, including stimulants, mood stabilizers, and neuroleptics, although their use may be "off label," that is, not specifically indicated for use with these disorders. In this case, prescriptive elements such as dosage, frequency, and duration are not readily available. Medications may be combined in order to manage the range of symptoms indicated, and each individual's response to medication must be evaluated with regard to both effectiveness and side effects, with adjustments made accordingly. For some individuals with more complex symptoms or medication needs, brief or extended hospitalization may be indicated in order for these medication adjustments to occur.

Gender and Cultural Considerations

Cultural differences from community to nation can influence the perception of these strongly behavioral-based disorders. A study by Biederman, Faraone, and Monuteaux (2002) noted an increased tendency toward ADHD in boys over girls living in environments with lower social class and other environment risks. This class difference may be further noted in a study of African American boys and girls from lower-income families who showed a greater tendency for earlier onset of conduct disorder (Kilgore, Snyder, & Lentz, 2000). Resources for intervention may be less readily available in these settings, and interventions may be resisted or unwelcomed by some.

Gender differences may be more difficult to determine. Disney, Elkins, McGue, and Iacono (1999) reported no significant gender differences toward development of substance abuse in adolescents diagnosed with conduct disorder. In a Nova Scotia study, Waschbusch and King (2006) noted that statistics regarding girls with ADHD or ODD may not reflect the actual prevalence of the disorder due to rater bias, when raters may not identify girls' behavior as being as significant as males', or the diagnostic criteria itself may reflect tendencies more prevalent among males (e.g., more physical aggression vs verbal aggression).

Intervention may also be culturally referenced, and therapists working with international or multicultural populations should consider these regionally or culturally specific beliefs and expectations during the intervention planning process. Curtis, Pisecco, Hamilton, and Moore (2006) notes differences in intervention between the United States and New Zealand, where it is believed that "academic failure or learning disorders" (p. 173) are at the root of these disorders. This shifts treatment to a teacher-focused model versus one in which counseling or behavioral intervention is primary.

Olfson, Gameroff, Marcus, and Jensen (2003) reported a higher rate of treatment among white than black children in the United States, although there is no conclusive information regarding this tendency, which could indicate either lack of access or lack of willingness to participate. Beliefs about behavioral management and family roles could influence these statistics. In the Virgin Islands (Dudley-Grant, 2001), treatment for conduct disorder and other similar disorders continues to emerge as this culture becomes increasingly influenced by Western beliefs and practices. Its predominantly black culture creates its own standards for family relationships that are less influenced by white or European standards.

Course

Because identification and treatment of ADHD and disruptive behavior disorders has been increasing over the past decade or more (Olfson et al, 2003), the course of these conditions remains somewhat uncertain. Anckarsater et al (2006) suggest that there may be many more associations between childhood ADHD and autism spectrum disorder with adult personality disorders and other conditions. Studies continue to investigate the prevalence of these conditions and patterns into adulthood. It might be helpful for the reader to reference Chapter 11.

Impact on Occupational Performance

Jackson and Arbesman (2005) developed occupational therapy practice guidelines for children with behavioral and psychosocial needs as part of a larger set of guidelines across several practice areas. These guidelines provide a good starting point when framing the role of occupational therapy with individuals challenged by attention deficit or disruptive behavior patterns. Information about using the occupational therapy process, including evidence-based

The Lived Experience

Three different lived experiences are included in this chapter so that the reader learns from the different perspectives of a child, an adult, and a parent.

Nate

Nate is a 9-year-old boy who attends the third grade and has changed schools twice this year, from a parochial school to two public schools, while trying to find the goodness of fit for his educational needs.

Q: What is a regular day like for you from the time you get up until the time you go to bed?

A: *On the weekends, it goes pretty good unless me and my friends get into a fight. 'Cause me and Mark always get into a fight. Sometimes we hit, but one day we got into a fight. I thought, "Let's talk about this . . . because if it gets any worse, someone's going to call the police." Actually what happens is Mark pretends like he is going to call the police, but he doesn't. Once we fought over a rake because we both wanted it. We were going to rake leaves, a big pile, so that we could take it into the street because we were helping an old gentleman. There was only one rake, and there was two garbage cans. After we got done fighting, I helped the older gentleman put the leaves into the garbage can and take it to the curb. We asked him, since he is elderly, and we felt bad he had to do all this work. When we got done, we got some candy and Skittles, and we got $1.25.*

I play with another friend. The only problem is that I also have an enemy in my neighborhood who lives right across the street. We are enemies because we're mostly not friends. He tricked me. Two boys wanted to hurt me; I don't know why, but they go to the same school as me. It is a bully school, but I don't get bullied anymore because I am a cool kid. At one time I was not a cool kid, but now I am a cool kid.

Q: How do you get to be a cool kid?

A: *I act more cool, and I hang out with Terrance. He is the boss of cool kids. Terrance, he is a cool kid, he's black, and he's like the head cool. In my school, there is a "no bully" sign everywhere because it's a top bully school. Hitting a teacher, the school will call the police. I've been in that situation.*

Q: What are the things you do at school that you really enjoy?

A: *Playing with my friend Todd. We play Army. Mostly he understands that I am always captain and he is a radio operator. Mostly the things I'm into instead of the Army is being a Navy Seal. I just want to be a captain. I've been looking it up online and watching Navy Seal stories on the military channel. I'm recording these shows. We just play this at home at night and sometimes on weekend mornings.*

Q: Tell me about your favorite class at school.

A: *Neither. I don't like anything but music and art. We draw in art, and there's these computer pianos and they are hooked up to the computer and you can play them, and they are computer lessons. I play my piano at home. I want an electric guitar for Christmas. I play "Ode to Joy"*
and half of "Secret Agent Man"—that one is really hard. I can play "Mad Man," which is like a half an hour song. I like to draw cars, engines, battleships, people. Mostly I have music one day, then gym and then art in a pattern.

Q: Do you get any special help at school?

A: *Sometimes. Like math help if I need help with that. I do times and fractions. I get to do more of these at Sylvan Learning Center. At school, they don't think I can do that (then he demonstrates how much he knows about multiplications, including knowing that any number multiplied by 1 equals that number and how any number multiplied by zero equals zero).*

I am reading a naval war book. Actually, all I like to do is read library books that are higher than third grade.

I want an electric bass so I can play funk and see how low it can get. I'd like to play with my friend who knows a lot of songs, and he gives me music. I can read music, and I like to figure out how to play the songs.

Q: This has been kind of a tough year at school. What do you think is going on?

A: *When I am working, I don't feel my ADHD. The only time I feel it is when I am at bed time. A lot of times, I think that my medicine is making my chest hurt. Sometimes I start crying, it feels so bad. It feels like nails are in it. But then it takes me a while to get to sleep. I take some meds at night and listening meds in the morning. They are different colors, and they both are listening meds. I'm not sure if they work. In the past, I didn't always take my meds, and we found a pile of pills when we moved my bed. It was a stupid thing. I got into trouble. I think when I don't take my meds, it seems like to me that it gets a little crummy. Sometimes it's out of control, and I don't even realize that I am doing things and I get into trouble.*

Q: If you could tell someone how they could help you and kids like you who have ADHD, what would you say?

A: *Or what questions you might ask?*

Q: Sure, what questions you might ask.

A: *How could I be good in school? Listen to the teacher. You can take your medicine. Don't catch the school on fire. If you find a lighter on the floor, don't even pick it up or touch it. I just tell the teacher it is there. On one of my bad days, they might call the police or fire department and take me to a foster home. I know what a foster home is. If I get suspended, I could go to the slammer. If I go to a foster home and got suspended, they could put me in jail. My aunt was in a foster home. I've heard stories about that. No bringing weapons to school—kids have brought real knives and a real gun. Do your homework. No bullying—about that, there's these second-grade kids. They got their side, and my side and Terrance's side. We are Americans. They go to the same school, and they are not on our side and they are not Americans. They don't know how to speak American. Terrance says we should take them down because they are not Americans. Terrance is really a sensitive kid. About who and what is messing with him. If he really wants to take them down, he could. Sometimes he's good. He mostly, me and him work together. We've done tests together.*

The Lived Experience—cont'd

Jeff

Jeff is a 23-year-old teaching assistant who is working to help students who struggle like him.

Q: What is a regular day like for you from the time you get up until the time you go to bed?

A: Busy! I get up, I take my medication, I make sure my room is nice and clean, I go to work for 8 hours, I come back home, take another dose of my Seroquel, then I just take it easy.

Q: How is this routine different from when you were younger and in school?

A: It is a lot different! I have to get up earlier than I did before. I was always in trouble, my parents had to take me back and forth to school when I was not allowed to take the bus or because I got expelled. Things have changed a lot.

Q: What were some things that you really enjoyed about school?

A: Learning. I loved doing class work and homework. I was the top in my class academically all the time and never got anything below a "B".

Q: Did you get any special help in school? If yes, why did you think that you were getting that help?

A: At my last two schools, I had a 1:1 aid because of the situations I was involved in while I was in the county schools. It was recommended by the superintendent of the county schools that if I were to go to another county school, I would need to have structured supervision by an adult with me to watch my behavior problems. At the time, I saw this as a punishment; I didn't like someone being my shadow and following me around to do everything I had to do. The only time I had my own time in school was in the bathroom.

Q: Looking back, is there anything that you would change about your school experience?

A: Yes, I would change the people that I hang around and doing the things that got me in trouble. I would have wanted to have a more pleasant school year instead of always being in trouble. Being in trouble meant cussing teachers out, flooding the bathroom toilets, poking at people's heads with pencils; I actually put tacks on one teacher's chair, a lot of things. I would get on the bus and start cussing, and when the bus driver told me not to, I would turn my headphones up loud just to get on the aide's nerves. I liked to "nitpick" and pick on kids to get attention. I would break the bus rules by drinking soda and use my phone just to make them mad; just for them to say something.

Q: Looking back, what do you think was the most helpful assistance you received at school? How did that assistance prepare you for what you are doing now?

A: That's a hard one. It was the staff at my last two schools. They were more hands on than the county teachers were. The county teachers just gave you the work and expected you to do it and that's it. At Forbush and Hanna Moore, there were more adults around and more supervision. When you had a question, they would answer it right then and there. The classrooms were smaller, so they had more ability to keep your attention. In the county schools, there

were 25 to 30 kids in there asking multiple questions at the same time. I also had the money management budgeting class with you, which helped me a lot. I had Dr. T while I was at school. I still see him now. We have a development plan for me with goals to work on for each year. Having the development plan and seeing the therapist and psychiatrist regularly has been very helpful.

Q: What is the development plan?

A: This helps me with controlling my impulses, the urges to make bad choices when I have a lot of unstructured time, to focus my time; like if I wanted to do something that would get me in trouble with the law, my plan tells me to look at the photo of the jail, which would remind me to stay out of trouble.

Q: What is the most difficult thing that you are having to deal with as an adult with ADHD? And as a working adult with ADHD?

A: It is a lot harder as an adult. Now you have bills to take care of, you have work responsibilities, you have to make sure you get there on time, you have a lot more responsibilities to deal with that you wouldn't have in school because your parents are mainly focused on you in school. I feel like I have my ADHD managed to where I can be successful and I am doing something that I like. I am interacting with a bunch of people, even though some of them have an attitude problem. I had to deal with that in school, so I have a better feeling as an adult how I can deal with it. As an adult, I am better able to stop and think. If I did the things that I used to do in school now and in the real world, you will end up going to jail. As a kid, you basically get a slap on the hand and Mom and Dad help you deal with it, but once you turn 18 it is in the hands of the courts.

Q: If you could tell someone something about how they could better help others with ADHD, what would you tell them?

A: With ADHD, it is going to be a struggle. You have to learn the basics of the diagnosis. If you are a parent, you can't just say that my kid has a disorder and ignore it and let someone else deal with it. The child will be spending a lot of time with the parent, so the parent will need to learn how to deal with the issues; there is treatment out there, plenty of medications to try, there are plenty of assistance and strategies.

Q: What have you learned over the years about your diagnosis?

A: I learned that, as a child, the diagnosis that I had was always getting me into trouble, constantly. I was doing horrible things, things that other kids wouldn't do. I also learned that I have a short attention span and have tried to deal with that better as an adult. I try to think of things that interest me the most, then my attention span seems to expand more than what is was in school. In school, they would give me work that I could finish in 5 minutes, then I had the rest of the class time to make fun of people and get into constant trouble. Keeping myself busy with things that interest me helps.

Continued

The Lived Experience—cont'd

Jan Fitzgerald, Executive Director, Parent to Parent of NYS

Parent to Parent is an organization developed by parents of children with special needs to provide information, advocacy, and support to others facing the same types of challenges each of its member families has encountered. Jan Fitzgerald, executive director of Parent to Parent of New York State, has worked diligently to ensure that each of her sons, especially her son John, has the opportunities he deserves. Here she shares the legacy of the countless parents who have helped create a more promising future for children with special needs. Her lesson is one that each clinician should consider as we work with families and individuals. Supporting hope and dreams can enable not only personal victories, but also policy.

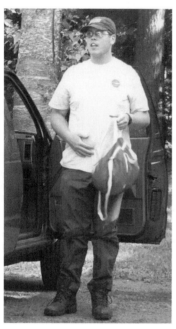

Jan's son John working for the New York State Department of Environmental Conservation.

When I started to think about what I was going to write, my first thought was about Burt Blatt and his book *Christmas in Purgatory*. If there is anything that reminds us of the past history of what care looked like for people with developmental disabilities, it is his books. If you have not heard of him or read his books, they are a must read for any parent. They are a reminder of what was reality for people with disabilities.

"We stand on the strong shoulders of those before us." I had never heard that statement until I entered the disability world. It has been used in other circles, but it certainly makes sense for us, doesn't it? We can only build on the successes of the past accomplished by those before us.

We all know parents who have paved the way for us and for our children. Many had few choices, and all made sacrifices to make life better for people with developmental disabilities and for the parents of people with disabilities. Their perseverance included the educational services we consider an entitlement.

Their determination included striving for a place to live other than in an understaffed ward in an institution and activities to fill a person's day so they do not sit idle. Things we consider an expectation.

We cannot forget the parents before us. Thank them for their strong shoulders and for their endless hours of advocacy. When you meet a parent who has come before you, thank them for their work. We would not be here now if it wasn't for them.

Parents before me knew that there had to be a better way. They believed in human dignity and that all people have abilities to build on. I believe this, too, and am grateful that my son has had the educational and social opportunities he has had. My next hope is that he will actually have a choice in employment. And that John will have a best friend, just like my other sons have. My hope is that someday everyone will recognize that people with developmental disabilities need fun and joy in their lives.

We have come so far, and yet we still have so far to go.

As our newer and younger parents come forward and become the parents who others turn to, we welcome them and also thank them. We offer our shoulders to those who follow us.

Remember that whenever a vision of possibility for people with disabilities has been expanded, at least one parent was involved with vision long before professionals were. We can never stop dreaming of making life better.

Our dream at Parent to Parent is that no parent will be alone; we cannot stop being there for other parents and for each other.

As challenging as things sometimes are, remember to show gratitude, practice forgiveness, and welcome the newcomer. Thank you.

---

assessment and treatment approaches, is outlined for specific diagnoses and setting. Because much is yet to be learned, occupational therapists focus on functional outcomes for individuals within their given context, while tying approaches to much needed research and reflection on occupational therapy theoretical foundations.

Each developmental stage or transition will present a new challenge to the individual with attention deficit disorder or other disruptive behavior disorders. Changes in body systems related to development (puberty, adulthood, aging, and menopause), weight gain/loss, and illness can influence the effectiveness of medications and require the individual to

seek medical attention. Early identification of these changes can prevent a crisis or need for hospitalization.

Individuals with disorders that are manifested through anxiety, aggression, or distress when their sense of control is threatened (conduct/oppositional defiant) may find themselves unable to follow protocols in the classroom or workplace, such as arriving on time or taking directions from others. People with attention deficit may be intimidated by new settings and routines or fail to recognize changes in the environment or its expectations. This may restrict their ability to adjust to a new classroom as a child, or to a new workplace or job type as an adult.

Similarly, difficulty following societal rules can result in ongoing legal issues that may ultimately lead to incarceration. In each case, the ability to assess future environments, plan ahead, and develop coping and/or self-management strategies is the key to success. Adult services may further emerge as research follows younger individuals diagnosed with attention deficit and behavioral disorders into adulthood.

Individuals with attention deficit disorder and other disruptive disorders do not fall easily into a ready-made assessment protocol. Each individual will present with unique characteristics, and the first sign that there is a problem may be poor performance on standardized assessments. These individuals have often had experiences that challenge their self-esteem and motivation, so the climate of assessment can be intimidating for them from the start. Several factors to consider when a referral is received include the reason for referral, age of the individual, previous assessments, and history of intervention.

If the referral occurs before the individual has experienced a lot of failure, the evaluation process can be more comprehensive and often more valid. When a referred individual has a long history of failure or a trauma history, the assessment process becomes more challenging. Observation, interviews, and assessment of processing, including sensory processing, may reveal the most useful assessment information. No assessment should proceed without gathering a thorough history and developing rapport with the individual. The nature of these disorders creates a climate in which skill deficits are most pronounced during times of stress. Although performance under stress is also a valuable piece of evaluative information, this will not present a good foundation for future work or goal setting if it is the therapist's entry into the occupational therapy process. Note that individuals with ODD or conduct disorder will often present a resistant front, and good clinical observation skills may be the therapist's best source of information in these cases. It is important to note again that later assessment may reveal more telling information, but a less formal initial approach will gain the most. Figure 8-1 provides an example of an occupationally based assessment process from screening to goal-setting for children and adults with attention and disruptive behavior disorders.

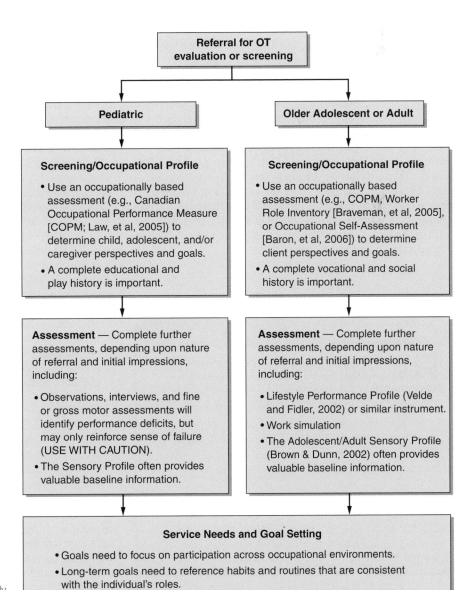

FIGURE 8-1. Example of an occupationally based assessment process—from screening to goal-setting—for children and adults affected by attention and disruptive behavior disorders.

Cognitive Impairment

Cognitive performance deficits in individuals with attention deficit include both processing and executive functions. This results in difficulties in both interpreting environmental cues and executing desired responses (Scheres et al, 2004). Information sorting and retrieval may be most challenging and, when coupled with a tendency toward impulsivity, can result in situations that put the individual at risk of injury or embarrassment. The individual may jump up or surge ahead of others as the cues to "wait one's turn" are lost amidst other information. Receptive and expressive language skills may be impaired, and individuals may interject unrelated or seemingly irrelevant information into conversations or appear unknowledgeable, disinterested, or insensitive when key elements of information are lost.

It is important for occupational therapists to identify the areas of greatest functional concern in order to maximize the effects of intervention. The Alert Program (Williams & Shellenberger, 1996) has been implemented with the adolescent population (Barnes, Beck, Vogel, Grice, & Murphy, 2003) as a means of providing combined cognitive and sensory strategies in order to enable emotionally challenged adolescents to cope more effectively with environmental demands. A series of awareness activities help adolescents identify how their body responds to the environment, such as what makes them calm, agitated, focused, etc. They then consider and try out various types of input (sensory tools or strategies) that help them adjust their body's response to the demands of specific situations. Decisions regarding what works are often part of the team process, with the adolescent, therapist, caregiver, and educators contributing to the analysis. Finding a means to efficiently provide these resources and measure their effect is an ongoing challenge within the fast-paced academic environment. See Chapter 18 for more detailed information.

Evidence-Based Practice

Research continues into the relationship between childhood attentional and conduct disorders and adult conditions.

➤ Occupational therapists need to consider transitional readiness for older students entering higher education or the workforce (Brollier, Shepherd, & Markley, 1994; Martin, 2005; Spear, 2007).

Brollier, C., Shepherd, J., & Markley, K. (1994). Transition from school to community living. *American Journal of Occupational Therapy, 48,* 346–353.

Martin, A. (2005). The hard work of growing up with ADHD. *American Journal of Psychiatry, 162,* 1043–1044.

Spear, S. (2007). Adult education: What's OT got to do with it? American Occupational Therapy Association. *Mental Health Special Interest Section Quarterly, 30*(2), 1–3.

Motor Impairment and Sensory Processing

A review by White (2005) suggests that investigation using instruments such as the Assessment of Motor and Process Skills can provide useful information regarding task process deficits in individuals with attention deficit, as well as the role that cortisol and other neurotransmitters play in task performance outcomes. This may further support investigations into related disorder types. It is important to note that underlying attentional deficits, anxiety, depression, or related symptoms may cause the appearance of motor impairment, which may resolve when the underlying condition is in better control. It is also important to consider medication side effects in relation to motor function and make this consideration a priority when discussing the course of treatment with the physician. Adjustments in medication can result in remarkable improvement or loss of function. Occupational therapy can provide valuable insight toward the most effective outcome.

One of the key components of intervention that has been a focus of occupational therapy is **sensory processing disorder** (Miller, 2006). Stemming from theories of sensory integration first postulated by Ayres (2005), this area of research and intervention focuses on the individual's ability to work with information from internal stimuli (i.e., the body's own processing rhythm and the external environment, including sights, sounds, touch, etc). This allows for a bottom-up view of the child's processing challenges, noting the inability to access executive functions if lower-level brain systems are in distress or unable to filter and interpret effectively.

The Sensory Profile (Brown & Dunn, 2002; Dunn 1997), an instrument that has been developed in forms appropriate for children, adolescents, and adults, can help categorize ways in which the individual responds to the sensory environment. The degree to which an individual responds to the environment and seeks or avoids interaction with the environment can help define the environments and activities in which he or she may be most comfortable and those that may cause the greatest distress. This information can further lead to the development of interventions that help modulate these responses to a more "typical" level or develop strategies to help the individual cope with their sensitivities in ways that enable function (e.g., wearing clothing that does not feel uncomfortable, using white noise or headphones to help manage auditory sensitivity).

In her book, *The Out-of-Sync Child: Recognizing and Coping With Sensory Processing Disorder,* Carol Kranowitz (2005) supports this view of the challenging child, providing concepts and resources to parents, educators, and clinicians as they support children on their quest toward participation. Note that the use of the term "sensory processing" in this text replaces "sensory integration" from Kranowitz and Silver (1998). Occupational therapists continue to investigate how sensory processing affects function and how applications of sensory techniques, such as the application of weight for proprioceptive input during activity, may enable greater self-management and attention (Honaker & Rossi, 2005). See Chapter 20 for more information about assessment and intervention.

Evidence-Based Practice

Published studies have focused on an individual's ability to engage in tasks (Honaker & Rossi, 2005; Segal et al, 2005; White, 2005). Additional studies have looked at factors influencing engagement, including sensory processing and decreased executive function (Miller, 2006). Results indicate that

➤ Occupational therapists should assess barriers to attention, including sensory processing, cognitive processing, and social perception and skills.

➤ Occupational therapists should evaluate task demands in order to facilitate development of compensatory strategies (Barnes, Beck, Vogel, Grice, & Murphy, 2003).

Barnes, K. J., Beck, A. J., Vogel, K. A., Grice, K. O., & Murphy, D. (2003). Perceptions regarding school-based occupational therapy for children with emotional disturbances. *American Journal of Occupational Therapy, 57,* 337–340.

Honaker, D., & Rossi, L. M. (2005). Proprioception and participation at school: Are weighted vests effective? Appraising the evidence, part 2. *Sensory Integration Special Interest Section Quarterly, 28*(4), 1–4.

Miller, L. J., with Fuller, D. A. (2006). *Sensational Kids: Hope and Help for Children With Sensory Processing Disorder (SPD).* New York: Putnam.

Segal, R., Hinojosa, J., Addonizio, C., Borisoff, D., Inderies, L., & Lee, J. (2005). Homework strategies for children with attention deficit hyperactivity disorder. *OT Practice, 10*(17), 9–12.

White, B. P. (2005). Behavioral and physiologic response measures of occupational task performance: A preliminary comparison between typical children and children with attention disorder. *American Journal of Occupational Therapy, 59,* 426–436.

Work and Adult Engagement

There is much to be learned regarding the influence of attention deficit and behavioral disorders into adulthood. Individuals struggling with work roles and engagement may benefit from occupational therapy strategies. Spear (2007) suggests that a battery of occupational therapy assessments may reveal barriers to both adult education and employment in much the same way as educational challenges are noted in children and adolescents. She further cites the need to explore occupational therapy roles in work or adult education settings. Brollier, Shepherd, and Markley (1994) made the case that occupational therapy services need to shift attention with older students toward management of adult roles and implementation of compensatory strategies if needed. (See Chapter 50.)

Medications

The most common medications associated with treatment of ADHD are the stimulants. These medications increase the levels of dopamine in the brain, although the exact mechanism by which they influence brain activity in ADHD is still under investigation (Findling, Aman, Eerdekens, Derivan, & Lyons, 2004; Pliszka et al, 2006; Sharfritz, Marchione, Gore, Shaywitz, & Shaywitz, 2004; Volkow & Swanson, 2003). Concerns exist regarding the relationship between medication use and other substance abuse because methylphenidate is a stimulant (Disney et al, 1999). In addition, there are concerns regarding people with ADHD who have not received treatment, in that they have more legal and social impairments (D. Pate, personal communication, 2009).

Further concerns regarding immediate response to treatment include psychotic or manic symptoms (Ross, 2006), overstimulation, or development of dependency and abuse of the prescribed methylphenidate (Volkow, 2006). Attention to the medication's therapeutic effect and whether a "go" versus "stop" response is responsible for improved "go" performance (i.e., is it the individual's ability to make the decision [improved process speed and sorting] or to "stop" undesired responses that enables the most functional performance?) may help refine medication choices and use (Pliszka et al, 2006).

Beyond the use of stimulants such as methylphenidate (Concerta, Ritalin), other medications include antidepressants and mood stabilizers, clonidine (Catapres), and other psychotropic medications. Depending on the specific diagnosis (ADHD, conduct disorder, ODD, etc) and individual symptoms, medications may be administered singly or in combination in order to achieve the most functional therapeutic result.

The U.S. Food and Drug Administration (2007) mandated that drug manufacturers issue more specific information about medication use. Guidelines such as these help assure that prescription guidelines are geared toward this specific population.

Concern regarding proper dosage and reporting of side effects is ongoing, especially because most of the individuals receiving medication for these disorders are children of varied ages with a mixed presentation of signs and symptoms.

Summary

The increasingly complex demands of community, work, and educational settings puts a high demand on individuals' ability to focus, receive, and interpret information, as well as make sound behavioral judgments that enable productive engagement. The additional challenges that individuals with attention deficit and disruptive behavior disorders face, although not insurmountable, require specialized evaluation and management. When unmanaged, these disorders can lead to dysfunction that endures throughout a lifetime, restricting work, interpersonal relationships, and engagement in the most meaningful occupations.

Occupational therapy's comprehensive focus on sensorineural, cognitive, motor, and psychosocial functions, as well as awareness of the lifestyle considerations in medication management, provide a dynamic perspective to the individual; the family; and the treatment, educational, or vocational team. Occupational therapists can employ a variety of assessment tools and integrative strategies to help develop plans that provide the individual with a greater sense of control and ability to select and participate in meaningful occupations of both necessity and choice.

Active Learning Strategies

1. Review of Narratives

- Reread Nate, Jeff, and Jan's first person narratives in this chapter. Note where the messages are similar or in sync with one another. Note where they are different from one another.
- Identify the challenges that might be addressed by an occupational therapy practitioner.
- Comment on the strategies that might be employed that seem to be effective related to home, school, social, and work environments.

 Write in your **Reflective Journal** about the lessons you have learned by reading these three narratives and how this might affect your future practice.

2. Classroom Observation

- Compile a list of sensory components (auditory, olfactory, gustatory, visual, tactile, proprioceptive, kinesthetic). List primary cognitive sequential skills (attention, intake, recognition, etc). List primary motor processes, including praxis (ideation, motor planning, etc).
- Using your lists, visit typical classrooms, and for each daily activity (including transitions), identify the sensory, cognitive, and motor skills required for each. Completing this activity with a partner or team may help you catch more of the details.
- Pay careful attention to the way in which directions are given, what knowledge or sequencing ability is assumed, and how behavioral expectations are reinforced.
- Compare and contrast the demands across grade levels and appropriate strategies for inclusion of students with attention and disruptive behavior disorders in these settings.

3. Planned Distractions

Work in teams or groups to
- Select a variety of "distractions" that you could use in class to challenge your classmates' ability to focus during an activity.
- Create or select an unfamiliar multistep activity that involves assembly, calculation, creativity, etc, providing enough materials for several others to complete the task.
- Set up the environment with your distractions and have other groups attempt to complete your task when the directions are provided.

- Evaluate your success.
  - Discuss factors that made tasks harder to perform.
  - Discuss skills individuals tried to or successfully used to complete the task.

4. Filtering Sensory Stimulation

Go to a particularly busy community setting and
- Make a list of all sensory stimuli you can note, sense by sense.
  - Note pattern of stimulation.
  - Note frequency of stimulation.
- Make a list of all social tasks individuals may engage in within this environment.
- Consider adaptations for an individual with difficulty filtering sensory stimulation and/or responding to social cues.

 Describe the experience in your **Reflective Journal**.

Reflective Questions

Reflect on how you felt after one of these activities.
For the classroom observation:
- How did the setting influence your comfort and/or your observations?
- If you had been in a different setting, how might the experience have changed?
- Do you have personal memories of this grade level and its demands that may have influenced your observations?
For the planned distractions:
- If you were the classroom "disruptor," how did you develop your role? What factors did you consider when demonstrating these challenges?
- If you were trying to complete an activity or focus during distraction, did you employ specific strategies? If so, what were they, and did they work? How did you feel during this time (i.e., challenged, frustrated, etc)?
- If you were observing others during complex tasks completed with distractions, consider times when you may have faced similar challenges and how these may have made you feel.
For the filtering sensory stimulation:
- Describe your personal comfort level in busy community settings.
- Describe a time when you have been in particularly challenging community situations, and reflect on how this made you feel.
- Have you ever lost control, become angry, agitated, etc? If not, what helped you cope?

Resources

Community Resources
- **Attention Deficit Disorder Association (ADDA)**
  PO Box 7557
  Wilmington, DE 19803-9997
  Phone/Fax: 800-939-1019
  Web site: http://www.add.org/

- **National Resource Center on ADHD, Children and Adults With Attention Deficit/Hyperactivity Disorder (CHADD)**
  8181 Professional Place, Suite 150
  Landover, MD 20785
  Telephone: 800-233-4050
  Web site: http://www.chadd.org/

- **U.S. Department of Health and Human Services, Substance Abuse and Mental Health Services Administration (SAMHSA)**
PO Box 2345
Rockville, MD 20847
Toll-free: 800-789-2647
Fax: 240-221-4295
TDD: 866-889-2647
Web site: http://mentalhealth.samhsa.gov/
Publications:
"Children's Mental Health Facts: Children and Adolescents With Conduct Disorder" (available at: http://mentalhealth.samhsa.gov/publications/allpubs/Ca-0010/default.asp)
- **The American Academy of Child and Adolescent Psychiatry (AACAP)**
3615 Wisconsin Avenue, NW
Washington, DC 20016-3007
Phone: 202-966-7300
Fax: 202-966-2891
Web site: http://www.aacap.org
Publications:
"Children With Oppositional Defiant Disorder" (available at: http://www.aacap.org/cs/root/facts_for_families/children_with_oppositional_defiant_disorder)
"Conduct Disorder" (available at: http://www.aacap.org/cs/root/facts_for_families/conduct_disorder)

References

American Psychiatric Association. (2000). *Diagnostic and Statistical Manual of Mental Disorders* (4th ed., text revision). Washington, DC: Author.

Anckarsater, H., Stahlberg, O., Larson, T., Hakansson, C., Jutblad, S., Nicklasson, L., Nyden, A., et al. (2006). The impact of ADHD and autism spectrum disorders on temperament, character, and personality development. *American Journal of Psychiatry, 163,* 1239–1244.

Ayres, A. J. (2005). *Sensory Integration and the Child: 25th Anniversary Edition.* Los Angeles: Western Psychological Services.

Barnes, K. J., Beck, A. J., Vogel, K. A., Grice, K. O., & Murphy, D. (2003). Perceptions regarding school-based occupational therapy for children with emotional disturbances. *American Journal of Occupational Therapy, 57*(3), 337–341.

Baron, K., Kielhofner, G., Iyenenger, A., Goldhammer, V., & Wolenski, T. (2006). Occupational Self Assessment, Version 2.2. Chicago, IL: MOHO Clearinghouse.

Biederman, J., Faraone, S. V., & Monuteaux, M. C. (2002). Differential effect of environmental adversity by gender: Rutter's index of adversity in a group of boys and girls with and without ADHD. *American Journal of Psychiatry, 159,* 1556–1562.

Braveman, B., Robson, M., Velozo, C., Kielhofner, G., Fisher, G., Forsyth, K., & Kershbaum, J. (2005). Worker Role Interview, Version 10.0. Chicago, IL: MOHO Clearinghouse.

Brollier, C., Shepherd, J., & Markley, K. (1994). Transition from school to community living. *American Journal of Occupational Therapy, 48,* 346–353.

Brown, C., & Dunn, W. (2002). *Adolescent/Adult Sensory Profile.* San Antonio, TX: The Psychological Corp.

Chandler, J. (2008, February 20). *Oppositional Defiant Disorder (ODD) and Conduct Disorder (CD) in Children and Adolescents: Diagnosis and Treatment.* Available at: http://jamesdauntchandler.tripod.com/ODD_CD/oddcdpamphlet.pdf (accessed October 27, 2009).

Curtis, D. E., Pisecco, S., Hamilton, R. J., & Moore, D. W. (2006). Teacher perceptions of classroom interventions for children with ADHD: A cross-cultural comparison of teachers in the United States and New Zealand. *School Psychology Quarterly, 21*(2), 171–196.

Disney, E., Elkins, I., McGue, M., & Iacono, W. (1999). Effects of ADHD, conduct disorder, and gender on substance use and abuse in adolescents. *American Journal of Psychiatry, 156,* 1515–1521.

Dudley-Grant, G. R. (2001). Eastern Caribbean Family Psychology with conduct-disordered adolescents from the Virgin Islands. *American Psychologist, 56*(1), 47–57.

Dunn, W. (1997). The Sensory Profile: A discriminating measure of sensory processing in daily life. *American Occupational Therapy Association Sensory Integration Special Interest Section Quarterly, 20*(1), 1–3.

Findling, R. L., Aman, M. G., Eerdekens, M., Derivan, A., & Lyons, B. (2004). Long-term, open-label study of risperidone in children with severe disruptive behaviors and below-average IQ. *American Journal of Psychiatry, 161,* 677–684.

Honaker, D., & Rossi, L. M. (2005). Proprioception and participation at school: Are weighted vests effective? Appraising the evidence, part 2. *Sensory Integration Special Interest Section Quarterly, 28*(4), 1–4.

Jackson, L., & Arbesman, M. (2005). *Occupational Therapy Practice Guidelines for Children With Behavioral and Psychosocial Needs (AOTA Practice Guidelines).* Bethesda, MD: AOTA Press.

Kilgore, K., Snyder, J., & Lentz, C. (2000). The contribution of parental discipline, parental monitoring, and school risk to early-onset conduct problems in African American boys and girls. *Developmental Psychology, 36*(6), 835–845.

Kranowitz, C. S. (2005). *The Out-of-Sync Child: Recognizing and Coping With Sensory Processing Disorder* (rev. ed.). New York: Perigee.

Kranowitz, C. S., & Silver, L. B. (1998). *The Out-of-Sync Child: Recognizing and Coping With Sensory Integration Disorder.* New York: Perigee.

Law, M., Baptiste, S., Carswell, A., McColl, M.A., Polatjko, H., & Pollock, N. (2005). *COPM: Canadian Occupational Performance Measure* (4th ed.) Ottawa, Ontario: Canadian Association of Occupational Therapy.

Martin, A. (2005). The hard work of growing up with ADHD. *American Journal of Psychiatry, 162,* 1043–1044.

Miller, L. J., with Fuller, D. A. (2006). *Sensational Kids: Hope and Help for Children With Sensory Processing Disorder (SPD).* New York: Putnam.

Olfson, M., Gameroff, M. J., Marcus, S. C., & Jensen, P. S. (2003). National trends in treatment of attention deficit hyperactivity disorder. *American Journal of Psychiatry, 160*(6), 1071–1077.

Pliszka, S. R., Carlson, C. L., & Swanson, J. M. (1999). *ADHD With Co-morbid Disorders: Clinical Assessment and Management.* New York: Guilford Press.

Pliszka, S. R., Glahn, D. C., Semrud-Clikeman, M., Franklin, C., Periz, R., Xiong, J., et al. (2006). Neuroimaging of inhibitory control areas in children with attention deficit hyperactivity disorder who were treatment naïve or in long-term treatment. *American Journal of Psychiatry, 163,* 1052–106.

Ross, R. G. (2006). Psychotic and manic like symptoms during stimulant treatment of attention deficit hyperactivity disorder. *American Journal of Psychiatry, 163,* 1149–1152.

Scheres, A., Oosterlaan, J., Geurts, H., Morein-Zamir, S., Meiran, N., Schut, H., Vlasveld, L. & Sergeant, J. A. (2004). Executive functioning in boys with ADHD: Primarily an inhibition deficit? *Archives of Clinical Neurology, 19,* 569–594.

Searlight, H. R., Rottnek, F., & Abby, S. L. (2001). Conduct disorder: Diagnosis and treatment in primary care. *American Family Physician, 63,* 1579–1588.

Sharfritz, K. M., Marchione, K. E., Gore, J. C., Shaywitz, S. E., & Shaywitz, B. A. (2004). The effects of methylphenidate on neural systems of attention in attention deficit hyperactivity disorder. *American Journal of Psychiatry, 161,* 1990–1997.

Shea, S., Gordon, K., Hawkins, A., Kawchuk, J., & Smith, D. (2000). Pathology in the Hundred Acre Wood: A neurodevelopmental perspective on A.A. Milne. *Canadian Medical Association Journal, 163*(12), 1557–1559.

Spear, S. (2007). Adult education: What's OT got to do with it? *American Occupational Therapy Association Mental Health Special Interest Section Quarterly, 30*(2), 1–3.

U.S. Department of Health and Human Services. (1999). *Mental Health: A Report of the Surgeon General.* Rockville, MD: Author.

U.S. Food and Drug Administration (FDA). (2007, September 17). "AHRQ and FDA to Collaborate in Largest Study Ever of Possible Heart Risks With ADHD Medications." FDA News Release. Available at: http://www.fda.gov/NewsEvents/Newsroom/PressAnnouncements/2007/ucm108983.htm (accessed October 27, 2009).

Velde, B., & Fidler, G. (2002). *Lifestyle Performance: A Model for Engaging the Power of Occupation.* Thorofare, NJ: Slack Inc.

Visser, S. N., & Lesesne, C. A. (2005). Mental health in the United States: Prevalence of diagnosis and medication treatment for attention-deficit/hyperactivity disorder—United States, 2003. Centers for Disease Control and Prevention. *Morbidity and Mortality Weekly Report, 54,* 842–847.

Volkmar, F. (2005). Toward understanding the basis of ADHD. *American Journal of Psychiatry, 162,* 1043–1557.

Volkow, N. D. (2006). Stimulant medications: How to minimize their reinforcing effects? *American Journal of Psychiatry, 163,* 359–361.

Volkow, N. D., & Swanson, J. M. (2003). Variables that affect the clinical use and abuse of methylphenidate in the treatment of ADHD. *American Journal of Psychiatry, 160,* 1909–1918.

Waschbusch, D. A., & King, S. (2006). Should sex-specific norms be used to assess attention-deficit/hyperactivity disorder or oppositional defiant disorder? *Journal of Consulting and Clinical Psychology, 74*(1), 179–185.

White, B. P. (2005). Behavioral and physiologic response measures of occupational task performance: A preliminary comparison between typical children and children with attention disorder. *American Journal of Occupational Therapy, 59,* 426–436.

Williams, M., & Shellenberger, S. (1996). *How Does Your Engine Run? A Leader's Guide to the Alert Program for Self-Regulation.* Albuquerque, NM: Therapy Works.

Intellectual Disabilities

Katie Alexander

> "*S*uccess is to be measured not so much by the position that one has reached in life as by the obstacles which he has overcome while trying to succeed.
>
> —Booker T. Washington

Introduction

Occupational therapists have the opportunity to work with individuals with developmental disabilities in many contexts. Because many developmental disabilities are identified early in life, occupational therapists working in early intervention are among the first to develop and share a comprehensive understanding of a child. They work alongside the family and other caregivers to identify barriers to participation and, through client-centered intervention, foster optimal participation, minimize disability, and promote a solid foundation on which future progress can be built. Occupational therapists may also work in school or community settings, serving students later in childhood. The therapeutic process remains the same, but the social and task expectations of the many contexts in which children live, play, and learn shift as a child gets older. The transition from adolescence into adulthood presents a new context that is rich with opportunity to foster community participation.

Occupational therapists who work in early childhood, school systems, and mental health are likely to serve an individual because of his or her developmental disability. However, an occupational therapist in settings such as physical rehabilitation may serve an individual with a developmental disability primarily due to physical impairment, for example, from trauma; in this case, the presence of an intellectual disability will have a significant affect on intervention decisions. In all cases, each individual with a developmental disability will have his or her own preferences, strengths, difficulties, expectations, and goals.

This chapter highlights the heterogeneity of intellectual disabilities. Although the diagnosis is simple and straightforward, there are a multitude of causes and the resulting severity and impact on occupational functioning varies widely among people with intellectual disabilities. This chapter also provides information on the prevalence, gender- and culture-specific influences, medications, and environmental factors that affect occupational performance.

Description of the Disorder

Developmental disorders include a heterogeneous group of genetic, biological, disease, injury, and yet unknown mechanisms that lead to a significant cognitive impairment that results in commensurate difficulty with independent participation in daily life. This dyad of impairments has most recently been identified as an **intellectual disability**, replacing the term "mental retardation," which is included in the *Diagnostic and Statistical Manual of Mental Disorders, Fourth Edition, Text Revision* (DSM-IV-TR). Therefore, throughout this chapter, with the exception of the summary of the DSM-IV-TR criteria, the term "intellectual disability" is used.

Intellectual disabilities represent one of the most frequent sources of disability in childhood (Stromme & Magnus, 2000). Some individuals with an intellectual disability have difficulty from birth, allowing for early detection and immediate intervention, whereas other individuals function well until later in life; still others develop typically until an external event causes injury to the central nervous system. Some individuals with intellectual disabilities can work independently, earn a salary that is above the mean income, own a home, marry, and have children, whereas others may require assistance for all activities of daily living.

All individuals with an intellectual disability are at risk for secondary physical and mental health concerns, but they also face significant barriers to health-care access (Krahn, Hammond, & Turner, 2006). Occupational therapists specialize in client-centered, contextually relevant service provision. They are well positioned to promote self-determination and self-advocacy among individuals with intellectual disabilities, while developing compensatory, skill acquisition, and preventative interventions that promote optimal participation in the community and optimum health and wellness.

DSM-IV-TR Criteria

As identified by the DSM-IV-TR, three basic criteria must be met in order for an individual to be diagnosed with mental retardation (American Psychiatric Association [APA], 2000). Because mental retardation is a developmental disorder, the onset of difficulties must occur prior to 18 years of age. In addition, an individual must present with impairments in both intellectual and adaptive functioning. With regard to intellectual functioning, the DSM-IV-TR requires that an individual obtain an IQ (Rahman, Iqbal, Bunn, Lovel, & Harrington, 2004) score of approximately 70 or below (at least approximately 2 standard deviations below the mean), which reflects significantly subaverage functioning (APA, 2000). The DSM-IV-TR defines adaptive functioning as an individual's ability to meet the performance expectations set forth by a particular culture, society, and/or community in accordance with the individual's chronological age (APA, 2000). The areas of adaptive functioning that are relevant to the diagnostic criteria include communication, self-care, social/interpersonal skills, self-direction, health, safety, work, functional academic skills, leisure, home living, and use of community resources. An individual must demonstrate significant difficulties in at least two of these areas.

The DSM-IV-TR has identified four degrees of severity and a diagnostic category for mental retardation, severity unspecified (APA, 2000). The severity assessment is based on intellectual functioning, and the four degrees of severity include (APA, 2000) (Fig. 9-1):

1. Mild mental retardation (IQ level 50–55 to approximately 70)
2. Moderate mental retardation (IQ level 35–40 to 50–55)
3. Severe mental retardation (IQ level 20–25 to 35–40)
4. Profound mental retardation (IQ level below 20–25)

A diagnosis of mental retardation, severity unspecified is most appropriate when there is a strong clinical impression of mental retardation, but an individual's IQ cannot be assessed formally due to interfering variables (e.g., too great an impairment, behavioral difficulty, infancy) (APA, 2000). Box 9-1 summarizes the core DSM-IV-TR diagnostic criteria for mental retardation.

Etiology

There are hundreds of different causal pathways that can lead to some degree of intellectual disability. Most of these causal pathways are known, but many others continue to elude research. The known pathways include those that are genetic, malformation related, external prenatal, paranatal (between (−1 and +4 weeks), and postnatal (Wilska & Kaski, 1999). The unknown pathways include those related to central nervous system pathology and those that are yet unclassified (Wilska & Kaski, 1999). Recent years have yielded an expanding fund of research exploring the etiology of mental retardation; the findings of these studies will help sculpt the

> **BOX 9-1** ■ **DSM-IV-TR Diagnostic Criteria for Mental Retardation**
>
> ■ Significantly subaverage intellectual functioning: based on an individually administered, culturally unbiased IQ measure, an IQ score of approximately 70 or below
> ■ Concurrent deficits in at least two areas of adaptive functioning
> ■ Onset prior to 18 years of age
>
> From American Psychiatric Association. (2000). *Diagnostic and Statistical Manual of Mental Disorders* (4th ed., text revision). Arlington, VA: Author.

range of therapeutic, both prevention and treatment, options for individuals with an intellectual disability (Leonard & Wen, 2002; Raymond & Tarpey, 2006; Wilska & Kaski, 1999). To date, the leading cause of preventable intellectual disability is iodine deficiency, which primarily affects underdeveloped nations (Delange, 2001).

Genetic Causes

There are more than 1,000 known genetic contributions to the expression of intellectual disabilities (Chelly, Khelfaoui, Francis, Cherif, & Bienvenu, 2006). Taken together, genetics account for roughly 35% of the cases (Hou, Wang, & Chuang, 1998; Stromme & Magnus, 2000). There are three primary mechanisms for the genetic etiology of intellectual disabilities: chromosomal (e.g., trisomy 21, 13, and 18; Prader-Willi syndrome; Angelman syndrome), genetic mutations (e.g., tuberous sclerosis, phenylketonuria [PKU], Tay-Sachs disease, fragile X syndrome), and multifactorial (e.g., familial, neural tube defects) (Chelly et al, 2006; Hou et al, 1998; Wilska & Kaski, 1999).

Down syndrome is the leading genetic cause of intellectual disability, representing 14% to 15% of all cases (Bower, Leonard, & Petterson, 2000). In addition, current studies have identified that the majority of single genes that lead to the expression of an intellectual disability is located on the X chromosome (Raymond & Tarpey, 2006) (Fig. 9-2). Fragile X is one example of an X-linked chromosomal abnormality, and it is the most heritable of all causes (Hou et al, 1998). In addition, heritable disorders account for approximately 8% to 18% of the genetic cases of intellectual disability (Hou et al, 1998; Stromme & Magnus, 2000).

Malformation-Related Causes

There are several conditions that lead to central nervous system malformation, termed **malformation syndromes** (e.g., Dandy-Walker malformation, schizencephaly, holoprosencephaly, lissencephalia). These syndromes are a product of complex and varied etiologies, and together represent approximately 12% of all cases of intellectual disability (Stromme & Magnus, 2000).

External Prenatal Causes

External prenatal causes of intellectual disability account for approximately 4.5% of all cases. Primarily, these cases are a result of toxic agents and disease to which a fetus is exposed in utero. They can include alcohol, drugs, and ToRCH (*Tox*oplasmosis, *R*ubella, *C*ytomegalovirus, *H*erpes virus) infections (Stromme & Magnus, 2000).

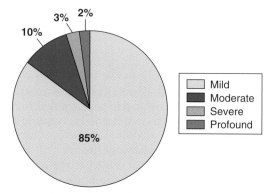

FIGURE 9-1. Level of severity prevalence. *Data from American Psychiatric Association. (2000). Diagnostic and Statistical Manual of Mental Disorders (Fourth edition, Text Revision). Arlington, VA: Author.*

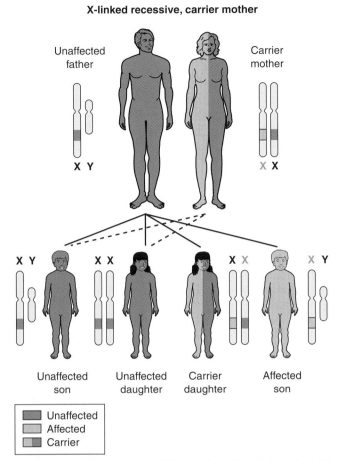

X-linked recessive, carrier mother

Unaffected father

X Y

Carrier mother

X X

X Y — Unaffected son

X X — Unaffected daughter

X X — Carrier daughter

X Y — Affected son

Unaffected
Affected
Carrier

FIGURE 9-2. Transmission of X-linked disabilities. A daughter with one mutated X chromosome can have only mild or no expression of fragile X because she has another nonmutated X chromosome. Males with a mutated X chromosome will always be affected. *Courtesy of the U.S. National Library of Medicine.*

Paranatal Causes

The paranatal period is similar to the perinatal period, but Wilska and Kaski (1999) specified that this period includes the time from birth through the fourth week of life. Approximately 5% to 10% of all cases of intellectual disability result from an event occurring during the paranatal period (Hou et al, 1998; Stromme & Magnus, 2000). Of these events, asphyxia is the most common cause (Hou et al, 1998). Hypoxic-ischemic encephalopathy, periventricular hemorrhage, meningitis, septicemia, and complications related to prematurity are also relatively common causes of intellectual disabilities during this period (Hou et al, 1998).

Postnatal Causes

A Centers for Disease Control and Prevention (CDC; 1996) study determined that events during the postnatal period of life account for approximately 4.5% of all cases of intellectual disability. In this study, the CDC found that there are three primary postnatal events that result in intellectual disabilities: injury, infectious disease, and chronic disease.

The greatest contributing cause to the postnatal etiology of intellectual disability is also the most preventable.

Injuries result in approximately 55.8% of all postnatal causes of intellectual disabilities; the most frequent of these events is child abuse (approximately 18.2%). Following this, motor vehicle collisions, falls, and near drowning are among the most typically cited injury-related causes of intellectual disability. Infectious disease contributes to approximately 34.5% of all postnatal cases, with the most frequent diseases including bacterial meningitis and encephalitis. Chronic disease is the third most common postnatal cause of intellectual disabilities (approximately 9% of postnatal causes), most commonly brain tumor and stroke.

Children with postnatally acquired intellectual disabilities are more likely to have multiple disabilities than children who have intellectual disabilities of a different etiology. This can include sensory impairments, such as blindness or hearing loss, as well as significant motor impairments that require the use of a wheelchair.

Unknown Causes

The remaining roughly 34% to 39% of cases of intellectual disability have an unknown etiology; however, the prevalence of individuals with intellectual disability of an unknown etiology varies tremendously depending on the study, its population sample, and diagnostic process (Leonard & Wen, 2002). It is a subject of increasing research attention, but this research is in its infancy. There is well-established evidence that certain risk factors can contribute to intellectual disabilities of an unknown etiology, and these risk factors are detailed in the next section (Croen, Grether, & Selvin, 2001). An unknown etiology is identified most frequently among individuals with mild intellectual disability as compared with other degrees of severity (Hou et al, 1998).

Other Risk Factors

In addition to biological and environmental risk factors, there are maternal factors associated with an increased risk for intellectual disability. Mothers who have completed less than a ninth-grade level of education are 20% more likely to have a child with an intellectual disability (Campbell, Broman, Nichols, & Leff, 1998). A maternal IQ of less than 70 is also associated with an increased risk. Younger maternal age is associated with a risk for mild intellectual disabilities, whereas older maternal age is associated with a risk for severe intellectual disabilities.

In addition, maternal smoking during pregnancy is associated with a 50% increase in the prevalence of intellectual disability, typically with an unknown cause (Drews, Murphy, Yeargin-Allsopp, & Decoufle, 1996). Furthermore, the more a pregnant female smokes, the greater her risk for having a child with an intellectual disability—a finding that is not associated with other sociodemographic risk factors (Drews et al, 1996). In total, approximately one-third of cases of intellectual disability among children of smokers can be attributed to maternal smoking (Drews et al, 1996).

Low birth weight is directly associated with an increased risk for intellectual disability. A birth weight of less than 1,000 grams presents the greatest level of risk and poses a higher risk for severe intellectual disability as opposed to mild intellectual disability (Chapman, Scott, & Stanton-Chapman, 2008).

The prevalence of intellectual disability is higher for individuals from families who are of low socioeconomic status, are poor, and/or have less education. There are also reports that maternal smoking is related to having a child with an intellectual disability. In addition, a mother with an IQ below 70 is more likely to have a child with an intellectual disability (Campbell et al, 1998; Drews et al, 1996). Furthermore, postnatal, preventable injury is a significant etiology after birth (CDC, 1996). Occupational therapists can work with individuals who are at risk in the following ways:

➤ Occupational therapists can work with individuals and caregivers to provide information and establish a setting that promotes optimal maternal health and wellness.

➤ Occupational therapists can work with consumers who have young children to ensure that the home environment is safeguarded against the typical dangers that place infants and young children at risk.

Campbell, B. W., Broman, S. H., Nichols, P. L., & Leff, M. (1998). Maternal and neonatal risk factors for mental retardation: Defining the "at-risk" child. *Early Human Development, 50*(2), 159–173.

Centers for Disease Control and Prevention (CDC). (1996). Postnatal causes of developmental disabilities in children aged 3–10 years—Atlanta, Georgia. *Morbidity and Mortality Weekly Report, 45*(6), 130–134.

Drews, C. D., Murphy, C. C., Yeargin-Allsopp, M., & Decoufle, P. (1996). The relationship between idiopathic mental retardation and maternal smoking during pregnancy. *Pediatrics, 97*(4), 547–553.

Neurological Factors

Due to the diversity of causes of intellectual disability, there is a commensurate heterogeneity in the neurology of intellectual disability, positioning it as one of the most neurobiologically heterogeneous disorders in existence. Neurological differences that give rise to an intellectual disability can include any combination of anatomical, neurochemical, and cellular mechanisms. For example, in some cases, there is a significant malformation of some area of the brain (e.g., Dandy-Walker malformation, in which the cerebellar vermis fails to develop), whereas someone with mild intellectual disabilities may have intact anatomical structures (Chelly et al, 2006).

A review of the neurological findings that correlate with genetic and environmental etiologies is outside the scope of this chapter. However, there is strong evidence that some cases of intellectual disability are related to poor neuronal connectivity and abnormal synapse structure (Chelly et al, 2006). Abnormalities related to neuronal communication can compromise neural plasticity and render the brain less able to process information. In this way, an individual's central nervous system prevents the individual from experiencing the typical intellectual development that is expected during childhood and adolescence.

Prevalence

Through a population-based study, the CDC reported a prevalence estimate of 12 per 1,000 individuals living with an intellectual disability (Bhasin, Brocksen, Avchen, & Van Naarden Braun, 2006). As such, intellectual disabilities represent the most prevalent source of disability currently identified worldwide (Stromme & Magnus, 2000). Of the individuals who are diagnosed with an intellectual disability, a majority (85%) have mild mental retardation (APA, 2000).

Although the CDC provides a population-based study with strong methodology for sampling the population and identifying the disorder, it is important to note that prevalence estimates can vary, depending on the study as a product of several variables, including study methodology, population sample, definition of intellectual disability, population age, and methods of diagnosis (Leonard & Wen, 2002).

Course

The diagnostic criteria for intellectual disability require an onset of impairment prior to 18 years of age. However, the age and mode of onset are directly related to etiology and degree of severity (APA, 2000). The onset of intellectual disability may begin in utero (e.g., Down syndrome), early in childhood (e.g., Rett's disorder), or at some unforeseen time in development (e.g., traumatic brain injury). In addition, research indicates that individuals with severe intellectual disabilities are more likely to be diagnosed earlier in life than those with mild intellectual disabilities (Drews, Yeargin-Allsopp, Decoufle, & Murphy, 1995).

The course of mental retardation is directly related to both the underlying pathology and environmental factors, such as environmental stimulation, education, and support (APA, 2000). Intellectual disability may be a life-long disorder and relatively static, or it may respond to circumstances or intervention, such as in cases of mild intellectual disability in which the individual acquires adaptive functioning skills that exceed the bounds of the diagnostic criteria (Hall et al, 2005). Many individuals with intellectual disabilities enjoy a life rich with social relationships, productive employment, and participation in the community (Hall et al, 2005).

Gender Differences

In the case of mental retardation, males outnumber females at a ratio of approximately 1.5:1 (Bhasin et al, 2006; Hou et al, 1998). This ratio can be partly attributed to the etiology of those intellectual disabilities associated with X-linked disorders (e.g., fragile X syndrome) (Bhasin et al, 2006).

Culture-Specific Information

The prevalence of intellectual disabilities correlates with maternal race, as well as socioeconomic and maternal educational status (less than a high school education) (Leonard & Wen, 2002). Approximately 44% to 50% of all cases of intellectual disability are present in families with low socioeconomic status (SES), and low SES primarily correlates with mild intellectual disability (Campbell et al, 1998; Drews et al, 1995).

Consistently, epidemiologic studies indicate that African American males comprise the group most frequently diagnosed with intellectual disability, which is more than two times the prevalence established for males who are Caucasian (Bhasin et al, 2006). This trend is common across all degrees of severity; however, males who are African American are diagnosed with mild mental retardation four times more frequently than males who are Caucasians (Bhasin et al, 2006). In addition, children who are African American are more likely to be diagnosed with mild intellectual disability of unspecified cause (Drews et al, 1995).

There is some evidence to indicate that children from minority cultures are more likely to score poorly on IQ tests due to socially different behavior and culturally inappropriate IQ testing (Yeargin-Allsopp, Drews, Decoufle, & Murphy, 1995). Culturally inappropriate IQ testing can lead to invalid IQ scores, possibly leading to an incorrect diagnosis of intellectual disability; this may account for the overrepresentation during school age of children who are African American (Yeargin-Allsopp et al, 1995).

In current research, the risk factors associated with race (e.g., an individual who is African American) include maternal age at delivery, economic status, and maternal education, which has led to the conclusion that much of the increased prevalence or identification among the population of people who are African American is preventable (Yeargin-Allsopp et al, 1995).

Impact on Occupational Performance

The severity of the intellectual disability contributes to the impact on occupational performance. For individuals with mild intellectual disability, participation in all areas of occupational performance is often possible. Conversely, individuals with a severe intellectual disability will be challenged across all areas of occupational performance. In addition, the comorbidities associated with intellectual disability, such as losses in hearing or eyesight and mobility impairments, can also have a significant impact on occupational performance. The next section discusses the impact of intellectual disability on health and adaptive skills.

Health

Individuals with intellectual disabilities are significantly more likely to have poorer health than their peers without disabilities (Emerson & Hatton, 2007; Janicki et al, 2002; Kerr et al, 2003). This health disparity is directly related to the complicated interaction of several variables, including genetics, social circumstances, environment, individual behavior, and healthcare access (Krahn et al, 2006). At one time, health problems among individuals with intellectual disabilities were considered inherent to the disorder, but current research has yielded the following conceptual reframing.

Individuals with intellectual disabilities experience health conditions that cluster in three primary categories: associated, comorbid, and secondary conditions (Krahn et al, 2006). **Associated conditions** include those that are directly related to the etiology of the primary impairment (e.g., early dementia, heart defects, low muscle tone), whereas **comorbid conditions** are diseases that are unrelated to the primary condition but co-occur with the associated condition (e.g., influenza, glaucoma, breast cancer) (Krahn et al, 2006). **Secondary conditions** are those diseases that an individual with an intellectual disability experiences at a higher rate than the general population and, in many cases, are preventable (e.g., hypertension, obesity, depression) (Krahn et al, 2006).

The fact that many of the health conditions are preventable or treatable indicates that individuals with intellectual disabilities could lead healthier lives. However, improved health for people with intellectual disabilities requires action on the part of caregivers, occupational therapists and other service providers, individuals with intellectual disabilities, and society. Specific health areas to address include physical health, obesity and underweight, and mental health. See Chapter 46 for additional information on assessment and intervention.

Physical Health

The physical health of individuals with intellectual disabilities is fraught with increased risk for disease, general health problems, and obesity (Janicki et al, 2002; Krahn et al, 2006). Individuals with intellectual disabilities present with relatively higher rates of disorders of the skin, respiratory disorders, urinary infections, psychoses, cardiac disease, arthritis, renal failure, and diabetes (e.g., Janicki et al, 2002; Kerr et al, 2003). Furthermore, individuals with intellectual disabilities demonstrate compromised nutritional states, including difficulty with chewing, aspiration, and food refusal, which contribute to overall poor health (Kerr et al, 2003). These general health conditions are accompanied by deterioration of vision and hearing that is typically underdiagnosed and unaddressed. In addition, individuals with intellectual disabilities have significantly higher rates of poor dental hygiene, missing teeth, and decay (Lewis, Lewis, Leake, King, & Lindemann, 2002).

Sensory impairments represent another area of health in which individuals with intellectual disabilities of all degrees of severity experience these impairments at a significantly higher rate than people without intellectual disabilities (Carvill, 2001; Evenhuis et al, 2001). It is also more likely that individuals with intellectual disabilities will have a sensory impairment that goes undetected and unaddressed (Evenhuis et al, 2001; Kerr et al, 2003). Individuals with severe and profound intellectual disabilities have the highest prevalence of sensory impairment, including visual (e.g., blindness), auditory, and combined impairments (Evenhuis et al, 2001). People with Down syndrome who are at least 50 years of age are most at risk for visual impairment, and individuals with intellectual disabilities are more likely to experience deteriorating vision with age (Evenhuis et al, 2001). Hearing impairments are most common among individuals with Down syndrome and those with a severe or profound degree of intellectual disability (Evenhuis et al, 2001).

Sensory impairments are directly correlated to quality of life and an ability to detect other health problems early; therefore, individuals with intellectual disabilities should receive routine, formal vision and hearing assessments (Kerr et al, 2003).

Occupational therapists can address many of these conditions by providing skills training interventions aimed at improving health promotion behaviors. In the case of sensory impairments, occupational therapists can be involved in modifying the environment to compensate for reduced vision or hearing. Health problems for people with intellectual disabilities frequently persist undetected for reasons primarily related to health-care access and living situation, both of which are reviewed in this chapter.

The Lived Experience

A teacher provided this narrative, describing several children and how they became "teachers" by providing lessons of building on strengths.

Years ago, a teacher spoke with me about the accommodations that she made for a student in her class whose vision impairment was severe enough to require that he read using Braille and navigate his world using mobility training strategies designed to mobilize his other senses. She said, "Everything that I do for Charlie makes my lessons and teaching better for the other students in my class." I have remembered this comment over decades of work with students who have a variety of developmental differences. I feel strongly that what we do for these students often represents the best teaching models that we can bring to our instruction of any group of students.

As a group, students who are developmentally different require that we notice how they learn best, that is, the thinking paths that are most productive for each, the outcome formats that best represent knowledge and understanding, and how each might best advocate for his or her own success. "What works" as the starting place for any instruction or intervention often provides a pathway to possibilities that may be masked by overattention to weaknesses. Here are a few examples.

Alex is a young man of 23 years who reads at the third- to fourth-grade level and regularly communicates independently with family and friends via e-mail, notes, and letters. At age 8, he could not read. Looking at print appeared to be almost physically painful for him, as though letters had thorns on them that pricked his eyes. He did, however, have exquisite sound discrimination, could identify instruments heard on tape by type and name, sing any song he heard with perfect pitch, and identify subtle sound differences in words presented to him auditorily. Alex learned to read by spelling, by first listening to the sounds in words and then recording and reading them.

Angel provides another example. Coming in from recess, a group of students reported an event that occurred on the playground. In answer to the question, "How do you know that?" they responded, "Angel told us." Angel was a student who could not articulate consonants and whole words. She could, however, make vowel sounds that, in combination with expressive inflection, rendered her communication comprehensible to those who paid attention. She was a communicator. The other students taught us to listen.

Matt, at age 14, developed a set of behaviors designed to help him avoid reading at all costs. He was unable to sit for more than 2 or 3 minutes at a task. He tore up materials and turned over furniture. His behaviors often required that he leave the room to protect the learning environment and even the safety of other students. On examination, however, Matt demonstrated the ability to read every sign in the building and to navigate Internet sites with considerable skill. Using these skills as starting points, he acquired enough confidence to tolerate learning skills that rendered him a functional reader in familiar vocational and leisure contexts.

As a teenager, Ann continued to be inconsistent in identifying coins after years of instruction and practice. When the task was defined functionally to focus on coins with clear physical differences (quarter and dime) and meaningful application (use in vending machines), she mastered the skill and was able to use it to purchase snacks independently.

Through work with these students and many others, I have learned the power of helping students identify functional and meaningful applications for their strengths. From this point of competence, they gain the confidence necessary to take risks in areas that are more challenging and to believe in their own capabilities. They become able.

Obesity and Underweight

Current literature indicates that, in developed nations, children and adults with intellectual disabilities demonstrate a significantly higher prevalence of obesity. These findings include individuals who are overweight, obese, and morbidly obese. The prevalence of obesity is higher among individuals who live independently or with family, can eat and drink unaided, are female, have Down syndrome, and/or have mild or moderate intellectual disabilities (Bhaumik, Watson, Thorp, Tyrer, & McGrother, 2008; Emerson, 2005; Rimmer & Wang, 2005; Rimmer & Yamaki, 2006). Women who are African American with an intellectual disability are at the highest risk for obesity (Rimmer & Wang, 2005; Rimmer & Yamaki, 2006). Poor health, high need for assistance, chronic pain, extreme fatigue, and mobility impairments are all associated with obesity and pose significant additional risks for individuals with intellectual disabilities (Rimmer & Wang, 2005; Rimmer & Yamaki, 2006). Of the factors that contribute to the increased prevalence of obesity, the most significant variables are living in the community, poor nutrition, and decreased physical activity (Emerson, 2005; Rimmer & Yamaki, 2006).

Occupational therapists are beginning to assume a role in weight loss programs (Brown, Goetz, Van Sciver, & Sullivan, 2006) and are poised to address obesity issues in people with developmental disabilities. In fact, the American Occupational Therapy Association has issued a position paper on obesity and occupational therapy (Clark, Reingold & Salles-Jordan, 2007). Occupational therapists can play a unique role in obesity prevention and weight loss due to our expertise related to daily activities. Occupational therapists can work to incorporate new habits and modify environments to support healthy eating and increased physical activity.

Individuals with intellectual disabilities are also at increased risk for being underweight, which poses yet another health risk (Emerson, 2005). Women who have severe to profound intellectual disabilities and do not have Down syndrome are most at risk for weighing too little (Bhaumik et al, 2008; Emerson, 2005). In this case, occupational therapists may evaluate feeding issues (e.g., problems with swallowing) and create interventions to increase the intake of calories.

Mental Health

Mental health concerns occur at a greater frequency among adults and children with intellectual disabilities as compared with adults and children without intellectual disabilities. Specifically, children and adolescents have a higher prevalence of conduct disorder, anxiety disorder, hyperactivity, and pervasive developmental disorders (Emerson, 2003). There is no evidence to indicate that individuals with intellectual disabilities have a higher prevalence of depressive disorders, eating disorders, or psychosis (Emerson, 2003; Kerr et al, 2003). However, there is a significant risk that the mental health needs of individuals with intellectual disabilities will not be addressed because they may present with unspecific behaviors that are attributed to the intellectual disability, so further evaluation is neglected (Kerr et al, 2003; Krahn et al, 2006).

Occupational therapists should consider potential mental health issues when working with people with intellectual disabilities, as well as be sensitive during evaluation to behaviors that might indicate anxiety, hyperactivity, or other mental health problems.

Adaptive Skills

To meet the criteria for a diagnosis of intellectual disability, an individual must demonstrate significant differences in at least two areas of adaptive functioning. Even though each individual presents with unique areas of strength and need, there are some trends related to development and degree of intellectual disability severity (Pratt & Greydanus, 2007). The following specific adaptive skills are addressed in this section: social skills, language and communication, mobility, and community participation.

Social Skills

Individuals with intellectual disabilities demonstrate significant differences with regard to social skills development and social participation (de Bildt et al, 2004; Hall et al, 2005). In early development, individuals with mild intellectual disabilities are more likely to demonstrate social skills development that approximates that of their peers; however, in adolescence, as social interaction becomes more complex and nuanced, they will begin to demonstrate more difficulty (de Bildt, Kraijer, Sytema, & Minderaa, 2005; de Bildt, Serra, et al, 2005).

Even in the presence of social skills impairment, there is evidence that individuals with intellectual disabilities are able to establish meaningful and satisfactory social relationships, although their relationships are fewer in number than individuals without a disability (Hall et al, 2005). Although individuals with severe (moderate to profound) intellectual disabilities are unlikely to marry, 73% of individuals with mild intellectual disabilities do marry, and 62% have children (Hall et al, 2005). Importantly, the more severe an individual's degree of intellectual disabilities, the less likely that he or she has reliable sources of help (Hall et al, 2005). Occupational therapists can provide interventions to support the development of social skills and create environments that promote relationships with others.

Language and Communication

There is evidence that individuals who have intellectual disabilities with different underlying etiologies (e.g., different syndromes, type of CNS injury) will demonstrate differing language development profiles that are commensurate with the intellectual disability etiology (Price, Roberts, Vandergrift, & Martin, 2007). However, there are some trends related to degrees of severity.

For example, individuals with mild intellectual disabilities are likely to develop speech, but may have some difficulty with pragmatic language or more abstract, sophisticated language (Pratt & Greydanus, 2007). Individuals with moderate intellectual disabilities will have more deficits in receptive and expressive communication (Pratt & Greydanus, 2007). People with severe intellectual disabilities may develop some speech early in life and basic levels of expressive and receptive language, whereas individuals with profound intellectual disabilities are unlikely to develop speech and will demonstrate limited receptive and expressive communication (APA, 2000; Pratt & Greydanus, 2007).

In a recent study of individuals with moderate to greater intellectual disability severity, receptive language skills were a significant area of difficulty for most: 54% understood some conversation, 33% understood only single words, and 13% were considered unable to comprehend speech (Kerr et al, 2003). There were also notable difficulties with expressive language: 40% could speak in sentences, 30% spoke only single words, and 30% did not have verbal speech (Kerr et al, 2003).

Often, speech therapists are the primary provider of language and communication skills, but occupational therapists are also involved in this area of adaptive skills. Occupational therapists may use adaptive equipment to support participation in daily activities. Adaptive equipment can include communication boards or electronic augmented communication devices. In addition, the occupational therapist may be involved in helping the individual with intellectual disability increase verbalizations or use sign language within the context of specific occupations that are important to the individual. See Chapter 21 for more information on assessment and intervention.

Mobility

An individual's mobility, in part, is determined by the etiology of his or her intellectual disability. However, individuals with severe or profound intellectual disabilities are more likely to experience impaired mobility. A recent study that included a population sample with a relatively high prevalence of moderate to profound intellectual disability found that 60% could walk without assistance and 66% had independent hand use (Kerr et al, 2003). Restrictions in mobility can interfere with self-care activities such as feeding, dressing, and toileting, as well as prevent the individual from traveling from one place to another, including within or between rooms at home. Again, assistive devices can increase independence for some individuals, although others may be unable to effectively use more complex technology such as electric wheelchairs or scooters.

Community Participation

Individuals with intellectual disabilities are capable of living meaningful lives in the community. With mild intellectual disabilities, independent life in the community is likely, but some supports may be necessary for targeted areas of household management (Hall et al, 2005) such as money management or home repairs. Individuals with moderate intellectual disabilities will most likely live in semi-independent living settings. For those with severe intellectual disabilities, assistance and supervision will foster participation in most activities of daily living, whereas individuals with profound mental retardation will require continuous help and supervision for all self-care (Pratt & Greydanus, 2007). Taken together, it is more likely that a person with severe or profound intellectual disability will require a highly structured or nursing-oriented living setting (APA, 2000).

Rates of employment among individuals with intellectual disabilities are lower than those of individuals without intellectual disabilities, and people who have mild intellectual disabilities are significantly more likely to participate in employed work than those with severe (moderate to profound) intellectual disabilities (Hall et al, 2005). However, approximately 13% of individuals with mild intellectual disabilities are able to earn above the median income of the population sampled in Europe (Hall et al, 2005). Individuals with intellectual disabilities are more likely to participate in manual labor and earn less money than people who do not have intellectual disabilities (Hall et al, 2005). Individuals with moderate intellectual disabilities require close employment supervision to secure successful participation in the workforce (Pratt & Greydanus, 2007). With vocation-oriented education, they are able to participate in unskilled or semiskilled work in structured, supervised vocation settings (APA, 2000). It is unlikely that individuals with severe to profound intellectual disabilities will be able to participate in a vocation (APA, 2000).

Using task analysis skills, occupational therapists can assist with making good job matches based on the interests and skills of the individual with intellectual disability. Occupational therapists can also make suggestions to the employer for reasonable accommodations to increase successful performance on the job. Coworkers and supervisors can benefit from education to support inclusion and good work performance. Particularly useful may be training in how to best provide instruction for job duties. See Chapters 18, 47, and 50 for more information on assessment and intervention.

Environmental Factors Contributing to Problems With Occupational Performance

Intellectual disabilities and other comorbidities have an impact on occupational performance; however, environment factors can also significantly interfere with optimal occupational performance. Health-care access, poverty, and maltreatment are common concerns for people with intellectual disabilities.

Health-Care Access

Poor access to health care contributes significantly to the poorer health of individuals with intellectual disabilities, and living in the community appears to contribute to reduced health-care access (Krahn et al, 2006; Lewis et al, 2002). Individuals who live in the community experience significantly poorer health and greater rates of obesity than those who live in more structured, supervised settings (Lewis et al, 2002). In part, supervised settings frequently include medical care, providing built-in access to health services that individuals living in the community must establish for themselves. For example, individuals with intellectual disabilities who live in the community are less likely than

---

Evidence-Based Practice

Individuals with intellectual disabilities experience difficulty engaging in daily life, including self-care, social, and leisure activities, as well as participation in work and school.

➤ Children with intellectual disabilities have less positive early school experiences, as indicated by multiple indices of adaptation to school. Fostering early social skills may be an important target for increasing the positive adaptation to school for young children, especially those with intellectual disabilities. Intervention should target both family education activities and child-centered intervention, attending closely to the development of a partnership between the family and school to ensure a smooth transition (McIntyre, Blacher, & Baker, 2006).

➤ Each individual with an intellectual disability presents with a unique constellation of areas of strength and need. Occupational therapists should carefully conduct assessments to secure a comprehensive, contextually relevant foundation on which to build intervention that fosters the success of the individual as well as any caregivers (as applicable).

McIntyre, L. L., Blacher, J., & Baker, B. L. (2006). The transition to school: Adaptation in young children with and without intellectual disability. *Journal of Intellectual Disability Research, 50*(5), 349–361.

those who live in supervised settings to have a personal physician (Lewis et al, 2002).

Another variable in the network of factors that contribute to poor health is the fact that individuals with intellectual disabilities have less access to preventative care (Krahn et al, 2006). For example, these individuals are less likely to receive vaccinations, obtain screening for diseases such as HIV, have a mammogram, or receive a Pap smear (Lewis et al, 2002). This significant absence of preventative care places the health of people with intellectual disabilities at significant risk.

In addition to inadequate preventative care, physicians are unlikely to dedicate enough time to individuals with intellectual disabilities to allow a comprehensive medical assessment, and many physicians are not adequately prepared to work with this population (Lewis et al, 2002). Furthermore, there is some evidence to indicate that general physicians are reluctant to work with individuals with intellectual disabilities (Lewis et al, 2002), and there is evidence that individuals with intellectual disabilities are not referred to specialists as often as necessary (Kerr et al, 2003).

Besides the environmental and provider factors that affect the health of individuals with intellectual disabilities, there are factors related to the individual that also have an impact on health-care access. Frequently, there are physical barriers to participating in health-care appointments (e.g., transportation, assistance) (Krahn et al, 2006). In addition, there are caregiver variables related to high rates of staff turnover and inaccurate assessment of health-care needs (Kerr et al, 2003). For example, a personal attendant may assess that an individual's vision is only mildly poor, but a formal assessment reveals significant visual impairment. In this way, routine assessment is critical in order to rule out the risk of this type of error. Furthermore, the behaviors that frequently result from an intellectual disability or its underlying etiology can interfere with comprehensive and accurate medical assessment (Kerr et al, 2003).

Poverty

There is a complex relationship among poverty, health, and intellectual disability. Poverty is a significant factor in the prevalence of intellectual disabilities, the health of those individuals, and the socioeconomic status (SES) of families who support them. Individuals who live in poverty are at higher risk for having children with intellectual disabilities (Emerson, 2007). In addition, low SES accounts for 31% of the increased risk for poor health among people with intellectual disabilities (Emerson & Hatton, 2008).

Families who support an individual with an intellectual disability are at significantly higher risk of descent into poverty and are unlikely to emerge from it (Emerson, 2007). Families face a combination of direct and indirect sources of poverty. The support of an individual with an intellectual disability requires financial resources (**direct source** of poverty), such as therapy and special equipment. In addition, the burden of care required for individuals with severe intellectual disabilities results in a higher prevalence of mothers who do not work outside the home (**indirect source** of poverty) (Emerson, 2007; Loprest & Davidoff, 2004). Exposure to poverty in childhood is directly related to decreased health, well-being, opportunity, and experiences,

Evidence-Based Practice

Individuals with intellectual disabilities experience poorer physical and mental health, which is partly related to barriers to health-care access (Krahn, Hammond, & Turner, 2006).

➤ Occupational therapists can work with individuals and with care providers to support physicians in understanding the nature of an individual's impairment, which could promote a more comprehensive and accurate medical assessment.

➤ Occupational therapists can work with agencies and with families to ensure that a person with an intellectual disability has a relationship with critical primary care providers (e.g., physician, dentist, optometrist).

➤ Occupational therapists can work with caregivers to establish a home environment and daily life patterns that promote physical health and emotional well-being. This work is particularly important for individuals who live in the community as opposed to structured, supervised facilities (Lewis, Lewis, Leake, King, & Lindemann, 2002).

Krahn, G. L., Hammond, L., & Turner, A. (2006). A cascade of disparities: Health and health care access for people with intellectual disabilities. *Mental Retardation and Developmental Disabilities Research and Reviews, 12*(1), 70–82.

Lewis, M. A., Lewis, C. E., Leake, B., King, B. H., & Lindemann, R. (2002). The quality of health care for adults with developmental disabilities. *Public Health Report, 117*(2), 174–184.

and children with intellectual disabilities are at higher risk of these circumstances (Emerson, 2007).

Maltreatment

In a review of the prevalence research from 1995 to 2005, Horner-Johnson and Drum (2006) noted that individuals with intellectual disabilities are the victims of maltreatment at a significantly higher prevalence than individuals without disabilities (Horner-Johnson & Drum, 2006). In addition, there is some evidence to indicate that individuals with intellectual disabilities are the victims of maltreatment at a greater prevalence than people with other disabilities (Horner-Johnson & Drum, 2006).

The types of maltreatment that have been documented include sexual, physical, and emotional abuse; neglect; financial exploitation; and over- and undermedication (Murphy, O'Callaghan, & Clare, 2007). The perpetrators can be both acquaintances and staff members (Murphy et al, 2007). Incidents of maltreatment have a deleterious effect on individuals with intellectual disabilities that results in observable differences in their participation and emotional well-being, regardless of the severity of intellectual disability (Murphy et al, 2007). However, there is evidence that individuals do demonstrate some recovery in subsequent months (Murphy et al, 2007).

Occupational therapists need to act as advocates when maltreatment is suspected, and reporting of such incidents is essential. Occupational therapists can work with individuals who have experienced maltreatment to reduce the long-term effects of trauma. Increasing a sense of safety, providing the individual with skills to say no or report maltreatment, and eliminating shame and guilt associated with past events are important strategies for victims of abuse.

Medications

There is no pharmacological treatment that addresses the fundamental cognitive deficits of intellectual disabilities (Handen & Gilchrist, 2006). However, there is evidence that individuals with intellectual disabilities can benefit from psychotropic medications in order to ameliorate the behavioral symptoms and psychiatric conditions that frequently accompany the disorder (Handen & Gilchrist, 2006). A recent study established that individuals with intellectual disabilities are the most overmedicated population of individuals with mental disorders, but research has only just begun to explore the effectiveness of medications for this population (Holden & Gitlesen, 2004).

Recent clinical trends indicate that approximately 27% to 35% of persons with intellectual disabilities are prescribed at least one psychotropic medication (Aman, Sarphare, & Burrow, 1995; Holden & Gitlesen, 2004). Of the medications prescribed, antipsychotic medications are the most common, followed by antianxiety, antidepressant, and anticonvulsant medications (Spreat & Conroy, 1998). More recently, an atypical antipsychotic, risperidone (Risperdal) has become the medication of choice for individuals with intellectual disabilities (Deb & Unwin, 2007; Spreat, Conroy, & Fullerton, 2004). The prescription of antipsychotic medication is associated with mental health problems, violence toward others, adaptive behavior, screaming/yelling/crying behavior, hyperactivity, and age (Spreat & Conroy, 1998). Notably, the severity of an intellectual disability does not predict medication use (Holden & Gitlesen, 2004).

Risperidone

Of the psychotropic medications currently in use for individuals with intellectual disabilities, risperidone is the only medication that has been the subject of randomized controlled trials (RCTs). These studies provide evidence that risperidone is effective and well tolerated for these individuals (Aman, De Smedt, Derivan, Lyons, & Findling, 2002; Gagiano, Read, Thorpe, Eerdekens, & Van Hove, 2005). Specifically, significant gains in the area of severely disruptive

behavior (e.g., aggression, destruction) result from a relatively low dosage compared with that required for the treatment of psychosis (Gagiano et al, 2005; Snyder et al, 2002). In addition, these treatment benefits are not affected by diagnosis, presence or absence of attention deficit-hyperactivity disorder, or IQ (Snyder et al, 2002). Of the side effects documented, weight gain and drowsiness were the most prevalent and problematic (Snyder et al, 2002). Although other atypical antipsychotic medications may be useful for individuals with intellectual disabilities, there is not yet enough evidence to empirically support their use (Deb & Unwin, 2007).

Other Medications

In a review of the literature, Handen and Gilchrist (2006) conclude that the available data indicate that individuals with intellectual disabilities respond to psychotropic medication similarly to individuals who do not have intellectual disabilities. However, the literature that evaluates the effectiveness and safety of antidepressants, mood stabilizers, antianxiety drugs, and opioid antagonists for individuals with intellectual disabilities is sparse, and incorporates weak methodology and small sample sizes (Deb & Unwin, 2007). Although these drugs may be useful for individuals with intellectual disabilities, Handen and Gilchrist (2006) advise that physicians exercise the following cautions when prescribing psychotropic medications: close monitoring, use of lower dosages, and more gradual dosage increases than would be applied to the typically developing population.

Summary

Intellectual disabilities have a great impact on society because of their prevalence and their profound effect on both the physical and psychosocial health of those individuals with the disability. By appreciating the heterogeneity of intellectual disabilities and understanding the influence on occupational performance, occupational therapists can play a significant role in enhancing daily life for individuals with intellectual disabilities at all ages.

Active Learning Strategies

1. Get to Know Someone

To best understand the lived experience of an individual with an intellectual disability, assume an active role in the life of someone who has an intellectual disability. For example, find a group home that serves individuals with intellectual disabilities at which you can volunteer for at least half a day and schedule an interview with one of the group home managers. Ensure that you have an opportunity to support an individual with self-care, home maintenance, and an activity in the community. In advance, use the information in this chapter to create a structured interview with the group home manager.

Reflective Questions

- In what ways did the individual encounter success in his or her day? In what ways did he or she encounter difficulty?

- What actions did you take to facilitate success? When was the best course of action to do nothing?
- What are the moments you would "do over" if you could? Why?
- What were the discrepancies between the caregiver/individual's desired roles and activities, and what was actually possible for him or her?
- Is there anything that would need to be done differently at this group home in order to promote self-determination, independent participation, and/or optimum health and wellness? What?

 In your **Reflective Journal**, describe your experience.

Resources

Books

- Bernstein, J. (2007). *Rachel in the World: A Memoir.* Chicago: University of Illinois Press.
- Defrain, J., Campbell, J. S., & Dahl, S. (2006). *We Cry Out: Living With Developmental Disability.* Lincoln, NE: iUniverse.
- Drew, C. J., & Hardman, M. L. (2006). *Intellectual Disabilities Across the Lifespan* (9th ed.). Upper Saddle River, NJ: Prentice Hall.
- Odom, S. L., Horner, R. H., Snell, M. E., & Blacher, J. (2007). *Handbook of Developmental Disabilities.* New York: Guilford Press.

Organizations

- The ARC of the United States (the world's largest community-based organization of and for individuals with intellectual and developmental disabilities): www.thearc.org
- American Association on Intellectual and Developmental Disabilities: www.aaidd.org
- Division on Developmental Disabilities, Council for Exceptional Children: www.dddcec.org
- National Down Syndrome Society: www.ndss.org
- Learning about intellectual disabilities and health: http://www.intellectualdisability.info/

References

Aman, M. G., De Smedt, G., Derivan, A., Lyons, B., & Findling, R. L. (2002). Double-blind, placebo-controlled study of risperidone for the treatment of disruptive behaviors in children with sub-average intelligence. *American Journal of Psychiatry, 159*(8), 1337–1346.

Aman, M. G., Sarphare, G., & Burrow, W. H. (1995). Psychotropic drugs in group homes: Prevalence and relation to demographic/psychiatric variables. *American Journal of Mental Retardation, 99*(5), 500–509.

American Psychiatric Association (APA). (2000). *Diagnostic and Statistical Manual of Mental Disorders* (4th ed., text revision). Arlington, VA: Author.

Bhasin, T. K., Brocksen, S., Avchen, R. N., & Van Naarden Braun, K. (2006). Prevalence of four developmental disabilities among children aged 8 years—Metropolitan Atlanta Developmental Disabilities Surveillance Program, 1996 and 2000. *Morbidity and Mortality Weekly Report. Surveillance Summaries, 55*(1), 1–9.

Bhaumik, S., Watson, J. M., Thorp, C. F., Tyrer, F., & McGrother, C. W. (2008). Body mass index in adults with intellectual disability: Distribution, associations and service implications: A population-based prevalence study. *Journal of Intellectual Disability Research, 52*(pt 4), 287–298.

Bower, C., Leonard, H., & Petterson, B. (2000). Intellectual disability in Western Australia. *Journal of Paediatrics and Child Health, 36*(3), 213–215.

Brown, C., Goetz, J., Van Sciver, A., & Sullivan, D. (2006). A psychiatric rehabilitation approach to weight loss. *Psychiatric Rehabilitation Journal, 29,* 267–273.

Campbell, B. W., Broman, S. H., Nichols, P. L., & Leff, M. (1998). Maternal and neonatal risk factors for mental retardation: Defining the "at-risk" child. *Early Human Development, 50*(2), 159–173.

Carvill, S. (2001). Sensory impairments, intellectual disability and psychiatry. *Journal of Intellectual Disability Research, 45*(6), 467–483.

Centers for Disease Control and Prevention (CDC). (1996). Postnatal causes of developmental disabilities in children aged 3–10 years—Atlanta, Georgia. *Morbidity and Mortality Weekly Report, 45*(6), 130–134.

Chapman, D. A., Scott, K. G., & Stanton-Chapman, T. L. (2008). Public health approach to the study of mental retardation. *American Journal of Mental Retardation, 113*(2), 102–116.

Chelly, J., Khelfaoui, M., Francis, F., Cherif, B., & Bienvenu, T. (2006). Genetics and pathophysiology of mental retardation. *European Journal of Human Genetics, 14*(6), 701–713.

Clark, F., Reingold, F. S., & Salles-Jordan, K. (2007). Obesity and occupational therapy: Position paper. *American Journal of Occupational Therapy, 61,* 701–703.

Croen, L. A., Grether, J. K., & Selvin, S. (2001). The epidemiology of mental retardation of unknown cause. *Pediatrics, 107*(6), E8.

de Bildt, A., Kraijer, D., Sytema, S., & Minderaa, R. (2005). The psychometric properties of the Vineland Adaptive Behavior Scales in children and adolescents with mental retardation. *Journal of Autism and Developmental Disorders, 35*(1), 53–62.

de Bildt, A., Serra, M., Luteijn, E., Kraijer, D., Sytema, S., & Minderaa, R. (2005). Social skills in children with intellectual disabilities with and without autism. *Journal of Intellectual Disability Research, 49*(pt 5), 317–328.

de Bildt, A., Sytema, S., Ketelaars, C., Kraijer, D., Mulder, E., Volkmar, F., & Minderaa, R. (2004). Interrelationship between Autism Diagnostic Observation Schedule–Generic (ADOS-G), Autism Diagnostic Interview–Revised (ADI-R), and the *Diagnostic and Statistical Manual of Mental Disorders* (DSM-IV-TR) classification in children and adolescents with mental retardation. *Journal of Autism and Developmental Disorders, 34*(2), 129–137.

Deb, S., & Unwin, G. L. (2007). Psychotropic medication for behaviour problems in people with intellectual disability: A review of the current literature. *Current Opinion in Psychiatry, 20*(5), 461–466.

Delange, F. (2001). Iodine deficiency as a cause of brain damage. *Postgraduate Medical Journal, 77*(906), 217–220.

Drews, C. D., Murphy, C. C., Yeargin-Allsopp, M., & Decoufle, P. (1996). The relationship between idiopathic mental retardation and maternal smoking during pregnancy. *Pediatrics, 97*(4), 547–553.

Drews, C. D., Yeargin-Allsopp, M., Decoufle, P., & Murphy, C. C. (1995). Variation in the influence of selected sociodemographic risk factors for mental retardation. *American Journal of Public Health, 85*(3), 329–334.

Emerson, E. (2003). Prevalence of psychiatric disorders in children and adolescents with and without intellectual disability. *Journal of Intellectual Disability Research, 47*(1), 51–58.

Emerson, E. (2005). Underweight, obesity and exercise among adults with intellectual disabilities in supported accommodation in Northern England. *Journal of Intellectual Disability Research, 49*(2), 134–143.

Emerson, E. (2007). Poverty and people with intellectual disabilities. *Mental Retardation and Developmental Disabilities Research Reviews, 13*(2), 107–113.

Emerson, E., & Hatton, C. (2007). Poverty, socio-economic position, social capital and the health of children and adolescents with intellectual disabilities in Britain: A replication. *Journal of Intellectual Disability Research, 51*(pt 11), 866–874.

Emerson, E., & Hatton, C. (2008). Self-reported well-being of women and men with intellectual disabilities in England. *American Journal of Mental Retardation, 113*(2), 143–155.

Evenhuis, H. M., Evenhuis, H. M., Theunissen, M., Denkers, I., Verschuure, H., & Kemme, H. (2001). Prevalence of visual and hearing impairment in a Dutch institutionalized population with intellectual disability. *Journal of Intellectual Disability Research, 45*(5), 457–464.

Gagiano, C., Read, S., Thorpe, L., Eerdekens, M., & Van Hove, I. (2005). Short- and long-term efficacy and safety of risperidone in adults with disruptive behavior disorders. *Psychopharmacology (Berlin), 179*(3), 629–636.

Hall, I., Strydom, A., Richards, M., Hardy, R., Bernal, J., & Wadsworth, M. (2005). Social outcomes in adulthood of children with intellectual impairment: Evidence from a birth cohort. *Journal of Intellectual Disability Research, 49*(pt 3), 171–182.

Handen, B. L., & Gilchrist, R. (2006). Practitioner review: Psychopharmacology in children and adolescents with mental retardation. *Journal of Child Psychology and Psychiatry, 47*(9), 871–882.

Holden, B., & Gitlesen, J. P. (2004). Psychotropic medication in adults with mental retardation: Prevalence and prescription practices. *Research in Developmental Disabilities, 25*(6), 509–521.

Horner-Johnson, W., & Drum, C. E. (2006). Prevalence of maltreatment of people with intellectual disabilities: A review of recently published research. *Mental Retardation and Developmental Disabilities Research Reviews, 12*(1), 57–69.

Hou, J. W., Wang, T. R., & Chuang, S. M. (1998). An epidemiological and aetiological study of children with intellectual disability in Taiwan. *Journal of Intellectual Disability Research, 42*(pt 2), 137–143.

Janicki, M. P., Davidson, P. W., Henderson, C. M., McCallion, P., Taets, J. D., Force, L. T., Sulkes, S. B., Frangenberger, E., & Ladrigan, P. M. (2002). Health characteristics and health services utilization in older adults with intellectual disability living in community residences. *Journal of Intellectual Disability Research, 46*(4), 287–298.

Kerr, A. M., McCulloch, D., Oliver, K., McLean, B., Coleman, E., Law, T., Beaton, P., Wallace, S., Newell, E., & Eccles, T. (2003). Medical needs of people with intellectual disability require regular reassessment, and the provision of client- and carer-held reports. *Journal of Intellectual Disability Research, 47*(2), 134–145.

Krahn, G. L., Hammond, L., & Turner, A. (2006). A cascade of disparities: Health and health care access for people with intellectual disabilities. *Mental Retardation and Developmental Disabilities Research and Reviews, 12*(1), 70–82.

Leonard, H., & Wen, X. (2002). The epidemiology of mental retardation: Challenges and opportunities in the new millennium. *Mental Retardation and Developmental Disabilities Research Reviews, 8*(3), 117–134.

Lewis, M. A., Lewis, C. E., Leake, B., King, B. H., & Lindemann, R. (2002). The quality of health care for adults with developmental disabilities. *Public Health Report, 117*(2), 174–184.

Loprest, P., & Davidoff, A. (2004). How children with special health care needs affect the employment decisions of low-income parents. *Maternal and Child Health Journal, 8*(3), 171–182.

Murphy, G. H., O'Callaghan, A. C., & Clare, I. C. (2007). The impact of alleged abuse on behaviour in adults with severe intellectual disabilities. *Journal of Intellectual Disability Research, 51*(Pt 10), 741–749.

Pratt, H. D., & Greydanus, D. E. (2007). Intellectual disability (mental retardation) in children and adolescents. *Primary Care, 34*(2), 375–386; abstract ix.

Price, J., Roberts, J., Vandergrift, N., & Martin, G. (2007). Language comprehension in boys with fragile X syndrome and boys with Down syndrome. *Journal of Intellectual Disability Research, 51*(pt 4), 318–326.

Rahman, A., Iqbal, Z., Bunn, J., Lovel, H., & Harrington, R. (2004). Impact of maternal depression on infant nutritional status and illness: A cohort study. *Archives of General Psychiatry, 61*(9), 946–952.

Raymond, F. L., & Tarpey, P. (2006). The genetics of mental retardation. *Human Molecular Genetics, 15*(spec no 2), R110–R116.

Rimmer, J. H., & Wang, E. (2005). Obesity prevalence among a group of Chicago residents with disabilities. *Archives of Physical Medicine and Rehabilitation, 86*(7), 1461–1464.

Rimmer, J. H., & Yamaki, K. (2006). Obesity and intellectual disability. *Mental Retardation and Developmental Disabilities Research Reviews, 12*(1), 22–27.

Snyder, R., Turgay, A., Aman, M., Binder, C., Fisman, S., & Carroll, A. (2002). Effects of risperidone on conduct and disruptive behavior disorders in children with subaverage IQs. *Journal of the American Academy of Child and Adolescent Psychiatry, 41*(9), 1026–1036.

Spreat, S., & Conroy, J. (1998). Use of psychotropic medications for persons with mental retardation who live in Oklahoma nursing homes. *Psychiatric Services, 49*(4), 510–512.

Spreat, S., Conroy, J. W., & Fullerton, A. (2004). Statewide longitudinal survey of psychotropic medication use for persons with mental retardation: 1994 to 2000. *American Journal of Mental Retardation, 109*(4), 322–331.

Stromme, P., & Magnus, P. (2000). Correlations between socioeconomic status, IQ and aetiology in mental retardation: A population-based study of Norwegian children. *Social Psychiatry and Psychiatric Epidemiology, 35*(1), 12–18.

Wilska, M., & Kaski, M. (1999). Aetiology of intellectual disability— The Finnish classification: Development of a method to incorporate WHO ICD-10 coding. *Journal of Intellectual Disability Research, 43*(pt 3), 242–250.

Yeargin-Allsopp, M., Drews, C. D., Decoufle, P., & Murphy, C. C. (1995). Mild mental retardation in black and white children in metropolitan Atlanta: A case-control study. *American Journal of Public Health, 85*(3), 324–328.

Eating Disorders

Laura C. Lock and Geneviève Pépin

> "Starvation is control. Control is tough. Bones are beautiful when thin isn't enough.
>
> —Anonymous, World Wide Web, 2006

Introduction

Many people struggle to understand the behaviors associated with eating disorders such as anorexia and bulimia nervosa. Eating disorders have been superficially labeled as "slimming diseases," but these conditions are not in the least superficial. People experiencing these disorders are tortured with self-rejection and emotional difficulties linked to the demands of adult roles and relationships (Broussard, 2004; Crisp, 2006a). They experience a constant struggle to eat in a normal, healthy way, resulting in "overcontrolled" or "out of control" eating patterns that become maladaptive coping mechanisms. They develop maladaptive eating and lifestyle habits due to limited stress management, psychological, social, and life skills (Kloczko & Ikiugu, 2006; Martin, 1998; National Institute for Clinical Excellence [NICE], 2004).

These conditions are on the increase (American Psychiatric Association [APA], 2006). Individuals with eating disorders struggle to feel acceptable and competent within their cultural, familial, and/or social environment, which they perceive as threatening, unsupportive, or dissatisfying (Stice, Maxfield, & Wells, 2003; Surgenor, Maguire, Russell, & Touyz, 2007; Tozzi, Sullivan, Fear, McKenzie, & Bulik, 2003). Their low self-esteem evokes intense distress, which is alleviated by the relentless pursuit of an idealized thin identity and accompanying maladaptive lifestyle (Cohen, Kristal, Neumark-Sztainer, Rock, & Neuhouser, 2002). Their pursuit provides meaning, purpose, and satisfaction, albeit maladaptive, and leads to significantly compromised physical and mental health, social isolation, and impaired quality of life (de la Rie, Noordenbos, Donker, & van Furth, 2007; Hoek, 2006; Nordbo, Espeset, Gulliksen, Skarderud, & Holte, 2006; Rusca, 2003). In essence, people with eating disorders experience difficulties with identity and competence that result in impaired motivation to participate in adaptive everyday self-care, work, and leisure activities.

This chapter describes the symptomatology, etiology, and impact of anorexia nervosa and bulimia nervosa. It also explains how these conditions affect occupational participation, which is defined as "engagement in work, play or activities of daily living, that are part of one's socio-cultural context, and that are desired and/or necessary to one's well-being" (Kielhofner, 2002, p. 114). It outlines the role of occupational therapy, which aims to help people with eating disorders experience health and wellness via participation in adaptive, meaningful activity (Wilcock, 1998). It also highlights challenges inherent in the treatment of individuals with eating disorders, including change resistance, psychosocial impairment, and comorbid mental disorders, and physical risk factors such as suicide attempts and mortality (Blinder, Cumella, & Sanathara, 2006; Calvo, Alba, Serva, & Pelaz, 2001; Stice, 2002a).

Description of Eating Disorders

Eating disorders are considered disorders of the mind and body, characterized by the intense fear of being fat, which leads to an obsessive quest for thinness (Garfinkel, 2002; Kinoy, 2001; Thompson & Smolak, 2001). Eating disorders can be considered on a spectrum—with anorexia at one end, bulimia at the other—and many unhealthy and potentially dangerous eating habits (e.g., dieting, binge eating, purging, overexercising) falling between the two extremes.

Eating disorders were first described in the late 17th century by Richard Morton, in a paper published in 1689 in which he presented two cases of what would become known as anorexia nervosa (Goldbloom, 1997). Other clinical cases were described in the mid-1800s by other physicians, including Charles Laseque and William Gull. Gull's work concluded that anorexia nervosa was not only self-starvation associated with different traditions and cultures, but also a psychological disorder (Gordon, 2000). Following that, little information can be found about anorexia and other disordered eating behaviors during the 1920s and 1930s (Brumberg, 2000). The following decades saw literature addressing psychoanalytic interpretations of eating disorders and, particularly, anorexia nervosa, but it was in the 1970s with Hilde Bruch's work that more literature concerning eating disorders and more persons presenting with eating disorders became known (Gordon, 2006).

Eating disorders are on the increase in North America and elsewhere in the world (APA, 2006). North American statistics present eating disorders as the mental illness with the highest mortality rate (Harbottle, Birmingham, & Sayani, 2008). More precisely, it is the third most prevalent chronic disease among adolescents, with numerous and severe consequences (APA, 2000a; Health Canada, 2002). As an example, in Canada between 1987 and 1999, there were 34% more hospitalizations of girls younger than 15, and a 29% increase was noted among young women ages 15 to 24 years (Health Canada, 2002).

Traditionally, eating disorders have been associated with industrialized countries and Western culture. However, literature suggests an increase in the number of cases of eating disorders in other parts of the world such as Japan, China, Mexico, and Fiji (Becker, Burwell, Gilman, Herzog, & Hamburg, 2002; Huon , Mingyi, Oliver, & Xiao, 2002; Kazutoshi et al., 2000; Toro et al., 2006). Also, although eating disorders are more frequent in adolescent girls and women, more males are now struggling with these disorders (Andersen, 2001; Crisp, 2006b). Eating disorders are spreading to diverse communities with differing race, gender, and socioeconomic status, although higher socioeconomic status presents a higher risk (Soh, Touyz, & Surgenor, 2006).

Anorexia Nervosa

Anorexia nervosa is described as the intense fear of being fat, a disturbance of body image, and an obsession with food and thinness, associated with the refusal to maintain a normal weight for one's age and height (Garfinkel, 2002; Wilson, 2005). This obsession translates into severe food restriction and extreme weight control behaviors, which lead to major weight loss (Health Canada, 2002; National Institute of Nutrition [NIN], 2001).

DSM-IV-TR Criteria

Because anorexia develops most often during adolescence, it is sometimes difficult to differentiate between normal growth and developmental changes and the development of the eating disorder. Weight loss is often noted at the time of pubertal menarche, and growing concerns about appearance and body image are common. Therefore, specific diagnostic criteria have been developed by the American Psychiatric Association in the *Diagnostic Statistical Manual of Mental Disorders, Fourth Edition, Text Revision* (DSM-IV-TR) (APA, 2000b). Detailed criteria are listed in Box 10-1.

BOX 10-1 ▓ DSM-IV-TR Criteria for Anorexia Nervosa

1. Refusal to maintain body weight at or above a minimally normal weight for age and height (e.g., weight loss leading to maintenance of body weight less than 85% of that expected, or failure to make expected weight gain during periods of growth, leading to body weight less than 85% of that expected).

2. Intense fear of gaining weight or becoming fat, even though underweight.

3. Disturbance in the way in which one's body weight or shape is experienced, undue influence of body weight or shape on self-evaluation, or denial of the seriousness of the current low body weight.

4. Amenorrhoea (in women) (i.e., the absence of at least three consecutive menstrual cycles).

From American Psychiatric Association. (2000). *Diagnostic and Statistical Manual of Mental Disorders* (4th ed.). Washington, DC: Author.

The intense fear of being fat and a distorted body image are specific traits of anorexia. In fact, individuals with anorexia are often thin to the point of emaciation, but they do not recognize this. As a result, they become or remain obsessed with food and weight. They count calories, engage in vigorous exercise, and tend to isolate themselves in order to continue these self-reinforcing behaviors.

The diagnosis of anorexia nervosa also requires that the person be significantly underweight, which is a major distinction between anorexia and bulimia. **Body mass index (BMI)** is often used to determine if someone is underweight. BMI is calculated by dividing an individual's weight (in kilograms) by the square of his or her height (in meters). Normal BMI ranges between 20 and 25, and anorexia is diagnosed at less than 17.5. A BMI below 13 indicates a life-threatening disorder.

Subtypes

There are two subtypes of anorexia nervosa: **restricting type** and **binge eating/purging type**. An individual with the restricting type will not engage in binge eating or purging behaviors such as self-induced vomiting (Gleaves, Miller, Williams, & Summers, 2000; NIN, 2001). Instead, these individuals will decrease their food intake dramatically and continuously, leading to a striking weight loss. Individuals with the binge eating/purging type of anorexia regularly engage in binge eating or purging behavior (Gleaves et al., 2000; NIN, 2001). Approximately one-half of people with anorexia develop the restricting type, and the other half engages in binge eating and purging behaviors (Andersen, 2001; APA, 2000a; Pomerleau, Ratté, Boivin, & Brassard, 2001). However, recent studies showed that between 8% and 62% of individuals with an initial diagnosis of anorexia will develop bulimic-like symptoms during the course of their illness (Bulik, Reba, Siega-Riz, & Reichborn-Kjennerud, 2005).

Prevalence

Anorexia nervosa affects approximately 1% of Western populations, the mortality rate is close to 15%, and individuals with anorexia nervosa as a group have a life span 25 years shorter than the general population (Harbottle et al., 2008). There are indications that anorexia is on the rise, with a North American study indicating that by age 13 years, 80% of girls and 10% of boys have been on diets with the precise intent to lose weight because they are dissatisfied with their appearance (Striegel-Moore & Smolak, 2001).

Course

Epidemiological studies report that anorexia most frequently starts between the ages of 14 and 25, with a peak age of onset that varies between 15 and 19 years (Bulik et al., 2005; Health Canada, 2002; Wilson, 2005). The literature suggests that approximately 90% of people diagnosed with anorexia are female (APA, 2000a; Striegel-Moore & Smolak, 2001). However, more cases are now found in women past adolescence, and authors have cited that up to 5% of individuals with anorexia nervosa are older than 25 years of age (NIN, 1993; Pomerleau et al., 2001).

Several psychological and physical comorbidities are observed in individuals with anorexia (APA, 2000a; Garfinkel, 2002; Thompson & Smolak, 2001). The most frequent psychological factors are depression, anxiety, obsessive-compulsive disorders, personality disorders, and mood disorders (APA, 2000a; Garfinkel, 2002; Health Canada, 2002; NIN, 2001). The malnourishment and food restriction observed in anorexia are believed to lead to many physical problems, including the following (APA, 2000b, 2006; Beumont, 2002; Health Canada, 2002):

- Hypothermia (a lower than normal body temperature)
- Bradycardia (an abnormally slow heart rate) and risk of cardiac failure
- Amenorrhea (absence of a period) or irregular menses
- Edema
- Loss of muscle tone and muscle mass
- Osteoporosis and other skeletal problems
- Hormonal problems
- Skin problems
- Brittle nails and hair, hair loss, and lanugo (a fine, white hair that helps keep the body warm)
- General decrease in bodily functions
- Metabolic, biochemical, renal, and gastrointestinal problems
- Generalized weakness

Fortunately, most physical problems abate when the individual resumes healthy eating habits. However, osteoporosis is irreversible. Finally, deaths from anorexia are most often due to cardiac arrest secondary to severe food restriction or suicide (APA, 2000b, 2006; Beumont, 2002; Hoek, 2006).

Bulimia Nervosa

Bulimia, which is found at the other end of the eating disorder spectrum, can also be a life-threatening disorder. Despite an apparently normal weight, the disorder shares the psychopathological fear of fatness with anorexia. However, an essential distinction in the clinical presentation is the presence of episodes of binging that are associated with different forms of purging and inappropriate compensatory behavior such as abuse of laxatives and diuretics (APA, 2000a; Beumont, 2002). Binge eating episodes imply consumption of an abnormally large amount of food associated with the intense fear of being unable to stop or control the binge eating episodes. These episodes are combined with attempts to rid the body of the food by engaging in self-induced vomiting, excessive use of laxatives or diuretics, excessive exercise, or fasting (APA, 2000a; Beumont, 2002; Thompson & Smolak, 2001). The binging and purging episodes are typically undertaken in utmost secrecy, and often result in rapid weight gains and losses. Moreover, an overwhelming feeling of guilt and shame follows each episode (APA, 2000a; Beumont, 2002; Thompson & Smolak, 2001).

DSM-IV TR Criteria

Symptomatology of bulimia is characterized by recurrent binge eating episodes and frenetic compensatory behaviors. Just as with anorexia nervosa, specific diagnostic criteria define bulimia (APA, 2000b). These criteria are listed in Box 10-2.

It is important to understand that the amount of food eaten during a binge eating episode is usually, but not always, larger than what another person would normally eat. For most, it is far more than nibbling during the day or eating between meals. The mean caloric intake during a binge eating episode ranges between 3,031 and 4,479 kcal,

---

BOX 10-2 ■ DSM-IV-TR Criteria for Bulimia

1. Recurrent episodes of binge eating. The episode of binge eating is characterized by both of the following:
   a. Eating, in a discrete period of time (e.g., within any 2-hour period), an amount of food that is definitely larger than most people would eat during a similar period of time and under similar circumstances
   b. A sense of lack of control over eating during the episode
2. Recurrent compensatory behavior in order to prevent weight gain, such as self-induced vomiting, misuse of laxatives, diuretics, or other medications, fasting, or excessive exercise.
3. The binge eating and compensatory behaviors both occur, on average, at least twice a week for 3 months.
4. Self-evaluation is unduly influenced by body shape and weight.
5. The disturbance does not occur exclusively during episodes of anorexia nervosa.

---

making the amount of food taken unambiguously large (Keel, Mayer, & Harnden-Fisher, 2001; NIN, 2001). For others, it is the feeling of being "out of control" with food intake that represents a binge. Usually, the person eats very quickly; hence, the duration of the episode is usually short (NIN, 2001).

Subtypes

There are two distinct subtypes of bulimia: purging and nonpurging. In the purging type, the individual engages in behaviors such as self-induced vomiting and excessive use of laxatives and diuretics (APA, 2000b; Gleaves et al., 2000). In the nonpurging type, the person will not purge, but engages in other compensatory behaviors, such as intense exercising and fasting (APA, 2000b; Gleaves et al., 2000). In either case, these behaviors are often linked to a lack of impulse control (Engel et al., 2005; Steiger, 2004; Wonderlich, Crosby, et al., 2005), which points to another distinction between bulimia and anorexia. Whereas bulimia is associated with impulsivity, anorexia is often linked with perfectionism and control, although impulsive features can also coexist.

Prevalence

Bulimia, having been officially recognized more recently than anorexia in 1979, has fewer available statistics. However, it has been estimated that approximately 4% of the population suffers from bulimia (Andersen, 2001; APA, 2000b; Garfinkel, 2002; Ratté & Pomerleau, 2001). A recent study of 2,881 individuals with bulimia nervosa found a lifetime prevalence rate of 2.3%; 76% fit the purging subtype and 24% the nonpurging subtype (Keski-Rahkonen et al., 2008). The study also found a 5-year clinical recovery rate of 55%, but most symptoms are long standing, and recovery is gradual.

Course

Most cases of bulimia are found in females, starting in late adolescence or early adulthood (APA, 2000b; Garfinkel, 2002). Several psychological comorbidity factors and other health problems are associated with this complex disorder (APA, 2000b, 2000b; Garfinkel, 2002; Health Canada, 2002;

Thompson & Smolak, 2001). The most common psychological factors are mood disorders combined with impulsive actions, such as drug and alcohol abuse, self-harm, sexual disinhibition, or shoplifting. Anxiety and personality disorders are also common (Engel et al., 2005; Steiger, 2004; Wonderlich, Crosby, et al., 2005). Problems that occur as a result of binging, purging, and other weight control strategies are renal problems and electrolytic imbalance (potassium, sodium), leading to headaches, dizziness, loss of balance, and gastrointestinal problems. These problems are mostly due to repeated vomiting (NIN, 2001). Moreover, the most serious complication related to excessive vomiting is hypokalemia (low blood potassium levels), which can cause cardiac problems. Furthermore, excessive vomiting leads to loss of teeth enamel, dental problems, swelling of salivary glands, chronic sore throat, and irritated vocal cords and deep mouth structures. Excessive use of laxatives can lead to intestinal problems and metabolic imbalance (APA, 2000a; Pomerleau et al., 2001).

Etiology

Eating disorders are multifactorial, and understanding the complex etiology can require comprehensive intervention approaches (Andersen, 2001; APA, 2000a; Garfinkel, 2002; Wilson, 2005). Indeed, several factors interacting with each other are considered potential causes of the development of eating disorders. Figure 10-1 illustrates the multifactorial aspect of these disorders. As shown, predisposing factors are believed to increase the vulnerability of a person to an eating

disorder in the presence of precipitating factors (Lilenfeld, Wonderlich, Riso, Crosby, & Mitchel, 2006; Sassaroli & Ruggiero, 2005; Westerberg, Edlund, & Ghaderi, 2008). Precipitating factors, such as stressful life events, are often described as "the last straw" by clients. The interaction between predisposing and precipitating factors is believed to lead to the development of an eating disorder. Once the disorder has developed, perpetuating factors keep the person in the cycle of restrictions and compulsions, therefore maintaining the illness.

Predisposing Factors

Predisposing factors are believed to increase the individual's vulnerability to develop an eating disorder.

Personality

Characteristics that promote the development of a fragile and anxious personality increase the risk of an individual developing an eating disorder. Many personality characteristics differ, depending on the eating disorder (Pomerleau et al., 2001; Steiger & Israël, 2000), and are presented in Table 10-1.

Other psychological factors related to both eating disorders involve insecure attachments and separation-individuation problems (Gleaves et al, 2000; Striegel-Moore & Smolak, 2001). In fact, identity formation depends on the ability to move through the separation-individuation continuum of normal development. It allows individuals to experiment, learn, identify, evaluate, and compare before deciding what and whom to become (Striegel-Moore & Smolak, 2001). Tension between the need to belong and the desire to be

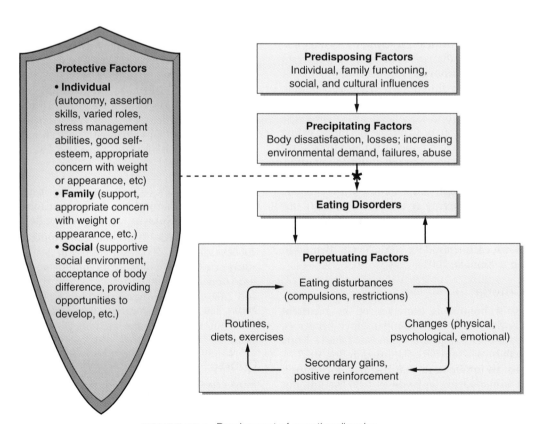

FIGURE 10-1. Development of an eating disorder.

Table 10-1 ● **Personality Characteristics and Eating Disorders**

Eating Disorder	Common Personality Characteristics
Anorexia nervosa	• Compulsivity and perfectionism • Desire to conform • Lack of initiative and spontaneity • Introversion and limited expression of emotions • Tendency to avoid risks, danger, and emotions • High need for validation from others • Excessive self-control • Impaired ability to permit self-gratification
Bulimia nervosa	• Impulsivity • Seeking sensory stimulations and/or heightened mood states (e.g., substance use, self-harm, sexual relationships) • Extroversion • Inadequate self-control • Impaired ability to cope with delayed or denied self-gratification

independent is influential in eating disorder development (Striegel-Moore & Smolak, 2001). Moreover, low self-esteem, difficulties in identity formation, negative self-image, and difficulty in establishing fulfilling and meaningful relationships are believed to put people at risk for developing eating disorders (Striegel-Moore, Seeley, & Lewinsohn, 2003; Striegel-Moore & Smolak, 2001).

Biology

There is an important body of literature concerning biology and its links to eating disorders, including strong evidence that indicates that serotonin plays a role in the development of eating disorders (Engel et al., 2005; Steiger, 2004; Wonderlich et al., 2005). More precisely, on the one hand, serotonin dysregulation (i.e., variability in the concentration levels of serotonin and alteration in its functions) contributes to different signs and symptoms of eating disorders (Engel et al., 2005; Steiger, 2004; Wonderlich et al., 2005). On the other hand, evidence shows that dieting can result in reduced brain serotonin synthesis, leading to more serotonergic dysregulation, which creates a vicious circle in which eating disorder symptomatology is maintained (Steiger, 2004). Moreover, some personality traits, such as impulsivity and perfectionism, have been linked to variations in serotonin level (Steiger, 2004). Finally, increasing evidence links traumatic stress, such as child abuse, to altered serotonin activity (Engel et al., 2005, Steiger, 2004; Wonderlich et al., 2005). The specific mechanisms of these interactions is still being investigated, but current evidence is strong and suggests promising theoretical and clinical implications for understanding and treating eating disorders.

Family Functioning

There are claims in the literature that there is a genetic contribution to eating disorders (APA, 2002a, 2002b; Pomerleau et al., 2001). Thus, families of individuals with eating disorders should be studied with attention. Genetic and hereditary studies indicate that children of parents who have had eating disorders are at higher risk of developing eating

disorders (Kaye et al., 2008). The same findings apply to twin studies, which demonstrated that, when one twin has an eating disorder, the other twin is at higher risk of developing eating difficulties of his or her own (Garner & Garfinkel, 1997; Gleaves et al., 2000; Pomerleau et al., 2001). A recent review compared data from family and twin studies and concluded that there is a concordance rate of 26% for bulimia and 35% for anorexia in monozygotic twins (Ross, 2006).

When one family member experiences an eating disorder, the entire family system is affected. Interactions within the family system can influence the development of an eating disorder, just as eating disorders can influence the family's functioning and its dynamic (Kinoy, 2001). However, specific family characteristic can increase an individual's sensitivity to develop an eating disorder (Gleaves et al., 2000; Striegel-Moore & Smolack, 2001; Thompson & Smolack, 2001; Vandereycken, 2002):

■ Alcohol and/or drug abuse in the family
■ Family violence
■ Sexual abuse
■ Overvaluing of appearance and thinness
■ Eating habits organized around diets and food restriction
■ Lack of opportunity to develop one's independence and autonomy
■ Overprotectiveness
■ Rigidity
■ Excessive or absence of parental control

Social and Cultural Influences

Increasing evidence indicates that social and cultural influences play an important role in the development of eating disorders (Berg, 2001; Gleaves et al., 2000; Kinoy, 2001; Stice, 2002b; Striegel-Moore & Smolak, 2001). Increasingly, social pressures glorify thinness and associate it with success and happiness. Social reinforcement and cultural norms value people on the basis of physical appearance and place value on obtaining the perfect body (Kinoy, 2001; Stice, 2002b). The image of Western women promoted in the media influences body image and self-esteem. It sanctions thinness as beauty. Despite the fact that most fashion magazine photos are altered to fit certain standards, girls and women still aspire to them as symbols of beauty and happiness. This sends the message that to be popular and successful, one must be strikingly thin (Drench, Noonan, Sharby, & Hallenborg Ventura, 2007). Also, being overweight is associated with laziness and lack of discipline. People who are overweight can be alienated, rejected by society, and subject to discrimination (Puhl & Brownell, 2002).

The media promotes an ever thinner body type (Stice, 2002b). In fact, over the past several decades, top models, actresses, and other cultural female icons have become significantly thinner (Stice, 2002b). In addition, controlling weight and refraining from eating certain foods is perceived as showing strength and determination (Berg, 2001). To someone with low self-esteem, the pressure to be thin that is promoted by the mass media, in combination with body dissatisfaction, can increase feelings of inadequacy and trigger a cycle of food restriction and dieting.

Precipitating Factors

Negative perceptions and thoughts about oneself, one's appearance, the environment, and/or the future can precipitate the development of disordered and unhealthy eating habits, which can eventually result in an eating disorder. A comment on one's body or appearance, a failure, a defeat or a setback, a relationship break-up, or major stress can all precipitate an eating disorder (Striegel-Moore & Smolack, 2001; Wilkins, 1998). A specific environmental event linked to eating disorder vulnerability is changes in school from one level to another (e.g., moving from primary school to high school, or from high school to college or university) because students must adapt to a new environment with new demands and higher expectations (Striegel-Moore & Smolack, 2001; Wilkins, 1998). A study of high school students found that eating disorders were highly related to substance use (Pisetsky, Chao, Diencer, May, & Striegel-Moore, 2008). Although the exact nature of the relationship is unknown, substance abuse may increase vulnerability to eating disorders.

Importantly, no single event will lead to an eating disorder; rather, it involves the interactions between multiple factors that significantly increase the risk of developing an eating disorder (Pomerleau et al., 2001; Striegel-Moore & Smolack, 2001).

Perpetuating Factors

Once an eating disorder has developed, the early changes are often satisfying and seen as improvement by people around the individual, whether family members, peers, or even a stranger. Indeed, it is common to hear someone being complimented on his or her new figure and weight loss. Unfortunately, comments of that sort reinforce the disordered eating attitudes and behaviors in people who are already vulnerable (Andersen, 2001; APA, 2000a; Kinoy, 2001). Consequently, the vulnerable individual will develop strategies to maintain the weight loss and/or increase the restriction and obsessive thoughts about weight and appearances (Gleaves et al., 2000; Striegel-Moore & Smolack, 2001). Also, the effects of fasting and food restrictions can contribute to the development of cognitive distortions that perpetuate the disorder. For example, the individual thinks of him- or herself as strong and in control, as demonstrated by the ability to restrict food intake.

Protective Factors

Although rarely addressed in the literature, **protective factors** are now considered when looking at the development of eating disorders (Thompson & Smolak, 2001). These factors can be grouped in individual, family, and social categories. Hence, developing protective factors can play an important role in preventing the developmental process of eating disorders, as shown in Figure 10-1. Protective factors include (Thompson & Smolak, 2001)

- Assertion skills, independence, and autonomy
- Opportunity to invest in a variety of roles (e.g., student, friend, club member, worker)
- Ability to use stress management techniques
- Positive self-esteem
- Family environment that is not overly concerned with appearance, beauty, and thinness
- Family relationships that allow the person to develop a sense of belonging and individuation
- Social environment that is not overly concerned with beauty and thinness

These protective factors can guide families and healthcare specialists in the development of prevention strategies.

Gender Differences

Research shows that eating disorders are most common in females, although up to 10% of individuals with anorexia are male, and recent studies demonstrate that men experience bulimia more commonly than anorexia (Andersen, 2002; NIN, 1993; Weltzin et al., 2005). When compared with females, males have a stronger tendency to use compulsive exercise rather than different purging methods for weight control (Weltzin et al., 2005). The age of onset in males ranges from 17 and 24, indicating a later onset than females (Crisp, 2006a; NIN, 1993). As is the case in females with eating disorders, the risks of developing anorexia or bulimia are greater when a male's professional and personal recognition is linked to his body (Hulley & Hill, 2001; Wertheim, 1992).

Occupations in which aesthetics are directly linked to success increase the risk of developing an eating disorder (Baum, 2006; Crisp, 2006b). The same applies in sports in which athletes must maintain a specific weight or low body fat is an advantage (Baum, 2006). Occupations and sports with a greater risk for eating disorders in women include ballet, modeling, figure skating, diving, swimming, gymnastics, and rowing, whereas wrestling and horse racing are particularly associated with male anorexia nervosa (Andersen, Bartlett, Morgan, & Brownell, 1995; Hulley & Hill, 2001; Wertheim, 1992). In the latter, male jockeys are more at risk than their female counterparts because women tend to be naturally lighter and smaller (Baum, 2006; Hulley & Hill, 2001). In wrestling, a lower weight allows the individual to participate in a weight class in which he may have a greater advantage. In males, it seems that weight loss is more motivated by the desire to achieve an athletic performance than by an obsession with weight and thinness, as is the case in women (Andersen et al., 1995).

Other predisposing factors that are more common in males than females include being raised in a family with parents who have a mental illness and conflicts regarding sexual identity (Andersen, 2002; Andersen et al., 1995; Crisp, 2006a; Herzog, Bradburn, & Newman, 1990; Schneider & Agras, 1987; Wertheim, 1992). Apparently, fear about possible homosexuality can prompt anorexia as a defense mechanism (Crisp, 2006a).

Approximately twice as many females as males are regularly on a diet because of ambivalent attitude and feelings toward food, weight, and appearance. Generally speaking, females are less satisfied with their weight than males (Kiefer, Rathmanner, & Kunze, 2005; Weltzin et al., 2005). Furthermore, 18% of females and 5% of males will have carried out at least one diet in the course of their adolescence due to overconcern with weight and appearance (Kiefer et al., 2005). Consequently, in adolescence, there is an increased risk of developing an eating disorder over time.

The Lived Experience

Katharine Wealthall

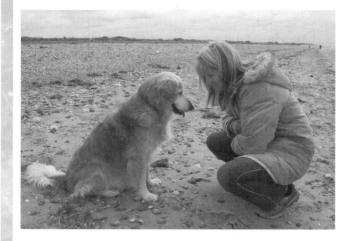

Katharine Wealthall, a young British woman, describes the experience of reaching life in recovery from anorexia nervosa in extracts from her book, Little Steps: Surviving Anorexia and Bulimia Nervosa.

I am an anorexic. I have anorexia nervosa. Existing within the illness is a terrifying horror. It makes little sense and yet the sufferer feels trapped by thoughts, feelings and associated behaviors . . . regardless of how damaging and dangerous they are.

During my most serious bout of anorexia (in its obvious physical form) I could see what was happening and I wanted it over before it began, and yet it was like looking at someone else, I was utterly powerless to halt the destruction. It was as though there were two sides to me: the positive rational side and its negative, irrational counterpart, Even now in recovery, I still experience this conflict . . . the mind of someone with an eating disorder becomes closed off to hearing or seeing situations for what they really are. The brain behaves in such a way that only the negative perception of any given circumstance is acknowledged. To put it in more simple terms, ask any person with an eating disorder if a glass is half full or half empty—the glass is always half empty! It is as though the person is not allowed to feel happy or to feel good about themselves, even if they are able to value aspects of their lives, these things are masked by the negativity.

I have always been so lucky with many aspects of my life but I always experience enormous guilt about that. The profoundly negative mindset and the consequent illness just did not allow me to feel I was worthy of anything positive. There are certain patterns of thinking that are evident within the majority of sufferers whilst in the illness. These include: an intense dislike for themselves (developing into the need to hurt/punish themselves), the belief of being a failure . . . of not being good enough at anything, the feeling that they have nothing to offer and nothing of worth to say and the belief that they are responsible for the well-being of those around them and the power to fix all that is wrong. It is interesting to note that all these thoughts, feelings and beliefs are ones that are constantly demanding far too much of any one person.

The need for perfection, if it is evident, is seen in absolute terms. Nothing less is satisfactory. When aiming for such impossibly high standards it is obvious to objective observers that such perfection is unattainable and yet those in the illness are simply not allowed to rest from striving to achieve it.

I have often referred to my own recovery as being like a child trapped in an adult body; people who meet me make the normal assumptions you would of an adult and I have normal adult responsibilities. For me, however, every day is a battle to cope with the way the world works and being a responsible adult in normal ways, for example, not hurting myself if things go wrong, not feeling to blame/responsible if things are difficult for others.

Although I am in recovery and am working to achieve this normality, I can vividly remember the intense fear of what it would be like without the illness; indeed I still experience that fear now that I am living it. For a period of my treatment I felt as though I wasn't anybody without the illness that had defined and controlled me all my life. It takes time to rebuild, to relearn but it can be done. Therefore, to further emphasise, a reluctance to leave the illness is not the sufferer wanting to be ill . . . it is the fear of what is to come and being ready to find out. Sufferers must be constantly reassured that it will be worth finding out who they can be, what their life could be like. Those close to them must keep sight of the real person and do all they can to keep affirming that reality.

Even on really black days when it would be so much easier to stop fighting and allow it to just consume me again I have to remember that I have gotten this far for a reason and I have to find out what that is . . . to do that I have to stay well, stay safe. I am slowly beginning to realise that I don't just owe it to the people that love me: I owe it to myself too.

I have anorexia nervosa. I am an anorexic. But that is not all I am.

Reprinted with permission from Wealthall, K. (2005). *Little Steps: Surviving Anorexia and Bulimia Nervosa.* Brentwood, UK: Chipmunka.

Cultural Differences

Eating disorders and, particularly, idealization of thinness have long been associated with Western cultures and, within the United States, most prevalent in European Americans. However, recent studies debunk this conventional wisdom. In a large study comparing individuals from several different Eastern and Western countries, there were no differences in body image discrepancy or eating pathology (Rubin, Gluck, Knoll, Lorence, & Geleibter, 2008). Similarly, a study of college students in the United States found no differences in disordered eating behavior among African American, European American, and Latina American students (Rich & Thomas, 2008).

Prognosis

Current knowledge about eating disorders allows for the identification of factors that influence the outcomes of anorexia nervosa and bulimia. Literature yields evidence that duration of illness, importance that the individual assigns to the weight loss, successive inefficient treatment, and presence of comorbid personality disorders are factors associated with a poor outcome (Berkman, Lohr, & Bulik, 2007; Pomerleau et al., 2001). More specifically, outcomes of anorexia are believed to be worse when the disorder is coupled with depression, mood and anxiety disorders, limited social functioning and contacts, and substance abuse. However, a younger age of onset is associated with a better outcome (Bulik et al., 2005). Factors associated with poor outcomes in bulimia are similar to those related to anorexia. Depression, mood disorders, and substance abuse are common to both illnesses, whereas lack of impulse control is specific to bulimia (Bulik et al., 2005).

Other evidence specific to anorexia and bulimia shows that between 40% and 50% of individuals with anorexia, and 50% of people with bulimia, can expect to fully recover and see their symptoms disappear over time (APA, 2000a; Health Canada, 2002; Ratté & Pomerleau, 2001). Approximately 30% of people with eating disorders will experience an improvement in their condition, but will face relapses and residual symptoms (Sullivan, 2002). Last, in 20% of cases of anorexia and bulimia, the illness will become severe and enduring (Sullivan, 2002). In other words, these individuals will still meet some diagnostic criteria and will experience enduring symptoms and ongoing resistance to change. Of that last percentage, between 5% and 10% of persons with anorexia nervosa will die (Ratté & Pomerleau, 2001).

Another longitudinal study looking at a 20-year follow-up period revealed a mortality rate of 15% to 20% for persons with anorexia nervosa (Sullivan, 2002). These findings contradict a recent study conducted over a 12-year period with 103 women with anorexia nervosa (Fichter, Quadflieg, & Hedlund, 2006). The results suggest that 27.5% of the participants had a good outcome, 25.3% an intermediate outcome, 39.6% had a poor outcome, and 7.7% (or 7 persons) were deceased (Fichter et al., 2006). Fichter et al. defined the categories of outcomes. A "good outcome" implied that the participants maintained a body weight within the normal range and experienced regular menstrual cycles. Participants reached an "intermediate outcome" when their body weight reached normal ranges, but was not maintained, and/or when they experienced menstrual irregularities. Finally, a poor outcome was noted when participants' body weight never reached a normal range, leading to serious health concerns, and when menstruation was absent or virtually absent (Fichter et al., 2006). These findings highlight a smaller proportion of persons presenting a good outcome or full recovery from the disorder and a much higher percentage of persons with a poor outcome.

Psychological Influences That Affect Occupational Participation

People with eating disorders experience difficulties participating in self-care, productivity, and leisure occupations, particularly if the activities involve eating or interactions with others (Gogarty & Brangan, 2004; Harries, 2005; Lock, 2000). Psychological factors, which are usually preconscious, impair the individuals' **volition**, with pathologically disabling consequences (Cohen et al., 2002) (Fig. 10-2). Volition refers to a person's motivation for action and different occupations (Kielhofner, 2008). It can be defined as "a pattern of thoughts and feelings about oneself as an actor in one's world which occur as one anticipates, chooses, experiences and interprets what ones does" (Kielhofner, 2008, p. 16). Five key cognitive concepts commonly affecting motivation in persons with eating disorders have been identified by Cooper, Whitehead, and Boughton (2004). These constructs negatively impact the individual's volition, thus impairing the person's motivation to engage in occupational and social activities that are perceived as stressful. These constructs are

1. Overvaluation of weight, shape, and their control
2. Mood intolerance
3. Core low self-esteem
4. Perfectionism
5. Interpersonal problems

Overvaluation of Weight, Shape, and Their Control

Individuals with eating disorders judge their self-worth largely, or even exclusively, in terms of weight and shape, as well as their ability to control them (Fairburn & Harrison, 2003, p. 408). They perceive their bodies as worthy of criticism, which precipitates avoidance of social interaction, social eating, and body-centric activities (Gogarty & Brangan, 2004).

Mood Intolerance

People with eating disorders find it difficult to tolerate negative emotions that are part of the normal experience of adult occupations, roles, responsibilities, and relationships (Fryer, Waller, & Kroese, 1997; Holtkamp, Müller, Heussen, Remschmidt, & Herpertz-Dahlmann, 2005; Waller et al., 2003). This construct is linked to lack of self-acceptance; fear of rejection from others; and impaired emotional, social, and life skills. Participating in maladaptive weight minimization activities allows the person to avoid or alter negative emotions, increase personal control, and reinforce acceptability and self-competence (Crisp, 2006a; Nordbo et al., 2006). For example, a person with an eating disorder may avoid dating because of a fear of rejection. Dietary restriction or binging/purging and other comorbid behaviors provide distraction and assist with mood regulation and stress relief (Bloks & van Furth, 2004; Paul, Schroeter, Dahme, & Nutzinger, 2002). However, people with bulimia feel overwhelming guilt after binging.

Core Low Self-Esteem

Low self-esteem, which has been described as a combination of limited self-liking and self-competence, has a significant impact on occupational performance (Bardone, Perez, Abramson, & Joiner, 2003; Halvorsen & Heyerdahl, 2006; Stoffel, 1993; Surgenor et al., 2007). Low self-esteem is a central theme in the development of eating disorders. The

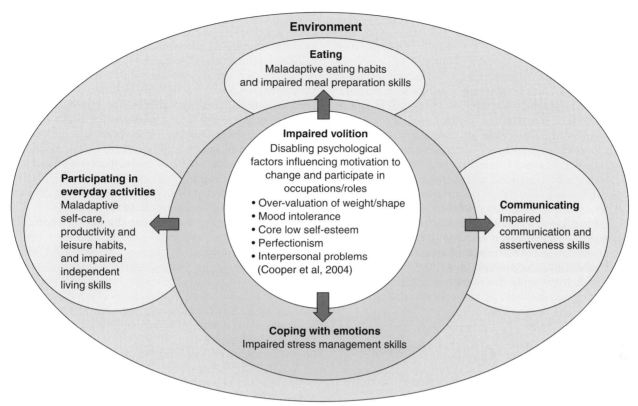

FIGURE 10-2. Difficulties experienced by people with eating disorders that impact occupational participation.

individual's perceived inability to feel acceptable or cope within their social or occupational environment is fueled by distorted beliefs and cognitions (Barris, 1987; Bers & Quinlan, 1992; Jone, Harris, & Leung, 2005) about themselves, others, and life in general. This mind-set precipitates avoidance of certain adaptive occupations that are perceived as threatening or dissatisfying, such as trying out for a sports team or accepting a promotion (Gogarty & Brangan, 2004).

Perfectionism

Most individuals with eating disorders have unrealistically high personal standards and believe they are unacceptable and unlovable unless they are perfect (Striegel-Moore, Silberstein, & Rodin, 1993). Eating is linked to greed or fat, which symbolize unacceptability, leading to self-rejection and erroneously expected rejection from others (Lock, 2006; Strauman, Vookes, Berenstein, Caiken, & Higgins, 1991). Perfectionism is strived for in the individual's daily performance at work and school, at home, and with friends and family. The inability to achieve perfection leads to a sense of failure and shame (Bouley & Sadik, 1992; Forbush, Heatherton, & Keel, 2007; Shafran, Cooper, & Fairburn, 2002). This shame is alleviated through the maladaptive pride linked to weight minimization or other maladaptive achievements associated with striving for the perfect body (Skarderud, 2007).

Interpersonal Problems

Social anxiety and interpersonal difficulties, which are often linked to insecure early attachments, conflict, or trauma (e.g., neglect, abuse), can lead to impoverished relationships

(Hernandez, 1995; Mangweth et al., 2005; Troisi et al., 2006). Sufferers often drift into social isolation due to impaired social confidence and preoccupation with self-presentation (Hinrichsen, Wright, Waller, & Meyer, 2003; Striegel-Moore et al., 1993). Negative social comparison leads to social withdrawal and fear of romantic encounters and physical intimacy (Jarry, Polivy, Herman, Arrowood, & Pliner, 2006). The limited social and emotional coping skills of people with eating disorders often fall short of the demands of the social environment.

Impact on Occupational Performance

Attempts to differentiate between anorexia and bulimia can be misleading when focusing on occupational performance because both disorders can lead to similar occupational performance issues. Individuals can also experience both anorexic and bulimic episodes (Beumont & Touyz, 2003; Collier & Treasure, 2004; NICE, 2004). Both conditions share the struggle to achieve satisfactory relationships and to develop a strong sense of self-esteem and a positive identity. However, there are areas of functioning that are different.

The most significant difference between anorexia and bulimia is the anorexic's phobic avoidance of normal body weight, shape, and function (Crisp, 2006a). Anorexia can be described as a way of coping with problems of identity or avoidance of adult role expectations (Halmi, 2005; Nordbo et al., 2006). Individuals with anorexia often demonstrate competence and accomplishment, particularly in academic and task performance (Barris, 1986), but exhibit impairment in areas of social-leisure performance and family relations (Thompson & Schwartz, 1982). They hold abnormal beliefs regarding guilt, perceive themselves as less competent than others, and expect less success (Bers & Quinlan, 1992). Individuals with a diagnosis of anorexia, who also exhibit impulsive features, share functional difficulties commonly demonstrated by individuals with bulimia (Ward, Campbell, Brown, & Treasure, 2003).

Individuals with bulimia are often attracted to occupations and roles that involve challenge, risk, and sexuality (Culbert & Klump, 2005; Diaz-Marsa, Carrasco, & Saiz, 2000). They seek gratification, comfort, approval from others, and success, but struggle to tolerate dissatisfaction, discontentment, frustration, discomfort, loss, and social responsibility (Broussard, 2004). They often find social, leisure, and work activities stressful, although many are high achievers within their employment role. They may also struggle to perform roles as spouse, parent, and family member (Johnson & Berndt, 1983).

Individuals with eating disorders face several challenges that impact on occupational participation, including

- Maladaptive eating habits and impaired meal preparation skills
- Maladaptive lifestyle habits and impaired independent living skills
- Impaired communication and assertion skills
- Impaired stress management skills
- Resistance to change

Maladaptive Eating Habits and Impaired Meal Preparation Skills

Maladaptive food consumption and problematic meal preparation skills are common primary difficulties in individuals with eating disorders (Martin et al., 1999; Shah, Passi, Bryson, & Agras, 2005; Sysko, Walsh, Schebendach, & Wilson, 2005). Eating evokes extreme anxiety (Cohen et al., 2002), and individuals struggle to identify "normal" healthy meals and accurate portion sizes (Abeydeera, Willis, & Forsyth, 2006). They restrict food intake or avoid digestion of food and have a very narrow range of foods that they feel safe eating. They often use eating as a mechanism to manage their emotions (Lindeman & Stark, 2001). Vegetarianism is common, possibly as another means of weight control (Gilbody, Kirk, & Hill, 1999). Meals are often eaten excessively slowly or inappropriately fast, sometimes in abnormal, ritualistic, or socially inappropriate ways (Boschi et al., 2003; Tappe, Gerberg, Shide, Rolls, & Anderson, 1998). Food may be cut into tiny pieces or contaminated with excessive condiments to ensure the experience of eating is self-punitive. Many have no experience of eating three balanced meals per day in their lifetime. Although many individuals have advanced cooking skills, others have none (Lock, 2000). Shopping for food can sometimes take hours. Social situations requiring public eating are either avoided or followed by purging to avoid absorption of calories (Martin, 1998).

Maladaptive Lifestyle Habits and Impaired Independent Living Skills

Other challenges faced by individuals with eating disorders include the participation in maladaptive self-care, productivity, and leisure occupations, and difficulties with independent living (Harries, 2005; Lock, 2000; NICE, 2004). Typical maladaptive activities include pathological dieting, exercise, obsession-compulsive routines, mirror gazing, and body checking (Collier & Treasure, 2004; Cooper et al., 2004; Davis et al., 1998; Pearlstein, 2002; Shafran, Fairburn, Robinson, & Lask, 2004). Domestic, educational, and vocational activities can be undertaken to excess to the extent that adaptive interests become subordinate (Barris, 1986; Lock, 2000). For example, individuals may work extreme hours and, in doing so, avoid social and leisure occupations. Overly restrained or impulsive spending may also be a feature of individuals with eating disorders. Personal grooming activities may be undertaken either to excess or neglected. Dressing is often used to camouflage the emaciated body (Gogarty & Brangan, 2004).

People with eating disorders can also exhibit a decreased interest in vocational and social pursuits, and their lives often lack a sense of meaning and purpose (Barris, 1987; Henderson, 1998). They become obsessed with eating-disordered and eating-focused thoughts, and leave little time and energy for anything else. For example, participation in maladaptive activities associated with maintaining the eating disorder can result in a narrowing repertoire of daily occupations and, ultimately, occupational deprivation and imbalance as the eating-disordered behavior becomes the person's major life role (Gold, 2004; Helbig & McKay, 2003). These self-reinforcing occupations lead to the development of a maladaptive occupational identity (Roth, 1986). For example, a client in treatment within the St. George's Eating Disorders Service in London stated, "My eating disorder used to be my job."

Impaired Communication and Assertion Skills

Difficulties with interpersonal communication are also significant (Takahashi, Takahashi, Hisamura, & Miyaoka, 2005). Contributory factors include social anxiety, body image disturbance, conflict avoidance, and perceived ineffectiveness (Hinrichsen et al., 2003; Larson & Johnson, 1981; Lilenfield et al., 2006). Individuals struggle with making and sustaining effective relationships, asserting their needs and views, managing conflict, and expressing difficult feelings, especially anger (Geller, Cockell, & Goldner, 2000; Henderson, 1998). Individuals with bulimia or anorexia often demonstrate marked frustration, intolerance, and sometimes an aggressive, alienating communication style, which can lead to impaired relationships and negatively impact their employment record and social relationships (Hillert, Staedtke, & Wise, 2002; Treasure, Smith, & Crane, 2007).

Impaired Stress Management Skills

The pervasive difficulty that compounds all other challenges is the individual's limited ability to manage stress. Individuals struggle to cope with their emotional responses to the demands of their social and occupational roles (Fryer et al., 1997; Martin, 1998). This impairs their self-competence and motivation to participate in adaptive activities that are perceived as risky. They are psychologically disabled by subconscious negative beliefs about their acceptability to others and ability to cope. For example, an individual who receives a negative comment from a supervisor at work may overgeneralize and catastrophize the comment such that the job is now seen as impossible. The person may then quit the job to escape further stress and also avoid looking for new work.

Resistance to Change

Most individuals with an eating disorder present as significantly resistant to change (Calvo et al., 2001). Many perceive their symptoms as a lifestyle choice rather than a clinical problem (Meenan, 2003). Enhancing readiness to change is vital to enable these individuals to accept the challenges of learning new coping, living, and social skills (Killick & Allen, 1997; Treasure & Bauer, 2005). Prochaska and DiClemente's (1983) Transtheoretical Model of Change is a useful tool for identifying a client's readiness to change (Collins, 2005).

The model suggests that individuals move through a number of stages when embarking on any form of behavioral change (Fig. 10-3). These stages are as follows:

1. Precontemplation
2. Contemplation
3. Determination
4. Action
5. Maintenance

Before an individual even considers change, this person is said to be in the **precontemplation stage** of change. During that stage, the person resists change because he or she cannot see any reason to change the behaviors (Treasure et al., 2007). When the individual starts to consider changing, he or she moves into the **contemplation stage**. The person is still unsure about embarking on change, but considers the pros and cons of changing some behaviors. Then he or she progresses through the **determination stage** of change. In this stage, the person considers change and recognizes the challenges, while building a determination to at least start to change some of the behaviors. Hopefully, determination will lead to the **action stage** of change, which indicates he or she is implementing behavioral change. The final stage is identified as the **maintenance stage**, when the individual is learning to maintain the changes that he or she has implemented. The person consolidates and builds on the skills he or she has learned (Treasure et al., 2007).

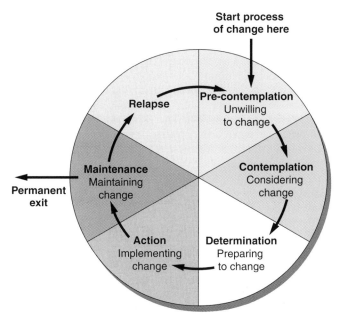

FIGURE 10-3. Stages of change according to Prochaska and DiClemente's (1983) Transtheoretical Stages of Change model.

Evidence-Based Practice

Evidence supports the use of cognitive behavioral therapy (NICE, 2004; Wilson, 2005) and motivational interviewing (Cassin, von Ranson, Heng, Brar, & Wojtowicz, 2008), particularly in reducing binge eating. Motivational enhancement, which is an adaptation of motivational interviewing applied to eating disorders (Treasure & Schmidt, 2001; Vitousek, Watson, & Wilson, 1998), is cited as a promising new treatment for anorexia nervosa focused on promoting readiness to change (Kaplan, 2002; NHS Quality Improvement Scotland [QIS], 2006). Group treatment is cited as an important means of therapy (Bell, 2003; Kalodner & Coughlin, 2004; NHS QIS, 2006; Zipfel et al., 2002).

➤ Occupational therapists can use cognitive behavioral approaches in combination with occupation-based activities to address distorted thinking related to body image, self-esteem, and perfectionism, as well as difficulties engaging in adaptive self-care, productivity, and leisure occupations.

➤ Occupational therapists can use cognitive behavioral approaches in combination with occupation-based activities to address distorted thinking related to body image, self-esteem, and perfectionism, as well as difficulties engaging in adaptive self-care, productivity, and leisure skills.

➤ Motivational interviewing (more recently described within the eating disorders literature as motivational enhancement) (Dean, Touyz, Rieger, & Thornton, 2008; Feld, Woodside, Kaplan, Olmsted, & Carter, 2001) is important when trying to engage the reluctant client into therapy.

➤ Motivational enhancement is important when trying to enhance readiness to change in change-resistant clients.

➤ Group-based treatment, including experiential and psychoeducative occupation-focused activities, are recommended.

Bell, L. (2003). What can we learn from consumer studies and qualitative research in the treatment of eating disorders? *Eating & Weight Disorders, 8*(3), 181–187.

Cassin, S. E., von Ranson, K. M., Heng, K., Brar, J., & Wojtowicz, A. E. (2008). Adapted motivational interviewing for women with binge eating disorder: A randomized controlled trial. *Psychology of Addictive Behaviors, 22*, 417–425.

Dean, H. Y., Touyz, S. W., Rieger, E., & Thornton, C. E. (2008). Group motivational enhancement as an adjunct to inpatient treatment for eating disorders: A preliminary study. *European Eating Disorders Review, 16*(4), 256–267.

Feld, R., Woodside, D. B., Kaplan, A. S., Olmsted, M. P., & Carter, J. C. (2001). Pretreatment motivational enhancement therapy for eating disorders: A pilot study. *International Journal of Eating Disorders, 29*(4), 393–400.

Kalodner, C. R., & Coughlin, J. W. (2004). Psychoeducational and counseling groups to prevent and treat eating disorders and disturbances. In W. J. L. DeLuca, D. A. Gernty, & M. T. Riva (Eds.), *Handbook of Group Counselling and Psychotherapy* (pp. 481–496). Thousand Oaks, CA: Sage.

Kaplan, A. S. (2002). Psychological treatments for anorexia nervosa: A review of published studies and promising new directions. *Canadian Journal of Anorexia Nervosa, 4*(3), 235–242.

National Institute for Clinical Excellence (NICE). (2004, January). "Eating Disorders: Core Interventions in the Treatment and Management of Anorexia Nervosa, Bulimia Nervosa and Related Eating Disorders." Clinical Guideline 9. London: Author. Available at: http://www.nice.org.uk/nicemedia/pdf/cg009niceguidance.pdf (accessed November 1, 2009).

NHS Quality Improvement Scotland (QIS). (2006, November). *Eating Disorders in Scotland: Recommendations for Management and Treatment.* Available at: http://www.nhshealthquality.org/nhsqis/files/EATDISORDER_REP_NOV06.pdf (accessed November 1, 2009).

Treasure, J., & Schmidt, U. (2001). Ready willing and able to change: Motivational aspects of the assessment and treatment of eating disorders. *European Eating Disorders Review, 9*, 4–18.

Vitousek, K. B., Watson, S., & Wilson, G. T. (1998). Enhancing motivation for change in treatment-resistant eating disorders. *Clinical Psychology Review, 18*, 391–420.

Wilson, G. T. (2005). Psychological treatment of eating disorders. *Annual Review of Clinical Psychology, 1*, 439–465.

Zipfel, S., Reas, D. L., Thornton, C., Olmsted, M. P., Williamson, D. A., Gerlinghoff, M., Herzog, W., & Beumont, P. J. (2002). Day hospitalisation programs for eating disorders: A systematic review. *International Journal of Eating Disorders, 31*(2), 105–117.

Intervention

Treatment is offered within inpatient, day patient, outpatient, and community-based settings, depending on the severity of the disorder and risk factors. Interventions should be multidisciplinary. The team provides services, including psychiatric, medical, nursing, dietetic, psychology, psychotherapy, family therapy, physical therapy (physiotherapy), and occupational therapy interventions (Royal Australian and New Zealand College of Psychiatrists, 2004). Clients with life-threatening conditions (usually measured with a BMI below 13) require specialist inpatient care, often with nasogastric tube feeding. In most treatment programs, clients receive nutritional counseling, pharmacotherapy, interpersonal or psychodynamic psychotherapy, and family therapy (Fairburn & Brownell, 2002; Luborsky, 1984; Martin, 1998; Vitousek & Gray, 2005). Cognitive behavior therapy is often a primary component of the treatment because it has a strong evidence base for treating eating disorders (Mitchell, Agras, & Wonderlich, 2007; NICE, 2004). There is also much interest in the effect of unassisted and assisted self-help (Mitchell et al., 2007).

Self-Help and Support Groups

Many individuals with eating disorders seek help outside the professional realm through self-help programs or support groups. These approaches may serve as a primary intervention or as maintenance after professional intervention. Self-help can take the form of books, workbooks, or CD-ROMs, and many such programs use a cognitive behavioral approach. In a review of self-help programs, Sysko and Walsh (2007) found that self-help was more beneficial than no treatment, but studies have not been conducted comparing self-help to professional intervention.

Support groups can take the form of face-to-face meetings or online groups that offer support and information to people with eating disorders (Darcy & Dooley, 2007). Evidence, even if limited, about the efficacy of support groups for eating disorders, especially in cases of bulimia nervosa, is promising (Banasiak, Paxton, & Hay, 2005; Crow et al., 2006; Ljotsson et al., 2007; Perkins, Murphy, Schmidt, & Williams, 2006; Schmidt et al., 2007).

General Principles of Intervention

Treatment interventions must be tailored to the client's presenting risk factors and readiness to change. The client may choose treatment that leads to full "recovery" (symptom abatement) or "harm reduction" (staying ill safely), or he or she may require "intensive care" interventions. To fully address the complexity of eating disorders, treatment must focus on the following three elements:

1. **Physical harm reduction** via weight gain and/or symptom interruption to minimize risk. Some individuals may be unwilling to participate in treatment if the expectation is full recovery. Therefore, a focus on harm reduction serves as a means of engaging the client and addressing the most dangerous behaviors.
2. **Cognitive reconstruction** via individual and/or group therapy to improve ego strength, conflict resolution, personal identity, and self-acceptance at normal body weight.

3. **Psychosocial functional enablement** via individual and/or group psychoeducative, creative, and experiential occupation-focused activities to improve occupational performance and perceived self-competence.

Occupational therapy provides the functional enablement component, with a focus on developing motivation to participate in adaptive occupations that are perceived as risky; replacing unhealthy routines with healthy ones; and improving task performance skills, that is, improving volition, habituation, and performance capacity using therapeutic activity, as described within the Model of Human Occupation (Kielhofner, 2008).

Occupational therapy also assists with cognitive reconstruction. Clients' distorted cognitions about their acceptability and competence can be supportively challenged within experiential and psychoeducative occupation-focused activities, using cognitive behavioral interventions. When clients experience supportive cognitive challenge and skills enhancement within activities that they associate with rejection or failure, this promotes the development of self-acceptance and self-competence. By providing a range of activities that provide positive experiences, occupational therapists help develop clients' interpretation processes and performance abilities concurrently, leading to a stronger and more positive identity (Breden, 1992; Kielhofner, 2008).

Treatment should address eating behavior and attitudes regarding weight and shape, and focus on wider psychosocial issues, with the goal of weight gain and symptom abstention (NICE, 2004, p. 89). Enhancing psychosocial functioning includes the improvement of the following skills:

- Eating and meal preparation skills (Gogarty & Brangan, 2004; Kloczko & Ikiugu, 2006; NICE, 2004)
- Lifestyle and independent living skills (Abeydeera et al., 2006; Lim & Agnew, 1994; Lock, 2000; NICE, 2004)
- Communication and assertion skills (Gogarty & Brangan, 2004; Martin, 1998; NHS Quality Improvement Scotland [QIS], 2006; Stoffel, 1993)
- Stress management skills (Gogarty & Brangan, 2004; Henderson, 1998; NHS QIS, 2006; Stoffel, 1993)

Specific Occupational Therapy Interventions

Several frames of references that are familiar to occupational therapists are cited as efficacious in the literature, in particular the Model of Human Occupation, combined with cognitive behavioral therapy (Beck, Rush, Shaw, & Emery, 1979; Fairburn & Brownell, 2002; Henderson, 1998; Kielhofner, 2008; Lim & Agnew, 1994). The psychoanalytic approach is recommended when using creative or projective interventions (Harries, 2005; Lim & Agnew, 1994; Luborsky, 1984). Motivational enhancement, which is an adaptation of motivational interviewing, applied to eating disorders and focused on promoting readiness to change, is cited as a promising new treatment (Geller, 2002; Kaplan, 2002; Kotler, Boudrea, & Devlin, 2003; Miller & Rollnick, 2002; Pung, 2004; Treasure & Schmidt, 2001; Vitousek, Watson, & Wilson, 1998). It is particularly useful for individuals who are highly ambivalent about change. This approach is particularly relevant for clients with a life-threatening condition and those who need to learn how to stay ill safely, as well as for adolescents who are usually in treatment because their parents mandate it. Individuals with an eating disorder clearly prefer collaborative interventions (Geller, Brown, Zaitsoff, Goodrich, & Hastings, 2003). Bell (2003, p. 183) states that clients consider supportive, empathetic relationships (by professionals or nonprofessionals) to be essential.

Occupational therapists may consider implementing the following interventions:

- Menu planning and meal preparation
- Lifestyle redesign and independent living skills
- Communication and assertion training
- Stress management
- Leisure activities
- Projective art
- Crafts
- Relapse prevention
- Body image improvement

Menu Planning and Meal Preparation

The literature suggests that enabling clients to eat effectively is essential (Lock, 2000; Martin, 1998; Matusevich, Garcia, Gutt, de la Parra, & Finkelstein, 2002). This includes helping the client develop the following skills (Bell, 2003; Vanderlinden, Buis, Pieters, & Probst, 2007) (also see Chapter 47):

- Planning, shopping for, preparing, and eating cooked meals within a therapeutic group setting
- Planning menus in advance of preparing the meal, which trains the client to disconnect food intake from mood management
- Using dietetically approved portion guidelines when planning menus
- Cooking, if cooking skills are limited
- Serving themselves correct portion sizes and discarding leftovers
- Eating in company and in public places in a more socially acceptable way, at a normal speed (including restaurant, buffet, and take-out meal practice)
- Managing the distress evoked by eating the meal
- Recognizing that learning to eat a healthy diet is important

Lifestyle Redesign and Independent Living Skills

Enabling clients to identify and participate in meaningful, *adaptive* self-care, productivity, and leisure activities is important (Abeydeera et al., 2006; Lim & Agnew, 1994; Lock, 2006). Helping them discover "higher values" and interests beyond the pursuit of an idealized identity is vital (de la Rie et al., 2007; Hammell, 2004). Attention to difficulties performing independent living skills may be required, such as finding accommodation, using public transportation, booking cinema tickets, and navigating the public library (Breden, 1992). The demands of a healthy lifestyle must match the client's emotional coping skills and other abilities to avoid relapse. Improving their social network is recommended (Aime, Sabourin, & Ratté, 2006). Clients state that their quality of life is enhanced by discovering a sense of belonging, purpose, and "self," often including participation in work, education, and leisure activities, as well as competency in life skills (Cockell, Zaitsoff, & Geller, 2004; de la Rie et al., 2007; Keski-Rahkonen & Tozzi, 2005). They claim that these help maintain change and reduce risk of relapse following treatment. An adapted form of lifestyle redesign, as described within the empirically supported Well Elderly Study (Jackson, Carlson, Mandel, Zemke, & Clark, 1998), is highly applicable. In brief, this includes enabling clients to identify their maladaptive occupations and replace these with adaptive occupations.

Communication and Assertion Training

Communication and assertion training is widely cited as helpful (Cockell et al., 2004; Gogarty & Brangan, 2004; Harries, 2005). Takahashi and Kosaka (2003) claim that social skill training helps maintain motivation for therapy, reduces anxiety, and improves self-esteem. Role-play can be used to effectively enhance interpersonal skills (Lock, 2000). (Also see Chapter 21.)

Stress Management

Enabling clients to manage their stress response related to their occupational and social demands, including anxiety, anger, and mood management, is cited as essential (Deffenbacher, Oetting, & DiGiuseppe, 2002; NICE, 2004; Robert-McComb, 2001). Training them to acknowledge feelings and express emotions promotes the development of better coping strategies, decreases inner conflicts, and limits the disordered eating habits and their impact on occupational performance (Cockell et al., 2004; Pépin, Boulard, & Bergeron, 2004). (Also see Chapter 22.)

Projective Art

The literature suggests that the use of projective art is efficacious in enabling clients to identify and express difficult feelings, unravel problems of identity, and promote self-image and spontaneity (Harries, 1992; Martin, 1998). Projective art can include a variety of media, such as paint, clay, or sculpture. The therapist may provide some direction (e.g., portray a particular feeling) or may be more open ended, allowing the individual to create and then discuss the meaning of the completed project (Levick, 2005).

Crafts

Participation in craftwork is cited as useful to enhance intrapersonal, relational, and functional performance skills, as well as personal growth (Bailey, 1986; Breden, 1992; Harries, 1992, 2005; Martin, 1998; Matusevich et al., 2002; Meyers, 1989; Stoffel, 1993). Authors have identified that participating in craft activity can improve

- Self-esteem, through creative expression
- Self-competence, through mastery of creative projects
- Clinical perfectionism, by learning imperfection tolerance related to creative projects
- Interpersonal skills
- Quality of life, during and following treatment, by participation in spontaneous social interaction within a group setting

Relapse Prevention

Anorexia and bulimia nervosa are both chronically relapsing conditions (Stice, 2002a). Relapse prevention is cited as efficacious to overcome addictive behavior and decreased self-efficacy and confidence about maintaining the changes achieved during treatment (Collins, 2005; Kaplan, 2002; Orimoto & Vitousek, 1992). Lock (2000) describes an occupation-focused adaptation of the Relapse Prevention model (Marlatt & George, 1984) for clients with eating disorders. This includes training clients to participate in meaningful adaptive occupation using adaptive coping strategies, by means of an easy to remember acronym—"PLEASE":

P = PLAN your daily activity and meals.

L = LOOK OUT for "triggers" (i.e., things that can precipitate eating disordered behavior).

E = EAT three meals a day (one of them cooked with dessert, plus snacks, using prescribed portion sizes).

A = ASSERT your needs and wants with others.

S = SEEK SUPPORT from others.

E = EXPRESS your feelings, rather than act them out through eating disordered behavior.

Body Image Improvement

Interventions such as psychoeducation, cognitive behavioral techniques, and the use of mirror exposure and video feedback are cited as methods to reduce body dissatisfaction (Farrell, Shafran, & Lee, 2006; Shearsmith-Farthing, 2001; Trevan-Hawke, 1985). (Also see Chapter 19.)

Adapting Interventions

Interventions for clients within the early stages of change must be adapted to emphasize a motivational enhancement approach. Potentially distressing interventions, such as meal cookery, projective art, and body image improvement, are contraindicated for these clients. Building a strong therapeutic alliance with the client is crucial (Bell, 2003).

Adolescent Interventions

Adolescent clients require age-appropriate versions of adult interventions that incorporate a highly motivational approach (Bridges, 1993; Kloczko & Ikiugu, 2006). For example, establishing rapport and using interventions that capitalize on the adolescent's interests and strengths are important. Occupation-focused family interventions are also helpful, for example, enabling an adolescent to cook and eat with her mother and other family members. It is important to teach family, peers, and significant others to limit their demands on the client. It is also vital to shift the focus of interaction away from food because it will increase resistance to change or the disordered thoughts and behaviors. If family members and other individuals with whom the client regularly interacts increase their knowledge and understanding of eating disorders, they will be better able to act supportively. As a result, tensions will decrease as behaviors and attitudes that exacerbate symptoms gradually disappear (Pépin et al., 2004).

Medication

Medical management of eating disorders is challenging. However, there seems to be a consensus that antidepressants have a role to play in the treatment of bulimia. Various classes of antidepressants have been used, but serotonin reuptake inhibitors appear to be the drug of choice (Mitchell et al., 2007; Walsh, 2002). Although they can reduce binge eating and purging, the long-term effects of using these drugs need more investigation (NICE, 2004). They are used when concurrent depression or depressive symptomatology is present, as well as when depression is not alleviated when the eating disorder symptoms subside. Limited evidence regarding the use of pharmacotherapy in the treatment of anorexia nervosa is available (NICE, 2004). More often, drugs are used to treat the comorbid conditions. In all cases, medication should be carefully monitored and used with caution, and it should never be the sole source of treatment (APA, 2006; Walsh, 2002). Other common treatments for individuals with eating disorders include nutritional counseling, family therapy, and cognitive behavioral therapy (Mitchell et al., 2007; Vitousek & Gray, 2005).

Summary

Eating disorders have a complex etiology and, although there are effective interventions, some individuals with eating disorders may struggle with certain symptoms for most of their lives. Occupational therapists can enable individuals with eating disorders to eat, participate in adaptive activity, communicate, and manage stress effectively. Therapeutic activities must provide opportunities for clarification of adaptive values, enhanced self-esteem, increased tolerance of emotion and imperfection, and positive interpersonal experiences. Enhancing readiness to change must be ongoing. The goal is the improvement of the client's sense of identity and competency, at a normal body weight.

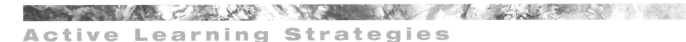

Active Learning Strategies

1. Changing Your Behavior

Think of a problematic behavior in yourself that you find hard to change. You might need to clean your home more, study more, watch less television, or go to bed earlier. You may struggle to exercise regularly or drink less alcohol. You may find it hard to keep in regular contact with family or friends. Take another look at the Transtheoretical Model of Change (Prochaska & DiClemente, 1983) shown in Figure 10-3, and determine which stage of change describes where you are in relation to your problematic behavior.

Now, follow these instructions:

1. Set a specific, measurable, achievable, realistic, time-limited goal to address your problematic behavior.

2. Define what additional resources, including support from others, you would need for you to move into the "action" stage of change to address this behavior.

3. Attempt to reach your goal every day for a week.

4. Write down your reflections on your experiences at each stage.

5. Consider how difficult change must be for people who have used maladaptive coping strategies for years.

 Describe the experience in your **Reflective Journal**.

Resources

Books

- *Eating Disorders and Obesity: A Comprehensive Handbook*, 2nd edition, 2002, edited by C. G. Fairburn and K. D. Brownell. New York: Guilford Press.
- *Handbook of Eating Disorders: Theory, Treatment and Research*, 1995, by J. Treasure and D. Szmulker. Hoboken, NJ: Wiley
- *Eating Disorders, Food, and Occupational Therapy*, 1998, by Joan E. Martin. London: Whurr.
- *Anorexia Nervosa: Let Me Be*, 1995, by A. H. Crisp. East Sussex, UK: Lawrence Erlbaum Associates.
- *Anorexia: The Wish to Change*, 2001, by A. H. Crisp, N. Joughin, C. Halek, and C. Bowyer. East Sussex, UK: Psychology Press.
- "Health Promotion in Eating Disorders: The Contribution of the Occupational Therapist," 2005, by Priscilla Harries. In *Health Promoting Practice: The Contribution of Nurses and Allied Health Professionals*, edited by A. Scriven. Basingstroke: Palgrave Macmillan.
- "Reoccupying the Preoccupied: Occupational Therapy for Sufferers of Eating Disorders," 2000, by Laura C. Lock. In *Eating Disorders: A Multi-Professional Approach*, edited by T. Hindmarsh. London: Whurr.
- *Getting Better Bite by Bite*, 1996, by U. Schmidt and J. Treasure. Florence, KY: Psychology Press.
- *Cognitive Behavioral Therapy for Eating Disorders: A Comprehensive Treatment Guide*, 2007, by G. Waller, H. Cordery, E. Corstorphine, H. Hinrichsen, R. Lawson, V. Mountford, and K. Russell. Cambridge: Cambridge University Press.
- *Little Steps: Surviving Anorexia and Bulimia Nervosa*, 2005, by K. Wealthall. Brentwood, UK: Chipmunka.
- *Anorexia Nervosa: A Survival Guide for Families, Friends and Sufferers*, 1997, by J. Treasure. Florence, KY: Psychology Press.
- *Eating Disorders: The Journey to Recovery Workbook*, 2001, by L. J. Goodman and M. Villapiano. Philadelphia, PA: Brunner-Routledge.

Organizations and Websites

- **b-eat or Eating Disorders Association:** UK-based charitable organization that provides information, help, and assistance to clients, caregivers, and professionals.
103 Prince of Wales Drive
Norwich, NR1 1DW
United Kingdom
Website: http://www.b-eat.co.uk/Home.

- **Mirror Mirror:** Self-help organization for clients. www.mirror-mirror.org
- **National Eating Disorders Association (NEDA):** 603 Stewart Street, Suite 803
Seattle, WA 98101
E-mail: info@NationalEatingDisorders.org
Website: www.edap.org

References

Abeydeera, K., Willis, S., & Forsyth, K. (2006). Occupation focused assessment and intervention for clients with anorexia nervosa. *International Journal of Therapy and Rehabilitation, 13*(7), 296.

Aime, A., Sabourin, S., & Ratté, C. (2006). The eating disorders spectrum in relation with coping and interpersonal functioning. *Eating and Weight Disorders, 11*(2), 66–77.

American Psychiatric Association (APA). (2000a). Practice guideline for the treatment of patients with eating disorders (revision). *American Journal of Psychiatry, 157* (1 Suppl), 1–39.

American Psychiatric Association (APA). (2000b). *Diagnostic and Statistical Manual of Mental Disorders* (4th ed., text revision). Washington, DC: Author.

American Psychiatric Association (APA). (2006). "Developing a Treatment Plan for the Individual Patient." Available at: http://www.psychiatryonline.com/context.aspx?aID=138866 (accessed March 5, 2010).

Andersen, A. E. (2001). Progress in eating disorders research. *American Journal of Psychiatry, 158*(4), 515–518.

Andersen, A. E. (2002). Eating disorders in males. In C. G. Fairburn & K. D. Brownell (Eds.), *Eating Disorders and Obesity: A Comprehensive Handbook* (pp. 188–192). New York: Guilford Press.

Andersen, R. E., Bartlett, S. J., Morgan, G. D., & Brownell, K. D. (1995). Weight loss, psychological and nutritional patterns in competitive male body builders. *International Journal of Eating Disorders, 18*(1), 49–57.

Bailey, M. K. (1986). Occupational therapy for patients with eating disorders. *Occupational Therapy in Mental Health, 6*(1), 89–116.

Banasiak, S. J., Paxton, S. J., & Hay, P. (2005). Guided self-help for bulimia nervosa in primary care: A randomized controlled trial. *Psychology Medicine, 35*, 1283–1294.

Bardone, A. M., Perez, M., Abramson, L. Y., & Joiner, T. E., Jr. (2003). Self-competence and self-liking in the prediction of change in bulimic symptoms. *International Journal of Eating Disorders, 34*(3), 361–369.

Barris, R. (1986). Occupational dysfunction and eating disorders: Theory and approach to treatment. *Occupational Therapy in Mental Health, 6*(1), 27–45.

Barris, R. (1987). Relationships between eating behaviours and person/environment interactions in college women. *Occupational Therapy Journal of Research, 7*(5), 273–288.

Baum, A. (2006). Eating disorders in male athlete. *Sports Medicine, 36*(1), 1–6.

Beck, A. T., Rush, A., Shaw, B., & Emery, G. (1979). *Cognitive Therapy of Depression.* New York: Guilford Press.

Becker, A. E., Burwell, R. A., Gilman, S. E., Herzog, D. B., & Hamburg, P. (2002). Eating behaviours and attitudes following prolonged exposure to television among ethnic Fijian adolescent girls. *British Journal of Psychiatry, 180,* 509–514.

Bell, L. (2003). What can we learn from consumer studies and qualitative research in the treatment of eating disorders? *Eating & Weight Disorders, 8*(3), 181–187.

Berg, F. M. (2001). *Women Are Afraid to Eat.* Hettinger, NJ: Healthy Weight Network.

Berkman, N., Lohr, K. N., & Bulik, C. M. (2007). Outcomes of eating disorders: A systematic review of the literature. *International Journal of Eating Disorders, 40*(4), 293–309.

Bers, S. A., & Quinlan, D. M. (1992). Perceived-competence deficit in anorexia nervosa. *Journal of Abnormal Psychology, 101*(3), 423–431.

Beumont, P. J. (2002). Clinical presentation of anorexia nervosa and bulimia nervosa. In C. G. Fairburn & K. D. Brownell (Eds.), *Eating Disorders and Obesity: A Comprehensive Handbook* (pp. 162–110). New York: Guilford Press.

Beumont, P. J. V., & Touyz, S. W. (2003). What kind of illness is anorexia nervosa? *European Child & Adolescent Psychiatry, 12*(suppl 1), 20–24.

Blinder, B. J., Cumella, E. J., & Sanathara, V. A. (2006). Psychiatric co-morbidities of female inpatients with eating disorders. *Psychosomatic Medicine, 68*(3), 454–462.

Bloks, H., & van Furth, E. F. (2004). Coping strategies and recovery in patients with a severe eating disorder. *Eating Disorders, 12,* 157–169.

Boschi, V., Siervo, M., D'Orsi, P., Margiotta, N., Trapenese, E., Basile, F., Nasti, G., Papa, A., Bellini, O., & Falconi, C. (2003). Body composition, eating behaviour, food-body concerns and eating disorders in adolescent girls. *Annals of Nutrition and Metabolism, 47*(6), 284–293.

Bouley, B., & Sadik, C. (1992). In patient treatment of eating disorders within a cognitive-behavioural framework. *Occupational Therapy Practice, 3*(2), 1–11.

Breden, A. K. (1992). Occupational therapy and the treatment of eating disorders. *Occupational Therapy in Health Care, 8*(2–3), 49–68.

Bridges, B. (1993). Occupational therapy evaluation for patients with eating disorders. *Occupational Therapy in Mental Health, 12*(2), 79–89.

Broussard, B. B. (2004). Women's experience of bulimia nervosa. *Journal of Advanced Nursing, 49*(1), 43–50.

Brumberg, J. J. (2000). *Fasting Girls: The History of Anorexia Nervosa.* New York: Vintage Books.

Bulik, C. M., Reba, L., Siega-Riz, A. M., & Reichborn-Kjennerud, T. (2005). Anorexia nervosa: Definition, epidemiology, and cycle of risk. *International Journal of Eating Disorders, 37*(suppl), S2–S9 ; discussion S20–S21.

Calvo, S. R., Alba, F. V., Serva, G.I., & Pelaz, S. (2001). Processes of change and resistance to change in eating disorders according to J. O. Prochaska & C. DiClemente's model. *Clinica y Salud, 12*(2), 237–251.

Cassin, S. E., von Ranson, K. M., Heng, K., Brar, J., & Wojtowicz, A. E. (2008). Adapted motivational interviewing for women with binge eating disorder: A randomized controlled trial. *Psychology of Addictive Behaviors, 22,* 417–425.

Cockell, S. J., Zaitsoff, S. L., & Geller, J. (2004). Maintaining change following eating disorder treatment. *Professional Psychology: Research and Practice, 35*(5), 527–534.

Cohen, J. H., Kristal, A. R., Neumark-Sztainer, D., Rock, C. L., & Neuhouser, M. L. (2002). Psychological distress is associated with unhealthy dietary practices. *Journal of the American Dietetic Association, 102*(5), 699–704.

Collier, D. A., & Treasure, J. L. (2004). The aetiology of eating disorders. *British Journal of Psychiatry, 185,* 363–365.

Collins, R. L. (2005). Relapse prevention for eating disorders and obesity. In G. A. Marlaat & M. Dennis (Eds.), *Relapse Prevention: Maintenance Strategies in the Treatment of Addictive Behaviours* (2nd ed., pp. 248–275). New York: Guilford Press.

Cooper, M., Whitehead, L., & Boughton, N. (2004). Eating disorders. In J. Bennett-Levy, G. Butler, M. Fennell, A. Hackman, M. Mueller, & D. Westbrook (Eds.), *Cognitive Behaviour Therapy: Science and Practice Series, Oxford Guide to Behavioural Experiments in Cognitive Therapy* (pp. 267–284). London: Oxford University Press.

Crisp, A. (2006a). In defence of the concept of phobically driven avoidance of adult body weight/shape/function as the final common pathway to anorexia nervosa. *European Eating Disorders Review, 14,* 189–202.

Crisp, A. (2006b). Anorexia nervosa in males: Similarities and differences to anorexia nervosa in women. *European Eating Disorder Review, 14,* 163–167.

Crow, S., Nyman, J. A., Agras, W. S., Halmi, K., Fairburn, C. G., & Mitchell, J. (2006). "Cost-Effectiveness of Stepped-Care Treatment for Bulimia Nervosa." Paper presented at the Eating Disorders Research Society, August 31, Port Douglas, Australia.

Culbert, K. M., & Klump, K. L. (2005). Impulsivity as an underlying factor in the relationship between disordered eating and sexual behaviour. *International Journal of Eating Disorders, 38*(4), 361–366.

Darcy, A. M., & Dooley, B. (2007). A clinical profile of participants in an on-line support group. *European Eating Disorders Review, 15,* 185–195.

Davis, C., Kaptein, S., Kaplan, A. S., Olmsted, M. P., Woodside, D., & Blake, M. D. (1998). Obsessionality in anorexia nervosa: The moderating influence of exercise. *Psychosomatic Medicine, 60*(2), 192–197.

de la Rie, S., Noordenbos, G., Donker, M., & van Furth, E. (2007). The patient's view on quality of life and eating disorders. *International Journal of Eating Disorders, 40*(1), 13–20.

Deffenbacher, J. L., Oetting, E. R., & DiGiuseppe, R. A. (2002). Principles of empirically supported interventions applied to anger management. *Counselling Psychologist, 30*(2), 262–280.

Diaz-Marsa, M., Carrasco, J. L., & Saiz, J. (2000). A study of temperament and personality in anorexia and bulimia nervosa. *Journal of Personality Disorder, 14*(4), 352–359.

Drench, M. E., Noonan, A. C., Sharby, N., & Hallenborg Ventura, S. (2007. *Psychosocial Aspects of Health Care* (2nd ed.). Upper Saddle River, NJ: Prentice Hall.

Engel, S. G., Corneliussen, S. J., Wonderlich, S. A., Crosby, R. D., le Grange, D., Crow, S., Klein, M., Bardone-Cone, A., Peterson, C., Joiner, T., Mitchell, J. E., & Steiger, H. (2005). Impulsivity and compulsivity in bulimia nervosa. *International Journal of Eating Disorders, 38*(3), 244–251.

Fairburn, C. G., & Brownell, K. D. (2002). *Eating Disorders and Obesity: A Comprehensive Handbook* (2nd ed.). New York: Guilford Press.

Fairburn, C. G., & Harrison, P. J. (2003). Eating disorders. *The Lancet, 361*(9355), 407–417.

Farrell, C., Shafran, R., & Lee, M. (2006). Empirically evaluated treatments for body image disturbance: A review. *European Eating Disorders Review, 14*(5), 289–300.

Fichter, M. M., Quadflieg, N., & Hedlund, S. (2006). Twelve-year course and outcome predictors of anorexia nervosa. *International Journal of Eating Disorders, 39*(2), 87–100.

Forbush, K., Heatherton, T. F., & Keel, P. K. (2007). Relationships between perfectionism and specific disordered eating behaviours. *International Journal of Eating Disorders, 40*(1), 37–41.

Fryer, S., Waller, G., & Kroese, B. S. (1997). Stress, coping and disturbed eating attitudes in teenage girls. *International Journal of Eating Disorders, 22*(4), 427–436.

Garfinkel, P. E. (2002). Classification and diagnosis of eating disorders. In C. G. Fairburn & K. D. Brownell (Eds.), *Eating Disorders and Obesity: A Comprehensive Handbook* (pp. 155–161). New York: Guilford Press.

Garner, D. M., & Garfinkel, P. E. (1997). *Handbook of Treatment for Eating Disorders* (2nd ed.). New York: Guilford Press.

Geller, J. (2002). What a motivational approach is and what a motivational approach isn't: Reflections and responses. *European Eating Disorders Review, 10,* 155–160.

Geller, J., Brown, K. E., Zaitsoff, S. L., Goodrich, S., & Hastings, F. (2003). Collaborative versus directive interventions in the treatment of eating disorders: Implications for care providers. *Professional Psychology Research and Practice, 34*(4), 406–413.

Geller, J., Cockell, S. J., & Goldner, E. M. (2000). Inhibited expression of negative emotions and interpersonal orientation in anorexia nervosa. *International Journal of Eating Disorders, 28,* 8–19.

Gilbody, S. M., Kirk, S. F. L., & Hill, A. J. (1999). Vegetarianism in young women: Another means of weight control? *International Journal of Eating Disorders, 26*(1), 87–90.

Gleaves, D., Miller, K., Williams, T., & Summers, S. (2000). Eating disorders: An overview. In K. J. Miller & J. S. Mizes (Eds.), *Comparative Treatments for Eating Disorders* (pp. 1–49). New York: Springer.

Gogarty, O., & Brangan, J. (2004). The lived body experience of women with eating disorders: A phenomenological study of the perceived impact of body image disturbance on occupational performance. *Irish Journal of Occupational Therapy, 33*(2), 11–19.

Gold, M. S. (2004). Eating disorders, overeating, and pathological attachment to food: Independent or addictive disorders? *Journal of Addictive Diseases, 23*(3), 1–118.

Goldbloom, D. (1997). The early Canadian history of anorexia nervosa. *Canadian Journal of Psychiatry, 42,* 163–167.

Gordon, R. A. (2000). *Eating Disorders: Anatomy of a Social Epidemic* (2nd ed.). Malden, MA: Blackwell.

Halmi, K. (2005). Psychopathology of anorexia nervosa. *International Journal of Eating Disorders, 37,* 20–21.

Halvorsen, I., & Heyerdahl, S. (2006). Girls with anorexia nervosa as young adults: Personality, self-esteem and life satisfaction. *International Journal of Eating Disorders, 39*(4), 285–293.

Hammell, K. W. (2004). Dimensions of meaning in the occupations of daily life. *Canadian Journal of Occupational Therapy, 71*(5), 296–305.

Harbottle, E. J., Birmingham, C. L., & Sayani, F. (2008). Anorexia nervosa: A survival analysis. *Eating and Weight Disorders, 13,* e32–e34.

Harries, P. (1992). Facilitating change in anorexia nervosa: The role of occupational therapy. *British Journal of Occupational Therapy, 55*(9), 334–339.

Harries, P. (2005). Health promotion in eating disorders: The contribution of the occupational therapist. In A. Scriven (Ed.), *Health Promoting Practice: The Contribution of Nurses and Allied Health Professionals.* Basingstroke: Palgrave Macmillan.

Health Canada. (2002). *A Report on Mental Illnesses in Canada.* Ottawa, ON: Government of Canada.

Helbig, K., & McKay, E. (2003). An exploration of addictive behaviours from an occupational perspective. *Journal of Occupational Science, 10*(3), 140–145.

Henderson, S. (1998). Frames of reference utilized in the rehabilitation of individuals with eating disorders. *Canadian Journal of Occupational Therapy, 66*(1), 43–51.

Hernandez, J. (1995). The concurrence of eating disorders with histories of child sexual abuse among adolescents. *Journal of Child Sexual Abuse, 4*(3), 73–85.

Herzog, D. B., Bradburn, I. S., & Newman, K. (1990). Sexuality in males with eating disorders. In A. E. Andersen (Ed.), *Males With Eating Disorders* (pp. 40–53). New York: Brunner/Mazel.

Hillert, A., Staedtke, D., & Wise, K. (2002). Anorexia and bulimia nervosa: Symptoms, therapeutic approaches, relationship to work. *Arbeitsmedizin Sozialmedizin Umweisltmedizin, 37*(6), 271–278.

Hinrichsen, H., Wright, F., Waller, G., & Meyer, C. (2003). Social anxiety and coping strategies in the eating disorders. *Eating Behavior, 4,* 117–126.

Hoek, H. W. (2006). Incidence, prevalence and mortality of anorexia nervosa and other eating disorders. *Current Opinion in Psychiatry, 19*(4), 389–394.

Holtkamp, K., Müller, B., Heussen, N., Remschmidt, H., & Herpertz-Dahlmann, D. (2005). Depression, anxiety and obsessionality in long-term recovered patients with adolescent-onset anorexia nervosa. *European Child & Adolescent Psychiatry, 14*(2), 106–110.

Hulley, A., & Hill, A. (2001). Eating disorders and health in elite women distance runners. *International Journal of Eating Disorders, 30*(3), 312–317.

Huon, G., Mingyi, Q., Oliver, K., & Xiao, G. (2002). A large-scale survey of eating disorder symptomatology among female adolescents in the People's Republic of China. *International Journal of Eating Disorders, 32*(2), 192–205.

Jackson, J., Carlson, M., Mandel, D., Zemke, R., & Clark, F. (1998). Occupation in lifestyle redesign: The Well Elderly Study Occupational Therapy program. *American Journal of Occupational Therapy, 52*(5), 326–336.

Jarry, J. L., Polivy, J., Herman, C. P., Arrowood, A. J., & Pliner, P. (2006). Restrained and unrestrained eater's attributions of success and failure to body weight and perception of social consensus: The special case of romantic success. *Journal of Social and Clinical Psychology, 25*(8), 885–906.

Johnson, C., & Berndt, D. J. (1983). Preliminary investigation of bulimia and life adjustment. *American Journal of Psychiatry, 140*(6), 774–777.

Jone, C., Harris, G., & Leung, N. (2005). Core beliefs and eating disorder recovery. *European Eating Disorders Review, 13*(4), 237–244.

Kaplan, A. S. (2002). Psychological treatments for anorexia nervosa: A review of published studies and promising new directions. *Canadian Journal of Anorexia Nervosa, 4*(3), 235–242.

Kaye, W. H., Bulik, C. M., Plotnicov, K., Thornton, L., Devlin, B., Fichter, M. M., Treasure, J., Kaplan, A., Woodside, D. B., Johnson, C. L., Halmi, K., Brandt, H. A., Crawford, S., Mitchell, J. E., Strober, M., Berrettini, W., & Jones, I. (2008). The genetics of anorexia nervosa collaborative study: Methods and sample description. *International Journal of Eating Disorders, 41,* 289–300.

Kazutoshi, N., Masaharu, Y., Osamu, Y., Yoshiaki, K., Kensuke, M., Toshiyuki, S., Koji, S., & Shinichi, N. (2000). Prevalence of anorexia nervosa and bulimia nervosa in a geographically defined area in Japan. *International Journal of Eating Disorders, 28*(2), 173–180.

Keel, P. K., Mayer, S. A., & Harnden-Fisher, J. H. (2001). Importance of size in defining binge eating episodes in bulimia nervosa. *International Journal of Eating Disorders, 29*(3), 294–301.

Keski-Rahkonen, A., Hoek, H. W., Linna, M. S., Raevuori, A., Sihvola, E., Bulik, C. M., Rissanen, A., & Kaprio, J. (2008). Incidence and outcomes of bulimia nervosa: A nationwide population based study. *Psychological Medicine, 8,* 1–9.

Keski-Rahkonen, A., & Tozzi, F. (2005). The process of recovery in eating disorder sufferers' own words: An internet-based study. *International Journal of Eating Disorders, 37*(suppl), S80–S86.

Kiefer, I., Rathmanner, T., & Kunze, M. (2005). Eating and dieting differences in men and women. *Journal of Men's Health and Gender, 2*(2) 194–201.

Kielhofner, G. (2002). *A Model of Human Occupation: Theory and Application,* (3rd ed.). Baltimore: Lippincott Williams & Wilkins.

Kielhofner, G. (2008). *A Model of Human Occupation: Theory and Application* (4th ed.). Baltimore: Lippincott Williams & Wilkins.

Killick, S., & Allen, C. (1997). "Shifting the balance": Motivational interviewing to help behaviour change in people with bulimia nervosa. *European Eating Disorders Review, 5*(1), 33–41.

Kinoy, B. P. (2001). *Eating Disorders: New Directions in Treatment and Recovery* (2nd ed.). New York: Columbia University Press.

Kloczko, E., & Ikiugu, M. N. (2006). The role of occupational therapy in the treatment of adolescents with eating disorders as perceived by mental health therapists. *Occupational Therapy in Mental Health, 22*(1), 63–83.

Kotler, L. A., Boudrea, G. S., & Devlin, M. J. (2003). Emerging psychotherapies for eating disorders. *Journal of Psychiatric Practice, 9*(6), 431–441.

Larson, R., & Johnson, C. (1981). Anorexia nervosa in the context of daily experience. *Journal of Youth and Adolescence, 10*(6), 455–470.

Levick, M. F. (2005). Using drawings in assessment and therapy: A guide for mental health professionals (2nd ed.). *Art Therapy, 22*(3), 165–167.

Lilenfeld, L. R. R., Wonderlich, S., Riso, C. P., Crosby, R., & Mitchel, J. (2006). Eating disorders and personality: A methodological and empirical review. *Clinical Psychology Review, 26*(3), 299–320.

Lim, K. Y., & Agnew, P. (1994). Occupational therapy with eating disorders: A study on treatment approaches. *British Journal of Occupational Therapy, 57*(8), 309–314.

Lindeman, M., & Stark, K. (2001). Emotional eating and eating disorder psychopathology. *Eating Disorders, 9*, 251–259.

Ljotsson, B., Lundin, C., Mitsell, K., Carlbring, P., Ramklint, M., & Ghaderi, A. (2007). Remote treatment of bulimia nervosa and binge eating disorders: A randomized trial of Internet assisted cognitive behavioural therapy. *Behaviour Research and Therapy, 45*, 649–661.

Lock, L. C. (2000). Reoccupying the preoccupied: Occupational therapy for sufferers of eating disorders. In T. Hindmarsh (Ed.), *Eating Disorders: A Multi-Professional Approach* (pp. 70–87). London: Whurr.

Lock, L. C. (2006). "Fat" is a political and psychological issue. An invited response to Adrian Glyn Pacey's article: "Fat Is a Political Issue, Not Psychological." *Mental Health Occupational Therapy, 11*(2), 61–64.

Luborsky, L. (1984). *Principles of Psychoanalytic Psychotherapy: A Manual for Supportive-Expressive Treatment.* New York: Basic Books.

Mangweth, B., Hausmann, A., Danzl, C., Walch, T., Rupp, C. I., Biebl, W., Hudson, J. I., & Pope, H. G. (2005). Child body-focused behaviours and social behaviours as risk factors of eating disorders. *Psychotherapy and Psychosomatics, 74*, 247–253.

Marlatt, G. A., & George, W. H. (1984). Relapse prevention: Introduction and overview of the model. *British Journal of Addiction, 79*(3), 261–273.

Martin, A. R., Nieto, J. M. M., Jimenez, M. A. R., Ruiz, J. P. N., Vazquez, M. C. D., Fernandez, Y. C., Gomez, M. A. R. G., & Fernandez, C. C. (1999). Unhealthy eating behaviour in adolescents. *European Journal of Epidemiology, 15*(7), 643–648.

Martin, J. E. (1998). *Eating Disorders, Food, and Occupational Therapy.* London: Whurr.

Matusevich, D., Garcia, A., Gutt, S., de la Parra, I., & Finkelstein, C. (2002). Hospitalization of patients with anorexia nervosa: A therapeutic proposal. *Eating and Weight Disorders, 7*(3), 196–201.

Meenan, A. L. (2003). Eating disorders: Lifestyle choice or clinical problem? *American Family Physician, 63*(1), 41.

Meyers, S. K. (1989). Occupational therapy treatment of an adult with an eating disorder: One woman's experience. *Occupational Therapy in Mental Health, 9*(1), 33–47.

Miller, W. R., & Rollnick, S. (1991). *Motivational Interviewing: Preparing People to Change Addictive Behavior.* New York: Guilford Press.

Miller, W. R., & Rollnick, S. (2002). *Motivational Interviewing: Preparing People to Change Addictive Behavior.* (2nd ed.) New York: Guilford Press.

Mitchell, J. E., Agras, S., & Wonderlich, S. (2007). Treatment of bulimia nervosa: Where are we and where are we going? *International Journal of Eating Disorders, 40*(2), 95–101.

National Institute for Clinical Excellence (NICE). (2004, January). "Eating Disorders: Core Interventions in the Treatment and Management of Anorexia Nervosa, Bulimia Nervosa and Related Eating Disorders." Clinical Guideline 9. London: Author. Available at: http://www.nice.org.uk/nicemedia/pdf/cg009niceguidance.pdf (accessed November 1, 2009).

National Institute of Nutrition (NIN). (1993). "Giving Adolescents a Fighting Chance Against Eating Disorders." *Healthy Bites*, (Winter), *163*.

National Institute of Nutrition (NIN). (2001). "Adolescents Neglected in Fight Against Eating Disorders." Available at: http://www.nin.ca/public_html/Media/Archives/newsfeb_93.html (accessed August 19, 2001).

NHS Quality Improvement Scotland (QIS). (2006, November). *Eating Disorders in Scotland: Recommendations for Management and Treatment.* Available at: http://www.nhshealthquality.org/nhsqis/files/EATDISORDER_REP_NOV06.pdf (accessed November 1, 2009).

Nordbo, R. H. S., Espeset, E. M. S., Gulliksen, K. S., Skarderud, F., & Holte, A. (2006). The meaning of self-starvation: Qualitative study of patients' perception of anorexia nervosa. *International Journal of Eating Disorders, 39*(7), 556–564.

Orimoto, L., & Vitousek, K. B. (1992). Anorexia nervosa and bulimia nervosa. In P. Wilos (Ed.), *Principles and Practice of Relapse Prevention* (pp. 85–127). New York: Guilford Press.

Paul, T., Schroeter, K., Dahme, B., & Nutzinger, D. O. (2002). Self-injurious behaviour in women with eating disorders. *American Journal of Psychiatry, 159*(3), 408–414.

Pearlstein, T. (2002). Eating disorders and co-morbidity. *Archives of Women's Mental Health, 4*, 67–78.

Pépin, G., Boulard, M., & Bergeron, F. (2004). *Guide conseil pour les proches de personnes atteintes de troubles des conduites alimentaires.* Sherbrooke, QC: Éditions du CRP.

Perkins, S. S. J., Murphy, R. R. M., Schmidt, U. U. S., & Williams, C. (2006). Self-help and guided self-help for eating disorders. *Cochrane Database of Systematic Reviews*, Issue 3. Art. No.: CD004191. DOI: 10.1002/14651858.CD004191.pub2.

Pisetsky, E. M., Chao, Y. M., Diencer, L. C., May, A. M., & Streigel-Moore, R. I. (2008). Disordered eating and substance use in high school students: Results from the Youth Risk Behavior Surveillance System. *International Journal of Eating Disorders, 41*, 464–479.

Pomerleau, G., Ratté, C., Boivin, S., & Brassard, A. (2001). *Anorexie et boulimie: Comprendre pour agir.* Boucherville, Québec: Gaëtan Morin.

Prochaska, J., & DiClemente, C. C. (1983). Stages and processes of self-change in smoking: Towards an integrated model of change. *Journal of Consulting and Clinical Psychology, 51*, 390–395.

Puhl, K. R., & Brownell, D. (2002). Stigma, discrimination, and obesity. In C. G. Fairburn & K. D. Brownell (Eds.), *Eating Disorders and Obesity: A Comprehensive Handbook* (pp. 108–112). New York: Guilford Press.

Pung, M. A. (2004). Motivational interviewing in the reduction of risk factors for eating disorders: A pilot study. *Dissertation Abstract International: Section B: Science and Engineering, 65*(6B), 3178.

Ratté, C., & Pomerleau, G. (2001). Troubles des conduites alimentaires: Anorexie mentale et boulimie. In D. A. Gagnon (Éds.), *Démystifier les maladies mentales: Les troubles de l'enfance et de l'adolescence.* Boucherville, Québec: Gaëtan Morin.

Rich, S. S., & Thomas, C. R. (2008). Body mass index, disordered eating behaviour and acquisition of health information: Examining ethnicity and weight related issues in a college population. *Journal of American College Health, 56*, 623–628.

Robert-McComb, J. J. (2001). *Eating Disorders in Women and Children: Prevention, Stress Management and Treatment.* Boca Raton, FL: CRC Press.

Ross, C. A. (2006). Overestimates of the genetic contribution to eating disorders. *Ethical Human Psychology and Psychiatry, 8*(2), 123–131.

Roth, D. (1986). Treatment of the hospitalised eating disorder patient. *Occupational Therapy in Mental Health, 6*(1), 67–87.

Royal Australian and New Zealand College of Psychiatrists. (2004). Australian and New Zealand clinical guideline for the treatment of anorexia nervosa. *Australian and New Zealand Journal of Psychiatry, 38*(9), 659–670.

Rubin, B., Gluck, M. E., Knoll, C. M., Lorence, M., & Geleibter, A. (2008). Comparison of eating disorders and body image disturbances between Eastern and Western countries. *Eating and Weight Disorders, 13,* 73–80.

Rusca, R. (2003). An existentialist approach to anorexia nervosa. *American Journal of Psychotherapy, 57*(4), 491–498.

Sassaroli, S., & Ruggiero, G. M. (2005). The role of stress in the association between low self esteem, perfectionism and worry and eating disorders. *International Journal of Eating Disorders, 37,* 135–141.

Schmidt, U., Lee, S., Beecham, J., Perkins, S., Treasure, J., Yi, I., et al. (2007). A randomized controlled trial of family therapy and cognitive behavioural therapy guided self-care for adolescents with bulimia nervosa and related disorders. *American Journal of Psychiatry, 164,* 591–598.

Schneider, J. A., & Agras, W. S. (1987). Bulimia in males: A matched comparison with females. *International Journal of Eating Disorders, 6,* 235–242.

Shafran, R., Cooper, Z., & Fairburn, C. G. (2002). Clinical perfectionism: A cognitive-behavioural analysis. *Behaviour Research and Therapy, 40*(7), 773–791.

Shafran, R., Fairburn, C. G., Robinson, P., & Lask, B. (2004). Body checking and its avoidance in eating disorders. *International Journal of Eating Disorder, 35*(1), 93–101.

Shah, N., Passi, V., Bryson, S., & Agras, W. S. (2005). Patterns of eating and abstinence in women treated for bulimia nervosa. *International Journal of Eating Disorders, 38*(4), 330–334.

Shearsmith-Farthing, K. (2001). The management of altered body image: A role for occupational therapy. *British Journal of Occupational Therapy, 64*(8), 387–392.

Skarderud, F. (2007). Shame and pride in anorexia nervosa: A qualitative descriptive study. *European Eating Disorders Review, 15,* 81–97.

Soh, N. L., Touyz, S. W., & Surgenor, L. J. (2006). Eating and body image disturbances across cultures: A review. *European Eating Disorders Review, 14,* 54–65.

Steiger, H. (2004). Eating disorders and the serotonin connection: State, trait and developmental effects. *Journal of Psychiatry and Neuroscience, 29*(1), 20–29.

Steiger, H., & Israël, M. (2000). "Personality Pathology in the Eating Disorder Sufferer: A Practice-Oriented Guide." Paper presented at the 9th International Conference on Eating Disorders, New York, May 4–9.

Stice, E. (2002a). Risk and maintenance factors for eating pathology: A meta-analytic review. *Psychological Bulletin, 128*(5), 825–846.

Stice, E. (2002b). Sociocultural influences on body image and eating disturbance. In C. G. Fairburn & K. D. Brownell (Eds.), *Eating Disorders and Obesity: A Comprehensive Handbook* (pp. 103–107). New York: Guilford Press.

Stice, E., Maxfield, J., & Wells, T. (2003). Adverse effects of social pressure to be thin on young women: An experimental investigation of the effects of' "fat talk." *International Journal of Eating Disorders, 34*(1), 108–117.

Stoffel, V. C. (1993). Women's self esteem issues in substance misuse and eating disorders. *Occupational Therapy Practice, 4*(20), 12–18.

Strauman, T. L., Vookes, J., Berenstein, V., Caiken, S., & Higgins, E. T. (1991). Self-discrepancies and vulnerability to body dissatisfaction and disordered eating. *Journal of Personality and Social Psychology, 61*(6), 946–956.

Striegel-Moore, R., Seeley, J. R., & Lewinsohn, P. M. (2003). Psychosocial adjustment in young adulthood of women who experienced an eating disorder during adolescence. *Journal of American Academy of Child and Adolescent Psychiatry, 42,* 587–593.

Striegel-Moore, R., & Smolak, L. (2001). *Eating Disorders: Innovative Directives in Research and Practice.* Washington, DC: American Psychology Association.

Striegel-Moore, R. H., Silberstein, L. R., & Rodin, J. (1993). The social self in bulimia nervosa: Public self-consciousness, social anxiety and perceived fraudulence. *Journal of Abnormal Psychology, 102*(2), 297–303.

Sullivan, P. (2002). Course and outcomes of anorexia nervosa and bulimia. In C. G. Fairburn & K. D. Brownell (Eds.), *Eating Disorders and Obesity: A Comprehensive Handbook* (pp. 226–230). New York: Guilford Press.

Surgenor, L. J., Maguire, S., Russell, J., & Touyz, S. (2007). Self-liking and self-competence: relationship to symptoms on anorexia nervosa. *European Eating Disorders Review, 15,* 139–145.

Sysko, R., & Walsh, B. T. (2007). A critical evaluation of the efficacy of self help intervention for the treatment of bulimia nervosa and binge eating disorder. *International Journal of Eating Disorders, 41,* 97–112.

Sysko, R., Walsh, B. T., Schebendach, J., & Wilson, G. T. (2005). Eating behavior among women with anorexia nervosa. *American Journal of Clinical Nutrition, 82,* 296–301.

Takahashi, M., & Kosaka, K. (2003). Efficacy of open social skills training in inpatients with mood, neurotic and eating disorders. *Psychiatry and Clinical Neurosciences, 57*(3), 295–302.

Takahashi, M., Takahashi, E., Hisamura, M., & Miyaoka, H. (2005). Communication skills of anorexics. In. P. I. Swain (Ed.), *Trends in Eating Disorders Research* (pp. 109–122). Hauppauge, NY: Nova Biomedical Books. *Trends in Eating Disorders Research,* 109–122.

Tappe, K. A., Gerberg, S. E., Shide, D. J., Rolls, B. J., & Anderson, A. E. (1998). Videotape assessment of changes in aberrant meal-time behaviours in anorexia nervosa after treatment. *Appetite, 30*(2), 171–184.

Thompson, J. K. (2006). Group treatment of eating disorders: The Toronto Hospital's Eating Disorder program model. *Psych-CRITIQUES.*

Thompson, J. K., & Smolak, L. (2001). *Body Image, Eating Disorders, and Obesity in Youth: Assessment, Prevention, and Treatment.* Washington, DC: American Psychological Association.

Thompson, M. G., & Schwartz, D. M. (1982). Life adjustment of women with anorexia nervosa and anorexic-like behaviour. *International Journal of Eating Disorders, 1*(2), 47–60.

Toro, J., Gomez-Peresmitré, G., Sentis, J., Vallés, A., Casulà, V., Castro, J., Pineda, G., Leon, R., Platas, S., & Rodriguez, R. (2006). Eating disorders and body image in Spanish and Mexican female adolescents. *Social Psychiatry and Psychiatric Epidemiology, 41*(7), 556–565.

Tozzi, F., Sullivan, P. F., Fear, J. L., McKenzie, J., & Bulik, C. (2003). Causes and recovery in anorexia nervosa: The patient's perspective. *International Journal of Eating Disorders, 33*(2), 143–154.

Treasure, J., & Bauer, B. (2005). Assessment and motivation. In J. Treasure, U. Schmidt, & E. van Furth (Eds.), *The Essential Handbook of Eating Disorders* (pp. 103–116). West Sussex, UK: Wiley.

Treasure, J., & Schmidt, U. (2001). Ready willing and able to change: Motivational aspects of the assessment and treatment of eating disorders. *European Eating Disorders Review, 9,* 4–18.

Treasure, J., Smith, G., & Crane, A. (2007). *Skills-Based Learning for Caring for a Loved One With an Eating Disorder: The New Maudsley Method.* London: Routledge.

Trevan-Hawke, J. A. (1985). Body image disturbance: An issue of anorexia nervosa. *American Journal of Occupational Therapy, 32*(1), 3–9.

Troisi, A., Di Lorenzo, G., Alcini, S., Nanni, R. C., Di Pasquale, C., & Siracusano, A. (2006). Body dissatisfaction in women with eating disorders: Relationship to early separation anxiety and insecure attachment. *Psychosomatic Medicine, 68*(3), 449–453.

Vandereycken, W. (2002). Families of patients with eating disorders. In C. G. Fairburn & K. D. Brownell (Eds.), *Eating Disorders and Obesity: A Comprehensive Handbook* (pp. 215–220). New York: Guilford Press.

Vanderlinden, J., Buis, H., Pieters, G., & Probst, M. (2007). Which elements in the treatment of eating disorders are necessary ingredients in the recovery process? A comparison between the patient's and therapist's view. *European Eating Disorders Review, 15,* 357–365.

Vitousek, K. B., Watson, S., & Wilson, G. T. (1998). Enhancing motivation for change in treatment-resistant eating disorders. *Clinical Psychology Review, 18,* 391–420.

Vitousek, K. M., & Gray, J. A. (2005). Eating disorders. In G. O. Gabbard, J. S. Beck, & J. Holmes (Eds). *Oxford Textbook of Psychotherapy* (pp. 177–202). New York: Oxford University Press.

Waller, G., Babbs, M., Milligan, R., Meyer, C., Ohanian, V., & Leung, N. (2003). Anger and core beliefs in the eating disorders. *International Journal of Eating Disorders, 34*(1), 118–124.

Walsh, T. (2002). Pharmacological treatment of anorexia nervosa and bulimia nervosa. In C. G. Fairburn & K. D. Brownell (Eds.), *Eating Disorders and Obesity: A Comprehensive Handbook* (pp. 325–329). New York: Guilford Press.

Ward, A. M. D., Campbell, I. C., Brown, N., & Treasure, J. (2003). Anorexia nervosa subtypes: Differences in recovery. *Journal of Nervous and Mental Disease, 191*(3), 197–201.

Weltzin, T., Weisensel, N., Franczyk, D., Burnett, K., Klitz, C., & Bean, P. (2005). Eating disorders in men: Update. *Journal of Men's Health and Gender, 2*(2), 186–193.

Wertheim, E. H. (1992). Psychosocial predictors of weight loss behaviours and binge eating in adolescent girls and boys. *International Journal of Eating Disorders, 12,* 151–160.

Westerberg, J., Edlund, B., & Ghaderi, A. (2008). A longitudinal study of eating attitudes, BMI, perfectionism, asceticism and family climate in adolescent girls and their parents. *Eating and Weight Disorders, 13,* 64–72.

Wilcock, A. A. (1998). Reflections on doing, being and becoming. *Canadian Journal of Occupational Therapy, 65*(5), 248–256.

Wilkins, J. (1998). Quatre temps pour mieux comprendre l'anorexie. *Le Clinicien, March,* 45–49.

Wilson, G. T. (2005). Psychological treatment of eating disorders. *Annual Review of Clinical Psychology, 1,* 439–465.

Wonderlich, S. A., Crosby, R. D., Joiner, T., Peterson, C., Bardone-Cone, A., Klein, M., Crow, S., Mitchell, J. E., le Grange, D., Steiger, H., Kolden, G., Johnson, F., & Vrshek, S. (2005). Personality subtyping and bulimia nervosa: Psychopathological and genetic correlates. *Psychological Medicine, 35*(5), 649–657.

Wonderlich, S. A., Lilenfeld, L. R., Riso, L. P., Engel, S., & Mitchell, J. E. (2005). Personality and anorexia nervosa. *International Journal of Eating Disorders, 37*(suppl), S68–S71.

Personality Disorders

Christine Urish

❝ *I know what it's like to want to die. How it hurts to smile. How you try to fit in but you can't. How you hurt yourself on the outside to try to kill the thing on the inside.*
—Susanna Kaysen (1993), from her autobiography *Girl, Interrupted*

Introduction

The behaviors associated with personality disorders are familiar to everyone. Think of a time when you saw an individual who behaved in a manner that drew attention (e.g., dressed in a peculiar fashion), or one who engaged in a behavior that many others would find uncomfortable (e.g., reclusive behavior with a lack of interaction with friends). What types of behavior are consistent with a diagnosis of personality disorder, as defined by the *Diagnostic and Statistical Manual of Mental Disorders, Fourth Edition, Text Revision* (DSM-IV-TR) (American Psychiatric Association [APA], 2000)?

For an individual to receive a diagnosis of personality disorder, the associated behaviors must be enduring and severe enough that they interfere with functioning and/or present significant distress to the individual. These behaviors often result in labeling the client as "difficult"; however, by understanding personality disorders, the client is more likely to receive the respect and services he or she deserves.

Because of the associated functional impairments, occupational therapists can play an essential role in assisting persons with personality disorders (Cara, 1992). Functional impairments may be observed in instrumental activities of daily living (IADLs), work, leisure, and social participation. They may also be evident in cognitive and psychosocial areas, such as the inability to develop effective interpersonal and coping skills, and the emotion regulation required to live independently and successfully as a full participant in the community (Reed, 2001). Occupational therapists are skilled at working with individuals in recovery and are challenged to embrace the Person-Environment-Occupation model as central to recovery in mental illness (Merryman & Riegel, 2007).

This chapter provides a description of each personality disorder, a discussion of the controversy associated with diagnosing these disorders, and specific information for occupational therapists related to the impact of personality disorders on functioning and intervention.

Description of the Disorder

A personality disorder is "an enduring pattern of inner experience and behavior that deviates markedly from the expectations of the individual's culture, is pervasive and inflexible, has an onset in adolescence or early adulthood, is stable over time, and leads to distress or impairment" (APA, 2000, p. 685).

Every person has a unique personality that consists of a particular combination of traits. **Traits** are typically distinguished from **states.** Traits are enduring characteristics that exist across situations, whereas states are associated with a specific point in time and circumstance. For example, in the case of anxiety, an individual may be anxious about an upcoming exam. This individual is experiencing a state of anxiety. However, an individual who is described more generally as a "worrier" has trait anxiety.

Traits can be both adaptive and maladaptive, and in many cases, the functionality of the trait depends on the situation. For example, an individual with a trait of introversion may function well in most situations, but find it difficult to enjoy a social event with unfamiliar people. Traits affect the way an individual addresses problems in life and are the foundation for understanding differences within individual personalities (Livesley, 2003). Each personality disorder is distinguished by a particular set of traits that have become maladaptive.

An individual with a personality disorder demonstrates traits that are significantly different from the norm (Fischler & Booth, 1999). These traits are pervasive, often affecting all life areas, and are not easily amenable to change. "They influence the range, intensity, consistency, and appropriateness of emotional responses; they can lead to emotional pain and distress. They can affect impulse control and judgment. They are evident in the way the person thinks about self, others and events. They can ruin interpersonal relationships, including work" (Fischler & Booth, 1999, p. 79).

According to the DSM-IV-TR, there are 10 specific personality disorders: schizoid, schizotypal, paranoid, antisocial, borderline, histrionic, narcissistic, avoidant, dependent, and obsessive-compulsive. The personality disorders are coded on Axis II of the multiaxial system of the DSM-IV-TR (APA, 2000). Personality disorders are frequently overlooked, especially in individuals with an Axis I condition, so placement on Axis II promotes adequate attention for diagnosis and treatment. An unfortunate outcome has been that many health insurance companies do not provide coverage for Axis II disorders.

High impairment in social role functioning is the hallmark of a personality disorder diagnosis, with borderline and antisocial personality disorders typically presenting with the greatest dysfunction (Lenzenweger, Lane, Loranger, & Kessler, 2007). However, individuals rarely seek treatment for a personality disorder; rather, individuals often present in a clinical setting due to an Axis I condition such as major depression or an anxiety disorder because personality disorders are often comorbid with Axis I conditions (Lenzenweger et al., 2007; Grant et al, 2004; Roth & Fonagy, 2005). In addition, clients may meet the criteria for more than one personality disorder, which can make intervention more challenging (Ward, 2004).

Personality disorders are most often diagnosed in persons age 18 or older, but can be diagnosed in children if the symptoms have been present for longer than 1 year. One exception to this rule relates to the diagnosis of antisocial personality disorder, which cannot be diagnosed in individuals younger than 18 years (APA, 2000).

DSM-IV-TR Criteria

The DSM-IV-TR criteria for personality disorder are listed in Box 11-1.

The 10 personality disorders are organized into three clusters (Table 11-1) (APA, 2000). The three clusters are distinguished by the predominant traits of the diagnoses within a cluster. Specific diagnostic criteria are provided for each individual disorder. Occupational therapists should consult this criteria prior to assessment selection, treatment planning, and intervention, and are encouraged to use the activities and resources available at the end of the chapter to promote occupational function.

Table 11-1 ● DSM-IV-TR Personality Disorder Clusters

Cluster	Personality Disorder Diagnosis
Cluster A	• Paranoid personality disorder • Schizoid personality disorder • Schizotypal personality disorder
Cluster B	• Antisocial personality disorder • Borderline personality disorder • Histrionic personality disorder • Narcissistic personality disorder
Cluster C	• Avoidant personality disorder • Dependent personality disorder • Obsessive-compulsive personality disorder

Cluster A: Paranoid, Schizoid, and Schizotypal Personality Disorders

Individuals who present with Cluster A personality disorders (paranoid, schizoid, schizotypal) are characterized with traits related to discomfort in interpersonal situations and relationships, emotionally distant, isolative, distrustful, and suspicious. The expression of emotion by individuals in Cluster A is restricted (Ward, 2004). Individuals diagnosed with Cluster A personality disorders tend to interpret the intentions and actions of others as negative (Roth & Fonagy, 2005). The DSM-IV-TR criteria for paranoid personality disorder are listed in Box 11-2.

The DSM-IV-TR criteria for schizoid personality disorder are listed in Box 11-3.

The DSM-IV-TR criteria for schizotypal personality disorder are listed in Box 11-4.

BOX 11-1 ■ DSM-IV-TR Criteria for a Personality Disorder

A. An enduring pattern of inner experience and behavior that deviates markedly from the expectations of the individual's culture. This pattern is manifested in two (or more) of the following areas:

1. Cognition (i.e., ways of perceiving and interpreting self, other people, and events)
2. Affectivity (i.e., the range, intensity, lability, and appropriateness of emotional response)
3. Interpersonal functioning
4. Impulse control

B. The enduring pattern is inflexible and pervasive across a broad range of personal and social situations.

C. The enduring pattern leads to clinically significant distress or impairment in social, occupational, or other important areas of functioning.

D. The pattern is stable and of long duration, and its onset can be traced back at least to adolescence or early adulthood.

E. The enduring pattern is not better accounted for as a manifestation or consequence of another mental disorder.

F. The enduring pattern is not due to the direct physiological effects of a substance (e.g., drug of abuse, medication) or a general medical condition (e.g., head trauma).

From American Psychiatric Association. (2000). *Diagnostic and Statistical Manual of Mental Disorders* (4th ed.). Washington, DC: Author.

BOX 11-2 ■ DSM-IV-TR Criteria for Paranoid Personality Disorder

A. A pervasive distrust and suspiciousness of others such that their motives are interpreted as malevolent, beginning by early adulthood and present in a variety of contexts, as indicated by four (or more) of the following:

1. Suspects, without sufficient basis, that others are exploiting, harming, or deceiving him or her
2. Is preoccupied with unjustified doubts about the loyalty or trustworthiness of friends or associates
3. Is reluctant to confide in others because of unwarranted fear that the information will be used maliciously against him or her
4. Reads hidden demeaning or threatening meanings into benign remarks or events
5. Persistently bears grudges (i.e., is unforgiving of insults, injuries, or slights)
6. Perceives attacks on his or her character or reputation that are not apparent to others and is quick to react angrily or counterattack
7. Has recurrent suspicions, without justification, regarding fidelity of spouse or sexual partner

B. Does not occur exclusively during the course of schizophrenia, a mood disorder with psychotic features, or another psychotic disorder and is not due to the direct physiological effects of a general medical condition.

From American Psychiatric Association. (2000). *Diagnostic and Statistical Manual of Mental Disorders* (4th ed.). Washington, DC: Author.

BOX 11-3 ■ DSM-IV-TR Criteria for Schizoid Personality Disorder

A. A pervasive pattern of detachment from social relationships and a restricted range of expression of emotions in interpersonal settings, beginning by early adulthood and present in a variety of contexts, as indicated by four (or more) of the following:

1. Neither desires nor enjoys close relationships, including being part of a family
2. Almost always chooses solitary activities
3. Has little, if any, interest in having sexual experiences with another person
4. Takes pleasure in few, if any, activities
5. Lacks close friends or confidants other than first-degree relatives
6. Appears indifferent to the praise or criticism of others
7. Shows emotional coldness, detachment, or flattened affectivity

B. Does not occur exclusively during the course of schizophrenia, a mood disorder with psychotic features, another psychotic disorder, or a pervasive developmental disorder and is not due to the direct physiological effects of a general medical condition.

From American Psychiatric Association. (2000). *Diagnostic and Statistical Manual of Mental Disorders* (4th ed.). Washington, DC: Author.

BOX 11-4 ■ DSM-IV-TR Criteria for Schizotypal Personality Disorder

A. A pervasive pattern of social and interpersonal deficits marked by acute discomfort with, and reduced capacity for, close relationships as well as by cognitive or perceptual distortions and eccentricities of behavior, beginning by early adulthood and present in a variety of contexts, as indicated by five (or more) of the following:

1. Ideas of reference (excluding delusions of reference)
2. Odd beliefs or magical thinking that influences behavior and is inconsistent with subcultural norms (e.g., superstitiousness; belief in clairvoyance, telepathy, or "sixth sense"; in children and adolescents, bizarre fantasies or preoccupations)
3. Unusual perceptual experiences, including bodily illusions
4. Odd thinking and speech (e.g., vague, circumstantial, metaphorical, overelaborate, stereotyped)
5. Suspiciousness or paranoid ideation
6. Inappropriate or constricted affect
7. Behavior or appearance that is odd, eccentric, or peculiar
8. Lack of close friends or confidants other than first-degree relatives
9. Excessive social anxiety that does not diminish with familiarity and tends to be associated with paranoid fears rather than negative judgments about self

B. Does not occur exclusively during the course of schizophrenia, a mood disorder with psychotic features, another psychotic disorder, or a pervasive developmental disorder.

From American Psychiatric Association. (2000). *Diagnostic and Statistical Manual of Mental Disorders* (4th ed.). Washington, DC: Author.

Cluster B: Antisocial, Borderline, Histrionic, and Narcissistic Personality Disorders

The traits associated with Cluster B personality disorders (antisocial, borderline, histrionic, narcissistic) include excessive and unstable expression of emotions, maladaptive interpersonal relationships, and a disregard for the needs and right of others (Roth & Fonagy, 2005; Ward, 2004). The DSM-IV-TR criteria for antisocial personality disorder are listed in Box 11-5.

The DSM-IV-TR criteria for borderline personality disorder are listed in Box 11-6.

The DSM-IV-TR criteria for histrionic personality disorder are listed in Box 11-7.

The DSM-IV-TR criteria for narcissistic personality disorder are listed in Box 11-8.

Cluster C: Avoidant, Dependent, and Obsessive-Compulsive Personality Disorders

Cluster C personality disorders include avoidant, dependent, and obsessive-compulsive personality disorders. The primary trait associated with Cluster C personality disorders is anxiety. This anxiety may stem from fear of rejection or humiliation, the need to be taken care of, or a preoccupation with perfection (Ward, 2004). Social discomfort, a sense of helplessness, the inability to make decisions, and perfectionism and inflexibility are characteristic of individuals diagnosed with Cluster C disorders (Roth & Fonagy, 2005). The DSM-IV-TR criteria for avoidant personality disorder are listed in Box 11-9.

The DSM-IV-TR criteria for dependent personality disorder are listed in Box 11-10.

The DSM-IV-TR criteria for obsessive-compulsive personality disorder are listed in Box 11-11.

BOX 11-5 ■ DSM-IV-TR Criteria for Antisocial Personality Disorder

A. There is a pervasive pattern of disregard for and violation of the rights of others occurring since age 15 years, as indicated by three (or more) of the following:

1. Failure to conform to social norms with respect to lawful behaviors as indicated by repeatedly performing acts that are grounds for arrest
2. Deceitfulness, as indicated by repeated lying, use of aliases, or conning others for personal profit or pleasure
3. Impulsivity or failure to plan ahead
4. Irritability and aggressiveness, as indicated by repeated physical fights or assaults
5. Reckless disregard for safety of self or others
6. Consistent irresponsibility, as indicated by repeated failure to sustain consistent work behavior or honor financial obligations
7. Lack of remorse, as indicated by being indifferent to or rationalizing having hurt, mistreated, or stolen from another

B. The individual is at least age 18 years.

C. There is evidence of conduct disorder with onset before age 15 years.

D. The occurrence of antisocial behavior is not exclusively during the course of schizophrenia or a manic episode.

From American Psychiatric Association. (2000). *Diagnostic and Statistical Manual of Mental Disorders* (4th ed.). Washington, DC: Author.

BOX 11-6 ■ DSM-IV-TR Criteria for Borderline Personality Disorder

A pervasive pattern of instability of interpersonal relationships, self-image, and affects, and marked impulsivity beginning by early adulthood and present in a variety of contexts, as indicated by five (or more) of the following:

1. Frantic efforts to avoid real or imagined abandonment

   Note: Do not include suicidal or self-mutilating behavior covered in Criterion 5.

2. A pattern of unstable and intense interpersonal relationships characterized by alternating between extremes of idealization and devaluation

3. Identity disturbance: markedly and persistently unstable self-image or sense of self

4. Impulsivity in at least two areas that are potentially self-damaging (e.g., spending, sex, substance abuse, reckless driving, binge eating).

   Note: Do not include suicidal or self-mutilating behavior covered in Criterion 5.

5. Recurrent suicidal behavior, gestures, or threats, or self-mutilating behavior

6. Affective instability due to a marked reactivity of mood (e.g., intense episodic dysphoria, irritability, or anxiety usually lasting a few hours and only rarely more than a few days)

7. Chronic feelings of emptiness

8. Inappropriate, intense anger or difficulty controlling anger (e.g., frequent displays of temper, constant anger, recurrent physical fights)

9. Transient, stress-related paranoid ideation or severe dissociative symptoms

From American Psychiatric Association. (2000). *Diagnostic and Statistical Manual of Mental Disorders* (4th ed.). Washington, DC: Author.

BOX 11-8 ■ DSM-IV-TR Criteria for Narcissistic Personality Disorder

A pervasive pattern of grandiosity (in fantasy or behavior), need for admiration, and lack of empathy, beginning by early adulthood and present in a variety of contexts, as indicated by five (or more) of the following:

1. Has a grandiose sense of self-importance (e.g., exaggerates achievements and talents, expects to be recognized as superior without commensurate achievements)

2. Is preoccupied with fantasies of unlimited success, power, brilliance, beauty, or ideal love

3. Believes that he or she is "special" and unique and can only be understood by, or should associate with, other special or high-status people (or institutions)

4. Requires excessive admiration

5. Has a sense of entitlement (i.e., unreasonable expectations of especially favorable treatment or automatic compliance with his or her expectations)

6. Is interpersonally exploitative (i.e., takes advantage of others to achieve his or her own ends)

7. Lacks empathy: is unwilling to recognize or identify with the feelings and needs of others

8. Is often envious of others or believes that others are envious of him or her

9. Shows arrogant, haughty behaviors or attitudes

From American Psychiatric Association. (2000). *Diagnostic and Statistical Manual of Mental Disorders* (4th ed.). Washington, DC: Author.

BOX 11-7 ■ DSM-IV-TR Criteria for Histrionic Personality Disorder

A pervasive pattern of excessive emotionality and attention seeking, beginning by early adulthood and present in a variety of contexts, as indicated by five (or more) of the following:

1. Is uncomfortable in situations in which he or she is not the center of attention

2. Interaction with others is often characterized by inappropriate sexually seductive or provocative behavior

3. Displays rapidly shifting and shallow expression of emotions

4. Consistently uses physical appearance to draw attention to self

5. Has a style of speech that is excessively impressionistic and lacking in detail

6. Shows self-dramatization, theatricality, and exaggerated expression of emotion

7. Is suggestible (i.e., easily influenced by others or circumstances)

8. Considers relationships to be more intimate than they actually are

From American Psychiatric Association. (2000). *Diagnostic and Statistical Manual of Mental Disorders* (4th ed.). Washington, DC: Author.

BOX 11-9 ■ DSM-IV-TR Criteria for Avoidant Personality Disorder

A pervasive pattern of social inhibition, feelings of inadequacy, and hypersensitivity to negative evaluation, beginning by early adulthood and present in a variety of contexts, as indicated by four (or more) of the following:

1. Avoids occupational activities that involve significant interpersonal contact because of fears of criticism, disapproval, or rejection

2. Is unwilling to get involved with people unless certain of being liked

3. Shows restraint within intimate relationships because of the fear of being shamed or ridiculed

4. Is preoccupied with being criticized or rejected in social situations

5. Is inhibited in new interpersonal situations because of feelings of inadequacy

6. Views self as socially inept, personally unappealing, or inferior to others

7. Is unusually reluctant to take personal risks or to engage in any new activities because they may prove embarrassing

From American Psychiatric Association. (2000). *Diagnostic and Statistical Manual of Mental Disorders* (4th ed.). Washington, DC: Author.

BOX 11-10 ▪ DSM-IV-TR Criteria for Dependent Personality Disorder

A pervasive and excessive need to be taken care of that leads to submissive and clinging behavior and fears of separation, beginning by early adulthood and present in a variety of contexts, as indicated by five (or more) of the following:

1. Has difficulty making everyday decisions without an excessive amount of advice and reassurance from others
2. Needs others to assume responsibility for most major areas of his or her life
3. Has difficulty expressing disagreement with others because of fear of loss of support or approval

   Note: Do not include realistic fears of retribution.
4. Has difficulty initiating projects or doing things on his or her own (because of a lack of self-confidence in judgment or abilities rather than a lack of motivation or energy)
5. Goes to excessive lengths to obtain nurturance and support from others, to the point of volunteering to do things that are unpleasant
6. Feels uncomfortable or helpless when alone because of exaggerated fears of being unable to care for him- or herself
7. Urgently seeks another relationship as a source of care and support when a close relationship ends
8. Is unrealistically preoccupied with fears of being left to take care of him- or herself

From American Psychiatric Association. (2000). *Diagnostic and Statistical Manual of Mental Disorders* (4th ed.). Washington, DC: Author.

BOX 11-11 ▪ DSM-IV-TR Criteria for Obsessive-Compulsive Personality Disorder

A pervasive pattern of preoccupation with orderliness, perfectionism, and mental and interpersonal control, at the expense of flexibility, openness, and efficiency, beginning by early adulthood and present in a variety of contexts, as indicated by four (or more) of the following:

1. Is preoccupied with details, rules, lists, order, organization, or schedules to the extent that the major point of the activity is lost
2. Shows perfectionism that interferes with task completion (e.g., is unable to complete a project because his or her own overly strict standards are not met)
3. Is excessively devoted to work and productivity to the exclusion of leisure activities and friendships (not accounted for by obvious economic necessity)
4. Is overconscientious, scrupulous, and inflexible about matters of morality, ethics, or values (not accounted for by cultural or religious identification)
5. Is unable to discard worn-out or worthless objects even when they have no sentimental value
6. Is reluctant to delegate tasks or to work with others unless they submit to exactly his or her way of doing things
7. Adopts a miserly spending style toward both self and others; money is viewed as something to be hoarded for future catastrophes
8. Shows rigidity and stubbornness

From American Psychiatric Association. (2000). *Diagnostic and Statistical Manual of Mental Disorders* (4th ed.). Washington, DC: Author.

Dimensional Models of Personality

The 10 personality disorders described previously have overlapping criteria and similar traits across categories, and it is often the case that an individual is diagnosed with more than one personality disorder (Livesley, 2003). The DSM-IV-TR (APA, 2000) system of diagnosis for personality disorders has received significant criticism for compartmentalizing the traits into discrete diagnoses, when in actuality each person is characterized by multiple personality traits of different levels of intensity. Consequently, critics of the DSM-IV-TR system have proposed a dimensional model of personality. The dimensional model is more capable of capturing the uniqueness of the individual.

One of the most commonly described dimensional models is the five-factor model. It is argued by proponents that the five-factor model demonstrates clinical validity that categories in the DSM-IV-TR do not. Research has indicated that the five-factor model provides a mechanism for understanding personality symptomatology as "maladaptive variants of personality traits" (Costa & Widiger, 2002, p. 80).

The five-factor model, refined and further developed by Costa and McCrae (1990), is based on analyses of personality inventories such as the Neuroticism-Extroversion-Openness Personality Inventory, whereas other models have been based on dictionary definitions of terms (Millon & Davis, 2000). This model considers an individual's behavior across five dimensions: neuroticism, extroversion, openness to experience, agreeableness, and conscientiousness (Table 11-2), ranking each from high to low in order to present a hierarchical structure. A disorder exists when traits (typically extremes on a dimension) are associated with difficulties in the areas of work and social participation (Fischler & Booth, 1999). For example, someone who is highly agreeable may have difficulty disciplining an employee, whereas someone with low agreeability may be so distrusting of others that making friends is nearly impossible.

The five-factor model views psychological health across the entire configuration of the person's characteristics and potentials to those in the environment where the person functions (Millon & Davis, 2000). This holistic approach provides a comprehensive method for examining the individual's function and dysfunction in areas of occupation for the occupational therapy practitioner.

Table 11-2 ▪ Dimensions of the Five-Factor Model

Dimension	Description
Neuroticism	Emotional instability or inclination toward unpleasant emotions, such as anxiety, anger, depression, self-consciousness, impulsivity, and vulnerability
Extroversion	Sociability, talkativeness, energetic, and expressions of affect; others refer to this dimension as surgency
Openness to experience	Appreciates experiences for their own sake; curious, adventurous, creative, and unconventional
Agreeableness	Compassionate, good natured, trusting, helpful, forgiving, and altruistic
Conscientiousness	Self-disciplined, persistent, and motivated in goal-directed behavior

The Lived Experience

Dawn, a 25-Year-Old Woman

I am a person diagnosed with borderline personality disorder, although that is not a very good name for the condition. Some people want to call it emotional intensity disorder, or emotional dysregulation disorder, and I think this is a good idea. People don't understand what I am dealing with when they hear "borderline personality disorder." They may think that I am bordering on becoming violent or that my personality is horrible and that they should stay as far away from me as possible.

The truth is that I feel emotions very strongly and sometimes get distracted by them or fooled by them into believing that the way I feel about things is automatically the way that things really are. Sometimes many thoughts go through my head and I get caught up worrying about bad things that might happen, regretting bad things that already have happened, or obsessing about everything that is wrong with the world. Sometimes I am so mentally exhausted from thinking so many thoughts and experiencing emotions so strongly that I am physically tired and just want to be able to relax or sleep.

Trying to relax can be a problem, too. It is often difficult to stop the flow of thoughts or numb the pain of the emotions in order to concentrate on anything else. Activities that don't require a lot of effort to focus on and "lose myself" in, like talking to others, video games, or watching movies, can help bring relief. Other times, I rely on more negative ways of coping, like using self-harming behaviors or eating food that is full of sugar, starch, or fat.

I am frequently lonely and want more than anything to be accepted and loved by others. It is not easy to feel good about myself if no one else does. When someone criticizes me or hurts me, I tend to believe that the negative things they say about me are true and that I deserve to get hurt. I am also inclined to take it personally when I think people are trying to criticize me, even if that is not their intention, sometimes even if they are not talking about me or have never even met me, like things said on television or written in books. I struggle to trust people again once they have hurt me.

The best way that someone can help me is to understand that I am an individual and actually get to know me instead of just assuming that I am the same as somebody else. Also, positive reinforcement can go a long way while negative reinforcement only supports my suspicions that I am a horrible person and that I can't do anything right. Simply listening to me, believing what I say, and acknowledging my suffering is very powerful. I really want others to know that I am trying as hard as I can.

I want to get married, finish college, and get a job. I'd like to be more productive and continue to contribute to the world, but most of all I hope to be satisfied with my life and to truly like myself.

Etiology

Research into the etiology of personality disorders explores genetic disposition, biological factors, and environmental factors (Mullins-Sweatt & Widiger, 2007).

Genetic Factors

There is growing evidence that individuals with personality disorders are more likely to have relatives with the same personality disorder or a personality disorder from the same cluster. A large twin study in Norway has provided much of the evidence, finding a genetic relationship for Cluster A personality disorders, with schizotypal personality disorder having the strongest genetic association (Kendler et al., 2006).

The Norwegian twin study also found that Cluster B personality disorders had a heritability between 24% and 38%, with antisocial personality disorder and borderline personality disorder more closely related to each other than to histrionic and narcissistic personality disorder (Torgersen et al., 2008). Finally, the Norwegian study found that Cluster C personality disorders were moderately heritable, with obsessive-compulsive personality disorder distinct from dependent and avoidant personality disorders (Reichborn-Kjennerud et al., 2007).

Additional research shows that individuals with borderline personality disorder are 5 to 10 times more likely to have a first-degree relative with borderline personality disorder (APA, 2000; New, Triebwasser, & Charney, 2008). A genetic link is also suggested in individuals diagnosed with antisocial personality disorders, as evidenced in studies of children who were adopted at a young age and had a birth parent with antisocial personality disorder (Kaylor, 1999).

Biological Factors

The biological basis of personality disorders can be attributed to hormones, platelet monoamine oxidase, and neurotransmitters. Individuals who exhibit impulsive symptoms associated with personality disorders have higher levels of the hormones testosterone, 17-estradiol, and estrone than individuals who do not exhibit these symptoms (Saddock & Saddock, 2007).

Levels of 5-hydroxyindoleacetic acid, a metabolite in serotonin, was found to be lower in persons who had attempted suicide and in individuals who were impulsive and aggressive, behaviors often demonstrated by persons with personality disorders. When prescribed a selective serotonin reuptake inhibitor (SSRI) such as Prozac, changes in some of the character traits of personality were observed. Depression, impulsiveness, and rumination were decreased, and an increased sense of general well-being was reported (Saddock & Saddock, 2007). The efficacy of the medication provides further support for the association of lower levels of serotonin and certain personality traits.

In addition, the amygdala, which signals fear and danger, was found to be overactive in persons with borderline personality disorder, and the prefrontal cortex, which is responsible for higher-order thinking and can affect the behavioral response of the amygdala, seems underactive (Borderline Personality Disorder Resource Center, 2006). When the difficult behaviors associated with personality disorders are understood within the context of biological vulnerabilities, it is possible that stigma may be reduced. The individual is no longer seen as being intentionally difficult, but someone that is struggling with challenging emotions and inadequate coping skills.

Environmental Factors

Although biological and genetic factors predispose an individual to a diagnosis of personality disorder, one cannot underestimate the role of the environment. Events that occur early in life may have a profound impact on the individual later in life. For example, a large percentage (40%–71%) of persons diagnosed with borderline personality disorder have been sexually abused, often by a noncaregiver (Zanarini, 2000). Research continues to examine the impact of the combination of medications, behavioral interventions, and childhood abuse and stress on brain hormones (National Institute of Mental Health, 2008).

In addition, an individual who is already at risk for personality disorder due to genetic and biological factors may be vulnerable to negative environmental factors to which they are exposed as a youth (Mental Health America, 2006). Persons diagnosed with borderline personality disorder are often in environments where their needs go unmet (Linehan, 1993). According to Linehan, emotions are not validated, such as the crying child who is told that he or she is overreacting and should stop crying. This invalidating environment yields an adult who demonstrates difficulty with emotional regulation and may respond erratically and inappropriately to life experiences that may not trouble others (Linehan, 1993).

Familial psychopathology has a direct effect on borderline personality pathology over and beyond the influence of environment (Bradley, Jenei, & Westen, 2005); however, continued research into the etiology of all personality disorders needs to be conducted.

Prevalence

Personality disorders are pervasive in the general population, with studies showing that between 13.2% and 14.8% of American adults have been diagnosed with at least one personality disorder (14.8% = 30.8 million individuals) (Lenzenweger et al., 2007; Grant et al, 2004).

A survey of 5,692 individuals by the National Comorbidity Study Replication identified the following prevalence estimates on completion of a survey of 5,692 individuals:

- Cluster A = 5.7%
- Cluster B = 1.5%
- Cluster C = 6.0%
- Any personality disorder = 9.1% (Lenzenweger et al., 2007)

Course

Personality disorders are chronic conditions (Fischler & Booth, 1999; Ward, 2004) that are typically diagnosed in adolescence or early adulthood (APA, 2000). Children can be diagnosed with a personality disorder if the behaviors have been present for more than 1 year, with the exception of antisocial personality, which cannot be diagnosed in individuals younger than 18 years (APA, 2000). Antisocial and borderline personality disorders are noted to become less evident or remit with age; this is not the case with other personality disorders such as obsessive-compulsive and schizotypal personality disorders (APA, 2000).

Research evidence exists to support the effectiveness of interventions for individuals with personality disorder, yet most individuals with personality disorders are reluctant to seek and remain in treatment (Linehan, 1993; Paris, 2005; Roth & Fonagy, 2005). Therefore, one of the biggest challenges in setting a more positive course involves engaging the individual in treatment.

Gender Differences

The risk of avoidant, dependent, and paranoid personality disorders is higher in women than men (Grant et al, 2004). Borderline personality disorder is also diagnosed more predominately in females (APA, 2000). In contrast, the risk of antisocial personality disorder is higher in men than in women. There were no gender risk differences identified in obsessive-compulsive, schizoid, and histrionic personality disorders (Grant et al, 2004).

Culture-Specific Information

Because the diagnostic criteria for personality disorders dictates that the individual's behavior must be outside the social norm for the culture, it is essential to consider the client's ethnic, cultural, and social background when determining a personality disorder diagnosis (APA, 2000). A culture of individualism, patriarchy, and media violence was identified as a cultural context positive for the development of antisocial personality disorder (Kaylor, 1999) because it promotes personality traits in which the individual disregards the rights of others and views violent behavior as acceptable.

A practitioner unfamiliar with a client's habits, customs, religious preferences, or political views may view the person as demonstrating behavior indicative of a personality disorder that is in fact in line with their cultural norms. For example, a woman from a highly patriarchal culture may exhibit characteristics consistent with dependent personality disorder when these behaviors are consistent with the expectations from her background. It is of utmost importance that the health-care provider gather additional information from someone familiar with the person's cultural background (APA, 2000).

Impact on Occupational Performance

Personality disorders are mental illnesses, and the symptoms of the diagnosis can affect occupational performance, including social participation, activities of daily living, IADLs, work, and leisure. Specifically, emotional modulation and coping have the ability to affect any area of occupational performance and are of concern for practitioners working with individuals diagnosed with personality disorders. It is essential for occupational therapists to work as part of a team to facilitate occupational performance by addressing impairments in social participation, emotional regulation skills, and coping skills.

Social Participation

Clients diagnosed with personality disorders have difficulty with social participation due to limited interpersonal skills (Roth & Fonagy, 2005). The particular problem varies with the diagnosis (Livesley, 2003; Ward, 2004). As a whole, individuals with Cluster A personality disorders appear odd and eccentric, are suspicious and distrusting, and lack interest in social contact. In general, the Cluster B personality disorders include intense emotions, lack of empathy, and unpredictable behaviors that interfere with socialization. More specifically, individuals with antisocial personality disorder are aggressive, individuals with narcissistic and histrionic personality disorder desire high levels of attention, and people with borderline personality disorder tend to categorize individuals as all good or all bad and have highly unstable relationships. Individuals diagnosed with personality disorders often experienced negative interactions and environments early in life, which have impaired their ability to trust in adulthood (Kaylor, 1999). Working with clients diagnosed with personality disorder to improve their communication and interaction skills may facilitate improved social participation in the community and with family and friends (see Chapter 21).

Emotional Modulation

Clients with personality disorders (especially Cluster B) may have difficulty effectively modulating their emotions and responding to situations with appropriate affect. This means that the individual moves quickly and unpredictably from positive to negative emotions and tends to express emotions intensely. On the one hand, individuals with strong personalities are often engaging, charismatic, and fun to be around when experiencing positive emotions. However, crying outbursts, yelling, and aggressive and impulsive behaviors are also common. Due to the extreme variations in emotions, clients may discontinue treatment abruptly or prematurely. The practitioner should try to engage the client in treatment to yield maximum benefit (Livesley, 2003; Stone, 2003). Note that younger clients often demonstrate more impulsivity and irrational behavior than older clients.

The impulsive behavior and difficulty with emotion modulation can yield clients who engage in self-harming behavior. Clients may act out in this way as an attempt to self-soothe (Linehan, 1993) and express uncomfortable emotions (Hart, 2007). Self-harming behavior may manifest through cutting, biting, burning, scratching, picking, or hair pulling, and most often occurs on the skin of the upper extremity. This behavior has been described as a mechanism of release for unresolved emotional pain and is often used as a coping

strategy. Occupational therapists can work with individuals using interventions such as dialectical behavior therapy (DBT) to improve emotion modulation skills (see Chapter 24).

Practitioners need to be aware of their own emotional responses to Cluster B behaviors. Clients may demonstrate manipulative behavior and test professional boundaries and limits. Practitioners need to be aware of these facts and monitor their own emotional state to ensure their therapeutic ability with clients who have this diagnosis (Ward, 2004).

Coping

Clients with personality disorders often have limited skills in coping with daily life challenges, especially in the area of interpersonal relationships. Practitioners should be aware of the potential for substance use and make appropriate referrals should they suspect this as an area of concern (Ward, 2004). Situations that may mildly irritate the average individual can cause a great deal of emotional discomfort and distress to the individual diagnosed with a personality disorder.

Clients with Cluster C personality disorders may experience difficulty with coping because it relates to making decisions and anxiety. These clients often have very low self-esteem and feel as if they are unable to function without the assistance of others (Ward, 2004). Consequently, these personality traits interfere with the individual's ability to fully participate in work, leisure, and social opportunities. For example, the individual with dependent personality disorder may have the knowledge to work in a supervisory capacity, but the inability to make independent decisions keeps him or her in a lower-level position. High levels of interpersonal sensitivity as seen in avoidant personality disorder or a need to control can make interpersonal rela-

---

Evidence-Based Practice

Lack of effective social skills in persons with personality disorder has been reported extensively in the research (Roth & Fonagy, 2005; Sperry, 1999).

➤ Occupational therapists can use their expertise in therapeutic use of self to assist client in development of effective social skills.

➤ Occupational therapists can use their expertise to assist clients in using assertive communication to increase communication and interaction skills that are essential for social participation in the community, with family and with peers or friends.

Roth, A., & Fonagy, P. (2005). *What Works for Whom: A Critical Review of Psychotherapy Research* (2nd ed.). New York: Guilford Press.

Sperry, L. (1999). *Cognitive Behavior Therapy of DSM-IV Personality Disorders: Highly Effective Interventions for the Most Common Personality Disorders*. New York: Brunner-Routledge.

PhotoVoice

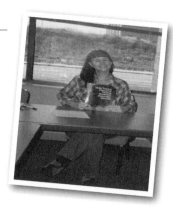

Recovery is DBT to me. DBT is dialectical behavior therapy for borderline personality disorder. There is DBT individual therapy and DBT group therapy. The group therapy teaches you how to use DBT skills. Amy Hammer (shown in photo) is the group facilitator. Amy does an excellent job of keeping the group on task when learning DBT skills. I never have to worry about subjects being discussed that are distressing to me. My individual DBT therapist is Kay Hoffsommer. She has taught me to use DBT skills in my life experiences. Kay also goes on about wanting me to build a life worth living. She works with me on closing the door to suicide. Kay has taught me it's okay to need people and it's okay to need her. And if seeing her is self-soothing to me, it's okay. I used to get overwhelmed really easy, and I didn't know what to do. But I know now. I have skills to use, and it feels good.

tionships challenging. The occupational therapist can help the individual with personality disorders have more successful and satisfying occupational performance by promoting more positive coping skills (see Chapter 22).

Medications

Research on the use and effectiveness of medications to treat personality disorders is limited. There are no medications that "cure" personality disorders, but some medications can provide temporary relief of symptoms (Thompson, 1998). There are no clear pharmacological interventions of choice for individuals with personality disorder (Roth & Fonagy, 2005; Triebwasser & Siever, 2007). Individuals with Cluster A personality disorders who experience cognitive, perceptual, or thought disorder may benefit from a low-dose antipsychotic (Ward, 2004) (see Chapter 14). Individuals with Cluster B

personality disorders who exhibit symptoms of mood lability, depression, or interpersonal sensitivity may be prescribed a mood stabilizer or antidepressant (see Chapter 12). Research suggests that a low-dose antipsychotic and mood stabilizer may decrease suicidal behavior in individuals with borderline personality disorder (Triebwasser & Siever, 2007). To treat the symptoms of Cluster C personality disorders, such as anxiety, obsessive thinking, and inhibited behaviors, SSRIs or related antidepressants may be prescribed, in addition to short-term use of benzodiazepines (Ward, 2004).

Although pharmacological agents are available to treat the symptoms of personality disorders, the results of intervention are limited. It appears that, despite the implementation of evidence-based pharmacotherapy, individuals diagnosed with a personality disorder typically continue to experience symptoms in one or more areas within the diagnostic criteria (Triebwasser & Siever, 2007). Medications do not come without side effects, and practitioners should be aware of adverse effects so they may assist in client education and ensure client compliance with a medication regime.

Occupational Therapy Interventions

Occupational therapy intervention in working with individuals diagnosed with personality disorders is multifaceted. Occupational therapists must understand defense mechanisms used by persons with personality disorders. "The unconscious mental processes that the ego uses to resolve conflicts" (Nott, 2005, p. 487); these defense mechanisms include splitting, denial, repression, and projection. If the therapist is not aware of and attending to the potential defense mechanisms demonstrated by the individual from the start, therapeutic intervention and the individual's progress toward goal attainment could be hindered (Nott, 2005).

The general focus of occupational therapy intervention with individuals diagnosed with personality disorder includes mood stabilization due to often extreme fluctuations; appropriate feeling expression; increased self-concept, self-esteem, insight, and judgment; and the development of appropriate interpersonal relationships, effective coping strategies to deal with life stressors and feelings of anxiety, conflict resolution skills, social skills, and assertive communication skills (Nott, 2005).

Establishing a Therapeutic Relationship

Therapeutic relationship is the key in working with persons diagnosed with personality disorder (Livesley, 2003). Four strategies that can be used, regardless of the practitioner's theoretical orientation and of individual differences in client personality and psychopathology, include the following:

1. Building and maintaining a collaborative relationship—Because individuals with personality disorder are often reluctant to engage in treatment, establishing trust is an important first step.
2. Consistency in treatment—Maintaining trust and addressing the pervasive nature of personality disorders requires intervention that is predictable. It is also important that all treatment providers are working collaboratively toward the same goals.

3. Validation—Individuals with personality disorders need to know that their feelings are real and that the therapist recognizes the difficulty in changing ingrained patterns of behavior.

4. Building and maintaining motivation for change—Often the most challenging of the principles, therapists can help the individual identify positive outcomes that would be associated with a change in behavior (Livesley, 2003).

Addressing Occupational Dysfunction

Occupational therapy interventions need to focus on addressing deficits in areas of occupation. The most common area of difficulty, across all personality disorders, is in interpersonal skills (Livesley, 2003; Ward, 2004). Clients with personality disorder also demonstrate difficulty with affect modulation and appropriate expression of emotion, specifically clients diagnosed with Cluster B personality disorders (Ward, 2004). Occupational therapists can address these challenges by engaging the client in life skills groups where they have the opportunity to develop new ways of adapting to problems and can expand their coping skills (Cara, 1992). DBT is commonly used to address maladaptive behaviors associated with borderline personality disorder (Linehan, 1993) (see Chapter 24).

Individuals diagnosed with Cluster C personality disorders experience anxiety in some form (Ward, 2004). Occupational therapy intervention can decrease feelings of anxiety by engaging the client in relaxation activities (see Chapter 22), as well as in simple graded tasks that can facilitate success and increase self-esteem (Cara, 1992).

Clients with personality disorders in each of the three clusters experience difficulties with work. Occupational therapists can address work by examining the tasks required and the client skills available to complete the task. Some clients may benefit from supported employment interventions (see Chapter 50).

Clients with Clusters A and C personality disorders may experience difficulties in the area of leisure due to the interpersonal nature of many leisure activities and the anxiety they may feel in engaging in unstructured leisure activities.

Occupational therapists can address these difficulties by engaging the client in group games and activities that allow the client to experience a sense of fun (Cara, 1992).

Prevention of Personality Disorders

Using a developmental approach, intervention can be directed toward prevention of personality disorders. This is evidenced in the findings of Raine, Mellingen, Liu, Venables, and Mednick (2003), who observed that children who were engaged in an environmental enrichment program demonstrated decreased rates of diagnosis of schizotypal personality disorder and antisocial behavior in young adulthood. The environmental enrichment program included three elements: nutrition, education, and physical exercise.

Occupational therapists have a role in prevention and could be involved in such enrichment programs. At this time, more research needs to be conducted on the treatment potential and impact a dynamic developmental approach (including environmental enrichment) could have as an intervention for personality disorders (Fonagy, 2007; Raine et al., 2003). As a result, it is presently more common to address symptoms of personality disorder through the use of interpersonally directed therapy.

Summary

Although occupational therapists rarely work in a setting in which personality disorders are the primary admitting condition, the pervasiveness of the disorder means that occupational therapists will work with people with personality disorders regardless of the work setting. However, these individuals are often dismissed or labeled as difficult because of their troubling interpersonal behaviors or limited coping skills. For truly holistic treatment, the occupational therapist with a working knowledge of personality traits and related interventions can provide the best care. Rather than dismissing a client, the occupational therapist can adapt communication styles and intervention approaches to promote successful outcomes.

Active Learning Strategies

1. Assessment and Intervention: Planning for Personality Disorders Through the Use of Feature Films

Visit one of the websites listed here and choose a feature film depicting a movie character with a personality disorder. Rent the film from your local video rental store or secure the film through interlibrary loan, as some libraries have feature films in their holdings.

Psychiatric Bulletin: Teach Psychiatry Through Cinema:

http://pb.rcpsych.org/cgi/content/full/27/11/429

Movies and Mental Illness: Psychology, Psychiatry, and the Movies:

http://moviesandmentalillness.blogspot.com/

 After viewing the film, identify what behaviors the client demonstrates that would indicate a personality disorder. Consider the following questions in your **Reflective Journal**.

Reflective Questions
- In what setting might an occupational therapist see a client with this diagnosis?
- Would the client's primary diagnosis be personality disorder or some other Axis I diagnosis?
- Identify the areas of occupation negatively affected by the movie character due to his or her behavior.
- What performance skills are affected by the movie character's personality disorder?

- What roles does the movie character possess? Are they impacted by the character's diagnosis? If so, in what way are they impacted? As an occupational therapist, how would you address the movie character?
- What are the movie character's routines? Are they impacted by the character's personality? If so, in what way?
- How does context affect the movie character throughout the film?
- Are there specific activities that are especially difficult or challenging for the movie character? As an occupational therapist, how would you address this?
- What occupational therapy frame of reference would you choose to use?
- You've conducted an occupational profile with the movie character and have ascertained that difficulties exist in interpersonal skills, coping skills, and adaptation, as well as IADLs, work, and leisure. What occupational therapy assessment(s) would you choose?
- Which occupational therapy intervention approach(es) would you use if you were providing intervention to this movie character based on the behavior demonstrated in the movie?

2. Vocational Impact of Personality Disorders

Choose a job about which you have extensive knowledge that you have held during your lifetime. Complete an activity analysis of the job based on one of the personality disorder diagnoses. What activities within the job might a person with a diagnosis of personality disorder have difficulty with? How could you assist the person with a personality disorder in being successful in this job? Would it be possible for them to be successful in the occupation, or would the demands of the tasks required by the job be too challenging without support or intervention?

 Describe the experience in your Reflective Journal.

Reflective Questions

- What impact does the diagnosis of a personality disorder have on a person, his or her vocational occupation, and the potential environments in which he or she may choose to work?
- What impact would the personality disorder have on the person's work experience? Refer to Fischler and Booth (1999) for assistance.
- How would understanding and memory, concentration and persistence, and social interaction and adaptation be affected by the person's behavior in a work setting?

- Identify some strategies and accommodations from which an individual diagnosed with a personality disorder or who presents with specific personality traits may benefit. Again, consult Fischler and Booth (1999) for assistance. Also consider consulting the Job Accommodation Network for vocational accommodations for psychiatric conditions: http://www.jan.wvu.edu/media/Psychiatric.pdf

3. Mindfulness

Mindfulness is a significant component of intervention in working with clients diagnosed with borderline personality disorder and a key concept in Dr. Marsha Linehan's DBT. Go to http://www.youtube.com/watch?v=3nwwKbM_vJc and participate in the Mindfulness Meditation led by Dr. Jon Kabat-Zinn, the author of *Full Catastrophic Living.*

 Describe the experience in your Reflective Journal.

Reflective Questions

- What are your thoughts of mindfulness as presented by Dr. Kabat-Zinn?
- What did you feel as you were meditating?
- Have you meditated in the past? How was this experience similar or different?
- What was most challenging about the experience?
- Were you able to increase your sense of awareness during the experience? In what area(s)?
- What problems might a client encounter when trying to become more aware of his or her experience by paying attention to his or her breath through meditation? What could you do as an occupational therapist to assist the client in developing skill in the area of meditation?

4. Matching Behavior to Diagnosis

Visit the following website and review the behaviors of each person planning to attend a party:

http://www-usr.rider.edu/~suler/perdis.html

After reviewing each person, identify which behaviors match the diagnostic criteria of personality disorders. If the individuals described in the party story appeared in your clinic, what would be your process with them as an occupational therapist?

 Use the questions from the first learning activity (Feature Films) to guide your reflections in your Reflective Journal.

Resources

Books
- Bockian, N. R., & Jongsma, A. E. (2001). *The Personality Disorders Treatment Planner.* New York: John Wiley & Sons.
- Linehan, M. (1993). *Skills Training Manual for Treating Borderline Personality Disorder.* New York: Guilford Press.

Educational Videos
- *Back from the Edge*—a landmark documentary-style short film (2006). Available from the Borderline Personality Disorder Resource Center at http://www.bpdresourcecenter.org

- From Chaos to Freedom Skills Training Videos by Dr. Marsha Linehan (http://www.behavioraltech.com/products/list.cfm?category=Videos)
  - Tape 1: Crisis Survival Skills, Part One: Distracting and Self-Soothing
  - Tape 2: Crisis Survival Skills, Part Two: Improving the Moment and Pros and Cons
  - Tape 3: From Suffering to Freedom: Practicing Reality Acceptance
  - Tape 4: This One Moment: Skills for Everyday Mindfulness

Organizations
- BPDCentral—Borderline Personality Disorder Information and Support: http://www.bpdcentral.com
- Borderline Personality Disorder Resource Center: http://www.bpdresourcecenter.org/
- Cleveland Clinic—Dependent Personality Disorder: http://my.clevelandclinic.org/disorders/Personality_Disorders/hic_Dependent_Personality_Disorder.aspx
- Mental Health America—Factsheet: Personality Disorders: http://www.nmha.org/index.cfm?objectId=C7DF8E96-1372-4D20-C87D9CD4FB6BE82F
- Mayo Clinic—Personality Disorders: http://www.mayoclinic.com/health/personality-disorders/DS00562
- National Alliance on Mental Illness: http://www.nami.org
- National Institute of Mental Health—Borderline Personality Disorder: http://www.nimh.nih.gov/health/publications/borderline-personality-disorder.shtml
- Treatment and Research Advancements, National Association for Personality Disorders (TARA): http://www.tara4bpd.org

References

American Psychiatric Association (APA). (2000). *Diagnostic and Statistical Manual of Mental Disorders* (4th ed., text revision). Arlington, VA: Author.

Borderline Personality Disorder Resource Center. (2006). *Back From the Edge: Living and Recovering From Borderline Personality Disorder.* White Plains, NY: Author.

Bradley, R., Jenei, J., & Westen, D. (2005). Etiology of borderline personality disorder: Disentangling the contributions from intercorrelated antecedents. *Journal of Nervous & Mental Disease, 193*(1), 24–31.

Cara, E. (1992). Neutralizing the narcissistic style: Narcissistic personality disorder, self-psychology and occupational therapy. *Occupational Therapy in Mental Health, 8,* 135–156.

Costa, P. T., & McCrae, R. R. (1990). Personality disorders and the five factor model of personality. *Journal of Personality Disorders, 4,* 362–371.

Costa, P. T., & Widiger, T. A. (Eds.). (2002). *Personality Disorders and the Five Factor Model of Personality* (2nd ed.). Washington, DC: American Psychological Association.

Fischler, G., & Booth, N. (1999). *Vocational Impact of Psychiatric Disorders.* Gaithersburg, MD: Aspen.

Fonagy, P. (2007). Personality disorder. *Journal of Mental Health, 16*(1), 1–4.

Forsyth, K., with Salamy, M., Simon, S., & Kielhofner, G. (1998). "The Assessment of Communication and Interaction Skill (ACIS) Version 4.0." Available at: http://www.moho.uic.edu/assess/acis.html (accessed November 2, 2009).

Gilliam, J. E. (1994). *Work Adjustment Inventory: Measures of Job Related Temperament.* Austin, TX: PRO-ED.

Grant, B. F., Stinson, F. S., Dawson, D. A., Chou, P., Ruan, J., & Pickering, R. P. (2004). Co-occurrence of 12 month alcohol and drug use disorders and personality disorder in the United States: Results from the National Epidemiologic Survey on Alcohol and Related Conditions. *Archives of General Psychiatry, 61,* 361–368.

Hart, B. G. (2007). Cutting: Unraveling the mystery behind the marks. *AAOHN Journal, 55*(4), 161–168.

Kaylor, L. (1999). Antisocial personality disorder: Diagnostic, ethical and treatment issues. *Issues in Mental Health Nursing, 20,* 247–258.

Kaysen, S. (1993). *Girl Interrupted.* New York: Vintage Books.

Kendler, K. S., Czajkowski, N., Tambs, K., Torgersen, S., Aggen, S. H., Neale, M. C., & Reichborn-Kjennerud, T. (2006). Dimensional representations of a DSM-IV Cluster A personality disorders in a population based sample of Norwegian twins: A multivariate study. *Psychological Medicine, 36,* 1583–1591.

Lenzenweger, M. F., Lane, M. C., Loranger, A. W., & Kessler, R. C. (2007). DSM-IV personality disorders in the National Comorbidity Survey Replication. *Biological Psychiatry, 62*(6), 553–564.

Linehan, M. M. (1993). *Cognitive-Behavioral Treatment of Borderline Personality Disorder.* New York: Guilford Press.

Livesley, W. J. (2003). *Practical Management of Personality Disorder.* New York: Guilford Press.

Mental Health America. (2006). "Fact Sheet: Personality Disorders." Available at: http://www.nmha.org/go/information/get-info/personality-disorders (accessed January 28, 2010).

Merryman, M. B., & Riegel, S. K. (2007). The recovery process and people with serious mental illness living in the community: An occupational therapy perspective. *Occupational Therapy in Mental Health, 23*(2), 51–73.

Millon, T., & Davis, R. (2000). *Personality Disorders in Modern Life.* New York: John Wiley & Sons.

Mullins-Sweatt, S. N., & Widiger, T. A. (2007). Million's dimensional model of personality disorders: A comparative study. *Journal of Personality Disorders, 21*(1), 42–57.

National Institute of Mental Health. (2008). "Borderline Personality Disorder." Available at: http://www.nimh.nih.gov/health/publications/borderline-personality-disorder-fact-sheet/index.shtml (accessed January 28, 2010).

New, A. S., Triebwasser, J., & Charney, D. S. (2008). The case for shifting borderline personality disorder to Axis I. *Biological Psychiatry* [epub ahead of print].

Nott, A. (2005). Understanding and treating people with personality disorders in occupational therapy. In R. Crouch & V. Alers (Eds.), *Occupational Therapy in Mental Health* (4th ed.). London: Whurr.

Paris, J. (2005). Recent advances in the treatment of borderline personality disorder. *Canadian Journal of Psychiatry, 50*(8), 435–441.

Raine, A., Mellingen, K., Liu, J., Venables, P., & Mednick, S. A. (2003). Effects of environmental enrichment at ages 3–5 years on schizotypal personality and antisocial behavior at age 17–23. *American Journal of Psychiatry, 160*(9), 1627–1635.

Reed, K. L. (2001). *Quick Reference to Occupational Therapy* (2nd ed.). Gaithersburg, MD: Aspen.

Reichborn-Kjennerud, T., Czajkowski, N., Neale, M. C., Orstavik, R. E., Torgersen, S., Tambs, K., Roysamb, E., Harris, J. R., & Kendler, K. S. (2007). Genetic and environmental influences on dimensional representations of DSM-IV cluster personality disorders: A population-based multivariate twin study. *Psychological Medicine, 37,* 645–653.

Roth, A., & Fonagy, P. (2005). *What Works for Whom: A Critical Review of Psychotherapy Research* (2nd ed.). New York: Guilford Press.

Saddock, B. J., & Saddock, V. A. (2007). *Kaplan & Saddock's Synopsis of Psychiatry: Behavioral Sciences/Clinical Psychiatry.* Philadelphia: Lippincott Williams & Wilkins.

Stone, M. H. (2003). Borderline patients at the border of treatability: At the intersection of borderline, narcissistic, and antisocial personalities. *Journal of Psychiatric Practice, 9*(4), 279–290.

Thompson, P. M. (1998). "In Transition: Treating Personality Disorders." Available at: http://www.armchair.com/aware/trnsit11.html (accessed September 7, 2006).

Torgersen, S., Czajkowski, N., Jacobson, K., Reichborn-Kjennerud, T., RØysamb. E., Neale, M. C., & Kendler, K. S. (2008). Dimensional representations of DSM-IV Cluster B personality disorders in a population-based sample of Norwegian twins: A multivariate study. *Psychological Medicine, 38,* 1617–1625.

Triebwasser, J., & Siever, L. J. (2007). Pharmacotherapy and personality disorders. *Journal of Mental Health, 16*(1), 5–50.

Ward, R. K. (2004). Assessment and management of personality disorders. *American Family Physician, 70*(8), 1505–1512.

Zanarini, M. C. (2000). Childhood experiences associated with the development of borderline personality disorder. *Psychiatric Clinics of North America, 23*(1), 89–101.

Mood Disorders

Nancy W. Spangler

> "People ask, "Why would a funny man be depressed?"
>
> My answer is, "Why not?"
>
> Humorists (also people in show business, writers, and artists) are funny to cover up the hurts they have suffered as children. When the humor fails to work for them, they have a depression.... The price I paid for success was that by building a wall around me, no one could penetrate my real feelings. The scars of childhood were always there, and I was a fool to think I could get away with humor forever.
>
> —Art Buchwald, *Too Soon to Say Goodbye*, 2006

Introduction

"Like a gray mist turning into a heavy, dark shroud" is how Susan (a pseudonym) described her first episode of major depression. She hardly noticed it creeping up on her. What she did notice was how much effort it took to complete the work that typically came so easily to her. A highly creative person, Susan was valued by her employer, the owner of a small public relations firm, for her brilliant ideas and her strong work ethic. Her first experience with depression eroded her abilities, making every decision difficult and merely getting out of bed a horrible labor.

When her boss finally confronted her, asking where her typical sparkle had gone, Susan melted into a puddle of sobs and apologies. The strength of her emotion shocked and disappointed her even further, but it was a familiar signal to her boss, who had experienced a depression of his own just a few months earlier. Her boss suggested she visit with a therapist who had helped him out of his distress. Susan began psychotherapy and took antidepressant medications for several months. Her work rebounded, and her mood brightened until she began a project with a particularly difficult client. The stress of her interactions brought back her irrational thoughts of inadequacy, and the dark shroud began creeping over her again. It was her boss who first noticed her symptoms returning, and this time he was quicker in saying something to her and reminding her of the available resources for support. Eventually, Susan learned to recognize signals earlier herself and apply self-management strategies to reduce the disabling aspects of her chronic condition.

Susan's story is just one example of the impact of **mood disorders** on daily living. Everyone experiences changes in moods, typically ranging from sad to happy to somewhere in between, depending on one's circumstances. For people with mood disorders, however, the mood fluctuations go beyond the typical and may have little or no relation to the person's current circumstances.

Researchers are just beginning to understand mood disorders—the mechanisms by which they affect the brain and behavior, their true prevalence, and how treatments actually work. What we do know is that the impact of mood disorders can be devastating. In fact, mood disorders are a leading cause of disability worldwide and a common cause of suicide for all age groups, including children and older adults (Bhatia & Bhatia, 2007; Bould, 2005). Depression and bipolar disorder, like other mental illnesses, are often stigmatizing conditions, and, unfortunately, individuals often choose not to seek care of any kind (Kanter, Rusch, & Brondino, 2008).

A variety of treatments are available, however, and treatment is effective for many people. Occupational therapists can play an important role in helping people with mood disorders—to recognize and understand the disorder, to seek treatment, and to prevent or better manage symptoms as they live, work, learn, and play.

Description of the Disorder

Mood disorder is the umbrella term that encompasses conditions in which individuals experience an extreme in the continuum of typical moods—from the low, sad, unpleasant mood of **unipolar depression** to the elevated, elated, energized mood of mania. Those individuals who experience both ends of the continuum are known as having **bipolar disorder.**

Mood disorders frequently occur in conjunction with other mental conditions, such as anxiety and personality disorder, and with medical illnesses, such as heart disease, cancer, chronic pain, asthma, and diabetes, thus contributing to their tendency to be disabling (Carnethon et al, 2007; Pincus & Pettit, 2001; Schatzberg, 2004). Mood disorders are also associated with substance abuse problems. The U.S. Surgeon General (U.S. Department of Health and Human Services, 1999) and the World Health Organization (2002) identified depression as a major public health problem that is growing in severity.

DSM-IV-TR Criteria

Although the term **depression** is well recognized and commonly used by the general public to mean a sad mood and something nearly everyone has experienced, the full range of symptoms necessary for a diagnosis of **clinical depression** are not well known by the layperson. The true meaning of bipolar disorder is also elusive to many people. The American Psychiatric Association (APA) provides criteria in the *Diagnostic and Statistical Manual of Mental Disorders, Fourth Edition, Text Revision* (DSM-IV-TR) (APA, 2000) for specific features for diagnosing depressive disorders, bipolar disorders, and their milder forms or subtypes.

Episodes

The DSM-IV-TR begins by describing **episodes,** or distinct periods and features of mood disturbance. For example, a depressed mood and loss of interest or pleasure in life activities (**anhedonia**) for at least 2 weeks are the main characteristics of a **depressive episode** (Box 12-1). An abnormally elevated, expansive, or irritable mood for at least 1 week, in conjunction with other criteria, such as inflated self-esteem or grandiosity, decreased need for sleep, rapid speech, psychomotor agitation, and involvement in high-risk activities, characterizes a **manic episode** (Box 12-2). These depressive and manic episodes are not diagnoses themselves; rather, they are used as building blocks for the various forms of mood disorders.

Mixed episodes are characterized by rapid changes in moods occurring nearly daily. **Hypomanic episodes** are similar to manic episodes, with periods of elevated, expansive, or irritable mood, but symptoms are at a lower intensity and without marked impairment in social or occupational functioning. Hypomania may even include brief periods of high efficiency or creativity.

Some depressive episodes are further specified based on notable behavioral features as either **melancholic** or **atypical subtype**. For example, an episode may be labeled as melancholic when its features include loss of pleasure in nearly all activities and/or lack of pleasure even when something good happens, along with such symptoms as early morning wakenings, increased depression in the morning, marked weight loss, excessive guilt, and psychomotor retardation or agitation. In contrast, an atypical depressive episode includes mood brightening with positive events and neurovegetative functions that are reversed from the melancholic (e.g., appetite is increased, sleep is excessive, the person may feel leaden paralysis as if he or she is unable to move). Symptoms are worse at night in atypical depression, and the individual is highly sensitive to rejection by others.

BOX 12-1 ■ DSM-IV-TR Criteria for Major Depressive Episode

A. Five (or more) of the following symptoms have been present during the same 2-week period and represent a change from previous functioning; at least one of the symptoms is either (1) depressed mood or (2) loss of interest or pleasure.

1. Depressed mood most of the day, nearly every day, as indicated by either subjective report (e.g., feels sad or empty) or observation made by others (e.g., appears tearful). *Note:* In children and adolescents, can be irritable mood.

2. Markedly diminished interest or pleasure in all, or almost all, activities most of the day, nearly every day (as indicated by either subjective account or observation made by others).

3. Significant weight loss when not dieting, or weight gain (e.g., a change of more than 5% of body weight in a month), or decrease or increase in appetite nearly every day. *Note:* In children, consider failure to make expected weight gains.

4. Insomnia or hypersomnia nearly every day.

5. Psychomotor agitation or retardation nearly every day (observable by others, not merely subjective feelings or restlessness or being slowed down).

6. Fatigue or loss of energy nearly every day.

7. Feelings of worthlessness or excessive or inappropriate guilt (which may be delusional) nearly every day (not merely self-reproach or guilt about being sick).

8. Diminished ability to think or concentrate, or indecisiveness, nearly every day (either subjective account or as observed by others).

9. Recurrent thoughts of death (not just fear of dying), recurrent suicidal ideation without a specific plan, or a suicide attempt or specific plan for committing suicide.

B. The symptoms do not meet criteria for a mixed episode.

C. The symptoms cause clinically significant distress or impairment in social, occupational, or other important areas of functioning.

From American Psychiatric Association. (2000). *Diagnostic and Statistical Manual of Mental Disorders* (4th ed.). Washington, DC: Author.

BOX 12-2 ■ DSM-IV-TR Criteria for Manic Episode

A. A distinct period of abnormally and persistently elevated, expansive, or irritable mood, lasting at least 1 week (or any duration if hospitalization is necessary).

B. During the period of mood disturbance, three (or more) of the following symptoms have persisted (four if the mood is only irritable) and have been present to a significant degree:

1. Inflated self-esteem or grandiosity

2. Decreased need for sleep (e.g., feels rested after only 3 hours of sleep)

3. More talkative than usual or pressure to keep talking

4. Flight of ideas or subjective experience that thoughts are racing

5. Distractibility (i.e., attention too easily drawn to unimportant or irrelevant external stimuli)

6. Increase in goal-directed activity (either socially, at work or school, or sexually) or psychomotor agitation

7. Excessive involvement in pleasurable activities that have a high potential for painful consequences (e.g., engaging in unrestrained buying sprees, sexual indiscretions, or foolish business investments)

C. The symptoms do not meet criteria for a mixed episode.

D. The mood disturbance is sufficiently severe to cause marked impairment in occupational functioning or in usual social activities or relationships with others, or to necessitate hospitalization to prevent harm to self or others, or there are psychotic features.

From American Psychiatric Association. (2000). *Diagnostic and Statistical Manual of Mental Disorders* (4th ed.). Washington, DC: Author.

Psychotic features may be present with depressive or manic episodes and are described as being congruent or incongruent with the current mood state. In other words, mood congruent psychotic features during a depressive episode are delusions or hallucinations consistent with depressive themes (e.g., inadequacy, guilt, death, punishment). Mood incongruent symptoms during depression may include thought broadcasting and delusions of control. During manic episodes, mood congruent psychotic features are those consistent with mania (e.g., inflated self-worth, power, or specialness), whereas mood incongruent features would include persecutory delusions and delusions of being controlled. A number of studies found increased rates of psychotic features in bipolar disorder versus unipolar depression (Goes et al, 2007). Furthermore, patients who present with psychotic features initially in unipolar depression are more likely to experience a manic episode at some point compared with individuals without psychotic features.

Mood disorders with postpartum onset may be diagnosed if onset occurs within 4 weeks after childbirth. Although "baby blues" are common 3 to 7 days after birth and consist of increased crying, anxiety, and insomnia, more serious symptoms can characterize episodes or disorders with postpartum onset, including psychotic hallucinations and/or delusions, and can increase the risk of the mother harming herself or her baby.

Disorders

Mood disorders are classified according to the type of episode or combination of episodes experienced by the individual.

Depressive Disorders

A person who experiences a **major depressive disorder** has one or more instances of a major depressive episode, but no occurrence of a manic episode; thus, the disorder is considered **unipolar**, or occurring on just one side of the affective spectrum. (*Note:* Clinicians frequently use the terms "unipolar depression" and "clinical depression" interchangeably to describe major depressive disorder, with unipolar referring to one end of the bipolar spectrum.)

Although the actual experience of depression can vary widely in its features and severity of symptoms, people with major depression are more likely to experience pain and physical illness along with decreased physical, social, and role functioning. Up to 15% of people with severe depression will die by suicide (APA, 2000).

Some people with major depressive disorder experience only a single episode, whereas others have a recurrence even after many years without symptoms. Still other individuals have clusters of frequently recurring episodes over the course of a lifetime, some in association with particular seasons. Each episode increases the odds of recurrent episodes, and the severity of the first episode predicts persistent episodes, as does chronic medical illness (Robinson & Sahakian, 2008). If full criteria for a major depressive episode have been met continuously for at least 2 years, the condition is considered chronic.

Dysthymic Disorder

Dysthymic disorder, or **dysthymia,** shares similar features with major depressive disorder, but symptoms are less severe and must be present chronically (a period of at least 2 years) rather than episodically. In children, irritability may be observed more than depressed mood. Feelings of inadequacy, guilt, and excessive anger are commonly experienced in dysthymia, along with periods of social withdrawal and reduced activity or productivity.

Bipolar Disorders

There are three primary types of bipolar disorder: bipolar I, bipolar II, and cyclothymia.

Bipolar I disorder is characterized by one or more manic episodes or mixed episodes (i.e., frequent fluctuations between low and expansive mood). Many individuals will experience major depressive episodes as well, but this is not required for bipolar I diagnosis. Bipolar I is highly recurrent (in more than 90% of people), and the number of lifetime manic and depressive episodes is higher for bipolar I than for major depressive disorder (APA, 2000). Those people with four or more recurring episodes within a given year (called "rapid cycling pattern") generally have a poorer prognosis.

Bipolar II disorder is characterized by one or more major depressive episodes and at least one hypomanic episode. Significant impairment in important areas of life function must be experienced to reach diagnostic criteria, but the impairment typically occurs during the depressive episodes, not the hypomanic ones. In fact, although the hypomania may not be evident to the individual, it can be troubling to family, friends, and/or coworkers. As with bipolar I, recurrence and rapid cycling in bipolar II are more likely to predict lower levels of function.

Cyclothymic disorder is a chronic (at least 2-year period) mood disturbance that is characterized by fluctuating hypomanic symptoms and depressive symptoms that are not of sufficient number or severity to reach criteria for either manic episodes or major depressive episodes. Although people can function adequately during hypomanic periods, marked impairment may occur, particularly due to unpredictable mood changes and social difficulties that result. The differential diagnosis between cyclothymic disorder and borderline personality disorder may be difficult, and both may be diagnosed if criteria are met for each.

(Readers should refer to the DSM-IV-TR (2000) for a full description of subtypes and specifiers for major depressive disorder and bipolar disorder.)

Etiology

There is growing evidence that the etiology of mood disorders is complex, with interacting contributions from biological, genetic, psychosocial, and environmental factors. In fact, some of the subtypes of mood disorders may actually reflect distinct neurobiological differences, explaining why certain treatments are effective for some people, but not for others.

Studies were conducted in the 1950s on the biological causes of mood disorders when medications used for treating other conditions were also found to have an impact on levels of depression and symptoms of mania. Researchers noting associated changes in the noradrenergic and serotonergic systems of the brain theorized that depression resulted from decreased availability of the neurotransmitters norepinephrine and/or serotonin, whereas mania resulted

The Lived Experience

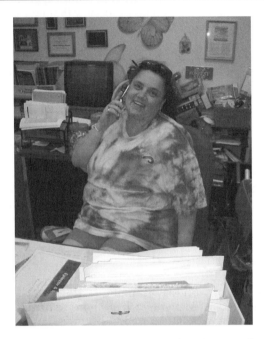

Kelly: Not an Ordinary Little Girl

I may not be every mother's dream for her little girl. I was always different from the other kids, and I knew it. Growing up was difficult. I went to a school for children with special learning disabilities because I was diagnosed with hyperkinetic behavior and put on Ritalin. I stayed in this school until I was in 8th grade. Then I went on to a private school. My parents were told I couldn't make it in public school because of my behavior and academic record. I managed to get through until 11th grade and was then asked to leave the following year because I wasn't making it there either. So back to public school I went, and the roller coaster rides began.

As I got older, the problems and the mania got bolder, and I needed to run. The day the gate opened was the day I had my first real roller coaster ride. I was flying high and nobody knew why. At the age of 18, I was hospitalized for the first time and was diagnosed with manic depression or, in other words, cyclothymia, which is always manic.

I had a wonderful doctor, Dr. Stevenson, and he explained that I had a chemical imbalance that could be helped with medication. This was my first attempt at any mood-altering drug. My life changed dramatically, I was actually able to sit down and concentrate for the first time, and my life was a bit easier, for a while. The medication made me feel better, and then I would stop taking it because I felt "normal." Boy did that change; as soon as the medication was out of my system, I was back on another HIGH. The rides got rougher and rougher, and I was put back into the hospital again. I can remember my Mom and Dad were always there at my side, and anything that needed to be done to make me better was not a problem, they did whatever it took. Knowing that over and over we would be back on this ride again, but they never gave up. I may not be every mother's dream for her little girl, but I knew I didn't deserve this crazy life.

I know there are lulls in every storm, but one will happen again. In my life when it rained it poured, and I knew there will

always be another rollercoaster ride and a collision up ahead. They took a bigger toll on my life every time I came back through, trying to stop it or at least slow it down. Almost too painful to even keep fighting back, I knew I needed another line of attack. Always experimenting off to another special doctor to see . . . take this pill with that one and come back to see them in a month or three . . . just call if these don't work, there is more we can try, and that we did. My life was in shambles, and I didn't have a clue that all I needed to do was take the medications and I would be fine.

Among all the diagnoses, I had another problem—I was a drug addict, I self-medicated with marijuana, and then harder drugs. They made me feel okay, but never in control of my life. Hospitals, doctors, psychs, and shrinks, together we would go, hands held tight like a link. We (my parents and I) refused to give up on this fight; we were gonna get my life right.

With hospitals and rehabs, we finally did something right. At the age of 30-something, we found Wyandot Mental Health, and I found a doctor who would listen to me and diagnose me right. He was great, and he knew all the answers to the questions of why I never felt right. He gave me hope that my life could change and that I was important in my fight. My mental illness was not me, I was me, and it just happened to be part of me. This gave me a whole new outlook on life and what I was to become. I may not be every mother's dream for her little girl, but now we were getting answers and solutions for the problems I have had all my life.

I began going to the drop-in center at Wyandot Mental Health and making friends and going to classes that taught me about my disease. It taught me that I could be normal, in my world. That there were others who lived with the voices and all that I had endured in my life. I began to speak out, not just for me but for many others that I encountered. I had become an advocate for the mentally ill and for myself. I was finally given the guidance to GROW. That I did. I went to classes and lectures and absorbed every thing I could, and people began to see the change in me, I was also given medication that helped, and my drug addiction was going away. I became involved in SIDE, which is the consumer-run organization in my state. I was given the opportunity to help facilitate groups and educate my friends. This was very empowering because it gave me the opportunity to see them grow and become advocates for themselves.

I have been with the mental health center for a number of years and have bloomed and helped others. This is my passion for my life. Today, I am Vice President of SIDE, Inc, and have gained the most important of friends in my life. I have many diagnoses: manic depression, schizophrenia, and agoraphobia, and they are controlled by medications. Today, I am living instead of just existing. I thank the good Lord above and a special thanks to my parents and the people who believed in me and never gave up. I will continue my road to recovery, with hope that I can be an inspiration to others that followed through that door of mental illness. I may not be every mother's dream for her little girl, but thank you for choosing me and never closing the door. Dedicated to all my friends that I have met on life's highways.

from excess activity of the noradrenergic system (Kandel, Schwartz, & Jessell, 2000). In other words, too little neural firing occurred in depression, and too much occurred in mania due to this neurochemical imbalance. Subsequently, numerous medications have been developed (see Medications section) that are highly effective for many people with depressive and bipolar disorders.

However, the neural mechanisms behind the so-called "chemical imbalance" associated with mood disorders, as well as the impact of antidepressant and mood-stabilizing medications, have not been well understood. Researchers studying the impact of psychosocial stress theorize that depression occurs as the result of prolonged or recurring stress responses that disrupt the **hypothalamic-pituitary-adrenal (HPA) axis,** which is highly important in gastrointestinal and immune system functioning (Kandel et al, 2000).

The HPA axis is a regulatory network that operates in response to stress and consists of chemical messengers that prepare the body for the "fight-or-flight response" and then a return to homeostasis, or relaxation, when the threat has been removed. One of these chemicals, cortisol, travels through the bloodstream and acts on bodily organs and tissues (Adinoff, Iranmanesh, Veldhuis, & Fisher, 1998). The hippocampus has an inhibitory effect on the HPA axis, and the amygdala has an excitatory effect (Nestler et al, 2002). People with depression exhibit a disturbance in this neuroendocrinologic function, which is identified by excessive secretion of cortisol from the adrenal cortex of the kidney (Kandel et al, 2000). This hypercortisolism affects structures in the hippocampus, which fail to relay signals to constrain the stress response.

Repeated reactivity to chronic stress is theorized to lower the threshold for a depressive episode (Pariante & Miller, 2001; Shumake & Gonzalez-Lima, 2003). With the advent of newer neuroimaging and neurometabolic techniques and sophisticated genetic studies, neural systems have been identified and additional theories generated. Research suggests that genetic vulnerability and experiencing early life stressors may contribute to depression through neural changes in certain brain circuits, most notably the limbic-cortical circuits (Fuchs, Czeh, Koke, Michaelis, & Lucassen, 2004).

Depression

The contribution of stress in depression has been supported by both behavioral and genetic studies. In studies of interactions between mothers with depression and their infants, depressed mothers were more likely to be angry, sad, or intrusive in face-to-face interaction or to be poorly timed, lacking synchrony in the communication loop (Tronick, 1989). Infants, in turn, were less able to calm themselves and showed more crying or withdrawing in response to such stressors. Babies of mothers with depression have higher levels of the stress hormone cortisol, lower levels of the neurotransmitters dopamine and serotonin, asymmetries in frontal lobe functioning, more signs of distress, and more sleeping difficulties (Field, Diego, & Hernandez-Reif, 2006). Thus, difficulty in adapting to stress, modulating negative affective states, and regulating emotions may make these infants vulnerable to depressive episodes in the future. Occupational therapists can play a role in prevention by addressing parenting issues among mothers with depression.

Such differences in emotion processing are believed to affect cognitive development in infants and young children, and may result in cognitive vulnerability to stress from environmental challenges (Seligman, 1991). Cognitive distortions and exaggerated responses to stress are frequently seen in adults with depression, can result in feelings of helplessness and despair, and are frequently a focus of cognitive behavioral psychotherapy, a common and effective intervention for depression.

Children who have experienced early loss of a parent, early parental neglect, or sexual abuse are at greater risk of depressive disorders, yet not all children of mothers with depression end up experiencing depression themselves. This has led to studies of resilience to determine what factors may help vulnerable children in developing coping strategies and avoiding psychosocial disorders (Rutter, 2006).

An interaction between vulnerability to depression and stressful life experiences was also found by genetic researchers (Caspi et al, 2003). The genetic vulnerability appears to impact the *5-HTT* gene, which is responsible for transport and reuptake of serotonin. People with at least one copy of the short form gene were more likely to become depressed in response to stressful life events. This genetic variability may be responsible for amygdala-mediated hyperresponsiveness seen in certain young children in reaction to frightening faces and encoding of painful memories, possibly increasing stress sensitivity in adulthood (Hariri et al, 2005).

The impact of emotional stress is seen in the **limbic-cortical circuit,** or neural pathways between the brainstem, amygdala, hippocampus, hypothalamus, and cingulate gyrus, and connections through the dorsolateral prefrontal, lateral orbitofrontal, and anterior cingulate circuits to the cortex (Kandel et al, 2000). The limbic-cortical circuit modulates arousal and alerting behaviors in organisms, and allows for storage and retrieval of memories to enable approach/avoidance behaviors. These structures interact in survival activities, such as eating, drinking, and reproduction, as well as during social interaction, emotion regulation, and activities related to pleasure and ego satisfaction. The amygdala and the nucleus accumbens are involved in processing memories with emotional associations and may, in turn, mediate the anhedonia, anxiety, and reduced motivation commonly seen in people with depression (Nestler et al, 2002). Depressive neurovegetative symptoms, such as sleep dysregulation, reduced energy, changes in appetite, and reduced interest in sex, may also implicate involvement of the hypothalamus, the body's regulator of internal homeostasis.

In summary, impairments in brain areas in the limbic-cortical circuits appear to be those most affected by depression. These areas regulate emotional and cognitive functioning, memory, concentration, sleep, appetite, mood, and motivation, and contribute to social interests and self-worth.

Bipolar Disorder

The etiology of bipolar disorder is less clear than that of depression. Genetic transmission is highly likely because first-degree relatives have a 5- to 10-fold greater risk of bipolar disorder than the general population, and the disorder is found concurrently in 80% to 90% of monozygotic (identical) twins versus 15% of dizygotic (fraternal) twins (Craddock & Jones, 2001). Although the particular gene site or sites have not been identified, multiple genes are likely to be involved. In both major depressive and bipolar disorders, it is likely that genetic influences on neurotrophic factors (or growth and nourishment of brain cells), which allow adaption to stress, are involved (Rosa et al, 2006).

Major life events that cause emotional stress may serve to precipitate symptoms of bipolar disorder as in depressive disorders, and differences in HPA axis functioning and neurotransmission are seen in both. In bipolar disorder, insufficient transport of sodium and potassium ions into neurons causes transmission to occur too readily. Prefrontal cortex activity is reduced during the depressive phase, and an increase in this region is observed during mania (Kandel et al, 2000).

Prevalence

Depression is a highly prevalent condition that affects approximately 7% of adult men and 12% of women each year in the United States, and nearly one in five Americans in their lifetime (Blazer, Kessler, McGonagle, & Swartz, 1994; Kessler et al, 2003; Regier et al, 1993). Within the workforce, the prevalence of depressive disorders is estimated at 9% (Stewart, Ricci, Chee, Hahn, & Morganstein, 2003). Depression occurs about twice as often in women as in men and tends to be more common among individuals who are younger than 45 years of age, of lower socioeconomic status, and separated or divorced (Pincus & Pettit, 2001).

Lifetime prevalence of bipolar disorder is approximately 1%, but subthreshold rates are estimated to be over twice as high (2.5%) and to cause significant role impairment (Merikangas et al, 2007). Rates of diagnosing bipolar disorder in children and adolescents appear to be sharply rising (Moreno et al, 2007), but it is undetermined whether this is due to an actual increase in the disorder, increased recognition that the disorder could exist in children, or a change in diagnosing patterns (e.g., instead of attention deficit disorder, which has overlapping symptoms).

Course

The average age for onset of major depressive disorder is the mid-20s, but depression can occur at any time during the life span. As described previously, infants as young as 3 months of age have been observed to be sensitive and reactive to expressions of flat or negative affect that are common to mothers with depression; they, in turn, exhibit symptoms of social withdrawal and difficulty with emotion regulation (Ashman, Dawson, & Panagiotides, 2008). In contrast to the symptoms of depression listed in the DSM-IV-TR (APA, 2000), behaviors of young children with depressive disorders may include irritable mood, decreased social interaction, and diminished interest or pleasure in typical activities for the child's age (Zeanah, 2000).

Depression is highly recurrent, and the more episodes one has had, the more likely the condition will remain chronic without subsiding. With each occurrence, there is a greater risk of psychosocial limitations, work impairment, and worsening of other medical conditions, thus the more disabling each episode is likely to become (Hirschfeld, Lewis, & Vornick, 2003). Therefore, the importance of early treatment, including occupational therapy, to prevent subsequent episodes and occupational performance impairment is essential. Figure 12-1 shows a painting by a participating artist at the Northern Initiative for Social Action.

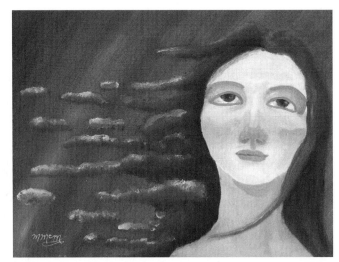

FIGURE 12-1. Artwork titled "Shining Through" by Meredith McMaster, participating artist at Northern Initiative for Social Action.

Although depression is not a normal consequence of aging, it does commonly co-occur with other medical illnesses associated with aging, such as heart disease, diabetes, stroke, cancer, and Parkinson's disease, and is often overlooked and untreated (National Institutes of Mental Health, 2003). It also frequently occurs with loss of a spouse or other social support or loss of vision, mobility, or functional abilities. In older people with depression, symptoms may include irritability, pacing, and restlessness.

About 65% of adults with bipolar disorder describe symptoms of bipolar disorder with onset prior to age 19 (Perlis et al, 2004). Episodes may recur after years with none. More frequent cycling of episodes is associated with declining functional abilities.

Suicide is completed by about 15% of people who were formerly hospitalized for depression (Angst, Angst, & Stassen, 1999). The high energy and elation of mania combined with low mood of depression in people with mixed episodes puts them at particular risk (Box 12-3).

Evidence-Based Practice

Early detection helps people access appropriate treatment and reduces severity and recurrence of symptoms in people with mood disorders (Druss, Rosenheck, Desai, & Perlin, 2002; Hirschfeld, Calabrese, et al, 2003).

➤ Occupational therapists can help educate workplace managers about the impact of depression and bipolar disorder.

➤ Occupational therapists can implement screenings for employees to enhance early detection and treatment.

➤ Occupational therapists can provide training in resilience and stress management.

Druss, B. G., Rosenheck, R. A., Desai, M. M., & Perlin, J. B. (2002). Quality of preventive medical care for patients with mental disorders. *Medical Care, 40*(2), 129–136.

Hirschfeld, R. M., Calabrese, J. R., Weissman, M. M., Reed, M., Davies, M. A., Frye, M. A., Keck, P. E. Jr., Lewis, L., McElroy, S. L., McNulty, J. P., & Wagner, K. D (2003). Screening for bipolar disorder in the community. *Journal of Clinical Psychiatry, 64*(1), 53–59.

Alcohol is used by up to 40% of those with mood disorders, often as a means of self-medication (Merikangas, 1998). Left untreated, substance abuse typically worsens the course of mood disorders, affects social relationships, and reduces functional abilities.

BOX 12-3 ▨ Suicide

Suicide, frequently associated with mood disorders, is particularly troublesome because of the emotional suffering experienced by surviving family members and friends, and the disabling effects on people who attempt suicide. Suicide rates vary by age, gender, and ethnic groups, but in general suicide occurs most frequently in males and tends to peak in adolescence and old age.

There are a number of risk factors that are associated with suicide, as well as protective factors that reduce the likelihood of suicide.

Risk Factors for Suicide

Biopsychosocial Risk Factors
- Mental disorders, particularly mood disorders, schizophrenia, anxiety disorders, and certain personality disorders
- Alcohol and other substance use disorders
- Hopelessness
- Impulsive and/or aggressive tendencies
- History of trauma or abuse
- Some major physical illnesses
- Previous suicide attempt
- Family history of suicide

Environmental Risk Factors
- Job or financial loss
- Relational or social loss
- Easy access to lethal means
- Local clusters of suicide that have a contagious influence

Sociocultural Risk Factors
- Lack of social support and sense of isolation
- Stigma associated with help-seeking behavior
- Barriers to accessing health care, especially mental health and substance abuse treatment
- Certain cultural and religious beliefs (e.g., the belief that suicide is a noble resolution of a personal dilemma)
- Exposure to, including through the media, and influence of others who have died by suicide

Protective Factors for Suicide

- Effective clinical care for mental, physical, and substance use disorders
- Easy access to a variety of clinical interventions and support for help-seeking
- Restricted access to highly lethal means of suicide
- Strong connections to family and community support
- Support through ongoing medical and mental health care relationships
- Skills in problem-solving, conflict resolution, and nonviolent handling of disputes
- Cultural and religious beliefs that discourage suicide and support self-preservation

Source: U.S. Department of Health and Human Services, Substance Abuse and Mental Health Services Administration. (2001). *National Strategy for Suicide Prevention: Goals and Objectives for Action.* Rockville, MD: Public Health Service.

Gender- and Culture-Specific Information

Depression is twice as prevalent in females as in males, but bipolar disorder occurs about evenly in men and women (Regier et al, 1993).

Depression and bipolar disorder, like many medical conditions, are associated with lower socioeconomic status (Murray & Lopez, 1997). It is not known, however, whether socioeconomic factors play a causal role in the etiology of mood disorders or whether the disorders reduce work opportunities and thereby reduce socioeconomic levels. Because stress is theorized as a factor in increased occurrence of mood disorders in vulnerable individuals, the fact that stress is associated with low socioeconomic status is important to consider. Poor young women of all ethnic groups and single mothers appear to be at greatest risk of developing depression (Brown & Moran, 1997; Miranda & Green, 1999).

Individuals from non-Caucasian cultures are less likely to seek treatment for depression. The STAR*D (Sequenced Treatment Alternatives to Relieve Depression) study found a much higher attrition rate (individuals that chose not to stay in treatment) for African Americans, Latinos, and other non-Caucasian groups (Warden et al, 2008). Another study found that African Americans sought mental health services for depression 50% less often than whites, and the number one reason for not seeking care was stigma (Cruz, Pincus, Harman, Reynolds, & Post, 2008). Acculturation can also contribute to depression. One study examining acculturation among college students of Asian and Latino descent found high rates of depression (Hwang & Wood, 2009). The depression was associated with a lack of family support that resulted from distancing themselves during acculturation and greater conflict with family members.

Impact on Occupational Performance

Mood disorders can range from mild to severe, but, in general, their impact can be pervasive and disabling if symptoms are recurrent and untreated. Occupational therapists can play an important role in addressing occupational performance problems associated with mood disorders. Individuals with depression may show poor self-esteem and low motivation,

---

Evidence-Based Practice

People with mood disorders can learn to recognize symptoms of relapse earlier and better manage their conditions (Perry, Tarrier, Morriss, McCarthy, & Limb, 1999).

➤ Occupational therapists can provide materials and teach programs to help people recognize triggers and symptoms for enhancing self-management.

➤ Occupational therapists can encourage appropriate care-seeking.

Perry, A., Tarrier, N., Morriss, R., McCarthy, E., & Limb, K. (1999). Randomised controlled trial of efficacy of teaching patients with bipolar disorder to identify early symptoms of relapse and obtain treatment. *British Medical Journal, 318,* 149–153.

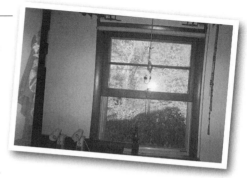

whereas those experiencing manic episodes may have exaggerated self-esteem and difficulty completing and finishing tasks (Christiansen & Baum, 1997). Areas frequently affected include cognitive (solving problems, making decisions, remembering, concentrating), behavioral (motivation, task completion) social (withdrawal, eye contact, listening skills, interpersonal conflicts), and physiological (sleep difficulties, restlessness, fatigue). Daily routines for sleep, meals, self-care, and social relationships are often disrupted, particularly in individuals experiencing manic episodes. Such difficulties can greatly impact performance in school, work, home, and community (Bilsker, Gilbert, Myette, & Stewart-Patterson, 2004).

For women with postpartum depression, numerous roles may be compromised in both the mother and her baby. Esdaile and Olson (2004) refer to co-occupational roles being affected. These may include comforting and self-comforting, feeding and eating, and getting to sleep and remaining asleep. Such difficulties can greatly affect bonding and social role development. Addressing the role of parenting becomes important for the occupational therapist to meet the needs of both the mother and the baby.

Both depressive disorders and bipolar disorders may affect effectiveness in school and work roles when cognitive and social skills are affected. At work, supervisors and coworkers are often the first to notice symptoms occurring or recurring when work skills begin to deteriorate (Bilsker et al, 2004). People with mood disorders are at increased risk of accidents and job loss.

In one large workplace study (Kessler et al, 2006), workers with bipolar disorder had higher work loss than those with major depressive disorder due to more severe and persistent episodes of depression rather than to manic or hypomanic symptoms. The authors suggest employers participate in coordinated workplace trials for screening and treating both bipolar disorder and major depressive disorder. If people with bipolar disorder are untreated or treatment is inappropriate, about 88% of these individuals remain unable to work, 68% have conflicts with family and friends, and 55% have financial difficulties (Hirschfeld et al, 2003). Feelings of high energy without the need for sleep are common during mania, yet lack of sleep over time may contribute to cognitive declines and even psychotic symptoms. Hallucinations and paranoia of manic episodes are often confused with schizophrenia. Occupational therapists can play an important role in helping people with mood disorders continue to be successful in the workplace.

The stigma that exists for depression is often due to the hidden nature of the disorder and misunderstandings that surround it (Bilsker et al, 2004). Research also suggests that stigma affects people who care for individuals with mood disorders, even when the person's symptoms are in remission (Gonzalez et al, 2007). This may affect social withdrawal, altered role expectations, and occupational choices for all family members. (For more information, see Chapter 28.)

Treatment

The most common forms of treatment for mood disorders are psychopharmacology (Tables 12-1 and 12-2) and behavioral therapy.

Medications for Depressive Disorders

The first class of medications used to treat depression was the **monoamine oxidase inhibitors (MAOIs).** MAOIs are effective, but have significant side effects, including dangerous interactions with common foods and risk of death with overdose. Another older class of medications, **tricyclic antidepressants (TCAs),** inhibits the uptake of serotonin and noradrenaline. These medications have numerous adverse side effects as well. Although MAOIs and TCAs are rarely used today, they may be effective in people with depression that is unresponsive to other treatments (Kandel et al, 2000; Mann, 2005).

The mainstay of depression treatment is now second-generation antidepressant drugs, called **selective serotonin reuptake inhibitors (SSRIs)** and **serotonin and norepinephrine reuptake inhibitors (SNRIs).** These medications have become well-established treatments with fewer side effects for most patients (Compton & Nemeroff, 2006), which tends to increase

Table 12-1 ● Commonly Used Medications for Depression

Class	Examples
Selective serotonin reuptake inhibitors (SSRIs)	• Citalopram (Celexa) • Escitalopram (Lexapro) • Fluoxetine (Prozac) • Paroxetine (Paxil, Paxil CR) • Sertraline (Zoloft)
Serotonin and norepinephrine reuptake inhibitors (SNRIs)	• Duloxetine (Cymbalta) • Venlafaxine, extended release (Effexor XR)
Other second-generation antidepressants	• Bupropion XL (Wellbutrin XL) • Mirtazapine (Remeron)

Table 12-2 ● **Commonly Used Medications for Bipolar Disorder**

Class	Examples
Mood stabilizers	• Lithium carbonate (Eskalith, Lithobid, Lithonate, Lithotabs)
Anticonvulsants	• Carbamazepine (Tegretol) • Divalproex sodium (Depakote, Depakote ER) • Gabapentin (Neurontin)

adherence to medication recommendations. Many side effects, such as insomnia, drowsiness, and nausea, subside over 4 to 6 weeks, but sexual side effects (decreased sex drive, lack of orgasm, and delayed ejaculation) are a common reason for discontinuing these medications. These medications work by blocking reuptake of serotonin and/or norepinephrine.

SNRIs, as the name implies, inhibit reuptake of both serotonin and norepinephrine. One such medication, duloxetine (Cymbalta), is also prescribed to relieve the physical pain that commonly occurs with depression. Bupropion (Wellbutrin), an atypical antidepressant, inhibits reuptake of both norepinephrine and dopamine, but may have other actions as well.

Researchers noted that it took several weeks to initiate mood elevation and behavioral changes in patients; therefore, theories developed to explain the delay in the antidepressants' action focus on neurogenesis (formation of new neurons), neurotrophic effects (proteins that help nourish neuronal tissue), neuronal connectivity and plasticity (formation of new synapses), and information processing (Castren, 2004; Perera et al, 2007).

The landmark STAR*D study, which looked at symptom management, found that not all patients initially respond to treatment, but they may with augmentation (the addition or replacement of another antidepressant) (Insel, 2006; Trivedi et al, 2006). Just one-third of patients responded to the first SSRI they received (Phase I). In Phase II, of the 70% who did not respond, another 25% to 30% did respond to a different or additional medication and, in about one-half of cases, supplemental psychotherapy. Most patients typically required 6 to 10 weeks of treatment to reach full remission of symptoms, which was the goal of treatment. Patient use of self-assessment tools may also have been helpful for increasing awareness of symptoms.

Medications for Bipolar Disorder

Lithium carbonate has been considered the gold standard for treatment of bipolar disorder since 1949 (Kandel et al, 2000). Although the precise mechanism is not known, lithium is effective in reducing manic symptoms and in stabilizing moods. Continued use helps prevent recurrence of manic and, to a lesser extent, depressive episodes. Lifelong use is recommended for many individuals, even in the absence of symptoms. Side effects include weight gain, nausea, slowing of cognitive functions, polyuria (passing large amounts of urine), polydipsia (ingesting large amounts of liquids), tremor, and metallic taste.

Anticonvulsants, including Tegretol, Depakote, and Neurontin, are also effective as mood stabilizers and help with reducing psychotic symptoms in acute mania and severe depression (Kandel et al, 2000). These medications may work by reducing neuronal cell membrane excitability and by affecting the γ-aminobutyric acid (GABA) systems. Additional

anticonvulsants and antipsychotics are being studied as possible treatments for mania.

Physicians typically prescribe multiple medications for bipolar disorder to both reduce depressive symptoms and stabilize manic symptoms. This can result in unpredictable side effects, and patient compliance with medication regimens is a problem. Goldberg and colleagues (2007), however, found that use of a mood stabilizer alone was just as effective as a mood stabilizer and an antidepressant, and, in fact, antidepressants may exacerbate existing manic symptoms.

Psychosocial Interventions

The most common forms of psychosocial interventions used currently for treatment of mood disorders are cognitive behavior therapy (CBT) and interpersonal psychotherapy (IPT). Both approaches are highly structured and relatively brief (12–16 weeks). Additional training is needed to understand the theory and techniques associated with these approaches, but occupational therapists are well suited to use these approaches within the context of daily life.

Cognitive Behavioral Therapy

Cognitive behavioral therapy (CBT) is based on work by Aaron Beck, who described depression as being related to distorted beliefs and faulty thinking patterns, which, in turn, affect emotions and behaviors (Beck, 1999). Beck theorized that humans develop schemas, or core beliefs, through early life experiences. CBT centers on uncovering distorted beliefs and faulty thinking patterns, and practicing alternative cognitive and behavior patterns.

(Refer to Chapter 19 for more detailed information about CBT and the role of occupational therapy.)

Interpersonal Psychotherapy

Interpersonal psychotherapy (IPT) is focused on clients' problems in interpersonal and social functioning as a means of symptom relief. The client's social functioning is discussed in relation to four areas:

- Grief and loss (e.g., death, miscarriage)
- Role disputes (e.g., conflicts with spouse or coworker)
- Role transitions (e.g., divorce or becoming a parent)
- Interpersonal deficits (e.g., social and communication skills)

A variant of IPT, called **interpersonal and social rhythm therapy (IPSRT),** has been used successfully for those individuals with bipolar disorder (Frank, 2005). In IPSRT, additional emphasis is placed on developing stable rhythms for daily routines, such as sleeping and eating, and social roles as a parent, spouse, worker, etc. Triggers for rhythm disruption are identified. The emphasis on daily routines is particularly compatible with the domain of concern of occupational therapy. See Chapter 47 for more information on IPSRT.

Other Treatments

Although controversial, **electroconvulsive therapy (ECT)** is an effective treatment for depression that has been used since the 1940s (APA, 2001). Its current use is primarily for individuals with severe depression that does not respond to

Two forms of psychotherapy, cognitive behavior therapy (CBT) and interpersonal psychotherapy (IPT), have well-established bodies of evidence supporting effectiveness in treating depression in adults (Lau, 2008). In a series of studies looking at treatment of people with bipolar disorder, intensive psychotherapy in addition to medication has helped more than medication and brief therapy alone (Morris et al, 2005).

➤ Occupational therapists trained in CBT can help clients increase attention to personally relevant emotional and environmental stimuli that are encoded and retrieved as negative associative memories, and thus serve to trigger stress responses and depressive moods. Helping clients change ineffective thinking patterns that repeatedly reverberate through cortical circuits may help the client reduce maladaptive behaviors that interfere with occupational roles and increase effective behaviors.

➤ Occupational therapists trained in IPT can work with clients on improving social networks, role transitions, interpersonal disputes, social deficits, and maladaptive response to grief.

➤ Occupational therapists trained in IPSRT can help clients stabilize daily routines, wake/sleep cycles, and important relationships.

Lau, M. A. (2008). New developments in psychosocial interventions for adults with unipolar depression. *Current Opinion in Psychiatry, 21*(1), 30–36.

Morris, C. D., Miklowitz, D. J., Wisniewski, S. R., Giese, A. A., Thomas, M. R., & Allen, M. H. (2005). Care satisfaction, hope, and life functioning among adults with bipolar disorder: Data from the first 1000 participants in the Systematic Treatment Enhancement Program. *Comprehensive Psychiatry, 46*(2), 98–104.

other treatments. ECT typically involves 6 to 12 repeated administrations of a low-intensity electrical stimulus to elicit a generalized seizure. Patients are completely anesthetized, and muscle relaxants prevent excessive limb movement. The treatment is used most frequently in patients with severe treatment-refractive depression, depression with psychotic features, and patients who are suicidal. ECT is highly effective in elevating mood, and its effects have a more rapid onset than antidepressant medications. A number of patients experience cognitive side effects initially following ECT. These include impairments in attention, orientation, concentration, and memory. Other side effects include mild headache, nausea, and vomiting. The majority of patients report improved long-term cognitive function, however.

The precise therapeutic mechanism of ECT is not well known; however, neurogenesis, or creation of new neurons, in the hippocampus has been noted following ECT. Therefore, enhanced connectivity of brain circuits may be one result of the repeated procedure (Perera et al, 2007).

Summary

The prevalence and disabling effects of mood disorders result in a serious public health concern. However, both medications and psychosocial interventions have demonstrated efficacy for mood disorders. Occupational therapists can play a larger role in the prevention and treatment of mood disorders by providing intervention strategies that help people engage or re-engage in meaningful occupations.

Active Learning Strategies

1. Self-Reflection

Most of us have experienced some symptoms of depression, elation, or even mania at some points in our lives. Reflect on a particularly difficult time in your life. What were your emotions like? Did you have difficulty regulating your emotions, feeling tearful, etc? Were you irritable? What strategies did you try to handle your emotions?

Reflective Questions

● What was your cognitive processing like? Did you have difficulty concentrating or making decisions? Did your mind seem to race, or were your thoughts sluggish and slow?
● Were you able to enjoy your typical activities, or was it difficult to feel pleasure and joy in life?
● What seemed to help lift your mood? Being around people? Scheduling some activities to get your mind focused on something else?
● What were your daily habits like? Did you have regular sleeping patterns? Eating patterns? Exercise? Drug/alcohol use? What did it feel like if you were off your typical pattern?
● Medications often take several weeks before even beginning to have an effect, and 4 to 6 weeks for substantial symptom relief. Think of a time you had to wait weeks for something you really wanted. How did you feel? How did you cope?

 Describe your thoughts in your **Reflective Journal**.

2. Ordinary People

Read the novel *Ordinary People* (Guest, 1976) and/or watch the movie by the same name. This story describes a family struggling to return to ordinary life following the accidental death of their son, Buck, and the suicide attempt of his brother, Conrad.

● Conrad is depicted as having self-absorption, chronic agitation, and numbness, or lack of feeling. He isolates himself from family and friends. How different are these behaviors from typical teens? How might these symptoms affect Conrad's typical occupational roles? What additional symptoms might parents look for in teens they suspect of having depression?
● Conrad's family frowns on public displays of emotion, but his psychiatrist points out, "People who keep stiff upper lips find that it's damn hard to smile." How might this excessive self-control impact Conrad's ability to recover from the guilt and anger he feels over his brother's death? What role could CBT play in Conrad's recovery?

Resources

Organizations

- American Academy of Family Physicians: http://familydoctor.org
- American Psychiatric Association (APA): www.psych.org
- Centers for Disease Control and Prevention, Suicide Prevention: http://www.cdc.gov/ViolencePrevention/suicide/index.html
- Depression and Bipolar Support Alliance (DBSA): www.dbsalliance.org, 1-800-826-3632
- Mental Health America (formerly National Mental Health Association): www.nmha.org
- The MoodGYM Training Program: www.moodgym.anu.edu.au
- National Alliance on Mental Illness (NAMI): www.nami.org, 1-800-950-6264
- National Institute of Mental Health (NIMH): www.nimh.nih.gov, 1-800-969-6642
- American Foundation for Suicide Prevention (AFSP): www.afsp.org
- Substance Abuse and Mental Health Services Administration (SAMHSA): www.samhsa.gov

References

Adinoff, B., Iranmanesh, A., Veldhuis, J., & Fisher, L. (1998). Disturbances of the stress response: The role of the HPA axis during alcohol withdrawal and abstinence. *Alcohol Health and Research World, 22*(1), 67–72.

American Psychiatric Association (APA). (2000). *Diagnostic and Statistical Manual of Mental Disorders* (4th ed., text revision). Washington, DC: Author.

American Psychiatric Association (APA). (2001). *The Practice of Electroconvulsive Therapy: Recommendations for Treatment, Training and Privileging (A Task Force Report on Electroconvulsive Therapy)* (2nd ed.). Washington, DC: Author.

Angst, J., Angst, F., & Stassen, H. H. (1999). Suicide risk in patients with major depressive disorder. *Journal of Clinical Psychiatry, 60*(suppl 2), 57–62; discussion 75–56, 113–116.

Ashman, S. B., Dawson, G., & Panagiotides, H. (2008). Trajectory of maternal depression over 7 years: Relations with child psychophysiology and behavior and role of contextual risks. *Developmental Psychopathology, 29*, 55–77.

Beck, A. T. (1999). Beyond belief: A theory of modes, personality, and psychopathology. In D. A. Clark & A. T. Beck (Eds.), *Scientific Foundations of Cognitive Theory and Therapy of Depression* (pp. 1–25). New York: Wiley & Sons.

Bhatia, S. K., & Bhatia, S. C. (2007). Child and adolescent depression. *American Family Physician, 75*, 73–80.

Bilsker, D., Gilbert, M., Myette, T. L., & Stewart-Patterson, C. (2004). *Depression and Work Function: Bridging the Gap Between Mental Health Care and the Workplace.* Mental Health Evaluation and Consultation Unit, Vancouver, BC: University of British Columbia.

Blazer, D., Kessler, R., McGonagle, K., & Swartz, M. (1994). The prevalence and distribution of major depression in a national community sample: The National Comorbidity Survey. *American Journal of Psychiatry, 151*, 979–986.

Bould, S. (2005). A population health perspective on disability and depression in elderly women and men. *Journal of Aging and Social Policy, 17*, 7–24.

Brown, G. W., & Moran, P. M. (1997). Single mothers, poverty and depression. *Psychological Medicine, 27*(1), 21–33.

Buchwald, A. (2006). *Too Soon to Say Goodbye.* New York: Random House.

Carnethon, M. R., Biggs, M. L., Barzilay, J. I., Smith, N. L., Vaccarino, V., Bertoni, A. G., Arnold, A., & Siscovich, D. (2007). Longitudinal association between depressive symptoms and incident type 2 diabetes mellitus in older adults: The cardiovascular health study. *Archives of Internal Medicine, 167*(8), 802–807.

Caspi, A., Sugden, K., Moffitt, T. E., Taylor, A., Craig, I. W., Harrington, H., McClay, J., Mill, J., Martin, J., Braithwaite, A., & Poulton, R. (2003). Influence of life stress on depression: Moderation by a polymorphism in the 5-HTT gene. *Science, 301*(5631), 386–389.

Castren, E. (2004). Neurotrophic effects of antidepressant drugs. *Current Opinion in Pharmacology, 4(1)*, 58–64.

Christiansen, C., & Baum, C. (Eds.). (1997). *Occupational Therapy: Enabling Function and Well-Being* (2nd ed.). Thorofare, NJ: Slack.

Compton, M. T., & Nemeroff, C. B. (2006). Depression and bipolar disorder (electronic version). *ACP Medicine.* Available at: http://www.acpmedicine.com/bcdecker/newrxdx/rxdx/dxrx1302.htm (accessed February 1, 2010).

Craddock, N., & Jones, I. (2001). Molecular genetics of bipolar disorder. *British Journal of Psychiatry, 41*(suppl), S128–S133.

Cruz, M., Pincus, H. A., Harman, J. S., Reynolds, D. F., & Post, E. P. (2008). Barriers to care-seeking for depressed African Americans. *International Journal of Psychiatry in Medicine, 38*, 71–80.

Druss, B. G., Rosenheck, R. A., Desai, M. M., & Perlin, J. B. (2002). Quality of preventive medical care for patients with mental disorders. *Medical Care, 40*(2), 129–136.

Esdaile, S. A., & Olson, J. A. (2004). Mothering Occupations: Challenge, Agency and Participation. Philadelphia: F A Davis Co.

Field, T., Diego, M., & Hernandez-Reif, M. (2006). Prenatal depression effects on the fetus and newborn: A review. *Infant Behavior Development, 29*(3), 445–455.

Frank, E. (2005). *Treating Bipolar Disorder: A Clinician's Guide to Interpersonal and Social Rhythm Therapy.* New York: Guilford Press.

Fuchs, E., Czeh, B., Koke, M. H., Michaelis, T., & Lucassen, P. J. (2004). Alterations of neuroplasticity in depression: The hippocampus and beyond. *European Neuropsychopharmacology: The Journal of the European College of Neuropsychopharmacology, 14*(suppl 5), S481–S490.

Goes, F. S., Sadler, B., Toolan, J., Zamoiski, R. D., Mondimore, F. M., Mackinnon, D. F., & Schweizer, B.; Bipolar Disorder Phenome Group, Raymond Depaulo, J., Jr., & Potash, J. B. (2007). Psychotic features in bipolar and unipolar depression. *Bipolar Disorders, 9*(8), 901–906.

Goldberg, J. F., Perlis, R. H., Ghaemi, S. N., Calabrese, J. R., Bowden, C. L., Wisniewski, S., Miklowitz, D. J., Sachs, G. S., & Thase, M. E. (2007). Adjunctive antidepressant use and symptomatic recovery among bipolar depressed patients with concomitant manic symptoms: Findings from the STEP-BD. *American Journal of Psychiatry, 164*(9), 1348–1355.

Gonzalez, J. M., Perlick, D. A., Miklowitz, D. J., Kaczynski, R., Hernandez, M., Rosenheck, R. A., Culver, J. L., Ostacher, M. J., & Bowden, C. L. (2007). Factors associated with stigma among caregivers of patients with bipolar disorder in the STEP-BD study. *Psychiatric Services (Washington, DC), 58*(1), 41–48.

Guest, J. (1976). *Ordinary People.* New York: Penguin Books.

Hariri, A. R., Drabant, E. M., Munoz, K. E., Kolachana, B. S., Mattay, V. S., Egan, M. F., & Weinberger, D. R. (2005). A susceptibility gene for affective disorders and the response of the human amygdala. *Archives of General Psychiatry, 62*(2), 146–152.

Hirschfeld, R. M., Calabrese, J. R., Weissman, M. M., Reed, M., Davies, M. A., Frye, M. A., Keck, P. E. Jr., Lewis, L., McElroy, S. L., McNulty, J. P., & Wagner, K. D. (2003). Screening for bipolar disorder in the community. *Journal of Clinical Psychiatry, 64*(1), 53–59.

Hirschfeld, R. M., Lewis, L., & Vornik, L. A. (2003). Perceptions and impact of bipolar disorder: How far have we really come? Results of the national depressive and manic-depressive association 2000 survey of individuals with bipolar disorder. *Journal of Clinical Psychiatry, 64*(2), 161–174.

Hwang, W. C., & Wood, J. J. (2009). Acculturative family distancing: Links with self reported symptomatology among Asian Americans and Latinos. *Child Psychiatry and Human Development, 40*, 123–138.

Insel, T. R. (2006). Beyond efficacy: The STAR*D trial. *American Journal of Psychiatry, 163*(1), 5–7.

Kandel, E. R., Schwartz, J. H., & Jessell, T. M. (2000). *Principles of Neural Science* (4th ed.). New York: McGraw-Hill.

Kanter, J. W., Rusch, L. C., & Brondino, M. J. (2008). Depression self stigma: A new measure and preliminary findings. *Journal of Nervous and Mental Disease, 196,* 663–670.

Kessler, R. C., Akiskal, H. S., Ames, M., Birnbaum, H., Greenberg, P., Hirschfeld, R. M., Jin, R., Merikangas, K. R., Simon, G. E., & Wang, P. S. (2006). Prevalence and effects of mood disorders on work performance in a nationally representative sample of U.S. workers. *American Journal of Psychiatry, 163*(9), 1561–1568.

Kessler, R. C., Berglund, P., Demler, O., Jin, R., Koretz, D., Merikangas, K. R., et al. (2003). The epidemiology of major depressive disorder: Results from the National Comorbidity Survey Replication (NCS-R). *Journal of the American Medical Association, 289*(23), 3095–3105.

Lau, M. A. (2008). New developments in psychosocial interventions for adults with unipolar depression. *Current Opinion in Psychiatry, 21*(1), 30–36.

Mann, J. J. (2005). The medical management of depression. *New England Journal of Medicine, 353*(17), 1819–1834.

March, J., Silva, S., Petrycki, S., Curry, J., Wells, K., Fairbank, J., Burns, B., Domino, M., McNulty, S., Vitiello, B., & Severe, J. (2004). Fluoxetine, cognitive-behavioral therapy, and their combination for adolescents with depression: Treatment for Adolescents with Depression Study (TADS) randomized controlled trial. *Journal of the American Medical Association, 292*(7), 807–820.

Merikangas, K. R., Akiskal, H. S., Angst, J., Greenberg, P. E., Hirschfeld, R. M., Petukhova, M., & Kessler, R.C. (2007). Lifetime and 12-month prevalence of bipolar spectrum disorder in the National Comorbidity Survey Replication. *Archives of General Psychiatry, 64*(5), 543–552.

Merikangas, K. R., Mehta, R. L., Molnar, B. E., Walters, E. E., Swendsen, J. D., Aguilar-Gaziola, S., Bijl, R., Borges, G., Caraveo-Anduaga, J. J., Dewit, D. J., Koloday, B., Vega, W. A., Wittchen, H. U., & Kessler, R. C. (1998). Co-morbidity of substance use disorders with mood and anxiety disorders: Results of the International Consortium in Psychiatric Epidemiology. *Addictive Behaviors, 23,* 893–907.

Miranda, J., & Green, B. L. (1999). The need for mental health services research focusing on poor young women. *Journal of Mental Health Policy and Economics, 2*(2), 73–80.

Moreno, C., Laje, G., Blanco, C., Jiang, H., Schmidt, A. B., & Olfson, M. (2007). National trends in the outpatient diagnosis and treatment of bipolar disorder in youth. *Archives of General Psychiatry, 64*(9), 1032–1039.

Morris, C. D., Miklowitz, D. J., Wisniewski, S. R., Giese, A. A., Thomas, M. R., & Allen, M. H. (2005). Care satisfaction, hope, and life functioning among adults with bipolar disorder: Data from the first 1000 participants in the Systematic Treatment Enhancement Program. *Comprehensive Psychiatry, 46*(2), 98–104.

Murray, C. J., & Lopez, A. D. (1997). Alternative projections of mortality and disability by cause 1990–2020: Global Burden of Disease study. *Lancet, 349*(9064), 1498–1504.

National Institutes of Mental Health (NIMH). (2003). "Older Adults and Mental Health." Available at: http://www.nimh.nih.gov/health/topics/older-adults-and-mental-health/index.shtml (accessed November 3, 2009).

Nestler, E. J., Barrot, M., DiLeone, R. J., Eisch, A. J., Gold, S. J., & Montegggia, L. M. (2002). Neurobiology of depression. *Neuron, 34,* 13–25.

Pariante, C. M., & Miller, A. H. (2001). Glucocorticoid receptors in major depression: Relevance to pathophysiology and treatment. *Biological Psychiatry, 49*(5), 391–404.

Perera, T. D., Coplan, J. D., Lisanby, S. H., Lipira, C. M., Arif, M., Carpio, C., Spitzer, G., Santarelli, L., Scharf, B., Hen, R., Rosoklija, G., Sackeim, H. A,. & Dwork, A. J. (2007). Antidepressant-induced neurogenesis in the hippocampus of adult nonhuman primates. *Journal of Neuroscience, 27*(18), 4894–4901.

Perlis, R. H., Miyahara, S., Marangell, L. B., Wisneiewski, S. R., Ostacher, M., DelBello, M. P., Bowden, C. L., Sadis, G. S., & Nierenberg, A. A. (2004). Long-term implication of early onset in bipolar disorder: Data from the first 1000 participants in the Systematic Treatment Enhancement Program for Bipolar Disorder (STEP-BD). *Biological Psychiatry, 55*(9), 875–881.

Perry, A., Tarrier, N., Morriss, R., McCarthy, E., & Limb, K. (1999). Randomised controlled trial of efficacy of teaching patients with bipolar disorder to identify early symptoms of relapse and obtain treatment. *British Medical Journal, 318,* 149–153.

Pincus, H. A., & Pettit, A. R. (2001). The societal costs of chronic major depression. *Journal of Clinical Psychiatry, 62*(suppl 6), 5–9.

Regier, D. A., Narrow, W. E., Rae, D. S., Manderscheid, R. W., Locke, B. Z., & Goodwin, F. K. (1993). The de facto mental and addictive disorders service system: Epidemiologic catchment area prospective 1-year prevalence rates of disorders and services. *Archives of General Psychiatry, 50*(2), 85–94.

Robinson, O. J., & Sahakian, B. J. (2008). Recurrence in major depressive disorder: A neurocognitive perspective. *Psychological Medicine, 38,* 315–318.

Rosa, A. R., Frey, B. N., Andreazza, A. C., Cereser, K. M., Cunha, A. B., Quevedo, J., Santin, A., Gottfried, C., Goncalves, C. A., Vieta, E., & Kapczinski, F. (2006). Increased serum glial cell line-derived neurotrophic factor immunocontent during manic and depressive episodes in individuals with bipolar disorder. *Neuroscience Letters, 407*(2), 146–150.

Rutter, M. (2006). Implications of resilience concepts for scientific understanding. *Annals of the New York Academy of Sciences, 1094,* 1–12.

Schatzberg, A. F. (2004). The relationship of chronic pain and depression. *Journal of Clinical Psychiatry, 65*(suppl 12), 3–4.

Seligman, M. E. (1991). *Learned Optimism.* New York: Alfred A. Knopf.

Shumake, J., & Gonzalez-Lima, F. (2003). Brain systems underlying susceptibility to helplessness and depression. *Behavioral and Cognitive Neuroscience Reviews, 2*(3), 198–221.

Stewart, W. F., Ricci, J. A., Chee, E., Hahn, S. R., & Morganstein, D. (2003). Cost of lost productive work time among US workers with depression. *Journal of the American Medical Association, 289*(23), 3135–3144.

Trivedi, M. H., Fava, M., Wisniewski, S. R., Thase, M. E., Quitkin, F., Warden, D., Ritz, L., Nierenberg, A. A., Lebowitz, B. D., Biggs, M. M., Luther, J. F., Shores-Wilson, K., & Rusha, J. (2006). Medication augmentation after the failure of SSRIs for depression. *New England Journal of Medicine, 354*(12), 1243–1252.

Tronick, E. Z. (1989). Emotions and emotional communication in infants. *American Psychologist, 44,* 112–119.

U.S. Department of Health and Human Services. (1999). "Mental Health: A Report of the Surgeon General." Available at: www.surgeongeneral.gov/library/mentalhealth/home.html (accessed November 3, 2009).

Warden, D., Rush, A. J., Wisniewski, S. R., Lesser, I. M., Kornstein, S. G., Balasubramani, G. K., Thase, M. E., Preskorn, S. H., Nierenberg, A. A., Young, E. Q., Shores-Wilson, K., & Trivedi, M. H. (2008). What predicts attrition in second step medication treatments for depression?: A STAR*D report. *International Journal of Neuropsychopharmacology, 9,* 1–15.

World Health Organization. (2002). *The World Health Report 2002: Reducing Risks, Promoting Healthy Life.* Geneva: Author.

Zeanah, C. H., Jr. (Ed.). (2000). *Handbook of Infant Mental Health* (2nd ed.). New York: Guilford Press.

Anxiety Disorders

Janis Davis

> "Neither comprehension nor learning can take place in an atmosphere of anxiety.
>
> —Rose Kennedy

Introduction

Anxiety disorders are the most common of all psychiatric disorders, affecting approximately 40 million adults or 18% of people in the United States aged 18 and older in a given year (National Institute of Mental Health [NIMH], 2006; World Health Organization [WHO], 2001). And like most psychiatric disorders, anxiety has been part of the human condition since the beginning of recorded history. Footage from the early 1900s reveals the scurry of people on an unpaved city street (Markowitz, 1998). On the film, the announcer explained that, in the midst of new inventions and emerging modern conveniences, people complained that life was moving too fast, and physicians lamented that the stress of modern life was causing a constellation of symptoms, such as insomnia, headaches, exhaustion, and anxiety (Markowitz, 1998).

Despite, or possibly because of, modern conveniences, technology, and daily life in the 21st century, anxiety is still part of the personal experience for millions of people worldwide (WHO, 2001). One recent study reported that 47% of visits to a family physician in the United States involve an emotional component, and 11% of visits were prompted by anxiety or nervousness (Kerr, 2003). A fear response is essential to human survival; it moves us to action. For example, a beeping horn causes you to move out of the way of oncoming traffic, or anxiety about an upcoming test compels you to study. Although evolution naturally selects the anxious gene, a prolonged state of anxiety is maladaptive to the human organism.

Regardless of the setting, occupational therapists will frequently work with people who experience anxiety. In some cases, the individual will meet the criteria for an anxiety disorder, but in other situations the individual may be experiencing situational anxiety associated with a distressing situation. Consequently, it is important for occupational therapists to understand anxiety disorders, the stress response, how anxiety affects occupational performance, and intervention approaches to address anxiety.

Description of the Disorder

It is normal for an individual to be slightly anxious before an important job interview, but it is not normal to experience an overwhelming and prolonged state of fear that interferes with daily functioning. The common characteristic of anxiety disorders is the inappropriate expression of fear (Bear, Connors, & Paradiso, 2001). **Anxiety** can range from relatively mild feelings of uneasiness to immobilizing terror. As an adaptive response to threatening or harmful stimuli, anxiety results in the defensive symptoms of hyperarousal, as well as increased autonomic responses, such as increased heart rate, blood pressure, and respiration (Takahashi, 2002). The physiological response rapidly yields to a protective behavioral reaction commonly known as the "fight, flight, or freeze" response. Anxiety becomes pathological when this protective behavioral response is prolonged and inappropriate to the actual threat level of the environment, compromising the individual's ability to function. If left untreated, anxiety disorders can develop into serious medical illnesses that can become chronic and severe.

There are several types of anxiety disorders, each with its own set of etiologies, symptoms, course, and prognosis. These include

- Panic disorder
- Agoraphobia
- Generalized anxiety disorder
- Obsessive-compulsive disorder
- Posttraumatic stress disorder
- Social phobia
- Specific phobia
- Substance-induced anxiety disorder
- Anxiety disorder due to a general medical condition

DSM-IV-TR Criteria

Anxiety disorders include the nine discrete disorders listed previously, all of which are characterized by fear. Some anxiety disorders go hand in hand, such as panic disorder and agoraphobia.

Panic Attack and Panic Disorder

In the DSM-IV-TR (APA, 2000), **panic disorder** is the diagnosis, but **panic attack** describes the specific symptoms that have to occur. Panic disorder requires that an individual experience recurring panic attacks; however, panic attacks may not develop into a disorder if they occur infrequently. The detailed DSM-IV-TR (APA, 2000) diagnostic criteria for panic attack are listed in Box 13-1.

BOX 13-1 ▧ DSM-IV-TR Criteria for Panic Attack and Panic Disorder

Panic Attack

A panic attack is defined as a discrete period of intense fear or discomfort, in which four (or more) of the following symptoms developed abruptly and reached a peak within 10 minutes:

1. Palpitations, pounding heart, or accelerated heart rate
2. Sweating
3. Trembling or shaking
4. Sensations or shortness of breath or smothering
5. Feeling of choking
6. Chest pain or discomfort
7. Nausea or abdominal distress
8. Feeling dizzy, unsteady, lightheaded, or faint
9. Derealization (feelings of unreality) or depersonalization (being detached from oneself)
10. Fear of losing control or going crazy
11. Fear of dying
12. Paresthesias (numbness or tingling sensation)
13. Chills or hot flashes

Note: A panic attack is not the disorder.

Panic Disorder

A. Both (1) and (2):
   a. Recurrent, unexpected panic attacks
   b. At least one of the attacks has been followed by 1 month (or more) of one (or more) of the following:
      i. Persistent concern about having additional attacks
      ii. Worry about the implications of the attack or its consequences (e.g., losing control, having a heart attack, "going crazy")
      iii. A significant change in behavior related to the attacks

   Panic disorder is further specified as with or without agoraphobia, depending on whether the individual meets the criteria for agoraphobia.

From American Psychiatric Association. (2000). *Diagnostic and Statistical Manual of Mental Disorders* (4th ed.). Washington, DC: Author.

BOX 13-2 ▧ DSM-IV-TR Criteria for Agoraphobia

A. Anxiety about being in places or situations from which escape might be difficult (or embarrassing), or in which help may not be available in the event of having an unexpected or situationally predisposed panic attack or paniclike symptoms. Agoraphobic fears typically involve characteristic clusters of situations that include being outside the home alone; being in a crowd or standing in a line; being on a bridge; and traveling in a bus, train, or automobile.

B. The situations are avoided (e.g., travel is restricted) or else are endured with marked distress or anxiety about having a panic attack or paniclike symptoms, or require the presence of companion.

Note: Agoraphobia is not a diagnosis, but is used as a specifier for panic disorder when it accompanies the condition.

From American Psychiatric Association. (2000). *Diagnostic and Statistical Manual of Mental Disorders* (4th ed.). Washington, DC: Author.

BOX 13-3 ▧ DSM-IV-TR Criteria for Generalized Anxiety Disorder

A. Excessive anxiety and worry (apprehensive expectation), occurring more days than not for at least 6 months, concerning a number of events or activities (e.g., work or school performance).

B. The person finds it difficult to control the worry.

C. The anxiety and worry are associated with three (or more) of the following six symptoms (with at least some symptoms present for more days than not for the past 6 months). *Note:* Only one item is required in children.
   a. Restlessness or feeling keyed up or on edge
   b. Being easily fatigued
   c. Difficulty concentrating or mind going blank
   d. Irritability
   e. Muscle tension
   f. Sleep disturbance (difficulty falling or staying asleep, or restless unsatisfying sleep)

D. The focus of the anxiety and worry is not confined to features of an Axis I disorder.

E. The anxiety, worry, or physical symptoms cause clinically significant distress or impairment in social, occupational, or other important areas of functioning.

From American Psychiatric Association. (2000). *Diagnostic and Statistical Manual of Mental Disorders* (4th ed.). Washington, DC: Author.

Agoraphobia

Panic attacks are commonly associated with **agoraphobia,** which is literally translated from Greek as "fear of the marketplace." Agoraphobia is often mistaken for fear of open spaces or crowds, but it has more to do with the fear of having a panic attack in public and the resulting humiliation and dependence that the attack may cause. The detailed DSM-IV-TR (APA, 2000) diagnostic criteria for agoraphobia are listed in Box 13-2.

Generalized Anxiety Disorder

Generalized anxiety disorder (GAD) is manifested by persistent and excessive worrying about many developmental life tasks. Persons with GAD may worry about job performance, money, partnerships, or health, for example. The detailed DSM-IV-TR (APA, 2000) diagnostic criteria for GAD are listed in Box 13-3.

Obsessive-Compulsive Disorder

Obsessive-compulsive disorder (OCD) is another anxiety disorder that can lead to suffering and impairment. With this disorder, an individual may fear, for example, that he or she is "losing his or her mind," his or her child is in danger, or his or her house will burn down. These thoughts can lead to compulsive checking behaviors, such as returning to check the stove several times before leaving the house. The detailed DSM-IV-TR (APA, 2000) diagnostic criteria for OCD are listed in Box 13-4.

Posttraumatic Stress Disorder

Posttraumatic stress disorder (PTSD) is unique among anxiety disorders due to its association with a terrifying or life-threatening event. Impairment is often the result of re-experiencing the event either in dreams or flashbacks, or avoidance of specific places or situations. For example, children from a war zone who live in a refugee camp may dream of ambulance sirens and roaring tanks, and avoid loud places in their environment. The detailed DSM-IV-TR (APA, 2000) diagnostic criteria for PTSD are listed in Box 13-5.

Social Phobia

Social phobia is different from PTSD, yet it also involves avoidance behaviors. For example, an individual may be extremely fearful of talking with strangers, eating alone in a restaurant, or speaking in public. The detailed DSM-IV-TR (APA, 2000) diagnostic criteria for social phobia are listed in Box 13-6.

Specific Phobia

An individual who is excessively afraid or persistently worries about a specific situation, natural event, or object may

---

BOX 13-4 ■ DSM-IV-TR Criteria for Obsessive-Compulsive Disorder

A. Either obsessions or compulsions:

Obsessions as defined by (1), (2), (3), and (4):

a. Recurrent and persistent thoughts, impulses, or images that are experienced, at some time during the disturbance, as intrusive and inappropriate and that cause marked anxiety or distress

b. The thoughts, impulses, or images are not simply excessive worries about real life problems

c. The person attempts to ignore or suppress such thoughts, impulses, or images, or to neutralize them with some other thought or action

d. The person recognizes that the obsessional thoughts, impulses, or images are a product of his or her own mind (not imposed from without as in thought insertion)

Compulsions as defined by (1) and (2):

a. Repetitive behaviors (e.g., hand washing, ordering, checking) or mental acts (e.g., praying, counting, repeating words silently) that the person feels driven to perform in response to an obsession, or according to rules that must be applied rigidly.

b. The behaviors or mental acts are aimed at preventing or reducing distress, or preventing some dreaded event or situation; however, these behaviors or mental acts either are not connected in a realistic way with what they are designed to neutralize or prevent or are clearly excessive.

B. At some point during the course of the disorder, the person has recognized that the obsessions or compulsions are excessive or unreasonable. *Note:* This does not apply to children.

C. The obsessions or compulsions cause marked distress, are time consuming (take more than 1 hour a day), or significantly interfere with the person's normal routine, occupational (or academic) functioning, or usual social activities or relationships.

Specify if:

With Poor Insight: if, for most of the time during the current episode, the person does not recognize that the obsessions and compulsions are excessive or unreasonable.

From American Psychiatric Association. (2000). *Diagnostic and Statistical Manual of Mental Disorders* (4th ed.). Washington, DC: Author.

BOX 13-5 ■ DSM-IV-TR Criteria for 309.81 Posttraumatic Stress Disorder

A. The person has been exposed to a traumatic event in which both of the following were present:

i. The person experienced, witnessed, or was confronted with an event or events that involved actual or threatened death or serious injury, or a threat to the physical integrity of self or others.

ii. The person's response involved intense fear, helplessness, or horror. *Note:* In children, this may be expressed instead by disorganized agitated behavior.

B. The traumatic event is persistently reexperienced in one (or more) of the following ways:

i. Recurrent and intrusive distressing recollections of the event, including images, thoughts, or perceptions. *Note:* In young children, repetitive play may occur in which themes or aspects of the trauma are expressed.

ii. Recurrent distressing dreams of the event. *Note:* In children, there may be frightening dreams without recognizable content.

iii. Acting or feeling as if the traumatic event were recurring (includes a sense of reliving the experience, illusions, hallucinations, and dissociative flashbacks episodes, including those that occur on awakening or when intoxicated). *Note:* In young children, trauma-specific reenactment may occur.

iv. Intense psychological distress at exposure to internal or external cues that symbolize or resemble an aspect of the traumatic event.

v. Physiological reactivity on exposure to internal or external cues that symbolize or resemble an aspect of the traumatic event.

C. Persistent avoidance of stimuli associated with the trauma and numbing of general responsiveness (not present before the trauma), as indicated by three (or more) of the following:

i. Efforts to avoid thoughts, feelings, or conversations associated with the trauma

ii. Efforts to avoid activities, places, or people that arouse recollections of the trauma

iii. Inability to recall an important aspect of the trauma

iv. Markedly diminished interest or participation in significant activities

v. Feeling of detachment or estrangement from others

vi. Restricted range of affect (e.g., unable to have loving feelings)

vii. Sense of foreshortened future (e.g., does not expect to have a career, marriage, children, a normal life span).

D. Persistent symptoms of increased arousal (not present before the trauma), as indicated by two (or more) of the following:

i. Difficulty falling or staying asleep

ii. Irritability or outbursts of anger

iii. Difficulty concentrating

iv. Hypervigilance

v. Exaggerated startle response

E. Duration of the disturbance (symptoms in Criteria B, C, and D) is more than 1 month.

F. The disturbance causes clinically significant distress or impairment in social, occupational, or other important areas of functioning.

From American Psychiatric Association. (2000). *Diagnostic and Statistical Manual of Mental Disorders* (4th ed.). Washington, DC: Author.

BOX 13-6 ■ DSM-IV-TR Criteria for Social Phobia

A. A marked and persistent fear of one or more social or performance situations in which the person is exposed to unfamiliar people or to possible scrutiny by others. The individual fears that he or she will act in a way (or show anxiety symptoms) that will be humiliating or embarrassing. *Note:* In children, there must be evidence of the capacity for age-appropriate social relationships with familiar people, and the anxiety must occur in peer settings, not just in interactions with adults.

B. Exposure to the feared social situation almost invariably provokes anxiety, which may take the form of a situationally bound or situationally predisposed panic attack. *Note:* In children, the anxiety may be expressed by crying, tantrums, freezing, or shrinking from social situations with unfamiliar people.

C. The person recognizes that the fear is excessive or unreasonable. *Note:* In children, this feature may be absent.

D. The feared social or performance situations are avoided or are endured with intense anxiety or distress.

E. The avoidance, anxious anticipation, or distress in the feared social or performance situation(s) interferes significantly with the person's normal routine, occupational (academic) functioning, or social activities or relationships, or there is marked distress about having the phobia.

F. In individuals younger than 18 years, the duration is at least 6 months.

From American Psychiatric Association. (2000). *Diagnostic and Statistical Manual of Mental Disorders* (4th ed.). Washington, DC: Author.

BOX 13-7 ■ DSM-IV-TR Criteria for Specific Phobia

A. Marked and persistent fear that is excessive or unreasonable, cued by the presence or anticipation of a specific object or situation (e.g., flying, heights, animals, receiving an injection, seeing blood).

B. Exposure to the phobic stimulus almost invariably provokes an immediate anxiety response, which may take the form of a situationally bound or situationally predisposed panic attack. *Note:* In children, the anxiety may be expressed by crying, tantrums, freezing, or clinging.

C. The person recognizes that the fear is excessive or unreasonable. *Note:* In children, this feature may be absent.

D. The phobic situation(s) is avoided or is endured with intense anxiety or distress.

E. The avoidance, anxious anticipation, or distress in the feared situation(s) interferes significantly with the person's normal routine, occupational (or academic) functioning, or social activities or relationships, or there is marked distress about having the phobia.

F. In individuals younger than 18 years, the duration is at least 6 months.

From American Psychiatric Association. (2000). *Diagnostic and Statistical Manual of Mental Disorders* (4th ed.). Washington, DC: Author.

be diagnosed with specific phobia. As with other anxiety disorders, the individual may suffer a great deal if, for example, they are afraid of flying, storms, or certain animals. The detailed DSM-IV-TR (APA, 2000) diagnostic criteria for specific phobia are listed in Box 13-7.

Etiology

Because anxiety disorders are heterogeneous, the etiologies of the different types of anxiety disorders differ. An understanding of the stress response and its underlying physiological, neuroanatomical, and neurochemical mechanisms is key. Studies in animals and humans reveal genetic, structural and functional neuroanatomical, neurotransmitter, cognitive and psychological, and environmental factors as causes of anxiety (NIMH, 2006).

Stress

Anxiety cannot be understood without an appreciation for the stress response and the underlying physiological, neuroanatomical, and neurochemical mechanisms that are activated when an individual perceives threat. Hans Selye developed the concept of the stress response in the 1950s (Pinel, 2005). As Selye observed human reactions to threat or insult, he noticed similar physiological sequelae, which he termed the **general adaptation syndrome**.

Selye noticed that the physiological response followed logical stages:

1. The central nervous system (CNS) is aroused, and the fight-or-flight mechanism begins to defend against noxious stimuli.

2. A stage of adaptation mobilizes major muscles, respiration, and the senses in order to fight or flee.

3. The third and final stage is one of exhaustion, marked by compensatory mechanisms that interfere with homeostasis (McCance & Huether, 2002).

Selye speculated that the stage of exhaustion was responsible for the onset of diseases he termed **diseases of adaptation**. When the organism remains in a state of fight or flight for too long and does not return to homeostasis, the physiological responses of the sympathetic branch of the CNS will ultimately lead to anxiety disorders or, even worse, impairment of the immune response and even organ and heart failure (McCance & Huether, 2002).

Genetic Factors

Twin studies provide evidence for a strong genetic component in anxiety disorders and comorbidity rates of anxiety, depression, and eating disorders (Silberg & Bulik, 2005; van Beijsterveldt, Verhulst, Molenaar, & Boomsma, 2004). In addition, genes appear to influence the organism's ability to cope with stress and anxiety, and account for variations in coping styles (Kozak, Strelau, & Miles, 2005). van Beijsterveldt and colleagues (2004) found that 43% to 53% of the variance of anxiety problems in twins were explained by genetic factors, and 19% to 28% of variance was accounted for by shared environmental factors.

This twin study investigated the genetic contribution to variation in coping with stressful situations and identified four coping styles: task oriented, emotion oriented, social diversion, and distraction. Evidence was found for genetic variance; however, no single genetic factor was shared by all coping styles (van Beijsterveldt et al, 2004).

There is also evidence for a genetic component for specific anxiety disorders. For example, with panic disorder,

The Lived Experience

Susan

Susan Giles is a 32-year-old mother of two. After moving to a suburb of Chicago with her husband for his new job, her world began to crumble. In her own words, Susan tells her story of struggling with overwhelming panic in the midst of a perfect life.

I had everything—a loving husband, two beautiful children, a beautiful home near Chicago, wonderfully fun friends, and a thriving social life. Then one day I remember standing at my sink looking out the window. I felt a tingling in my legs. I don't remember why, but I moved into a small bathroom off the kitchen, closed the door, and held my head. I thought I was going crazy. I literally felt I was losing my mind. I felt nauseous and disoriented. After that episode, I started having a strange feeling about the world. It appeared grey and devoid of colors and light. I would sit on the rocking chair on my front porch and stare at my little 4-year-old playing in the yard. I had no desire to leave my house for fear I would lose my mind in the middle of the grocery store or while talking to other mothers at my children's preschool. Later, I learned the word for what I was experiencing: agoraphobia.

A friend recommended a psychiatrist who diagnosed me with panic attacks. After talking with him, I realized that I had always had some anxiety. As a child, I had frequent stomachaches at school. Once, during a Halloween parade when I was around 3 or 4, I was attacked by a large boy and thrown to the ground. I also recalled being molested by a babysitter's brother when I was around the same age. The psychiatrist told me that these early childhood experiences may have made me vulnerable to anxiety later in life. He put me on Xanax and an antidepressant. I only took the Xanax when I felt overwhelmed with anxiety. I remember once my husband needed me to go on a business trip with him to Mexico and how I fretted over the decision. I wasn't sure I could cope. I ended up going and found myself sitting on the bed in the hotel room just panicking for no reason. I had to call my psychiatrist, and he talked me into calming down so that I could go to dinner with my husband's associates. I just remember the amount of suffering. It was terrible, and no one in my family understood what I was going through.

individuals with no family history of anxiety have a 2% to 6% risk of acquiring the disorder, whereas individuals with a family history of panic disorder are at 20% higher risk for developing the disorder (Takahashi, 2002). Panic disorder generally begins in childhood and adolescence. OCD also begins in childhood and has a strong familial link.

Structural and Functional Neuroanatomical Factors

Studies focused on neurological causes of anxiety implicate two key centers in the brain that regulate memory storage and emotions: the hippocampus and amygdala. Both animal and human studies verify that fear circuitry is located in the amygdala (Debiec & LeDoux, 1996). Sensory information is sent to the amygdala, where it is projected to the hypothalamus, which in turn activates the sympathetic nervous system. It is this hypothalamic-pituitary-adrenocortical (HPA) axis that activates a defensive response in an individual who experiences fear.

Functional magnetic resonance imaging (fMRI) has revealed that a dysregulation of the HPA axis is associated with anxiety disorders (Bear et al, 2001). Neuroimaging studies have found a reduction in the size of the hippocampus in individuals with PTSD, which is believed to be precipitated by the damaging effects of glucocorticoids. Excessive levels of glucocorticoids brought on by chronic exposure to stress can actually lead to atrophy and dendrite loss in the hippocampus (Debiec & LeDoux, 2004).

In addition to structural changes in the hippocampus, chronic fear can trigger dramatic glucose utilization in the frontal cortex. This hypermetabolism or hyperfrontality has been associated with OCD (Greenberg et al, 1997). Neuroimaging reveals extremely active frontal areas in individuals with untreated OCD. This hypermetabolism is believed to lead to the repetitive thoughts and behaviors that are resistant to control by the rational brain (Hollander, 1996).

Neurotransmitters

Stressful stimuli activate a cascade of hormones and neurotransmitters that contribute to the behavioral response of anxiety. When an individual experiences extreme fear or panic, the hormone cortisol, a glucocorticoid, is released from the adrenal gland that sits above the kidney. The job of cortisol is to prepare the body for fight or flight; thus, its release leads to increased blood pressure and blood sugar levels. Elevated cortisol levels, however, suppress the immune system and, as mentioned previously, are implicated in the physiological distress associated with anxiety disorders.

Neurotransmitters are also implicated in the development of social phobia, panic disorder, and PTSD. The brain's GABA-benzodiazepine (BZ) receptor system is implicated in panic disorder and GAD. GABA is a well-known inhibitor of presynaptic transmission in the brain. GABA supports emotional modulation by producing a calming effect when an individual is faced with a stressful situation. A disruption in the ability of GABA to bind to receptor sites in the frontal cortex contributes to the pathology in persons with anxiety disorders (Takahashi, 2002).

Cognitive and Psychological Factors

Cognitive and psychological factors also play a significant role in the development of anxiety disorders. For example, the cognitive model of panic disorder purports that only individuals who misinterpret physical and psychological symptoms associated with panic will develop panic disorders (Chambless, Beck, Gracely, & Grisham, 2000). This misinterpretation of threat can lead to cognitive distortions associated with anxiety. Cognitive distortions arise when the individual perceives a threat to be overwhelming to the personal resources needed to manage the threat (Kendall, Kortlander, Chansky, & Brady, 1992). For example, a parent whose teenager gets her first speeding ticket may perceive this event as catastrophic and overwhelming. This cognitive distortion will result in an imbalance between the parent's perceived ability to cope and the actual situational demand. Anxiety is often the result of this type of cognitive distortion.

Associated with cognitive distortions are cognitive schemas or ways of perceiving the world (Mumma, 2004). Cognitive schemas carry with them core beliefs, rules, and attitudes about specific situations and give rise to automatic thoughts. For example, an individual with anxiety may hold the dysfunctional schema that "other people will always take advantage of me." This schema will in turn promote automatic thoughts that feed anxiety, such as "I have to always protect myself" or "other people are to be feared."

Culture-related cognitive schemas such as simpatico and collectivism in the Latino culture are implicated in the development of anxiety disorders (Varela et al, 2004). These cognitive schemas may lead some to refrain from bothering others with their problems, exacerbating the symptoms associated with anxiety. The difference in child-rearing practices with a focus on others in Eastern cultures versus the self in Western cultures may also affect the way that social phobias are manifested (Chang, 1997). (See Culture-Specific Information section.)

Environmental Factors

Other anxiety disorders, such as PTSD, are rooted in experiencing traumatic life events. PTSD has been diagnosed in individuals who have experienced a major stressor(s) or traumatic event that was perceived as life-threatening and involved intense emotions such as fear, helplessness, and horror. These types of events include natural disasters, war, acts of violence, and accidents, all of which can lead to development of an anxiety disorder (Terr, 1988; van der Kolk, 1994).

In one study, pediatric emergency care providers reported that as many as 80% of injured children will develop at least one symptom of acute stress response within weeks of the incident, placing them at risk for PTSD (Ziegler, Greenwald, DeGuzman, & Simon, 2005). There are, however, individuals who are more susceptible to PTSD than others. Persons with a history of depression or panic disorder are more vulnerable to PSTD after experiencing a traumatic event than are persons who have no psychiatric history. An examination of female and male Vietnam veterans (King, King, Foy, Keane, & Fairbank, 1999) suggests that resilience factors help mitigate the stress response to a war zone. For both men and women in Vietnam, a strong and functional support system, as well as the personality trait of hardiness (which includes optimism and a tendency to see challenges as something to master), were found to be the most important mediators of

PTSD. For women, an unstable family life and early trauma history had the largest effect on PTSD (King et al, 1999).

Prevalence

Anxiety disorders affect approximately 40 million adults or 18% of people in the United States aged 18 and older in a given year (NIMH, 2006; WHO, 2001). One study of approximately 9,000 individuals in the United States found lifetime prevalence estimates for anxiety disorders to be at 28.8% (Barclay, 2005). The study also found the median age of onset for anxiety disorders to be much younger (11 years) than the age of onset for substance use (20 years) and mood disorders (30 years).

GAD is one of the most prevalent psychiatric disorders documented in the United States and is associated with significant levels of psychosocial dysfunction. Primary care settings report prevalence rates to be as high as 5% to 10% for GAD.

Ziegler et al (2005) found that emergency room physicians underestimate the likelihood of the development of PTSD in children, although studies reveal an overall prevalence rate of PTSD in children to be 13% to 45% after surviving traumatic events.

Gender Differences

Women are at a significantly higher risk than men for anxiety disorders (Barclay, 2005). According to the U.S. Surgeon General (U.S. Department of Health and Human Services, 1999), women may be at higher risk due to their perception of a wide range of life events as stressful. In addition, the WHO (n.d.) sights gender-specific risk factors for women, such as socioeconomic disadvantage, gender-based violence, subordinate social status, and responsibilities for the care of others.

Studies also report gender differences for persons diagnosed with GAD (Steiner et al, 2004). Women had a 5% prevalence rate in a 12-month period compared with a 2.4% prevalence rate for men. Among individuals with no other primary psychiatric disorders, GAD prevalence was 2.4% for women and 0.9% for men (Steiner et al, 2004). Of the 5% of people with agoraphobia in the United States, women are twice as likely to be diagnosed as men. OCD is reported equally in men and women (Bear et al, 2001).

In addition, the symptoms and consequences of symptoms vary in men and women. For example, Foot and Koszycki (2004) found that women with panic disorder fear the physical consequences of anxiety more than men. Women also report more symptoms during panic attacks than men.

PhotoVoice

This is a picture of the doorway to outside. To me, this is my doorway to recovery. It lets me know how far I've come and how far I still have to go—it shows me all the beautiful things outside and inside. The doorway to outside reminds me that if I feel trapped there's always an exit or two to get out. The doorway to my recovery is an ongoing process for life. I can see the fear in my eyes every time I have come from outside, but I have to push on for my recovery to work for me.

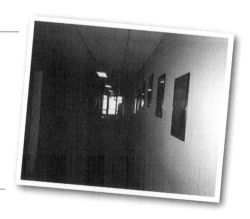

Culture-Specific Information

Epidemiological data and cross-cultural research verify the existence of anxiety disorders in many cultures (Chang, 1997; Kofler, 1997; Mizuta et al, 2005; Tseng, 2003; Tsuang, Tohen, & Zahner, 1995; Varela et al, 2004). The stressors that lead to anxiety can differ depending on the sociocultural environment; thus, culture can produce stress, alter its perception, influence coping mechanisms, and control resources for recovery (Tseng, 2003). Contributions to stress and anxiety from the cultural environment can include (Tseng, 2003)

- Cultural beliefs (e.g., breaking a taboo can cause voodoo death)
- Cultural demands (e.g., academic achievement or the restricted life of a widow)
- Discrimination of immigrant groups or separation from family members during war
- Rapidly changing value systems (e.g., a young adult wants to break away from the regulated choice of a mate)

A large-scale international investigation focusing on individuals who visited general health-care facilities identified prevalence rates for anxiety disorders in 14 countries (Tseng, 2003) and found variations in prevalence of anxiety disorders. For example, in South America, rates were high (22.6%), whereas in Turkey and China, rates for anxiety were low (0.9% and 1.9%, respectively). In the United States, studies have been conducted on different cultural groups (Tseng, 2003). In the 1980s, a study of Caucasian Americans, African Americans, and Hispanic Americans reported lifetime prevalence rates for panic disorder, OCD, and GAD. Results for panic were 1.62% for Caucasian Americans, 1.31% for African Americans, and 0.87% for Hispanic Americans; for OCD, 2.63% for Caucasian Americans, 2.31% for African Americans, and 1.82% for Hispanic Americans; and for GAD, 1.64% for Caucasian Americans, 2.74% for African Americans, and 0.86% for Hispanic Americans.

Many cultures share the same types of anxiety-provoking events in daily life. For example, the lifetime prevalence of traumatic events in young Japanese women is comparable to rates found in women in Western countries—37% to 92% (Mizuta et al, 2005). African American and Caucasian American women report similar lifetime sexual assault rates of 19% and 18%, respectively (Ramos, Carlson, & McNutt, 2004). There may be differences, however, in cultural experience in terms of the types and perceived severity of traumatic events. Terheggen, Stroebe, and Kleber (2001) report that Tibetan refugees in India associated their three most profound traumatic events with religion rather than personal dangers. For example, "witnessing the destruction of religious signs" was endorsed by 95% of respondents as the worst possible event that could happen to a Tibetan (Terheggen et al, 2001).

There are also cultural differences in the expression of the symptoms of anxiety disorders. Mexican and East Asian parents share similarities in parenting patterns that may lead to more anxiety in children in these countries, yet there is less expression of distress (Chang, 1997; Vandervoort, Divers, & Madrid, 1999; Varela et al, 2004). In Latino cultures, collectivism and simpatico are cultural constructs that promote interdependence, empathy, respect, agreement with the group, and personal sacrifices (Varela et al, 2004). **Collectivism** is a frame of reference whereby an individual's behavior and worth are determined by the valued group. Thus, the family's thoughts, feelings, and actions bring worth to individual family members, and individuals who asserts their own thoughts, feelings, and actions do so at the risk of alienation from the group. **Simpatico** is the ability to empathize with others and remain agreeable, even if it means personal sacrifice (Varela et al, 2004). Latino cultures tend to value controlling, restrictive, and primarily physical rather than verbal parenting styles, promoting dependent and obedient children. This type of parenting style is linked to avoidance of psychological issues, leading to children who are anxious. Research suggests that this type of parenting, along with the cultural stigma of mental illness, result in Mexican American and Mexican children reporting more physiological anxiety symptoms and worry symptoms than European American children (Varela et al, 2004)

The DSM-IV-TR (APA, 2000) includes a listing of culture-bound syndromes, which are psychiatric illnesses that are confined to a particular culture. Some of these culture-bound syndromes are typified by anxious symptomatology. **Susto** is described as a folk illness associated with Latino cultures. Similar to PTSD, susto occurs after an individual experiences a shocking or frightening experience. The belief is that the situation is so frightening that it causes the soul to leave the body. This leads to physical symptoms such as trouble sleeping, loss of appetite, muscle pain, gastrointestinal problems, and vertigo. Some evidence suggests a neurological component related to fear (Bourbonnais-Spear et al, 2007). Susto is often treated by a healer known as a curandera.

In Japan, a condition known as **taijinkyofusho**, abbreviated as TKS, is comparable to social phobia in the West (Chang, 1997). However, the phobia in TKS is manifested as fear of offending others, whereas in Western cultures social phobia most often involves a fear of embarrassment or humiliation. Chang (1997) suggests that the differences are due to child-rearing practices. In Eastern cultures, scolding a child involves pointing out how the behavior affects others, including the current family as well as ancestors. In Western cultures, the focus of scolding tends to focus on how the child as an individual did something wrong.

Caution must be exercised when interpreting research on cultural differences and similarities. Sociopolitical events situate a particular culture within a unique historical timeframe, shaping values, beliefs, and attitudes. For example, data collected on anxiety in Germany immediately after the fall of the Berlin Wall may distort the prevalence rates in that country. Therefore, any investigation into a culture's bearing on health must take into consideration the political, economic, and social climate that influences the population.

Within this framework, however, researchers and consumers of research must not confound a multitude of variables with culture in cross-cultural research. For example, Tseng (2003) suggests that many early cross-cultural studies confounded results by failing to focus on culture alone; rather, they included factors beyond cultural ones that potentially could contribute to pathology. Biology, economic level, social class, and religious beliefs are variables that must be taken into consideration when studying anxiety. In addition, cultures use different methodologies and analyses of data that are unique and culturally bound, making cross-cultural comparisons difficult. Translation of instruments is critical because translation of words can carry different meanings in different cultures. For example, the German words for fear (furcht) and anxiety (angst) are used interchangeably in German culture (Kofler, 1997). And some Western psychological constructs, such as stranger anxiety, may not exist in certain cultures (Van Dam-Baggen, Kraaimaat, & Elal, 2003).

Social phobia has only recently entered the lexicon of psychiatry in the United States, most likely due to an increase in diagnostic attention on the part of clinicians (Tseng, 2003). In Japan, the disorder has been recorded since the turn of the 20th century, when Japanese psychiatrics began treating persons with a "disorder of fear of interpersonal relations" (Tseng, 2003). So prevalent was this social anxiety that Morita Therapy, a particular treatment for social phobia, was developed. Chang (1997) asserts that the idea of social harmony lies at the heart of East Asian culture; the culture holds the fundamental belief of benevolent human nature. Japanese society is oriented around a hierarchically organized, interdependent, harmonious structure (Chang, 1997). In Japan, social phobia is associated with feelings of embarrassment and dysmorphic concerns with intermediately familiar persons, such as coworkers, neighbors, or classmates. In contrast, individuals in Western cultures are more socially phobic with strangers in open, public places (Tseng, 2003). Emotional expression and coping styles will vary among cultures. In the treatment of anxiety, it is critical to understand the central role that belief systems play in the development of anxiety disorders and their impact on occupational performance.

Course

Untreated, anxiety disorders can become chronic and unremitting. The course of the various types of anxiety disorders varies in terms of age of onset, severity, gender, and functional impairment. The mean age of onset of social phobia has been reported to be 14 years of age; it has a chronic, unremitting course associated with a pervasive detrimental impact on daily functioning (Kerr, 2003). The course for GAD may extend for 20 years or longer, with low rates of remission (Keller, 2003). OCD is also chronic and may occur as young as 6 years of age (Farrell & Barrett, 2006). The course of PTSD varies between individuals and is highly influenced by the type of traumatic event and the characteristics of the individual. In addition, PTSD is associated with the comorbid conditions of major depression and substance abuse disorders. Predictors of poorer outcomes in PTSD are greater initial severity, greater anger, and more negative interpretations of symptoms (Speckens, Ehlers, Hackmann, & Clark, 2005).

Several researchers have studied childhood experiences as predictors of the development of anxiety disorders. Phillips, Hammen, Brennan, Najman, and Bor (2002) found that early childhood adversity (even as early as maternal prenatal stress) was more likely to predict anxiety as opposed to depressive disorders in adolescence. A large Finnish study found that children who are the victims of bullying are at greater risk for anxiety disorders in early adulthood (Sourander et al, 2007). And family dysfunction was related to less favorable treatment outcomes in children with anxiety disorders (Crawford & Manassis, 2001). All told, these studies suggest a preventive role for occupational therapists, particularly those working in early intervention and schools who are in a position to address these early risk factors for anxiety disorders.

Impact on Occupational Performance

Occupational performance refers to the individual's ability to plan and carry out roles and tasks that support engaging in meaningful activities. Anxiety disorders create a substantial burden on the occupational performance of individuals, families, and society. Measurements of quality of life are commonly used to assess an individual's subjective sense of well-being. The term "quality of life" not only encompasses complex aspects of life that are unquantifiable, but also includes objective indicators of health status and life context (Mendlowicz & Stein, 2000). Anxiety disorders significantly compromise quality of life and psychosocial functioning. In turn, anxiety hinders learning by interrupting cognition and affective and psychomotor functioning (Bastable, 2003; Rapaport, Clary, Fayyad, & Endicott, 2005). The economic costs for anxiety disorders include hospitalization, psychiatric and nonpsychiatric care, psychotropic medications, absenteeism from work, loss of productivity, and suicide (Lapine, 2002). Individuals with PTSD are at a significantly higher risk for diminished well-being, consistent employment, and physical health and limitations than individuals without PTSD (Mendlowicz & Stein, 2000).

Moderate levels of impairment in functional ability in individuals with social phobia have been reported by Kerr (2003). Social phobia can result in functional impairments in educational status, financial status, employability, marital status, and social supports. For example, an individual with social phobia may refuse to attend work or family events with a spouse, causing disruption in the marriage. Others may be impaired in the workplace when they cannot face strangers in a meeting or speak in public.

Although occupational therapists have not played a major role in treating anxiety disorders in the United States, our knowledge of occupational performance provides us with the expertise to address the impact of the disorder on daily life. Occupational therapists should assess and provide interventions for individuals experiencing occupational performance problems related to anxiety and, in doing so, can improve their quality of life.

Physical Impairments

Studies have documented the toll that PTSD takes on physical health even decades after the precipitating event (Neria & Koenen, 2003). In fact, PTSD was the main predictor of long-term physical responses to combat stress reaction in soldiers (Neria & Koenen, 2003). Brackbill et al. (2006) studied survivors of collapsed or damaged buildings during the September 11, 2001, attack on the World Trade Center in New York City. Those exposed to the dust and debris cloud had the worst outcomes, with two-thirds reporting respiratory problems, and the same number reporting mental health problems. The relationship between the physical and mental health issues are difficult to untangle.

Panic disorder is another condition in which high rates of comorbid physical illnesses exist. Cardiac patients with panic disorder experience greater pain and poorer overall health (Bringager, Arnesen, Friis, Husebye, & Dammen, 2008). People with panic attacks are also at a significantly greater risk for physical illness, and the combination of the two conditions compounds the level of disability (Marshall, Zvolensky, Sachs-Ericsson, Schmidt, & Bernstein, 2008). Occupational therapists, with their training in both physical and mental health, are uniquely qualified to address the challenges associated with conditions in which anxiety disorders co-occur with physical illnesses.

Cognitive Impairments

Elevated anxiety levels can alter cognitive functioning and the way information is processed in the brain. These alterations can take place as early as infancy, which is a time of critical structural and functional organization of the brain. Children, youth, and adults who experience a state of hyperarousal have difficulty following directions, recalling what has been heard, and making sense out of what they have heard (Perry, n.d.; Wood, 2006). This state of intense arousal can impair the ability to concentrate on academic tasks due to disruption in the left hippocampal area, which is associated with memory storage. Children and adults who have been traumatized have lower memory volume in the hippocampal areas of the brain than do nontraumatized individuals, leading to a decrease in short-term and verbal memory (Perry, n.d.; Steele, 2002). Farrell and Barrett (2006) report that, in the case of OCD, disruptive cognitive processes appear to worsen across the developmental trajectory. Occupational therapists can create interventions that modify the cognitive demands or create adaptations to support successful performance for individuals with anxiety disorders experiencing cognitive impairments.

Psychosocial Impairments

Anxiety disrupts engagement in meaningful occupations because individuals, for example, may quit attending church or community activities. Relationships may be disrupted when individuals decline to share in family activities and events involving friends and coworkers. Anxiety disorders appear to disrupt career development by restricting educational experiences and interfering with employment (Waghorn, Chant, White, & Whiteford, 2005). In children, anxiety and phobic disorders, excluding PTSD, are atypical and generally arise from fears associated with specific objects or events, such as animals, separation from parents or others, and dying, resulting in disruption of occupational performance at home, school, and in social situations (Stein & Cutler, 2002). A sense of hopelessness is also common with anxiety disorders, which contributes to susceptibility to depression.

Occupational therapists are first and foremost concerned with occupational performance. When occupational performance issues exist—whether they be at home, work, or school, or in social situations—it is important that the occupational therapists consider anxiety as a prevailing factor. When anxiety is present, the occupational therapist should then employ interventions that reduce anxiety so that the individual can experience successful engagement in meaningful occupations.

Evidence-Based Practice

The cognitive behavioral frame of reference has been identified in the literature as the primary framework for the psychological treatment of anxiety disorders (Morrison, Bradley, & Western, 2003; Stein & Cutler, 2002).

➤ Occupational therapists should use the cognitive behavioral frame of reference with its emphasis on the elimination of irrational thoughts, cognitive restructuring, and behavioral rehearsal to facilitate mastery over trauma (Stein & Cutler, 2002).

➤ Occupational therapists can use cognitive behavioral interventions for children whose anxiety is interfering with academic performance (Wood, 2006).

➤ Occupational therapists should also consider expressive therapies supported by a psychodynamic frame of reference for people with anxiety disorders (Stein & Cutler, 2002).

Morrison, K. H., Bradley, R., & Western, D. (2003). The external validity of controlled clinical trials of psychotherapy for depression and anxiety: A naturalistic study. *Psychology and Psychotherapy: Theory, Research, and Practice, 76,* 109–132.

Stein, F., & Cutler, S. K. (2002). *Psychosocial Occupational Therapy: A Holistic Approach.* Albany, NY: Delmar.

Wood, J. (2006). Effect of anxiety reduction on children's school performance and social adjustment. *Developmental Psychology, 42,* 345–349.

Treatment

Individuals who suffer from anxiety disorders have several treatment options. Antianxiety medications and cognitive behavioral therapy (CBT) are standard approaches with strong research efficacy for treating anxiety, as well as the behavioral and psychosocial responses to fear, in children, adolescents, and adults (Nash & Hack, 2002; Takahashi, 2002). Approaches to intervention are discussed only briefly, with more extensive discussion of occupational therapy interventions appearing in other chapters of this text.

Medications

The most commonly used medications for anxiety disorders are benzodiazepines (BZs) and certain antidepressants, such as selective serotonin reuptake inhibitors (SSRIs) and tricyclic antidepressants (TCAs). SSRIs, which are antidepressants, are considered first-line medications for treatment of anxiety; these include Prozac (fluoxetine), Paxil (paroxetine), Luvox (fluvoxamine), Zoloft (sertraline), and Celexa (citalopram). SSRIs also have both antiobsessional and antipanic effects. BZs are not considered first-line medication; rather, they are generally used as an adjunct to antidepressants for less responsive individuals. Examples of benzodiazepines include Xanax (alprazolam) and Ativan (lorazepam). A major concern with BZs is their potential for physiological and psychological dependence. In addition, abrupt withdrawal from BZs has been implicated in a withdrawal syndrome resulting in rebound anxiety, insomnia, diarrhea, and light sensitivity (Takahashi, 2002).

Other Medical Treatments

Other medical treatments are sometimes used for the treatment of OCD. Case reports suggest that electroconvulsive therapy (ECT) may be effective in reducing symptoms of OCD in patients with comorbid major depression. Repetitive transcranial electromagnetic stimulation (rTMS) is a newer technology that is being applied to psychiatric disorders. rTMS involves the application of variable magnetic fields to areas of the brain and was found in one study to decrease compulsive urges for up to 8 hours after treatment (Greenberg et al, 1997).

Psychosocial Intervention Approaches

Psychosocial intervention approaches that occupational therapists might use in addressing anxiety include CBT, relaxation therapy, and expressive writing. CBT is often used to treat anxiety disorders and has extensive evidence to support its efficacy (Shearer, 2007). In some cases, CBT is used in conjunction with medication; however, in some situations, and particularly with panic disorder, medications can interfere with the treatment approach. The CBT approach to panic disorder involves having the individual approach situations that cause anxiety and reduce the catastrophizing associated with the event. When medications are used to eliminate anxious feelings, this makes it difficult to implement this technique effectively. For the treatment of anxiety disorders, CBT typically includes education in the fear cycle and the challenging of distorted cognitions related to fear. For more detailed information about CBT, refer to the Chapter 19.

Relaxation therapy is another approach used for the treatment of anxiety disorders. In some cases, such as phobias, the individual practices relaxation during exposure to the feared object or event. There are many different approaches to relaxation, including deep breathing, meditation, visualization, and progressive muscle relaxation. Surprisingly, there is limited research, and the results are equivocal when it comes to the application of relaxation to anxiety disorders (Conrad & Roth, 2007; Toneatto & Nguyen, 2007). Chapter 22 provides more information on intervention to address stress management.

When dealing with traumatic events, there is some evidence that writing about the event can lead to better understanding and acceptance of the occurrence (Pennebaker & Chung, 2007). Writing and journaling is discussed in more detail in Chapter 6.

Summary

Anxiety disorders are prevalent and, although it may not be the presenting condition for which the client is referred, there are many situations in which the occupational therapist will encounter people with anxiety disorders. For example, an individual dealing with traumatic injuries may experience comorbid PTSD, and a socially anxious child may have problems with academic performance. Individuals in pain are often anxious. And the therapy session itself may invoke a fear response in some individuals. This chapter provides information that the occupational therapist can use to obtain better outcomes by understanding anxiety, the fear response, and its affect on occupational performance.

Active Learning Strategies

People with anxiety suffer a great deal psychologically. They sometimes feel as though they are "losing their minds," and this creates more anxiety. Extreme fear presents people with many barriers. They may avoid people, places, or specific situations; they may feel trapped inside their own bodies and minds. They also often feel alone. It is difficult to simulate anxiety. One way to try to understand this disorder is to place yourself in a vulnerable position, such as attending a church of a different ethnic group by yourself or going alone to an activity involving strangers. Other ways to understand anxiety include reading first-hand accounts and watching films. Choose from one of the following activities to gain a better understanding of anxiety disorders:

1. Attend Alone

- A church service of an ethnic group other than your own
- A festival full of strangers
- A gay or lesbian activity if you are heterosexual

 Describe the experience in your **Reflective Journal**.

2. Read one of the following books:

- *Jailbird* by Kurt Vonnegut
- *The Pleasure of My Company* by Steve Martin
- *Everworld* series by K. A. Applegate

3. View one of the following films:

- "As Good As it Gets" starring Jack Nicholson
- "The Aviator" starring Leonardo DiCaprio
- "Matchstick Men" starring Nicholas Cage
- "What About Bob" starring Bill Murray

Reflective Questions

Reflect on how you felt after one of these activities. Consider the following questions:

- What feelings were aroused in you when you were alone among strangers?
- What did you fear would happen to you?
- What if these feelings were magnified 1,000%? What would that feel like?
- How did the characters in the book or film suffer?
- What types of occupations were impaired due to their anxiety disorder?

Resources

Organizations

- Anxiety Disorders Association of America, Panic Disorder (Panic Attack): www.adaa.org/GettingHelp/AnxietyDisorders/Panicattack.asp
- National Alliance for the Mentally Ill (NAMI): www.nami.org
- Freedom From Fear: www.freedomfromfear.org
- Panic Anxiety Disorder: www.panicanxietydisorder.org

Educational Videos

- Public Broadcasting Service (PBS): www.pbs.org
- Stanford Health Library: http://healthlibrary.stanford.edu/

Books

- *Why Zebras Don't Get Ulcers* by Robert Sapolsky (New York: Holt and Company, 2004)
- *Hope and Help for Your Nerves* by Claire Weekes (New York: Signet Paperback, 1969)
- *Coping With Anxiety: 10 Simple Ways to Relieve Anxiety, Fear, and Worry* by E. J. Bourne and C. Garano (Oakland, CA: New Harbinger, 2002)

References

American Psychiatric Association (APA). (2000). *Diagnostic and Statistical Manual of Mental Disorders* (4th ed., text revision). Washington, DC: Author.

Barclay, L. (2005). "Half of Americans May Meet DSM-IV Criteria for a Mental Disorder During Their Lifetime." Available at: http://www.medscape.com/viewarticle/506348 (accessed November 16, 2009).

Bastable, S. B. (2003). *Nurse as Educator: Principles of Teaching and Learning for Nursing Practice.* Sudbury, MA: Jones and Bartlett.

Bear, M. F., Connors, B. W., & Paradiso, M. A., (2001). *Neuroscience: Exploring the Brain* (3rd ed.). Philadelphia: Lippincott.

Bourbonnais-Spear, N., Awad, R., Merali, Z., Maquin, P., Cal, V., & Arnason, J. T. (2007). Ethnopharmacological investigation of plants used to treat *susto,* a folk illness. *Journal of Ethnopharmacology, 109,* 380–387.

Brackbill, R. M., Thorpe, L. E., DiGrande, L., Perrin, M., Sapp, J. H., Wu, D., et al. (2006). Surveillance for World Trade Center disaster health effects among survivors of collapsed and damaged buildings. *Morbidity and Mortality Weekly Report, 55*(SS02), 1–18.

Bringager, C., Arnesen, H., Friis, S. Husebye, T., & Dammen, T. (2008). A long-term follow-up study of chest pain patients: Effect of panic disorder on mortality, morbidity, and quality of life. *Cardiology, 110,* 8–14.

Bull, B. C., Arnesen, H., Friis, S., Husebye, T., & Dammen, T. (2008). A long-term follow-up study of chest pain patients: Effect of panic disorder on mortality, morbidity, and quality of life. *Cardiology, 110*(1), 8–14.

Chambless, D. L., Beck, A. T., Gracely, E. J., & Grisham, J. R. (2000). Relationship of cognitions to fear of somatic symptoms: A test of the cognitive theory of panic. *Depression and Anxiety, 11,* 1–9.

Chang, S. C. (1997). Social anxiety (phobia) and East Asian culture. *Depression and Anxiety, 5,* 115–120.

Conrad, A., & Roth, W. T. (2007). Muscle relation therapy for anxiety disorders: It works but how? *Journal of Anxiety Disorders, 21,* 243–264.

Crawford, M. A., & Manassis, K. (2001). Familial predictors of treatment outcome in childhood anxiety disorders. *Journal of the American Academy of Child and Adolescent Psychiatry, 40,* 1182–1189.

Davis, J. (1999). Effects of trauma on children: Occupational therapy to support recovery. *Occupational Therapy International, 6,* 126–142.

Debiec, J., & LeDoux, J. E., (2004). Fear and the brain. *Social Research, 71,* 807–818.

Debiec, J., & Le Doux, J. E. (1996). *The emotional brain.* New York: Simon & Schuster.

Farrell, L., & Barrett, P. (2006). Obsessive-compulsive disorder across developmental trajectory: Cognitive processing of threat in children, adolescents, and adults. *British Journal of Psychology, 97,* 95–114.

Foot, M., & Koszycki, D. (2004). Gender differences in anxiety-related traits in patients with panic disorder. *Depression and Anxiety, 20,* 123–130.

Greenberg, B. D., George, M. S., Martin, J. D., Benjamin, J., Schlaepfer, T. E., Altermus, M., et al. (1997). Effect of prefrontal repetitive transcranial magnetic stimulation in obsessive-compulsive disorder: A preliminary study. *American Journal of Psychiatry, 154,* 867–869.

Hollander, E. (1996). Obsessive-compulsive disorder–related disorders: The role of selective serotonergic reuptake inhibitors. *International Clinical Psychopharmacology, 11,* 75–87.

Keller, M. B. (2003). The lifelong course of social anxiety disorder: A clinical perspective. *Acta Psychiatrica Scandinavica, 108,* 85–95.

Kendall, P. C., Kortlander, E., Chansky, T. E., & Brady, E. U. (1992). Comorbidity of anxiety and depression in youth: Treatment implications. *Journal of Consulting and Clinical Psychology, 60,* 869–880.

Kerr, M. (2003). "Social Anxiety Disorder Much More Prevalent Than Previously Thought." Available at: http://www.medscape.com/viewarticle/462578 (accessed November 16, 2009).

King, D. W., King, L. A., Foy, D. W., Keane, T. M., & Fairbank, J. A. (1999). Posttraumatic stress disorder in a national sample of female and male Vietnam veterans: Risk factors, war-zone stressors, and resilience-recovery variables. *Journal of Abnormal Psychology, 108*(1), 164–170.

Kofler, A. (1997). Fear and anxiety across continents: The European and the American way. *Innovation: The European Journal of Social Sciences, 10,* 381–404.

Kozak, B., Strelau, J., & Miles, J. N. V. (2005). Genetic determinants of individual differences in coping styles. *Anxiety, Stress, and Coping, 18,* 1–15.

Lapine, J. P. (2002). The epidemiology of anxiety disorders: Prevalence and social costs. *Journal of Clinical Psychiatry, 63,* 4–8.

Markowitz, A. (Producer). (1998). "In Search of Ourselves: A Science Odyssey." [Television broadcast]. Boston: Public Broadcasting Service.

Marshall, E. C., Zvolensky, M. J., Sachs-Ericsson, N., Schmidt, N. B., & Bernstein, A. (2008). Panic attacks and physical health problems in a representative sample: Singular and interactive associations with psychological problems, and interpersonal and physical disability. *Journal of Anxiety Disorders, 22,* 78–87.

McCance, K. L., & Huether, S. E. (2002). *Pathophysiology: The Biologic Basis for Disease in Adults and Children.* St. Louis, MO: Mosby.

Mendlowicz, M. V., & Stein, M. B. (2000). Quality of life in individuals with anxiety disorders. *American Journal of Psychiatry, 157,* 669–682.

Mizuta, I., Ikuno, T., Shimai, S., Hirotsune, H., Ogasawara, M., Ogawa, A., Honaga, E., & Inoue, Y. (2005). The prevalence of traumatic events in young Japanese women. *Journal of Traumatic Stress, 18,* 33–37.

Morrison, K. H., Bradley, R., & Western, D. (2003). The external validity of controlled clinical trials of psychotherapy for depression and anxiety: A naturalistic study. *Psychology and Psychotherapy: Theory, Research, and Practice, 76,* 109–132.

Mumma, G. H. (2004). Validation of idiosyncratic cognitive schema in cognitive case formula. *Psychological Assessment, 16,* 211–230.

Nash, L. T., & Hack, S. (2002). The pharmacological treatment of anxiety disorders in children and adolescents. *Expert Opinion on Pharmacotherapy, 3,* 555–571.

National Institute of Mental Health (NIMH). (2006). "Anxiety Disorders." Available at: http://www.nimh.nih.gov/publicat/numbers.cfm#Anxiety (accessed November 15, 2009).

Neria, Y., & Koenen, K. C. (2003). Do combat stress reaction and posttraumatic stress disorder relate to physical health and adverse health practices? An 18-year follow-up of Israeli war veterans. *Anxiety, Stress, and Coping, 16,* 227–239.

Pennebaker, J. W., & Chung, C. K. (2007). Expressive writing, emotional upheavals, and health. In H. S. Friedman & R. C. Silver (Eds.), *Foundations of Health Psychology* (pp. 263–284). New York: Oxford University Press.

Perry, B. (n.d.). "Violence and Childhood: How Persisting Fear Can Alter the Developing Child's Brain." [A Special Child Trauma Academy Web Site version of Perry, B. D. (2001b). The neurodevelopmental impact of violence in childhood. In D. Schetky & E. Benedek (Eds.), *Textbook of Child and Adolescent Forensic Psychiatry* (pp. 221–238). Washington, DC: American Psychiatric Press.] Available at: http://www.childtrauma.org/ctamaterials/vio_child.asp (accessed November 15, 2009).

Phillips, N. K., Hammen, C. L., Brennan, P. A., Najman, J. M., & Bor, W. (2002). Early adversity and prospective prediction of depression and anxiety disorders in adolescents. *Journal of Abnormal Child Psychology, 33,* 13–24.

Pinel, P. J. (2005). *Biopsychology.* Boston: Allyn & Bacon.

Ramos, B. M., Carlson, B. E., & McNutt, L. A. (2004). Lifetime abuse, mental health, and African American women. *Journal of Family Violence, 19,* 153–164.

Rapaport, M. H., Clary, C., Fayyad, R., & Endicott, J. (2005). Quality of life impairment in depressive and anxiety disorders. *American Journal of Psychiatry, 162,* 1171–1178.

Shearer, S. L. (2007). Recent advances in the understanding and treatment of anxiety disorders. *Primary Care Clinics in Office Practice, 34,* 475–504.

Silberg, J. L., & Bulik, C. M. (2005). The developmental association between eating disorders symptoms and symptoms of depression and anxiety in juvenile twin girls. *Journal of Child Psychology and Psychiatry, 46,* 1317–1326.

Sourander, A., Jensen, P., Ronning, J. A., Niemela, S., Helenius, H., Sillanmaki, L., Kumpulaiken, K., Piha, J., Tamminen, T., Moilanen, I., & Almquist, F. (2007). What is the early adult outcome of boys who bully or are bullied in childhood? The Finnish "From a Boy to a Man" study. *Pediatrics, 120,* 397–404.

Speckens, A. E. M., Ehlers, A., Hackmann, A., & Clark, D. M. (2005). Changes in intrusive memories associated with imaginal reliving in post traumatic stress disorder. *Journal of Anxiety Disorders, 20,* 328–341.

Steele, W. (2002). Trauma's impact on learning and behavior: A case for intervention in schools. *Trauma and Loss: Research and Interventions, 2*(2), 34–47.

Stein, F., & Cutler, S. K. (2002). *Psychosocial Occupational Therapy: A Holistic Approach.* Albany, NY: Delmar.

Steiner, M., Allgulander, C., Ravindran, A., Kosar, H., Burt, T., & Austin, C. (2004). Gender differences in clinical presentation and response to sertraline treatment of generalized anxiety disorder. *Human Psychopharmacology, 20,* 3–13.

Takahashi, L. K. (2002). Neurobiology of schizophrenia, mood disorders, and anxiety disorders. In K. L. McCance & S. E. Huether (Eds.), *Pathophysiology: The Biologic Basis for Disease in Adults and Children* (5th ed., pp. 550–564). St. Louis, MO: Mosby.

Terheggen, M. A., Stroebe, M. S., & Kleber, R. J. (2001). Western conceptualizations and Eastern experience: A cross-cultural study of traumatic stress reactions among Tibetan refuges in India. *International Society for Traumatic Stress Studies, 14,* 391–403.

Terr, L. (1988). Childhood traumas, an outline and overview. In G. S. Everly & J. M. Lating (Eds.), *Psychotraumatology: Key Papers and Core Concepts in Posttraumatic Stress* (pp. 301–319). New York: Plenum.

Toneatto, T., & Nguyen, L. (2007). Does mindfulness meditation improve anxiety and mood symptoms: A review of the controlled research. *Canadian Journal of Psychiatry, 52,* 260–266.

Tseng, W. S. (2003). *Clinician's Guide to Cultural Psychiatry.* San Diego: Academic Press.

Tsuang, M. I., Tohen, M., & Zahner, G. E. P. (1995). *Textbook in Psychiatric Epidemiology.* New York: Wiley & Sons

U.S. Department of Health and Human Services (1999). *Mental health: A report of the Surgeon General.* Rockville, MD: U.S. Department of Health and Human Services.

van Beijsterveldt, C. E. M., Verhulst, F. C., Molenaar, P. C. M., & Boomsma, D. I. (2004). The genetic basis for problem behavior in five-year-old Dutch twin pairs. *Behavior Genetics, 34,* 229–242.

Van Dam-Baggen, R., Kraaimaat, F., & Elal, G. (2003). Social anxiety in three Western societies. *Journal of Clinical Psychology, 59,* 673–686.

van der Kolk, B. A. (1994). The body keeps the score: Memory and the evolving psychobiology of posttraumatic stress. *Harvard Review Psychiatry, 1,* 253–265.

Vandervoort, D., Divers, P. P., & Madrid, S. (1999). Ethno-culture, anxiety, and irrational beliefs. *Current Psychology, 18,* 287–893.

Varela, R. E., Vernberg, E. M., Sanchez-Sosa, J. J., Riveros, A., Mitchell, M., & Mashunkashey, J. (2004). Anxiety reporting and culturally associated interpretation biases and cognitive schemas: A comparison of Mexican, Mexican American, and European American families. *Journal of Clinical Child and Adolescent Psychology, 33,* 237–247.

Waghorn, G., Chant, D., White, P., & Whiteford, H. (2005). Disability, employment, and work performance among people with ICD-10 anxiety disorders. *Australian and New Zealand Journal of Psychiatry, 39,* 55–66.

WHO (n.d.) Gender and women's health. Retrieved from http://www.who.int/mental_health/prevention/genderwomen/en/ on April 2, 2010.

Wood, J. (2006). Effect of anxiety reduction on children's school performance and social adjustment. *Developmental Psychology, 42,* 345–349.

World Health Organization (WHO). (2001). Chapter 2: Burden of mental and behavioural disorders. In *The World Health Report 2001—Mental Health: New Understanding, New Hope* (pp. 19–46). Geneva, Switzerland: Author.

World Health Organization (WHO). (n.d.). "Gender and Women's Mental Health." Available at: http://www.who.int/mental_health/prevention/genderwomen/en/ (accessed November 15, 2009).

Ziegler, M. F., Greenwald, M. H., DeGuzman, M. A., & Simon, H. K. (2005). Posttraumatic stress responses in children: Awareness and practice among a sample of pediatric emergency care providers. *Pediatrics, 115,* 1261–1267.

Schizophrenia

Catana Brown

> "Yes, I too sense danger everywhere, each morning and all day. It's hard for me to get out of bed, to go out of the house, to talk to people. It's hard just to get dressed and get outside and function. I'm afraid of people, of change. I'm sensitive to sunlight and noise. I never watch the news or read a newspaper because it frightens me.
>
> —Anonymous, 1983, p. 152, a pharmacy student with schizophrenia

Introduction

Anyone who has seen the movie or read the book, *A Beautiful Mind,* has an appreciation for how schizophrenia disrupts the life of the individual, as well as the lives of those close to the person (Nasar, 2001). The brilliant mathematician, John Nash, was tormented by hallucinations and paranoid delusions, which resulted in divorce, unemployment, and multiple involuntary hospitalizations. Yet, eventually, John Nash was awarded the Nobel Prize for his work on game theory, was reunited with his wife, and held a position as a senior research mathematician at Princeton University.

As remarkable as John Nash's life may be, it is not unlike the story of recovery that can be told by many ordinary people who have lived with schizophrenia. Despite the illness and the associated stigma, people with schizophrenia are creating lives characterized by hope and dreams for the future. By better understanding the illness and recognizing the uniqueness of each individual, occupational therapists can become facilitators of the recovery process.

Description of the Disorder

Schizophrenia is a multifaceted and complex disorder. Unlike anxiety disorders, in which anxiety is the core symptom, or major depression, in which the central symptom is depressed mood, it is difficult to identify specific traits that are shared by all people with schizophrenia. In fact, there is disagreement and controversy as to the cardinal features of schizophrenia and its subtypes (Tsuang, Stone, & Faraone, 2000).

The symptoms of schizophrenia are often classified as positive or negative. **Positive symptoms** represent aberrations in behavior or behavior that is not typically present in other individuals, such as hallucinations, delusions, disorganized thinking, and disorganized behavior. With positive symptoms, perceptions and thoughts assume a richness and idiosyncratic meaning that is often disturbing or even terrifying to the individual who experiences them. In contrast, **negative symptoms** are the absence of typical function, such as flat affect, social withdrawal, and difficulty initiating activity.

Negative symptoms have a greater impact on functioning and are related to early onset, poor outcomes, and cognitive impairment (Crow, 1995; Milev, Ho, Arndt, & Andreason, 2005). Some research findings indicate that negative symptoms are associated with structural brain abnormalities, whereas positive symptoms are related to neurochemical disturbances (Crow, 1995). In summary, the symptoms of schizophrenia include unwelcome additions to and subtractions from the lived experience.

Although psychosis (delusions and hallucinations) is often equated with schizophrenia, negative symptoms are just as prevalent and can be even more debilitating. Furthermore, it seems that no two individuals with schizophrenia are the same. For example, one person with a diagnosis of schizophrenia may have prominent paranoid delusions, whereas another person with the same diagnosis may have no delusions, but a flat affect and speech that is difficult to follow. Some individuals experience significant improvement in symptoms over time, whereas others plateau or get worse. Some individuals with schizophrenia have significant cognitive impairments, and others do not. The heterogeneity of schizophrenia makes the illness equally perplexing and fascinating. In fact, some argue that schizophrenia is not a single disorder, but a "collection of unrelated or partially related disorders" (Heinrichs, 1993, p. 222).

DSM-IV-TR Criteria

To meet the criteria for schizophrenia, an individual must have at least two of the following symptoms for at least 1 month (American Psychiatric Association [APA], 2000):

- Delusions
- Hallucinations
- Disorganized speech
- Disorganized or catatonic behavior
- Negative symptoms

These symptom criteria represent the acute phase of the illness. The psychotic symptoms of delusions and hallucinations represent one symptom dimension of schizophrenia. **Delusions** are distortions in thought or false beliefs,

The Lived Experience

Samantha, a young Native American woman, tells her own story. Samantha recently moved into an apartment, where she lives with her two cats, Diamond and Rio. As you will read, a connection to God and writing poetry are central components of Samantha's recovery journey. In addition to her story, Samantha shares one of her poems.

Walking on a Good Road
by Samantha Blessington

It has been hard walking on a good road. There have been so many ups and downs, stresses, trials, tribulations, and many more disturbing things that have been in my life. There have been detours and temptations, tempting me to take the no outlet roads that only lead to self-destruction, hate, greed, and self-pity. The many obstacles I have faced to become a better person have strengthened my spirit. If it was not for the creator, I would be lifeless and left without a clue. I confide in my God to help me cope with the many stresses life brings and the stresses I take on by being mentally ill. God helps me walk through life on a good road. Poetry inspired me to dig deep into my soul to get in tune with my inner self. It has helped me cope with grieving for loved ones, anger, and anxiety. Without my coping skills, I don't think I could of made it this far. Forgiveness has been an important part of my life. Forgiving people who have done me wrong has freed my spirit. Holding grudges only brought me anger, bitterness, and hate. It also messed with my ability to trust.

I was born mentally ill, and my mother knew it right away. I was first hospitalized for my symptoms when I was 6 years old. I have been raped, molested, and beaten by older peers. I strived for a better life. Many bad things have happened to me, but I try to focus on the good things in life. Life is a path to salvation. We start clueless, make mistakes, and learn from them. We face obstacles, dead ends, and one-ways that tear our spirits down, but we can have faith to overcome the obstacles. We can have faith and God shows us the right way to walk on a good road. We have a purpose on this earth. We all do. Coping with our feelings is the first step to recovery.

To Give Up

To give up is to let my past take control,
To give up is to let hate overcome my soul,
To give up is to give up on myself,
To give up is to think of me and no one else,
To give up is to let God out of my life,
To give up is to let go of what I call paradise,
To give up is to not have faith in who I am,
To give up is to lose the sense of knowing who I really am,
But to have faith is to take control,
To have faith is to purify my soul,
To have faith is to free my spirit,
To have faith is to know I'm not there but to know I am near it,
To have faith is to know God is near,
To have faith is to be able to shed a tear,
To love is to know I am loved too,
To love is to know I can stay true,
But to give up is to lose,
And to give up is to know my faith I have refused.

---

whereas **hallucinations** are distortions in perception. The two are often related. For example, an individual with schizophrenia can have an auditory hallucination (i.e., "hear voices"). These voices may tell the individual that he or she is under surveillance by the FBI, so the individual develops a paranoid delusion that there are "bugs" in the apartment and spies are all around. Delusions can be classified as bizarre or nonbizarre. A **nonbizarre delusion** is a belief that in actuality is untrue, but is in the realm of possibility. The example of being under surveillance by the FBI is a nonbizarre delusion. A **bizarre delusion** is outside the realm of possibility, for example, believing that one did not start out as a baby, but evolved from an amoeba.

In addition to the symptom criteria, a diagnosis of schizophrenia requires a marked decline in function since the onset of the illness. The detailed DSM-IV-TR diagnostic criteria for schizophrenia are listed in Box 14-1.

Subtypes of Schizophrenia

The heterogeneous nature of schizophrenia has led to numerous attempts to subtype the disorder; this has been an arduous and frustrating endeavor because there is great variability in symptomatology, course, and outcome among individuals with the disorder. The DSM-IV-TR lists five subtypes, which are described in Table 14-1:

- Paranoid
- Disorganized
- Catatonic
- Undifferentiated
- Residual

Studies that attempt to differentiate the different DSM-IV-TR subtypes in terms of prognosis, etiology, and cognitive function tend to find few differences between the subtypes (Hill, Ragland, Gur, & Gur, 2001; Seaton, Allen, Goldstein, Kelley, & van Kammen, 1999). Therefore, the reliability and validity of the DSM-IV-TR subtypes is not well established, and they are often viewed primarily as descriptive (Andreason, 1987). One exception is the paranoid versus nonparanoid distinction. In general, the course and prognosis for individuals with paranoid schizophrenia is better than for individuals with the nonparanoid subtypes. Individuals with paranoid schizophrenia are typically less cognitively impaired (Zalewski, Johnson-Selfridge, Ohriner, Zarella, & Seltzer, 1998). They tend to develop the disorder later in life, have fewer hospitalizations, are more socially competent, and are more likely to marry (Nicholson & Neufeld, 1993).

BOX 14-1 ▪ DSM-IV-TR Criteria for Schizophrenia

A. Characteristic symptoms

Two (or more) of the following, each present for a significant portion of time during a 1-month period (or less if successfully treated):

1. Delusions
2. Hallucinations
3. Disorganized speech
4. Grossly disorganized or catatonic behavior
5. Negative symptoms (e.g., affective flattening, alogia, avolition)

Note: Only one Criterion A symptom is required if delusions are bizarre or hallucinations consist of a voice keeping up a running commentary on the person's behavior or thoughts, or two or more voices conversing with each other.

B. Social/occupational dysfunction

For a significant portion of the time since the onset of the disturbance, one or more major areas of functioning, such as work, interpersonal relations, and self-care, are markedly below the level achieved prior to the onset.

C. Duration

Continuous signs of the disturbance persist for at least 6 months. This 6-month period must include at least 1 month of symptoms that meet Criterion A and may include periods of prodromal or residual symptoms.

D. Significant mood disorder must not be present

E. Psychotic symptoms must not be associated with substance abuse or general medical conditions

Source: From American Psychiatric Association (2000). *Diagnostic and Statistical Manual of Mental Disorders* (4th ed.). Washington, DC: Author.

Symptom Clusters

In an effort to better understand the symptoms associated with schizophrenia and to identify possible subtypes, many researchers use statistical techniques to identify clusters of symptoms. Different studies indicate different symptom dimensions, but several studies support three distinct symptom clusters: psychotic, disorganized, and negative (Andreason et al, 1995; Liddle, Barnes, Morris, & Haque, 1989). In the three-cluster model, positive symptoms are divided into psychotic and disorganized symptom clusters, and negative symptoms comprise the third cluster. These symptom clusters suggest that, if an individual has one of the symptoms within a symptom cluster, he or she is more likely to have the other symptoms within that same cluster.

Although these symptom clusters may be regarded as subtypes, the prevailing view is that the symptom clusters represent dimensions of the disorder (Andreason & Carpenter, 1993). That is, subtypes represent a categorical distinction, and each individual fits into only one subtype. However, from a dimensional perspective, there is overlap among individuals, and the emphasis is on the degree to which an individual experiences symptoms in each of the dimensions. For example, an individual with schizophrenia can have predominant symptoms in just the psychotic dimension, or he or she can have predominant symptoms in both the psychotic and disorganized dimensions. urther details about the symptoms in each cluster are provided in Table 14-2.

Cognitive Subtypes

Although cognitive impairments are not part of the diagnostic criteria for schizophrenia, problems in cognition have been recognized since the earliest classifications of the disorder by Kraepelin (1919) and Bleuler (1911). Similar to

Table 14-1 ● **DSM-IV-TR Criteria for Schizophrenia Subtypes**

Subtype	Description
Paranoid type	A. Preoccupation with one or more delusions or frequent auditory hallucinations. B. *None* of the following is prominent: 1. Disorganized speech 2. Disorganized or catatonic behavior 3. Flat or inappropriate affect
Disorganized type	A. *All* of the following are prominent: 1. Disorganized speech 2. Disorganized behavior 3. Flat or inappropriate affect B. Criteria are not met for catatonic type.
Catatonic type	The clinical picture is dominated by *at least two* of the following: 1. Motoric immobility as evidenced by catalepsy (including waxy flexibility) or stupor 2. Excessive motor activity (purposeless and not influenced by external stimuli) 3. Extreme negativism or mutism 4. Peculiarities of voluntary movement as evidenced by posturing, stereotyped movements, prominent mannerisms, or prominent grimacing 5. Echolalia or echopraxia
Undifferentiated type	The presence of symptoms that meet Criterion A of schizophrenia, but that do not meet criteria for the paranoid, disorganized, or catatonic type.
Residual type (used when there has been at least one episode of schizophrenia, but the current clinical picture is without prominent psychotic symptoms)	A. Absence of prominent delusions, hallucinations, disorganized speech, and grossly disorganized or catatonic behavior. B. There is continuing evidence of the disturbance as indicated by the presence of negative symptoms or two or more symptoms listed in Criterion A for schizophrenia present in an attenuated form (e.g., odd beliefs, unusual perceptual experiences).

Source: From American Psychiatric Association (2000). Diagnostic and Statistical Manual of Mental Disorders (4th ed.). Washington, DC: Author.

Table 14-2 ● Schizophrenia Symptom Clusters

Symptom Clusters	Symptoms
Psychotic symptoms	• *Hallucinations*—A disturbance of perception. A perceptual experience that occurs in the absence of a sensory stimulus. Hallucinations can occur in any of the sensory modalities, but auditory hallucinations are the most common in schizophrenia. • *Delusions*—A disturbance in thought that involves a false belief. It is important to take into account a person's cultural and educational background in determining whether a belief is delusional.
Negative symptoms	• *Alogia*—Speech that is characterized by limited spontaneity, reduced amount, or impoverished content. • *Flat affect*—Reduced intensity of emotional expression and response as evidenced through a lack of facial expression, gesturing, and voice inflection. • *Avolition*—Difficulty initiating and carrying out goal-directed behavior. • *Anhedonia*—Inability to experience pleasure. Individuals no longer enjoy activities that were previously pleasurable. • *Attentional impairment*—Difficulty concentrating or screening out irrelevant information.
Disorganized symptoms	• *Disorganized*—Speech that is difficult to understand and includes symptoms such as loose associations, neologisms, magical thinking, and difficulty with abstraction. • *Disorganized or bizarre behavior*—Includes abnormal motor behavior or engagement in purposeless or odd behaviors. • *Inappropriate affect*—Affect that is not consistent with speech or situation, or smiling and giggling for no apparent reason.

the studies of symptoms, several researchers have used a battery of cognitive tests to identify cognitive clusters within groups of people diagnosed with schizophrenia (Goldstein, 1994; Goldstein & Shemansky, 1995; Heinrichs & Awad, 1993). Similar to the symptomatology, a great deal of heterogeneity exists in both the types of impairments and the degrees to which individuals with schizophrenia experience cognitive impairments.

Two distinct categories become apparent from the cluster analyses: a subgroup of serious cognitive impairment and one of intact cognitive function. There are also middle clusters that are less distinct but represent moderate cognitive impairment with specific areas of cognitive dysfunction, such as slowed psychomotor speed. In a study in which cognitive clusters were associated with symptom clusters, greater cognitive impairment was found among people with negative and disorganized symptoms than people with primarily psychotic symptoms (Hill et al, 2001). More specifically, executive function impairments were common across all symptom dimensions, and memory impairments were particularly pronounced in people with disorganized symptoms. (Cognitive function is further explained later in the chapter.) Attentional and psychomotor impairments were common in both the disorganized and negative symptom dimensions.

Etiology

Research into the etiology of schizophrenia explores genetic factors, prenatal factors, structural neuroanatomical differences, functional neuroanatomical differences, neurotransmitters, and diathesis stress.

Genetic Factors

Family, adoption, and twin studies provide evidence that there is a genetic contribution to schizophrenia. Twin studies indicate that there is a remarkably higher concordance rate in schizophrenia for identical twins when compared with nonidentical twins, 46% and 14%, respectively (Cardno, Rijsdijk, Sham, Murray, & McGuffin, 2002). However, because the concordance rate for identical twins is far from 100%, it is possible that the genetic

vulnerability for schizophrenia goes unexpressed in some individuals. It is also possible that some individuals develop the disorder without a genetic predisposition.

Currently, there is research investigating the specific chromosomes that are associated with the disorder. Genetic models suggest that schizophrenia is **polygenetic** (i.e., a combination of genes must be present for the disorder to be expressed). Therefore, the search for the specific genetic link is much more difficult. Some studies suggest that the genetic vulnerability is not specific to schizophrenia, but that there is a general genetic vulnerability for psychosis (Cardno et al, 2002; Potash, Willour, Chieu, Simpson, & MacKinnon, 2001). The expression of the genes can then take the form of schizophrenia, schizoaffective disorder, or a mood disorder with psychotic features such as bipolar disorder.

Prenatal Factors

There is evidence that events affecting fetal development are related to the subsequent diagnosis of schizophrenia. Individuals with schizophrenia are more likely to have a history

---

Evidence-Based Practice

Several published studies have explored the role of cognition in overall community functioning for people with schizophrenia. The results indicate that cognitive functioning is an important factor in successful community functioning.

➤ Occupational therapists should assess cognition in people with schizophrenia and determine whether cognition is interfering with community functioning.

➤ Occupational therapists should consider ways to remediate or compensate for cognitive impairments when providing interventions for people with schizophrenia.

Green, M. F. (1996). What are the functional consequences of neurocognitive deficits in schizophrenia? *American Journal of Psychiatry, 153,* 321–330.
Green, M. F., Kern, R. S., Braff, D. L., & Mintz, J. (2000). Neurocognitive deficits and functional outcome in schizophrenia: Are we measuring the "right stuff"? *Schizophrenia Bulletin, 26,* 119–136.

of obstetric complications, particularly complications that involve oxygen deprivation (Cannon et al, 2000). Maternal viral infection resulting in prenatal exposure to the flu or rubella is also associated with an increased risk for schizophrenia (Brown, Cohen, Harkavy-Friedman, & Babulas, 2001; Murray, Jones, O'Callaghan, & Takei, 1992).

Structural Neuroanatomical Differences

Although there is no definitive neuroanatomical abnormality that is associated with schizophrenia, consistent findings arise when groups of individuals with schizophrenia are studied and compared with individuals without schizophrenia. One of the most frequent findings in people with schizophrenia is enlargement of the cerebral ventricles. Associated with this finding is an increase in cerebrospinal fluid in the ventricles and a decrease in cortical gray matter. Research suggests that neural cell loss close to the ventricles accounts for this enlargement (Pfefferbaum, Lim, Rosenbloom, & Zipursky, 1990). This particular abnormality is associated with poorer outcomes in schizophrenia. There is also evidence of a smaller thalamus and smaller hippocampus in individuals with schizophrenia (Baare, van Oel, Pol, Schnack, & Durston, 2001; Schmajuk, 2001). It appears that these brain changes occur before the onset of schizophrenia and may begin in adolescence.

Neurodevelopmental and neurodegenerative theories of schizophrenia provide different perspectives as to the cause of the disorder (Allin & Murray, 2002). From a neurodevelopmental perspective, subtle structural abnormalities exist in the brains of individuals with schizophrenia at birth. Support for the neurodegenerative theory comes from studies indicating reduction in gray matter volume over time (DeLisi, 1999; Rapoport, Giedd, Blumenthal, Hamburger, & Jeffries, 1999). It is likely that both neurodevelopmental and neurodegenerative processes contribute to the etiology of schizophrenia.

Functional Neuroanatomical Differences

In addition to structural abnormalities, individuals with schizophrenia differ from their control counterparts in functional brain activity. One of the most often cited findings in functional brain imaging in schizophrenia is hypofrontality (Hill et al, 2004). Hypofrontality, which is indicated by reduced cerebral blood flow or metabolism in the frontal lobe of the brain, is associated with **executive dysfunction** (higher-level cognitive impairments) in schizophrenia. Studies investigating frontal lobe activity during rest and when the individual is engaged in a cognitive activity find that people with schizophrenia have less frontal lobe activation than non–mentally ill controls.

Neurotransmitters

The "dopamine hypothesis" of schizophrenia is one of the oldest theories related to the cause of schizophrenia. This theory was initiated in the 1950s, when antipsychotics were first used to treat schizophrenia. The antipsychotic drugs block dopamine activity and reduce psychotic symptoms. Furthermore, drugs that increase dopamine activity, such as amphetamines, can trigger a psychotic episode (Carlsson, 1988). More recently, studies of dopamine in the brain of individuals with schizophrenia do not support excess dopamine, but instead suggest that individuals with schizophrenia have a

higher number of dopamine receptors, particularly in the basal ganglia (Kestler, Walker, & Vega, 2001).

Although it is widely accepted that psychotic symptoms respond to drugs that block dopamine activity, it is also acknowledged that the "dopamine hypothesis" does not sufficiently account for the spectrum of impairments associated with the disorder. More recently, other neurotransmitters such as y-aminobutyric acid (GABA) and serotonin have been implicated in the etiology of schizophrenia, but their association with the symptoms of schizophrenia is less clear.

Diathesis Stress

The diathesis stress theory proposes that exposure to stress is required for individuals who are biologically predisposed to schizophrenia to go on to express the disorder. There is strong evidence that environmental stress is associated with the onset of schizophrenia and that stressful life events can lead to a worsening of symptoms for individuals who are already diagnosed (Norman & Malla, 1993). In a seminal study, Brown and Birley (1968) found that 46% of individuals with schizophrenia reported a stressful life event in the 3-week period before a psychotic episode. This was compared with 14% in a sample of controls. For individuals with schizophrenia, it is particularly important to take into account the impact of events such as a change in apartment, job interview, or financial problems, and to provide additional supports during these stressful life events.

People with schizophrenia may have difficulty managing stress for biological reasons (Corcoran, Gallitano, Leitman, & Malaspina, 2001). An adaptive biological system that is capable of managing stress is dependent on efficient cortisol regulation. Cortisol dysregulation can lead to negative long-term effects, including memory impairment. There is evidence that some individuals with schizophrenia experience cortisol dysregulation (i.e., higher than normal levels of cortisol are present in the blood at baseline). When under stress, individuals with schizophrenia take longer to experience a reduction in cortisol levels. High levels of cortisol can lead to atrophy of the hippocampus, which can subsequently cause memory impairments. High levels of cortisol in individuals with schizophrenia have been associated with symptom severity, cognitive impairments, and poorer prognosis (Walker & Diforio, 1997). Furthermore, heightened cortisol release can intensify dopamine activity, resulting in an exacerbation of symptoms.

Evidence-Based Practice

Stressful life events can lead to an exacerbation of symptoms in people with schizophrenia (Norman & Malla, 1993).

➤ Occupational therapists can help individuals with schizophrenia consider ways to reduce exposure to stress.

➤ Occupational therapists can assist individuals with schizophrenia in developing coping methods to manage stress.

➤ Occupational therapists can create additional supports when individuals with schizophrenia are experiencing stressful life events.

Norman, R. M. G., Scholten, D. J., Malla, A. K., & Ballageer, T. (2005). Early signs in schizophrenia spectrum disorders. *Journal of Nervous and Mental Disease, 193*, 17–23.

Prevalence

The DSM-IV-TR reports a prevalence rate of 0.5% to 1% of the population (APA, 2000); however, a systematic review of studies of schizophrenia prevalence suggest this is an overestimate and that the lifetime prevalence for schizophrenia is closer to 4 persons in 1,000 (Saha, Chant, Welham, & McGrath, 2005). The prevalence rates are relatively stable across cultures, although the prognosis may vary in different countries.

Course

Schizophrenia is typically first diagnosed during the early 20s (Walker, Kestler, Bollini, & Hochman, 2004). The age of onset can be particularly devastating because this is a time when most people are establishing significant adult relationships and worker roles. However, schizophrenia can develop at any age, but it is rarely diagnosed before adolescence. Late-onset schizophrenia is more common in women.

Before meeting the criteria for schizophrenia, most individuals have a prodromal period lasting for weeks or months in which there are nonspecific changes in behavior and experiences. The **prodromal period** is the time between the emergence of early signs of the illness and the point at which the diagnostic criteria for the disorder are met. Some of the most frequently noted early signs of schizophrenia are impairments in role functioning and social withdrawal (Norman, Scholten, Malla, & Ballageer, 2005). For example, there may be problems at work or school, or the individual may begin avoiding friends and family. Other common symptoms include mood changes, odd thinking and perceptual experiences, disrupted sleep, and poor appetite.

Retrospective studies indicate that a vulnerability to the disorder exists even in childhood. That is, even though a diagnosis of schizophrenia typically does not occur until the late teens or early 20s, when looking back to childhood, there may have been subtle signs of a problem. Home movies and interviews reveal delays in motor development and problems with social adjustment (Walker & Lewine, 1990; Walker, Savoie, & Davis, 1994).

Individuals experiencing their first psychotic symptoms (typically referred to as "first episode schizophrenia") are typically not diagnosed or treated for 1 year or more (Beiser, Erickson, Fleming, & Iaconon, 1993). There is some evidence that the longer a person goes without treatment, the poorer the treatment response (Haas, Garratt, & Sweeney, 1998). Consequently, some people advocate for the initiation of medication during the prodromal period (Kablinger & Freeman, 2000). Although highly controversial, it is theoretically possible that early medication treatment can decrease or delay brain dysfunction and alter the course of the disorder. One of the main problems with preventive treatment of schizophrenia is determining the severity of prodromal symptoms that warrant early intervention.

Moreover, psychosocial treatment may be just as important and effective as medication in first episode schizophrenia. In a Finnish study (Lehtinen, Aaltonen, Koffert, Rakkolainen, & Syvalahti, 2000), individuals with first episode schizophrenia received either antipsychotic medications according to usual practice or minimal medication and psychosocial intervention. In the 2-year study, many patients in the psychosocial intervention group received no medication at all, yet the outcomes of this group were as good or better than the medication group.

When Emil Kraepelin first described dementia praecox in 1919 (the disorder that later came to be known as schizophrenia), he depicted the course of the illness as one of progressive decline. This view became so prevalent that the *Diagnostic and Statistical Manual for Mental Disorders, Third Edition* included the following description: "A complete return to premorbid functioning is unusual—so rare, in fact, that some clinicians would question the diagnosis. However, there is always the possibility of full remission or recovery, although its frequency is unknown. The most common course is one of acute exacerbations with increasing residual impairment between episodes" (APA, 1981, p. 185).

Although longitudinal studies indicate that this description of the course of schizophrenia is inaccurate, it is not uncommon, even today, for mental health professionals to question the schizophrenia diagnosis when an individual is in remission. A landmark study by Harding, Brooks, Ashikaga, Strauss, and Breier (1987) led to a new understanding of the prognosis of schizophrenia. The study, which began in the mid-1950s, followed 82 individuals who met the DSM-III criteria for schizophrenia for 20 to 25 years. The results indicated that, like other characteristics of schizophrenia, there was great heterogeneity in the functional outcomes of the participants. Furthermore, instead of a downward course, the study found that 73% "led a moderate to very full life," 81% were "able to meet basic needs," 68% "displayed slight or no symptoms," and 44% were "employed in the past year" (p. 732).

The recognition that individuals with schizophrenia can and often do improve is exemplified by the Remission in Schizophrenia Working Group, which was assigned the task of developing a definition of remission in schizophrenia (Andreason et al, 2005). They distinguished recovery from remission. According to the working group, *recovery* involves community living, whereas *remission* is focused on symptom reduction. Remission was defined as a score of mild or less for delusions, hallucinations, thought disorder, bizarre behavior, flat affect, social withdrawal, and lack of spontaneity, as measured by standardized symptoms scales. The minimum time period to meet the criteria of remission is 6 months. Defining recovery was not part of the consensus conference.

Gender Differences

There is a slightly higher incidence of schizophrenia in males, and schizophrenia is generally less severe for females than it is for males (Tamminga, 1997). Females have a later age of onset, require fewer hospitalizations, respond better to medications, and have better outcomes. The mean age of onset for males is around 21, whereas for females it is 27.

There are several theories explaining gender differences in schizophrenia. It may be that deviant behavior is more acceptable in females than it is for males (Goldstein & Kreisman, 1988), that estrogen is protective (Hafner, 2003), or that greater hemispheric bilaterality in females reduces the cognitive dysfunction (Flor-Henry, 1985). In terms of symptomatology, females are more likely to have mood symptoms and paranoid delusions, and males are more likely to have negative symptoms.

Culture-Specific Information

Cultural considerations are essential in distinguishing psychotic experiences from commonly held cultural beliefs. For example, in certain religions, it is a typical religious experience to hear the voice of God or believe in virgin birth. In carefully controlled studies, there are no major race-related differences in the prevalence of schizophrenia in the United States (Regier, 1991). However, in clinical populations, there tend to be biases in diagnosing minority groups (Strakowski, Shelton, & Kolbrener, 1993). Typically, schizophrenia is overdiagnosed in minority groups, but one study found that African Americans were more likely and Latinos were less likely to receive a schizophrenia diagnosis when compared with European American individuals (Minsky, Vega, Miskimen, Gara, & Escobar, 2003). In addition, individuals from minority groups are less likely to receive best practice interventions for schizophrenia (Copeland, Zeber, Valenstein, & Blow, 2003; Wells, Klap, Koike, & Sherbourne, 2001). From a worldwide perspective, there appear to be differences in outcomes for people with schizophrenia in developed and developing countries (Jablensky et al, 1992; Thara, 2004). Perhaps surprisingly, individuals with schizophrenia in developing countries have better outcomes. For example, the marriage and employment rates are higher in these countries.

Impact on Occupational Performance

Schizophrenia is recognized as a serious mental illness and, as such, the illness can interfere with successful occupational performance. In addition, the social consequences of schizophrenia such as stigma and poverty are just as or even more significant in terms of their impact on daily life.

Cognitive Impairments

Although cognitive impairments are not part of the diagnostic criteria of schizophrenia, impaired cognitive functioning is a core feature of the disorder. Cognitive impairments precede the diagnosis and often persist after psychotic symptoms have remitted. In fact, cognitive dysfunction is more strongly associated with functional impairment than symptoms, particularly the positive symptoms of schizophrenia. Cognitive impairments tend to worsen with illness onset, but there does not appear to be a progression of the deficit over time (Heaton et al, 2001) (i.e., the cognitive impairment remains fairly stable). As noted previously, there is a great deal of heterogeneity in the degree to which individuals experience cognitive impairments. Some individuals with schizophrenia have serious cognitive impairments, and some have intact cognitive function, with most individuals falling somewhere in between (Goldstein, 1994; Goldstein & Shemansky, 1995; Heinrichs & Awad, 1993).

The study of cognition and schizophrenia is extensive and long. Large meta-analyses reveal that measures of cognition are more effective at distinguishing people with schizophrenia from health controls than brain imaging results (Heinrichs, 2005). Generally, the meta-analyses found

people with schizophrenia had scores almost a full standard deviation lower than controls on tests of cognition.

Cognitive impairments in schizophrenia include problems with attention, memory, and executive function (Spaulding, Reed, Poland, & Strozbach, 1996). In terms of attentional impairments, individuals with schizophrenia often have difficulty screening out irrelevant information. When the amount of information in the environment exceeds the processing ability of the individual, information processing becomes inefficient and erratic. Individuals with schizophrenia also have trouble sustaining attention over time.

Individuals with schizophrenia have relatively intact short-term memory, except in demanding conditions or in the presence of distractors (Spaulding et al, 1996). For example, individuals with schizophrenia typically perform well if they are required to remember only a few items for a short period of time. However, a hallmark of cognitive impairment in schizophrenia is difficulty with working memory (Barch, 2003), or the ability to manipulate information in the brain for short periods of time. For example, when an individual is grocery shopping, he or she must remember which items from a list have already been found and placed into a cart and which items still remain on the list. Barch argues that working memory dysfunction is a result of disturbances in executive functioning.

Executive function (Spaulding et al, 1996) refers to higher-level cognitive processing and includes abilities such as organization, planning, conceptual flexibility, and problem-solving. People with schizophrenia are less likely to develop and use scripts or habit patterns when involved in familiar situations. For example, most people have a "script" for making an appointment and then going to get a haircut. There are certain steps to follow and social expectation in this situation. Although many people are unaware of the fact that they are following a script, the person with schizophrenia has more trouble drawing up the steps and rules of the script to carry out the task. In unfamiliar situations, individuals with schizophrenia have even more trouble making sense of the environment and determining what they already know about the situation. Individuals with schizophrenia find it particularly difficult to make changes in behavior, and require more feedback and a higher level of certainty before making a change. Obviously, this has important implications for intervention, suggesting that useful and concrete feedback, along with reassurance, should be regularly provided.

There is increasing interest in factors that predict functional outcomes. The first major review found that cognition was more important than symptoms in predicting outcome (Green, 1996). In another important review of cognition and function in schizophrenia, Green, Kern, Braff, and Mintz (2000) divided functional outcomes into three categories: (1) success in psychosocial rehabilitation programs, (2) laboratory or simulated measures of social and instrumental skills, and (3) broader measures of community outcome. The review indicates that cognition is clearly related to functional outcomes, although the cognitive predictors vary by type of outcome. The strongest results (meaning at least four studies supported the finding) indicated that verbal memory was related to all outcomes, whereas executive function was related to broader community outcomes, and sustained attention was related only to the laboratory measures of skills. Previous studies have relied on cross-sectional designs in which current cognitive and functional status was assessed at a single point in time. A stronger design using longitudinal methods studying people over 4- and 7-year time periods also found cognition related to function (Kurtz, Moberg, Ragland, Gur, & Gur, 2005; Milev et al, 2005).

Clearly, it is important that cognition be addressed when considering interventions directed toward community living. Skills training and environmental modification should take into account the specific cognitive impairments that are common in schizophrenia.

Health and Wellness

Individuals with schizophrenia have much higher rates of morbidity and mortality than the general population. For example, people with schizophrenia are four times more likely to die from serious cardiac events than the general population (Enger, Weatherby, Reynolds, Glasser, & Walker, 2004) and have a 20% shorter life expectancy (Newman & Bland, 1991). Two studies examining lifestyle practices found that people with schizophrenia had poorer health practices, including limited physical activity, poor diets, less interpersonal support, and beliefs that health was not within their control (Brown, Birstwistle, Roe, & Thompson, 1999; Holmberg & Kane, 1999). In addition, people with schizophrenia are less likely to report physical symptoms to health-care providers. Even greater concerns exist today with the increasing evidence that atypical antipsychotics increase the risk for both type II diabetes and weight gain in an already vulnerable population. The combination of poor lifestyle behaviors and the side effects of most psychiatric medications (particularly Clozaril and Zyprexa) contribute to obesity and diabetes in people with schizophrenia (Wirshing, 2004).

High rates of smoking present another health risk. It is estimated that people with schizophrenia have rates of cigarette smoking that are at least two times and possibly more than three times greater than the general population (Grant, Hasin, Cou, Stinson, & Dawson, 2004).). There are several factors that contribute to these rates, including the potential for nicotine to reduce negative symptoms, cognitive deficits, and sensory processing abnormalities (George et al, 2000). Smoking-related deaths contribute to the excess mortality in schizophrenia.

Severe oral diseases are highly prevalent in this population. Many drugs used to treat schizophrenia have oral side effects. These include severe dry mouth, tardive dyskinesia, and acute dystonic reactions that affect the mouth, tongue, and other head and neck muscle groups. Dry mouth is a particular concern because dryness of the oral tissues increases the rate and severity of periodontal disease and tooth decay. In addition, it can make wearing of dentures impossible (King, 1998). Poor oral hygiene directly correlates with the severity of mental illness, which can influence the severity of periodontal disease and cavities (Chalmers, Smith, & Carter, 1998).

One positive finding from the few intervention studies that do exist is that people with schizophrenia can benefit from health promotion programs. In two separate studies using somewhat different approaches to smoking cessation, a statistically significant number of participants remained abstinent, with one group's cessation rates equal to those of individuals without a psychiatric illness in a similar program

(Addington, el Guebaly, Campbell, Hodgins, & Addington, 1998; George et al, 2000). Behavioral weight reduction programs for people with psychiatric disabilities also indicate that people with schizophrenia can lose weight with dietary reduction and behavior modification (as reviewed in Brown, Goetz, Van Sciver, & Sullivan, 2006; and Faulkner, Soundy, & Lloyd, 2003). Occupational therapists should consider the impact of poor health on occupational performance and contribute to programs that focus on lifestyle changes.

Stigma and Other Social Issues

Stigma is possibly the greatest barrier to successful and satisfying community living for people with schizophrenia. One review found the people with mental illness were discriminated against in instances of housing, jobs, and social interaction (Hinshaw & Cicchetti, 2000). Interestingly, recent evidence suggests that a greater belief in a biological cause of the disorder is associated with increased stigma (Read & Harry, 2001). This may be due to the view that a biological disorder is permanent. These findings are important because many antistigma campaigns promote understanding mental illness as a brain disease.

It is well established that the term "mental illness" carries a stigma, but Mann and Himelein (2004) conducted a study to determine if some mental illnesses were more stigmatizing than others, specifically schizophrenia and depression. They found stigmatization of schizophrenia was significantly higher than stigmatization of depression. They also found that people who believed that treatment could be effective had less stigmatizing attitudes. Corrigan et al (2001) examined different methods of changing stigmatizing attitudes and found that contact with people with mental illness is more effective than education or protest. The contact is most effective when the relationship is equal and there are opportunities for informal interaction.

Most individuals with schizophrenia live in poverty. Poverty presents another major barrier to community living. It is likely that many of the poor functional outcomes associated with schizophrenia are due to the effects of poverty (Cohen, 1993). For example, people with schizophrenia are less likely to have their own cars and have additional barriers

---

Evidence-Based Practice

There is research evidence that individuals with schizophrenia are less likely to engage in healthy lifestyle behaviors (Brown, Birtwistle, Roe, & Thompson, 1999; Holmberg & Kane, 1999). In combination with other factors, such as limited access to health care and the side effects of medications, this leads to high levels of morbidity and mortality (2004).

➤ Occupational therapists can use their expertise to design and implement interventions that support the development of habits that promote health.

Brown, S., Birtwistle, J., Roe, L., & Thompson, C. (1999). The unhealthy lifestyle of people with schizophrenia. *Psychological Medicine, 29*, 697–701.

Holmberg, S. K., & Kane, C. (1999). Health and self-care practices of persons with schizophrenia. *Psychiatric Services, 50*(6), 827–829.

to using public transportation. Consequently, employment and any other instrumental activity of daily living that takes place outside the home can be challenging. Meeting basic needs for food and shelter is a regular struggle. It is essential to consider the social barriers of stigma and poverty during both the assessment and intervention process of occupational therapy.

Interventions

Intervention for individuals with schizophrenia typically consists of psychosocial interventions and medication.

Psychosocial Interventions

Psychosocial interventions typically do not target schizophrenia per se, but there are several evidence-based interventions that are intended for individuals with serious mental illness of which schizophrenia is a primary diagnosis. The Substance Abuse and Mental Health Services Administration identified five evidenced-based practices for community mental health. These practices are described and toolkits are provided on their website at http//:mentalhealth.samhsa.gov. They include the following:

- Illness Management and Recovery
- Assertive Community Treatment
- Family Psychoeducation
- Supported Employment
- Integrated Dual Diagnosis Treatment

Illness Management and Recovery is a group or individual program that helps individuals with serious mental illness set personal goals, live healthier lives, and understand and manage their symptoms (Mueser et al, 2006). Assertive Community Treatment is a form of intensive case management that provides supports and skills training in the individual's natural environment (Krupa et al, 2005). Family Psychoeducation works with the family and the consumer to provide information about mental illness and teach interaction skills that reduce stress within the family (Lincoln, Wilhelm, & Nestoriuc, 2007). Supported Employment is designed to place individuals quickly in jobs of their choosing, while providing the necessary supports, accommodations, and training to facilitate success at work (Moll, Huff, & Detwiler, 2003). Integrated Dual Diagnosis Treatment is designed for co-occurring mental illness and substance abuse (Brunette & Mueser, 2006). Both concerns are treated in the same setting using a stagewise approach that includes

motivational treatment and substance abuse counseling. These approaches are all aimed at enhancing occupational performance for individuals with schizophrenia.

These interventions are discussed in greater detail in subsequent chapters (e.g., supported employment is covered in Chapter 42). Furthermore, Parts III and IV include specific intervention approaches for specific occupations or environments. Each chapter includes information that is relevant for schizophrenia intervention. For example, Chapter 47 provides information on how to teach skills to people with serious mental illness and how to modify environments to support occupational performance in these areas.

Medications

The pharmacological treatment of schizophrenia is based primarily on antipsychotic medications. Antipsychotic medication can be divided into two classes: **typical antipsychotics** (also called first generation or conventional) and **atypical antipsychotics** (also referred to as second generation). The first antipsychotic medication was Thorazine (chlorpromazine) (Julien, 2004). Introduced in 1952, it was first noticed that Thorazine had a calming effect on people with schizophrenia. Later, psychiatrists recognized that it also reduced hallucinations and delusions. Other common typical antipsychotics include Haldol (haloperidol) and Prolixin (fluphenazine). The typical antipsychotics are dopamine antagonists, which work primarily by blocking D2 receptors in the brain. Dopamine receptors bind the neurotransmitter, dopamine, to the presynaptic cell. Five dopamine receptors have been identified—D1, D2, D3, D4, and D5—but they are generally classified as two types: D1 like (includes D1 and D5) or D2 like (includes D2, D3, and D4). The density of D1 and D2 receptors varies in different parts of the brain. The typical antipsychotics are most effective in reducing the positive symptoms of schizophrenia; however, because typical antipsychotics block D2 receptors, they have many harmful side effects.

As shown in Figure 14-1, managing a wide array of medications becomes a regular part of daily life for people with serious mental illness.

The typical antipsychotics have many side effects, including sedation, sun sensitivity, anticholinergic effects (dry mouth, constipation, blurred vision), and orthostatic hypertension. However, the most serious side effects involve movement disorders, which result from the blockage of dopamine in the basal ganglia. Movement disorders include Parkinson-like side effects, akathisia (serious motor restlessness), acute dystonic reaction (a sustained contraction of the muscles of the neck, mouth, and tongue), and tardive dyskinesia. Tardive

PhotoVoice

I dread when 8 o'clock comes around because I know I have to take my handful of pills, which practically makes me gag. After I take my pills, they make me shake. I want to talk to my doctor to cut down on the amount of pills I take. I hope to find a doctor that will take the time to listen to me about the side effects and about how the pills are making me feel.

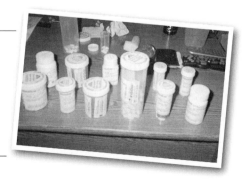

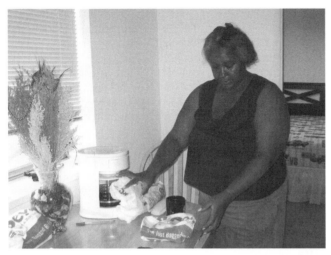

FIGURE 14-1. Managing a wide array of medications becomes a regular part of daily life for people with serious mental illness. This is challenging for Lagina, who lives alone.

dyskinesia occurs after long-term treatment with antipsychotic medication and involves involuntary movements, usually of the mouth and tongue.

The first atypical antipsychotic was Clozaril (clozapine) (Remington, 2003). Clozaril is often effective for individuals who have not responded to other medications. However, it is not used as a first-line drug because of the particularly serious side effect of agranulocytosis (a significant reduction in the number of circulating white blood cells), making the individual highly susceptible to infection. If left untreated, the risk of dying from agranulocytosis is very high. Approximately 1% to 2% of people taking Clozaril will develop agranulocytosis; therefore, individuals who take Clozaril must have regular blood monitoring. Other atypical antipsychotics include Risperdal (risperidone), Zyprexa (olanzapine), Seroquel (quetiapine), Geodon (ziprasidone), and Abilify (aripiprazole).

The differences between typical and atypical antipsychotics are complex and not fully understood (Remington, 2003). The atypical antipsychotics have a greater affinity for D1 receptors than D2 receptors. The atypical antipsychotics also block dopamine at the D2 sites, but the blockage occurs for a shorter period of time with atypical antipsychotics. D1 receptors are more prominent in the frontal lobe, and D2 receptors are more prevalent in the basal ganglia. This may account for the reduction in movement disorders with atypical antipsychotics and for possible improvements in cognition and negative symptoms. In addition to acting as a dopamine antagonist, most atypical antipsychotics are also serotonin antagonists. One theory is that blocking serotonin may help modulate dopamine activity.

Atypical antipsychotics are generally better tolerated than the typical antipsychotics and, for this reason, are more commonly prescribed (Barnes & Joyce, 2001). Tardive dyskinesia is rare with the atypical antipsychotics, as are other movement disorders, because these drugs have less affinity for dopamine blockage in the basal ganglia, but instead block dopamine in other areas of the brain. However, the atypical antipsychotics still have serious side effects. The anticholinergic effects of dry mouth, blurred vision, and constipation are common, and Clozaril and Zyprexa, in particular, are associated with significant weight gain and diabetes.

There is some evidence that atypical antipsychotics may reduce the cognitive impairment in schizophrenia. In a review, Barnes and Joyce (2001) concluded that the atypical antipsychotics were superior to typical antipsychotics in improving cognition; however, there appears to be specific cognitive advantages for each medication. For example, Clozaril seems especially effective in improving verbal fluency, whereas Risperdal has a greater effect on memory.

Summary

Schizophrenia presents many challenges given the psychosis, negative symptoms, and cognitive impairments inherent with the diagnosis. In addition, environmental factors such as stigma, medication side effects, and poverty contribute additional difficulties. However, stories of people with schizophrenia provide messages of hope and empowerment. The recovery model that has emerged from these stories has helped in the reframing of occupational therapy practice such that productive and satisfying community living is now the expectation and not the exception for individuals with schizophrenia.

Active Learning Strategies

People with schizophrenia experience many barriers to participation that are separate from the direct effects of the illness. Most people with schizophrenia live in poverty; consequently, many resources that others take for granted can present major obstacles to successful and satisfying community living. For example, many people are unable to afford a car and rely on public transportation or rides from others to get to where they need to go. Public transportation in some communities is limited or nonexistent and may be complex or stressful for someone with a serious psychiatric disability. Other issues may include having enough money for essential living expenses such as rent and food. Complete one of the following activities to appreciate external barriers to community living.

1. Public Transportation

If public transportation is available in your community, use it to get to an appointment. Take note of issues such as safety, convenience, schedules, exposure, frustration, etc, during the activity.

Describe the experience in your
Reflective Journal.

2. Food Stamps

Go to http://www.fns.usda.gov/fsp/applicant_recipients/fs_Res_Ben_Elig.htm and calculate how much money you would have per day based on your family size. Feed yourself and your family, if applicable, for 1 day on a food stamp budget without using any ingredients you have on hand. Consider satisfying your family's satiety, achieving a balanced diet, and providing a variety of food choices when completing this activity.

Reflective Questions
- What kinds of information did you need to carry out these tasks? How did you go about acquiring this information?
- What skills did you need to successfully complete the tasks? Did you feel competent when executing the tasks?

- Did you ask for help from others? If so, were others helpful?
- What was most challenging?
- What feelings did you experience?
- What would it be like if you had to rely on public transportation or food stamps all the time?
- Would the cognitive impairments associated with schizophrenia make these tasks more difficult? In what ways?
- How might auditory hallucinations affect your experience?
- If you were feeling paranoid, how would the experience differ?
- Do you think stigma would play a role in your ability to carry out these tasks if people knew you had schizophrenia?

 Describe the experience in your
Reflective Journal.

Resources

Books
- Nasar, S. (2001). *A Beautiful Mind.* New York: Simon & Schuster.
- Schiller, L., & Bennett, A. (1996). *The Quiet Room: A Journey Out of the Torment of Madness.* New York: Warner Books.
- Sheehan, S. (1983). *Is There No Place on Earth for Me?* New York: Vintage.

Educational Videos
- "West 47th Street"—PBS: http://www.pbs.org/pov/west47thstreet/
- "Secret Life of the Brain: Part 3: The Teenage Brain"—PBS: http://www.pbs.org/wnet/brain/episode3/index.html
- "Schizophrenia: Surviving the World of Normals"—Wellness Reproductions: www.wellness-resources.com

Organizations
- Institute for the Study of Human Resilience: www.bu.edu/resilience
- National Alliance for Research on Schizophrenia and Depression (NARSAD): www.narsad.org
- National Alliance on Mental Illness (NAMI): www.nami.org
- National Empowerment Center: www.power2u.org
- Schizophrenia.com: www.schizophrenia.com

References

Addington, J., el Guebaly, N., Campbell, W., Hodgins, D. C., & Addington, D. (1998). Smoking cessation treatment for patients with schizophrenia. *American Journal of Psychiatry, 155,* 974–976.

Allin, M., & Murray, R. (2002). Schizophrenia: A neurodevelopmental or neurodegenerative disorder? *Current Opinion in Psychiatry, 15,* 9–15.

American Psychiatric Association (APA). (1981). *Diagnostic and Statistical Manual of Mental Disorders* (3rd ed.). Washington, DC: Author.

American Psychiatric Association (APA). (2000). *Diagnostic and Statistical Manual of Mental Disorders* (4th ed., text revision). Washington, DC: Author.

Andreason, N. C. (1987). The diagnosis of schizophrenia. *Schizophrenia Bulletin, 13,* 9–22.

Andreason, N. C., Arndt, S., Alliger, R., Miller, D., & Flaum, M. (1995). Symptoms of schizophrenia. Methods, meanings and mechanism. *Archives of General Psychiatry, 52,* 341–351.

Andreason, N. C., & Carpenter, W. T. (1993). Diagnosis and classification of schizophrenia. *Schizophrenia Bulletin, 19,* 199–214.

Andreason, N. C., Carpenter, W. T., Kane, J. M., Lasser, R. A., Marder, S. R., & Weinberger, D. R. (2005). Remission in schizophrenia: Proposed criteria and rationale for consensus. *American Journal of Psychiatry, 162,* 441–449.

Anonymous. (1983). Schizophrenia: A pharmacy student's view. *Schizophrenia Bulletin, 9,* 152–155.

Baare, W. G., van Oel, C. J., Pol, H., Schnack, H. G., & Durston, S. (2001). Volumes of brain structures in twins discordant for schizophrenia. *Archives of General Psychiatry, 58,* 33–40.

Barch, D. M. (2003). Cognition in schizophrenia: Does working memory work? *Current Directions in Psychological Science, 12,* 146–150.

Barnes, T. R. E., & Joyce, E. M. (2001). Antipsychotic drug treatment: Recent advances. *Current Opinion in Psychiatry, 14,* 25–37.

Beiser, M., Erickson, D., Fleming, J. A. E., & Iaconon, W. G. (1993). Establishing the onset of psychotic illness. *American Journal of Psychiatry, 150,* 1349–1354.

Bleuler, E. (1911). *Dementia Praecox or the Group of Schizophrenia.* Leipzig, Germany: Deuticke.

Brown, A. S., Cohen, P., Harkavy-Friedman, J., & Babulas, V. (2001). Prenatal rubella, premorbid abnormalities, and adult schizophrenia. *Biological Psychiatry, 49,* 473–486.

Brown, C., Goetz, J., Van Sciver, A., & Sullivan, D. (2006). A psychiatric rehabilitation approach to weight loss. *Psychiatric Rehabilitation Journal., 29,* 267–273.

Brown, G. W., & Birley, J. L. T. (1968). Crisis and life change and the onset of schizophrenia. *Journal of Health and Social Behavior, 9,* 203–214.

Brown, S., Birtwistle, J., Roe, L., & Thompson, C. (1999). The unhealthy lifestyle of people with schizophrenia. *Psychological Medicine, 29,* 697–701.

Brunette, M. F., & Mueser, K. T. (2006). Psychosocial interventions for long term management of patients with serious mental illness and co-occurring substance use disorders. *Journal of Clinical Psychiatry, 67*(suppl 7), 10–17.

Cannon, T. D., Rosso, I. M., Hollister, J. M., Bearden, C. E., Sanchez, L. E., & Hadley, T. (2000). A prospective cohort study of genetic and perinatal influences in schizophrenia. *Schizophrenia Bulletin, 26,* 351–366.

Cardno, A. G., Rijsdijk, F. V., Sham, P. C., Murray, R. M., & McGuffin, P. (2002). A twin study of genetic relationships between psychotic symptoms. *American Journal of Psychiatry, 159,* 539–545.

Carlsson, A. (1988). The current status of the dopamine hypothesis in schizophrenia. *Neuropsychopharmacology, 1,* 179–186.

Chalmers, J. M., Smith, D., & Carter, K. D. (1998). A multidisciplinary dental program for community-living adults with chronic mental illness. *Special Care Dentistry, 18*(5), 194–201.

Cohen, C. I. (1993). Poverty and the course of schizophrenia: Implications for research and policy. *Hospital & Community Psychiatry, 44,* 951–958.

Copeland, L. A., Zeber, J. E., Valenstein, M., & Blow, F. D. (2003). Racial disparity in the use of atypical antipsychotic medications among veterans. *American Journal of Psychiatry, 160,* 1817–1822.

Corcoran, C., Gallitano, A., Leitman, D., & Malaspina, D. (2001). The neurobiology of the stress cascade and its potential relevance for schizophrenia. *Journal of Psychiatric Practice, 7,* 3–14.

Corrigan, P. W., River, L. P., Lundin, R. K., Penn, D. L., Uphoff-Wasowski, K., Campion, J., Mathisen, J., Gagnon, C., Bergman, M., Goldstein, H., & Kubiak, M. A. (2001). Three strategies for changing attributions about severe mental illness. *Schizophrenia Bulletin, 27,* 187–195.

Crow, T. J. (1995). Brain changes and negative symptoms in schizophrenia. *Psychopathology, 28,* 18–21.

DeLisi, L. E. (1999). Regional brain volume change over the lifetime course of schizophrenia. *Journal of Psychiatric Research, 33,* 535–541.

Enger, C., Weatherby, L., Reynolds, R. F., Glasser, D. B., & Walker, A. M. (2004). Serious cardiovascular events and mortality among patients with schizophrenia. *Journal of Nervous and Mental Disease, 192,* 19–27.

Faulkner, G., Soundy, A. A., & Lloyd, K. (2003). Schizophrenia and weight management: A systematic review of interventions to control weight. *Acta Psychiatrica Scandinavica, 108,* 324–332.

Flor-Henry, P. (1985). Psychiatric aspects of cerebral lateralization. *Psychiatric Annals, 15,* 429–433.

George, T. P., Ziedonis, D. M., Feingold, A., Pepper, W. T., Satterburg, C. A., Winkel, J., Rounsaville, B. J., & Kosten, T. R. (2000). Nicotine transdermal patch and atypical antipsychotic medications for smoking cessation in schizophrenia. *American Journal of Psychiatry, 157,* 1835–1842.

Goldstein, G. (1994). Cognitive heterogeneity in psychopathology: The case of schizophrenia. In P. Vernon (Ed.), *The Neuropsychology of Individual Differences* (pp. 209–233). New York: Academic Press.

Goldstein, G., & Shemansky, W. J. (1995). Influences on cognitive heterogeneity in schizophrenia. *Schizophrenia Research, 9,* 49–58.

Goldstein, J. M., & Kreisman, D. (1988). Gender, family environment and schizophrenia. *Psychological Medicine, 18,* 861–872.

Grant, B. F., Hasin, D. S., Chou, S. P., Stinson, F. S., & Dawson, D. A. (2004). Nicotine dependence and psychiatric disorders in the US. Results from the national epidemiological survey on alcohol and related conditions. *Archives of General Psychiatry, 61,* 1107–1115.

Green, M. F. (1996). What are the functional consequences of neurocognitive deficits in schizophrenia? *American Journal of Psychiatry, 153,* 321–330.

Green, M. F., Kern, R. S., Braff, D. L., & Mintz, J. (2000). Neurocognitive deficits and functional outcome in schizophrenia: Are we measuring the "right stuff"? *Schizophrenia Bulletin, 26,* 119–136.

Haas, G. L., Garratt, L. S., & Sweeney, J. A. (1998). Delay to first antipsychotic medication in schizophrenia: Impact on symptomatology and clinical course of illness. *Journal of Psychiatry Research, 32,* 151–159.

Hafner, H. (2003). Gender differences in schizophrenia. *Psychoneuroendocrinology, 28*(suppl 2), 17–54.

Harding, C. M., Brooks, G. W., Ashikaga, T., Strauss, J. S., & Breier, A. (1987). The Vermont longitudinal study of persons with severe mental illness, II: Long term outcome of subjects who retrospectively met DSM-III criteria for schizophrenia. *American Journal of Psychiatry, 144,* 727–735.

Heaton, R. K., Gladsjo, J. A., Palmer, B. W., Kuck, J., Marcotte, T. D., & Jeste, D. V. (2001). Stability and course of neuropsychological deficits in schizophrenia. *Archives of General Psychiatry, 58,* 24–32.

Heinrichs, R. W. (1993). Schizophrenia and the brain: Conditions for a neuropsychology of madness. *American Psychologist, 48,* 221–233.

Heinrichs, R. W. (2005). The primacy of cognition in schizophrenia. *American Psychologist, 60,* 229–242.

Heinrichs, R. W., & Awad, A. G. (1993). Neurocognitive subtypes of chronic schizophrenia. *Schizophrenia Research, 9,* 49–58.

Hill, K., Mann, L., Laws, K. R., Stephenson, I., Nimmo-Smith, I., & McKenna, P. J. (2004). Hypofrontality in schizophrenia: A meta-analysis of functional imaging studies. *Acta Psychiatrica Scandinavica, 110*(4), 243–256.

Hill, S. K., Ragland, J. D., Gur, R. C., & Gur, R. E. (2001). Neuropsychological differences among empirically derived clinical subtypes of schizophrenia. *Neuropsychology, 15,* 492–501.

Hinshaw, S. P., & Cicchetti, D. (2000). Stigma and mental disorder: Conceptions of illness, public attitudes, personal disclosure and social policy. *Development and Psychopathology, 12,* 555–598.

Holmberg, S. K., & Kane, C. (1999). Health and self-care practices of persons with schizophrenia. *Psychiatric Services, 50*(6), 827–829.

Jablensky, A., Sartorius, N., Ernberg, G., Anker, M., Korten, A., Cooper, J. E., Day, R., & Bertelsen, A. (1992). Schizophrenia: Manifestations, incidence and course in different cultures: A World Health Organization ten country study. *Psychological Medicine Monograph Supplement, 20,* 1–97. [Erratum in: *Psychological Medicine Monograph Supplement* 1992 Nov;22(4):following 1092.]

Julien, R. M. (2004). *A Primer of Drug Action* (9th ed.). New York: WH Freeman.

Kablinger, A. S., & Freeman, A. M. (2000). Prodromal schizophrenia and atypical antipsychotic treatment. *Journal of Nervous and Mental Disease, 133,* 642–652.

Kestler, L. P., Walker, E., & Vega, E. M. (2001). Dopamine receptors in the brains of schizophrenia patients: A meta-analysis of the findings. *Behavioral Pharmacology, 12,* 355–371.

King, K. (1998). Dental care of the psychiatric patient. *New Zealand Dental Journal, 94,* 72–82.

Kraepelin, E. (1919). *Dementia praecox and paraphrenia.* Chicago: Chicago Medical Book Co.

Krupa, T., Eastabrook, S., Hern, L., Lee, D., North, R., Percy, K., von Briesen, B., & Wing, G. (2005). How do people who receive assertive community treatment experience this service? *Psychiatric Rehabilitation Journal, 29*(1), 18–24.

Kurtz, M. M., Moberg, P. J., Ragland, J. D., Gur, R. C., & Gur, R. E. (2005). Symptoms versus neurocognitive test performance as predictors of psychosocial status in schizophrenia: A 1- and 4-year prospective study. *Schizophrenia Bulletin, 31*(1), 167–174.

Lehtinen, V., Aaltonen, J., Koffert, T., Rakkolainen, V., & Syvalahti, E. (2000). Two-year outcome in first-episode psychosis treated according to an integrated model. Is immediate neuroleptisation always needed? *European Psychiatry, 12,* 312–320.

Liddle, P. F., Barnes, T. R., Morris, D., & Haque, S. (1989). Three syndromes in chronic schizophrenia. *British Journal of Psychiatry, 7*(suppl), 119–122.

Lincoln, T. M., Wilhelm, K., & Nestoriuc, Y. (2007). Effectiveness of psychoeducation for relapse, symptoms, knowledge, adherence and functioning in psychotic disorders: A meta-analysis. *Schizophrenia Research, 96*(1–3), 232–245.

Mann, C. E., & Himelein, M. J. (2004). Factors associated with stigmatization of persons with mental illness. *Psychiatric Services, 55,* 185–187.

Milev, P., Ho, B. C., Arndt, S., & Andreason, N. C. (2005). Predictive values of neurocognition and symptoms on functional outcome in schizophrenia: A longitudinal first-episode study with 7-year follow-up. *American Journal of Psychiatry, 162,* 495–506.

Minsky, S., Vega, W., Miskimen, T., Gara, M., & Escobar, J. (2003). Diagnostic patterns in Latino, African American and European American psychiatric patients. *Archives of General Psychiatry, 60,* 637–644.

Moll, S., Huff, J., & Detwiler, L. (2003). Supported employment: Evidence for a best practice intervention in psychosocial rehabilitation. *Canadian Journal of Occupational Therapy, 70,* 298–310.

Mueser, K. T., Meyers, P. S., Penn, D. L., Clancy, R., Clancy, D. M., & Salyers, M. P. (2006). The Illness Management and Recovery Program: Rationale, development and preliminary findings. *Schizophrenia Bulletin, 32*(suppl), S32–S43.

Murray, R. M., Jones, P. B., O'Callaghan, E., & Takei, N. (1992). Genes, viruses and neurodevelopmental schizophrenia. *Journal of Psychiatric Research, 26,* 225–235.

Nasar, S. (2001). *A Beautiful Mind.* New York: Simon & Schuster.

Newman, S. C., & Bland, R. C. (1991). Mortality in a cohort of patients with schizophrenia: A record linkage study. *Canadian Journal of Psychiatry, 36,* 239–245.

Nicholson, I. R., & Neufeld, R. W. (1993). Classification of the schizophrenias according to symptomatology: A two-factor model. *Journal of Abnormal Psychology, 102,* 259–270.

Norman, R. M., & Malla, A. K. (1993). Stressful life events and schizophrenia. I: A review of the research. *British Journal of Psychiatry, 162,* 161–166.

Norman, R. M. G., Scholten, D. J., Malla, A. K., & Ballageer, T. (2005). Early signs in schizophrenia spectrum disorders. *Journal of Nervous and Mental Disease, 193,* 17–23.

Pfefferbaum, A., Lim, K., Rosenbloom, M., & Zipursky, R. B. (1990). Brain magnetic resonance imaging: Approaches for investigating schizophrenia. *Schizophrenia Bulletin, 16,* 452–476.

Potash, J. B., Willour, V. L., Chieu, Y. F., Simpson, S. G., & MacKinnon, D. F. (2001). The familial aggregation of psychotic symptoms in bipolar disorder pedigrees. *American Journal of Psychiatry, 158*(8), 1258–1264.

Rapoport, J. L., Giedd, J. N., Blumenthal, J., Hamburger, S., & Jeffries, N. (1999). Progressive cortical change during adolescence in childhood-onset schizophrenia: A longitudinal magnetic resonance imaging study. *Archives of General Psychiatry, 56,* 649–654.

Read, J., & Harry, N. (2001). The role of biological and genetic causal beliefs in the stigmatisation of "mental patients." *Journal of Mental Health, 10*(2), 223–235.

Regier, D. A. (1991). *Psychiatric Disorders in America: The Epidemiologic Catchment Area Study.* New York: Free Press.

Remington, G. (2003). Understanding antipsychotic "atypicality": A clinical and pharmacological moving target. *Journal of Psychiatry & Neuroscience, 28,* 275–284.

Saha, S., Chant, D., Welham, J., & McGrath, J. (2005). A systematic review of the prevalence of schizophrenia. *PLoS Medicine, 2*(5), e141.

Schmajuk, N. A. (2001). Hippocampal dysfunction in schizophrenia. *Hippocampus, 11,* 599–613.

Seaton, B. E., Allen, D. N., Goldstein, G., Kelley, M. E., & van Kammen, D. P. (1999). Relations between cognitive and symptom profile heterogeneity in schizophrenia. *Journal of Nervous and Mental Disease, 187,* 414–419.

Spaulding, W. D., Reed, D., Poland, J., & Storzbach, D. M. (1996). Cognitive deficits in psychotic disorders. In P. W. Corrigan & S. C. Yudofsky (Eds.), *Cognitive Rehabilitation for Neuropsychiatric Disorders* (pp. 129–166). Washington, DC: American Psychiatric Press.

Strakowski, S. M., Shelton, R. C., & Kolbrener, M. L. (1993). The effects of race and comorbidity on clinical diagnosis in patients with psychosis. *Journal of Clinical Psychiatry, 54,* 186–192.

Tamminga, C. A. (1997). Gender and schizophrenia. *Journal of Clinical Psychiatry, 58*(suppl 15), 33–37.

Thara, R. (2004). Twenty year course of schizophrenia: The Madras longitudinal study. *Canadian Journal of Psychiatry, 49,* 564–569.

Tsuang, M. T., Stone, W. S., & Faraone, S. V. (2000). Toward reformulating the diagnosis of schizophrenia. *American Journal of Psychiatry, 157,* 1041–1050.

Walker, E., Kestler, L., Bollini, A., & Hochman, K. M. (2004). Schizophrenia: etiology and course. *Annual Review of Psychology, 55,* 401–430.

Walker, E., & Lewine, R. J. (1990). Prediction of adult-onset schizophrenia from childhood home movies of the patients. *American Journal of Psychiatry, 147,* 1052–1056.

Walker, E., Savoie, T., & Davis, D. (1994). Neuromotor precursors of schizophrenia. *Schizophrenia Bulletin, 20,* 441–452.

Walker, E. F., & Diforio, D. (1997). Schizophrenia: A neural diathesis-stress model. *Psychological Review, 104,* 667–685.

Wells, K., Klap, R., Koike, A., & Sherbourne, C. (2001). Ethnic disparities in unmet need for alcoholism, drug abuse, and mental health care. *American Journal of Psychiatry, 158,* 2027–2032.

Wirshing, D. A. (2004). Schizophrenia and obesity: Impact of antipsychotic medications. *Journal of Clinical Psychiatry, 65*(suppl 18), 13–26.

Zalewski, D., Johnson-Selfridge, M. T., Ohriner, S., Zarella, K., & Seltzer, J. C. (1998). A review of neuropsychological differences between paranoid and non-paranoid schizophrenia patients. *Schizophrenia Bulletin, 24,* 127–145.

Substance-Related Disorders

Carol Haertlein Sells, Virginia Carroll Stoffel, and Heidi Plach

> "Who has woe? Who has sorrow? Who has strife? Who has complaints?
>
> Who has needless bruises? Who has bloodshot eyes?
> Those who linger over wine.
> Do not gaze at wine when it is red, when it sparkles in the cup, when it goes down smoothly!
> In the end it bites like a snake and poisons like a viper.
>
> — *The Bible,* Proverbs 23:29–32

Introduction

Alcohol. It has its own MySpace site. It is the title of a song. There are hundreds of books and dozens of movies about it—from the classic films *The Lost Weekend* and *Days of Wine and Roses* to the more contemporary *When a Man Loves a Woman.*

And then there are drugs, which have made their own mark in the movie business, appearing in familiar titles such as *Easy Rider* and the works of Cheech and Chong, and more recently, *The Basketball Diaries* and *The Big Lebowski.* In addition, more than 100 music artists are identified as being prodrugs, on the basis that they have at least one song about marijuana or other drugs (Drugs-Plaza, n.d.). A recent report indicates that one-third of the top 279 songs on the Billboard charts in 2005 made reference to alcohol or drugs (Primack, Dalton, Carroll, Agarwal, & Fine, 2008), confirming their pervasiveness in popular society.

Alcohol and drugs. The mere mention can bring longing to those who use, abuse, and depend on them; smiles to those who have used and survived; tears to those whose lives have been disrupted or destroyed; and frowns to those who have tried to tackle the effects of drugs on their own lives and the lives of others. Substance-related disorders can affect all aspects of functioning included in the domain of occupational therapy, but have a particular impact on individual client factors, performance patterns and skills, contexts, and all areas of occupation (American Occupational Therapy Association [AOTA], 2008). Occupational therapists provide important services to individuals, families, and communities that are affected by substance use, abuse, and dependence by determining occupational needs, providing assessment and interventions, and developing primary and secondary prevention programs (Stoffel & Moyers, 2004).

Description of the Disorder

Substance-related disorders primarily involve the use and abuse of alcohol and illicit drugs. These disorders are pervasive in American society and presented an economic cost of $246 billion in 1992, the most recent year for which data are available (Harwood, 2000). Costs are typically measured in lost productivity for the individual and his or her household, medical costs, and crime. Assuming that costs stayed the same, and factoring in inflation, the economic burden in 2005 was $342 billion (National Institute on Alcohol Abuse and Alcoholism [NIAAA], 2007), which translates to $1,344 for every man, woman, and child in the United States.

According to the 2006 National Survey on Drug Use and Health (NSDUH), approximately one-half of all Americans aged 12 and older used alcohol (125 million people), and 8.3% used illicit drugs (20.4 million people) (Substance Abuse and Mental Health Services Administration [SAMHSA], 2007). Alcohol use is defined as having at least one drink in the past 30 days (sips do not count); similarly, drug use is defined as one use in the past 30 days. Substance use varies considerably across the population, but use of both alcohol and illicit drugs is highest among 18- to 25-year-olds, with illicit drug use and abuse rates higher in males.

Substance-related disorders are characterized by varying degrees of tolerance, withdrawal symptoms, relapse, and psychological and physical consequences (American Psychiatric Association [APA], 2000). Disruption in meaningful activities across all areas of occupation can result. Life roles are typically unfulfilled: the college student misses classes and eventually flunks out; the parent neglects homemaking responsibilities and children suffer; or the wife or husband ignores work responsibilities and is fired, causing a loss of financial stability and considerable family upheaval. Substance-related disorders do not discriminate by age, gender, race, ethnicity, religious affiliation, geographic location, or socioeconomic status. All segments of society are potentially vulnerable to the consequences of substance-related disorders, which range from fetal alcohol syndrome (FAS) to heroin addiction, making them among the most serious health problems facing our nation (SAMHSA, 2007).

The NSDUH (and its earlier forms as the National Household Survey on Drug Abuse), the primary data system for collecting incidence and prevalence information about alcohol and illicit drug use in the United States, tracks the following categories of illicit drugs:

- Marijuana or cannabis (including hashish)
- Cocaine (including crack)
- Heroin (opioids)
- Hallucinogens (including LSD, PCP, peyote, mescaline, mushrooms, and "ecstasy")
- Inhalants
- Psychotherapeutics (including nonmedical use of prescription-type pain relievers, tranquilizers, stimulants [including methamphetamines], and sedatives) (SAMHSA, 2007)

In this chapter, the terms **drugs** and **illicit drugs** refer to these categories of drugs unless otherwise indicated.

DSM-IV-TR Criteria

According to the *Diagnostic and Statistical Manual of Mental Disorders, Fourth Edition, Text Revision* (DSM-IV-TR), substance-related disorders include a wide range of behaviors and conditions ranging from alcohol abuse to exposure to toxins (APA, 2000). This chapter emphasizes **substance use disorders**, specifically those substances (alcohol and the illicit drugs identified previously) that most often have the widest impact on occupational performance. The DSM-IV-TR criteria for **substance-induced disorders**, that is, disorders related to substance intoxication and withdrawal, are also briefly reviewed here.

Substance use disorders are classified as either abuse or dependence. The DSM-IV-TR criteria for **substance dependence**, the more serious condition, is described in Box 15-1. The symptoms of dependence are similar across the substances, although differences exist (e.g., withdrawal is not specified as a symptom of hallucinogens) (APA, 2000). The key feature of dependence is continued use of the substance in the face of major life disruptions, such as losing a job or marital status due to the negative effects of substance use.

In contrast, **substance abuse** is characterized by use that does not reach the level of tolerance or withdrawal, but consistently results in negative consequences, such as arriving home late, missing family events, or having a fight while under the influence. The DSM-IV-TR criteria for substance abuse is found in Box 15-2.

The substance-induced disorders of intoxication and withdrawal may be evident in clients seen by occupational therapists in a wide variety of settings. The symptoms of **substance intoxication** are typically reversible and are associated with both substance abuse and dependence. They may last for hours or days after use has ceased and the substance is no longer identifiable via body fluid tests (e.g., urine). The most notable characteristic of substance intoxication are changes in the areas of behavior, mood, and cognition secondary to the effect of the substance on central nervous system (CNS) function. They occur shortly after the substance is ingested and cannot be attributed to other medical or psychiatric health–related conditions. The symptoms of intoxication stop when use of the substance ceases (APA, 2000). The DSM-IV-TR criteria for substance intoxication are outlined in Box 15-3.

PhotoVoice

Barriers—We all have them. I've had to overcome a lot to get where I am—drugs, smoking cigarettes, drinking. Barriers block us from achieving our goals in life.

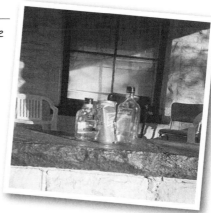

Success—My success is better seen through my artwork and my wellness toolbox. My attitude is changing things that I can change.

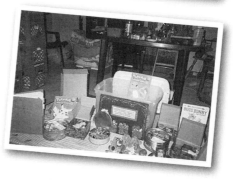

Substance withdrawal, which results when use of the substance decreases or stops, is closely associated with dependence. When use of the substance decreases or stops, the changes in behavior and physiology cause distress to the user with cravings to resume use. There are significant changes in one's ability to engage in occupational behaviors. Like intoxication, the symptoms cannot be attributed to other health conditions, although the presence of other illnesses or disease may mask or exacerbate withdrawal symptoms.

Detailed information about the DSM-IV-TR diagnostic criteria for substance withdrawal is found in Box 15-4.

It is important to note that the acceptable and legal use of substances (e.g., "social drinking" among adults older than 21, appropriate medical use of prescription and over-the-counter medications) should not be confused with the patterns of tolerance, withdrawal, and negative consequences that are symptomatic of abuse or dependence. It is the repeated episodes of intoxication that typically differentiate acceptable use from a disorder.

Subtypes of Substance-Related Disorders

According to the DSM-IV-TR, subtypes of substance-related disorders include alcohol, drugs of abuse, side effects of medications, and toxin exposure (APA, 2000, p. 191). Alcohol and illicit drugs are the focus of this chapter, but there are other comorbid conditions closely associated with substances that are discussed in the literature. Subtypes of substance-related disorders reviewed here are alcohol use, drug use, co-occurring mental illness, fetal alcohol spectrum disorder (FASD), and substance-related problems associated with medical conditions and physical disabilities, given that these are the most common subtypes that occupational therapy practitioners might experience in their clinical practice.

It is worth noting that caffeine and nicotine addictions commonly occur with other substance-related disorders. Unfortunately, they are not typically addressed in substance abuse treatment programs because the acute psychosocial and biological consequences associated with alcohol and drug abuse and dependence typically take precedence. Substance-related disorders may also involve abuse of multiple substances (e.g., cocaine use coupled with alcohol to reduce the anxiety caused by the cocaine). **Polysubstance dependence** is diagnosed when an individual abuses at least three types of substances, excluding caffeine and nicotine, and suffers the consequent functional impairments without one substance dominating the pattern of use (APA, 2000).

Alcohol Use

Alcohol use disorders are classified by the amount of alcohol consumed. For example, a "low-risk" male drinker has no more than 4 drinks on any single day and no more than 14 drinks per week (for women, no more than 3 drinks on any day and no more than 7 drinks per week) (NIAAA, 2009). Drinking more than these daily and weekly limits is

The Lived Experience

A Cocktail of Emotions: Loving a Parent With Alcoholism

Alcoholism is a disease that affects the whole family. Like a hangover, it can make all of its members sick—sick with a cocktail of emotions that consist of worry, guilt, anxiety, fear, frustration, loss, disappointment, and sadness. Family members learn about the disease through the perspective of the person using because it clearly affects their lifestyle and wellness. In my case, it was evident that as long as my father consumed alcohol, his life would be consumed by its consequences. What was not always visible was how my father's addictive behaviors could affect my wellness or transform the typical roles in a father–daughter relationship.

It is important for me to begin with sharing the positive side of my father because, all too often, the damaged path of alcoholism can make people lose sight of the person that exists outside the disease. First and most important, my dad always reminded me that I was loved. This was done in many ways, such as a hug or saying, "I love you" in person, by mail, or on the phone. It was also done through fun activities like camping, fishing, snowmobiling, or learning to drive stick shift. He also showed me how little things were big things in the grand scheme of life. He did this by taking time out to train, watch, and play with dogs; taking a walk in the woods; and visiting with others, especially family. We had quality visits with my grandparents, great-grandparents, aunts, and uncles that included reminiscing and joke-telling over a game of cards. Last, he taught me that material things were nothing compared to the gift of conversation. These are the strengths in character that made the consequences of alcohol use that much more of a devastating loss.

Unfortunately, I also have painful memories of how my dad's alcohol use interfered with our time together. From a young age, I recognized the unbreakable loyalty that my father had to alcohol. It was like his best friend. It was someone he could depend on, someone he couldn't get enough of, someone he would sacrifice anything to protect. In some ways, this relationship made me jealous. It was the arch rival I would battle for my dad's time. Often this "best friend" would win and my dad would choose to be with him over me, or he would bring his "best friend" along to events, knowing that alcohol was an uninvited guest. This was the case during important times in my life such as holidays, graduations, and other special occasions. It was not uncommon to get a phone call from my dad shamefully admitting that he could not be a part of the gathering because he had been drinking. I would be crushed and he knew it. It hurt more to know that my dad felt just as much sadness and disappointment, but could not change his behavior and would then take solace in a bottle of beer. At the same time, I would bottle up my feelings in order to function and try to enjoy the occasion despite my sadness. Sometimes my dad would be present but would be under the influence of alcohol (his uninvited guest). On the one hand, I felt relieved that my dad was with me; I knew he was safe and that he tried to be part of the family event. On the other hand, I felt fear. The unpredictability was unnerving;

I didn't know how he would act, how others would respond, and I didn't understand why he could not just be sober. The effect of my dad's drinking was ironic. To him, drinking was pleasurable and made him feel good. To me (and anyone who loved him), his drinking was unpleasant and made me feel sick. The amount of concern I had was exhausting. Typically, a parent is the one who worries about their child; in my case, the roles were reversed. I've been saying prayers for my dad's safety for as long as I can remember.

Role reversal was present in many situations. Parents usually put their own agenda aside to attend to their children's needs, interests, and so forth. When one has a parent with alcoholism, often the needs of the child are put aside to attend to the behaviors and addiction needs of the parent. An example of this was turning the focus of a family party from a celebration of my accomplishment to an intervention for my father. At the time, I was not concerned about myself; I just wanted my dad healthy. My family did their best to support me and tried to keep the celebration going amid the intervention, but when the cake of burning candles arrived, my wish was for my dad to get better.

Another instance of role reversal included wanting to avoid bars or to avoid spending too much time there. This was atypical because, while at a bar with my dad, my brother and I received a lot of attention from him and the other patrons. They fed us candy bars, sodas, chips, and loads of quarters to play pinball or darts. What kid wouldn't like that? Of course, it eventually got tiresome, and I knew that my dad's famous line of, "One more," meant at least "two more" and that his drinking was an activity that would eventually lead to more problems. As a child I was aware of the dangers of drinking and driving. Fortunately, my mom, older brother, and extended family played an important role with my safety. They would make arrangements so that I would have a safe ride home. Unfortunately, this could not always be controlled. One night, shortly after my dad dropped us off, he put his vehicle in a ditch. My brother and I wanted to keep our dad safe and, when we could, we drove. At age 14, my brother was caught driving my father home because he thought it was the more responsible thing to do.

These troubling circumstances would sometimes initiate intervention. My father's temporary residence at halfway houses would not only be respite for his drinking, but also for my worries. I would feel hopeful when my dad sought out the path of sobriety. I trusted that without alcohol's interference, we could just enjoy our time together. This proved to be true, but unfortunately not forever. Eventually, my father would once again choose to live a life in which drinking was a primary occupation. From my father's perspective, that occupation brought him life, and, from my perspective, it threatened to take his life. At one point, my father began using alcohol so regularly and excessively that when he was detained on an emergency, the absence of alcohol provoked a delirium tremor, causing a violent seizure where he cut up his tongue. I thought that this would be rock bottom, but as I mentioned earlier, there was an unbreakable loyalty to alcohol. Because of this loyalty and the consequent

Continued

problems, my hope began to fade, and I expected that if things were going right, something was likely to go wrong. I started to realize that no matter how much encouragement and support was provided, my father's relationship with alcohol was non-negotiable.

As a teenager, I realized I was unsuccessful with attempting to "fix" my dad, so unknowingly I began pouring my helping energy into troubled boys of my age. Like my relationship with my father, I was caring too much and feeling somehow responsible for helping. Through support, education, and literature, I learned that my behavior had a name—"codependency." Fortunately, I learned to let go of the exhausting caregiver effort in my relationships and started channeling my energy back into taking care of myself. I believe because of this knowledge, I took charge of not falling into the startling statistics that indicated that by being a child of a parent with alcoholism, I was at a high risk of marrying an alcoholic.

As an adult, I developed more skills to protect myself from my father's continued use of alcohol. I set up boundaries that minimized my exposure to my dad's drinking, but even with this, I could not be immune to the hurt and pain from his drinking. Like 15 years prior, our relationship would be compromised by his inability to refrain from using. On one occasion, I eagerly looked forward to hosting dinner at my new apartment, only to find myself pacing and investigating the whereabouts of my father. Later, I would learn that he had been arrested for driving under the influence, instead of having a nice evening of conversation over a home-cooked meal. This made me furious on so many

levels. I was angry for having my guard down and being so hopeful that my father would show up as promised, angry for realizing that his drinking was so out of control that it took precedence over any regard for my efforts and feelings, and angry for his disregard of the safety of himself and others (something that was opposite of his appreciative, sensitive, humane character). It was times like this that I questioned how much more I could take. The alternative of having no relationship was one I thought about, but I believed that it would be more devastating than dealing with the raw emotions of addiction.

Because of forced sobriety for several years, my relationship with my father was free of crisis, allowing an opportunity to reconnect with the father I knew existed. During our sober visits, I felt lucky to be in his company. He was the dad I kept in my heart and in my prayers; he was generous with his few resources, full of compassion, easy to talk to, fun to be around, showed his good sense of humor and made me laugh, preserved family memories through story-telling, and expressed a genuine interest in the lives of people he loved. I believe that my dad has made a valuable contribution to my life and still have hope that he will continue to do so.

This hope comes with caution because I am aware of the reality that my father must *want* to pursue a sober life, which will be no small feat. However, as of today, he has expressed a genuine willingness to be a part of a 6-month rehabilitation program for alcohol and other mental health treatment. For tonight, this brings me a sense of peace. For the future, my serenity is dependent on how I choose to take care of myself.

considered "at-risk" or "heavy" drinking, where the potential to suffer harm such as injuries, health problems, birth defects, or alcohol use disorders is increased. Amount is typically measured based on a common definition of a "unit" of an alcohol beverage, referred to as a standard drink (DuFour, 1999). One standard drink contains 0.5 to 0.6 fluid ounces (1.2 Tablespoons) of absolute ethanol, which is equal to 12 ounces of beer or wine cooler; 8 to 9 ounces of malt liquor; 5 ounces of table wine; 3 to 4 ounces of fortified wine (e.g., sherry or port); 2 to 3 ounces of a cordial, liqueur, or aperitif; and 1.5 ounces of spirits (whiskey, gin, vodka) (Fig. 15-1). Measures of standard drinks are always approximate, given the many types, brands, and containers of alcohol beverages. There is often more than one standard drink in a common size container. For example, a 16-ounce beer, or pint of beer, equals 1.3 standard drinks, so three bottles of beer are actually considered to be 4 standard drinks.

Alcohol use disorders are also categorized by patterns of consumption, including the frequency and quantity of drinking, as well as when, where, and with whom alcohol is consumed. Terms used to describe drinking patterns include abstainer, infrequent, moderate, responsible, social, frequent, high-risk, heavy, and binge drinker. Unfortunately, there are no clear, universally accepted definitions for most of these terms, and some are used interchangeably and inaccurately. The Dietary Guidelines for Americans, which are developed and revised every 5 years by the U.S. Department

of Health and Human Services and the U.S. Department of Agriculture (2005), define moderation as one drink per day for women and no more than two drinks per day for men. The NIAAA clinical guidebook, *Helping Patients Who Drink Too Much* (2005a), defines a heavy drinking day as four or more alcoholic beverages for women and five or more for men younger than age 65.

As a subtype of alcohol use disorder, "moderate" drinking has received the most attention from the popular media. The release of any research report suggesting the positive benefits of consuming a popular substance such as chocolate, caffeine, or alcohol typically draws a spot on the evening news. Research on middle-age to older adults over the past decade supports a positive relationship between light to moderate alcohol consumption (smaller amounts consumed several times a week as compared with the same amount on fewer occasions) and reduction in risk factors for coronary heart disease regardless of sex, age, smoking habits, and body mass index as compared with nondrinkers or heavy drinkers (NIAAA, 2003). Unfortunately, many moderate drinkers may periodically be heavy drinkers. It has been reported that any episode of heavy drinking significantly increases the risk of heart disease (Murray et al, 2002). Other suggested health-related benefits of light to moderate alcohol use are under ongoing scrutiny by researchers; at this time, the previously suggested moderate drinking guideline is the safest one for most adults to follow.

What Is a Standard Drink?

A standard drink is any drink that contains about 14 grams of pure alcohol (about 0.6 fluid ounces or 1.2 tablespoons). Below are standard drink equivalents as well as the number of standard drinks in different container sizes for each beverage. These are approximate, as different brands and types of beverages vary in their actual alcohol content.

Standard Drink Equivalents	Approximate Number of Standard Drinks In:
BEER or COOLER	
12 oz. ~5% alcohol	• 12 oz. = 1 • 16 oz. = 1.3 • 22 oz. = 2 • 40 oz. = 3.3
MALT LIQUOR	
8-9 oz. ~7% alcohol	• 12 oz. = 1.5 • 16 oz. = 2 • 22 oz. = 2.5 • 40 oz. = 4.5
TABLE WINE	
5 oz. ~12% alcohol	• a 750 mL (25 oz.) bottle = 5
80-proof SPIRITS (hard liquor)	
1.5 oz. ~40% alcohol	• a mixed drink = 1 or more* • a pint (16 oz.) = 11 • a fifth (25 oz.) = 17 • 1.75 L (59 oz.) = 39

*Note: Depending on factors such as the type of spirits and the recipe, one mixed drink can contain from one to three or more standard drinks.

FIGURE 15-1. What is a standard drink? *From the National Institute on Alcohol Abuse and Alcoholism (n.d.). "What Is a Standard Drink?" Available at: http://pubs.niaaa.nih.gov/publications/Practitioner/pocketguide/pocket_guide2.htm (accessed November 17, 2009).*

Five subtypes of alcohol dependence have been empirically derived based on clinical characteristics of 1,484 alcohol-dependent respondents to a national survey (Moss, Chen, & Yi, 2007). The two most impaired groups (about 30% of the sample) demonstrated substantial rates of multigenerational alcohol dependence and the largest number of other psychiatric and drug use disorders with subsequent impaired psychosocial functioning. Members of these two groups were also most likely to seek help and were most likely to be seen by occupational therapists in alcohol treatment programs.

A comparably sized group (31% of the sample) consisted primarily of at-risk young adult drinkers commonly seen on college campuses and throughout society. Members of this group exhibited low rates of co-occurring disorders (CODs), psychosocial dysfunction, and multigenerational alcohol dependence; moderately high levels of occasional heavy drinking; and limited help-seeking behaviors.

The remaining 40% of participants in this survey displayed low to medium levels of CODs with higher psychosocial function, late onset with low rates of periodic heavy drinking, and moderate levels of help-seeking.

Drug Use

The subtypes of drug use disorder are less defined in the literature than the subtypes of alcohol use, mainly because of the vast number and types of abused drugs. They are not typically categorized by amount or patterns of use, but are often delineated by the category of drug (see list of illicit drugs noted previously), prescription or nonprescription drugs, age of users, and use by gender. An extensive discussion about subtypes of drug use is beyond the scope of this chapter. However, it is worth noting that classifications of drug use change as new drugs are created and become available. For example, methamphetamine was previously included in questions about prescription-type drugs in the NSDUH, but was redefined as a stimulant in the 2006 version (SAMHSA, 2007). There are also shifts in drug use trends. For example, club drugs such as ecstasy reached their peak of popularity in the 1990s; in more recent years, oxycodone has become increasingly popular (SAMHSA, 2007). Overall, there was a national peak in drug use in the late 1970s, followed by a decrease in the 1980s and an increase in the 1990s; use has remained relatively stable for the past decade (Compton, Thomas, Conway, & Colliver, 2005).

Methamphetamine, or meth, is an interesting drug to review for its many classifications of use. Pharmaceutical methamphetamine is a Schedule II prescription drug used for limited medical treatment of narcolepsy and attention deficit disorder. It is also easily produced illicitly from common ingredients (including pseudoephedrine, drain cleaner, and ammonia) and is a readily available and highly addictive stimulant (NIDA, 2006). Meth abuse and addiction has become a worldwide epidemic in the past decade, and abusers and addicts cross age groups, genders, races, and socioeconomic levels. In the United States, it can be categorized geographically, with use in the western states about three times higher than use in the Midwest and five times higher than use in the Northeast (SAMHSA, 2007).

Another subtype of drug use disorder is based on substance-induced mental disorders (APA, 2000). These include substance-induced delirium, persisting dementia, persisting amnesic disorder, psychotic disorder, mood disorder, anxiety disorder, sexual dysfunction, and sleep disorder, although not all drugs are associated with all conditions (e.g., amphetamines are not associated with persisting dementia or persisting amnesic disorder). There must be clear symptoms of drug-induced intoxication or withdrawal (or, in some cases, both) within approximately a 4-week time period for these diagnostic categories to be considered.

Finally, there are other substances outside the illicit drug categories identified in the NSDUH that are addictive and can lead to dependence and occupational impairment. These include anabolic steroids, nitrate inhalants or "poppers," nitrous oxide ("laughing gas"), catnip, betel nut, kava, and over-the-counter and prescription drugs (APA, 2000). The reader is urged to use the resources at the end of this chapter to learn more about these and other drugs and their potential impact on occupational therapy practice across the spectrum of health conditions.

Co-occurring Mental Illness

Co-occurring disorder (COD) is the term used to describe a person with a concurrent substance-related disorder and mental disorder. Chapter 16 is devoted to this condition. Note that comorbid substance use and mental illness are also frequently referred to in the literature as dual diagnosis (Tiet & Mausbach, 2007).

The 2006 NSDUH (SAMHSA, 2007) identifies serious psychological distress (SPD) and/or major depressive episode along with substance use/dependence/abuse as comorbid conditions. (Note that because the NSDUH is completed by a noninstitutionalized population, people with severe mental illnesses in inpatient or residential care facilities are excluded.) Of the 5.6 million adults (18 years and older) who reported having both SPD and a substance use disorder, almost one-half received no treatment, and only 8.4% received treatment for both conditions.

One of the challenges in treating COD is the necessity for independent establishment of both diagnoses before individuals can receive appropriate interventions. A recent report reviewed 59 studies of psychosocial and medication treatments and found that there is no documented treatment that is effective for CODs of substance use and one of the following mental disorders: depression, anxiety disorder, schizophrenia, bipolar disorder, severe mental illness, and nonspecified mental illness (Tiet & Mausbach, 2007). Existing treatments known to reduce psychiatric symptoms or decrease substance use tend to be effective for patients with CODs, but the success of integrated treatment is unclear.

A co-occurring diagnosis of substance-related disorder is more prevalent in individuals already diagnosed with a severe mental illness (e.g., schizophrenia or bipolar disorder) than with other mental illness (RachBeisel, Scott, & Dixon, 1999). Substance abuse by individuals with severe mental illness results in a wide range of adverse consequences, including poorer prognosis, higher costs due to greater use of acute psychiatric services, low compliance with treatment regimens, and overall decreased occupational functioning.

Fetal Alcohol Spectrum Disorder

Women of child-bearing age who drink are at risk for having a baby that has been affected by their alcohol use. Although women who know they are pregnant drink at rates considerably lower than their nonpregnant peers (11.8% compared to 53%) (SAMHSA, 2007), any alcohol use during pregnancy puts infants at risk for a variety of conditions that fall under the umbrella of **fetal alcohol spectrum disorder (FASD)**. These conditions include FAS, alcohol-related neurodevelopmental disorder, and other alcohol-related birth defects, which manifest themselves in a wide range of behavioral, cognitive, physical, and health-related problems throughout childhood with carryover into

Evidence-Based Practice

Although there has been a decrease in the rate of alcohol use by pregnant women in recent years, including a 60% drop in binge drinking between 2004 and 2006 (from 10.6% to 4.6%) (SAMHSA, 2007), unplanned pregnancies still pose considerable risk for having a baby with fetal alcohol spectrum disorder (FASD). According to the National Organization on Fetal Alcohol Syndrome (n.d.b), unexpected pregnancies account for half of all new pregnancies in the United States, and many women do not realize that they are pregnant for weeks or even months. During this time, they may consume alcohol. For women who are alcohol abusers or dependent on alcohol, the fear that they may lose their children may prevent them from seeking prenatal care and treatment for their addiction.

➤ Occupational therapy practitioners should inquire about alcohol use with all female clients of child-bearing age, regardless of setting or health condition. When appropriate, refer them to local clinics to obtain contraceptives and community organizations that provide substance abuse treatment confidentially and at minimal charge.

➤ Occupational therapists working in school-based settings who may be working with children with FASD should be aware of the health status of the mother, and seek opportunities to offer encouragement and support if the mother appears to be using alcohol or is pregnant.

National Organization on Fetal Alcohol Syndrome (NOFAS). (n.d.b). "Factsheet: FASD: What the Health Care System Should Know." Available at: http://www.nofas.org/MediaFiles/PDFs/factsheets/healthcare.pdf (accessed November 17, 2009).

adulthood (Fetal Alcohol Spectrum Disorders Center for Excellence, 2008). According to the National Organization on Fetal Alcohol Syndrome (NOFAS) (n.d.a), prenatal alcohol use is the most preventable cause of retardation and birth defects in the United States.

Diagnostic criteria for FAS are growth deficiencies, a specific pattern of facial abnormalities (i.e., thin upper lip, elongated and flattened midface, an indistinct philtrum [the midline groove in the upper lip], small eye openings), and CNS disorders seen as developmental and intellectual delays. Confirmed maternal use of alcohol is not required for a diagnosis of FAS, but is required for the other conditions noted previously such as alcohol-related neurodevelopmental disorder. Magnetic resonance imaging can be used to confirm FAS by revealing structural anomalies in the brains of individuals.

According to NOFAS (n.d.a), FASD is seen in approximately 40,000 live births annually, or in 1 out of every 100 births. Fortunately, FASD is not a genetic condition, and women who have FAS or are affected by FASD will not pass it on to their babies. However, most experts believe that there is no safe level of alcohol use during pregnancy (NOFAS, n.d.b). Because the developmental issues that accompany FASD often result in the children being referred to occupational therapy in early intervention programs or school-based programs, occupational therapists working with infants and children and in settings that emphasize family-centered care may find this chapter to be helpful in w orking with parents whose alcohol or drug use (past or current) presents as an issue needing attention.

Physical Disabilities and Medical Conditions

Substance use contributes to the cause of disabilities for up to 40% to 80% of the population with spinal cord and traumatic brain injuries; it is also a major cause of disabilities for individuals aged 20 to 21 and puts college students at risk for contracting sexually transmitted diseases such as HIV infection (Substance Abuse Resources and Disability Issues [SARDI], 2007b).

In addition to being a major contributor to the onset of disability, substances are frequently used to cope with the daily life issues affected by disability, such as loss of roles, underemployment, dependence on others for activities of daily living, altered instrumental activities of daily living, and excess free time. In fact, substance-related disorders occur in people with physical disabilities at a rate almost double that of people without disabilities (SARDI, 2007b). The U.S. Department of Health and Human Services (UDHHS; n.d.) states that approximately 4.7 million people who have a disability also have a substance-related disorder.

Substances can be used as a form of self-medication to manage pain and other health problems. Prescription medications for a physical condition are also subject to abuse and, when mixed with alcohol and illicit drugs, can be especially dangerous. A recent study on alcohol use among college students with disabilities found that 50% of them abused alcohol (i.e., met the criteria for high-risk drinking), as compared with 43.2% for all college students (Jerabek, 2008). A study of 3,216 people with vision loss found that 40% were moderate to heavy drinkers compared to 25% of the general population (Nelipovich & Buss, 1991).

Whether it is the cause of disability or occurs after the disability is present, a substance-related disorder complicates and undermines adjustment to a physical disability and hinders healthy progress through normal stages of development (Koch, Nelipovich, & Sneed, 2002). Substance-related disorders can be overlooked by rehabilitation professionals focused on addressing the impairments associated with physical disabilities and may even be tolerated (O'Rourke, 1993; SARDI, 2007a). Although addressing both conditions concurrently is desirable, it can be particularly challenging to do so, especially when the individual shows little readiness to change his or her use of alcohol or other drugs, or is unaware of the link between their drinking and its interference with achieving rehabilitation goals.

Use of illicit drugs and alcohol can also compromise treatment of and recovery from other medical conditions, such as cardiovascular disease and respiratory and gastrointestinal conditions. It has been reported that alcohol ingestion contributes to 4% to 14% of medical admissions, and illicit drugs contribute to 6% to 13% of medical admissions (Canning, Marshall, Kennel-Webb, & Peters, 1999; Mordal, Bramness, Holm, & Morland, 2008).

When working with individuals with medical conditions in the acute care setting, the occupational therapist's role is to assess activities of daily living, cognitive function, and safety issues. A study by McQueen, Allan, and Mains (2006) explored the potential for occupational therapists to use the **motivational interviewing (MI)** techniques developed by Rollnick and Miller (1995) with people who screened positive for alcohol abuse in an acute medical setting in the United Kingdom. MI is a client-centered process whereby the therapist uses nonconfrontational highly empathic responses to explore and resolve ambivalence toward change (Miller & Rollnick, 2002). Results suggest that the participants in the group that received the MI intervention provided by occupational therapists were more likely to reduce their alcohol consumption as compared with those in the control group, who received an informational booklet. More important, the study confirmed that it was both feasible and effective for occupational therapists to provide MI in a medical setting. MI as an effective intervention for people with substance-related disorders is reviewed in Chapter 23.

Etiology

The causes and origins of substance-related disorders involve complex biological, psychological and social mechanisms. Etiological areas that should be considered for their impact on occupational performance include genetic factors, temperament, psychological theories, and sociocultural influences.

Genetic Factors

Genetic factors play a key role in determining an individual's risk factor for alcohol dependence. Individuals with close relatives who are alcohol dependent (e.g., biological parents and grandparents) are three to four times more likely to develop alcohol dependence themselves. The variance of risk is influenced by the number of relatives affected, the severity of their illness, and the biological closeness of the relationships (e.g., father vs. uncle). It is widely documented that there is a significantly higher risk for alcohol dependence in identical twins as compared to fraternal twins when one twin is dependent. Adopted children whose biological parents were alcohol dependent have a three to fourfold increase in risk for developing dependence, even though they are raised by adoptive parents (APA, 2000). A single gene has not been clearly associated with alcohol dependence, but it is likely that a variety of genetic factors make an individual more vulnerable (NIAAA, 2005b). There is research that suggests inherited cognitive factors such as memory, attention span, abstract thinking, and visual-spatial skills (frontal and temporal lobe functions) are predictive of the age of first drink and frequency of drinking to intoxication in young males (NIAAA, 2005b).

The research on genetic factors linked to dependence on the many different types of illicit drugs is much more complex and less well developed given the range and character of drug addiction (e.g., the casual, chronic use associated with marijuana vs. the rapid path to dependence and quick development of tolerance with cocaine). Overall, genetic factors, along with other biological factors, account for some of the risk associated with developing a substance-related disorder. However, they are likely less influential than social and cultural experiences and intrapersonal factors, including temperament, expectations of the effects of the substance, and mood.

Temperament

Longitudinal studies have documented the relationship between childhood and adolescent behavior problems (e.g., vandalism, aggression) and problems in adulthood, including substance-related dependence (NIAAA, 2005b). Youths who exhibit a "difficult" temperament, such as problems with self-regulation of emotion, decreased attention span, and low "soothability," may have less control over their behavior in adulthood, which may result in substance use, abuse, and dependence. Substance use may occur as a means of self-medicating the mild and undiagnosed problems associated with the stressors and anxiety of poor self-regulation. For example, an individual with a mild learning disability may react with impulsive behavior in the classroom, which leads to academic problems and his or her eventual dropping out of school, which in turn results in affiliation with gang members who abuse substances.

A study by occupational therapists on the abuse of substances by adults presenting with sensory modulation disorder (defined as hyper- or hyposensitivity to sensory input) found that 67% abused CNS depressant substances (e.g., benzodiazepines, hypnotic agents, opioids, alcohol), 18% abused CNS stimulants (e.g., cocaine, nicotine, ecstasy, LSD), and 15% used a combination of both (Quadling, Maree, Mountjoy, Bosch, & Kotkin, 1999). This research contributes to the knowledge base on the effect of individual characteristics of temperament on the development of a substance-related disorder in adulthood with a stronger likelihood for abuse of alcohol and other CNS depressants. Implications for accurate diagnosis and intervention for sensory modulation disorder in childhood are considerable for later onset of substance-related problems.

Psychological Theories

Explanations for the development of substance-related disorders based on psychological theories are extensive and influence the course of treatment. Behavioral and cognitive models are reviewed here.

Traditional behavioral theories propose that all behavior is learned and maintained through either operant or classical conditioning. With **classical conditioning**, drinking or using drugs is paired with a person, location, or time of day and develops into a conditioned response. The theory of **operant conditioning** assumes that substance use is paired with a stimulus such as stress or anger and is reinforced by a perceived calm and lowered emotional state (NIAAA, 2005b). In both instances, substance use is identified with the maintenance of cravings and development of tolerance or is positively reinforced by a "reward" for using. Negative consequences associated with use (e.g., hangovers, legal problems, interpersonal conflicts) have less impact because they occur at a later time and are removed from the positive rewarding effect of using.

Cognitive models used to explain substance-related disorders focus on the role of thoughts, beliefs, and feelings that precede substance use and sustain it. The individual's perception of use as either a positive or negative event is influenced by these cognitive factors and eventually sustained by conditioning processes. For example, one begins using alcohol based on the belief that it will enhance one's comfort in social situations, and that belief is reinforced throughout young adulthood by its availability and frequent use in new, unfamiliar social situations, such as college or a new job. As one moves into marriage and parenthood, where social situations become more familiar and comfortable, the perceived need and thus the social use of alcohol diminishes.

There is a body of literature that supports the impact of modeling (i.e., learning through observing and doing what others do both in real life and via the media) and one's experiences on the expectations that one has about using substances, especially alcohol (NIAAA, 2005b). These expectations, referred to as **expectancies**, have been identified in children and

are associated with the age of onset of drinking, plans to use alcohol, and drinking rates (NIAAA, 2005b). Although linked with positive reinforcers, such as tension reduction and social facilitation, positive expectancies are also identified with memory processes in that they are easily retrieved when in a new drinking situation, especially for individuals who use alcohol socially without experiencing compelling negative consequences. In other words, when a person drinks socially and only experiences relaxation and social connectedness with no negative consequences (e.g., saying or doing something embarrassing while under the influence), the positive expectancies are fairly automatic.

Sociocultural Influences

The relationship among family, peers and social environments, and substance-related behaviors and beliefs are well documented in the literature. It is less clear whether the multitude of relationships that have been examined are causal for substance use or merely associative. For example, does the young adult woman engage in high-risk drinking in college because of the alcohol dependence in her nuclear family, or does this experience influence her to abstain from drinking in college entirely? Is the relationship to use of alcohol different if the young adult is male rather than female? Environmental risk factors for substance-related disorders certainly exist, but there is tremendous variation as to their role in the development of the disorder at a later stage of life.

Research on the role of the family on substance-related disorders, particularly alcohol use, is complex (NIAAA, 2005b). Use of substances by parents, intimate partners, and siblings has been examined for its influence on the development of substance-related disorders in other family members, particularly children. Child-rearing practices, the centrality of substance use to family function, and the impact of substances on family members' ability to maintain key roles (e.g., parent as caregiver and provider) are all related to the development of substance use and abuse in others in the family (NIAAA, 2005b). Children who grow up in situations where substance abuse negatively affects family functioning are at greater risk for developing their own problems related to substance use. However, the influence of protective factors (e.g., extended family members who support the child, temperament of the child, maintenance of positive family rituals) may allow those who grow up in families with substance-related disorders to avoid and distance themselves from substance use throughout their childhood and adolescence, and into adulthood. In addition, family factors can be positively related to change in behavior where negligence of functions that support the integrity of the family (e.g., full-time employment of the father) create such hardship for loved ones that there is internal motivation to make and sustain changes in substance-related behaviors.

The onset of use of both alcohol and many illicit drugs is most likely to occur during the mid- to late teens (APA, 2000). This is both a developmental phenomenon (i.e., increased independence and valued peer approval) and a response to greater availability and societal tolerance (e.g., college drinking as a rite of passage). The 2006 NSDUH data supports this, reporting that the average age of first alcohol use among those aged 12 to 21 was 15.8 years (SAMHSA, 2007). Average age for first use of inhalants, PCP, marijuana, and LSD is 15.7, 16.3, 17.4, and 19.4 years, respectively. Adolescents report that their interest in using substances is influenced by expectancies of increased sociability, reduced anxiety and boredom, and the perceived positive experience of getting high (NIAAA, 2005b). The following Evidence-Based Practice box explores the influence of music. Close peer relationships factor in the initiation of use, and an individual whose best friend or other peer associations support use is predictive of the individual's future use. However, it is unclear whether these associations are the risk factor for use or whether the use of illicit substances based on other influences (e.g., family problems, co-occurring mental illness) results in peer associations that continue to support use (Deas & Thomas, 2002).

Young Adults and College Age

The use of alcohol among young adults, particularly college students, warrants a brief discussion, specifically in light of recent reports that drinking on college campuses is a serious health problem and occurs at epidemic proportions (National Center on Addiction and Substance Abuse, 2007; NIAAA, 2002b). Young adults aged 18 to 25 are, for the most part, identified with the heaviest use of alcohol and illicit drugs across all categories, particularly among males. It is well documented that many students enter college with their drinking habits already established. Interestingly, drinking among college-bound high school students is generally lower than their peers without plans for college, likely due to real and perceived pressure to achieve in academics, athletics, the arts, and so forth. However, once in the college environment, students who are enrolled full time drink at considerably higher rates (66.4% past month use) compared to their peers who are part-time college students or are not currently enrolled (54.1% past month use) (SAMHSA, 2007).

The factors that influence young adults to drink (personal, social, environmental), particularly on college campuses, are often continuations of influences from adolescence. The college environment is seen as a relatively safe place for young adults, yet periodic drinking at very high levels of intoxication is fairly common (up to 64% of all college students), and the consequences of drinking can have a serious impact on the drinker and those around them. Most academic years are tarnished with media reports of serious injuries and deaths within the ranks of college students, often associated with Greek organization rituals, celebrations around athletic events, and spring break outings. More common and seemingly less serious negative consequences, such as missed classes, hangovers, nausea and vomiting, depression, anxiety, memory loss, and relationship problems, can potentially have very serious life impacts when experienced cumulatively. Unintended sexual activity and sexual assaults are common occurrences on college campuses and are most often associated with the excessive use of substances, particularly alcohol. Roommates and friends experience the secondhand consequences of a peer who drinks to excess via excessive noise, physical caregiving, and emotional support when problems arise due to drinking. Almost all students who reside on a college campus face disrupted sleep and study and the potential for damaged property because of someone else's misuse of alcohol. The entire campus community—students, staff, and neighbors—suffers through the negative consequences of excessive drinking on college campuses across the United States (National Center on Addiction and Substance Abuse, 2007).

Evidence-Based Practice

There is research evidence of a relationship between substance use and aggression in young people who listen to certain types of music. Alcohol and drug use and aggressive behaviors were positively associated with listening to rap, techno and reggae music in a cross-sectional study of a diverse population of college students with typical drinking behavior (74% drank in past month) under age 25. Specifically, alcohol use disorder was significantly associated with *often* (subjectively defined) listening to heavy metal, punk, rap, reggae and rock music; higher scores on a sensation-seeking scale positively predicted frequency of alcohol, marijuana, and club-drug use and aggressive behavior

Music listening and preferences in music are established at increasingly younger ages (e.g., seeing elementary age children using portable listening devices such as iPODs).

➤ Occupational therapists who work with adolescents in any capacity, but particularly in substance abuse programs, should pay attention to the use of listening devices and the choices for music at recreational and other activities.

Chen, M., Miller, B. A., Grube, J. W., & Waters, E. D. (2006). Music, substance use, and aggression. *Journal of Studies on Alcohol, 67,* 372–381.

Evidence-Based Practice

A relationship has been found between drinking heavily in college (defined as three or more drinks at least 4 days per week, or five or more drinks in one sitting at least 2 days per week) and an increased amount of a biological marker for inflammation of the heart called C-reactive protein (CRP). The level of CRP associated with moderate risk of heart disease is between 1 and 3 milligrams per liter.

There were significant differences in CRP levels between students who were moderate drinkers (consumed two to five drinks 1 to 2 days per week) and those who drank heavily, with the average CRP level at 0.58 for moderate drinkers and 1.25 for heavy drinkers. Although this research was done on a nonrandom group of 25 college students, it suggests another reason to be concerned about the potential dangers associated with heavy drinking among college students. Campuses tend to focus on those risks that are most immediate, including academic and personal problems. A causative relationship between college drinking and heart disease could only be determined with a longitudinal study of students at college age and into middle age. However, if CRP levels prove to be predictive of future risk of heart disease, moderating drinking behaviors while in college might prove to be beneficial both now and in the future.

➤ Occupational therapists working with young adults, regardless of setting or medical condition, can caution them about the potential long-term risks associated with the periodic high-risk drinking common in this age group.

American Heart Association. (2007). "Drinking Heavily in College May Lead to Heart Disease Later in Life." Meeting Report, April 19. Available at: http://www.americanheart.org/presenter.jhtml?identifier=3047060 (accessed November 17, 2009).

Older Adults

Substance-related disorders, specifically alcohol-related disorders, in adults aged 65 and older are less studied and reported on than other segments of the U.S. population. Few older adults identify problems with substances in primary care visits or seek assistance in specialized alcohol treatment programs, so epidemiological data on this group is incomplete. An important consideration with older adults is the likelihood of problems created by using alcohol in combination with the use of prescription and over-the-counter medications.

Low-risk drinking limits for healthy adults aged 65 and older are no more than 3 drinks in a day and no more than 7 drinks in a week (NIAAA, 2005a). It was reported in a 1996 study of adults older than 60 that 15% of men and 12% of women regularly drank more than the NIAAA recommended guidelines at the time, which suggested less than 7 drinks per week for women and less than 14 drinks per week for men; 9% of men and 2% of women reported having more than 21 drinks per week (Adams, Barry, & Fleming, 1996). Although these figures may seem high, the vast majority of older adults do not drink at all (65%), and the remaining 20% drink modestly (i.e., within the recommended guidelines) and do not drink in risky situations such as prior to operating a car or boat (NIAAA, 2005b).

One of the challenges in identifying causes of alcohol-related problems in older adults is the difficulty in determining whether changes in occupational behaviors are related to alcohol misuse or to the onset of medical conditions. As the aging U.S. population continues to grow, with baby boomers moving into the 65 and older age group, the problems of detecting, understanding, and treating substance-related disorders in older adults will become more significant to society.

Prevalence

According to the 2006 NSDUH (SAMHSA, 2007), slightly more than one-half of all Americans aged 12 and older use alcohol. The breakdown by ages, as shown in Figure 15-2, shows an increase in alcohol use through ages 21 to 25, followed by a decrease in use for ages 26 and older.

The NSDUH also reports information about the nonmedical use of illicit drugs: marijuana (including hashish), cocaine (including crack), heroin, hallucinogens (including LSD, PCP, peyote, mescaline, mushrooms, and "ecstasy"), inhalants, and psychotherapeutics (the nonmedical use of prescription-type pain relievers, tranquilizers, stimulants such as methamphetamines, and sedatives) (SAMHSA, 2007). The percentage of Americans older than 12 who report illicit drug use (8.3%) has remained relatively stable since 2002. The most popular illicit drug is marijuana, which represents 72.8% of all drug use and is the only drug in use for 52.8% of users. It is used by 14.8% of the population older than 12 years and has the highest rate of use among young adults aged 18 to 25 years (16.3%) (SAMHSA, 2007). Additional information on prevalence and incidence from the 2006 NSDUH, and previous editions are available at http://www.oas.samhsa.gov/.

Course and Severity

The patterns of substance-related disorders vary widely based on the substance of abuse, age of onset, duration and intensity of use, and co-occurring conditions. As stated previously, the first episode of alcohol intoxication typically occurs in the mid-teen years. Several trajectories of use from adolescence into early adulthood have been described (NIAAA, 2005b):

- *Early-heavy*, with early onset and high frequency of drinking
- *Late-moderate*, with later onset and moderate frequency
- *Infrequent*, with early onset and low frequency
- *Abstainers/light users/non-bingers*

Most young people fall into one of the last two groups and have a low risk of future substance-related disorders (Maggs & Schulenberg, 2004/2005). The transition to adult roles of marriage and parenthood are influential in changing drinking behaviors; this occurrence is sometimes described as "maturing out" of problematic drinking (O'Malley, 2004/2005).

Alcohol abuse leads to dependence in a segment of the population and usually occurs by the late 30s. Dependence is not a life sentence and, among more highly functioning individuals, a 1-year abstinence rate occurs for 65% following treatment (APA, 2000). The course of dependence is characterized by times of remission and relapse, where a period of abstinence may be followed by an interval of controlled drinking that ultimately results in the resumption of heavy use and severe problems. This phenomenon of dependence, or addiction, to alcohol and other substances of misuse is increasingly understood to have a strong neurochemical base that may be linked to genetics (Gutman, 2006). This body of research suggests that the brain undergoes permanent neurochemical alterations that continue to trigger extreme cravings despite extended periods of abstinence. Neurochemical changes in the brain provide a basis for our understanding of the effectiveness of pharmaceutical treatment for addiction to substances (see Medications section) (Gutman, 2006).

Alcohol Use in the United States by Age

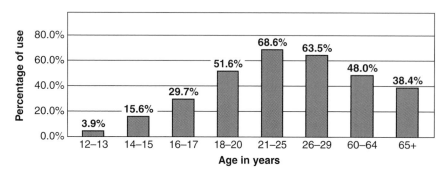

FIGURE 15-2. Alcohol use in the United States by age. *Data from Substance Abuse and Mental Health Services Administration (SAMHSA). (2007). Results From the 2006 National Survey on Drug Use and Health: National Findings. Office of Applied Studies, NSDUH Series H-32, DHHS Publication No. SMA 07-4293. Rockville, MD: Author.*

The course of abuse and dependence for the many types of illicit drugs varies greatly; in addition, little is known about the long-term course of use of several illicit drugs, including cocaine, opioids, hallucinogens, and inhalants (APA, 2000). The role of marijuana (cannabis) in different cultures and as a legal remedy for certain health conditions is a factor to consider when examining the processes that lead to its abuse and dependence. About 5% of the U.S. population report lifetime use of marijuana, with about 2 million new users annually (6,000 initiates per day) for the past 5 years (SAMHSA, 2007). Young people who develop dependence on marijuana are more likely to have co-occurring personality and conduct disorders. Marijuana is also frequently described as a "gateway" drug to other substance misuse, although the actual progression of this phenomenon is not well understood (APA, 2000). For drugs that can be smoked or used intravenously, the path from experimentation to abuse to dependence on illicit drugs is often rapid. Long-term dependence can have serious adverse mental and physical effects such that the user can no longer afford the financial, emotional, and physical costs to continue use and seeks treatment requiring total abstinence and lifestyle changes.

Gender Differences

There are differences between men and women in the use of substances; in general, males use alcohol and illicit drugs at higher rates than females. The characteristics of substance-related disorders (prevalence, course, etiology, interventions, etc) have historically been influenced by research on males. Although there are similarities in the substance-related experiences of men and women, there are also significant biological, social, environmental, and psychological differences. One area discussed previously in this chapter is the occurrence and prevention of fetal alcohol spectrum disorders, which is a uniquely female issue.

Males aged 12 and older consume alcohol at a higher rate than females (57% compared with 45.2%). Among young adults aged 18 to 25, the rates of use are 65.9% for men and 57.9% for women. The only switch in the ratio of male/female use occurs in youth aged 12 to 17, where 17% of females and 16.3% of males drink alcohol. Likewise, males aged 12 and older use illicit drugs at a higher rate than females (10.5% vs. 6.2%), with rates of marijuana use at twice the rate for males. Males are also twice as likely as females to abuse or be dependent on illicit substances (12.3% as compared to 6.3%) (all data from the 2006 NSDUH) (SAMHSA, 2007). Alcohol consumption affects females differently than men. Females usually have a smaller body mass than males, which explains some of the differences; however, dissimilar absorption rates and a greater ratio of body fat to water also play a role. When body mass and consumption rates are similar, females get more intoxicated than males because they metabolize alcohol differently due to smaller amounts of stomach enzymes and have higher concentrations of alcohol in their bloodstream due to less body water content (NIAAA, 2005b).

Women with alcohol dependence are more likely to come from a family in which a parent has a substance-related disorder, and they have twice the likelihood of experiencing sexual abuse in childhood compared to the broader population of women in general. The result is greater potential for

co-occurring mental illnesses, higher rates of partner violence, and less economic and social resources (e.g., divorced single parents with low incomes) (NIAAA, 2005b). Women are less represented in substance-related treatment programs, possibly due to fewer social and economic supports and child care issues. Once in treatment, they may be overwhelmed by guilt and low self-esteem, and be vulnerable to fears about loss of parental rights if they reveal too much information about their needs and problems. Women have better alcohol treatment outcomes in programs that personalize interventions and where they have choice; they may be more successful in treatment programs targeted specifically to women as compared to mixed-gender programs (NIAAA, 2005b).

Culture-Specific Information

Much of our knowledge about substance-related disorders is based on research and study of historically male populations that are predominantly white. Not surprisingly, though, differences in alcohol and illicit drug use, abuse and dependence across different ethnic, racial, and cultural groups have been identified, and thus result in differences in prevalence, course, etiology, interventions and so forth. Of course, individuals are more than their age, sex, race, or culture, so adoption of a client-centered approach will promote focus on the individual in treatment of substance-related disorders. Nonetheless, a client's ethnic and cultural (ethnocultural) background has an effect on their occupational behaviors and needs, and their achievement of intervention outcomes. There are substantial commonalities within ethnocultural groups; group affiliation is often a valued identity and resource for its members. As can be understood from the data reflected here, some groups might be protected from risky use due to intolerance of alcohol or other drugs, whereas other groups might be much more likely to be inclined toward risky levels of use.

Substance use data for different ethnocultural groups in the United States is organized around race, that is, the classification of people "on the basis of genetically transmitted physical characteristics" (Straussner, 2001, p. 5). According to the 2006 NSDUH, the racial group that consumes the most alcohol in people aged 12 and older is white (55.8%). Table 15-1 shows the rates for all U.S. racial groups.

Table 15-1 ● **Reported Alcohol Use by U.S. Racial Groups, Aged 12 and Older (%)**

Race	Reported Alcohol Use (%)
White	55.8
Two or more races	47.1
Hispanic	41.8
Black	40.0
American Indian/Alaska Native	37.2
Native Hawaiians/other Pacific Islander	36.7
Asian	35.4

Source: Substance Abuse and Mental Health Services Administration (SAMHSA). (2007). Results From the 2006 National Survey on Drug Use and Health: National Findings. Office of Applied Studies, NSDUH Series H-32, DHHS Publication No. SMA 07-4293. Rockville, MD.: author.

Use of illicit drugs by racial groups is a somewhat different picture, with the highest rate for age 12 and older among American Indians/Native Americans at 13.7%. Table 15-2 shows the illicit drug use rates for all U.S. racial groups.

Substance abuse or dependence was reported to be the highest among American Indians/Native Americans (19.0%). Rates of abuse or dependence for all U.S. racial groups are found in Table 15-3.

Rates of substance use by racial groups provide only a very small part of the picture of ethnic and culture differences. Within each racial group are dozens if not hundreds of different ethnocultural orientations. For example, white includes Irish, Quaker, and Jewish ethnicity. Patterns of use vary widely within ethnocultural groups and across the life span. Some groups may permit substance use at younger ages, revere it within elders, but frown on it during the middle adult years when it may disrupt function in key life roles. Some groups incorporate substances into important religious and cultural ceremonies, whereas others disapprove of any public use.

There are also significant differences in the effects of substances within the many ethnocultural groups. Some of these differences may be due to biological and genetic factors (e.g., differences that affect absorption and metabolism of alcohol) (NIAAA, 2002a). Others may be due to disparities in prevention resources and access to health care when difficulties with

substance use first emerge; by the time a problem is serious enough to warrant medical attention, it may be in an advanced state and much more difficult to treat. Individuals from historically underserved populations who seek services for substance-related disorders may encounter discrimination, language barriers, sexism, and inconsistent quality of care based on geographic locations (e.g., central city urban, reservation, rural). Ethnocultural competence is a responsibility of all occupational therapy practitioners; it is a complex, challenging concern for all areas of practice and is especially critical for services to people with substance-related disorders that may also co-occur with the many health conditions seen by occupational therapists.

Impact on Occupational Performance

Occupational therapists are concerned with the activities and routines that affect a person's ability to participate in meaningful occupational roles and achieve an overall state of health and well-being (AOTA, 2008). All areas of occupation identified in the *Occupational Therapy Practice Framework* (AOTA, 2008) may be affected by substance-related disorders, including

- Activities of daily living (ADL)
- Instrumental activities of daily living (IADL)
- Rest and sleep
- Education
- Work
- Play
- Leisure
- Social participation

Given that the DSM-IV-TR (APA, 2000) criteria for substance abuse and dependence includes a negative impact on occupational role performance, the occupational nature of substance use disorders is central to identifying how substances have affected an individual's life, as well as helping the individual seek recovery and improve his or her quality of life (Martin, Bliven, & Boisvert, 2008; Stoffel & Moyers, 2001, 2004, 2005; Yeager, 2000).

Occupational therapy practitioners work with people in their early recovery to find specific routines that support one's recovery from substance-related disorders. Such routines might make it possible to pursue meaningful occupational roles such as parenting, taking care of a pet, driving a car, maintaining personal finances, eating and exercising in a healthy manner, maintaining a home, or participating with a spiritual community. In addition, a change in substance use may affect one's ability to fall or stay asleep, or may affect the quality of one's rest. Performance in school and work often precipitates outside attention to the negative consequences of substance use disorders (missed classes or days at work; poor school or work performance; attention from teachers, supervisors, or peers due to performance issues), further underscoring the occupational nature of substance use disorders. Pursuit of playful activities that provide enjoyment, leisure exploration, and participation in nondrinking or using environments can also be early challenges to making healthy changes in occupational routines. Frequently, conscious and deliberate choices about the people and places where one engages in social and community participation need to be

Table 15-2 ● **Reported Illicit Drug Use by U.S. Racial Groups, Aged 12 and Older (%)**

Race	Reported Illicit Drug Use (%)
American Indian/Alaska Native	13.7
Black	9.8
Two or more races	8.9
White	8.5
Native Hawaiians/Other Pacific Islander	7.5
Hispanic	6.9
Asian	3.6

Source: Substance Abuse and Mental Health Services Administration (SAMHSA). (2007). Results From the 2006 National Survey on Drug Use and Health: National Findings. Office of Applied Studies, NSDUH Series H-32, DHHS Publication No. SMA 07-4293. Rockville, MD.: Author.

Table 15-3 ● **Reported Substance Abuse or Dependence by U.S. Racial Groups, Aged 12 and Older (%)**

Race	Reported Substance Abuse or Dependence (%)
American Indian/Alaska Native	19.0
Native Hawaiian/Other Pacific Islander	12.0
Two or more races	12.0
Hispanic	10.0
White	9.2
Black	9.0
Asian	4.3

Source: Substance Abuse and Mental Health Services Administration (SAMHSA). (2007). Results From the 2006 National Survey on Drug Use and Health: National Findings. Office of Applied Studies, NSDUH Series H-32, DHHS Publication No. SMA 07-4293. Rockville, MD.: Author.

considered, as continuing to spend time in drinking or using environments with former drinking and using friends might place the person with a substance use disorder at high risk for relapse. Use of substances is likely woven into the fabric of everyday life, as evidenced by the seemingly common examples highlighted in this paragraph, and needs to be extricated so that the person seeking recovery and health can rebuild his or her lifestyle and occupational routines.

Evidence-Based Practice

Occupational therapists with a background in mental health are more likely to ask questions to screen for problematic use of alcohol or other drugs and to offer direct intervention than therapists in physical rehabilitation or gerontology practice areas, who are more likely to refer the person to others for alcohol and other drug abuse (AODA) services or self-help groups (Thompson, 2007). Screening and brief intervention strategies have been suggested as appropriate for occupational therapy practitioners across all areas of practice (Martin & Bonder, 2004; McQueen, Allan, & Mains, 2006; Stoffel & Moyers, 2001, 2004, 2005; Thompson, 2007).

➤ Use of screening tools such as the CAGE-AID (Brown & Rounds, 1995; Ewing, 1984) or the Fast Alcohol Screening Test (Health Development Agency, 2002) can be used in conjunction with tools such as the Occupational Performance History Interview (Kielhofner, Henry, & Whalens, 1989) to determine whether occupational issues are related to substance use so that intervention planning can be more effectively constructed.

➤ Offering brief intervention in the form of feedback, referral to AODA services, menu of options regarding change in substance use, and information about how substance use affects a person's life should follow such screening and assessment (McQueen, Allan, & Mains, 2006; Moyers & Stoffel, 1999; Stoffel & Moyers, 2004, 2005).

Brown, R. L., & Rounds, L. A. (1995). Conjoint screening questionnaires for alcohol and drugs abuse. *Wisconsin Medical Journal, 94,* 135–140.

Ewing, J. A. (1984). Detecting alcoholism: The CAGE questionnaire. *Journal of the American Medical Association, 252,* 1905–1907.

Health Development Agency. (2002). *Manual for the Fast Alcohol Screening Test (FAST).* London: Health Development Agency and University of Wales College of Medicine.

Kielhofner, G., Henry, A. D., & Whalens, D. (1989). *Occupational Performance History Interview (OPHI).* Bethesda, MD: American Occupational Therapy Association.

Martin, P., & Bonder, B. (2004). Screening for substance abuse. *OT Practice, 9*(8), 25–27.

McQueen, J., Allan, L., & Mains, D. (2006). Brief motivational counseling for alcohol abusers admitted to medical wards. *British Journal of Occupational Therapy, 69,* 327–333.

Moyers, P. A., & Stoffel, V. C. (1999). Alcohol dependence in a client with a work-related injury. *American Journal of Occupational Therapy, 53,* 640–645.

Stoffel, V., & Moyers, P. A. (2001). *Occupational Therapy Practice Guidelines for Substance Use Disorder* (3rd ed.). Bethesda, MD: American Occupational Therapy Association.

Stoffel, V., & Moyers, P. A. (2005). Occupational therapy and substance use disorders. In E. Cara & A. MacRae (Eds.), *Psychosocial Occupational Therapy: A Clinical Practice* (2nd ed., pp. 446–473). Albany, NY: Delmar

Stoffel, V. C., & Moyers, P. A. (2004). An evidence-based and occupational perspective of interventions for persons with substance-use disorders. *American Journal of Occupational Therapy, 58,* 570–586.

Thompson, K. (2007). Occupational therapy and substance use disorders: Are practitioners addressing these disorders in practice? *Occupational Therapy in Health Care, 21*(3), 61–77.

Interventions

Treatment for substance-related disorders may occur in many locations, including hospitals, emergency rooms, drug or alcohol rehabilitation facilities, mental health centers, private medical or psychology offices, prisons, and self-help groups. Most people who receive substance use treatment obtain it at self-help groups (2.2 million people in 2006), followed by outpatient treatment in drug or alcohol rehabilitation facilities (1.6 million people) and outpatient treatment in mental health facilities (1.2 million people). Less than 2% of the population receives treatment for any kind of problem related to substance use, abuse, or dependence, and the majority (55%) of those who receive treatment get services for alcohol-related disorders versus treatment for all other substances combined. Self-reported barriers to receiving appropriate interventions are ranked as follows (all data from the 2006 NSDUH) (SAMHSA, 2007):

1. No health coverage or could not afford the cost
2. Not ready to stop using
3. Able to handle problem without treatment
4. No transportation or inconvenient
5. Might cause neighbors/community to have negative opinions
6. No program having type of needed treatment

The most effective interventions for substance-related dependence are a combination of psychosocial and pharmaceutical approaches. The psychosocial therapies address the beliefs, coping/stress management techniques, and social skills necessary to function without reliance on substances. Pharmaceutical approaches (i.e., medications) affect the neurochemistry of addiction to reduce the positive effects of the illicit substances and reduce cravings (Gutman, 2006). Individuals diagnosed with severe mental illness and a substance-related disorder have been examined for their receptiveness to interventions using motivational and cognitive therapies (Barrowclough et al, 2001; Carey, Carey, Maisto, & Purnine, 2002; Carey, Purnine, Maisto, & Carey, 2001). The findings of these studies support an integrated approach of traditional therapies (e.g., medication, outpatient follow-up, access to day treatment) with motivational and cognitive-based interventions that address readiness to change and responsibility for one's own treatment program.

Specific intervention techniques aimed at motivation, coping skills, cognitive beliefs, and communication and interaction skills associated with occupations are covered in other chapters in this text; medications used for substance-related disorders, stages of change and harm reduction, contingency management, Project*MAINSTREAM*, and 12-step group participation recommendations for occupational therapists are reviewed here.

Medications

The past decade has seen substantial research on the use of medications to combat substance-related dependence. Three oral medications (naltrexone, acamprosate, and disulfiram) and an injectable form of naltrexone have been approved for treatment of alcohol dependence in the United States. Naltrexone has shown to be effective in reducing drinking relapses in the first 3 months of use; it is also effective for opiate addiction because it blocks opiate receptors in the brain, thus reducing the perceived positive benefits of both alcohol and opiate use (NIAAA, 2005a). It does not affect the perceived positive benefits of other types of drugs, so polysubstance users are less likely candidates for naltrexone (Gutman, 2006). Its usefulness has also been demonstrated in a small study of patients with both bipolar disorder and alcohol dependence, with patients reporting that the number of days of alcohol use and cravings were significantly decreased (Brown, Beard, Dobbs, & Rush, 2006).

Acamprosate reduces unpleasant symptoms associated with abstinence such as insomnia, restlessness, and dysphoria. Research indicates that it is more effective with patients who are more dependent, who abstain for a longer period of time before it is used, and whose goal for treatment is complete abstinence; however, more research is needed (Anton et al, 2006; NIAAA, 2005a, 20005b). Disulfiram (Antabuse) works by inhibiting metabolism; if the user ingests alcohol while on disulfiram, he or she experiences flushing, nausea, and tachycardia. Compliance is limited if patients must self-administer the drug, but it is effective with those who are highly motivated to abstain or for use in high-risk drinking situations (NIAAA, 2005a).

Medications that mimic the drugs they replace are used to reduce cravings and prevent relapse (Gutman, 2006). Methadone, used to treat heroin addiction and the most well-known example of this type of medication, is controversial because it is also addictive but does not have the negative effects of the illicit opiates it replaces, such as overdose, mortality, and risk of infections. Wellbutrin works similarly for smoking cessation and does not have the negative quality of becoming addictive (Gutman, 2006). Two new medications for alcohol dependence, topiramate and baclofen, are still in clinical trials with promising results, but have not been approved for use (Johnson, 2008; DeSousa, 2010). With advances in the neurosciences, there is reason to be hopeful that new drugs will be developed and studied.

Combining medications with behavioral therapies to treat alcohol dependence has been examined in a large, multisite research study involving 1,383 participants (Anton et al, 2006). Study participants received naltrexone and/or acamprosate, medical management (nine sessions on adherence and abstinence) and combined behavioral interventions (CBIs) using motivational interviewing approaches in various combinations. A placebo group received only the behavioral intervention. Although all participants demonstrated increases in the amount of time they abstained from drinking (main outcome measure), those who received naltrexone or CBI had the best outcomes (Anton et al, 2006).

Stages of Change and Harm Reduction

Changing any behavior is complex and challenging, and requires internal motivation, commitment, and a realistic understanding of the steps of change. A model for changing health behaviors such as addictions is the **stages of change** model (DiClemente & Prochaska, 1998), also referred to as the transtheoretical model. It is often used in research and intervention programs for substance-related disorders to better understand and use different interventions at various points in the pattern of substance use. The model proposes that individuals go through a series of stages (*precontemplation, contemplation, preparation,* and *action*) to accomplish change. There are intervention strategies that match the thoughts, beliefs, and readiness for change at each stage (e.g., during *preparation,* the participant might identify an alternate afternoon activity in place of "happy hour"; attending the alternate activity would occur during the *action* stage). Stoffel and Moyers (2004) provide examples of how occupational therapy practitioners might apply the stages of change model in their interventions with persons who struggle with their use of substances in an effort to facilitate their readiness to change. For example, when a person is in the contemplation stage, he or she might be aware of how his or her alcohol or drug use has caused problems in his or her life. The occupational therapist might have him or her explore the full set of good and not so good things associated with his or her substance use as a means to explore a life without alcohol or drugs, thereby facilitating movement from contemplation to preparation for change.

Harm reduction is a public health philosophy that incorporates practical strategies that help reduce the negative consequences associated with drug use (Harm Reduction Coalition, n.d.; Marlatt, 1998). It is viewed by critics as being in opposition to abstinence and has been somewhat controversial. Harm reduction advocates believe that the neurochemistry of addiction may preclude abstinence and that some strategies for using drugs are safer than others. Harm reduction approaches have been incorporated into brief interventions for alcohol use, most notably in primary care settings, where a minimal amount of time with a patient is devoted to alcohol issues (Fleming & Manwell, 1999). The goal of using a harm reduction approach in primary care is to reduce the number of problems associated with alcohol use and increase the patients' readiness to change their behavior.

Contingency Management

Contingency management (CM) is an intervention strategy that, using the principles of operant conditioning, provides reinforcing consequences for substance-abusing individuals who meet treatment goals. It has been used since the 1960s in both alcohol and other drug programs, and several studies support its effectiveness in reducing substance use, improving treatment attendance, and reinforcing medication compliance and treatment goals (Higgins & Petry, 1999). A CM program typically provides vouchers that can be redeemed for desirable items, such as bus tokens, clothing, movie passes, or even more expensive electronics when treatment goals are met (e.g., clean urine sample). Costs can be a barrier to use, however, and Petry (2006) describes an alternate system at about half the cost in which patients have an opportunity to receive a prize based on a drawing. This system has received renewed interest in the past decade because its use has been reexamined and found to be effective with polydrug abusers (Petry, Alessi, Hanson, & Sierra, 2007; Vandrey, Bigelow, & Stitzer, 2007).

Project*MAINSTREAM*

Project*MAINSTREAM* (www.projectmainstream.net) is part of an interdisciplinary effort by the Health Resources and Services Administration (HRSA), the Association for Medical Education and Research in Substance Abuse (AMERSA), the

Substance Abuse and Mental Health Services Administration (SAMHSA), and Center for Substance Abuse Treatment (CSAT) to prepare health professionals to address the needs of clients with substance-related disorders in response to goals set forth in Healthy People 2010. Occupational therapy is 1 of 15 professions targeted for faculty development in substance abuse education.

The strategic plan behind the project is to provide a foundation for the development of interdisciplinary faculty; it identifies the core knowledge, competencies, and skills needed by health professionals to effectively identify, intervene, and refer individuals with substance-related disorders. Health-care professionals, the front line providers to most people with substance-related problems, do not regularly identify and diagnose these conditions because they lack the skills and knowledge. Project*MAINSTREAM* has developed a complete course syllabus, including readings, handouts, and slide presentations, that is available at no cost. Topics covered include prevention, screening, assessment, intervention, referral, community involvement, assisting children of substance-abusing parents, and assisting older adults with issues on cultural competency integrated throughout. This resource can be adapted as necessary and is an excellent follow-up for readers of this chapter.

12-Step Group Participation

Given that the majority of people who received help for their substance use disorders get it from self-help groups (SAMHSA, 2007), occupational therapists should familiarize themselves with groups such as Alcoholics Anonymous (AA), Cocaine Anonymous (CA), and Narcotics Anonymous (NA), as well as their locations, frequency of meetings, and traditions, so that they can encourage access to this fellowship of support for recovery. Twelve-step programs are often referred to as being based on spirituality and social support, both of which are understood as important to recovery. Stoffel and Moyers (2004) provide a variety of ways in which occupational therapy practitioners can provide encouragement and build a recovery lifestyle consistent with self-help group participation.

Summary

This chapter provides the reader with important information about how substance-related disorders affect the occupational lives of people who live with substance abuse and dependence. Occupational therapy provides a variety of options to restoring health and well-being by providing the person with meaningful alternatives to use of alcohol and other drugs. Helping facilitate the readiness to change through skillful use of motivational interviewing, facilitating coping, and encouraging exploration, as well as use of 12-step self-help groups to build a co mmunity of support for recovery from alcohol and drug use, are potential ways an occupational therapy practitioner might promote change.

Active Learning Strategies

1. Cost of College Drinking

Although most college students "mature out" of heavy episodic drinking that occurs while they are in college, there can be substantial costs to drinking excessively, including financial costs, emotional costs, and even costs in terms of extra calories.

Go to the National Institute on Alcohol Abuse and Alcoholism website at http://www.collegedrinkingprevention.gov/CollegeStudents/calculator/default.aspx, which is devoted to college drinking prevention. On this site,
- Use the calculators to calculate the costs of drinking.
- Learn more about college drinking through the other resources on the site, especially those devoted to college students.
- Check if your campus subscribes to e-CHUG (www.e-chug.com) for a personalized analysis of college drinking at your school.

2. Substance Use Rates Close to Home

Go to the website of the Office of Applied Studies of the Substance Abuse and Mental Health Services Administration at http://www.oas.samhsa.gov/. Use this site to learn about the rates of alcohol, tobacco, marijuana, and other drug use for the state in which you live.

3. Self-Reflection

 Use the following prompts to reflect on substance abuse disorders and then describe your thoughts in your **Reflective Journal**.

Reflective Questions
- How do you feel about illicit drug use?
- Has your opinion changed in recent years?
- How do you feel about workplace drug testing?
- How do you feel about use of performance-enhancing drugs by athletes?
- Ask your friends about these topics to learn what they think and why.

4. Self-Help Meetings

Attend an open meeting of Alcoholics Anonymous, Al-Anon, Narcotics Anonymous, or another self-help group in your area. Be sure that you only attend OPEN meetings, and be aware of the need to abide by confidentiality. Use the Yellow Pages in your community to locate a number for the local Alcoholics Anonymous (you might also find meeting information available online); call the number and ask for the location and time of an upcoming open meeting. Once you attend, familiarize yourself with the format of the meeting because you might need to describe a meeting to future clients who are early in their own recovery process.

 In your journal, reflect on how members welcome others into the fellowship of the recovery community. Note how people describe their involvement in these self-help groups and the impact it seems to have on their health and well-being.

5. Narrative Analysis

Read The Lived Experience narrative in this chapter (A Cocktail of Emotions: Loving a Parent With Alcoholism) and note how the writer's father's use of alcohol affected the occupations in which he engaged. Note how these changes also affected the writer and the significance of occupational role performance when her father was drinking and when he was not.

Resources

Organizations and Programs

- National Institute on Alcohol Abuse and Alcoholism (NIAAA)—social work curriculum on alcohol use disorders: Available at: http://pubs.niaaa.nih.gov/publications/l
- BACCHUS Network—information about drinking, sexual health, tobacco use, and wellness for college students: http://www.bacchusnetwork.org and http://www.bacchusgamma.org/
- ProjectMAINSTREAM—education resource for health professionals who want to learn more about substance use disorders: http://www.projectmainstream.net
- SAMHSA's National Registry of Evidence-based Programs and Practices (NREPP): http://www.nrepp.samhsa.gov/
- Substance Abuse Resources and Disability Issues (SARDI): http://www.med.wright.edu/citar/sardi/index.html
- Guide to Evidence-Based Practices on the Web: http://www.samhsa.gov/ebpwebguide/index.asp

References

Adams, W. L., Barry, K. L., & Fleming, M. F. (1996). Screening for problem drinking in older primary care patients. *Journal of the American Medical Association, 276,* 1964–1967.

American Heart Association. (2007). "Drinking Heavily in College May Lead to Heart Disease Later in Life." Meeting Report, April 19. Available at: http://www.americanheart.org/presenter.jhtml?identifier=3047060 (accessed November 17, 2009).

American Occupational Therapy Association (AOTA). (2008). Occupational therapy practice framework: Domain and process, 2nd edition. *American Journal of Occupational Therapy, 62,* 625–683.

American Psychiatric Association (APA). (2000). *Diagnostic and Statistical Manual of Mental Disorders* (4th ed., text revision). Washington, DC: Author.

Anton, R. F., O'Malley, S. S., Ciraulo, D. A., Cisler, R. A., Couper, D., Donovan, D. M., Gastfriend, D. R., Hosking, J. D., Johnson, B. A., LoCastro, J. S., Longabaugh, R., Mason, B. J., Mattson, M. E., Miller, W. R., Pettinati, H. M., Randall, C. L., Swift, R., Weiss, R. D., Williams, L. D., & Zweben, A. (2006). Combined pharmacotherapies and behavioral interventions for alcohol dependence. *Journal of the American Medical Association, 295,* 2003–2017.

Barrowclough, C., Haddock, G., Tarrier, N., Lewis, S. W., Moring, J., O'Brien, R., Schofield, N., & McGovern, J. (2001). Randomized controlled trial of motivational interviewing, cognitive behavior therapy, and family intervention for patients with comorbid schizophrenia and substance use disorders. *American Journal of Psychiatry, 158,* 1706–1713.

Brown, E. S., Beard, L., Dobbs, L., & Rush, A. J. (2006). Naltrexone in patients with bipolar disorder and alcohol dependence. *Depression and Anxiety, 23,* 492–495.

Brown, R. L., & Rounds, L. A. (1995). Conjoint screening questionnaires for alcohol and other drug abuse. *Wisconsin Medical Journal, 94*(3), 135–140.

Canning, U. P., Marshall, E. J., Kennel-Webb, S. C., & Peters, T. J. (1999). Substance misuse in acute general medical admissions. *Quarterly Journal of Medicine, 92,* 319–326.

Carey, K. B., Carey, M. P., Maisto, S. A., & Purnine, D. M. (2002). The feasibility of enhancing psychiatric outpatients' readiness to change their substance use. *Psychiatric Services, 53,* 602–608.

Carey, K. B., Purnine, D. M., Maisto, S. A., & Carey, M. P. (2001). Enhancing readiness-to-change substance abuse in persons with schizophrenia: A four-session motivation-based intervention. *Behavior Modification, 25,* 331–384.

Chen, M., Miller, B. A., Grube, J. W., & Waters, E. D. (2006). Music, substance use, and aggression. *Journal of Studies on Alcohol, 67,* 372–381.

Compton, W. M., Thomas, Y. F., Conway, K. P., & Colliver, J. D. (2005). Developments in the epidemiology of drug use and drug use disorders. *American Journal of Psychiatry, 162,* 1494–1502.

Deas, D., & Thomas, S. (2002). Comorbid psychiatric factors contributing to adolescent alcohol and other drug use. *Alcohol Research & Health, 26*(2), 116–121. Available at: http://pubs.niaaa.nih.gov/publications/arh26-2/116-121.htm (accessed November 17, 2009).

De Sousa, A. (2010). The pharmacotherapy of alcohol dependence: A state of the art review. In A. R. Singh and S. A. Singh (Eds.), *Psychopharmacology Today: Some Issues* (MSM, 8, Jan–Dec 2010, pp. 69–82.

DiClemente, C. C., & Prochaska, J. O. (1998). Toward a comprehensive, transtheoretical model of change: Stages of change and addictive behaviors. In W. R. Miller & N. Heather (Eds.), *Treating Addictive Behaviors: Processes of Change* (2nd ed., pp. 3–24). New York: Plenum Press.

Drugs-Plaza. (n.d.). "Marijuana Music." Available at: http://www.drugs-plaza.com/music.htm (accessed November 17, 2009).

DuFour, M. C. (1999). What is moderate drinking? Defining "drinks" and drinking levels. *Alcohol Research & Health, 23*(1), 5–14. Available at: http://pubs.niaaa.nih.gov/publications/arh23-1/05-14.pdf (accessed November 17, 2009).

Ewing, J. A. (1984). Detecting alcoholism: The CAGE questionnaire. *Journal of the American Medical Association, 252,* 1905–1907.

Fleming, M., & Manwell, L. B. (1999). Brief interventions in primary care settings: A primary treatment method for at-risk, problem, and dependent drinkers. *Alcohol Research & Health, 23*(2), 128–137. Available at: http://pubs.niaaa.nih.gov/publications/arh23-2/128-137.pdf (accessed November 17, 2009).

Gutman, S. A. (2006). Why addiction has a chronic, relapsing course. The neurobiology of addiction: Implications for occupational therapy practice. *Occupational Therapy in Mental Health, 22*(2), 1–29

Harm Reduction Coalition. (n.d.). "Principles of Harm Reduction." Available at: http://www.harmreduction.org/article.php?list=type&type=62 (accessed November 22, 2009).

Harwood, H. (2000). *Updating Estimates of the Economic Costs of Alcohol Abuse in the United States: Estimates, Update Methods, and Data*. Report prepared by The Lewin Group for the National Institute on Alcohol Abuse and Alcoholism. (Based on estimates, analyses, and data reported in Harwood, H., Fountain, D., and Livermore, G. *The Economic Costs of Alcohol and Drug Abuse in the United States 1992*. Report prepared for the National Institute on Drug Abuse and the National Institute on Alcohol Abuse and Alcoholism, National Institutes of Health, Department of Health and Human Services. NIH Publication No. 98-4327. Rockville, MD: National Institutes of Health, 1998.)

Health Development Agency. (2002). *Manual for the Fast Alcohol Screening Test (FAST)*. London: Health Development Agency and University of Wales College of Medicine.

Higgins, S. T., & Petry, N. M. (1999). Contingency management: Incentives for sobriety. *Alcohol Research & Health, 23*(2), 122–127. Available at: http://pubs.niaaa.nih.gov/publications/arh23-2/122-127.pdf (accessed November 17, 2009).

Jerabek, A. L. (2008). "Alcohol Use Among College Students With Disabilities: An Exploratory Study." Unpublished master's thesis, University of Wisconsin–Milwaukee.

Johnson, B. A. (2008). Update on neuropharmacological treatments for alcoholism: Scientific basis and clinical findings. *Biochemical Pharmacology, 75,* 34–56.

Kielhofner, G., Henry, A. D., & Whalens, D. (1989). *Occupational Performance History Interview (OPHI)*. Bethesda, MD: American Occupational Therapy Association.

Koch, S., Nelipovich, M., & Sneed, Z. (2002). Alcohol and other drug abuse as coexisting disabilities: Considerations for counselors serving individuals who are blind or visually impaired. *Review, 33*(4), 151–159.

Maggs, J. L., & Schulenberg, J. E. (2004/2005). Trajectories of alcohol use during the transition to adulthood. *Alcohol Research & Health, 28*(4), 195–201. Available at: http://pubs.niaaa.nih.gov/publications/arh284/195-201.htm (accessed November 17, 2009).

Marlatt, G. A. (1998). *Harm Reduction: Pragmatic Strategies for Managing High-Risk Behaviors*. New York: Guilford Press.

Martin, L. M., Bliven, M., & Boisvert, R. (2008). Occupational performance, self-esteem, and quality of life in substance addictions recovery. *OTJR: Occupation, Participation and Health, 28,* 81–88.

Martin, P., & Bonder, B. (2004). Screening for substance abuse. *OT Practice, 9*(8), 25–27.

McQueen, J., Allan, L., & Mains, D. (2006). Brief motivational counseling for alcohol abusers admitted to medical wards. *British Journal of Occupational Therapy, 69,* 327–333.

Miller, W. R., & Rollnick, S. (2002). *Motivational Interviewing: Preparing People to Change Addictive Behavior* (2nd ed.). New York: Guilford Press.

Mordal, J., Bramness, J. G., Holm, B., & Morland, J. (2008). Drugs of abuse among acute psychiatric and medical admission: Laboratory based identification of prevalence and drug influence. *General Hospital Psychiatry, 31,* 55–60.

Moss, H. B., Chen, C. M., & Yi, H. (2007). Subtypes of alcohol dependence in a nationally representative sample. *Drug and Alcohol Dependence, 91*(2–3), 149–158.

Moyers, P. A., & Stoffel, V. C. (1999). Alcohol dependence in a client with a work-related injury. *American Journal of Occupational Therapy, 53,* 640–645.

Murray, R. P., Connett, J. E., Tyas, S. L., Bond, R., Ekuma, O., Silversides, C. K., & Barnes, G. E. (2002). Alcohol volume, drinking pattern, and cardiovascular disease morbidity and mortality: Is there a U-shaped function? *American Journal of Epidemiology, 155,* 242–248.

National Center on Addiction and Substance Abuse. (2007, March). *Wasting the Best and Brightest: Substance Abuse at America's Colleges and Universities*. New York: Columbia University.

National Institute on Alcohol Abuse and Alcoholism (NIAAA). (2002a). Alcohol Alert: Alcohol and minorities, an update, 55. Bethesda, MD: U.S. Department of Health and Human Services, Public Health Service, National Institutes of Health. Retrieved 5/13/10 from http://pubs.niaaa.nih.gov/publications/aa55.htm

National Institute on Alcohol Abuse and Alcoholism (NIAAA). (2002b). A call to action: Changing the culture of drinking at US Colleges. Rockville, MD: Author. Retrieved 5/13/10 from http://www.collegedrinkingprevention.gov/NIAAACollegeMaterials/TaskForce/TaskForce_TOC.aspx

National Institute on Alcohol Abuse and Alcoholism (NIAAA). (2003, December 19). "State of the Science Report on the Effects of Moderate Drinking." Available at: http://pubs.niaaa.nih.gov/publications/ModerateDrinking-03.htm (accessed November 17, 2009).

National Institute on Alcohol Abuse and Alcoholism (NIAAA). (2005a). *Helping Patients Who Drink Too Much: A Clinician's Guide*. Washington, DC: Author. (accessed November 17, 2009).

National Institute on Alcohol Abuse and Alcoholism (NIAAA). (2005b). Social Work Curriculum on Alcohol Use Disorders. Bethesda, MD: Author. Retrieved 5/13/10 from http://pubs.niaaa.nih.gov/publications/Social/main.html

National Institute on Alcohol Abuse and Alcoholism (NIAAA). (2009). "Rethinking Drinking: Alcohol and Your Health." Available at: http://RethinkingDrinking.niaaa.nih.gov (accessed November 17, 2009).

National Institute on Drug Abuse (NIDA). (2005, August). "Prescription Drugs: Abuse and Addiction." National Institute on Drug Abuse Research Report Series. NIH Publication No. 05-4881. Available at: http://www.drugabuse.gov/PDF/RRPrescription.pdf (accessed November 17, 2009).

National Institute on Drug Abuse (NIDA). (2006, September). "Methamphetamine Abuse and Addiction." National Institute on Drug Abuse Research Report Series. NIH Publication No. 06-4210. Available at: http://www.drugabuse.gov/ResearchReports/methamph/Methamph.html (accessed October 12, 2007).

National Organization on Fetal Alcohol Syndrome (NOFAS). (n.d.a). "Factsheet: FASD: What Everyone Should Know." Available at: http://www.nofas.org/MediaFiles/PDFs/factsheets/everyone.pdf (accessed November 17, 2009).

National Organization on Fetal Alcohol Syndrome (NOFAS). (n.d.b). "Factsheet: FASD: What the Health Care System Should Know." Available at: http://www.nofas.org/MediaFiles/PDFs/factsheets/healthcare.pdf (accessed November 17, 2009).

Nelipovich, M., & Buss, E. (1991). Investigating alcohol abuse among persons who are blind. *Journal of Visual Impairment & Blindness, 85*(8), 343–345.

O'Malley, P. M. (2004/2005). Maturing out of problematic alcohol use. *Alcohol Research & Health, 28,* 202–204. http://pubs.niaaa.nih.gov/publications/arh284/202-204.htm

O'Rourke, G. C. (1993). Alcoholism as a secondary diagnosis: Treatment implications. *Occupational Therapy Practice, 4*(2), 19–23.

Petry, N. M. (2006). Contingency management treatments. *British Journal of Psychiatry, 189,* 97–98.

Petry, N. M., Alessi, S. M., Hanson, T., & Sierra, S. (2007). Randomized trial of contingent prizes versus vouchers in cocaine-using methadone patients. *Journal of Consulting and Clinical Psychology, 75,* 983–991.

Primack, B. A., Dalton, M. A., Carroll, M. V., Agarwal, A. A., & Fine, M. J. (2008). Content analysis of tobacco, alcohol and drugs in popular music. *Archives of Pediatric Adolescent Medicine, 162,* 169–175.

Quadling, A., Maree, K., Mountjoy, L., Bosch, G., & Kotkin, Z. (1999). An investigation into a relationship between sensory modulation disorder and substance abuse. *South African Journal of Occupational Therapy, 29*(1), 10–13.

RachBeisel, J., Scott, J., & Dixon, L. (1999). Co-occurring severe mental illness and substance use disorder: A review of recent research. *Psychiatric Services, 50,* 1427–1434.

Rollnick, S., & Miller, W. R. (1995). What is motivational interviewing? *Behavioural and Cognitive Psychotherapy, 23,* 325–334.

Stoffel, V., & Moyers, P. A. (2001). *Occupational Therapy Practice Guidelines for Substance Use Disorder* (3rd ed.). Bethesda, MD: American Occupational Therapy Association.

Stoffel, V., & Moyers, P. A. (2005). Occupational therapy and substance use disorders. In E. Cara & A. MacRae (Eds.), *Psychosocial Occupational Therapy: A Clinical Practice* (2nd ed., pp. 446–473). Albany, NY: Delmar.

Stoffel, V. C., & Moyers, P. A. (2004). An evidence-based and occupational perspective of interventions for persons with substance-use disorders. *American Journal of Occupational Therapy, 58,* 570–586.

Straussner, S. L. A. (2001). Introduction: Ethnocultural issues in substance abuse treatment—An overview. In S. L. A. Straussner (Ed.), *Ethnocultural Factors in Substance Abuse Treatment* (pp. 3–30). New York: Guilford Press.

Substance Abuse and Mental Health Services Administration (SAMHSA). (2007). *Results From the 2006 National Survey on Drug Use and Health: National Findings.* Office of Applied Studies, NSDUH Series H-32, DHHS Publication No. SMA 07-4293. Rockville, MD.: SAMHSA.

Substance Abuse Resources and Disability Issues (SARDI). (2007a). Substance abuse and students with disabilities: Little known facts. Available at: http://www.med.wright.edu/citar/sardi/brochure_facts.html (accessed February 16, 2010).

Substance Abuse Resources and Disability Issues (SARDI). (2007b). "Welcome to SARDI." Available at: http://www.med.wright.edu/citar/sardi/index.html (accessed July 24, 2008).

Thompson, K. (2007). Occupational therapy and substance use disorders: Are practitioners addressing these disorders in practice? *Occupational Therapy in Health Care, 21*(3), 61–77.

Tiet, Q. Q., & Mausbach, B. (2007). Treatments for patients with dual diagnosis: A review. *Alcoholism: Clinical and Experimental Research, 4,* 513–536.

U.S. Department of Health and Human Services. (n.d.). "Office on Disability—Substance Abuse and Disability: A Companion to Chapter 26 of Health People 2010." Washington, DC: Author. Available at: http://www.hhs.gov/od/about/fact_sheets/substance-abusech26.html (accessed November 17, 2009).

U.S. Department of Health and Human Services & U.S. Department of Agriculture. (2005). *Dietary Guidelines for Americans.* Washington, DC: Author.

Vandrey, R., Bigelow, G. E., & Stitzer, M. L. (2007). Contingency management in cocaine abusers: A dose–effect comparison of goods-based versus cash-based incentives. *Experimental and Clinical Psychopharmocology, 15,* 338–343.

Yeager, J. (2000). Functional implications of substance use disorders. *OT Practice, 5*(7), 36–39.

Co-Occurring Disorders

Penelope A. Moyers

> "They [treatment staff] worked mainly on substance abuse and I think they should split the time between mental health and substance abuse because I really honestly don't know anyone who has a substance abuse problem who doesn't have a mental problem.
> —Anonymous youth, Federation of Families for Children's Mental Health, 2001
>
> It was our responsibility as family members to put the two together, substance abuse and mental health. No one even offered to help us sort this out.
> —Anonymous parent, 2001, Federation of Families for Children's Mental Health, 2001

Introduction

In other Section 2 chapters, individual mental health diagnoses are described, highlighting the role of occupational therapy practitioners in delivering services to persons with resulting occupational performance issues. This chapter augments learning through the emphasis on persons who have at least one substance use disorder and one mental health disorder, otherwise referred to as co-occurring disorders (CODs).

The term *co-occurring disorder* is clarified because there is a history of confusing terminology. The epidemiology of COD is explored, noting a discrepancy between prevalence and intervention accessibility, which represents a legitimate public health crisis (Minkoff & Cline, 2004). In addition, the availability of professionals and peers who are trained to address both classes of disorders in an integrated manner is also problematic (McLellan & Meyers, 2004).

Occupational therapy practitioners require education and training in addressing the occupational performance problems and community participation of persons with CODs. This understanding can affect the ability of occupational therapy practitioners to improve existing programs and develop new prevention and intervention programs for persons with CODs that are fully integrated and address all problems of living related to the combination of diagnoses. These programs can facilitate recovery in which the person experiences positive interaction throughout everyday life, leading to successful community participation.

Description of the Disorder

Co-occurring disorder (COD) is the term used to describe persons who have one or more substance-related disorders and one or more mental disorders (Center for Substance Abuse Treatment [CSAT], 2006a), for example, an individual with bipolar disorder who also has an alcohol use disorder or a young adult with schizoaffective disorder who also has cocaine dependence.

A variety of terms for COD have been used in the past, including *dual diagnosis, mentally ill substance abuser,* and *mentally ill chemically dependent* (Table 16-1 includes a complete list), but the current accepted terminology is *persons with CODs*. Still, this term is not precise and can become distorted when users fail to clarify how the term is being used (CSAT, 2005a).

Some individuals benefit from intervention specifically designed for COD, but may not technically be classified as having a COD. This may be due to circumstances (e.g., the person with a mental illness has not used preferred substances because he or she was incarcerated and did not have access to mood-altering substances such as alcohol, marijuana, or cocaine) or motivation (e.g., the person with bipolar disorder wanted to get his or her driver's license back and so complies with substance-free expectation monitored by the court). To be identified as a person with a COD, the diagnosis of each disorder (mental and substance use) occurs when all criteria are present for each condition as spelled out in the *Diagnostic and Statistical Manual of Mental Disorders, Fourth Edition, Text Revision* (DSM IV-TR; American Psychiatric Association [APA], 2000).

Another potential factor contributing to the lack of clear diagnostic indicators in both mental and substance use disorder is that in a given agency, service provision may be only directed toward one condition (i.e., an agency that only works with people with mental illness). Therefore, no questions get asked about substance use unless the person presents as being under the influence of mood-altering substances.

However, it is important for persons at risk for CODs to receive the appropriate services, rather than be denied services until each diagnosis can be separately established (CSAT, 2005a). For example, an individual with a clearly recognized diagnosis in one domain (e.g., posttraumatic stress disorder [PTSD]) may at pretreatment display some signs and symptoms of an evolving disorder in the other domain (e.g., abuse of alcohol and marijuana as a means of regulating emotion) (CSAT, 2006a). Also, one of the disorders may resolve after

Table 16-1 ● **Alternative Terminology for Co-Occurring Disorders**

Abbreviation	Definition
MICA	Mentally ill chemical abuser
MICAA	Mentally ill chemically addicted or affected
MISA	Mentally ill substance abuser
MISU	Mentally ill substance using
CAMI	Chemically abusing mentally ill or chemically addicted and mentally ill
SAMI	Substance abusing mentally ill
MICD	Mentally ill chemically dependent
	Dually diagnosed
	Dually disordered
	Comorbid disorders
ICOPSD	Individuals with co-occurring psychiatric and substance disorders

diagnosis, but the need for integrated COD intervention is still important to prevent return of the resolved disorder and continued intervention for the remaining disorder. It is additionally important for persons with a **unitary disorder** (i.e., only one diagnosis, either a mental health diagnosis or a substance use disorder), such as substance dependence with suicidal ideation, which is a mental health symptom that increases in severity, to receive integrated COD services. Likewise, a person with a mental health disorder who is hospitalized because of substance intoxication should be considered for COD services, even though substance abuse or dependence has not been fully established.

Currently, because of reimbursement limitations, COD services are often not included for persons who abuse caffeine or who are nicotine dependent as the only substance use disorder, and the same is true for persons with impulse control disorders as the only mental health disorder. This is unfortunate because nicotine dependence has high rates of morbidity and mortality, and it co-occurs with other addictive and mental disorders (Grant, Hasin, Chou, Stinson, & Dawson, 2004). Caffeine abuse may not qualify an individual for COD services, unless the caffeine abuse triggers panic attacks in a person with agoraphobia (CSAT, 2006a).

Any definition of COD should address the goal of relieving the severity of symptoms, the limitations in occupational performance, and the restrictions in community participation that are typical of persons with mental health disorders and concomitant substance use disorders (CSAT, 2006c). Vulnerable individuals can inadvertently fail to receive the appropriate interventions because of the technical use of the term and arbitrary exclusion of certain drug classes or mental health diagnoses.

COD Conceptual Framework

The National Association of State Mental Health Program Directors (NASMHPD) and the National Association of State Alcohol and Drug Abuse Directors (NASADAD) (2000; NASADAD & NASMHPD, 2005) published a conceptual framework based on the original work of Ries (1993) to classify persons with CODs in terms of relative symptom severity rather than by diagnostic combinations and matched them to the system of care, also referred to as the Quadrant Model (Table 16-2).

Epidemiology

Kessler (2004) reported that the co-occurrence of mental disorders and substance use disorders is much higher than chance. The data from the 2006 National Survey on Drug Use and Health (NSDUH) (SAMHSA, 2007) indicated that there were 24.9 million adults aged 18 or older with serious psychological distress (SPD), or 11.3% of all adults. Of these adults with SPD, 22.3% were dependent on or abused alcohol and drugs (5.6 million adults with COD), compared with the 7.7% rate of substance use among adults without SPD. Note that SPD means having symptoms of a mental disorder, using a new process by which the NSDUH now collects data in the United States.

National Comorbidity Survey Replication (NCS-R) data are currently being analyzed; the most recent reports indicate 12-month prevalence rates of 26.2% for the presence of any mental disorder among the 9,282 adults surveyed, with 22% having two DSM-IV-TR diagnoses and 23% having three or more diagnoses. The mental disorders were categorized in four classes: anxiety, mood, impulse control, and substance use disorders (Kessler, Chiu, Demler, & Walters, 2005). Those

Table 16-2 ● **Categories of Co-Occurring Disorders and Locus of Care**

Category: Locus of Care	Level of Symptom Severity	Description
Category I: Primary health-care settings	Low for both	Less severe mental disorder/less severe substance disorder
Category II: Mental health system	High mental disorder/low substance disorder	More severe mental disorder/less severe substance disorder
Category III: Substance abuse system	Low mental disorder/high substance disorder	Less severe mental disorder/more severe substance disorder
Category IV: Joint alcohol and mental health systems, prisons, state hospitals, emergency rooms	High for both	More severe mental disorder/more severe substance disorder

Source: Adapted from National Association of State Alcohol and Drug Abuse Directors and the National Association of State Mental Health Program Directors. (2005). The Evolving Conceptual Framework for Co-Occurring Mental Health and Substance Abuse Disorders: Developing Strategies for Systems Change. Final Report of the NASMHPD NASADAD Task Force on Co-Occurring Disorders. Washington, DC, and Alexandria, VA: Authors; p. 3.

with more severe mental illness were more likely to have more than one diagnosis. However, Kessler et al (2005) additionally reported that, of persons with psychotic disorders, 9.9% also had alcohol abuse, 10.4% also had drug abuse, or 26.8% also had some type of substance-related disorder.

In the previous NCS, which was administered between 1990 and 1992, Kessler et al (1996) found 42.7% of persons with substance use disorders within the previous 12 months had at least one mental disorder, and 14.7% of persons with mental disorders in the previous 12 months had at least one substance use disorder. Approximately 51.4% of the respondents on the NCS with a lifetime substance use disorder met criteria for at least one lifetime mental disorder, with a similar percentage of 50.9% of the NCS respondents with a lifetime mental disorder also having a history of substance use.

From 2001 to 2002, the National Institute on Alcohol Abuse and Alcoholism conducted the National Epidemiologic Survey on Alcohol Related Conditions (NESARC) in persons aged 18 years and older (Grant, Moore, Shepard, & Kaplan, 2003) for the purpose of examining the prevalence of various DSM-IV-TR disorders and the way in which they co-occur. Results are shown in Table 16-3.

Because there are multiple national epidemiological studies, it is important to analyze the data to draw conclusions regarding what the data describe. There is evidence within these surveys to support the possibility of four probable mechanisms of action to explain the high rate of CODs (Kessler, 2004):

1. Mental disorders contribute to the onset and persistence of substance use disorders because of increased exposure to substances related to having a conduct disorder, disinhibition to experiment with substances because of having an impulse control disorder, and self-medication with substances because of having dysphoric mood.
2. Substance use disorders contribute to the onset and persistence of mental disorders through a combination of biological mechanisms, increased exposure to stress, and decreased access to coping resources.
3. There are common causes for both types of disorders involving genetic and environmental mechanisms, which lead these disorders to co-occur.
4. Survey methodological error makes some overestimation of CODs highly likely.

Complications of COD

There are complications often associated with CODs that are related to homelessness, incarceration, infectious diseases, trauma, and PTSD. From 1990 to 2000 (North, Eyrich, Pollio, & Spitznagel, 2004), homelessness in females with CODs increased from 14.3% to 36.7%, compared with homelessness in males with CODs, which increased from 23.2% to 32.2%. Women and families are the fastest growing among the homeless population (SAMHSA, 2003).

McNeil, Binder, and Robinson (2005) assessed the relationships between homelessness, mental disorder, and incarceration using the San Francisco County Jail system database and found that 78% of the homeless inmates with a severe mental disorder had co-occurring substance-related disorders. These inmates were also more likely to be charged with a violent crime when compared with other inmates. Even when compared with inmates charged with similar crimes who did not have a COD, they were more likely to be held in jail longer. Similarly, Hartwell (2004) found in Massachusetts that offenders with a COD on release had greater service needs for housing and for assessment of dangerousness. As a result, these offenders were more likely to return to correctional custody.

Another complication of CODs is the problem of infectious diseases. Tucker, Kanouse, Miu, Koegel, and Sullivan (2003) reported that, in a sample of persons infected with HIV who also had serious mental illness, problem drinking was associated with sexual activity and more sexual risk behaviors. Berger-Greenstein et al (2007) found that in 85 persons who abused substances and had HIV/AIDS, 72.9% met the criteria for a major depressive disorder. Meta-analyses have indicated that prevalence rates of depression are significantly higher among people living with HIV/AIDS than in the general population. Persons with AIDS appear to experience a faster progression of the disease and higher mortality rates when depression is a complicating factor (Leserman, 2003).

PTSD often occurs in the comorbidity of substance use and other psychiatric disorders (Brady & Sinha, 2005). A high proportion, or 20% to 30%, of individuals with substance use disorders meet criteria for PTSD (Back et al, 2000). Waldrop, Back, Verduin, and Brady (2007) found that the high-risk substance use triggers for persons with PTSD were typically in response to negative situations, such as unpleasant emotions and physical discomfort, when compared

Table 16-3 ● **National Epidemiologic Survey on Alcohol-Related Conditions (NESARC) Results**

Diagnosis	Comorbidity	Prevalence Within Previous 12 Months	Standard Error	Authors
Personality disorder (at least one)	Alcohol use disorder	16.4%	0.62	Grant, Stinson, Dawson, Chou, Ruan, et al (2006)
	Drug use disorder	6.5%	0.41	Grant, Stinson, Dawson, Chou, Ruan, et al (2006)
Alcohol use disorder	Personality disorder (at least one)	28.6%	1.00	Grant, Stinson, Dawson, Chou, Ruan, et al (2006)
Drug use disorder	Personality disorder (at least one)	47.7%	1.96	Grant, Stinson, Dawson, Chou, Ruan, et al (2006)
Mood disorder	Alcohol use disorder	17.30%	0.75	Grant, Stinson, Dawson, Chou, Dufour, et al (2006)
	Drug use disorder	6.9%	0.56	Grant, Stinson, Dawson, Chou, Dufour, et al (2006)
Anxiety disorder	Alcohol use disorder	13.02%	0.65	Grant, Stinson, Dawson, Chou, Dufour, et al (2006)
	Drug use disorder	4.58%	0.41	Grant, Stinson, Dawson, Chou, Dufour, et al (2006)

Source: Data from Grant, Stinson, Dawson, Chou, Dufour, et al (2006); Grant, Stinson, Dawson, Chou, Ruan, et al (2006).

with individuals without PTSD, who were more likely to cope during recovery with these milder forms of substance use triggers. In addition, individuals with cocaine dependence and PTSD tended to use cocaine not only in unpleasant situations, but also in pleasant situations, unlike people with alcohol dependence and PTSD. It is clear that persons with substance use disorders should be screened for trauma related to childhood abuse (Anderson, Teicher, Pocari, & Renshaw, 2002) because PTSD seems to play a role in the development of substance use disorders (Brady, Kileen, Brewerton, & Lucerini, 2000).

Course

The course of COD can involve remission, recovery, and relapse (CSAT, 2006a)—in any order. A person who is in **remission** no longer meets the DSM-IV-TR (APA, 2000) criteria for either or both the substance use disorder or the mental health disorder. Although there is an absence of distress from COD, a person in remission would likely benefit from intervention focusing on relapse prevention and improvement in occupational performance and community participation.

According to Lowinson, Ruiz, Millman, and Langrod (1992), **recovery** is more than the absence of distress from the COD; instead, it occurs when the person works on gaining information and self-awareness, and developing the skills necessary for living chemically free. Through this ongoing effort, the person is able to live, work, and fully participate in his or her community, despite any residual disability. Recovery implies that the person remains abstinent from use of substances and is able to successfully cope with any remaining mental health symptoms, while participating fully in meaningful life activities. Quality of life, health and wellness, a strengths perspective, hope, growth, and choice are all seen as important to recovery from mental illness and addictions (Gagne, White, & Anthony, 2007).

Relapse is considered a normal aspect of recovery and involves a return to active substance use or the return of disabling psychiatric symptoms after a period of remission (CSAT, 2006a). Return in one or both diagnostic categories may occur. Prior to relapse, warning signs are usually noticeable, and the person, friends, and family members can learn to recognize these signs and help reduce the impairment in person factors, the limitations in occupational performance, and restrictions in community participation that

result from a complete relapse. The person and family can implement appropriate health-care–seeking behaviors and a variety of useful coping strategies that include reengagement in healthy occupations.

Service Integration for COD

The quadrant model (referred to previously in this chapter, including Table 16-2) has been helpful in creating better understanding regarding the need for **service integration,** that is, integration of mental health and substance abuse services (NASADAD & NASMHPD, 2005). The level of integration among mental health and substance use disorder services becomes more imperative for individuals in category IV COD.

Traditionally, the mental health and substance abuse treatment systems have operated as separate and independent systems, both possessing different intervention philosophies, cultures, funding mechanisms, and administrative structures (CSAT, 2005a). To some degree, the COD conceptual framework (Table 16-2) can help providers determine the type of placement for intervention; however, without better integration of services, the diagnostic rating of less severe can change rapidly, thereby placing the person in the more severe category. Unfortunately, occupational therapy service provision is rarely integrated into COD intervention because the system for addressing substance use disorders often does not employ occupational therapy practitioners. Services can be rated in terms of their level of integration on a scale of more to less integration (CSAT, 2005a).

Levels of Integration

Different types of programs have varying levels of service integration for people with CODs. For example, **minimal coordination** of services means the service provider is aware of the COD and may be aware that the person is receiving help elsewhere for the other diagnostic category. One provider may have referred the client to another provider, but there is no contact between service providers, nor is there follow-up

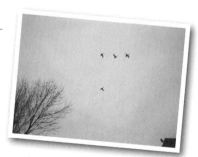

PhotoVoice

Oh, to fly free! My vision of recovery and a satisfying life includes a jubilant sense of freedom. Freedom to laugh and love, to sing, dance and create, to learn, to explore, to grow.

Evidence-Based Practice

It is important to understand the factors associated with substance abuse relapse and sustained recovery among persons with severe mental illness who live in urban areas. At the 6-month follow-up period, 68% of the 133 persons were in recovery, whereas 52% were in recovery at the 12-month follow-up period (Rollins, O'Neill, Davis, & Devitt, 2005). Older age (47 and older), holding jobs, and living in residential integrated intervention facilities were factors in sustaining recovery.

➤ Occupational therapists who work with urban-dwelling clients with co-occurring disorders can advocate for housing, job opportunities, and community supports needed to provide the optimal environment for recovery from their substance use disorder as well as their mental illness.

Rollins, A. L., O'Neill, S. J., Davis, K. E., & Devitt, T. S. (2005). Substance abuse relapse and factors associated with relapse in an inner-city sample of patients with dual diagnoses. *Psychiatric Services, 56,* 1274–1281.

between the providers. Minimal coordination can occur in programs that only provide services to people with addiction or mental health disorders (CSAT, 2006a).

The next level of integration is **consultation,** in which the service provider informally and occasionally communicates information about the person's status to the other providers. Often the referring service provider ensures that the person actually receives the recommended intervention from the other provider of care. Some addiction-only or mental health–only service providers may include a consultative component in their approach to care as a way to improve their client outcomes (CSAT, 2006a).

Collaboration is a prescribed process of integration in which there is planned communication and deliberate sharing of information. The providers of care may enter into a formal contractual relationship, delineating separate responsibilities for each diagnostic category (i.e., one provider addresses the mental health problem and the other addresses the substance use problem). Addiction-only or mental health–only service providers who take a collaborative approach to care greatly improve the recovery process of their clients with CODs (CSAT, 2006a).

Full integration is the ideal level of integration because it involves a single intervention plan that addresses both sets of conditions; in full integration, the care providers are trained in both substance abuse and mental health services (CSAT, 2006c). Not only are there formal contractual agreements when needed, but also all providers, ranging from a single provider to multiple providers, depending on the capacities of the programs to make available what is needed, share responsibility for the well-coordinated intervention process and outcome. For example, one service provider may be designated as the primary provider for inpatient services involving withdrawal from the substances and provision of immediate stabilization from the mental health condition, and another provider is responsible for the long-term recovery processes, including housing, community integration, and return to work.

Figure 16-1 illustrates the levels of integration of substance abuse and mental illness treatment services.

Some providers of full integration services would be considered **dual diagnosis capable** (American Society of Addiction Medicine [ASAM], 2001), meaning that, when admitting a client with a COD to a program that is primarily oriented to one diagnostic classification over the other, the personnel are appropriately trained and services are available to address the integrated assessment and intervention processes. This is in contrast to a **dual diagnosis enhanced program** (ASAM, 2001), in which a high level of integration exists, with no one orientation to a primary diagnostic category.

Screening, Assessment, and Intervention

During the screening, assessment, and intervention of clients with COD, there should be appropriate emphasis, guided by the client's presenting problems and conditions, on both the mental health and the substance use problems. In addition, for occupational therapy practitioners, the focus of screening, assessment, and intervention is on the occupational performance and participation issues that are uniquely related to the complications of CODs and their effect on person factors, occupational engagement and roles, skills, healthy patterns

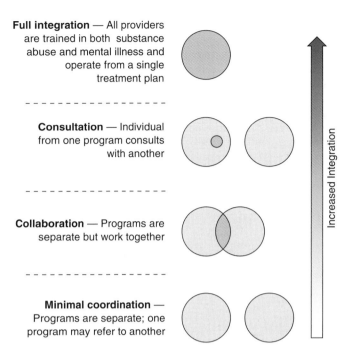

FIGURE 16-1. Levels of integration of substance abuse and mental illness treatment services.

and routines, and the environmental contexts that create barriers and supports for recovery (Stoffel & Moyers, 2004).

An **integrated screening** conducted in a brief manner at the point of first contact with the individual determines the likelihood of a COD and does not lead to a diagnosis; however, it determines whether there is a need for an in-depth integrated assessment and referral to a range of experts (CSAT, 2006a). Using the screening guidelines suggested by the CSAT (2006b) and outlined in the CSAT TIP 42 (CSAT, 2005a, 2007) is suggested. Additional occupational therapy screening provides information related to the occupational history of the individual and how it might have been affected by the potential co-occurring diagnoses, and determines whether a full occupational therapy assessment would be beneficial (Moyers & Stoffel, 2001).

The **integrated assessment** occurs when the person has screened positive for the presence or history of mental illness and a substance use history; in general, it focuses on whether there are CODs, delineates the specific diagnoses involved, determines the client's readiness for change, identifies the client's strengths and problem areas as they affect the process of recovery, and establishes the service needs of the person (CSAT, 2006a). The occupational therapist's role in the integrated assessment process is to determine the nature of what the person needs and wants to do; the extent of the occupational performance limitations, abilities, participation engagement, and restrictions; and the influence of the underlying person factors, performance skills, performance patterns, environmental contexts, and activity demands on overall performance (Stoffel & Moyers, 2004). The integrated assessment is typically ongoing due to the withdrawal, psychiatric and medical stabilization, and recovery processes, which create continuous changes in capability related to cognitive functioning and receptivity to help (CSAT, 2006a).

Integrated intervention occurs when all aspects of the co-occurring diagnostic conditions are addressed in a comprehensive plan, whether in a single or series of contacts over time. These services range from acute care to fostering long-term recovery. The occupational therapy practitioner's role is to address the occupational performance limitations and participation restrictions through a combination of skill building or retraining, establishment of routine performance patterns supportive of recovery, occupational and environmental modifications, and client and family educational strategies. Engagement in meaningful occupations within relevant social roles as part of recovery is a major method of intervention (Moyers & Stoffel, 2001; Stoffel & Moyers, 2004).

Special Settings

The need for screening, assessment, and intervention for CODs is not limited to programs that are specifically designed to address these problems. According to SAMHSA (2007), only half of persons with CODs receive formalized mental health or substance abuse services; therefore, the intervention process often must occur in other locations, such as within primary (e.g., physicians or clinics), acute (e.g., emergency rooms, trauma centers, intensive care), and specialty health-care services settings (e.g., rehabilitation or HIV/AIDS programs).

Jones et al (2004) determined that 74% of individuals with COD had a least one diagnosed chronic health problem, which typically comes to the attention of the primary care provider first. The high rate of concomitant health problems results partially from the effect of the substances on organ systems, as well as from the susceptibility to infectious diseases, such HIV/AIDS. Brady (2002) estimated that, of those patients seen in primary care settings, 20% have a current psychiatric disorder and 20% to 25% have a substance use disorder.

Two other common locations for integrated screening, assessment, and intervention are in the criminal justice system and social welfare settings. Because of possessing or selling controlled substances, persons with CODs frequently come in contact with the criminal justice system, involving police, corrections (jails and prisons), and court and probation officers. They may also come to the attention of police because of violent and bizarre behavior exacerbated by the use of substances and its negative effect on the expression of the symptoms of mental illness (Reuland, 2004). Unfortunately, access to integrated intervention or even access to intervention for substance use alone is often not provided within jails and prisons (CSAT, 2005b).

In terms of social welfare services, such as homeless services and community settings, access to integrated screening, assessment, and intervention is variable, depending on the community. North et al (2004) estimated that one third of homeless persons have CODs. Most homeless people do not have access to integrated intervention for CODs, which in turn leads to continued homelessness and further deterioration in occupational performance and community participation (SAMHSA, 2003).

Professionals who would benefit from information about the early warning signs of COD include parents, teachers, clergy, and employers. With some basic education and training, those individuals who come in contact with persons with CODs can refer them to integrated screening, assessment, and intervention programs.

Diagnostic Challenges

Case Study

A client receiving occupational therapy services for slipping and falling on the ice and sustaining a wrist fracture tells the occupational therapist that his wife left him and that "life is not worth living." The occupational therapist is concerned because the client is typically well dressed and groomed; on this visit, however, he is unshaven and slightly unkempt, and his breath smells of alcohol.

The occupational therapist begins asking him questions about his situation and discovers that he has been feeling "down" for the past week and has been feeling guilty over his marital situation. When the occupational therapist asks him about thoughts of suicide, the client admits he has been thinking about suicide and that these thoughts have become more frequent since his wife left. However, he does not have a plan and does not really want to hurt himself. He only wants his "old life back." When the occupational therapist tells the client she smells alcohol on his breath, the client states he has been drinking because he has not gone to work since his wife left. He states his drinking has helped to "ease the pain."

The occupational therapist is concerned for the client's safety and by the fact that he has not been going to his job as a computer programmer for a major corporation. He had just returned to work 3 weeks ago after a successful rehabilitation program focusing on physical occupational performance. Today was supposed to have been his final visit, primarily for follow-up to determine the impact of his work tasks on his wrist. Now, the therapist's primary goal is to get him immediate help for his suicidal ideation. The occupational therapist tells the client that she called the emergency room of the hospital and that she would walk him over to the service, unless he objected to going. She did not have to call security because he stated that he would go with her and that he was relieved she was going to help him.

While walking him to the ER, she starts wondering about the following issues: is her client clinically depressed in that he might have a major depressive episode, or are his feelings of "being down" related to his situation?

- Has the client given her information about the extent of his drinking? Could drinking have contributed to his marital problems, his feeling "down," or even to his falling on the ice?
- Were there any clues she might have missed in her initial health screening when he was first referred to the occupational performance outpatient service to suggest whether he has more than a grief reaction to his wife's leaving?
- Does he really have a drinking problem, depression, or both?
- What role will his mental health issues have in her efforts to help him not only return to work, but also to stay working successfully?

Although the role of occupational therapy practitioners is not to make mental health diagnoses, they are expected to refer clients to the appropriate health-care professionals and contribute relevant occupational performance information that will help diagnosticians to identify and answer those important mental health diagnostic questions illustrated in the case study. Once the client receives appropriate mental health services, the occupational therapy practitioner must incorporate appropriate mental health recovery interventions within the occupational therapy intervention plan. Occupational therapy practitioners often work in settings where the client is not currently being seen by any other medical personnel, or with clients who have not accessed help for long-standing mental health problems. In these cases, it would be even more important to make a referral to a health professional with a background in both mental health and substance abuse so that a full assessment and intervention plan can be carefully coordinated. It is clear that mental health status affects occupational performance and participation outcomes.

Substance-Related Mental Health Symptoms and Signs

Use of substances, whether alcohol or other drugs, affects brain functioning and may have an impact on the hormonal system, depending on the drug(s) used. Both the neurological and hormonal systems are involved in the development of mental health disorders (Koob, 2000). As a result, the substance misuse often manifests as a broad range of mental health symptoms, such as sadness or difficulty concentrating, or as signs, such as crying. These mental health symptoms and signs often prompt the person to seek initial help from mental health practitioners, or may cause the family to seek the advice of health-care professionals. The extent and nature of these mental health symptoms and signs depend on the most recent occurrence of substance use, the length of substance use over time, the frequency of use during a given time frame, and the quantity of use in a single instance (Shivani, Goldsmith, & Anthenelli, 2002).

In addition, mental health status is reliant on whether the person is currently intoxicated or in acute or protracted withdrawal. Also influencing the mental health signs and symptoms are the psychosocial stressors experienced, such as legal or financial problems, divorce or domestic trauma, housing instability, or difficulties related to unemployment. These stressors exacerbate the individual's mental health symptoms the longer and the more consistently the person uses substances.

Regardless of the factors influencing mental health status, the mental health signs and symptoms may fail to develop into a complete **syndrome.** A syndrome corresponds to the DSM-IV-TR (APA, 2000) diagnostic criteria used for classifying mental disorders in which the mental health symptoms and signs occur in a regular pattern within a discrete period of time. The substance-related mental health symptoms and signs may resolve on their own without specific intervention, other than the intervention targeted for recovery from the substance use. This latter intervention typically includes the initial goal of helping the client withdraw through safe medical management and maintenance of physical and psychological comfort.

Substance-Induced Mental Health Symptoms and Signs

In addition to the substance use disorders, the DSM-IV-TR (APA, 2000) describes several **substance-induced disorders**, such as delirium and mood disorder (Box 16-1). The critical factor for diagnosticians is that these substance-induced disorders are prominent and persistent *because of* the use of alcohol and drugs; that is, they are not due to a medical disorder or another mental health disorder (APA, 2000). To determine whether the mental health symptoms are substance induced, knowledge of onset of the symptoms, the client's history, physical examination, and laboratory findings is required.

Substance-induced disorders must occur within 4 weeks of the last use of or withdrawal from the alcohol and drug, and the symptoms must be beyond what would be expected from typical intoxication or withdrawal; that is, they endure longer than typical and are more severe (APA, 2000). However, it is difficult to differentiate substance-related signs and symptoms, as described previously, from substance-induced disorders. Generally, the induced disorder classifications are used to help the mental health professional group the signs and symptoms in order to enhance the likelihood of providing an intervention for the substance use for the person receiving mental health intervention. Substance-induced disorders are expected to resolve with recovery from the substance use disorder by helping promote abstinence and targeted intervention for mental health symptom reduction, such as training in deep breathing and medication for relaxation for individuals coping with anxiety disorders.

Substance Use Disorder and Independent Mental Health Disorders

Complicating diagnostic issues further is the question of how to determine whether the mental health signs and symptoms developed independently of the substance use. This is an important issue because independent mental health disorders contribute to increased vulnerability to substance-related problems (Schuckit et al, 1997) and complicate the substance use recovery process. Occupational therapists can provide information to assist in the diagnostic process. Through the occupational history, it may become clear how occupational performance has been affected by the mental health symptom clusters prior to, or only in conjunction with, substance use. Examining the occupational history during times of abstinence is particularly useful to identify the impact of any remaining mental health signs and symptoms when the person is substance free. Box 16-2 provides sample occupational history questions.

Certainly, knowledge of the client's family history of mental health problems is helpful to discern whether there is a strong likelihood of a COD. It is important for all health professionals who work with the client to monitor the client's behavior; in the case of occupational therapy, the client's occupational performance throughout the first 4 weeks of recovery is important to assess. Typically, substance-related and substance-induced mental health disorders resolve with recovery from using substances and with targeted mental health interventions. Independent mental health disorders may become more

BOX 16-1 ▓ Substance-Induced Disorders

Diagnoses

Substance intoxication: A reversible substance-specific syndrome (some substances produce identical syndromes) due to recent ingestion or exposure to a substance. Social and occupational performance is often disrupted during or shortly after use of the substance because of such behavior as belligerence, mood lability, and cognitive impairment characterized by impaired judgment (p. 116).

   Substance withdrawal: Cessation of or reduction of the substance in situations where the substance use has been heavy and prolonged leads to a substance-specific syndrome that affects occupational performance because of significant distress (p. 116).

   Substance-induced delirium: Involves a change of consciousness or reduced awareness of the environment occurring because of intoxication or withdrawal. There is difficulty to focus, sustain, or shift attention that occurs over a short period of time, fluctuating throughout the day (pp. 84–85).

   Substance-induced persisting dementia: There is evidence to suggest that memory and other cognitive impairments, which persist beyond the duration of withdrawal or intoxication, are etiologically related to the persisting effects of using substances. The memory impairment is manifested in inability to learn new information or recall previously learned information. The cognitive disturbances could include aphasia; apraxia; agnosia; and disturbances in executive functioning, such as planning, organizing, sequencing, and abstracting. Memory and cognitive impairments significantly affect social and occupational performance (p. 93).

   Substance-induced persisting amnestic disorder: There is evidence to suggest that memory impairment, which persists beyond the duration of withdrawal or intoxication, is etiologically related to the persisting effects of using substances. The memory impairment is manifested in inability to learn new information or recall previously learned information. The memory impairment significantly affects social and occupational performance and results in a decline from a previous level of functioning (p. 96).

   Substance-induced psychotic disorder: Hallucinations and delusions are prominent during or within a month of substance intoxication or withdrawal and do not occur exclusively during the course of a delirium. However, because some substances are considered hallucinogenic, to be diagnosed with this disorder, the person does not have insight that the hallucinations and delusions are substance induced. The person's pattern of substance use suggests that the onset of the hallucinations and delusion are etiologically related. The person's medical history should not show a history of non–substance use–induced hallucinations and delusions, nor should these symptoms persist beyond what would be expected during withdrawal or intoxication of the type and amount of substance used or the duration of use (pp. 163–164).

Substance-induced mood disorder: A disturbance of mood persists within a month of substance intoxication or withdrawal and does not occur exclusively during the course of a delirium. The depressed mood may involve diminished interest or pleasure in most activities. The mood could also be elevated, expansive, or irritable. The person's pattern of substance use suggests the onset of the mood disorder is etiologically related. The person's medical history should not show a history of a non–substance use–induced mood disorder, nor should these symptoms persist beyond what would be expected during withdrawal or intoxication of the type and amount of substance used or the duration of use (pp. 192–193). Social and occupational performances are typically affected.

   Substance-induced anxiety disorder: There is prominent anxiety, panic attacks, or obsessions or compulsions persisting within a month of substance intoxication or withdrawal, none of which occurs exclusively during the course of a delirium. The person's pattern of substance use suggests that the onset of the anxiety disorder is etiologically related. The person's medical history should not show a history of a non–substance use–induced anxiety disorder, nor should these symptoms persist beyond what would be expected during withdrawal or intoxication of the type and amount of substance used or the duration of use (pp. 224–225). Social and occupational performances are typically affected because the person may experience much distress.

   Substance-induced sexual dysfunction: There is significant sexual dysfunction creating distress and interpersonal difficulty persisting within a month of substance intoxication or withdrawal. The person's pattern of substance use suggests the onset of the sexual disorder is etiologically related. The person's medical history should not show a history of a non–substance use–induced sexual dysfunction, nor should these symptoms persist beyond what would be expected during withdrawal or intoxication of the type and amount of substance used or the duration of use. The sexual dysfunction is in excess of what would normally be expected during intoxication or withdrawal (pp. 253–254).

   Substance-induced sleep disorder: There is prominent disturbance in sleep that is severe enough for intervention developed within a month of substance intoxication or withdrawal, none of which occurs exclusively during the course of a delirium. The person's pattern of substance use suggests the onset of the sleep disorder is etiologically related. The person's medical history should not show a history of a non–substance use–induced sleep disorder, nor should these symptoms persist beyond what would be expected during withdrawal or intoxication of the type and amount of substance used or the duration of use. The sleep disorder is in excess of what would normally be expected during intoxication or withdrawal (pp. 278–279). Social and occupational performances are typically affected because the person may experience much distress.

Source: Adapted from American Psychiatric Association (APA). (2000). *Diagnostic and Statistical Manual of Mental Disorders* (4th ed., text revision). Washington, DC: Author.

BOX 16-2 ▓ Sample Occupational History Questions

1. When did the mental health symptoms first affect occupational performance? How was occupational performance affected?
2. When did symptoms of substance use first affect occupational performance? How was occupational performance affected?
3. How did substance use affect the mental health symptoms? Was there a change in occupational performance?
4. What effect did cessation of substance use have on the mental health symptoms? Was there a change in occupational performance?
5. What effect does a change in mental health status have in the substance use patterns? How does this change in pattern affect occupational performance?

evident as recovery proceeds and may indicate a necessary change in the intervention process to more strongly address the mental health issues of the client.

Impact on Occupational Performance

The revision to the *Occupational Therapy Practice Framework* (AOTA, 2008) is useful for analyzing how occupational therapy practitioners can approach their understanding of the potential occupational performance and participation problems of persons with CODs.

Occupation

Depending on the combination of diagnoses and the complexity of the activity demands, the existence of CODs without intervention negatively affects the performance of occupations or activities in all occupational areas, including

- Activities of daily living (e.g., bathing, grooming)
- Instrumental activities of daily living (e.g., taking care of others, home management)
- Rest and sleep
- Education
- Work
- Play
- Leisure
- Social participation (e.g., community, family)

Each of these activities requires (i.e., activity demands) a combination of performance skills, including sensory-perceptual, motor and praxis, emotional regulation, cognitive, and communication and social. Depending on the activity, the skills required could cause the person who has an untreated COD to have difficulty performing according to standard and within time frames, completing the activity, or beginning the activity in the first place. For example, a person with schizophrenia and marijuana abuse may not understand the directions for successful completion of an assigned work task and may be actively hallucinating to the extent that the person is unable to communicate his or her lack of understanding about what to do during the activity.

This type of performance limitation is especially true for those activities that are novel, rarely performed, complicated, or occur within distracting environments. Activities performed routinely or habitually within familiar roles (performance patterns) and within supportive environments may be completed properly, thus giving the impression the person is performing at a higher level than what is more indicative of his or her overall capability. Occupational performance may plummet when the person is asked to assume a new role with unfamiliar routines and activities performed in diverse environments.

Person

The person's skills may need to be developed to support performance and must be organized into habits and routines to ensure that they are mobilized regularly to meet expectations associated with the roles he or she assumes (e.g., parent, worker, family member). Skill performance also depends on intact underlying body structure and function, as well as other client factors such as values, beliefs, and spirituality. In terms of body function, the combination of mental disorders and substance use disorders affect the person's specific mental health functions (e.g., higher-level cognitive ability, attention, memory, perception, thought, sequencing complex movement, emotional, experience of self and time), as well as global mental health functions (e.g., consciousness, orientation, temperament and personality, energy and drive). Physical body function may be affected by the mental health disorder and its complications, partially related to medications, as well as by the drug(s) abused and resultant effects on the body's organ systems, including cardiovascular, neuromuscular, metabolic and digestive, and reproductive functions.

Typically, the person values the use of drugs and alcohol as a coping mechanism and believes these drugs of abuse will have a positive change on his or her life, such as improving his or her mental health condition. The person may not fully realize the negative impact of substance abuse and may attribute problems resulting from the substance use disorder to his or her situational problems or mental health status, or both. The person may also believe that the substances improve his or her spiritual relationship or replace an inadequately developed spirituality.

Environment

A variety of client contexts support or obstruct occupational performance, as well serve as supports or barriers to the substance using activity. Social and cultural environments may involve interaction with other people who abuse substances, and people in the community may also communicate negative views toward those with mental illness. The physical environment typically possesses a host of alcohol and drug cues (e.g., driving past a bar, seeing beer in the refrigerator, smelling the odor of marijuana). As a result, the person habitually responds to these cues with craving or an increased desire to use alcohol or drugs. This desire to use activates physiological and psychological expectations regarding the potentially positive experience associated with using (Moyers & Stoffel, 2001).

In addition to the environmental supports for substance use, the presence of prevention factors within a community

---

Evidence-Based Practice

Individuals with a coexisting substance use disorder and a mental health diagnosis were able to successfully complete vocational rehabilitation and achieve work functioning and employment outcomes (Drebing et al, 2002).

➤ It is important for occupational therapy practitioners to address the work goals of persons with co-occurring disorders.

Drebing, C. E., Fleitas, R., Moore, A., Krebs, C., Van Ormer, A., Penk, W., Seibyl, C., & Rosenheck, R. (2002). Patterns in work functioning and vocational rehabilitation associated with coexisting psychiatric and substance use disorders. *Rehabilitation Counseling Bulletin, 46*, 5–13.

The Lived Experience

Oil and Water

Try as you may, but oil and water will not mix, no matter how many variations in combining the two you attempt. This is analogous to mixing substances and mental illness, an infectious recipe that is destined to be disastrous. In the case of my loved one, the toxic dual was alcoholism and bipolar disorder.

As occupational therapists, we are often trained to document and communicate positives before the negatives; therefore, I will begin this narrative by illustrating the good person that exists in my loved one, despite the challenges presented in his life. My father has and always will hold a very special place in my world, and through my eyes, he is a very valuable person. He is someone who when well (not using alcohol or experiencing the extremes of bipolar disorder) is an absolute pleasure to have in one's company. He is intelligent, loving, sensitive, and charismatic, and has quick wit that is unmatched. He has the ability to strike up a conversation with anyone and treats all walks of life with kindness and respect as long as they demonstrate it in return.

Given the chronic nature of his disorders, I could write a book about the various relapses, exacerbations, crises, and periods of recovery. However, I can help you (the reader) develop an understanding of what this lifelong battle may look like by simply reviewing the past few months:

After serving 2 years in prison for drinking and driving (DUI), my father was released. Ahh, occupational freedom—a term I have used to describe the opportunity and ability to choose and participate in activities that are meaningful to an individual. For my father, the immediate occupational freedoms he partook in included riding in a car, rolling down the windows, and breathing the fresh air while listening to some classic rock. Next up was using cash to purchase a cup of coffee and a pack of cigarettes. All chosen activities that resulted in profound joy. My father and his family had high hopes to continue this positive exploration and attainment of meaningful activities. To list a few, my father wanted to play with my dog, eat a fish fry in good company, ride his horse for the first time, visit a friend who was battling cancer, secure housing, find work, and participate in family functions. So many plans and opportunities at his fingertips, yet so little resources, and, oh yes, let us not forget that he has two conditions that can seriously interfere with his newfound occupational freedoms.

Since my father was released from the state's custody without anything in place except a parole officer, my husband and I agreed to provide him immediate housing while he reconnected with the Veterans Administration (VA) and pursued a more permanent residence. My father also stayed with my brother and his wife, helping them recover and move things out of their home after a major flood ruined their basement and belongings. It was then that we noticed my father's bipolar disorder beginning to surface (after more than 2 years of stable mental health). Although medication compliant, mania persisted. He was disorganized, misplacing things, putting things in odd places, not sleeping, easily agitated, and feeling very anxious and stressed. One thing that temporarily soothed his anxieties and slowed things down for him was alcohol, an unhealthy option.

To make a long story short, he agreed to get help at the VA, but the emergency care was not equipped for addressing psychiatric emergencies. Within minutes of admission (hours from the time we arrived), my father was handcuffed and detained, absent of any previous freedoms. Fortunately, after about 1-month inpatient stay (and after much advocacy from the family), he started improving.

Adversity continued because my father had no place to live, and while I was on vacation, he was discharged from the VA to a motel room. He described hopeless feelings as "the walls were coming in on him." This made sense as his options were scarce. The motel bill was racking up, and he had no independence with transportation, which meant that cabs and bus fare were also heavily weighing on his mind. He was seeking resolution and staying in contact with me, but on one particular day I missed his phone call. Hours later, I called him back only to hear his condition to be in dire straits. He sounded beyond intoxicated, slurring his words, long pauses, difficulty tracking the conversation at first, and statements that concerned me about his mental health. The next morning he was admitted to an inpatient psychiatric facility.

He began to improve and had the mental strength to seek out all the resources he had. Fortunately, a landlord who remembered my father from years ago, welcomed him with open arms, and he found a quaint flat in a four-story home. I shared the news that he would be a grandpa for the first time, a special moment for my father as well as my husband and me. He worked hard to reestablish himself within the community, as he found work, visited the local American Legion post, went to the library, spent time with family and friends, helped out on the horse ranch, rode his horse for the first time, started physical therapy at the VA, obtained his occupational drivers license, and adopted a beautiful little puppy whom he adored and trained well. He was adhering to medications and remained sober at all family affairs.

As good as things were, I knew from past experiences that sometimes when things were for the most part going right something was bound to go wrong. What I could not believe was the speed of disaster. My uncle called me on a Sunday concerned that my father was getting sick and possibly drinking more. A few days later, I received a phone call that he my father was in a motor vehicle accident involving alcohol. My first reaction was denial; there was no way, he had been doing so well and had so much to look forward to (the grandbaby, the puppy, the prospect for work). The father I had spent time with over the past few months would never risk losing his freedoms for alcohol.

With saddened confirmation from my uncle, my next reaction was pure devastation. I knew what this meant...prison for years to come, as he was on a zero tolerance for alcohol. Now I felt the walls come in on me. All I could do was feel a profound sadness that I had never experienced before in my life. Sad because our relationship was now compromised, the greeting of his first grandchild would be robbed, and all the things he built to reestablish himself gone. What made me even sadder was thinking about how he must feel, how his life just spiraled out of control so quickly and now he is left with loss. How can someone who cares about life and those he loves risk losing it all?

The Lived Experience — cont'd

The only explanation I can come to is that my father was beginning to live as normal as possible and that he began to test whether he could have this "normal" life and an occasional drink on top of it. Regardless, it is my theory that the combination of alcohol (be it 1–2 drinks or 4–5 drinks) and my father's bipolar disorder were a recipe for disaster. Drinking countereffects his medications, consequently initiating his manic symptoms of bipolar disorder. In addition, there were environmental stressors present, albeit positive, but seemingly too stimulating.

Now we are faced with loss. In some ways I am grieving because I had so much hope. I had hope that with the help of my family, my father, and the system, we could defeat this thing called dual diagnosis or co-occurring disorders. However, I realize that the current system fails all parties involved, including individuals who have chronic injuries, families who love them, and the community who continues to be vulnerable to the state of those not adequately treated. Incarceration only temporarily controls the safety of individuals and communities. It does next to nothing to facilitate rehabilitation or provide hope for successful community living.

I am not denying the accountability that my father has in this mess, he plays the key role. However, I am hopeful that more attention is given to the complexities that co-occurring disorders demand. As for my relationship with my father, despite the sad circumstances, I am grateful that our relationship can continue to be one of support, hope, and love.

can affect the rate at which persons initiate alcohol and drug use. A community can remain healthy when it prevents problems related to alcohol and drug abuse and untreated CODs. Prevention depends on local government and organizational policies regarding alcohol and drug use. The community's ability to raise awareness of socially acceptable levels of alcohol use and make services available to persons with CODs is critically important. Drinking patterns can be modified when a community deliberately severs the relationship between drinking and community events, such as removing alcohol from a central role in the celebration of holidays and religious or cultural festivals (Moyers & Stoffel, 2010).

The local media plays a role in creating this community awareness and can work with the police to publicize enforcement of laws related to drinking and driving, drug trafficking and purchasing of illegal substances, public intoxication, and disorderly conduct. A healthy community is dependent on the collective engagement of its citizens in positive activities and occupations; thus, prevention strategies are incomplete unless the community ensures the availability of healthy and meaningful occupations for everyone, regardless of socioeconomic or mental health status. The presence of these prevention factors within a community determines the rate at which people initiate alcohol and drug use and seek help for untreated CODs (Moyers & Stoffel, 2009).

Intervention

A treatment improvement protocol (TIP 42), Substance Abuse Treatment for Persons with Co-occurring Disorders (CSAT, 2005a), identifies six main principles for organizing service delivery for persons with CODs, including

- Employing a recovery perspective
- Adopting a multiproblem viewpoint
- Developing a phased approach to treatment
- Addressing specific, real life problems early in treatment
- Planning for the client's cognitive and functional impairments
- Using support systems to maintain and extend treatment effectiveness (p. 38)

A recovery perspective views intervention as a long-term process that occurs in stages or phases, one requiring continuity of care over time. Phases include engagement in intervention, stabilization of mental health and substance use status, treatment, aftercare, and continuing care.

People with CODs have multiple interconnected problems that are often complex in nature and that typically involve such real life problems as housing, employment, consistent health care, and access to a support network. These real life problems and activity limitations are aggravated by cognitive impairments that can range from mild to severe, depending on the substance abused, the amount of the substance used per frequency and duration, and the nature of the mental health status. Consequently, the support needs of each person vary, with the most support needed for those individuals with severe cognitive impairments and activity limitations. Support systems should include a mutual self-help strategy in which people with CODs are encouraged to help one another with problem-solving, decision-making, and coping. In addition, support in interfacing with the community (religious, social, and community organizations) and with family and friends should occur.

Provision of intervention following the six guiding principles can lead to effective outcomes when the delivery of the program incorporates several key components (CSAT, 2005a). These components create the philosophy of a "no wrong door approach"; that is, how the person enters the health-care system, whether through the mental health system, the substance abuse system, or the medical system, does not determine whether the person will receive integrated services based on the six guiding principles. This philosophy requires access to integrated services, which in many communities if often limited due to funding, insurance coverage, availability of trained health-care professionals, and public policy.

Access begins with all health-care practitioners being trained to screen for symptoms of untreated mental illness and substance use disorders. Training must also include how to refer individuals to integrated services for further evaluation. Integrated evaluation additionally determines the appropriate level and combination of integrated services, whether they are provided inpatient, outpatient, or within-other-community

Evidence-Based Practice

Participants (*n* = 351) receiving inpatient intervention for co-occurring disorders (CODs) successfully attended Alcoholics Anonymous (AA) or Narcotics Anonymous (NA) self-help programs (Jordan, Davidson, Herman, & Boots Miller, 2002). Participants who were diagnosed with schizophrenia or schizoaffective disorder, combined with substance use disorders, most frequently, cocaine and alcohol abuse or dependence, comprised 50% of the sample. The other half of the participants with COD demonstrated rates of AA or NA attendance 10 months after hospitalization that were similar to those of persons with only substance use disorders; however, persons with COD involving schizophrenia or schizoaffective disorders specifically had significantly fewer days of AA or NA attendance.

➤ Occupational therapy practitioners should recommend self-help groups such as AA or NA to individuals with COD, while being aware that individuals' rates of attendance might vary.

➤ Encouraging attendance and engagement in the fellowship and acceptance of self-help groups can be beneficial for those with COD, despite the social participation limitations that might be associated with mental illness.

Jordan, L. C., Davidson, W. S., Herman, S. E., & Boots Miller, B. J. (2002). Involvement in 12-step programs among persons with dual diagnoses. *Psychiatric Services, 53,* 874–896.

programming. Health-care professionals must also be trained to provide integrated services using the six guiding principles. Services must be culturally sensitive to the values and beliefs of their clients, which may necessitate developing nontraditional models of care. For example, assisting a Native American to continue to participate in tribal pow-wows and ceremonies might be scheduled in coordination with attendance at AA meetings on and off the reservation. Services must be comprehensive enough and continuous to adequately address all phases of recovery.

These service delivery issues require occupational therapy practitioners in all practice areas to have the education and experience to, at the minimum, conduct integrated screenings to ensure that clients have access to integrated intervention. Those occupational therapy practitioners who work in the community and in mental health settings can broaden their education and experience by providing integrated evaluation and intervention. Advocacy efforts must be focused on developing the funding for and research of the role of occupational therapy in providing services, especially highlighting occupational therapy intervention with persons who have cognitive impairments, activity limitations, and restrictions participating in daily life activity in the community.

Summary

This chapter clarifies the meaning of the term "co-occurring disorders" as referring to persons who have at least one substance use disorder and a minimum of one mental disorder. The epidemiology of COD was explored, concluding with the need to simultaneously address both classes of disorders in an integrated manner. Occupational therapy practitioners are encouraged to take responsibility for improving research, training, insurance coverage, and evidence-based intervention programs for COD.

Occupational therapy practitioners require education and training to address the occupational performance problems and community participation of persons with CODs, thereby improving existing and developing new prevention and intervention programs.

Active Learning Strategies

1. How Co-Occurring Conditions Affect Occupational Performance

Choose a mental health diagnosis (schizophrenia, bipolar disorder, PTSD, or depression) and research how the symptoms and occupational performance would be complicated by a co-occurring substance use disorder. Use information from DSM-IV-TR (APA, 2000) to help you outline the symptoms of both the mental and substance use disorder. Explore how these co-occurring conditions might affect major occupational roles such as parent/spouse, worker, student, and leisure participant.

2. Case Study

Consider the following case and answer the reflective questions posed.

Case: Juanita M.

The client is a 32-year-old Hispanic woman who is married and has two daughters, one who is 6 years old and another who is 15 years old. Juanita has a 2-year history of cocaine and alcohol dependence, as well as major depression. She is currently taking antidepressants. Juanita reports that her husband of 20 years has shown an escalating tendency to physically and verbally abuse her and her oldest daughter. She and her children currently reside in a shelter for women who are in abusive relationships. The shelter has access to a variety of treatment programs to which Juanita and her children can be referred. Juanita is motivated to obtain and participate in treatment, including receiving legal help in leaving her husband and securing custody of their children, obtaining employment, and finding an appropriate living arrangement.

Reflective Questions
● What information would you need in order to have a more in-depth understanding of Juanita's case?
● What client factors might be involved as a result of Juanita's diagnoses?
● What occupational performance issues would you expect Juanita to have in addition to her legal, employment, and living arrangement concerns?
● What family issues will likely affect Juanita's recovery?
● What activity demands would support and inhibit Juanita's recovery?
● What contextual factors would support and inhibit Juanita's recovery?

Reflective Journal

Use the following prompts to reflect on COD, and then describe your thoughts in your Reflective Journal.
- Reflect on the way in which occupational therapy's principles of holism and client centeredness affect how occupational therapy practitioners can help persons with CODs.

- Reflect on the way in which occupational therapy practitioners can incorporate their understanding of the dynamic interaction among the person, environment, and activity as a foundation for designing integrated intervention programs for persons with CODs.

Resources

Websites
- Homelessness Resource Center: http://homelessness.samhsa.gov/
- SAMHSA's Co-Occurring Center for Excellence: http://coce.samhsa.gov/
- TIP 42: Substance Abuse Treatment for Persons With Co-Occurring Disorders: http://www.ncbi.nlm.nih.gov/books/bv.fcgi?rid=hstat5.chapter.74073
- TIP Curriculum (PowerPoint slides): http://www.kap.samhsa.gov/products/trainingcurriculums/tip42.htm

References

American Occupational Therapy Association (AOTA). (2008). *Occupational Therapy Practice Framework: Domain and Process* (2nd ed.). Bethesda, MD: Author.

American Psychiatric Association (APA). (2000). *Diagnostic and Statistical Manual of Mental Disorders* (4th ed., text revision). Washington, DC: Author.

American Society of Addiction Medicine (ASAM). (2001). *Patient Placement Criteria for the Treatment of Substance-Related Disorders: ASAM PPC-2R* (2nd rev. ed.). Chevy Chase, MD: Author.

Anderson, C. M., Teicher, M. H., Pocari, A., & Renshaw, P. F. (2002). Abnormal T2 relaxation time in the cerebellar vermis of adults sexually abused in childhood: Potential role of the vermin in stress-enhanced risk for drug abuse. *Psychoneuroendocrinology, 27,* 231–244.

Back, S., Dansky, B. S., Coffey, S. F., Saladin, M. E., Sonne, S., & Brady, K. T. (2000). Cocaine dependence with and without posttraumatic stress disorder: A comparison of substance use, trauma history and psychiatric comorbidity. *American Journal on Addictions, 9,* 51–62.

Berger-Greenstein, J. A., Cuevas, C. A., Brady, S. M., Trezza, G., Richardson, M. A., & Keane, T. M. (2007). Major depression in patients with HIV/AIDS and substance abuse. *AIDS Patient Care and STDs, 21,* 942–955.

Brady, K., & Sinha, R. (2005). Co-occurring mental and substance use disorders: The neurobiological effects of chronic stress. *American Journal of Psychiatry, 162,* 1483–1493.

Brady, K. T. (2002, September). Recognizing and treating dual diagnosis in general health care settings: Core competencies and how to achieve them. In M. R. Haack & H. Adger, Jr. (Eds.), *Strategic Plan for Interdisciplinary Faculty Development: Arming the Nation's Health Professional Workforce for a New Approach to Substance Use Disorders* (pp. 143–154). Providence, RI: Association for Medical Education and Research in Substance Abuse (AMERSA). Available at: http://www.projectmainstream.net/newsfiles/1134/SPACdocfinal.pdf (accessed November 22, 2009).

Brady, K. T., Kileen, T. K., Brewerton, T., & Lucerini, S. (2000). Comorbidity of psychiatric disorders and posttraumatic stress disorder. *Journal of Clinical Psychiatry, 61*(17), 22–32.

Center for Substance Abuse Treatment (CSAT). (2005a). *Substance Abuse Treatment for Persons With Co-Occurring Disorders.* Treatment Improvement Protocol (TIP) Series No. 42, DHHS Publication No. (SMA) 05-3992. Rockville, MD: Substance Abuse and Mental Health Services Administration.

Center for Substance Abuse Treatment (CSAT). (2005b). *Substance Abuse Treatment: Group Therapy.* Treatment Improvement Protocol (TIP) Series No. 41, DHHS Publication No. (SMA) 05-3991. Rockville, MD: Substance Abuse and Mental Health Services Administration.

Center for Substance Abuse Treatment (CSAT). (2006a). *Definitions and Terms Relating to Co-Occurring Disorders.* COCE Overview Paper 1, DHHS Publication No. (SMA) 06-4163. Rockville, MD: Substance Abuse and Mental Health Services Administration and Center for Mental Health Services.

Center for Substance Abuse Treatment (CSAT). (2006b). *Screening, Assessment, and Treatment Planning for Persons With Co-Occurring Disorders.* COCE Overview Paper 2, DHHS Publication No. (SMA) 06-4164 Rockville, MD: Substance Abuse and Mental Health Services Administration and Center for Mental Health Services.

Center for Substance Abuse Treatment (CSAT). (2006c). *Overarching Principles to Address the Needs of Persons With Co-Occurring Disorders.* COCE Overview Paper 3, DHHS Publication No. (SMA) 06-4165. Rockville, MD: Substance Abuse and Mental Health Services Administration.

Center for Substance Abuse Treatment (CSAT). (2007). *Substance Abuse Treatment for Persons With Co-Occurring Disorders Inservice Training.* DHHS Publication No. (SMA) 07-4262. Rockville, MD: Substance Abuse and Mental Health Services Administration.

Drebing, C. E., Fleitas, R., Moore, A., Krebs, C., Van Ormer, A., Penk, W., et al. (2002). Patterns in work functioning and vocational rehabilitation associated with coexisting psychiatric and substance use disorders. *Rehabilitation Counseling Bulletin, 46,* 513.

Federation of Families for Children's Mental Health. (2001). *Blamed and Ashamed: The Treatment Experiences of Youth With Co-occurring Substance Abuse and Mental Health Disorders and Their Families.* Alexandria, VA: Author. Available at: http://www.ffcmh.org/pdf/booksandguides/blamedashamed.pdf (accessed November 22, 2009).

Gagne, C., White, W., & Anthony, W. A. (2007). Recovery: A common vision for the fields of mental health and addictions. *Psychiatric Rehabilitation Journal, 31,* 32–37.

Grant, B. F., Hasin, D. S., Chou, P., Stinson, F. S., & Dawson, D. A. (2004). Nicotine dependence and psychiatric disorders in the United States. *Archives of General Psychiatry, 61,* 1107–1115.

Grant, B. F., Moore, T. C., Shepard, J., & Kaplan, K. (2003). *Source and Accuracy Sstatement: Wave 1 National Epidemiologic Survey on Alcohol and Related Conditions (NESARC).* Bethesda, MD: National Institute on Alcohol Abuse and Alcoholism.

Grant, B. F., Stinson, F. S., Dawson, D. A., Chou, S. P., Dufour, M. C., Compton, W., Pickering, R. P., & Kaplan, K. (2006). Prevalence and co-occurrence of substance use disorders and independent mood and anxiety disorders. *Alcohol Research & Health, 29,* 107–120.

Grant, B. F., Stinson, F. S., Dawson, D. A., Chou, S. P., Ruan, W. J., & Pickering, R. P. (2006). Co-occurrence of 12-month alcohol and drug use disorders and personality disorders in the United States. *Alcohol Research & Health, 29,* 121–130.

Hartwell, S. W. (2004). Comparison of offenders with mental illness only and offenders with dual diagnoses. *Psychiatric Services, 55,* 145–150.

Jones, D. R., Macias, C., Barreira, P. J., Fisher, W. H., Hargreaves, W. A., & Harding, C. M. (2004). Prevalence, severity and co-occurrence of chronic physical health problems of persons with serious mental illness. *Psychiatric Services, 55,* 1250–1257.

Jordan, L. C., Davidson, W. S., Herman, S. E., & Boots Miller, B. J. (2002). Involvement in 12-step programs among persons with dual diagnoses. *Psychiatric Services, 53,* 874–896.

Kessler, R. C. (2004). The epidemiology of dual diagnosis. *Biological Psychiatry, 56,* 730–737.

Kessler, R. C., Chiu, W. T., Demler, O. & Walters, E. E. (2005). Prevalence, severity, and comorbidity of 12-month DSM-IV disorders in the National Comorbidity urvey Replication. *Archives of General Psychiatry, 62,* 617–627.

Kessler, R. C., Nelson, C. B., McGonagle, K. A., Edlund, M. J., Frank, R. G., & Leaf, P. J. (1996). The epidemiology of co-occurring addictive and mental disorders: Implications for prevention and service utilization. *American Journal of Orthopsychiatry, 66,* 17–31.

Koob, G. F. (2000). Animal models of craving for ethanol. *Addiction, 95,* S73–S81.

Leserman, J. (2003). HIV disease progression: Depression, stress, and possible mechanisms. *Biological Psychiatry, 54,* 295–306.

Lowinson, J. H., Ruiz, P., Millman, R. B., & Langrod, J. G. (1992). *Substance Abuse: A Comprehensive Textbook.* Baltimore, MD: Williams & Wilkins.

McLellan A. T., & Meyers, K. (2004). Contemporary addiction treatment: A review of systems problems for adults and adolescents. *Biological Psychiatry, 56,* 764–770.

McNeil, D. E., Binder, R. L., & Robinson, J. C. (2005). Incarceration associated with homelessness, mental disorders and co-occurring substance abuse. *Psychiatric Services, 56,* 840–846.

Minkoff, K., & Cline, C. A. (2004). Changing the world: The design and implementation of comprehensive continuous, integrated systems of care for individuals with co-occurring disorders. *Psychiatric Clinics of North America, 27,* 727–743.

Moyers, P. A., & Stoffel, V. C. (2001). Community-based approaches for substance use disorders. In M. Scaffa (Ed.), *Occupational Therapy in Community-Based Practice Settings* (pp. 318–342). Philadelphia, PA: FA Davis.

Moyers, P. A., & Stoffel, V. C. (2010). Preventing substance abuse in adolescents and adults. In M. E. Scaffa, M. Reitz, & M. A. Pizzi, (Eds.), *Occupational Therapy in the Promotion of Health and Wellness.* (pp. 280–306). Philadelphia, PA: FA Davis.

National Association of State Alcohol and Drug Abuse Directors (NASADAD) and the National Association of State Mental Health Program Directors (NASMHPD) (2005). *The Evolving Conceptual Framework for Co-Occurring Mental Health and Substance Abuse Disorders: Developing Strategies for Systems Change.* Final Report of the NASMHPD-NASADAD Task Force on Co-Occurring Disorders. Washington, DC and Alexandria, VA: Authors.

National Association of State Mental Health Program Directors (NASMHPD) & National Association of State Alcohol and Drug Abuse Directors (NASADAD). (2000). *Financing and Marketing the New Conceptual Framework for Co-Occurring Mental Health and Substance Abuse Disorders: A Blueprint for Systems Change.* Alexandria, VA: Author.

North, C. S., Eyrich, K. M., Pollio, D. E., & Spitznagel, E. L. (2004). Are rates of psychiatric disorders changing over time in the homeless population? *American Journal of Public Health, 94,* 103–108.

Reuland, M. (2004, January). *A Guide to Implementing Police-Based Diversion Programs for People With Mental Illness.* Delmar, NY: Technical Assistance and Policy Analysis Center for Jail Diversion. Available at: http://gainscenter.samhsa.gov/pdfs/jail_diversion/PERF.pdf (accessed November 22, 2009).

Ries, R. K. (1993). The dually diagnosed patient with psychotic symptoms. *Journal of Addictive Diseases, 12,* 103–122.

Rollins, A. L., O'Neill, S. J., Davis, K. E., & Devitt, T. S. (2005). Substance abuse relapse and factors associated with relapse in an inner-city sample of patients with dual diagnoses. *Psychiatric Services, 56,* 1274–1281.

Schuckit, M. A., Tipp, J. E., Bergman, M., Reich, W., Hesselbrock, V. M., & Smith, T. L. (1997). Comparison of induced and independent major depressive disorders in 2,945 alcoholics. *American Journal of Psychiatry, 154,* 948–957.

Shivani, R., Goldsmith, R. J., & Anthenelli, R. M. (2002). Alcoholism and psychiatric disorders: Diagnostic challenges. *Alcohol Research & Health, 26,* 90–98.

Stoffel, V. C., & Moyers, P. A. (2004). An evidence-based and occupational perspective of interventions for persons with substance-use disorders. *American Journal of Occupational Therapy, 58,* 570–586.

Substance Abuse and Mental Health Services Administration (SAMHSA). (2003). *Blueprint for Change: Ending Chronic Homelessness for Persons With Serious Mental Illnesses and Co-Occurring Substance Use Disorders.* DHHS Publication No. SMA-04-3870. Rockville, MD: Author.

Substance Abuse and Mental Health Services Administration (SAMHSA). (2007). *Results From the 2006 National Survey on Drug Use and Health: National Findings.* Office of Applied Studies, NSDUH Series H-32, DHHS Publication No. SMA 07-4293. Rockville, MD: SAMHSA.

Tucker, J. S., Kanouse, D., E., Miu, A., Koegel, P., & Sullivan, G. (2003). HIV risk behaviors and their correlates among HIV-positive adults with serious mental illness. *AIDS and Behavior, 7,* 29–40.

Waldrop, A. E., Back, S. E., Verduin, M. L., & Brady, K. T. (2007). Triggers for cocaine and alcohol use in the presence and absence of posttraumatic stress disorder. *Addictive Behaviors, 32,* 634–639.

Dementia

Patricia Schaber

> "I live on the edge of fear and insecurity, and I am filled with uncertainty. . . . (p. 171) At some point, I will no longer experience the pain of watching my mind deteriorate to a point of incomprehension. The loved ones around me will have the unwelcome task to look after me and shelter me from harm. My burden is slight compared to that of the truly living (p. 102).
>
> —Thomas DeBaggio, 2002

Introduction

Little is certain about the condition of **progressive dementia** except that, at some point, as Thomas DeBaggio described, the person will "lose" his or her mind. As practitioners, we struggle in our attempt to define these individuals without a past that they remember or a future they can control. Pauline Boss, a prominent family social scientist, coined an apt term for the family experience of dementia—*ambiguous loss,* when the person is physically present but psychologically absent (Boss, 2006). Family members, friends, colleagues, and acquaintances experience a slow grieving process as they mourn the loss of the person they knew and rally to support the ever-changing person whom they are struggling to know. For the most part an insidious syndrome, dementia unleashes fear and challenges us to look carefully at the human condition and seek value and worth of each life lived.

Dementia is an acquired syndrome that results from a disease or disorder of the brain that affects cognition, or thinking, and memory. It disrupts perception, information processing, problem-solving, judgment, sequencing of tasks, recognition and naming of objects, mood and affect, writing and calculating, and other functions necessary to carry out daily activities (Abraham, 2005). The majority of dementias are progressive, indicating a gradual decline in the ability to care for oneself. In the later stages, the syndrome is characterized by behavioral difficulties, including aggression, agitation, and altered sleep/wake cycles that can necessitate 24-hour supervision and care.

The most common type of dementia is **Alzheimer's disease**, an age-related, neurological, degenerative disorder that predominately affects persons older than 65 years. Lewy body disease, vascular or multi-infarct dementia, frontotemporal lobe or Pick disease, Parkinson disease, Huntington disease, and normal pressure hydrocephalus are other dementing diseases or disorders that can affect a person in mid- to late life, precipitating an increasing need for care with age. Creutzfeldt-Jakob disease, HIV/AIDS-related dementia, brain tumors, brain trauma, infectious diseases, toxic exposure, and vitamin B12 deficiency are contributors to dementia that can occur throughout the life span. Symptoms of dementia in younger adults are frequently due to metabolic disorders, substance abuse, immune-mediated diseases, and infectious disease.

The increasing prevalence of dementia is a societal and economic problem that demands attention. As the average life span increases, so does the number of individuals and families who experience the effects of dementia in their everyday lives. The Alzheimer's Association predicts that by 2050, there will be 11 to 16 million persons with the disease in the United States, costing $148 billion a year (Hebert, Beckett, Scherr, & Evans, 2001). There are an estimated 34 million caregivers in America providing assistance for older adults for $5,531 out-of-pocket annually (National Alliance for Caregiving, 2007). Individuals need to plan for the supports required to maintain a quality of life in their later years, with the primary goal of preserving human dignity throughout the course of the syndrome until the end stage of life.

Dementia disrupts a person's ability to engage in daily activities. Occupational therapy is a cost-effective intervention for community-dwelling elders with dementia, with improved daily functioning and increased caregiver confidence (Graff et al, 2008). Behavioral issues related to dementia have been effectively treated in a home-based, occupational therapy program involving clients and family caregivers (Gitlin & Corcoran, 2005). Occupational therapy practitioners provide services to reduce the impact of declining cognition on performance of daily activities, modify the environment to enhance independent functioning, and engage the family caregivers in strategies to enhance optimal participation in life.

Description of the Disorder

Dementia is defined as "a loss of multiple acquired cognitive and emotional abilities sufficient to interfere with daily activities" (Goetz, 2003, p. 1158). As a syndrome, it manifests as a cognitive disorder resulting from one or more medical conditions. Dementia is characterized by multiple cognitive deficits, including a global decrease in intellect, memory, and executive function (Moore & Jefferson, 2004). Its etiology differentiates the degree of impairment, rate of progression, and manifestations of the symptoms of the dementia. The gradual or acute decline in abilities follows a predictable pattern:

- Thinking—progresses from using abstract thought processes to concrete processes to object centered
- Memory—initially presents with short-term memory impairment and advances to long-term memory impairment
- Problem-solving—challenges start with complex, high-impact decisions and progress to an inability to make simple decisions
- Calculating—noticeable problems with complex math procedures advance to errors in simple calculations
- Judgment—begins with a lack of awareness of factors in decision-making and progresses to an inattention to problem-solving processes

Most forms of dementia are chronic, **progressive**, and irreversible, with cognitive abilities declining with the course of the disease. Progressive dementias include Alzheimer's disease and vascular dementia, which make up 90% of all dementia-related disease, as well as Parkinson disease, Huntington disease, frontotemporal lobe dementia or Pick disease, and HIV/AIDS-dementia complex, which account for the remaining 10% (Moore & Jefferson, 2004). Although it is rare, some dementias are reversible; that is, if the related disease is resolved, the cognitive processes return to premorbid levels or improve. Reversible dementias include metabolic or endocrine deficiencies; toxic exposure such as alcohol or heavy metal poisoning; and hydrocephalus, specifically, normal pressure hydrocephalus. A recent meta-analysis revealed that, of the 9% of potentially reversible forms of dementia that have been identified, only 0.6% actually showed any signs of reversal (0.31% partial, 0.29% full) (Clarfield, 2003). In other words, 99.4% of the time, the dementing condition gets worse.

Other forms of dementia are nonprogressive, or static. With **static dementia**, such as that caused by traumatic brain injury (TBI), the degree of cognitive impairment can remain relatively stable for years.

The manifestation of a progressive type of dementia, such as Alzheimer's' disease, presents with a broad range of behaviors, most notably, short-term memory difficulty. Initially, the symptoms of memory impairment are masked by normal, age-related, declining rates of processing of information (Salthouse, 2000). Persons begin forgetting appointments, losing common objects such as keys and purses, or leaving the stove on. The difference from normal age-related decline is that these incidents become more noticeable, form a pattern of changed behavior from the primordial personality, and the individual and family members begin to voice concerns. Family members listen to the same question repeated in short succession and are often asked to repeat information that was provided 5 minutes earlier. Because short-term memory is affected earlier than long-term memory in the progression of the dementia, the person may rely on past experiences for topics of conversation. In late stage dementia, individuals may forget they are married, where they reside, or if they have children.

Dementia can include disruptions in language ability, usually initially presenting as word finding problems. Forgetting names of family members or common objects and having difficulty relating details of an incident can be early indicators of aphasia. Although it is normal behavior to occasionally forget a word or lose a train of thought, the incidence of word retrieval problems increases, and the family members begin to offer word options to complete a sentence. Visual-spatial perception may be affected, making it challenging to read a newspaper or engage in former hobbies. The individual may have difficulty attending to tasks; in fact, distraction may be so severe that the individual is unable to perform a sequential task such as setting the table. Motor planning may be affected, exemplified as difficulty signing checks or using a can opener.

A person with dementia may display emotional changes, such as anxiety or agitation, as their everyday tasks become more difficult. Higher-level thinking tasks such as financial management, becomes problematic, and frustration may escalate when balancing a checkbook or during monetary transactions. Loss of judgment may be observed in signs of personal neglect, mismatched clothing, or inappropriate outerwear for the weather. Personality changes and loss of former interests may lead family members to declare that the individual is "not the same person he or she used to be."

Behavioral events, termed **catastrophic reactions**, can occur in the later stages of dementia (Mace, 1990). These are emotional and physical reactions to tasks, such as yelling or hitting due to frustration with a task the person can no longer perform. These responses may concern family members when the person becomes frustrated with tasks that were formerly easy but are now difficult to execute. Sensory seeking or way finding behaviors create challenges for caregivers in restricting the person's mobility to safe or secure areas. Hallucinations or delusions with paranoia are not uncommon later in the syndrome; the person may make accusations, such as "Someone stole my purse" or "Someone took my wallet," or perseverate on a theme such as "There is someone in my room at night."

DSM-IV-TR Criteria

The essential feature for a diagnosis of dementia is memory impairment (Criterion A1) and one or more of the following cognitive disturbances (American Psychiatric Association [APA], 2000):

- Aphasia (Criterion A2a)
- Apraxia (Criterion A2b)
- Agnosia (Criterion A2c)
- Loss of executive function (Criterion A2d)

Four other criteria signify dementia. First, Criteria A1 and A2 must be "severe enough to cause significant impairment in social or occupational functioning." Second, the change must "represent a decline from the previous level of functioning" (APA, 2000, p. 148). Third, the cognitive changes are not due to a delirium. Fourth, the changes are not due to another Axis I psychiatric disorder.

Memory impairment is an inability to learn new information and/or recall past information. With mild memory impairment in the early stages of dementia, the individual may become frustrated with new learning or anxious when expected to take in new information. For example, changing a familiar route due to a detour in the road may cause confusion and fear of getting lost. In later stages, memory impairment is characterized by the inability to recall simple life details, such as home address, the names of family members, or a former career.

Aphasia is an "absence or impairment of the ability to communicate through speech, writing, or signs because of brain dysfunction" (Thomas, 1997, p. 132). Aphasia is characterized by a loss of memory for words (i.e., the person may know what he or she wants to say, but cannot find the words to say it). Individuals are unable to recall the names of common objects, and family members find themselves offering word options or cues to communicate. In the later stages of dementia, a person may use disconnected sentences or gibberish.

Apraxia, or the "inability to perform purposive movements although there is no sensory or motor impairment" (Thomas, 1997, p. 138), is evident in mid- to later stage dementia. The cognitive command to initiate and plan movement is impeded as clients struggle to, for example, put on a coat or drink a glass of water. Family members may initially guide the movement to get the task started, but eventually, in the later stages, the caregiver must provide moderate to full assistance with daily self-care.

Agnosia is a "loss of comprehension of visual, auditory, or other sensations although sensory sphere is intact" (Thomas, 1997, p. 52). The person is unable to interpret sounds, visual objects or images, tactile sensations, or time sequences. With agnosia, for example, a person may observe a set of keys and be unable to associate the object with its use. In later stages of dementia, individuals are unable to recognize faces or their own reflection in the mirror.

Disturbances in **executive function** are attributed to frontal lobe or subcortical pathway involvement. Executive function is the "ability to think abstractly and to plan, initiate, sequence, monitor, and stop complex behavior" (APA, 2000, p. 149). Impairment in executive function is manifest in difficulty with new tasks and multistep processes, calculations, word or number puzzles, planning and organizing, scheduling, and multitasking.

With dementia, the severity of impairment is determined by a report of the social and occupational activities that the person is unable to perform due to the condition. These activities (e.g., work, leisure, social interactions, instrumental activities of daily living [IADLs], activities of daily living [ADLs]) are dependent on the activity demands of the environment. With dementia, a high-demand environment, such as a work setting, may precipitate major life changes, whereas a low-demand environment may be easily adapted to the gradual changes in cognition. For example, a 55-year-old person with young or early onset Alzheimer's disease may need to leave a job with high cognitive demands, whereas a 67-year-old retired individual could continue home management tasks throughout the early stages of the disease.

The detailed *Diagnostic and Statistical Manual of Mental Disorders, Fourth Edition* (DSM-IV-TR) diagnostic criteria for dementia are listed in Box 17-1.

BOX 17-1 ■ DSM-IV-TR Criteria for Dementia

A. Characteristic symptoms: Criterion A1 must be present with one or more of Criterion A2.
Criterion A1—Memory impairment
Criterion A2—Aphasia, apraxia, agnosia, and loss of executive function

B. Social/occupational dysfunction: The Criteria A1 and A2 must be severe enough to cause a significant impairment in social or occupational functioning.

C. There must be a decline from previous function.

D. The cognitive deficits are not exclusively in the course of a delirium.

E. The cognitive disturbances are not due to another Axis I disorder (major depression, schizophrenia).

From American Psychiatric Association. (2000). *Diagnostic and Statistical Manual of Mental Disorders* (4th ed.). Washington, DC: Author.

Subtypes

The DSM-IV-TR lists three subtypes of dementia, which are described in Box 17-2. Subtypes of dementia are based on age of onset, behavioral factors, and co-occurring disorders:

- Early and late onset dementia is determined by the occurrence of the disease at or prior to age 65 or after age 65.
- Behavioral disturbances refer to those behaviors that require supervision for safety (e.g., way finding [formerly termed wandering], agitation, insomnia, aggression, extreme lethargy, socially inappropriate comments and behaviors [disrobing], psychosis). Psychosis manifests with hallucinations, delusions, or delusional misidentifications, and is more frequently present in later stages of Alzheimer's disease or with Parkinson disease and stroke (Rayner, O'Brien, & Shoenbachler, 2006).
- Dementia may be co-occurring with delirium or depression (see differentiation of dementia, delirium, and depression as follows).

The symptoms that characterize dementia can distinguish one etiology from another by degree and distinction based on where the degeneration begins in the brain; over time, as the disease spreads, the symptoms blend and render one type of dementia indistinguishable from another. Cortical dementias include Alzheimer's disease, characterized early on by executive dysfunction along with problems in declarative memory and language. **Executive function** involves foresight, planning, attention, and dexterity in task completion. **Declarative memory** involves conscious awareness of events and objects, including encoding, storing, and retrieving information (Manning, 2004). In cortical dementia, procedural or unconscious motoric memory may remain intact in the early stages, and the individual can be successful with familiar repetitive tasks through the later stages of the disease (Bares, 1998; Poe & Seifert, 1997).

Frontotemporal lobe dementia or **Pick disease** can be distinguished from Alzheimer's disease by the prominence of more definitive personality changes, aphasia, and disinhibition due to frontal lobe involvement (Solomon et al, 1995). There are other rare variants of Alzheimer's disease, including

primary progressive aphasia and **posterior cortical atrophy**. These are believed to originate in the parietal (language area) and occipital (visual area) lobes, respectively, and progress to the cortical region of the brain over time. Initial symptoms center on language problems or visual disturbances.

Subcortical dementias such as with **Huntington's** and **Parkinson's** disease are characterized by **bradykinesia** (slowed movement) and **bradyphrenia** (slowed thought), which also are seen in supranuclear palsy, multiple sclerosis, Wilson's disease, and HIV/AIDS-dementia (Cummings & Benson, 1984). These conditions involve subcortical basal ganglion structures, which support procedural memory rote skill performance (Levy, 2005, p. 318). Subcortical dementias include significant motor involvement, precipitating functional skill impairment. This is a distinguishing characteristic from cortical dementias such as Alzheimer's disease; apraxias are typically not seen in Alzheimer's disease until the later stages.

Dementias that involve motor areas of the cortex are Lewy body, corticobasal ganglionic degeneration, and progressive supranuclear palsy. **Lewy body dementia** is sometimes regarded as a variant of Alzheimer's' disease (Goldman, 2004). It is manifest in fluctuations in cognition, visual hallucinations, and parkinsonian motor signs (Goldman, 2004). Frequent falls due to motor involvement are characteristic of Lewy body dementia. **Corticobasal ganglionic degeneration**, a rare cause of dementia, is noted by a marked early phase apraxia or "alien hand" (unconscious movement). The visuospatial deficits and apraxia make it challenging to engage in daily tasks. **Progressive supranuclear palsy** is clinically seen as postural instability, along with falls and gait disturbances. The inability to gaze downward is an early sign. Oral motor involvement leads to dysarthria or speech disorders.

Vascular dementia is associated with the presence of cerebrovascular disease and risk factors, including hypertension, diabetes, hyperlipidemia, and smoking. The onset of vascular dementia is generally more abrupt or may present with a stepwise decline in cognition (Goldman, 2004). Individuals may be able to register information, but have difficulty with memory recall and retrieval. Motor involvement is common, such as limb flaccidity or spasticity, plantar extension, and gait disturbances. In some cases, neuroimaging can identify the cerebrovascular incident, thus distinguishing vascular dementia from other types of dementia.

Figure 17-1 shows Burt, a person with vascular dementia.

Etiology

Degenerative disorders are a major contributor to cognitive decline, although other diseases and disorders are associated with dementia. In fact, more than 50 diseases contribute to the development of cognitive decline (see Box 17-3 for additional etiologies). Because of the broad range of cortical changes related to dementing disorders, neuropathological features are not included in this chapter.

Conditions that precipitate reversible dementias include Wilson's disease, Hashimoto's encephalopathy, systemic lupus erythematosus, subdural hematoma, certain tumors (e.g., meningiomas, low-grade gliomas), normal pressure hydrocephalus, hyper- and hypothyroidism, and vitamin B12 and folate deficiency (Moore & Jefferson, 2004). These conditions can be diagnosed with lab tests, magnetic resonance imaging (MRI) scans, and medical examination.

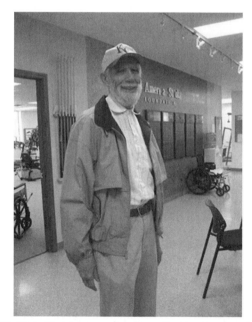

FIGURE 17-1. Burt has vascular dementia. He attends a American Stroke Foundation wellness center for people who have had strokes. Burt participates in activities such as "Wake Up Your Brain" and relaxation classes.

Prevalence

The most prevalent forms of dementia are age related, with Alzheimer's type dementia accounting for two-thirds of all dementias (Geldmacher, 2003). Vascular or multi-infarct dementia (stroke) accounts for the remaining one-third, along with other causes (Goetz, 2003). Age and onset are important factors in the diagnoses of dementia. Although 1% of people between the ages of 65 and 69 have probable dementia, the percentages rise with age to 9% of 80- to 84-year-olds (General Accounting Office, 1998). It is estimated that 30% to 50% of the elderly who are older than 85 years have some degree of dementia (Goetz, 2003; Moore & Jefferson, 2004).

Course

The course of dementia is determined by the underlying cause of the syndrome. Onset may be insidious, with subtle changes to memory difficulties, or abrupt with acute or dramatic changes, such as occur with TBI. The dementia may be relatively static (TBI or stroke) or progressive (Alzheimer's, Parkinson's, HIV). If the cause is determined to be progressive, the rate of decline can range from gradual to rapid, and the duration from diagnosis to death can range from 5 to 15 years. The rate of decline in Alzheimer's disease is generally steady and specific to the individual, and prognosis is based on the rate of decline in prior years projected into future years. If the dementia is due to a static condition, there may be some improvement, a stepwise decline, or a plateau in decline, although full recovery is rare.

Mild cognitive impairment is a diagnosis based on client- and family-corroborated report of memory difficulty, mild cognitive deficits in memory domains, and intact functional abilities (Manning, 2004). Mild cognitive impairment is believed to be an early, transitional stage prior to the onset of dementia (Gauthier et al, 2006). Caselli et al (2006) found that in longitudinal studies, about 10% to 15% of individuals diagnosed with mild cognitive impairment progress to Alzheimer's disease annually. The minor changes in memory may pose occasional problems with complex tasks such as financial management or driving in unfamiliar areas. Neuropsychological assessment can provide information on cognitive abilities in the absence of observable functional impairment.

Evaluation

Medical evaluation of dementia is important to determine the cause, treatment, and prognosis, as well as to facilitate education for the family members and primary caregivers in planning for the future. Evaluation of dementia begins with a history of symptoms from the client and family members. Important diagnostic information includes when the initial memory problems began and what events that occurred over the past 2 to 5 years were attributed to changes in cognitive function.

Progressive dementia is described using the terms early, middle, or late stage, reflecting duration of the condition or severity of the symptoms. There are models with which to stage the degree of dementia that reflect the course of the disease. The Allen Cognitive Level (ACL) Screen is used to rate dementia levels based on thought process: planning/abstract to goal directed/concrete to automatic/object centered (Allen, Kehrberg, & Burns, 1992; Burns, Mortimer, & Merchak, 1994). Burns developed the Cognitive Performance test (CPT), a cognitive functional assessment that scores individuals on the ACL six-level scale (6.0 as normal cognition and 1.0 as severe dementia), as shown in Box 17-4 (Burns, 2006) The Clinical Dementia Rating scale is used to track memory, orientation, judgment and problem-solving, community affairs, home and hobbies, and personal care (Morris, 1993). This scale identifies the levels as healthy (0), very mild impairment (0.5), mild (1.0), moderate (2.0), and severe (0.3). The Reisberg FAST Rating scale reverses the scale with 1.0 for normal cognition and 7.0 for severely impaired.

The clinical examination may include examination by a neurologist, psychiatrist, or geriatrician; structural neuroimaging such as MRI scans; laboratory exams; neuropsychological testing; occupational therapy evaluation; and social services or family therapy interviews. Imaging studies reveal the presence or absence of structural (tumor or stroke) changes and are proving to offer greater sensitivity to biomarkers for dementia diagnoses (Leon & Klunk, 2006). Laboratory tests may indicate a metabolic disorder, infectious disease, or HIV. Cerebrospinal fluid exam is used for stroke, encephalitis, or Creutzfeldt-Jakob diagnoses. Neuropsychological testing is used in the early stages of dementia and requires the individual to be alert and attentive for 2 to 3 hours. This testing can provide information regarding the nature and extent of the impairments and provide a baseline of cognition to measure change over time (Lezak, Howieson, & Loring, 2004).

The most common, evidence-supported, standardized cognitive screening assessment administered by many disciplines is the **Mini-Mental Status Examination** (MMSE), a verbally based test of global cognition (Folstein, Folstein, & McHugh, 1975). Weaker evidence supports the use of the Draw a Clock Test measuring cognitive and spatial domains (Wolf-Klein, Silverstone, Levy, & Brod, 1989) and Functional Assessment Questionnaire reporting levels of assistance with select IADLs (Pfeffer, Kurosaki, Harrah, Chance, &

BOX 17-4 ■ Cognitive-Functional Profiles

Level 6. Normal Functioning; Absence of Cognitive Functional Disability

Persons can use complex information to carry out daily activities with accuracy and safety.

Level 5. Mild Functional Decline; Beginning Deficits in Abstract Thought Processes

Persons begin to have difficulty using complex information or performing complex tasks, including job performance, managing finances, driving, meal preparation, shopping, or following a complex medication schedule.

Level 4.5. Mild to Moderate Functional Decline; Significant Deficits in Abstract Thought Processes

Abstract thought processes, including problem-solving, memory, judgment, reasoning, and planning ahead, are impaired. Persons participate in portions of complex tasks and show difficulties with simple tasks such as bathing, dressing, grooming, and occupying leisure time.

Level 4. Moderate Functional Decline; Use of Concrete Thought Processes

Abstract thought processes, including memory, judgment, reasoning, and planning ahead, are replaced by concrete thought processes. Familiar tasks such as dressing, grooming, and bathing

are remembered, but the quality of performance diminishes, and the task usually requires cues, setup, or initiation of task.

Level 3.5. Moderate Functional Decline; Deficits in Concrete Thought Process

Concrete task steps and direct prompting and cueing are needed to complete even simple tasks. Task objects may need to be handed to get the person started, and demonstration may be necessary for the person to perform the desired movements. Twenty-four-hour supervision is required to ensure safety.

Level 3. Moderate to Severe Functional Decline; Object-Centered Thought Processes

Task performance is sporadic with assistance needed to begin, sequence, and end tasks. The ability to use objects effectively is inconsistent, and caregivers may find it easier to do things for or to the person.

Level 2. Severe Functional Decline; Deficits in Object-Centered Thought Processes

The person requires total care but may cooperate in portions of tasks (i.e., holding up an arm for a sleeve or using a spoon or fingers to pick up foods). Resisting care is common.

Level 1. Late Stage Dementia

Basic walking and eating abilities are impaired; total care is required.

Filos, 1982). The MBRC Caregiver Strain Instrument looks at caregiver feelings toward providing care and restriction of caregiver activities (Bass, Noelker, & Rechlin, 1996). If the screening assessments reveal cognitive impairment (MMSE below 28 or any distortion in the clock drawing test), the occupational therapist conducts an evaluation that includes formal cognitive functional testing to determine the impact of the impairment on occupational performance.

A social services assessment is used to determine the needs and types of external resources available to support the individual in his or her living environment or to make recommendations for changes in the residential setting to meet the needs of the person and/or family. A family therapy interview determines the interactional needs of the family in adjusting to the diagnosis and designing a family care provider plan.

Differential Diagnosis

The stigma attached to degenerative brain disease is similar to the stigma around mental health diagnoses. This can prevent family members from seeking medical advice related to memory impairments and behavioral changes. The gradual decline in thinking or changes in personality are commonly attributed to depression or "ministrokes."

It is important to distinguish among the "three Ds": dementia, delirium, and depression. Symptoms may be similar, but the management approach varies depending on the condition. **Delirium** is an abrupt change in cognitive responses from one day to another characterized by confusion, delusions, and agitation. Delirium is manifested by an acute onset and requires immediate medical attention. Factors that contribute to delirium are dehydration, urinary tract infections,

drug reactions, and respiratory infections, all treatable conditions. Dementia can mask delirium and make it difficult to diagnose.

Depression is often a comorbid diagnosis in early stage dementia, as the individual grieves the gradual loss of cognitive abilities. Depression can resemble dementia in that it is characterized by the inability to concentrate or attend to a task, mental slowing, and apathy. The MMSE can help differentiate between depression and dementia because individuals with depression generally perform better on declarative memory tests. A single-item depression indicator, "Do you often feel sad or depressed?" is a brief, yet valid screening tool (Mahoney, 1994). Another tool, the Geriatric Depression scale, is a 15-item questionnaire used to screen for depression in the elderly (Sheikh & Yesavage, 1986). Five or more "yes" answers indicate the need for referral and further evaluation.

Table 17-1 identifies the symptoms that differentiate delirium, dementia, and depression. There is some overlap of symptoms and comorbidities; Table 17-1 identifies primary symptoms by degree that can generally be identified in textbook cases.

Other disorders that are similar to and distinguishable from dementia include amnesia, or memory impairment, without the other cognitive features (aphasia, apraxia, agnosia, and executive functioning). Substance intoxication or withdrawal can present as a dementia that reverses when the toxin is eliminated. Individuals with cognitive developmental disability are diagnosed before age 18, and cognition is relatively static unless there is a dual diagnosis with dementia. Extreme sleep deprivation can mimic memory loss, but even extreme untreated sleep apnea rarely causes significant cognitive impairment.

Table 17-1 ● **Differentiation of Delirium, Dementia, and Depression**

Symptoms and Features	Delirium	Dementia	Depression
Disorganized thought	X	X	
Altered consciousness	X		
Attention deficit	X	X	X
Global cognitive problems	X	X	
Memory loss		X	
Memory deficit	X		X
Perceptual/sensory disturbances (e.g., hallucinations)	X	X	
Sleep/wake disturbances	X	X	
Insomnia or hypersomnia			X
Disorientation	X	X	
Language disturbance (aphasia)		X	
Inability to motor plan (apraxia)		X	
Failure to identify objects (agnosia)		X	
Disturbance in executive functioning (i.e., planning, sequencing, organizing, abstracting)		X	
Use of MRI for Dx (to rule out other Dx)		X	
Secondary psychosis to other Dx	X	X	
Acute onset and fluctuating course of short duration	X		
Gradual onset and continuing cognitive decline		X	
Loss of sense of self	X	X	
Loss of continuity with life history	X	X	
Distortion of time and space, light and darkness	X	X	
Periods of amnesia	X		
Behavioral disturbance (e.g., wandering, agitation, aggression)	X	X	
Poor appetite or overeating			X
Fatigue and slowed responses			X
Low self-esteem			X
Poor concentration or difficulty making decisions			X
Feelings of hopelessness			X
Impairment in social, occupational, and daily function	X	X	X
Affective lability	X	X	X
Low motivation or diminished interest in activity			X
Depressed mood most of the day			X
Hx or presence of a major depressive episode of at least 2 weeks' duration			X
Reversible condition	X		X
Recurrent thoughts of death			X
Precipitating loss			X
Preoccupation with physical symptoms			X

Genetic Factors

There appears to be a genetic link for some forms of degenerative dementia. Risk factors for Alzheimer's disease include age and a first-degree relative with the disease. Families of Volga-German heritage have a gene mutation characteristic of early onset Alzheimer's (Levy-Lahad et al, 1994). Genes linked to Alzheimer's are found on chromosome 1, 14, and 21 (Down syndrome) for young or early onset forms and chromosome 19 for later onset where autopsies have shown pathologies consistent with this diagnosis (Small et al, 1997). Chromosomes 3 and 17q appear to have a familial link to frontotemporal lobe dementia (Widerholt, 2000). Creutzfeldt-Jakob disease has a familial variant, and Huntington's is an inherited disease. The family history is an important piece of the medical diagnosis.

Culture

Prevalence of causes of dementia varies with different cultural groups due to environmental influences, nutrition, education, life span, substance abuse, infection, and cerebrovascular disorders. Culture and language can be barriers to the accurate assessment of cognition when the person being evaluated is from a different culture or speaks a different language than the evaluator. Behavior that is unacceptable to a particular culture, such as uninhibited behavior, may be misinterpreted as confusion. Subcultures influenced by economic status or educational background may skew the behavioral assessment. It is important to consider the history and background of the individual prior to making assumptions about cognitive function. Using culturally sensitive assessment tools is important in the screening and diagnosing of cognitive impairments. One approach to minimize the language barrier is to include a translator throughout the evaluation and intervention process.

The care of persons with dementia in many non–Euro-American cultures is provided in the home setting by family members. With a filial responsibility to care for their elders, adult children are frequently primary caregivers. The therapist should be cautious about sharing information with appropriate parties and sensitive to the family dynamic in offering consultation and strategizing interventions.

Medication

There are few medications that treat the cognitive decline of dementia, and patients have reported mixed results. The acetylcholinesterase inhibitors or donepezil (Aricept), rivastigmine (Exelon), and galantamine (Razadyne) are the drugs of choice for Alzheimer's disease, Lewy body dementia, vascular dementia, and Parkinson's dementia (Abramowicz, 2007). These may cause gastrointestinal problems. Memantine (Namenda) is prescribed after the disease has advanced and may be used along with acetylcholinesterase inhibitor therapy. Although pharmacological interventions do not cure the disease, they are reported to slow the progression of cognitive decline in 30% to 50% of patients (Moore & Jefferson, 2004). Vitamin E has been investigated as a treatment for Alzheimer's disease, but results are inconclusive. Other pharmacological interventions are used to manage the symptoms of dementia. For example, antipsychotic medications are often used to treat agitation, aggression, delusions, and hallucinations. It is important to limit medications that can exacerbate cognitive impairment, such as anticholinergics. The preferred approach is to simplify the patient's medication regimen and ask a caregiver to closely monitor medication management.

Impact on Occupational Performance

Criteria for a diagnosis of dementia includes significant impairment in social or occupational functioning, a key area of occupational therapy intervention. Because of the broad range of conditions contributing to the diagnoses, the performance skills (motor, process, communication/interaction), performance patterns (habits, routines, roles) and client factors (body functions, body structures) are affected to various degrees throughout the progression of the disease. The evaluation is an analysis of occupational performance at one point in time, with an emphasis on identifying the environmental supports and barriers to participation in daily activities.

The focus of occupational therapy intervention is to determine the optimal types and amount of environmental supports to facilitate performance and to educate the caregiver on adaptations and strategies to achieve the desired goals. This section briefly describes the occupational therapy process. For more information on occupational therapy interventions with dementia, see Chapters 18 and 47.

Evaluation

The evaluation of occupation in clients with dementia begins with an occupational profile that includes a description of present performance in pertinent areas of occupation (e.g., ADL, IADL, work or volunteer, leisure, social participation, sleep). An interview format with the client and caregiver is useful to gain information about performance patterns (e.g., daily habits, routines, roles) and unique strengths that have been preserved or abilities that have been "overlearned." Information about changes in participation in IADLs and self-care can provide insight into the rate and degree of cognitive decline over time (Aitken, 1996). It is important to frame the client's experience in the context of the family and community in which the individual resides.

The initial interview is intended to draw out the individual's and caregiver's interests, values, and needs. Exploring the meaning the client attributes to his or her occupations is equally important. Observation of the client in his or her natural environment can provide more accurate information than a caregiver report. A critical appraisal of the client's context or environment will aid the therapist in identifying supports and barriers to performance.

Standardized assessments used in occupational therapy evaluation include screening tools, brief assessments, and comprehensive tests for functional cognition. In dementia, the focus of a standardized assessment is to measure the cognitive ability to perform rather than a direct assessment of skills, such as an ADL assessment. The ACL's leather lacing tool is designed to screen for cognitive functional limitations and predict functional performance levels (Allen et al, 1992). This information is useful for the therapist to select additional assessments based on the goals of intervention and the client's contextual factors.

An example of a brief occupational therapy assessment is the Kitchen Task Assessment, which identifies the cognitive support needed to complete a cooking task (Baum & Edwards, 1993). It rates task performance in six areas: initiation, organization, steps of task, sequencing, judgment and safety, and completion. The CPT involves observation of the individual in the performance of select tasks in a controlled context with standardized protocols (Burns, Mortimer, & Merchak, 1994). Cognitive functional assessment (CPT) scores are used to predict the level and quality of performance in IADL and ADL tasks and determine the amount of assistance required for safety and supervision in daily activities. The Performance Assessment of Self-Care Skills rates ADL and IADL performance in three areas: independence (amount of assist needed), safety, and adequacy (Rogers, Holm, Chisholm, Raina, & Toto, 2008). This assessment outlines the intervention plan in select areas of daily activities and measures change over time. The process scale of the Assessment of Motor and Process Skills (Fischer, 2003) can discriminate between those individuals who can live independently in the community and those who need assistance (Kizony & Katz, 2002).

The Lived Experience

Jim

My memories are slowly disappearing from places inhabited for so long. In themselves, memories do not compare with the great sagas of this century, the births, deaths, tumult, madness, great art and music, and the intense suffering of so many human beings. Our immortality, such as it may be, is not contained in what we dreamed or the secrets we kept; it is how our friends and loved ones remember us.

(DeBaggio, 2002, p. 207)

My mother was a very proper lady, an old-fashioned school teacher to be exact. She corrected my grammar at every turn and made sure my shirts were white and pressed. (To this day, I use starch on my shirts when I iron.) That is why when she began the journey into Alzheimer's disease, it was hard to watch her as she struggled to maintain her former habits of cleanliness. It was a long journey over many years. She never really talked to me about what she was experiencing. She was a very private person. But as her son and closest family member, I remember having that sense of knowing she was struggling with her mind; she did not want my help but as her needs increased, I made every effort to give her the dignity that I knew she deserved.

Mom was very active in the community and was what I like to call a professional volunteer. My father died shortly after my mother's 80th birthday. Because my other siblings had long ago moved away, she remained living alone in the house for the next 4 years. During that time, she continued to be very active in the community, volunteering at the hospital and nursing home, as well as participating in her book clubs and playing bridge several days a week. I lived 175 miles away and would visit about once a month or so and called her weekly. I began noticing some slight memory difficulties after a year or so and, although somewhat concerned because her only sister was suffering from Alzheimer's disease, she seemed to be functioning just fine and enjoying her independence. I did notice a few "dings" in the car but attributed that to parking lot incidents. It was 4 years after my father's death that a friend of hers called me to tell me that she was concerned about my mother's driving. She also reported that mother could no longer play bridge and forgot her car at the shopping mall. I began to make more frequent weekend trips to visit and realized later that she was going to great lengths to hide

what she must have known were the same dementia symptoms that her sister experienced. What a scary time this must have been for her.

Shortly after the friend's phone call, I started receiving nighttime telephone calls from mother telling me about "strangers in the house" and other frightening delusions. On one of my next visits, I took the car away from her and made arrangements to admit her into the nursing home where she had volunteered for the past 25 years. Mother agreed, but when the time came, she entered the nursing home kicking and screaming (almost literally, as she was in the real angry stage of the disease). After she settled in, the volunteer coordinator allowed her to wear her pink volunteer smock, and she would wander around the home helping with events as she had for years. Everyone knew and loved my mother there.

During that first year in the nursing home, when I visited we would talk for hours on end about the family. Gradually, she had more and more difficulty carrying on a conversation as her memory and cognitive skills declined. My visits changed from conversations to car rides and long walks along the Mississippi River. Once, I took her to JCPenney's to buy underwear, and she wandered away in the store when I was paying the clerk. That was the last excursion to the mall.

Toward the end, when I visited her in the long-term care center, she was unable to verbally communicate and did not recognize me. Intuitively, I knew she felt my presence and seemed calm during my visits. Being a little, frail lady, she would crawl into my lap and let me rock her like a child. I remember thinking that this is what she did for me so many years ago. On one particular visit, she pulled me to her bed and wanted me to lie next to her, with my arm around her, providing comfort and security. I think she was afraid and didn't want to be alone. Shortly after that, she left this world, gracefully, without a struggle, actually in her own proper way.

I experienced first-hand what Alzheimer's disease does to a vibrant, healthy human. As a son and caregiver, I experienced the pain, the frustration, and the helplessness that comes from not quite knowing what to do next. I also experienced the incredible bonds of family love as we cared for each other through the last years of my mother's journey. We were lucky that she really had no physical difficulties and she died, almost pain free, surrounded by her family shortly after her 86th birthday.

These are only a few select assessment tools that have been successfully used with the dementia population. Although there are numerous standardized assessments, it is important to view the testing results as one piece of the evaluation of performance and to consider all factors that affect occupational performance for the individual.

Performance Goals

The primary goal for occupational performance in clients with dementia is to ensure maximum engagement in occupation in a safe and supported environment over the course of

the disease. This may include altering the existing environment by increasing supports as the needs arise or changing the environment by a move to a more supportive residence. Early in the dementia, the client can participate in selecting performance goals for future anticipated needs, such as retirement activities, community mobility, financial management, and residential changes or institutional supports. Legal issues, including conservatorship or guardianship, power of attorney, health-care directives, and burial plans, can be put in place. In later stages, the family serves as a client proxy in the selection of goals and strategies to meet those goals.

The progressive nature of most cases of dementia means that those intervention strategies that work well at one stage may prove ineffective in the next stage. For example, memory aids such as calendars and planners may work in the early stage to compensate for memory difficulties; however, at some point, the person will be unable to locate the aid or remember to use it. New learning is difficult, so activity performance should draw on activity patterns that were well established prior to the onset of the dementia. The goal of therapy at any stage is to minimize the decline and adapt the activity demands so the person can continue to participate in activities that bring meaning and satisfaction.

Areas of Occupation

The areas of occupation that prove to be challenging initially for individuals with dementia are work or volunteer experiences that demand complex thinking and new learning. A person may withdraw from leisure activities that demand high cognitive skills (e.g., playing bridge) or have a hazardous component (e.g., cutting trees with a chain saw or hunting). Social participation often declines with language skills, and social circles diminish from clubs and civic groups to family and friends to immediate family members. In the early stages, the IADLs that present challenges are financial management, complex home maintenance tasks, and driving. Later, shopping, home making, meal preparation, and reading are difficult.

The middle stage of dementia presents challenges in ADLs, including bathing, dressing, grooming, and mobility. An aversion to bathing appears to be a common symptom and one for which family members often seek outside assistance. In dressing, there is a tendency to layer clothing or reuse soiled clothes. The individual may experience occupational deprivation due to an inability to self-initiate leisure activities and a limited desire to participate without encouragement.

Dementia in the later stages presents dependence in basic ADLs, including incontinence care and disturbances in sleep/wake patterns, two behaviors that serve as indicators for a change in residence. Interrupted sleep/wake cycles can lead to nighttime "way finding," or wandering, and a disruption in the primary caregiver's rest. Other key performance challenges are limited leisure and social participation because the person ultimately withdraws from most activities. The final stage is characterized by a refusal to eat.

Performance Skills

Motor signs are predictive of cognitive and functional decline in Alzheimer's disease, even though some individuals in the early stages have relatively strong motor skills (Scarmeas et al, 2005). With subcortical dementias and dementias that affect the motor cortex, the result is an unsteady gait and an increased risk for falls. In late stage dementia, the limited mobility skills and postural deterioration eventually contribute to the need for 24-hour care to counteract the propensity for contractures and decubiti.

Distorted sensory perceptions and an inability to reason can lead to catastrophic reactions. Although contraindicated in the majority of cases, in severe dementia, the use of physical or chemical restraints may be indicated as a last resort. Occupational therapy can provide strategies to reduce the use of restraints through sensory interventions or appropriately designed diversional activities.

Fatigue is a major problem with dementia. The energy required to continue daily tasks increases as the person's cognitive abilities decrease. Time becomes distorted, and the person is eternally living in the present. An inability to recognize environmental cues and impaired orientation to space may lead to way finding. Visual perceptions may be distorted, leading to hallucinations, delusions, and paranoia.

Communication deficits are unique to each person with dementia, affecting some more than others. Although some individuals remain articulate into later stages of the disease, others experience aphasia or word finding problems early on. Common difficult behaviors may be related to the inability to express oneself. Verbal behaviors include repeated questioning, arguing, inaccurate reasoning, social withdrawal, restlessness and agitation, screaming, and catastrophic reactions (Bimesser, 1997).

Performance Patterns

Habits, or overlearned activities, have been found to be useful to perpetuate performance in daily activities, especially grooming and dressing tasks. Although it is a frequently cited strategy, there is no conclusive evidence to support the establishment of routines for persons with dementia. Routines may help a caregiver organize the day in order to schedule some respite time and increase predictability of the external environment. Roles change dramatically; an individual who was the head of the household may move into a dependent role, and his spouse may move into a caregiving role. Families tend to rally and support the member with the disease, and roles emerge depending on the strengths and abilities of the individual members.

Activity Demands

The key to optimal participation in areas of occupation and minimizing behavioral disruptions is to adjust the activity demands to meet the client's capabilities. A person with dementia may feel anxious in unfamiliar surroundings or agitated by crowds. Frustration builds when the timing of activities is not adapted to his or her new pace or the activity requirements are too challenging to be successful. A starting point is a clear sense of what the client is capable of doing successfully and adjusting the activity demands accordingly.

Interventions

Three key areas of intervention for individuals with dementia are environmental intervention, caregiver education, and behavioral intervention. These areas encompass other intervention areas, such as communication, driving, feeding, and sleep.

Environmental Intervention

A key approach to intervention with persons with dementia is to adapt the environment to meet the changing needs. Establishing consistent performance contexts (e.g., physical and social environment) and reinforcing well-developed habits and routines can facilitate participation and ease the task of caregiving (Gitlin, Hauck, Dennis, & Winter, 2005; Graff et al,

2008). In an occupational therapy environmental skill building program, the intervention was to create an adaptive zone in which individual competence is equal to environmental demands (Corcoran et al, 2002; Gitlin, Corcoran, Winter, Boyce, & Hauck, 2001). This was accomplished by attending to the task objects and adapting the activities, designing appropriate social groups in a culturally sensitive environment, and adjusting the expectations for behavior. The goal was to improve quality of activity engagement and reduce behaviors that were barriers to participation.

Adapting the environment may involve modifying the home for maximum safety. For example, by installing grab bars, tub benches, or faucet extensions, the caregiver may be able to supervise a bathing activity with greater confidence. There are numerous home adaptations to increase security for a person who enjoys sensory seeking or way finding. Electronic monitoring devices, door alarms, pressure gates, and video intercoms are cost-effective measures that can be installed in the home. Additional safety features commonly considered are disconnecting a stove or installing a power switch, removal of appliances or replacement with those with an auto shut-off feature, faucet valves to prevent overflow, window gridlines on patio doors, and camouflaging exits (Warner, 2000).

Low-tech assistive devices can be effective in the early stages of dementia. These include calendars, list making, and note taking for memory aides. Medication boxes or alarm med boxes can be useful initially, but may be confusing to some individuals, especially those with cognitive decline. Seeking plausible alternatives to community mobility is recommended in the early stages to limit driving. In middle stages, maintaining a simplified schedule in a familiar environment with repetition and consistency may ease the responsibilities for caregivers.

During the later stages of dementia, environmental adaptations may include mealtime positioning and adaptive feeding strategies, along with nutritional monitoring. It is important to note that effective adaptations require trial and error; that is, what works for one individual may not be appropriate or effective with another individual. The intervention plan should be designed with consideration of the unique individual and family strengths and needs.

Caregiver Education

A home care, family-centered model can be an effective approach for persons with dementia (Corcoran, 1999). It is important to acknowledge that the caregiver "can be considered the hidden client in the caregiver–care receiver dyad" (Shaw, Kearney, Vause Earland, & Eckhardt, 2003, p. 1). More than 80% of clients with dementia are living in their homes with family members providing daily care (National Institute on Aging, 1999). Caregivers fill the role of collaborator in the intervention process as they identify the barriers and supports for occupational participation, adapt the environment, adjust the activity demands, and guide compensatory strategies. A person-centered care model in which the well-being of the caregiver is considered and supported through the intervention is essential (Ortigara, 2000). Consideration of the needs of the client as a family member and support for healthy family interactions within the caregiving relationship can be accomplished through appropriately designed, shared activities and adapting roles and expectations (Schaber, 2002).

Evidence-Based Practice

Due to the progressive nature of most dementing disorders, occupational therapy intervenes at intervals to adjust occupational demands to performance capacity. Occupational therapy has been proven effective in home- and community-based programs (Gitlin, Hauck, Dennis, & Winter, 2005; Graff et al, 2008). These programs include strategies such as establishing consistent performance contexts (physical and social environment), reinforcing well-developed habits and routines, creating an adaptive zone to ease environmental demands, attending to the task objects, adapting the activities, designing appropriate social groups in a culturally sensitive environment, and adjusting the expectations for behavior.

Occupational therapy intervention is designed to maximize participation in day-to-day occupations. Each stage of dementia reflects differing barriers to occupational performance (Corcoran, 2006).

Early stage challenges participation in select IADLs including driving and navigation errors (Uc, Rizzo, Anderson, Shi, & Dawson, 2004), medication administration, meal preparation, and managing finances.

➤ Occupational therapists can refer clients for driving evaluations for persons with cognitive changes (Shold Davis, 2003).

➤ Occupational therapists provide strategies and caregiver training in breaking down complex tasks such as personal finances, medication management, and meal preparation to identify portions of the task for the client to participate with success and to reduce caregiver stress (Dooley & Hinojosa, 2004).

Corcoran, M. A. (Ed.). (2006). *Neurorehabilitation for Dementia-Related Diseases*. (Neurorehabilitation Self-Paced Clinical Course Series, G. M. Giles, Series Senior Ed.). Bethesda, MD: American Occupational Therapy Association.

Dooley, N. R., & Hinojosa, J. (2004). Improving quality of life for persons with Alzheimer's disease and their family caregivers: Brief occupational therapy intervention. *American Journal of Occupational Therapy, 58*, 561–569.

Gitlin, L. M., Hauck, W. W., Dennis, M. P., & Winter, L. (2005). Maintenance of effects of the home environmental skill-building program for family caregivers and individuals with Alzheimer's disease and related disorders. *Journal of Gerontology, 60A*, 368–374.

Graff, M., Bernookj-Dassen, M., Zajec, J., Olde-Rikkert, M., Hoefnagels, W., & Dekker, J. (2008). Community occupational therapy is cost-effective for patients with dementia. *British Medical Journal, 33*, 134–138.

Shold Davis, E. (2003). Defining OT roles in driving. *OT Practice, 8*(1), 15–18.

Uc, E. Y., Rizzo, M., Anderson, S. W., Shi, Q., & Dawson, J. D. (2004). Driver route-following and safety error in early Alzheimer's disease. *Neurology, 14*, 832–827.

Caregiver training includes education about the disease or disorder, strategies to adapt activities or compensate for declining performance in areas of occupation, and communication training such as validation therapy (Feil, 1992, 1993). It is important for families to understand how to promote participation at present and plan for future care needs. This entails training in task breakdown to identify portions of IADLs that can be performed with support (e.g., meal preparation, housekeeping, grocery shopping, bill paying, leisure activities) or ADLs with assistance (e.g., clothing selection, dressing, grooming, bathing, toileting, eating, mobility).

Caregivers may need skill training in communication and strategies to facilitate ongoing interactions. The use of **validation** has been found to aid caregivers in interacting with persons with disorientation (Feil, 1992, 1993). This approach is used as a communication method to calm agitated older persons. The premise of validation is to probe into the lived experience of the individual rather than challenging his or her reality. As the person relates more about the disturbing event, the listener responds, validating the underlying feelings that are expressed. In a study by Friedman and Tappen (1991), a program of planned walking (vs. a conversation group) significantly increased the communication abilities of patients with Alzheimer's disease. Caregiver skills training can include modeling effective interactions with nonverbal clients, interpreting sensory cues and gestures.

Behavioral Intervention

In the early stages of dementia, a challenging behavior to manage is the tendency to get lost in familiar areas. This requires client training in the use of an aid such as a cell phone or lifeline system. A Safe Return program developed by the Alzheimer's Association helps identify individuals who are lost and do not have memory skills for self-identification.

To manage fatigue and maintain normal sleep/wake cycles, it is important to pace but encourage regularly scheduled activities to keep the person awake during the day. Suggestions to counteract sleep disturbances include (Duthie, 1998) the following:

- Avoid caffeine in the afternoon and evening.
- Limit fluids after dinnertime.
- Increase daily physical activity.
- Limit daytime napping (including napping in front of the television).
- Medical screening for other causes of insomnia, such as pain.

In the middle stages of dementia, structured activity programs in community centers, adult day services, assisted living, and memory care centers can provide leisure activities, physical exercise, social activities, cognitive stimulation, and respite for the caregiver. It may be helpful to familiarize the client with a program and staff early on and build the regular activity into the weekly schedule. It is important to provide a mix of daily activities that are within the client's ability level that have meaning and purpose.

In the mid- to later stages of the disease, clients with behavior problems are often referred to occupational therapists to explore nonpharmacological interventions for behavior management. Individualized interventions for catastrophic reactions can include offering reassurance, reminiscence, distraction, sensory stimulation, and calming procedures, such as rocking chairs, aviaries, manipulative tasks, music, massage, oral reading, dimmed lighting, and reducing clutter. Programs for incontinence care can include using external stimuli for finding the toilet or identifying behaviors that indicate the need to void.

These are only a few intervention strategies for persons with dementia. The progressive nature of most forms of dementia dictates that occupational therapists intervene periodically as changes occur throughout the course of the related disease. The occupational therapy practitioner can apply the person-environment-occupation model, considering the person with declining cognition, the environment with increasing supports, and the occupation with continuous adaptations for maximum engagement. Each client is unique, and intervention approaches should be individualized, considering both client and family needs. The therapist considers these needs in a culturally sensitive context, upholding the inherent dignity of the person during each stage. The goal of intervention, guided through creative, evidence-based occupational therapy practice, is maximum participation in occupation and increasing the quality of life for the client and caregiver.

Summary

There are few conditions that have a more pervasive effect on everyday life than dementia. Although the course of dementia is almost always a progressive decline, occupational therapists can still play a significant role in the lives of individuals with the disorder. When individuals lose their memory and other basic cognitive functions, it is challenging but important that the uniqueness of the individual as well as that person's dignity be maintained. By creating environments that support performance (which includes supporting the caregiver), individuals with dementia can continue to participate in valued occupations for longer periods of time.

Active Learning Strategies

1. Illustrating Movement Patterns

The experience of dementia, specifically Alzheimer's-type dementia, is that the world shrinks. First, long-distance travel becomes more challenging and distressing. Then, regular activities become more difficult, and people with dementia may require assistance and supervision when they venture out of their home. They discontinue driving in the early stages, yet may have difficulty using public transportation because it may require learning a new skill. So often, with dementia, days are filled with few activities and substituted with sleep and watching TV.

You can graphically represent a person's daily patterns of movements. Take a sheet of paper and draw your home in

the center. Now draw around your home all the places you have traveled to on a regular or occasional basis over the past month (e.g., a friend's house, a relative's house, work, school, church, grocery store, gym, shopping mall). Draw a line from your home to each place for each trip over the past 30 days; this indicates your movement patterns. The places you visit frequently will have many lines, and those places you visit less frequently will have fewer lines. Next, indicate on each line with a symbol if you walked, biked, drove a car, or took public transportation.

Look at your graphic, which should visually represent your world. Examine your movement patterns. What patterns can you identify? What places are meaningful? Who is present in those places? What do you do in each place? How do you travel between places?

Reflective Questions
Reflect on the world of a person with dementia.

- What places on your graphic would you eliminate if you had significant cognitive impairment?
- What would be the challenges to continuing your participation in some of those places?
- What mobility or transportation supports would you need to continue former movement patterns?
- What supports would you need to remain engaged in the activities you perform in that place?
- Which activities would you give up?
- Which activities could be added to substitute for the gap or void in your world?
- What would you suggest to counteract occupational deprivation? Select a place on your graphic and list the supports you would need to get to that place and what you would need to continue involvement in the activities there.

Reflective Journal

Describe the experience in your **Reflective Journal.**

2. Aging in Place

Family caregivers of individuals with dementia provide for their day-to-day needs. The term "aging in place" means that an elder can remain in his or her own community with services brought to him or her. Sometimes it is not feasible or possible for the person to remain at home with a family caregiver, but the person can live close to home and family. Identifying the optimal setting for an individual with cognitive decline is challenging. An important role for occupational therapy in the evaluation of an older adult with dementia is to determine the capabilities of the individual and the supports he or she may require to live in an optimal and safe environment. This requires the therapist to have knowledge of housing options and the supports provided with each option. Based on the evaluation results, the therapist would consult with family members to discuss options tailored to the functional needs of the individual.

Study the definitions and explanations of the various options for residential care, listed for the most part in a hierarchy from greatest independence (requiring no assistance) to dependence (requiring most assistance).

- Senior Housing Development (a large apartment complex for seniors, aged 55 or older, in which some services are available for a fee, such as light housekeeping, activities, transportation, meals, and laundry)
- Accessory Apartment (an apartment attached to a family home with a separate entrance for the elderly family member)
- Home Sharing (individuals or families share their home and provide board and care)
- Life Care Communities (housing with an entry fee that ensures the continuum of care for life from independent living to skilled nursing care)
- Assisted Living (housing complexes with efficiencies or one-bedroom apartments in which services are included in the cost of the room, such as light housekeeping, activities, transportation, meals, laundry, medication management, and security checks)
- Adult Day Services (day activity programs that provide supervision, some basic care, meals, and activities during daytime hours not at home)
- Memory Care Facilities (community facilities for individuals with dementia in which institutional care is provided by trained personnel)
- Long-Term Care Facilities or Skilled Nursing Facilities (facilities in which care is provided by nursing professionals with full care available 24 hours a day with locked units)

Now read the following two cases and make a professional decision regarding residential options for the client with dementia. You may do this exercise as an in-class or small group discussion.

Case 1: Jerome

Jerome is an 89-year-old widower who is staying with his son and daughter-in-law after a recent hip fracture. He and his family agree that he is no longer safe living alone on the farm. Jerome has some slight memory deficits, but is able to heat up a meal prepared by another person, able to complete his own self-care, and—with his medications set up by someone else—is able to take them independently. He no longer drives, is not comfortable grocery shopping, is not able to keep his house clean, and is not safe using his walker outside in winter. Jerome is very social and enjoys music and playing cards.

Case Analysis
- Senior Housing Development—Jerome might need more services than independent living senior apartments provide.
- Accessory Apartment—This is a good option if his son and daughter-in-law are able to provide minimal care, transportation, and daily monitoring.
- Home Sharing—This might be a good option if another adult is present during the day.
- Life Care Communities—This option may be too late for Jerome because entrance generally occurs prior to the need for assistance.
- Assisted Living—This might be a good option for Jerome because he will require monitoring for falls and medication setup; he needs meals offered and housekeeping services, and he may need encouragement to participate in group activities.
- Adult Day Services—Jerome may not need this level of service due to slight nature of his memory deficits.
- Long-Term Care Facilities or Skilled Nursing Facilities—Jerome does not need this level of service at this time.
- Memory Care Facilities—Jerome does not need this level of service because he only has slight memory deficits.

Case 2: Mabel

Mabel is a 86-year-old homemaker who lives with her husband, Irwin, who is 91. They live in a metropolitan area. With moderate dementia and diabetes, Mabel is no longer able to prepare meals, do laundry, clean the house, or drive. She needs full assistance with her medications, especially in order to manage her diabetes. Mabel and Irwin live in a small rambler that is adapted for her wheelchair. Irwin wants her to remain at home, but is stressed by the demands of providing care for his wife. She is combative with self-care tasks, especially bathing, and he is challenged by transferring her from her wheelchair to the commode alone.

Case Analysis

■ Senior Housing Development—Mabel would need more services than independent living senior apartments provide.

■ Accessory Apartment—No additional family members are mentioned in the case.

■ Home Sharing—Mabel would need more care than home sharing would provide.

■ Life Care Communities—This option may be too late for Mabel because entrance generally occurs prior to the need for assistance.

■ Assisted Living—This might be a good option for Irwin, but Mabel's care, including transfers and medication management, would be costly. She may need more care than this option could provide.

■ Adult Day Services—Mabel may benefit from daily service due to moderate nature of her memory deficits and possibility for nursing care with the service.

■ Long-Term Care Facilities or Skilled Nursing Facilities—Mabel may benefit from this level of service at this time; Irwin could live in assisted living in a nearby complex.

■ Memory Care Facilities—Mabel could benefit from this level of service because she has moderate memory deficits.

Resources

Assessment

• Folstein, M. F., Folstein, S. E., & McHugh, P. R. *The Mini-Mental State Examination.* Available at: www.minimental.com (accessed November 28, 2009).

Books

• Bowlby, C. (1993). *Therapeutic Activities With Persons Disabled by Alzheimer's Disease and Related Disorders.* Gaithersburg, MD: Aspen.

• Byers-Connon, S., Lohman, H., & Padilla, R. L. (Eds.). (2004). *Occupational Therapy With Elders* (2nd ed.). St. Louis, MO: Elsevier Mosby.

• Corcoran, M. (Ed.). (2003). *Geriatric Issues in Occupational Therapy.* Bethesda, MD: American Occupational Therapy Association Press.

• Glickstein, J. K. (1997). *Therapeutic Interventions in Alzheimer's Disease* (2nd ed.). Gaithersburg, MD: Aspen.

• The Hartford. (2003). *At the Crossroads: A Guide to Alzheimer's Disease, Dementia & Driving.* Hartford, CT: Author.

• Larson, K. O., Stevens, R. G., Pedretti, L., & Crabtree, J. L. (Eds.). (1996). *ROTE: The Role of Occupational Therapy With the Elderly.* Bethesda, MD: American Occupational Therapy Association Press.

• Lewis, S. C. (2003). *Elder Care in Occupational Therapy* (2nd ed.). Thorofare, NJ: Slack.

• Rosenfeld, M. S. (Ed.). (1997). *Motivational Strategies in Geriatric Rehabilitation.* Bethesda, MD: American Occupational Therapy Association Press.

• Warner, M. (2000). *The Complete Guide to Alzheimer's Proofing Your Home.* West Lafayette, IN: Purdue University Press.

Books: Autobiographical

• DeBaggio, T. (2002). *Losing My Mind: An Intimate Look at Life With Alzheimer's.* New York: Free Press.

• McGowin, D. F. (1993). *Living in the Labyrinth: A Personal Journey Through the Maze of Alzheimer's.* New York: Delacorte Press.

• Snyder, L. (1999). *Speaking Our Minds: Personal Reflections From Individuals With Alzheimer's.* New York: W.H. Freeman Press.

Films

• *Away From Her* (2006)
• *Complaints of a Dutiful Daughter* (1994)
• *Marvin's Room* (1996)
• *On Golden Pond* (1981)

Organizations

• AAN Guideline Summary for Clinicians: Detection, Diagnosis, and Management of Dementia: www.aan.com/professionals/practice/pdfs/dementia_guideline.pdf

• AAN Guideline Summary for Patients and Their Families: Alzheimer's Disease: www.aan.com/professionals/practice/pdfs/dem_pat.pdf

• Agency for Healthcare Research and Quality (AHRQ) Innovations Exchange: www.innovations.ahrq.gov (select diagnostic area for best practice guides)

• Alzheimer's Association: www.alz.org

• Alzheimer's Disease Education and Referral (ADEAR) Center: www.nia.nih.gov/alzheimers

• American Academy of Neurology (AAN): www.aan.com

• American Parkinson Disease Association Inc.: www.apdaparkinson.org

• Huntington's Disease Society of America: www.hdsa.org

• Minnesota Chapter, American Physical Therapy Association (MN APTA). (2007). "Stand Up and Be Strong! Falls Prevention Model." St. Paul, MN: Author.

• National Institute on Aging: www.nia.nih.gov

• National Library of Medicine, HIV/AIDS Information: http://sis.nlm.nih.gov/hiv/organizations.html

Catalogues

• Resources in Aging and Long-Term Care: www.healthpropress.com

References

Abraham, I. L. (2005). Dementia and Alzheimer's disease: A practical orientation. *Nursing Clinics of North America, 41,* 119–127.

Abramowicz, M. (Ed.). (2007). Drugs for cognitive loss and dementia. *Treatment Guidelines from the Medical Letter, 5*(54), 9–14.

Aitken, M. J. (1996). Common assessments in geriatric practice. *Gerontology Special Interest Section Newsletter, 19*(4), 1–3.

Allen, C., Kehrberg, K., & Burns, T. (1992). Evaluation instrument. In C. Allen, C. A. Earhart, & T. Blue (Eds.), *Occupational Therapy Treatment Goals for the Physically and Cognitively Disabled* (pp. 54–68). Rockville, MD: American Occupational Therapy Association.

American Psychiatric Association (APA). (2000). *Diagnostic and Statistical Manual of Mental Disorders* (4th ed., text revision). Washington, DC: Author.

Bares, K. (1998). "Neuropsychological Predictors of Functional Level in Alzheimer's Disease." Unpublished dissertation, Finch University of Health Sciences–Chicago Medical School.

Bass, D. M., Noelker, L. S., & Rechlin, L. R. (1996). The moderating influence of service use on negative caregiving consequences. *Journals of Gerontology, 51B,* S121–S131.

Baum, C., & Edwards, D. F. (1993). Cognitive performance in senile dementia of the Alzheimer's type: The Kitchen Task Assessment. *American Journal of Occupational Therapy, 47*(5), 431–436.

Bimesser, L. R. (1997). Treating dementia. *OT Practice, 2*(6), 16–21.

Boss, P. (2006). *Loss, Trauma, and Resilience: Therapeutic Work With Ambiguous Loss.* New York: WW Norton.

Burns, T. (2006). *The Cognitive Performance Test Manual.* Pequannock, NJ: Maddak.

Burns, T., Mortimer, J., & Merchak, P. (1994). Cognitive performance test: A new approach to functional assessment in Alzheimer's disease. *Journal of Geriatric Psychiatry and Neurology, 7,* 46–54.

Caselli, R. J., Beach, T. G., Yaari, R., & Reiman, E. M. (2006). Alzheimer's disease a century later. *Journal of Clinical Psychiatry, 67,* 1784.

Cecil, R. L., Goldman, L., & Bennett, J. (Eds.). (2004). *Cecil Textbook of Medicine* (22nd ed.). St. Louis, MO: WB Saunders.

Clarfield, A. M. (2003). The decreasing prevalence of reversible dementias. *Archives of Internal Medicine, 163,* 2219–2229.

Corcoran, M. (1999). *Occupational Therapy Practice Guidelines for Adults With Alzheimer's Disease.* Bethesda, MD: American Occupational Therapy Association Press.

Corcoran, M. A., Gitlin, L. N., Levy, L., Eckhardt, S., Vause Earland, T., Shaw, G., & Kearney, P. (2002). An occupational therapy home-based intervention to address dementia-related problems identified by family caregivers. *Alzheimer's Care Quarterly, 3,* 82–89.

Cummings, J. L., & Benson, D. F. (1984). Subcortical dementia: Review of an emerging concept. *Archives of Neurology, 41,* 874–879.

DeBaggio, T. (2002). *Losing My Mind: An Intimate Look at Life With Alzheimer's.* New York: Free Press.

Duthie, E.H. (1998). *Practice of Geriatrics* (3rd ed.). St. Louis, MO: WB Saunders.

Feil, N. (1992). *Validation: The Feil Method.* Cleveland, OH: Edward Feil Productions.

Feil, N. (1993). *The Validation Breakthrough: Simple Techniques for Communicating With People With Alzheimer's-Type Dementia.* Baltimore: Health Professions Press.

Fischer, A. (2003). *Assessment of Motor and Process Skills. Development, standardization and administration manual.* (5th ed., Vol. 1). Ft. Collins, CO: Three Star Press, Inc.

Folstein, M. F., Folstein, S. E., & McHugh, P. R. (1975). Mini-Mental State: A practical method for grading the cognitive state of patients for the clinician. *Journal of Psychiatric Research, 12,* 196–198.

Friedman, R., & Tappen, R. M. (1991). The effect of planned walking on communication in Alzheimer's disease. *Journal of the American Geriatrics Society, 39,* 650–654.

Gauthier, S., Reisberg, B., Zaudig, M., Petersen, R., Ritchie, K., Broich, K., Belleville, H., Brodaty, H., Bennett, D., & Chertkow, H. (2006). Mild cognitive impairment. *Lancet, 367,* 1262.

Geldmacher, D. S. (2003). *Contemporary Diagnosis and Management of Alzheimer's Disease.* Newtown, PA: Handbooks in Health Care.

General Accounting Office (GAO). (1998). *Alzheimer's Disease: Estimates of Prevalence in the United States, GAO/HEHS-98-16, January 28, 1998.* Washington, DC: Author.

Gitlin, L. M., & Corcoran, M. (2005). *Occupational Therapy and Dementia Care: The Home Environmental Skill-Building Program for Individuals and Families.* Bethesda, MD: American Occupational Therapy Association.

Gitlin, L. M., Corcoran, M., Winter, L., Boyce, A., & Hauck, W. W. (2001). A randomized, controlled trial of a home environment intervention: Effect on efficacy and upset in caregivers and on daily functioning of persons with dementia. *Gerontologist, 41,* 4–14.

Gitlin, L. M., Hauck, W. W., Dennis, M. P., & Winter, L. (2005). Maintenance of effects of the home environmental skill-building program for family caregivers and individuals with Alzheimer's disease and related disorders. *Journal of Gerontology, 60A,* 368–374.

Goetz, C.G. (Ed.). (2003). *Textbook of Clinical Neurology* (2nd ed.). St. Louis, MO: WB Saunders.

Graff, M., Bernookj-Dassen, M., Zajec, J., Olde-Rikkert, M., Hoefnagels, W., & Dekker, J. (2008). Community occupational therapy is cost-effective for patients with dementia. *British Medical Journal, 336,* 134–138.

Hebert, L. E., Beckett, L. A., Scherr, P. A., & Evans, D. A. (2001). Annual incidence of Alzheimer disease in the United States projected to the years 2000 through 2050. *Alzheimer Disease and Associated Disorders, 15,* 169–173.

Kizony, R., & Katz, N. (2002). Relationships between cognitive abilities and the process scale and skills of the Assessment of Motor and Process Skills (AMPS) in patients with stroke. *OTJR: Occupation, Participation, and Health, 22*(2), 82–92.

Levy-Lahad, E., Wijsman, E. M., Anderson, L., Goddard, K. A., Weber, J. L., Bird, T. D., & Schellenberg, G. D. (1995). A familial Alzheimer's disease locus on chromosome 1. *Science, 269,* 970–973.

Leon, M. J., & Klunk, W. (2006). Biomarkers for the early diagnosis of Alzheimer's disease. *Lancet, 5,* 198.

Levy, L. L. (2005). Cognitive aging in perspective. In N. Katz (Ed.), *Cognition and Occupation Across the Lifespan* (pp. 305–325). Bethesda, MD: American Occupational Therapy Association Press.

Lezak, M. D., Howieson, D. B., & Loring, D. W. (2004). *Neuropsychological Assessment* (4th ed.). New York: Oxford University Press.

Mace, N. L. (1990). The management of problem behaviors. In N. L. Mace (Ed.), *Dementia Care: Patient, Family & Community* (pp. 74–112). Baltimore: The Johns Hopkins University Press.

Mahoney, J. (1994). Screening for depression: Single question versus GDS. *Journal of the American Geriatrics Society, 42*(9), 1006–1008.

Manning, C. (2004). Beyond memory: Neuropsychologic features in differential diagnosis of dementia. *Clinics in Geriatric Medicine, 20,* 45–58.

Moore, D. P., & Jefferson, J. W. (Eds.). (2004). *Handbook of Medical Psychiatry* (2nd ed.). St. Louis, MO: Mosby.

Morris, J. C. (1993). Clinical Dementia Rating scale. *Neurology, 43,* 2412–2414.

National Alliance for Caregiving (NAC). (2007, November). *Evercare Study of Family Caregivers: What They Spend, What They Sacrifice.* NAC Report. Bethesda, MD: Author.

National Institute on Aging. (1999). *Progress Report on Alzheimer's Disease, 1999.* Bethesda, MD: National Institute of Health.

Ortigara, A. (2000). The heart of education and training: Person-centered care. *Alzheimer's Care Quarterly, 1,* 73–74.

Pfeffer, R. I., Kurosaki, T. T., Harrah, C. H., Chance, J. M., & Filos, S. (1982). Measurement of functional activities of older adults in the community. *Journal of Gerontology, 37,* 323–329.

Poe, M. K., & Seifert, L. S. (1997). Implicit and explicit tests: Evidence for dissociable motor skills in probable Alzheimer's dementia. *Perceptual and Motor Skills, 85,* 631–634.

Rayner, A., O'Brien, J., & Schoenbachler, B. (2006). Behavior disorders of dementia: Recognition and treatment. *American Family Physician, 73,* 647–652.

Rogers, J. C., Holm, M. B., Chisholm, D., Raina, K. D., & Toto, P. E. (2008). "Performance Assessment of Self-Care Skills: An Observational Clinical Tool to Measure Activity Performance." Presented at the American Occupational Therapy Association (AOTA) Conference, April 11, Long Beach, CA.

Salthouse, T. (2000). Aging and measures of processing speed. *Biological Psychology, 54,* 35–54.

Scarmeas, N., Albert, M., Brandt, J., Hadjigeorgiou, G., Papadimitriou, A., Dubois, B., Sarazin, M., et al. (2005). Motor signs predict poor performance outcomes in Alzheimer disease. *Neurology, 64*(10), 1696–1703.

Schaber, P. (2002). FIRO model: A framework for family centered care. *Physical & Occupational Therapy in Geriatrics, 20*(3/4), 1–18.

Shaw, G., Kearney, P. J., Vause Earland, T., & Eckhardt, S. M. (2003). Managing dementia-related behaviors. *Home & Community Health, Special Interest Section Quarterly, 10*(1) 1–4.

Sheikh, J. I., & Yesavage, J. A. (1986). Geriatric Depression scale (GDS): Recent evidence and development of a shorter version. In T. L. Brink (Ed.), *Clinical Gerontology: A Guide to Assessment and Intervention* (pp. 165–175). New York: Haworth Press.

Small, G. W., Noble, E. P., Matsuyama, S. S., Jarvik, L. F., Komo, S., Kaplan, A., Ritchie, T., Pritchard, M. L., Saunders, A. M., Conneally, P. M., Roses, A. D., Haines, J. L., & Pericak-Vance, M. A. (1997). D2 dopamine receptor A1 allele in Alzheimer disease and aging. *Archives of Neurology, 54*, 281–285.

Solomon, P. R., Brett, M., Groccia-Ellison, M. E., Oyler, C., Tomasi, M., & Pendlebury, W. W. (1995). Classical conditioning in patients with Alzheimer's disease: A multiday study. *Psychology of Aging, 10*, 248–254.

Thomas, C. L. (Ed.). (1997). *Taber's Cyclopedic Medical Dictionary.* Philadelphia: FA Davis.

Warner, M. L. (2000). *The Complete Guide to Alzheimer's Proofing Your Home.* West Lafayette, IN: Purdue Press.

Widerholt, W. C. (2000). *Neurology for Non-Neurologists.* Philadelphia: WB Saunders.

Wolf-Klein, G. P., Silverstone, F. A., Levy, A. P., & Brod, M. S. (1989). Screening for Alzheimer's disease by clock drawing. *Journal of the American Geriatrics Society, 37*, 730–734.

Zarit, J. M. (1980). Caregiver Burden scale. *Gerontologist, 20*, 649–655.

CHAPTER 18

Cognitive Skills

Catana Brown

> "Memory is a net; one finds it full of fish when he takes it from the brook; but a dozen miles of water have run through it without sticking.
>
> —Oliver Wendell Holmes

Introduction

In a classic and fascinating study, McGhie and Chapman (1961) interviewed individuals with "early" schizophrenia and asked them to describe, in their own words, recent changes in experiences. This study revealed that people with schizophrenia are aware of and can describe some of the challenges they face while trying to attend to and make sense of their world. Here are just a few quotes from the study:

> My concentration is very poor. I jump from one thing to another. If I am talking to someone, they only need to cross their legs or scratch their heads and I am distracted and forget what I was saying. I think I could concentrate better with my eyes shut. (p. 104)
>
> People just do things, but I have to watch first to see how you do things. I have to think out most things first and know how to do them, before I do them. When I am racing and am ready to get off the mark I have to think of putting my hands down in front of me and how to lift my legs before I can start. (p. 108)
>
> If I am reading I may suddenly get bogged down at a word. It may be any word, even a simple word that I know well. When this happens I can't get past it. It's as if I am being hypnotized by it. It's as if I am seeing the word for the first time and in a different way from anyone else. It's not so much that I absorb it, it's more like it's absorbing me. (p. 109)

These vivid descriptions indicate not only that cognition is challenging for people with schizophrenia, but also that it has an impact on their everyday life. The challenge for occupational therapists is to accurately assess cognitive impairments in clients with this and other mental illnesses, and then to create interventions that help people with cognitive impairments successfully carry out the things they need and want to do in their lives.

This chapter describes the different components that make up cognition, the assessments that occupational therapists can use to measure cognitive impairment, and practice models that support occupational performance by addressing cognitive concerns.

Cognition and Psychiatric Disabilities

Cognitive impairments are common in many psychiatric disabilities; for some clients, these impairments represent the core feature of their disorder. For example, **dementia** is distinguished by a significant deterioration in cognitive functioning. Alzheimer's dementia, the most common form of the disease, begins with impairments in recall memory and progresses to a total decline in cognitive and occupational performance (Knopman, Boeve, & Petersen, 2003; Small, Fratiglioni, Viitanen, Winblad, & Backman, 2000). Normal aging also results in decrements in cognitive ability. One study of adults aged 71 or older estimates that 22.2% of these adults have cognitive impairment without dementia (Plassman et al, 2008). **Attention deficit-hyperactivity disorder (ADHD)** is also considered a cognitive impairment; in addition to attentional problems, the disorder is characterized by deficits in inhibitory control and executive function. Despite normal IQ (Schuck & Crinella, 2005), **executive dysfunction** contributes to academic problems for children with ADHD (Biederman et al, 2004). Developmental disabilities are also primarily cognitive disorders. The *Diagnostic and Statistical Manual of Mental Disorders, Fourth Edition, Text Revision* (DSM-IV-TR; APA, 2000) criteria for mental retardation are based on an IQ below 85.

Other psychiatric disabilities that are characterized primarily by mood or psychotic symptoms are nevertheless associated with significant cognitive impairments. Although there is great heterogeneity in the severity and type of cognitive impairments in individuals with schizophrenia, deficits are noted across all areas of cognition, including attention, memory, and executive functions (Weickert & Goldberg, 2000), and these impairments can interfere with successful community living, employment, and socialization (Green, Kern, Braff, & Mintz, 2000). There are similar cognitive impairments in bipolar disorder (Kravariti, Dixon, Frith, Murray, & McGuire, 2005).

For the most part, the cognitive impairments in schizophrenia and bipolar disorder persist despite the acuity of the illness (Balanza-Martinez et al, 2005). In contrast, the cognitive impairments in depression seem to be most intense during acute phases of the illness (Majer et al, 2004), with attentional deficits most prominent.

The largest body of literature on cognitive impairments and psychiatric disabilities is related to schizophrenia. As a result, this chapter includes more examples related to this population; however, the reader will find relevant applications to many other psychiatric disabilities that involve cognitive impairments. Occupational therapists need to be familiar with the cognitive impairments associated with psychiatric disabilities so that these barriers to occupational performance can be addressed.

Components of Cognition

Cognition involves processes that are associated with perceiving, making sense of, and using information. Cognition is best understood by examining its components. The following information is organized around three cognitive components (and their related subcomponents): attention, memory, and executive function.

Attention

The world we live in is exploding with information. For a minute, consider the environment that you find yourself in right now. What are the sights, sounds, and feelings that are available to you? When you stop for a moment, do you notice things that you were previously unaware of, such as the ticking of a clock, the color of the carpet, and the feel of clothing against your skin?

There is so much information available to us at any given moment that it is impossible to attend to everything. Attention involves efficiently using cognitive resources to take in the information needed to accomplish a task. To be efficient, you must allocate cognitive resources to the entity that provides the most useful input. This can be challenging for anyone. Distractions in the environment interfere with the ability to focus on relevant information, screen out what is irrelevant, and maintain attention over time. For example, you may be trying to study while your roommate is watching TV or talking loudly on the telephone. You notice that your attention wanders from the study material to the television program. Or, you may be tired or preoccupied and unable to focus on the textbook that you are trying to read for tomorrow's class. You keep thinking about an argument that you had with a friend earlier that day.

Many things in the external environment and internal to the person compete for attentional resources. Specific aspects of attention, such as automatic and controlled processes, selective attention, divided attention, and vigilance, are described next.

Automatic and Controlled Processes

Many people have had the experience of "automatically" driving a familiar route. For the most part, you are unaware of the landmarks and do not really pay attention to the points at which you need to turn or the distance you are driving. You may describe this experience as being on "autopilot." This is an example of **automatic processing**. Contrast this situation with the experience of driving in an unfamiliar area on a rainy day while trying to locate an address. In this situation, there are intense attentional requirements, such as reading street signs, attending to distances, and noticing important landmarks. This is an example of **controlled processing**.

Reading also involves both automatic and controlled processes. As you are reading this sentence, you do not have to make sense of each word; rather, you automatically take in the word "sentence" without thinking about what it means. However, it takes mental effort to understand the sentences, paragraphs, and chapters of a textbook and to integrate this information so that you can use it during a test or occupational therapy practice situation.

Another example of an automatic task is walking. Most of us do not have to think about what muscles to move or how to move our bodies to walk. Yet, consider how the automatic process of walking changes dramatically for a person with a broken leg who is using crutches or a person who has had a stroke.

Most of the things people do are not purely automatic or controlled, but fall on a continuum. Posner and Snyder (1975) identified three criteria of automatic processing:

1. It is unintentional.
2. The activity or task is done without conscious awareness.
3. It does not interfere with other mental activity.

Generally, automatic tasks are highly familiar and practiced. Therefore, tasks that are extremely controlled initially can become automatic with practice. Typing on a keyboard and playing a musical instrument are good examples of tasks that require a great deal of conscious effort when learning, but can become automatic over time. The amount of practice necessary increases as the task becomes more complex. Although complex tasks can become automatic with enough practice, certain task characteristics interfere with automaticity. Highly unstable or irregular tasks such as social interaction can never be fully automatic.

Most of the time, automatic processing is adaptive and allows you to perform more tasks more efficiently. Automaticity facilitates the development of order and routine in life. However, there are instances in which automaticity leads to mistakes or even safety issues. For example, you may pick up the phone and automatically dial a familiar number rather than the intended new number. Or, more seriously, you may get in a car accident because you failed to notice a hazard in the road during your familiar driving route.

Individuals with developmental disabilities or schizophrenia can take longer or find it more difficult to establish automaticity. Occupational therapists need to consider interventions that incorporate repeated practice or simplify tasks so that the individual moves from controlled to automatic processing. With other disabilities, such as middle or late stage Alzheimer's disease, it may be impossible to establish new automatic patterns. In this case, environmental adaptations and assistance from others may be necessary.

Selective Attention

Selective attention involves sorting out and focusing on the relevant sensory stimuli in the environment. Selective attention is absolutely essential; without it, a person would be completely overwhelmed by all of the competing available input. One of the earliest descriptions of selective attention comes from Broadbent's (1958) **filter theory**. Filter theory suggests that there is a limit to the amount of information a person can attend to at any one point in time. Therefore, individuals use an "attentional filter" that lets in some information and blocks the rest. Only the information that is allowed in can be used later. The filter prevents people from experiencing information overload. However, for the filter to be effective, it must correctly select the important or relevant information and block what is not needed. Unfortunately, this does not always occur. For example, during a lecture you may miss something important because you are daydreaming or distracted by the conversation that is going on in the hallway.

Filter theory suggests that unattended messages are fully blocked and unattended; however, the work of Treisman (1960) suggests that some unattended information is weaker, but still available to the person. Her **attenuation theory** proposes that unattended information is not totally blocked, but is turned down. Treisman used dichotic listening studies to develop her theory. In these studies, participants wear earphones, and a different message is presented to each ear. Generally, the person is asked to ignore the message in one ear, while the attended to message is repeated aloud. Although these studies indicate that most of the unattended message is missed, certain characteristics are detected. For example, people typically notice if the gender of the speaker's voice changes or if their own name is inserted in the unattended message. This process may help people pick up on important cues and switch the focus of attention to something else.

Selective attention is involved in just about everything people do. The execution of daily occupations is more effective and efficient when the individual can attend to the relevant input and screen out what is irrelevant. Distracters can be external or internal. Noises and movement in the environment can distract our attention, as can thoughts, daydreams, and anxiety. Individuals with psychosis face another internal distraction: hallucinations. Auditory hallucinations or "voices" can be very difficult to inhibit and, therefore, present a significant attentional challenge. Reducing distractions is important to support improved attention; however, this may do little to diminish the interference of internal distractions. It is important to consider interventions that limit internal as well as external distractions. For example, stress reduction may reduce feelings of anxiety, and humming or wearing a single earplug helps some people reduce the impact of auditory hallucinations (Nelson, Thrasher, & Barnes, 1991).

Divided Attention

Selective attention implies that people work on one task at a time; however, everyday people engage in one or more tasks simultaneously, a process that is often called "multitasking." A mother might change her infant's diaper and, at the same time, watch her toddler play. When playing sports, a strong athlete can take a shot at the basket, while still attending to where the other players are located on the court. More recently, much consideration has been given to the **divided attention** required to drive and talk on the cell phone. How is it that people can carry out more than one task at a time? There are several different explanations as to how divided attention works (Galotti, 2004). One possibility is that individuals alternate their attention so that they move back and forth between the two tasks. Another explanation is that one of the two tasks is automatic and does not require conscious cognitive effort. Finally, specific practice performing the two tasks together may allow one to coordinate the execution of multitasking.

For the most part, individuals do better when focused on a single task. However, people can better manage two tasks at once when at least one of the tasks is automatic or when the two tasks have been practiced together. In a classic study by Spelke, Hirst, and Neisser (1976), individuals were asked to perform two controlled tasks: (1) reading for comprehension and (2) writing down dictated words. Participants practiced these tasks for 85 sessions. Eventually, the participants were able to perform both tasks simultaneously at the same level that they had initially performed each task alone. But remember it took 85 sessions to reach this proficiency!

The research on divided attention has implications for practice. For individuals with attentional impairments, tasks that require divided attention should be avoided. When divided attention tasks cannot be avoided, additional time is necessary, although this time may be reduced if extensive practice is provided.

Vigilance

Vigilance refers to the ability to sustain attention over time. Vigilance is similar to attention span and requires that the individual maintain a readiness to respond to a target stimulus. For example, a lifeguard must maintain attention to the activity in a pool to identify dangerous situations. When cooking, vigilance is necessary to watch what is happening to the food that is on the stove and make sure that it does not burn.

Vigilance, or the sensitivity to a target, wanes under certain conditions (See, Howe, Warm, & Dember, 1995). The passage of time results in deteriorating performance. Think about how your ability to pay attention becomes more difficult the longer the lecture goes. Also, the rate at which information is presented affects the ability to respond to a target. If the stimuli are presented very rapidly, the individual will have a higher rate of misses. For example, if someone recites an unfamiliar phone number very rapidly, you may miss some of the numbers. However, if the target occurs extremely infrequently, vigilance may also be impaired.

Vigilance is also problematic if the stimulus is difficult to detect. For example, it is easier to paint a wall if the new color contrasts significantly with the original color. It is also more difficult to remain vigilant if a large area must be monitored (e.g., watching children in the family room vs. a large playground). Strategies to support vigilance include incorporating frequent breaks, optimizing the rate at which information is presented, making the stimulus obvious, and limiting the area in which the stimulus can take place.

Memory

Like attention, memory is one of the most basic cognitive functions that is employed in virtually every daily life activity. There are times when you are very cognizant of the fact that you are drawing on your memory resources, such as while taking a test or trying to recall a phone number. However, as you will see, memory is also essential to reading a sentence and typing on the computer. The following discussion of memory is categorized in terms of short-term, long-term, and working memory.

Short-Term Memory

Short-term memories are held for only a matter of seconds or minutes. The classic paper by Miller (1956) indicates that most adults have a **short-term memory** capacity for about seven items, plus or minus 2. Chunks of items can often be remembered as a single item, allowing us to recall more information. For example, you may remember your social security number in terms of three separate chunks of information: XXX-XX-XXXX. If not rehearsed, information in short-term memory is lost in about 20 seconds (Peterson & Peterson, 1959).

Long-Term Memory

The capacity for **long-term memory** is unknown, but includes the accumulation of information over a lifetime. There are different taxonomies for categorizing types of memory, and this chapter distinguishes among semantic, episodic, and procedural memory.

Semantic memory is memory for facts. Much of the knowledge you acquire as an occupational therapy student is semantic memory (e.g., the origin and insertion of muscles, the names of specific assessments, the ethical principles of occupational therapy). Semantic memory tends to be created and forgotten relatively easy. However, there are many strategies that can be used to help us retain information. Shallow rehearsal, or repeating information, is the least effective method for remembering. **Deep processing**, which involves finding meaning in facts, results in better remembering. Examples of deep processing include answering questions about the information to be remembered (Craik & Tulving, 1975), identifying distinctiveness (Friedman, 1979), and relating information to one's self (Rogers, Kuiper, & Kirker, 1977).

Episodic memory is memory for events that have happened to you. It is organized temporally, or by when it occurred. When you recall something that happened to you, you may not remember the exact date, but you think of it in terms of the time and place it happened. Memories about a spring break vacation, a trip to the emergency room, or even thinking about what you had for dinner last night are all examples of episodic memory.

Procedural memory is memory about how to do something, such as how to ride a bike or how to bake a cake. Procedural memory takes longer to be created and is less susceptible to errors. Procedural memory is also more implicit, meaning it is less consciously accessible. For example, it is difficult to describe how to ride a bike. As occupational therapists, much of our work involves helping people establish procedural memories, whether it is establish new motor patterns or develop procedural memories for self-care tasks such as toothbrushing. Because procedural memories take longer to create, it is important to incorporate repeated practice into training when trying to establish new procedural memories.

Working Memory

Working memory involves short-term memory storage and active manipulation of new information; that is, the person is "working with" the information temporarily. Working memory allows you to hold several bits of information in your mind at the same time so that the information can be processed. If you have $5 in your pocket and order from a menu at a fast food restaurant, in your head you figure out which items you want to eat among the list, how much it will cost, and whether your selection fits within your budget. You may have to adjust your choices if your selection costs too much. You go through these steps not to memorize the menus, but so that you can accomplish the temporary daily living activity of placing an order. This is an example of working memory in action.

Alan Baddeley's (2002) model of working memory includes three components: the phonological loop, the visuospatial sketchpad, and the central executive. The **phonological loop** is analogous to inner speech or what you do when you talk yourself through a task. The **visuospatial sketchpad** plays a role in spatial orientation and problem-solving that involves visual input around locating objects and yourself. You use the visuospatial sketchpad to find your way around a building, as well as in smaller spaces such as the organization of words and sentences on a page. So the phonological loop maintains verbal information, and the visuospatial sketchpad works with visual information.

The **central executive** oversees the process, choosing and directing the flow of information. The central executive moves information in and out of short-term memory and integrates new information that is coming in with long-term memory stores.

Executive Function

The term **executive function** is commonly used to refer to higher-order cognitive skills; however, a specific definition for executive function is somewhat elusive. Executive skills can be distinguished from reflexive or automatic responses. They require a level of awareness and conscious effort. Executive function is required in situations that are new, conflicting, or complex (Godefroy, 2003), and includes skills such as conceptualization/categorization, schemas and scripts, problem-solving, decision-making, and metacognition. Executive function has often been associated with frontal lobe functioning; however, there is increasing recognition that multiple brain regions are involved in these higher-order skills (Palmer & Heaton, 2000).

Concept Formation and Categorization

Humans present knowledge in words and symbols. The basic unit of knowledge is the concept. There are concrete concepts, such as table, cat, and grass, and abstract concepts, such as democracy, hope, and creativity. Concepts establish order to a person's knowledge base. When confronted with new information, people relate new objects or ideas to previously existing concepts. Knowledge is further organized by grouping concepts into categories. For example, table falls into the category of furniture, whereas democracy may be categorized as a form of government. When creating categories, people define features of the category around prototypes (Sternberg, 2003). For example, when defining the category of bird, it may include features, such as it has feathers, it flies, and it lays eggs. However, exceptions can challenge these rules. For example, people think of an ostrich as a bird, yet it does not fly. These exceptions allow categories to remain flexible.

Concept formation and **categorization** are important skills for many daily life activities. For example, it is essential to know what is edible and safe to eat versus what is poisonous or toxic. When doing laundry, clothes are sorted into whites, delicates, and darks, and there can be consequences if a mistake is made such as adding bleach to the dark-colored clothes. People also categorize clothing in terms of what is worn when it is cold versus hot and what is appropriate to wear to work versus going out on a Friday night. Most of the concept formation and categorization people do is implicit. However, when working with individuals with cognitive impairments, the occupational therapist may need to make concepts and categories more explicit. For example, teaching grocery shopping skills may incorporate information on how items are categorized in the grocery store. The client may be taught what types of items are found in the section labeled dairy.

Schemas and Scripts

Schemas are mental representations that create structure out of related concepts. Schemas go beyond categories in that they include information about the relationship of a concept. For example, you have a schema about an airport, the terminals, the check-in counters, and security. A **script** is a type of schema that describes the sequence of events that you would expect to occur in a familiar activity (Schank & Abelson, 1977). If you are a frequent traveler, you have a schema for getting to the airport, checking in and receiving your boarding pass, going through security, boarding the plane, and finding your seat. Depending on the airports you have been through, you may or may not know how the process varies slightly according to the location.

Schemas and scripts help people integrate information and organize memories. However, schemas and scripts can result in memory mistakes, especially over time, because people tend to recall material in such a way that it is consistent with their schema (Wynn & Logie, 1998). In other words, people create inferences that may or may not be accurate. For example, you may remember a classmate being present during a particular lecture because this classmate is typically there; however, on that particular day, the classmate was sick and not present.

In intervention, the occupational therapist can create explicit scripts to help people with cognitive impairments sequence and negotiate the steps of complex activities. For example, you might write out the steps for preparing a frozen dinner in a microwave and post this list on the microwave itself.

Problem-Solving

The cognitive skill of problem-solving is what you use when you want to reach a certain goal, but you cannot immediately figure out the best pathway to that goal (Matlin, 2005). Problem-solving is a mental process that involves overcoming obstacles that interfere with goal attainment. The steps to problem-solving include the following:

1. Recognizing that there is a problem
2. Understanding the problem
3. Identifying strategies or solutions to resolve the problem
4. Evaluating the strategies
5. Selecting and carrying out a strategy
6. Evaluating the outcome

These steps can be applied to the following example of buying a textbook for a college course. You realize there is a problem when you go to the college bookstore and find that the bookstore has sold out of a required textbook. The problem is that you have a quiz in 2 weeks based on a reading assignment for the book that is unavailable. You imagine several different solutions, including asking the bookstore to order you a copy of the book, going online to order the book, or asking another student if you can borrow the book. The bookstore could take up to 2 weeks to get the book and borrowing the book will only be a short-term solution. You learn that you can get the book in 5 days if you order it online. You decide to order online, get the book, complete the reading, and get an A on the quiz. You did a good job of problem-solving that situation; however, next time you will go to the bookstore earlier in the semester.

Although individuals may have impairments in the skill of problem-solving per se, the ability to solve a particular problem is highly dependent on domain expertise. In other words, how much experience and knowledge do you have related to the specific situation? For example, someone with a lot of cooking expertise may be able to figure out how to substitute for missing key ingredients in a recipe, whereas a new cook may just have to abandon the task. For another example, compare your current abilities to do an Internet search with what it was like the first time.

Research examining differences between experts and novices when solving problems identifies particular characteristics that distinguish experts (Ericcson & Lehmann, 1996). Some characteristics of experts are as follows:

- Experts have well-organized and rich schemas related to the domain.
- Experts have better memory for information related to their area of expertise.
- Experts spend more time trying to understand the problem.
- Rather than using trial-and-error approaches to solve the problem, experts are more likely to devise a grand plan before starting to solve the problem.
- Experts have automated many scripts for problem-solving and solve problems more quickly and accurately.
- When presented with new information, experts are more flexible in adapting strategies.

Occupational therapists can help people with problem-solving difficulties by teaching the steps of the problem-solving process and working toward the establishment of expertise in a content area.

Decision-Making

How did you decide to study occupational therapy? What did you choose for breakfast this morning? Should you go out of town for spring break? How is it that people make so many decisions every day? Kahneman and Tversky (1996) suggest people use a small number of heuristics to guide decision-making. **Heuristics** are simple "rules of thumb" that help people make decisions quickly; unfortunately, heuristics can also lead to biased or incorrect decisions.

The **representativeness heuristic** suggests that people make decisions when something looks like a prototype or model you have come to expect. You might make decisions about what the weather is going to be like by looking outside the window or have expectations about the taste of an apple based on your prototype of an apple. According to the representative heuristic, people believe that random outcomes are more likely than orderly outcomes. For example, would you be surprised if your grocery bill rang up as exactly $100? You would probably be more likely to believe that the bill was accurate if it totaled $97.23.

The **availability heuristic** is used when people estimate frequency or make decisions based on how easy it is to think of an example. In a study by Ross and Sicoly (1979), spouses were asked to state which person performed the larger proportion of 20 different household chores. Both partners estimated performing 80% of the chores. This is an example of an availability heuristic because a person's own actions are the most available. Recent experience tends to bias decisions toward availability. For example, if you were recently sick after eating a particular food, you would probably not eat that same food the next day, but you might make a different decision in another 5 years. Familiarity also influences decisions. For example, if you know many people who have been successful in college, you are more likely to choose to go to college yourself.

In the **anchoring and adjustment heuristic**, people start with an anchor and then make adjustments with additional information. For example, you might start out estimating that it will take 4 hours to write a paper, but once 3 hours have passed and you are still researching the background, you make an adjustment to the estimate. People also use the anchoring and adjustment heuristic when making judgments about people. Certain stereotypes are applied when you meet a new person, but you make adjustments as you get to know the person better. Even though it is extremely useful, the main problem with the anchoring and adjustment heuristic is that people typically fail to make large enough adjustments.

Heuristics usually lead to accurate decisions; however, people can make better decisions when inherent biases are known. Occupational therapists can use techniques to help clients consider all possible options. When decision-making is overwhelming, it can be helpful to limit the number of options available.

Metacognition

Defined in a circular fashion, **metacognition** is cognition about your own cognition. Metacognition is an awareness of what you know and what you do not know. It includes anticipating your abilities to cognitively manage situations and recognizing errors as they occur. Metacognition is an important regulatory mechanism that helps people match their abilities with the tasks at hand. Individuals with cognitive impairments may lack metacognition, resulting in a lack of awareness of their own cognitive impairments.

Metacognition not only includes information about your own thinking, but includes metacognitive regulation or strategies for monitoring and managing others (Flavell, 1979). For example, students may rewrite or summarize their notes after a lecture. An employee may gauge the boss' mood and facial expressions to determine when and how to best ask for some time off. People can learn to approach tasks more metacognitively. A list of questions can be provided that promote a reflective approach (e.g., What should I do first? Am I going too fast or too slow? How am I doing?)

Thus far, this chapter describes cognitive components and provides general strategies for addressing impairments in the different areas of cognition. Table 18-1 shows a summary of these strategies. The intervention section of this chapter provides more detailed information on strategies organized according to cognitive practice models.

Table 18-1 ● **Strategies for Addressing Specific Areas of Cognitive Impairment**

Area of Cognitive Impairment	Intervention Strategy
Automatic processing	• Target tasks that have potential for automatic processing. • Simplify tasks and incorporate opportunities for consistent repeated practice.
Selective attention	• Remove irrelevant stimuli. • Enhance and intensify important information. • Use auditory and visual cues. • Address internal distractions such as anxiety and auditory hallucinations.
Divided attention	• If possible, separate tasks so that the individual does not need to divide attention. • Work toward making one or more tasks automatic. • Practice doing the two tasks together.
Vigilance	• Incorporate breaks. • Slow down the rate at which information is presented. • Make stimulus easy to detect.

Table 18-1 ● **Strategies for Addressing Specific Areas of Cognitive Impairment—cont'd**

Area of Cognitive Impairment	Intervention Strategy
Memory	• Chunk items together. • Create mnemonics. • Ask questions about the information. • Apply information to oneself. • Use memory aids such as calendars, checklists, and alarm clocks.
Working memory	• Simplify tasks. • Provide devices that can substitute or assist in the manipulation of information (e.g., calculators, maps).
Concept formation/categorization	• Provide cue sheet with category and exemplars. • Provide real world experiences/practice with concepts/categories.
Schemas and scripts	• Write out the steps of a task (or use pictures). • Create simple maps that include steps of the task. • Order objects (e.g., clothing for the day) in the sequence in which the task is carried out. • Repeatedly practice the sequence of a task.
Problem-solving	• Provide and practice problem-solving heuristics. • Prevent or eliminate common problems that occur with specific tasks.
Decision-making	• Limit the number of options. • Teach individual about potential biases in decision. • Teach individual to step back and think through important decisions. • Ask others for input when making important decisions.

Cognitive Assessment

Cognition is assessed by neuropsychologists who employ a number of different standardized measures, as well as by occupational therapists within the context of occupational performance.

Neuropsychological Testing

Neuropsychological testing uses standardized measures to assess specific cognitive abilities in the context of evaluating brain function. Neuropsychologists typically administer a comprehensive battery of tests that cover multiple components of cognition. Most neuropsychological tests have normative standards that consider age and educational achievement. There are hundreds of neuropsychological tests, and Table 18-2 describes some of the most common tests. More detailed information about these and other neuropsychological tests can be found in the classic text, *Neuropsychological Assessment*, by Lezak, Howieson, and Loring (2004). Information from the neuropsychological evaluation can be helpful to occupational therapists in determining a client's specific strengths and weaknesses related to cognitive functioning.

Cognitive Assessment in Occupational Therapy

Occupational therapy assessment is always conducted within the context of occupational performance. Cognition is critical for the performance of virtually every occupation, and cognition is a common impairment for many clients seen by occupational therapists. Consequently, cognitive assessment can be very useful in determining factors that might interfere with successful occupational performance. Occupational therapists may obtain assessment information about cognition from observation of performance, reports of the client or caregiver, neuropsychological reports, and administration of standardized cognitive measures. Standardized cognitive measures typically used by occupational therapists are based on functional tasks and/or everyday objects.

Test of Everyday Attention

The Test of Everyday Attention (Robertson, Ward, Ridgeway, & Nimmo-Smith, 1994) includes eight tasks, such as locating items on a map and searching a telephone directory, based on an imagined trip to Philadelphia. The tasks are designed to measure selective, sustained, alternating, and divided attention. Parallel forms are available to address practice effects. The measure has norms for adults aged 18 to 80. Test–retest reliability is adequate, and preliminary studies indicate that the measure discriminates individuals with stroke and traumatic brain injury (TBI) (Chan, 2000).

The Test of Everyday Attention for Children (Manley et al, 2001) assesses attention in children aged 6 to 16. This game-like assessment includes nine subtests that are similar to the adult measure in terms of cognitive requirements. The test takes about 1 hour to administer and includes parallel forms. In a study investigating the discriminant validity of the test, children with ADHD scored poorly on the tasks measuring sustained attention, but scored in the normal range on selective attention tasks (Manly et al, 2001).

The Lived Experience

The first part of this first-person narrative is written by the wife and caregiver of a man with Alzheimer's disease. This is followed by an account written by her husband. The story describes the very gradual progression of Alzheimer's. In addition, both accounts recognize the abilities that remain.

Narrative from Wife/Caregiver

"Where are we going?". . . . Again, "Where are we going?"

It all began with repeated questions. At first, it seemed that inattention was the problem (there had always been some of that!), but soon the excessiveness became apparent enough to convince me there was a problem. It was real—he just couldn't remember. When asked to do something his answer was usually, "in a little bit," and in that "little bit" of time, he had forgotten what he was to do. This was probably early 2003.

In our first visit to the doctor concerning his memory, he was given the oral "test" and did very well. I believe it was the date he couldn't remember. After our discussions and several visits, our doctor prescribed Aricept to help with his "memory loss." This was in October 2004.

Each time we visited the doctor, he was given "the test" and his abilities slipped a little. We spoke of more memory loss and finally the Alzheimer word came up—not really a diagnosis but a possibility. Namenda was added to his meds. MRIs, brain scans, etc, were given.

In the meantime, an Aging Brain Study was begun at Kansas University Medical Center, and we opted to be part of that. In it, 32 persons without problems and 32 persons with some dementia or early Alzheimer's were tested. There were discussions, questions by psychiatrists, physical tests, MRIs, blood tests, etc. We were involved in four sessions. He was very cooperative and happy to be involved in something that someday might help someone else. The neurologist there confirmed "early Alzheimer's."

Today, he is still forgetting most things, but is capable still of so much. This remains pretty much early stage for he still can work crossword puzzles; read books, magazines, and newspapers; and plays lots of solitaire on the computer.

We are trying to live one day at a time, still living in our home, for we know someday things will worsen and changes may have to be made.

Narrative From Client

I know that I have been diagnosed as having the early stages of Alzheimer's disease. However, I don't feel much difference. It is difficult to determine what ability or facility, if any, I am losing. Perhaps it is not a matter of loss, but instead a matter of decreasing abilities. Certainly, as we age, some of our abilities diminish. If I had to measure my abilities, I would think in terms of the following:

- Strength
- Agility
- Flexibility
- Quickness
- Memory
- Reasoning

Although I come up with four physical attributes, I could only think of two mental attributes. This is an intriguing problem for me. In how many ways can we describe and measure our abilities? I'm going to ponder that question for a day or two.

Rereading the above, I note that I left out sexual activity. Oh well. Also I failed to mention that my ability with short-term memory has diminished. I think I should also have included learning ability. That may be different from memory.

Table 18-2 ● **Names and Purposes of Common Neuropsychological Tests**

Test Name	Purpose of Test
Boston Naming test	Assesses aphasia through a set of cards with line drawings. The individual names the object on each card.
Continuous Performance tests	These tests require the individual to sustain attention over time while responding to a visual target. Conditions with and without distraction are included.
Controlled Oral Word Association test	A test of verbal fluency that requires the individual to name as many words as possible that begin with a specific letter.
Halstead-Reitan Neuropsychological Battery	A set of tests designed to provide an overall assessment of brain function. Assesses language, attention, motor speed, abstract thinking, memory, and spatial reasoning.
Rey-Osterrieth Complex Figure test	A complicated picture is presented. First, the individual copies the figure, and then the figure is drawn from memory.
Stroop test	Assesses attention and processing speed. Individuals read color words (e.g., red, green, blue) or name the color of the ink in which XXXs are printed. In the distracting condition, the word is written in a different color (e.g., the word red is printed in blue ink). The person is to name the ink color and not read the word.
Tower of London	An executive function test that involves moving objects on a peg with the fewest moves to reach a desired goal. Requires planning and strategy use.
Trail Making Tests A and B	A line is drawn linking consecutive letters or alternating between numbers and letters to assess attention and processing speed.
Verbal Learning tests (California or Rey)	Assess the ability to remember a list of words. The list is repeated several times to determine if the individual is able to remember more words with repetition. The California Verbal Learning test includes words that can be categorized.

Table 18-2 ● **Names and Purposes of Common Neuropsychological Tests—cont'd**

Test Name	Purpose of Test
Wechsler Adult Intelligence Scale and Wechsler Intelligence Scale for Children	Includes multiple subtest that result in summary measures of full scale, verbal, and performance IQ. Includes measures of memory, knowledge, problem-solving, calculation, abstract thinking, spatial orientation, planning, and processing speed.
Wechsler Memory Scale	Eighteen subtests of immediate and delayed recall and recognition memory. Includes verbal and nonverbal tasks.
Wisconsin Card Sorting test	Individuals sort cards according to different categories. Once a category is established, the sorting rule changes. Assesses executive functions.

Multiple Errands Test

The Multiple Errands test (Shallice & Burgess, 1991) is a measure of executive function that is administered in a shopping mall. Simple tasks are assigned, such as getting information about the times a particular service is available, purchasing items in a store, and getting oneself to an identified location at a prespecified time. In addition, specific rules are established, such as "No shop should be entered other than to buy something." The test is designed to test strategy use in an ecologically valid setting.

Shallice and Burgess (1991) studied individuals with brain injury who performed well on IQ tests and laboratory measures of executive function, and found that these individuals did poorly on the Multiple Errands test. They argue that tests such as the Multiple Errands test are more sensitive to subtle impairments of executive function that are common in neurological disorders. There is a simplified measure of the test (Alderman, Burgess, Knight, & Henman, 2003) and a measure that can be administered in a hospital setting (Knight, Alderman, & Burgess, 2002). The test has good inter-rater reliability, and both the simplified and hospital versions distinguished people with and without brain injury.

Loewenstein Occupational Therapy Cognitive Assessment

The Loewenstein Occupational Therapy Cognitive Assessment (LOTCA; Averbuch & Katz, 2005) assesses orientation, visual and spatial perception, visuomotor organization, and thinking operations. It includes 20 subtests and takes 30 to 50 minutes to administer. Each subtest is scored from 1 to 4 or 1 to 5, with the higher score representing better cognitive function. Norms are available for children aged 6 to 12 and adults aged 30 to 55 (Itzkovich, Elazar, Averbuch, & Katz, 2000). Inter-rater reliability of the measure has been estimated at 0.82 to 0.97, depending on the subtest (Katz, Itzkovich, Averbuch, & Elazar, 1989). The same study found that the LOTCA discriminated between individuals with brain injury, cerebrovascular accident, and a control group. A study comparing the Mini-Mental State Examination, the cognitive component of the Functional Independence Measure (FIM) and the LOTCA, found the LOTCA was better than the other two instruments at predicting functional outcome for individuals being treating for stroke (Zwecker et al, 2002).

Dynamic Occupational Therapy Cognitive Assessment for Children

The Dynamic Occupational Therapy Cognitive Assessment for Children (DOTCA-CH), based on the LOTCA, provides a dynamic approach to assessing cognitive impairments in children, which allows for the identification of strengths and impairments with the idea that the results can be used to develop a mediated learning intervention (see the Dynamic Interactional Approach) (Katz, Felzen, Tadmoor, & Hartman-Maeir, 2007). The measures include 22 subtests in the areas of orientation, spatial perception, praxis, visuomotor construction, and thinking operations. Initial support for inter-rater reliability, internal consistency, and construct validity exists.

Executive Function Performance Test

The Executive Function Performance test (EFPT) is a performance-based standardized assessment of cognition and executive function (Baum, Morrison, Hahn, & Edwards, 2003). The Kitchen Task Assessment, an earlier functional assessment test designed by Baum and Edwards (1993), was used as the prototype in developing the EFPT. The EFPT includes four standardized instrumental activity of daily living (IADL) tasks (cooking, telephone use, medication management, bill paying) that the client performs with graded cues provided by the therapist as needed. The EFPT serves three purposes: to determine which executive function components are deficient (initiation, organization, sequencing, judgment and safety, completion); to determine an individual's capacity for independent functioning; and to determine the type of assistance necessary for task completion. The EFPT has been validated in studies of individuals with stroke, multiple sclerosis, and schizophrenia (Baum et al, 2003, 2008; Goverover et al, 2005; Katz et al, 2007).

Assessments Associated With Toglia's Dynamic Interactional Approach

Toglia's (2005) assessments include both static and dynamic components. A static assessment captures an individual's performance at one moment in time. Dynamic assessment approaches are used to assess an individual's learning potential or ability to apply strategies to solve a problem. In a dynamic assessment approach, the individual is given instruction, cues, or strategies regarding how to perform the test.

Contextual Memory Test

The Contextual Memory test (CMT; Toglia, 2005) includes a subjective assessment of the individual's awareness of his or her memory ability and an objective assessment of memory. The awareness component asks the individual to predict his or her score. This is done at the beginning of the assessment and at different points throughout.

Part I of the objective assessment is the static assessment of memory. The test uses 20 drawings with either a restaurant or morning routine theme to assess recall memory. Each picture is presented for 90 seconds. After all 20 pictures are presented, the individual is asked to recall as many items as possible. After 15 to 20 minutes, the individual is asked to recall the items again. If the individual does poorly on Part I, then Part II, the dynamic assessment, is administered. The alternate theme of either restaurant or morning routine is presented. The individual is given cues about the theme of the pictures and instructed to analyze the overall context before attending to the specifics of each picture.

Several studies of the CMT examined discriminant validity. On the awareness component of the test, individuals with brain injury tend to overestimate their memory capacity and base their abilities on functioning prior to the brain injury (Toglia, 1993). The CMT did discriminate individuals with Alzheimer's disease (Gil & Josman, 2001) and children with brain injury (Josman, Berney, & Jarus, 2000).

Toglia Category Assessment

The Toglia Category Assessment (Toglia, 2005) uses a dynamic approach to assess categorization and conceptualization using everyday objects. Plastic utensils are sorted according to size (small or large), color (red, yellow, and green), and utensil type (knife, fork, and spoon). Once the utensils are sorted by one category (size, color, or type), the individual is asked to sort them again in a different way and then a third way. If the individual has difficulty with the sorting, cues are provided, such as alerting the individual to the differences of size, color, and type.

Assessments Associated with Allen's Cognitive Disabilities Practice Model

Allen Cognitive Level Test

The Allen Cognitive Level (ACL) Screen 5 uses a leather lacing task as a screening tool to determine cognitive level based on Allen's Cognitive Disability Practice Model (Allen et al, 2007). The first step, a running stitch, is used to establish criterion for levels 2 and 3 of the cognitive disability scale (Fig. 18-1). An individual achieves at least a level 3 if he or she can complete two running stitches. The next stitch is the whip stitch, which requires the individual to bring the lacing from front to back and keep it untwisted. A level 4 is achieved if the individual is

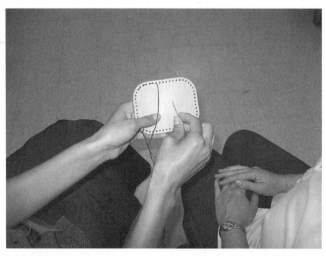

FIGURE 18-1. Administration of the Allen Cognitive Level test, the running stitch.

able to make at least two stitches without twisting the lace. The last stitch, the single cordovan, requires multiple steps. After a demonstration, the individual is asked to complete the stitch. The individual scores a 5 if he or she completes the stitch using trial-and-error problem-solving, and a level 6 is received if the individual uses deductive reasoning to correct an error. It is important that the tester be aware of potential biases in the test, particularly previous experience with needlecrafts. Penny, Mueser, and North (1995) found the ACL to be related to social competence in people with schizophrenia. In another study of schizophrenia, Secrest, Wood, and Tapp (2000) found relationships between the ACL and the Wisconsin Card Sorting test, and the ACL was associated with the Shipley Institute of Living scale in another sample of people with psychiatric disabilities (David & Riley, 1990).

Allen Diagnostic Module

The Allen Diagnostic Module (Earhart, 2006) is comprised of 24 craft projects with ACL ratings of 3.0 to 5.8. The craft activities can be used for both evaluation and treatment. Each craft activity is rated on the ACL scale. Specific observational criteria are established for each item, which allows the therapist to make more specific ratings. For example, instead of a 4.0, the individual can receive incremental ratings of 4.2, 4.4, and 4.6. By completing several craft activities, the therapists can combine observations and be more confident in a final score; however, the measure is limited in terms of psychometric reliability and validity testing.

Routine Task Inventory

The Routine Task Inventory (RTI; Allen, Earhart, & Blue, 1992) is an observational guide for 14 different activities of daily living (ADLs) that provides further verification of cognitive level. Performance of each task is described in terms of the ACL. For example, level 2 for bathing includes descriptions such as "may not try to wash self, or may resist the caregiver's help," whereas level 5 is described as "bathes without assistance, using shampoo, deodorant, and other desirable toiletries." The therapist may observe the individual performing the ADL or obtain information from a reliable caregiver. Studies of the RTI indicate it is correlated with the ACL (Heimann, Allen, & Yerxa, 1989; Wilson, Allen, McCormack, & Burton, 1989).

Dementia Screenings

Mini-Mental State Examination

The Mini-Mental State Examination (MMSE; Folstein, Folstein, & McHugh, 1975) is a widely used screening tool for assessing cognitive function in older adults. The MMSE assesses orientation, registration, attention, recall, and language. It is a quick measure that takes approximately 10 minutes to administer. Age-related norms are available (Crum, Anthony, Bassett, & Folstein, 1993). A score below 25 (out of a possible 30) is generally considered indicative of cognitive impairment (Anthony, LeResche, Niaz, Von Korff, & Folstein, 1982); however, the score should be interpreted in the context of the individual's age and education. A score of 25 or below would warrant further evaluation, as the MMSE is a screening tool.

Clock Drawing Test

The clock drawing test is another simple and quick screening measure of cognitive status. Like the MMSE it is most commonly used as a screening for cognitive impairment in older adults. The clock drawing test has several different variations of administration and scoring. In it earliest version (Goodglass & Kaplan, 1983), the procedures instruct individuals to mark 1:00, 3:00, 9:15, and 7:30 on four pre-drawn clock faces. One point is awarded for each correct placement of a hand, and one point is given for drawing the different lengths of the minute and hour hand.

The Alzheimer's Disease Cooperative Study Group (1999) scoring system uses a 5-point scale. One point each for drawing an approximately circular face, numbers in the correct order, symmetry and placement of numbers, presence of two hands, and hands showing correct time (Fig. 18-2). Sunderland et al (1989) developed a 10-point scale, and examples are provided for each level of scoring. The Tuokko, Jadjistavropoulos, Miller, and Beattie (1992) task involves clock drawing, clock setting, and clock reading.

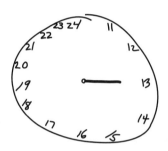

Scoring

Item	Points earned
1 point for clock circle	1
1 point for all numbers in correct order	1
1 point for symmetry and placement of numbers	0
1 point for two hands on clock	0
1 point for the correct time	0
Total	2

FIGURE 18-2. Sample clock drawing test. Note that there are different scoring systems available, but this system in common use suggests dementia if the individual scores 3 or lower.

In a review, Shulman (2000) noted that, across the various studies, the sensitivity and specificity rates of the clock drawing test average 85% with strong inter-rater reliability and good predictive validity. The measure is also sensitive to cognitive change. An epidemiological study of the clock drawing test with more than 13,000 participants suggests that the measure is more valid as a test of moderate to severe cognitive impairment and less sensitive to milder impairment (Nishiwaki et al, 2004). The measure is also sensitive to cognitive impairment in schizophrenia (Bozikas et al, 2002).

Intervention/Models and Techniques for Cognitive Impairment

In occupational therapy intervention, there are two primary approaches for addressing cognitive impairment: remediation and compensation. In the **remediation approach,** the cognitive impairment is targeted, and intervention is directed at improving a particular skill. In the **compensatory approach,** the therapist adapts the environment, task, or teaching method to compensate for the cognitive impairment. This separation is not always black and white, with some interventions combining both strategies. Several models of intervention that are relevant for occupational therapy practice are presented here, including cognitive remediation, integrated psychological therapy, dynamic interactional approach, cognitive adaptation, compensatory thinking techniques, cognitive disability practice model, errorless learning, reality orientation and validation therapy, and classroom and parental interventions for ADHD.

Cognitive Remediation

Cognitive remediation is aimed at improving or restoring specific cognitive skills, such as attention, memory, and problem-solving, so that the individual can more successfully engage in everyday occupations. The intervention techniques incorporate computer-based training, paper-and-pencil tasks, and group exercises that are incrementally graded for improving cognitive processes. Repetition and rehearsal are essential characteristics of cognitive remediation. Consequently, intervention sessions are frequent and often include homework exercises.

PhotoVoice

Extra-giant jumbo challenger jigsaw puzzle. When you've just dumped the pieces of a jigsaw puzzle onto the table, it may seem an impossible task to assemble them all into a picture like the one printed on the box. I often feel just as overwhelmed by situations and circumstances, and even the basic functions of living. A step in my recovery is learning to gain a measure of control through organizational skills: examining all of the pieces, sorting, evaluating, rearranging—dividing large into small, until I have a list of incremental steps that are much less intimidating to undertake.

—Willeta

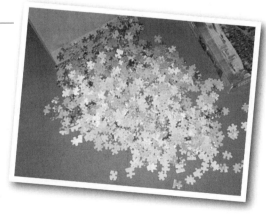

Cognitive remediation should target those cognitive areas that are known to be impaired. Because the type and severity of impairment can vary significantly among individuals with psychiatric disabilities, it is important that a careful assessment is conducted initially to identify the targets of intervention. Activities are selected that challenge the impaired cognition. For example, a letter cancellation task such as the one shown in Box 18-1 may be used to address selective attention and vigilance.

Similar tasks using auditory input can be presented. For example, the therapist may read a list of words and ask the client to indicate when he or she has heard a word that begins with the letter b. This could be graded to have the client indicate every time there is a word with the letter b in it.

Different tasks can be used to address other areas of attention, memory, and executive function. There are many commercially available packages providing cognitive remediation activities (see Resources section).

Several studies of cognitive remediation intervention for people with schizophrenia indicate improvement specific to the targeted impairment across all areas of cognitive impairment. For example, Medalia, Aluma, Tryon, & Merriam (1998) found that attention training for individuals with schizophrenia resulted in improvement on the Continuous Performance test. Likewise, in another study, memory improved on a target task but did not generalize to general measures of memory (Medalia, Revheim, & Casey, 2000). There is also evidence that cognitive remediation is effective in improving executive impairments in schizophrenia (Wykes, Reeder, Corner, Williams, & Everitt 1999). Cognitive remediation approaches also show promise for children with ADHD (Toplak, Connors, Shuster, Knezevic, & Parks, 2008). At this time, several reviews have been published on schizophrenia (Kurtz, Moberg, Gur, & Gur, 2001; McGurk, Twamley, Sitzer, McHugo, & Mueser, 2007; Pilling et al, 2002; Silverstein & Wilkniss, 2004; Twamley, Jeste, & Bellack, 2003) and ADHD (Toplak et al, 2008).

These reviews have differing levels of optimism for the intervention approach; however, they are critical of the ecological validity of the approach. In other words, studies suggest that individuals improve their skills on the target task, but these skills do not generalize to more general measures of cognitive functioning or, more important, to real-life functioning. For example, in the ADHD literature, the improvements in cognition may not translate into improved behaviors at school and home (Toplak et al, 2008).

Silverstein and Wilkniss (2004) argue that cognitive remediation should move away from focusing on isolated cognitive processes and focus on integrating cognitive activity. McGurk et al (2007) found that cognitive remediation resulted in better functional outcomes when combined with adjunctive psychiatric rehabilitation. This is consistent with Spaulding, Reed, Sulllivan, Richardson, and Weiler's (1999) suggestion that in schizophrenia recovery should not be based on specific processes, but rather the ability to recruit the necessary cognitive functions for a given task. Some efforts are being made toward enhancing the generalizability of cognitive remediation as discussed next with Integrated Psychological Therapy (Brenner, Hirsbrunner, & Heimberg, 1996) and the Dynamic Interactional Approach (Toglia, 2005).

Integrated Psychological Therapy

Integrated Psychological Therapy (IPT), developed by Brenner and colleagues (1996), uses a group format to provide hierarchically organized cognitive remediation activities for people with schizophrenia. The program is "integrated" so that cognitive impairments are addressed along with social and problem-solving skills. IPT consist of five subprograms: cognitive differentiation, social perception, verbal communication, social competence, and interpersonal problem-solving.

Cognitive differentiation targets attentional skills and conceptualization abilities using games such as card sorting and a variation of 20 questions. In *social perception*, group members view pictures of social situations and interpret or describe the situations. *Verbal communication* focuses on applying cognitive skills (e.g., paying attention) to conversation skills. The *social competence* subprogram uses role-play to practice behavioral social situations, and the final

---

BOX 18-1 ■ Letter Cancellation Task

Cross out each letter "b"

   d f r s b h q r s l t u b m n v b f a s b c t r o l b h a f h l b b o
p r s t u v
   l m j b o r s l f q r s b e w q o h t u v w s m u b l b n m b w u
y x y t o

The therapist then records both the amount of time it takes to complete the task and the number of errors (both missing the "b" and crossing out the incorrect letter). The therapist can also observe how the person goes about the task—for example, does the client use a systematic approach to scanning? If not, the therapist can provide the client with feedback on how to systematically scan from left to right.

The exercise is repeated until the individual becomes competent, at which point increasingly complex exercises are added. For example, the letter cancellation may involve only letters that are similar to the target, such as

   b p p d q b p d q p b b d d p b q q d p b q d p b q d b p p
d q b q p d b d d

Evidence-Based Practice

The research evidence on cognitive remediation suggests that the intervention does result in improvements on specific cognitive measures, but there is little evidence to support improvement in social or community functioning.

➤ If using cognitive remediation interventions, the occupational therapist should consider methods that facilitate generalization to everyday life.

Silverstein, S. M., & Wilkniss, S. M. (2004). At issue: The future of cognitive rehabilitation of schizophrenia. *Schizophrenia Bulletin, 30,* 679–692.

Toplak, M. E., Connor, L., Shuster, J., Knezevic, B., & Parks, S. (2008). Review of cognitive, cognitive behavioral and neural based intervention for attention deficit/hyperactivity disorder (ADHD). *Clinical Psychiatry Review, 28,* 801–823.

subprogram teaches an *interpersonal problem-solving* technique to apply to social situations.

Research on the efficacy of IPT in schizophrenia is inconsistent. Most studies suggest that IPT is more effective in improving basic cognitive functioning and not social skills, and some studies find no or limited cognitive improvement, whereas others identify associations between cognitive improvements and social competence (as reviewed by Wykes & van der Gaag, 2001).

Dynamic Interactional Approach

The Dynamic Interactional Approach (Toglia, 2005) considers the interplay of the person, activity, and environment. The focus of this approach is not cognitive subskills such as attention and memory, but the functional information processing capacity of the individual. This capacity is modifiable and varies as the activity, environment, and person change.

Instead of intervening at the cognitive skill level, intervention focuses on processing strategies and self-monitoring skills. For example, the Dynamic Interactional Approach would teach the client how to use a systematic and planned approach toward approaching a task. Characteristics of target activities are also considered in the intervention. Toglia (2005) describes the following activity parameters: familiarity, directions, distinctive features, degree of detail, contrast, background, context, amount, and arrangement. For example, with the task of paying a utility bill, the therapist would determine the individual's familiarity with a particular bill; the amount of information presented; the amount of detail and discrepancy between features that contribute to how easy it is to find the amount due, due date, etc; and then design an intervention based on this information.

The Dynamic Interactional Approach facilitates generalization by working on a strategy across different activities and situations that gradually change. For example, the strategy of anticipation can be taught to an individual who tends to engage in tasks impulsively. The client is taught to think about an activity before starting it and possibly answer questions such as, "What problems might this create for me, and what might I do if I run into difficulty?" This strategy would be practiced with increasingly difficult activities and in increasingly dissimilar environments. For someone who is easily distracted, the strategy could involve underlining, bolding, or listing the most important information.

The Dynamic Interactional Approach was originally designed for people with TBI, but has been applied to people with schizophrenia and children with learning disabilities and ADHD (Josman, 2005). Although there is a need for research to determine the efficacy of the approach, research has been done that supports the relevance of the model to people with schizophrenia. For example, a study with the Toglia Category Assessment found that people with schizophrenia performed similarly to people with brain injury (Toglia & Josman, 1994). When compared to health controls, individuals with schizophrenia had lower scores on the Contextual Memory Test (Josman, 1997) and used lower-order strategies (So, Toglia, & Donohue, 1997).

Cognitive Adaptation

Cognitive rehabilitation also involves strategies that adapt the environment or task to compensate for cognitive impairments. Because of the limitations of cognitive remediation, compensatory approaches are often used instead of or along with remedial strategies. Compensatory strategies include the use of adaptive devices as well as thinking techniques. A day planner is an example of an adaptive device, and the use of a memory mnemonic is a thinking technique.

Adapting Tasks and Environments

Task analysis and environmental assessment is the first step toward developing environmental adaptations. By understanding the components of a task, it is often possible to modify a task to compensate for cognitive impairments. For example, cooking tasks can be adapted by using pre-chopped ingredients, prepared foods, and simple recipes with limited steps and ingredients. Alternate methods may also be used to accomplish a task (e.g., money management may be simplified by using direct deposit and automatic bill paying systems available at most banks). Scripts can be created to help an individual sequence the steps of a task (Fig. 18-3).

Environmental adaptations often include the use of cues such as labels, signs, symbols, alarms, and beepers. Cabinets or drawers can be labeled to indicate contents. Signs that provide reminders can be placed in relevant locations; for example, a sign stating "don't forget your keys" may be place on the inside of the door. Alarm clocks and timers are used by most people to wake up in the morning or to time the baking of a cake, but more sophisticated systems are available to remind individuals to take their medication, follow a

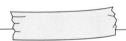

Toothbrushing

1. Remove the cap of the toothpaste.
2. Squeeze a pea-size ball of toothpaste on your toothbrush.
3. Wet the toothbrush under running water in your sink.
4. Brush your teeth for two minutes (use your timer).
5. Remember to brush front and back teeth and all surfaces, including your gums.
6. Rinse your mouth and the toothbrush.
7. Check your face in the mirror to make sure you've rinsed away all toothpaste.
8. Replace the cap on the toothpaste.
9. Return toothpaste and toothbrush to the medicine chest.

FIGURE 18-3. Sample script for toothbrushing.

self-care routine, and alert a caregiver that someone has left the house (see Resources section).

Calendars and day planners can be used to help provide reminders of appointments and daily schedules. Checklists are useful in helping establish routines. For example, individuals who have difficulty organizing housecleaning or feel overwhelmed by the task can use a weekly checklist to make housecleaning more manageable (Fig. 18-4).

Organizational strategies can be particularly useful in school-based practice for children with cognitive impairments such as ADHD or learning disabilities. One occupational therapist has created a system for keeping the student's desk organized by using a template placed in the storage section of the desk with labels for placement of the school-related objects such as books, pencil case, binders, etc (Gary Groening, personal communication, 2005).

Social supports provide another powerful compensatory tool. Family members or peers can provide reminders or cues. These same individuals may also perform a task alongside the client to act as a model. Naturally occurring community supports should also be considered. A friendly bus driver may be willing to help someone recognize their stop, a classmate can be a study partner, or the clerks at the grocery store may be available to help people locate items.

Cognitive Adaptation Training

Dawn Velligan, a psychologist collaborating with occupational therapists, has developed a manualized approach to the use of compensatory strategies for people with schizophrenia (Velligan, Mahurin, True, Lefton, & Flores, 1996; Velligan et al, 2000). Cognitive Adaptation Training uses a different set of strategies for apathetic versus disinhibited behaviors. Strategies to address apathetic behaviors focus on prompts and cues, such as creating checklists, using labels, and placing everyday objects such as toothbrushes within eyesight. Strategies to address disinhibited behavior involve the removal of distractions and organization of materials, such as removing out-of-season clothes from the closet and using colored bins to sort the laundry. A randomized controlled trial of the intervention found that, at the end of the study period, individuals in the cognitive adaptation training group had higher levels of global functioning and lower relapse rates.

Compensatory Thinking Techniques

Donald Meichenbaum (1979) was an early developer of compensatory thinking strategies. In teaching this strategy, the therapist demonstrates the process and then asks the client to talk him- or herself through a task. For example, in leaving the house for the morning, the self-talk may include "I'm checking to make sure that I've turned out all the lights and turned off the stove/oven. I've got my keys and my purse with me. I'm walking out the door and locking it. I'm placing my keys in the inside pocket of my purse so that I'll remember where they are." This strategy helps the individual attend to the task; think through the steps before acting on them; and, with repeated practice, supports the development of automatic processing. This approach has been used in schizophrenia (Meichenbaum & Cameron, 1973), older adults (Meichenbaum, 1979), and ADHD (Abikoff, 1991).

Another common thinking approach is to teach a series of questions or steps to help the individual self-monitor while working toward a goal. Levine et al (2000) developed Goal Management Training, which involves the following steps:

1. Stop
2. Define—what is the task or goal?
3. List—what are the steps?
4. Learn—do I know the steps? do I need to go back?
5. Check—am I doing what I planned to do?

Weekly Housecleaning Checklist

○ Sunday	Wash dishes	✗
Monday	Wash dishes	✗
	Take out garbage	✗
Tuesday	Wash dishes	✗
	Clean bathrooms	
Wednesday ○	Wash dishes	✗
	Dust	✗
Thursday	Wash dishes	
	Vaccum and sweep floors	
Friday	Wash dishes	✗
Saturday ○	Wash dishes	✗
	Laundry	

FIGURE 18-4. Sample weekly checklist for housecleaning.

Evidence-Based Practice

Adaptive approaches can help individuals successfully engage in daily activities by compensating for cognitive impairments. These approaches can involve changing the environment or employing compensatory thinking strategies.

➤ Environments can be simplified by removing distractions, incorporating visual or auditory cues, and organizing materials.

➤ Social supports, such as friends, family, and community members, can be included in the intervention process and serve as a compensatory cue or reminder.

➤ Occupational therapists can use self-monitoring strategies, like the one developed for the Cognitive Orientation to Daily Occupational Performance intervention, to help individuals with cognitive impairments stay focused on a task, use strategic thinking, and work toward a goal.

Abikoff, H. (1991). Cognitive training in ADHD children: Less to it than meets the eye. *Journal of Learning Disability, 24,* 205–209.

Miller, L. T., Polatjko, H. J., Missiuna, C., Mandich, A. D., & Macnab, J. T. (2001). A pilot trial of a cognitive treatment for children with developmental coordination disorder. *Human Movement Science, 20,* 183–210.

Velligan, D. I., Bow-Thomas, C. C., Huntzinger, C., Ritch, J., Ledbetter, N., Prihoda, T. J., & Miller, A. L. (2000). Randomized controlled trial of the use of compensatory strategies to enhance adaptive functioning in outpatients with schizophrenia. *American Journal of Psychiatry, 157,* 1317–1323.

The authors of Goal Management Training found this approach superior to a motor skills training program for people with TBI. They also describe a case study in which a woman with meningoencephalitis was taught meal planning using this method.

Similarly, in the Cognitive Orientation to Daily Occupational Performance (CO-OP), a four-step strategy is taught to help children work through motor tasks (Polatajko & Mandich, 2004). The steps include the following:

1. Goal—what do you want to do?
2. Plan—how will you go about doing it?
3. Do—carry out the plan
4. Check—did the plan work? does it need to be modified?

In a small randomized trial, Miller, Polatajko, Missiuna, Mandich, and Macnab (2001) found that the CO-OP method was more effective than treatment as usual in helping children with developmental coordination disorder achieve their goals. Sangster, Beninger, Polatajko, and Mandich (2005) found that children using CO-OP were able to identify more and better strategies for task success.

The use of thinking strategies is generally more effective if the individual has some awareness of his or her cognitive impairment. The person must also have the cognitive ability to learn and remember the steps of the strategy.

Cognitive Disability Practice Model

Claudia Allen (1996) suggests that cognitive remediation is not a reasonable goal for people with serious cognitive impairments. She developed the Cognitive Disability Frame of Reference as a framework for occupational therapists to use to create situations in which individuals with cognitive impairments can be successful. The model describes six hierarchical levels of cognitive functioning (Allen, Earhart, & Blue, 1992), as outlined in Table 18-3.

These six levels are further broken down into sublevels, such as Level 1.1, 1.2, etc, which make up the ACL scale.

When applying the model to intervention, the therapist begins with a detailed assessment. Using the Allen Cognitive Level Screen, the therapist assigns a cognitive level. The Allen Diagnostic Modules (Allen, Earhart, & Blue, 1993) are used to further verify the cognitive level. The intervention then focuses on providing activities in which the individual can succeed, with the goal of creating an environment that allows the individual the least restrictions while maintaining safety. Often, occupational therapists using the Cognitive Disability Frame of Reference create therapeutic groups based on cognitive levels. For example, clients at Level 3 might work with familiar tools and materials to create basic craft products.

Allen's Cognitive Disabilities Model was combined with Reisberg's theory of retrogenesis in the design of an interdisciplinary dementia program in a long-term care facility (Warchol, 2004). The occupational therapist works directly with the client and also consults with and provides training to other staff members so that they can implement strategies and supports that allow the individual to participate more successfully in the activities and dining programs.

Research related to this model suggests that the cognitive levels may be related to other cognitive measures, social competence, and community living status (Penny et al, 1995; Secrest et al, 2000; Wilson et al, 1989). There is limited

---

Table 18-3 ◉ **Cognitive Disability Frame of Reference—Hierarchical Levels of Cognitive Functioning**

Levels	Individual Characteristics	Therapist Responses
Level 1: automatic actions	Impaired awareness but person is conscious and has reflexive responses. Able to perform only very basic habits such as eating and drinking. Responses are primarily instinctive.	Use one-word commands. Provide familiar cues (e.g., place plate of food within view and hand individual a fork).
Level 2: postural actions	Aware of movements of their own muscles and joints. Watches movements of others. Seeks movements that are pleasurable or comfortable. May be resistive or easily agitated.	Imitate gross motor actions and simultaneously provide simple verbal directions (e.g., watch me, you try it). Focus is on gross motor movements.
Level 3: manual actions	Able to attend to the external environment, particularly tactile cues. Can use hands to manipulate materials. May include seemingly purposeless actions. Easily distracted.	Imitate manipulation of objects (e.g., brushing teeth). Provide repetitive practice of routine tasks. Use manually guided instruction.
Level 4: goal-directed actions	Can respond to visual motor cues. Attention is directed toward one cue at a time. Actions are more goal directed. Has difficulty correcting errors. Can attend a 1-hour group.	Provide visual demonstration. Limit instruction to one step at a time. Make all objects clearly visible. Provide visual comparisons so that individual knows what he or she is working toward. Situation-specific training is useful.
Level 5: exploratory actions	Concrete relations are understood, has trouble with abstraction. Uses exploratory actions, trial-and-error problem-solving. Does not anticipate problems.	Accompany visual demonstration with verbal explanation. Select or modify tasks to reduce problem-solving requirements. Use concrete explanations and examples. Assist with planning ahead.
Level 6: planned actions	Can make sense of symbolic cues and abstraction. Can plan ahead. Anticipates errors and engages in mental problem-solving. Pauses to think about potential problems.	Use verbal and written instruction, diagrams and drawings. Can carry out instructions from previous sessions.

research on the efficacy of the model as an intervention approach. A small pilot study of individuals with schizophrenia compared an intervention group that received treatment according to Allen's Cognitive Disabilities Model with a control group at a community activity center (Raweh, Holon, & Katz, 1999). The intervention group improved significantly more on the ACL, although both groups improved on the Routine Task Inventory.

Errorless Learning

Individuals with cognitive impairments such as Alzheimer's disease, schizophrenia, mental retardation, and learning disabilities often have difficulty learning new information. Learning is made more difficult by the inability to self-monitor. In other words, they may have difficulty recognizing mistakes and using feedback about these errors to change future performance. In this situation, the errors can intrude on correct response. For example, you may have had the experience of mistakenly learning the incorrect name for an individual. It then becomes more difficult to inhibit that mistake, and you have a tendency to still call that person by the wrong name. Errorless learning compensates for self-monitoring problems and prevents intrusive or perseverative errors.

When using errorless learning, the training process is structured so that mistakes are not allowed to occur or are kept to a minimum. The process has four parts (Kern et al, 2005):

1. The task is broken down into simple components.
2. The training starts with simple tasks with a high likelihood of success.
3. Increasingly difficult tasks are added, but at each level prompts cues and guided instruction are used until a high level of proficiency is attained.
4. Performance at each level is overlearned using repetitive, successful practice and positive reinforcement.

These steps are similar to many other rehabilitation strategies with the main difference being that mistakes are avoided.

Errorless learning is most easily applied to discrimination tasks such as learning names. For example, in a day treatment program for individuals with Alzheimer's, a goal may be established for group members to learn the names of the therapist and the four other people in the treatment group. In an "effortful" learning situation, the therapist might ask a group member to go around the circle and state the names of everyone in the group. However, this is likely to result in many mistakes. In an errorless learning approach, the therapist may use several strategies to help group members learn the names: going around the circle with each person saying his or her name aloud; having each person hold up a sign with his or her name on it so the group members can say the names aloud; showing photographs of the group members so the therapist can say each name aloud and ask each group member to repeat the name, etc. Once the therapist believes that an individual has learned a name, she might show a picture and say, "Don't guess if you're not sure, but if you do know, tell me the name of this person." A study using similar approaches with six individuals with early Alzheimer's disease found all six individuals were able to learn targeted everyday information, and five of the six maintained the information for 6 months (Clare et al, 2000).

Studies of errorless learning have demonstrated efficacy of this approach for individuals with developmental disabilities (Ducharme, Lucas, & Pontes, 1994; Lancioni & Smeets, 1986). For example, a single-subject design study examined the efficacy of errorless learning for three adults with developmental disabilities (Jerome, Frantino, & Sturmey, 2007). A 13-step task analysis was identified for teaching participants the requisite skills for accessing a Web site. All three participants were able to meet criterion for the 13 steps in 1 to 12 training sessions.

Furthermore, errorless learning has been successfully applied in schizophrenia to more complex activities such as work tasks (Kern, Liberman, Kopelowicz, Mintz, & Green, 2002) and social problem-solving (Kern et al, 2005). Giles (2005) describes using errorless learning in occupational therapy practice to teach washing and dressing skills. Tasks that are more difficult to teach using errorless learning strategies include those in which several behaviors or options are available, those for which the best response is highly dependent on previous responses, and those for which situational and contextual factors are variable and influence the preferred response. For example, teaching someone how to address an envelope is much easier using an errorless learning approach than teaching someone how to write a letter.

Reality Orientation and Validation Therapy

Reality orientation is a cognitive intervention that is used primarily for adults with dementia. It may be presented throughout the day as a continuous interaction technique or as a group meeting. The goal of reality orientation is to alleviate the disorientation associated with dementia. Common reality orientation techniques include the use of reality boards listing information such as the time, date, next meal, etc; name

Evidence-Based Practice

Although it is a relatively new area of research, studies of errorless learning suggest this approach can be beneficial for teaching new information to individuals with memory impairments such as Alzheimer's disease and schizophrenia, as well as developmental disabilities.

➤ When teaching new information to individuals with memory impairments, the occupational therapist should avoid intervention approaches that encourage trial-and-error learning or questioning that might lead to wrong answers.

➤ For individuals with memory impairments, the occupational therapist can construct interventions that incorporate repeated practice with accurate information and multiple methods of processing the same information so that new information is encoded correctly.

Clare, L., Wilson, B. A., Carter, G., Breen, K., Gosses, A., & Hodges, J. R. (2000). Intervening with everyday memory problems in dementia of Alzheimer type: An errorless learning approach. *Journal of Clinical and Experimental Neuropsychology, 22,* 132–146.

Jerome, J., Frantino, E. P., & Sturmey, P. (2007). The effects of errorless learning and backward chaining on the acquisition of Internet skills in adults with developmental disabilities. *Journal of Applied Behavioral Analysis, 40,* 185–189.

Kern, R. S., Green, M. F., Mitchell, S., Kopelowicz, A., Mintz, J., & Liberman, R. P. (2005). Extensions of errorless learning for social problem solving deficits in schizophrenia. *American Journal of Psychiatry, 162,* 513–519.

Kern, R. S., Liberman, R. P., Kopelowicz, A., Mintz, J., & Green, M. F. (2002). Applications of errorless learning on improving work performance in persons with schizophrenia. *American Journal of Psychiatry, 159,* 1921–1926.

tags and labels for rooms; reminiscence activities; and reminding people of names and situations. A randomized controlled trial of a program combining reality orientation and cognitive stimulation found significant improvement in cognition as measured by the Mini-Mental Status Exam and the Alzheimer's Disease Assessment Scale–Cognition (Spector et al, 2003). The study also found improvements in quality of life but not functional ability.

In contrast, validation therapy focuses on emotional and psychological components of the interactive process as opposed to factual information (Feil, 1989, 1993). Like reality orientation, validation therapy is used both as an interaction style and a group. The practice of validation therapy involves endorsing what is said rather than correcting factual errors. For example, a widow with dementia may express concern that she does not want to attend the occupational therapy group that day because she is afraid she will miss her husband when he comes to visit. Instead of correcting the client and explaining that her husband died several years ago, a validation therapy approach would look at confirming the feelings of the moment and might include a statement like "You really miss your husband, don't you?" The therapist might go on to assure the client that the therapist will make sure that the nursing staff knows where the client is going to be for the next hour should a visitor arrive.

In a group setting, some activities may resemble reality orientation (e.g., reminiscing about past events); however, a validation therapy group does not include orientation to factual information. Validation therapy groups typically follow a set format to establish familiarity within the group context. This may include initial greetings and singing a familiar song. An activity such as poetry reading or listening to music might be followed by refreshments and a closing. A controlled study compared the effectiveness of validation therapy, a social contact group, and usual care among nursing home residents with dementia (Toseland et al, 1997). The results indicated that individuals in the validation therapy group had a significant reduction in problem behaviors, but there was no difference in terms of use of psychotropic medication or physical restraints.

Classroom and Parental Interventions for Attention Deficit-Hyperactivity Disorder

Parental training and teacher consultation focus on the implementation of behavioral strategies at home and in the classroom (Pelham & Gnagy, 1999). Parental training includes information on how to attend, reward, and ignore behaviors; develop home reward systems; establish and enforce limits; assist with homework; and facilitate peer relationships. Similar strategies are used in the classroom and may include the provision of classwide interventions. Studies of these programs generally find improvements in ADHD behaviors (e.g., Anastopoulos, Shelton, & DuPaul, 1993; Klein & Abikoff, 1997) and school functioning when there is significant teacher contact (e.g., Pelham, Carlson, & Sams, 1993; Klein & Abikoff, 1997). Contingency management systems are generally a major component of classroom interventions. In one example, Rapport, Murphy, and Bailey (1980) used a flip-card system in which the child could earn up to 20 minutes of free time by staying on task. The teacher flipped a card down, and the child lost 1 minute whenever the teacher noticed the child was not working. This method was effective in increasing on-task behavior.

Occupational therapists have used environmental modifications that address sensory modulation issues to improve classroom performance for children with ADHD. Schilling, Washington, Billingsley, and Dietz (2003) compared two different classroom seating options (therapy balls and chairs) for children with ADHD. Therapy balls were fitted for each child so that the child sat comfortably with his or her feet flat on the floor and knees and hips flexed at a 90-degree angle. Using a single-subject design, time spent on the therapy ball as opposed to a chair resulted in more in-seat time and writing that was more legible. In another classroom study, students with ADHD wore weighted vests (VandenBerg, 2001). The deep pressure provided by the vest is believed to result in a calming effect. This single-subject designed study found increased on-task behavior when the vest was worn.

Summary

Cognitive impairments contribute to psychiatric disability across many different diagnoses. There is great variability in the type of impairment associated with a particular mental illness and within individuals. Careful assessment is important to determine the cognitive strengths and impairments for the individual and how cognition affects occupational performance. Unless an occupational performance problem is known, assumptions that link cognitive impairments with the inability to successfully engage in a particular occupation should be avoided. A strong assessment will aid the occupational therapist in selecting intervention approaches that best match the particular needs and wants of the individual.

Active Learning Strategies

1. Applying Practice Models to Different Diagnoses

This chapter describes several approaches for addressing cognitive impairments in people with psychiatric disabilities. Imagine that the following case study describes a client who was recently referred for occupational therapy.

Frank wants to prepare a simple lunch for himself at home; however, his family is concerned that he may not be safe in the kitchen, particularly when using the stove or oven. There are concerns that he may burn the food or himself, or that he may forget to turn off the stove or oven.

Now consider how your approach might differ depending on Frank's diagnosis. Which practice model would you select, and how would you go about designing an intervention if the diagnosis were as follows:

1. Early stage Alzheimer's disease, knowing that there will be a gradual and continual cognitive decline

2. Mild to moderate mental retardation, knowing that there is a stable intellectual impairment
3. Schizophrenia with moderate impairments in attention, memory, and executive function

What factors did you consider in selecting a practice model? Did you select a different practice model for each diagnosis, or did you think the same practice model could be used for more than one diagnosis?

Once you have selected a practice model, specifically describe two or three techniques that you would use to help Frank prepare a simple lunch at home.

How did you decide on these techniques? How are the techniques influenced by the practice model? Are there times that you would use the same technique for different reasons?

2. Designing Errorless Learning Interventions

The section on errorless learning explained that certain tasks are easier to teach using an errorless learning approach than others. Tasks that are more difficult to teach using errorless learning strategies include (1) those in which several behaviors or options are available, (2) those for which the best response is highly dependent on previous responses,

and (3) those in which situational and contextual factors vary and influence the preferred response.

If you were working with a client on money management, which of the following components would be most amenable to teaching using an errorless learning approach?
1. Identifying coins
2. Making change
3. Writing a check
4. Creating a budget

For those tasks that you identified as well suited to errorless learning, describe how you would go about designing a teaching session that would preclude mistake making by the client.

What are the steps involved in the particular task that you chose? Ask someone else to write up a list of the steps. Did the two of you come up with the same list? What does this tell you about analyzing a task? Would observing a person engaged in the activity make it easier to do a task analysis? Would the observation be different if the person had a disability?

Now that you have created the list of steps, how would you go about teaching the task using errorless learning principles? Try this out with a volunteer. What are the challenges to teaching when you do not let the person make an error?

Resources

Cognitive Retraining
- ATP II (Attention Process Training II) by Catherine A. Mateer and McKay Moore Sohlberg: www.nss-nrs.com/cgi-bin/WebObjects/NSS.woa/wa/Products/detail?id=1000113
- Brain and Memory Software Programs: www.rmlearning.com/MemorySoftware.htm
- Brain Train Cognitive Retraining Software: www.brain-train.com
- Brainwave–Revised by Kit B. Malia, Kristin C. Bewick, Michael J. Raymond, and Thomas L. Bennett: www.proedinc.com/customer/productView.aspx?ID=1294&SearchWord=brainwave
- Delahunty, A., & Morice, R. *The Frontal/Executive Program.* 2nd ed. Albury: Mental Health Unit, South-West NSW Health Districts.

Compensatory Devices
- Planning and Execution Assistant and Trainer (PEAT): www.brainaid.com
- Safe Home Products: www.safehomeproducts.com
- AbleData, a government-sponsored site that serves as a clearinghouse for assistive devices: www.abledata.com

Creating Safe Environments for People With Dementia
- Alzheimer's Association: http://www.alz.org/national/documents/brochure_homesafety.pdf

Cognitive Measures
- Allen, C. A., Austen, S. K., David, S. K., Earhart, C. A., McCraith, D. B., & Williams, L. R. (2007). *Manual for the Allen Cognitive Level Screen 5 and Large Cognitive Level Screen.* Colchester, CT: S & S Worldwide.
- Anderson, V., Manly, T., & Robertson, I. H. (1999). *Test of Everyday Attention for Children (TEA-CH).* Available at: http://www.nss-nrs.com/cgi-bin/WebObjects/NSS.woa/wa/Products/detail?id=1000087 (accessed November 29, 2009).
- Earhart, C. A. (2006). *Allen Diagnostic Module* (2nd ed.). Colchester, CT: S & S Worldwide.
- Folstein, M. F., Folstein, S. E., & McHugh, P. R. (2005). *Mini-Mental State Examination.* Lutz, FL: Psychological Assessment Resources. Available at: www.minimental.com (accessed November 29, 2009).

- Itzkovich, M., Elazar. B., Averbuch, S., & Katz, N. (2000). *LOTCA Manual* (2nd ed.). Wayne, NJ: Maddak.
- Lezak, M. D. (1995). *Neuropsychological Assessment.* New York: Oxford University Press.
- Ridgeway, V., Robertson, I. H., & Ward, T. (1996). *Test of Everyday Attention (TEA).* Available at: http://www.nss-nrs.com/cgi-bin/WebObjects/NSS.woa/wa/Products/detail?id=1000085 (accessed November 29, 2009).
- Toglia, J. P. (1993). *Contextual Memory Test.* San Antonio, TX: Psychological Corporation.
- Toglia, J. P. (1994). *Dynamic Assessment of Categorization Skills: The Toglia Category Assessment.* Pequannock, NJ: Maddak.

References

Abikoff, H. (1991). Cognitive training in ADHD children: Less to it than meets the eye. *Journal of Learning Disability, 24,* 205–209.

Alderman, N., Burgess, P. W., Knight, C., & Henman, C. (2003). Ecological validity of a simplified version of the Multiple Errands Shopping test. *Journal of the International Neuropsychological Society, 9,* 31–44.

Allen, C. K. (1996). *Allen Cognitive Level Test Manual.* Colchester, CT: S & S Worldwide.

Allen, C. A., Austen, S. K., David, S. K., Earhart, C. A., McCraith, D. B., & Williams, L. R. (2007). *Manual for the Allen Cognitive Level Screen 5 and Large Cognitive Level Screen.* Colchester, CT: S & S Worldwide.

Allen, C. K., Earhart, C. A., & Blue, T. (1992). *Occupational Therapy Treatment Goals for the Physically and Cognitively Disabled.* Bethesda, MD: American Occupational Therapy Association.

Allen, C. K., Earhart, C. A., & Blue, T. (1993). *Allen Diagnostic Module Manual.* Colchester, DT: S & S Worldwide.

Alzheimer's Disease Cooperative Study Group. (1999). "A Randomized, Double-Blind, Placebo-Controlled Trial to Evaluate the Safety and Efficacy of Vitamin E and Donepezil HCL (Aricept) to Delay Clinical Progression from Mild Cognitive Impairment (MCI) to Alzheimer's Disease (AD)." Protocol no. ADC-008.

American Psychiatric Association (APA). (2000). *Diagnostic and Statistical Manual of Mental Disorders* (4th ed., text revision). Washington, DC: Author.

Anastopoulos, A. D., Shelton, T. L., & DuPaul, G. J. (1993). Parent training for attention-deficit hyperactivity disorder: Its impact on parent functioning. *Journal of Abnormal Child Psychology, 21*, 581–596.

Anthony, J. C., LeResche, L., Niaz, U., Von Korff, M., & Folstein, M. (1982). Limits of the "Mini-Mental State" as a screening test for dementia and delirium in aging hospital patients. *Psychological Medicine, 12*, 397–408.

Averbuch, S., & Katz, N. (2005). Cognitive rehabilitation: A retraining model for clients with neurological disabilities. In N. Katz (Ed.), *Cognition and Occupation Across the Lifespan: Models for Intervention in Occupational Therapy* (pp. 113–138). Bethesda, MD: American Occupational Therapy Association.

Baddeley, A. D. (2002). Is working memory still working? *European Psychology, 7*(2), 85–97.

Balanza-Martinez, F., Tabares, Seisdedos, R., Selva-Vera, G., Martinez-Aran, A., Torrent, C., Salazar-Fraile, J., Leal-Cercos, L., Vieta, E., & Gomez Beneyto, M. (2005). Persistent cognitive dysfunctions in bipolar I disorder and schizophrenic patients: A 3-year follow-up study. *Psychotherapy and Psychosomatics, 74*, 113–119.

Baum, C., & Edwards, D. F. (1993). Cognitive performance in senile dementia of the Alzheimer's type: The Kitchen Task Assessment. *American Journal of Occupational Therapy, 47*, 431–438.

Baum, C., Morrison, T., Hahn, M., & Edwards, D. (2003). *Executive Function Performance Test: Test Protocol Booklet. Program in Occupational Therapy*. St. Louis, MO: Washington University School of Medicine.

Baum, C. M., Connor, L. T., Morrison, M. T., Hahn, M., Dromerick, A. W., & Edwards, D. F. (2008). The reliability, validity, and clinical utility of the Executive Function Performance test: A measure of executive function in a sample of people with stroke. *American Journal of Occupational Therapy, 62*(4), 446–455.

Biederman, J., Monuteaux, M. C., Doyle, A. E., Seidman, L. J., Wilens, T. E., Ferrero, F., Morgan, C. L., & Faraone, S. V. (2004). Impact of executive function defitis and attention deficit/hyperactivity disorder (ADHD) on academic outcomes in children. *Journal of Consulting and Clinical Psychology, 72*, 757–766.

Bozikas, V. P., Kosmidis, M. H., Kourtis, A., Gamvrula, K., Melissidis, P., Tsolaki, M., & Karavatos, A. (2002). Clock drawing test in institutionalized patients with schizophrenia compared with Alzheimer's disease patients. *Schizophrenia Research, 59*, 173–179.

Brenner, H. D., Hirsbrunner, A., & Heimberg, D. (1996). Integrated psychological therapy program: Training in cognitive and social skills for schizophrenia patients. In P. W. Corrigan & S. C. Yudofsky (Eds.), *Cognitive Rehabilitation for Neuropsychiatric Disorders* (pp. 329–348). Washington, DC: American Psychiatric Press.

Broadbent, D. E. (1958). *Perception and Communication*. Oxford: Pergamon Press.

Chan, R. C. K. (2000). Attentional deficits in patients with closed head injury: A further study to the discriminative validity of the Test of Everyday Attention. *Brain Injury, 14*, 227–236.

Clare, L., Wilson, B. A., Carter, G., Breen, K., Gosses, A., & Hodges, J. R. (2000). Intervening with everyday memory problems in dementia of Alzheimer type: An errorless learning approach. *Journal of Clinical and Experimental Neuropsychology, 22*, 132–146.

Craik, F., & Tulving, E. (1975). Depth of processing and the retention of words in episodic memory. *Journal of Experimental Psychology: General, 104*, 268–294.

Crum, R., Anthony, J., Bassett, S., & Folstein, M. (1993). Population based norms for the Mini-Mental Status Examination by age and educational level. *Journal of the American Medical Association, 269*, 2386–2391.

David, S. K., & Riley, W. T. (1990). The relationship of the Allen Cognitive Level test to cognitive abilities and psychopathology. *American Journal of Occupational Therapy, 44*, 493–497.

Ducharme, J. M., Lucas, H., & Pontes, E. (1994). Errorless embedding in the reduction of severe maladaptive behavior during interactive and learning tasks. *Behavior Therapy, 24*, 489–501.

Earhart, C. A. (2006). *Allen Diagnostic Module 2nd Edition: Manual*. Colchester, CT: S & S Worldwide.

Ericsson, K. A., & Lehmann, A. C. (1996). Expert and exceptional performance: Evidence of maximal adaptation to task constraints. *Annual Review of Psychology, 47*, 273–305.

Feil, N. (1989). Validation: An empathic approach to the care of dementia. *Clinical Gerontologist, 8*(3), 889–894.

Feil, N. (1993). *The Validation Breakthrough*. Baltimore: Health Professions Press.

Flavell, J. H. (1979). Metacognition and cognitive monitoring: A new area of cognitive-developmental inquiry. *American Psychologist, 34*, 906–911.

Folstein, M. F., Folstein, S. E., & McHugh, P. R. (1975). Mini-Mental State: A practical method for grading the cognitive state of patients for the clinician. *Journal of Psychiatric Research, 12*, 189–198.

Friedman, A. (1979). Framing pictures: The role of knowledge in automatized encoding and memory for gist. *Journal of Experimental Psychology: General, 108*, 316–355.

Galotti, K. M. (2004). *Cognitive Psychology: In and Out of the Laboratory* (3rd ed.). Belmont, CA: Wadsworth/Thomson Learning.

Gil, N., & Josman, N. (2001). Memory and metamemory performance in Alzheimer's disease and healthy elderly: The Contextual Memory test (CMT). *Aging Clinical Experimental Research, 13*, 309–315.

Giles, G. M. (2005). A neurofunctional approach to rehabilitation following severe brain injury. In N. Katz (Ed.), *Cognition and Occupation Across the Lifespan: Models for Intervention in Occupational Therapy* (pp. 139–165). Bethesda, MD: American Occupational Therapy Association.

Godefroy, O. (2003). Frontal syndrome and disorders of executive function. *Journal of Neurology, 250*, 1–6.

Goodglass, H., & Kaplan, E. (1983). *The Assessment of Aphasia and Related Disorders*. Philadelphia: Lea and Febiger.

Goverover, Y., Kalmar, J., Gaudino-Goering, E., Shawaryn, M., Moore, N. B., Halper, J., & DeLuca, J. (2005). The relation between subjective and objective measures of everyday life activities in persons with multiple sclerosis. *Archives of Physical Medicine and Rehabilitation, 86*, 2303–2308.

Green, M. F., Kern, R. S., Braff, D., & Mintz, J. (2000). Neurocognition and functional outcome in schizophrenia: Are we measuring the right stuff? *Schizophrenia Bulletin, 26*, 119–136.

Heimann, N., Allen, C. K., & Yerxa, E. (1989). The Routine Task Inventory: A tool for describing the functional behavior of the cognitively disables. *Occupational Therapy Practice, 1*, 67–74.

Itzkovich, M., Elazar, B., Averbuch, S., & Katz, N. (2000). *LOTCA Manual* (2nd ed.). Wayne, NJ: Maddak.

Jerome, J., Frantino, E. P., & Sturmey, P. (2007). The effects of errorless learning and backward chaining on the acquisition of Internet skills in adults with developmental disabilities. *Journal of Applied Behavioral Analysis, 40*, 185–189.

Josman, N. (1997). *Study of Differences in Metamemory in Chronic Schizophrenic Participants and Controlling the CMT*. Unpublished manuscript.

Josman, N. (2005). The dynamic interactional model in schizophrenia. In N. Katz (Ed.), *Cognition and Occupation Across the Lifespan: Models for Intervention in Occupational Therapy* (pp. 169–186). Bethesda, MD: American Occupational Therapy Association.

Josman, N., Berney, T., & Jarus, T. (2000). Evaluating categorization skills in children following severe brain injury. *Occupational Therapy Journal of Research, 20*, 241–255.

Kahneman, D., & Tversky, A. (1996). On the reality of cognitive illusions. *Psychological Review, 103*, 582–591.

Katz, N., Felzen, B., Tadmor, I., & Hartman-Maeir, A. (2007). Validity of the Executive Function Performance test (EFPT) in persons with schizophrenia: An occupational performance test. *Occupational Therapy Journal of Research, 27*, 44–51.

Katz, N., Itzkovich, M., Averbuch, S., & Elazar, B. (1989). Loewenstein Occupational Therapy Cognitive Assessment (LOTCA) battery for brain-injured patients: Reliability and validity. *American Journal of Occupational Therapy, 43,* 184–192.

Kern, R. S., Green, M. F., Mitchell, S., Kopelowicz, A., Mintz, J., & Liberman, R. P. (2005). Extensions of errorless learning for social problem solving deficits in schizophrenia. *American Journal of Psychiatry, 162,* 513–519.

Kern, R. S., Liberman, R. P., Kopelowicz, A., Mintz, J., & Green, M. F. (2002). Applications of errorless learning on improving work performance in persons with schizophrenia. *American Journal of Psychiatry, 159,* 1921–1926.

Klein, R. G., & Abikoff, H. (1997). Behavior therapy and methylphenidate in the treatment of children with ADHD. *Journal of Attention Disorders, 2,* 89–114.

Knight, C., Alderman, N., & Burgess, P. W. (2002). Development of a simplified version of the multiple errands test for use in hospital settings. *Neuropsychological Rehabilitation, 12,* 231-256.

Knopman, D. S., Boeve, B. F., & Petersen, R. D. (2003). Essentials of the proper diagnoses of mild cognitive impairment, dementia and major subtypes of dementia. *Mayo Clinic Proceedings, 78,* 1290–1308.

Kravariti, E., Dixon, T., Frith, C., Murray, R., & McGuire, P. (2005). Association of symptoms and executive function in schizophrenia and bipolar disorder. *Schizophrenia Research, 74,* 221–231.

Kurtz, M. M., Moberg, P. J., Gur, R. C., & Gur, R. E. (2001). Approaches to cognitive remediation of neuropsychological deficits in schizophrenia: A review and meta-analysis. *Neuropsychology Review, 11,* 197–210.

Lancioni, G. E., & Smeets, P. M. (1986). Procedures and parameters of errorless discrimination training with developmentally impaired individuals. *International Review of Research in Mental Retardation, 14,* 135–164.

Levine, B., Robertson, I. H., Clare, L., Carter, G., Hong, J., & Wilson, B. (2000). Rehabilitation of executive functioning: An experimental-clinical validation of goal management training. *Journal of International Neuropsychological Society, 6,* 299–312.

Lezak, M. D., Howieson, D. B., & Loring, D. (2004). *Neuropsychological Assessment.* New York: Oxford University Press.

Majer, M., Ising, M., Kunzel, H., Binder, E. B., Holsboer, F., Modell, S., & Zihl, J. (2004). Impaired divided attention predicts delayed response and risk to relapse in subjects with depressive disorders. *Psychological Medicine, 34,* 1453–1463.

Manly, T., Anderson, V., Nimmo-Smith, I., Turner, A., Watson, P., & Robertson, A. H. (2001). The differential assessment of children's attention: The Test of Everyday Attention for Children (TEA-Ch), normative sample and ADHD performance. *Journal of Child Psychology and Psychiatry, 42,* 1065–1081.

Manley, T., Robertson, I. H., Anderson, V., & Nimmo-Smith, I. (1999). *Test of Everyday Attention for Children (TEA-Ch).* London: Thames Valley Test Company.

Matlin, M. W. (2005). *Cognition* (6th ed). Hoboken, NJ: John Wiley Sons, Inc.

McGhie, A., & Chapman, J. (1961). Disorders of attention and perception in early schizophrenia. *British Journal of Medical Psychology, 34,* 103–116.

Medalia, A., Aluma, M., Tryon, W., & Merriam, A. E. (1998). Effectiveness of attention training in schizophrenia. *Schizophrenia Bulletin, 24,* 147–152.

Medalia, A., Revheim, N., & Casey, M. (2000). Remediation of memory disorders in schizophrenia. *Psychological Medicine, 30,* 1451–1459.

McGurk, S. R., Twamley, E. W., Sitzer, D. I., McHugo, G. J., & Mueser, K. T. (2007). A meta-analysis of cognitive remediation in schizophrenia. *American Journal of Psychiatry, 164,* 1791–1802.

Meichenbaum, D. (1979). *Cognitive Behavior Modification: An Integrative Approach.* New York: Plenum Press.

Meichenbaum, D., & Cameron, R. (1973). Training schizophrenics to talk to themselves: A means of developing attentional controls. *Behavior Therapy, 4,* 515–534.

Miller, G. A. (1956). The magical number seven, plus or minus two: Some limits on our capacity for processing information. *Psychological Review, 63,* 81–97.

Miller, L. T., Polatajko, H. J., Missiuna, C., Mandich, A. D., & Macnab, J. J. (2001). A pilot trial of a cognitive treatment for children with developmental coordination disorder. *Human Movement Science, 20,* 183–210.

Nelson, H. E., Thrasher, S., & Barnes, T. R. (1991). Practical ways of alleviating auditory hallucinations. *British Medical Journal, 9,* 327.

Nishiwaki, Y., Breeze, E., Smeeth, L., Bulpitt, C. J., Peters, R., & Fletcher, A. E. (2004). Validity of the clock-drawing test as a screening tool for cognitive impairment in the elderly. *American Journal of Epidemiology, 160,* 797–807.

Palmer, B. W., & Heaton, R. K. (2000). Executive dysfunction in schizophrenia. In T. Sharma & P. Harvey (Eds.), *Cognition in Schizophrenia* (pp. 51–72). Oxford, UK: Oxford University Press.

Pelham, W. E., Carlson, C., & Sams, S. E. (1993). Separate and combined effects of methylphenidate and behavior modification on boys with ADHD in the classroom. *Journal of Consulting and Clinical Psychology, 61,* 506–515.

Pelham, W. E., & Gnagy, E. M. (1999). Psychosocial and combined treatments for ADHD. *Mental Retardation and Development Disabilities Research Reviews, 5,* 225–236.

Penny, N. H., Mueser, K. T., & North, C. T. (1995). The Allen Cognitive Level test and social competence in adult psychiatric patients. *American Journal of Occupational Therapy, 49,* 420–427.

Peterson, L. R., & Peterson, M. J. (1959). Short-term retention of individual items. *Journal of Experimental Psychology, 58,* 193–198.

Pilling, S., Bebbington, P., Kuipers, E., Garety, P., Geddes, P., Martindale, B., Orbach, G., & Morgan, C. (2002). Psychological treatment in schizophrenia II: Meta-analyses of randomized controlled trials of social skills training and cognitive remediation. *Psychological Medicine, 32,* 783–791.

Plassman, B. L., Langa, K. M., Fisher, G. G., Heeringa, S. G., Weir, D. R., Ofstedal, M. D., Burke, J. R., Hurd, M. D., Potter, G. G., Rodgers, W. L., Steffens, D. C., McArdle, J. J., Willis, R. J., & Wallace, R. B. (2008). Prevalence of cognitive impairment without dementia in the United States. *Annals of Internal Medicine, 148,* 427–434.

Polatajko, H. J., & Mandich, A. (2004). *Enabling Occupation in Children: The Cognitive Orientation to Daily Occupational Performance (CO-OP) Approach.* Ottawa, Ontario: Canadian Association of Occupational Therapists.

Posner, M. I., & Snyder, C. R. R. (1975). Attention and cognitive control. In R. Solso (Ed.), *Information Processing and Cognition: The Loyola Symposium* (pp. 55–85). Hillsdale, NJ: Erlbaum.

Rapport, M. D., Murphy, A., & Bailey, J. S. (1980). The effects of a response cost treatment tactic on hyperactive children. *Journal of School Psychology, 18,* 98–111.

Raweh, D. V., Holon, R., & Katz, N. (1999). Treatment effectiveness of Allen's Cognitive Disabilities Model with adult schizophrenia outpatients: A pilot study. *Occupational Therapy in Mental Health, 14,* 65–77.

Robertson, I. H., Ward, T., Ridgeway, V., & Nimmo-Smith, I. (1994). *The Test of Everyday Attention.* Bury St. Edmund's, UK: Thames Valley Test Company.

Rogers, T., Kuiper, N., & Kirker, W. (1977). Self-reference and the encoding of personal information. *Journal of Personality and Social Psychology, 35,* 677–688.

Ross, M., & Sicoly, F. (1979). Egocentric biases in availability and attribution. *Journal of Personality and Social Psychology, 37,* 322–336.

Sangster, C. A., Beninger, C., Polatajko, H. J., & Mandich, A. (2005). Cognitive strategy generation in children with developmental coordination disorder. *Canadian Journal of Occupational Therapy, 72*, 67–77.

Schank, R. C., & Abelson, R. P. (1977). *Scripts, Plans, Goals and Understanding*. Hillsdale, NJ: Erlbaum.

Schilling, D. L., Washington, K., Billingsley, F. F., & Dietz, J. (2003). Classroom seating for children with attention deficit hyperactivity disorder: Therapy balls versus chairs. *American Journal of Occupational Therapy, 57*, 534–541.

Schuck, S. E. B., & Crinella, F. M. (2005). Shy children with ADHD do not have low IQs. *Journal of Learning Disabilities, 38*, 262–280.

Secrest, L., Wood, E. W., & Tapp, A. (2000). A comparison of the Allen Cognitive Level test and the Wisconsin Card Sorting test in adults with schizophrenia. *American Journal of Occupational Therapy, 54*, 129–133.

See, J. E., Howe, S. R., Warm, J. S., & Dember, W. N. (1995). Meta-analysis of the sensitivity decrement in vigilance. *Psychological Bulletin, 117*, 230–249.

Shallice, T., & Burgess, P. W. (1991). Deficits in strategy application following frontal lobe damage in man. *Brain, 114*, 727–741.

Shulman, K. I. (2000). Clock-drawing: Is it the ideal cognitive screening test? *International Journal of Geriatric Psychiatry, 14*, 548–561.

Silverstein, S. M., & Wilkniss, S. M. (2004). At issue: The future of cognitive rehabilitation of schizophrenia. *Schizophrenia Bulletin, 30*, 679–692.

Small, B. J., Fratiglioni, L., Viitanen, M., Winblad, B., & Backman, L. (2000). The course of cognitive impairment in preclinical Alzheimer disease: Three and 6 year follow-up of a population-based sample. *Archives of Neurology, 57*, 839–844.

So, Y. P., Toglia, J., & Donohue, M. V. (1997). A study of memory functioning in chronic schizophrenia patients. *Occupational Therapy in Mental Health, 13*, 1–23.

Spaulding, W. D., Reed, D., Sullivan, M., Richardson, C., & Weiler, M. (1999). Effects of cognitive treatment in psychiatric rehabilitation. *Schizophrenia Bulletin, 25*, 657–676.

Spector, A., Thorgrimsen, L., Woods, B., Royan, L., Davies, S., Butterworth, M., & Orrell, M. (2003). Efficacy of an evidence-based cognitive stimulation therapy programme for people with dementia. *British Journal of Psychiatry, 138*, 248–254.

Spelke, E., Hirst, W., & Neisser, U. (1976). Skills of divided attention. *Cognition, 4*, 215–230.

Sternberg, R. J. (2003). *Cognitive Psychology* (3rd ed.). Wadsworth.

Sunderland, T., Hill, J. L., Mellow, A. M., Lawlor, V. A., Gundersheimer, J., Newhouse, P. A., & Grafman, J. H. (1989). Clock drawing in Alzheimer's disease. A novel measure of dementia severity. *Journal of the American Geriatric Society, 37*, 724–729.

Toglia, J. P. (1993). *Contextual Memory Test*. San Antonio, TX: Psychological Corporation.

Toglia, J. P. (2005). A dynamic interactional approach to cognitive rehabilitation. In N. Katz (Ed.), *Cognition and Occupation Across the Lifespan: Models for Intervention in Occupational Therapy* (pp. 29–72). Bethesda, MD: American Occupational Therapy Association.

Toglia, J. P., & Josman, N. (1994). Preliminary reliability and validity study on the TCA. In J. P. Toglia (Ed.), *Dynamic Assessment of Categorization: TCA—The Toglia Category Assessment.*(pp. 8–10). Pequannock, NJ: Maddak.

Toplak, M. E., Connors, L., Shuster, J., Knezevic, B., & Parks, S. (2008). Review of cognitive, cognitive-behavioral and neural based interventions for attention deficit/hyperactivity disorder (ADHD). *Clinical Psychology Review, 28*, 801–823.

Toseland, R. W., Diehl, M., Freeman, K., Manzanares, T., Naleppa, M., & McCallion, P. (1997). The impact of validation group therapy on nursing home residents with dementia. *Journal of Applied Gerontology, 16*, 31–51.

Treisman, A. M. (1960). Contextual cues in selective listening. *Quarterly Journal of Experimental Psychology, 12*, 242–248.

Tuokko, H., Jadjistavropoulos, T., Miller, J. A., & Beattie, B. L. (1992). The clock test: A sensitive measure to differentiate normal elderly from those with Alzheimer disease. *Journal of the American Gerontological Society, 40*, 579–584.

Twamley, E. W., Jeste, D. V., & Bellack, A. S. (2003). A review of cognitive training in schizophrenia. *Schizophrenia Bulletin, 29*, 359–382.

VandenBerg, N. L. (2001). The use of a weighted vest to increase on-task behavior in children with attention difficulties. *American Journal of Occupational Therapy, 55*, 621–628.

Velligan, D. I., Bow-Thomas, C. C., Huntzinger, C., Ritch, J., Ledbetter, N., Prihoda, T. J., & Miller, A. L. (2000). Randomized controlled trial of the use of compensatory strategies to enhance adaptive functioning in outpatients with schizophrenia. *American Journal of Psychiatry, 157*, 1317–1323.

Velligan, D. I., Mahurin, R. K., True, J. E., Lefton, R. S., & Flores, C. V. (1996). Preliminary evaluation of cognitive adaptation training to compensate for cognitive deficits in schizophrenia. *Psychiatric Services, 47*, 415–417.

Warchol, K. (2004). An interdisciplinary dementia program model for long-term care. *Topics in Geriatric Rehabilitation, 20*, 59–71.

Weickert, T. W., & Goldberg, T. E. (2000). The course of cognitive impairment in patients with schizophrenia. In T. Sharma & P. Harvey (Eds.), *Cognition in Schizophrenia: Impairments, Importance and Treatment Strategies* (pp. 3–15). New York: Oxford University Press.

Wilson, D., Allen, C. K., McCormack, G., & Burton, G. (1989). Cognitive disability and routine task behaviors in a community-based population with senile dementia. *Occupational Therapy Practice, 1*, 58–66.

Wykes, T., Reeder, C., Corner, J., Williams, C., Everitt, B. (1999). The effects of neurocognitive remediation on executive processing in patients with schizophrenia. *Schizophrenia Bulletin, 25*, 291–307.

Wykes, T., & van der Gaag, M. (2001). Is it time to develop a new cognitive therapy for psychosis—Cognitive remediation therapy? *Clinical Psychology Review, 21*, 1227–1256.

Wynn, V. E., & Logie, R. H. (1998). The veracity of long-term memories—Did Bartlett get it right? *Applied Cognitive Psychology, 12*, 1–20.

Zwecker, M., Levenkrohn, S., Fleisig, Y., Zeilig, G., Ohry, A., & Adunsky, A. (2002). Mini-Mental State Examination, cognitive FIM instrument, and the Loewenstein Occupational Therapy Cognitive Assessment: Relation to functional outcome of stroke patients. *Archives of Physical Medicine and Rehabilitation, 83*, 342–345.

Cognitive Beliefs

Deane B. McCraith

> "Human beings can alter their lives by altering their attitudes of mind. . . . Be not afraid of life. Believe that life is worth living and your belief will help create the fact.
> —William James, pioneering American psychologist and philosopher, 1842–1910

Introduction

Is your glass half empty or half full? You may be asked this familiar question to determine if you are an optimist (glass half full) or a pessimist (glass half empty). Or, it may be asked as a rhetorical question, suggesting that there is more than one way to perceive, think about, and behave in a situation, depending on individuals' beliefs about themselves, others, and the world. Rosenfeld (1997), in his convincing argument on the importance of addressing psychosocial factors as part of physical rehabilitation, effectively illustrates the use of this expression in describing an occupational therapist's intervention with an older woman who was receiving treatment following hip replacement surgery.

> She made slow but steady progress in her rehabilitation. Despite improvements, however, she always focused on how much she still could not do. Her discouragement diminished her energy and effort. I pointed out her "glass half empty" way of seeing things. The woman readily admitted this but felt she could not change. With a contract to try, and persistent monitoring and substitution of more positive cognitions and statements, the patient was able to describe and to feel "the glass half full." "I just need a little assistance with the last 6 inches down to sitting, now," she said. "Six weeks ago, I needed two people to carry me from the wheelchair to the toilet!" (Rosenfeld, 1997, p. 35)

Rosenfeld noted that the patient's affect, efforts, and performance abilities improved dramatically as a result of the occupational therapist's willingness to listen to her judgmental thoughts about her performance and progress. The occupational therapist brought the impact of the woman's negative thinking to her attention, educated her about ways to substitute more positive thoughts and statements for her negative thoughts, and supported her in monitoring her thoughts in relation to her progress. This collaborative approach acknowledged the impact of the patient's beliefs and thoughts on her feelings and behavior and used cognitive behavior strategies to help her modify her thinking and attitudes. In addition, it addressed the woman's dysfunctional beliefs in the context of her rehabilitation and occupational performance goals. This chapter focuses on applying this cognitive behavioral approach in addressing clients' beliefs, psychosocial function, and occupational performance as part of the overall occupational therapy assessment and intervention process.

As occupational therapists, it is essential to listen to and address our clients' beliefs and thoughts about themselves, other people, and the world around them, including how beliefs both influence and are influenced by their occupational performance and quality of life. The importance of the relationship among behavior, feelings, and beliefs for occupational therapists is reflected in an early philosophical statement by Adolf Meyer (1977), a psychiatrist and founder of occupational therapy, who proposed that *"wholesome living"* was based on a program of *"wholesome doing, thinking, and feeling."* (p. 641) In contemporary occupational therapy literature and practice, there is strong support acknowledging the compatibility between the theory and practice of occupational therapy and most cognitive behavioral theories and therapies that focus on belief-oriented assessment and intervention (Bruce & Borg, 2002; Duncombe, 2005; Johnson, 1987).

Definition and Nature of Beliefs

Beliefs are among the most primitive and central of mental constructs, yet there is little agreement as to what they are or how they should be construed. In this chapter, the World Health Organization's (WHO's) International Classification of Functioning, Disability and Health (ICF; WHO, 2001) is used to define beliefs that are classified as *mental functions* within the *body functions* category. Beliefs and thoughts reside within the person, and both influence and arise from what a person perceives and the meaning that is attached to those perceptions. They are part of the cognitive content that is stored in memory, which can unconsciously or consciously affect the person. The *Occupational Therapy Practice Framework: Domain and Practice, 2nd edition (OTPF II)* extends the WHO-ICF definition to acknowledge that beliefs "may affect performance in areas of occupation" (American Occupational Therapy Association [AOTA], 2008, p. 630).

A number of psychological and educational theories recognize beliefs as basic to learning, health, and overall psychological well-being. Most of these formulations are grounded in the cognitive tradition. Although they can be distinguished from each other, there is general agreement regarding some basic assumptions about the nature of beliefs and their significance for human functioning.

Dynamic Nature of Beliefs

Beliefs and their dynamic interaction with emotions, physiologic reactions, behavior, and the environment comprise human functioning. Internal personal factors (e.g., beliefs, emotions, physiological reactions), behavior (e.g., actions, reactions), and external environmental factors (e.g., cultural, social, spiritual, physical contexts) all operate as interacting determinants that influence, and are influenced by, one another (e.g., Bandura, 1977, 1986; A. Beck, 1976; J. Beck, 1995; Dryden & Ellis, 2001; Meichenbaum, 1992).

Layers of Beliefs

Beliefs, operating at a deep structure level, influence the more surface structure of our thoughts, as well as our emotions and behavior. Beliefs are frequently conceptualized in terms of continuous, overlapping layers that might be visualized as "layers of an onion." Typically, conscious, "mindful," and more automatic "mindless" thoughts comprise the outermost or surface layers. These thoughts, consisting of actual words, images, or "self-talk" that go through our minds, are considered to be more accessible, flexible, and specific to a situation or person. The innermost layer is the storehouse for our most fundamental or core beliefs and philosophies, sometimes called **schema** (A. Beck, 1976; Meichenbaum, 1992), which serve as a cognitive "template" of absolutes about how we see ourselves, others, and the world. Although accessible if focused on in an effortful manner, these deeply rooted beliefs usually operate outside our conscious awareness. They are characterized as being more rigid, entrenched, and global. Various constructs, such as attitudes, values, and "rules for living," are sometimes used to label the intermediate layers. "Rules for living" tend to fit an "if . . . then" format (e.g., "If I do not do what others want me to do, they won't like me," "If I don't get all As, then I am a failure"). The beliefs that operate at the deepest structural level generate our surface thoughts. In turn, these surface thoughts often serve as a window to our underlying assumptions and rules for living, and to our deeper, more core beliefs. These layers of beliefs are outlined in Table 19-1.

In this chapter, the terms *beliefs* and *thoughts* are used interchangeably unless specifically distinguishing between core beliefs and automatic thoughts as described here.

Beliefs and Information Processing

Beliefs are instrumental in how we perceive and attach meaning to information from within ourselves and from the external environment. In this capacity, beliefs act as "filters" for the processing of information and events that we experience. They are basic to what we chose to perceive (see, hear, feel, smell), and how we appraise, interpret, and give meaning to the myriad of situations and experiences we encounter. From this cognitive perspective, it is not other people or external situations or events per se that determine how we feel and act; rather, how we feel and act is determined by how we chose to perceive and construe situations and events (A. Beck, 1976; Ellis, 1962; Meichenbaum, 1992). This perspective is supported by research that suggests that distortions in processing information about oneself and the environment are integral to many behavioral and psychological problems (see, for example, Goldfried & Davison, 1994).

Beliefs as Self-Fulfilling Prophecies

Beliefs, which are true or seem to be true for the believer, often act as self-fulfilling prophecies.

Beliefs represent one alternative among many, rather than the one true fact or rule agreed on by all. Although beliefs are not facts, for the believer, one's beliefs often carry the weight of "facts."

Regardless of what we believe, it is human nature to try to create consistency between our life and our beliefs. Once we believe something to be true, we tend to ignore counterexamples and options, choosing to perceive and accept only those events that verify our beliefs. Over time, as we generate more evidence from what we perceive and process, our beliefs become increasingly entrenched and more real thus leading to their own fulfillment. This process is referred to as a self-fulfilling prophecy (Madon, Guyll, Spoth, Cross, & Hilber, 2003).

For example, a person oversleeps and predicts, "Now, I'm probably going to have a lousy day." As a result, he feels irritable. When he gets to work, he is unusually argumentative and demanding with his coworkers, who in turn become annoyed with him, thus making his prediction of a lousy day

---

Table 19-1 ● **Layers of Beliefs**

		Example Situation: Student A and Student B Do Poorly on a Test	
Layer	**Description**	**Student A**	**Student B**
Automatic thoughts	Surface, peripheral; spontaneous, flexible, accessible, situational; arise from core beliefs	*"I'm a failure"*	*"I really blew off that test. I'd better study harder next time. I know I can do better."*
"Rules for living"	Intermediate assumptions, values, conditional "if. . .then. . ." rules; easier to test; arise from core beliefs	*"If people do well in school and get a good education, then they will be successful in a career."*	*"If people do well in school and get a good education, then they will be successful in a career."*
Core beliefs or schemas	Template of absolutes about self, others, world; rigid, global, entrenched	*"I am incompetent."*	*"I am competent."*

come true. His actions have fulfilled his prediction. In contrast, a person who espouses a positive prediction (e.g., "I'm going to have a great day") might act in ways that will actually make this prediction true.

The power of our beliefs to shape reality has long been emphasized in psychological theory and research (e.g., Harris & Rosenthal, 1985; Snyder & Stukas, 1999). The self-fulfilling role that beliefs play in human functioning also explains the quote by William James at the beginning of this chapter, "Believe that life is worth living and your belief will help create the fact." Even if we recognize that some of our beliefs have a fragile contact with any known larger reality, we are rarely motivated to challenge their truth or to change them unless they are clearly contributing to significant distress in our daily lives (Bandura, 1986).

Development of Beliefs

Beliefs develop beginning in early childhood and continue to develop throughout adulthood. From birth, infants absorb life experiences from interactions in the world and with other people, particularly primary caregivers. Because very young children have limited ways to choose or evaluate the accuracy and functionality of these early life experiences, they typically accept much of what they are told or experience about themselves (e.g., "You are stupid and incompetent," "You can achieve whatever you chose"). These experiences lead to certain "understandings" that become organized as fundamental beliefs about the self. For example, core beliefs determine whether we believe ourselves to be worthy of respect or worthless, competent or incompetent, fairly treated or victimized, or independent or helpless. In time, we also absorb and form beliefs about our relationships to others, the world, and the future. These early messages and fundamental beliefs contribute significantly to the development of our personality and to our adult views of self, other people, the world, and the future. In addition, our beliefs continue to form and change throughout our adult years as we are influenced by many internal and external factors, such as family and other role models, cultural and ethnic values, spiritual orientation, and the many other contexts and environments in which we function. However, unlike young children, as adults, we have the ability to choose, evaluate, modify, and replace our beliefs when they no longer meet our needs and interests (J. Beck, 1995).

Beliefs, Social Contexts, and Relationships

Beliefs affect our relationships, group affiliations, and society at large; and, in turn, these social contexts affect our beliefs. We function in many social contexts and relationships, such as interactions with family, friends, colleagues, and acquaintances in home, work, school, and leisure activities. At a broader level, we also function as members of our primary cultural group, our communities, and society at large. We affiliate with various groups based on our beliefs and the collective beliefs conveyed by the group. These affiliations and social transactions between ourselves and others serve to impart cultural, spiritual, relational, political, and many other beliefs, values, and attitudes that shape our views of ourselves, others, and society at large, as well as how we feel and behave, both individually and collectively. In like manner, our beliefs influence the persons and groups with whom we affiliate. Thus, our beliefs are both uniquely idiosyncratic and, at the same time, inseparably interrelated with the beliefs of those around us, of our culture, and of society (Bandura, 1986, 1997).

Occupational Therapy Perspective

From an occupational therapy perspective, our beliefs touch virtually every aspect of our daily lives as occupational beings—how we live and learn, work and play, care for ourselves, and participate with others as social beings. In addition, our view of the future, including our expectations, choices, goals, and motivation to engage in occupations, are linked to our beliefs about our capacities and our ability to do things that are important to us (e.g., see Baum & Christensen, 2005, p. 247; Keilhofner, 2002, pp. 48–50). When considering occupational performance from the perspective of the person-environment-occupation paradigm, beliefs that reside within the "person" affect the "person," as well as his or her interaction with the "environment" and with "occupations." Reciprocally, the "environment" and "occupations" also affect the "person" and, thus, the person's beliefs (Law et al, 1996).

To illustrate how these core assumptions about beliefs present themselves in daily life, imagine that you and several of your classmates are reading this book as part of a required occupational therapy course. In this context, each of you has a different emotional, physiological, and behavioral response

---

PhotoVoice

A basket of affirmation. I have learned that affirmation can be a wonderful tool in building and maintaining self-confidence and esteem. I collect quotations, and not some of my own thoughts, and keep them in this basket. Often, an "I can" affirmation will provide encouragement, but sometimes a reference to performance can carry the sting of recrimination. At those times, I find comfort in affirmations that speak of the value of being, especially those that remind me of God's love for me. The leaf in the basket is a reminder to look for the affirmations of life that abound in nature. One of the best things about finding a meaningful affirmation is the opportunity it brings to share it with a friend.

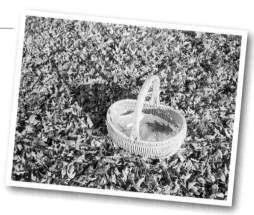

—Willeta

to this assigned activity (environmental event), based on the thoughts going through your mind as you begin to read. For example,

- Reader A thinks, "This book really makes sense. Finally, I have a guide for what I need to know and do to practice in mental health as an occupation-based occupational therapist!" Reader A feels excited and chooses to read beyond the assigned readings, making notes on key points.
- Reader B thinks, "There's so much detail to learn. If I don't learn it all, I'll never be a good therapist." Reader B, feeling anxious and overwhelmed, procrastinates and does not begin the assignment until he has time to take meticulous notes. He does not finish it before class, which further contributes to his emotional distress.

These student readers have different emotional and behavioral responses associated with their perceptions and thoughts about the reading assignment. The potential consequences of these responses are also likely to differ depending on the nature of each person's thoughts and perceptions. Furthermore, it is likely that each person's response is mediated by one or more rules for living, as well as by underlying core beliefs that probably developed early in their lives. For example, Reader B may hold fast to a core belief that he is incompetent, a belief that gives rise to the rule that "If I don't do everything perfectly, then I am incompetent." This belief may have been triggered by a physiological response, such as sweaty palms or rapid breathing. It is unlikely that he is consciously aware of this relationship between his physiological response and this core belief, or of its self-fulfilling nature. By putting off the assignment until he can do it "perfectly," he sets himself up to not meet his standards, reinforcing his core belief that he is incompetent. Furthermore, if this dysfunctional pattern repeats itself for other reading assignments and courses, not only does his belief become more entrenched, but also the consequences may be even greater. In contrast, Reader A's thoughts appear to support an optimal emotional and behavioral response for reaching her professional goals. She may have a core belief that she is competent, which gives rise to a rule for living such as, "If I complete assignments as best I can, then I will succeed." Although both Reader A and Reader B desire to do well, Reader A's beliefs and thoughts are more likely to lead her to continue to feel, act, and think in ways that fulfill her core belief, as well as meet her professional goals.

Adding an additional perspective, each student is likely to be influenced by past academic experiences, peer group affiliation, and other personal or environmental factors, such as cultural background, study environment, and previous academic success. If someone were to question the "truth" of their automatic thoughts or core beliefs, it is probable that most of them would strongly defend their position, particularly if it was supported by the beliefs of their peer group.

Impact of Beliefs on Mental Health and Illness

Our beliefs and thoughts affect all aspects of our functioning, whether we experience ourselves and our world from the perspective of a "glass half full or half empty," as optimists or pessimists, or somewhere in between. For individuals with medical or psychiatric illnesses, their beliefs have a profound influence on their healing, rehabilitation, and recovery, as well as on their occupational health and quality of life (Anthony, 1993). Research has demonstrated that believing rehabilitation and recovery are possible and that one can have quality of life, even with a disability, is critical for a successful therapy outcome (Landeen, Seeman, Goering, & Streiner, 2007; Sullivan, 1994). In addition, if individuals' beliefs and expectations do not support getting better when they are diagnosed with a physical or mental health problem, they are not likely to do all of the things that might help them get better, especially those things that may be difficult to do (Bandura, 1986). Stigmatizing beliefs about mental illness and recovery are particularly powerful (e.g., Landeen et al, 2007; Sullivan, 1994). Because they are so prevalent and have such a significant impact, a full chapter is devoted to this topic (see Chapter 28).

In her writings about being diagnosed with schizophrenia, Pat Deegan (1994) vividly illustrates the impact of mental illness and stigmatizing beliefs on her self-efficacy and recovery process. She describes the shattering of her hopes and dreams when she was told, at age 17, that she had an "incurable illness," schizophrenia, and that the best she could expect was to take her medications, keep her stress levels low, and perhaps work in a sheltered workshop. She characterized her deep feelings of despair as "a wound with no mouth, a wound so deep that no cry can emanate from it." For many years, she reports sitting and smoking cigarettes and refusing to participate, "to do anything." She attributed her despair and apparent "giving up" to the hopelessness of her prognosis, the demoralizing attitude of her doctor, and her resulting belief that "giving up seemed like [the only] solution when one lives without hope" (Deegan, 1994, p. 153).

The hypothesis put forth by cognitive models of psychopathology is that beliefs and distorted information processing constitute a vulnerability to a variety of psychiatric disorders. Following are descriptions of the specific cognitive belief profiles associated with four psychiatric disabilities: depression, anxiety disorders, eating disorders, and conduct disorders.

Depression

Depressive beliefs have been described as a cognitive triad that constitutes negative views about the self, the world, and the future (A. Beck, 1976). For example, individuals with depression are more likely to see themselves as incompetent, unlovable, and helpless; the world or environment as threatening and unsupportive; and the future as hopeless. This negatively biased predisposition causes the individual to interpret daily experiences from a world view of pessimism and self-deprecation. Negative thoughts such as "I'm such a loser," "Nobody loves me," and "I'll never amount to anything" result in unpleasant feelings and maladaptive behaviors.

Anxiety Disorders

Cognitive theories are also frequently used to understand anxiety disorders. The Intolerance of Uncertainty Model provides an explanation for chronic worry, which is a core symptom of generalized anxiety disorder (Dugas & Robichaud,

The Lived Experience

Martha's Story

Interviewer: Martha is going to share about her head injury and depression, and how OT contributed to her recovery. Martha, can you talk about your life before your head injury?

Martha: I'm a veterinarian. I was in the Air Force and did veterinary things and a lot of public health. I was very successful, very productive. I was the expert in my field. And I was married and had three great children. Well, I still have them.

Interviewer: And then you had a head injury.

Martha: I was goofing around and fell and hit my head. I needed stitches. They thought I had a mild concussion maybe. But that was all. They thought I was fine.

Interviewer: As we know, you weren't really fine. How did you come to realize this?

Martha: I'd go to work every day and just sit at my desk and shuffle papers. Things got gradually worse. I couldn't do what I used to be able to do. I ended up being hospitalized for depression and being suicidal. They figured out that I had a brain injury. Since then, a lot for me is figuring out what I can do and not feel awful, like I'm an idiot and worthless.

Interviewer: That sounds like a very difficult time for you. I know you worked with many professionals. What about occupational therapy? How did it contribute to your recovery?

Martha: When I was first in the hospital, I had an occupational therapist. She ran ADL groups and we did lots of arts and crafts. I didn't really associate it with how it was helping me until much later. But the things it did do was I could pick out something small and I could work on it and finish it and say well, you know, it might be a pot, a trivet, a quilt, but I did it. It got to be kind of fun. Let me see if I can do that or try this. Now I know that was the beginning of doing something and thinking maybe I could do something.

Interviewer: Doing arts and crafts in OT helped you begin to see that you could do some things. It got you engaged again in doing something enjoyable. It gave you hope.

Martha: Yes, but, I still hated it because I wanted to be home, and I wanted to be working, and I wanted to be taking care of my kids. I'd get to the point where OK, I have to just do it—work, take care of my kids. So I might try something like volunteering as a veterinarian, but I'd fall flat on my face and it would put me back. And then I'd think, "I'm stupid. I'll never be worth anything again. I should die." I didn't want to have to try to do things differently.

Interviewer: So you'd believe there was hope, but when you tried something and it didn't work, you would believe you were worthless again, sort of "all-or-nothing" thinking and beliefs about yourself. What helped you begin to try to do things differently?

Martha: Actually, I worked with an OT. I had to try to learn to catch my thinking and feeling before I got to trying to kill myself. Like, "If I can't do this right or how I used to, then I am worthless and I should die." I had to learn to

think, "Well, maybe I can't do this today but if I do just a small thing, that would be progress." I have trouble getting going to do things like taking showers, or using my date book, and grocery shopping so there was food in the house or paying bills. And my memory and planning things isn't good. I used this clock thing about "TICs" and "TOCs." Like, if I thought, "If I have to plan and write everything down, only an idiot would have to do that," that's, uh, a "TIC." So I had to think, "What is wrong about that thought?" Well, it's like all-or-nothing; if I can't be like I was before, I'm worthless. Like there's nothing in between. I had to see that thinking that way isn't helping me, but maybe the book does help. Even if I have to use it, that's better than being late and forgetting. That is the "TOC" part, thinking more realistically so my thoughts don't stop me from doing what might help. And then I'd try to use the book, and I wouldn't be late or forget, and I didn't have to think I was so stupid. And then I'd feel better, too.

Interviewer: It was a behavioral experiment that worked; you learned a new skill and also changed your thinking so that you felt better about yourself. Has OT helped in other ways?

Martha: Well, I carry a card that reminds me of what makes me worthy to live, the big things and the little things. I try to turn negatives into something that's at least a little positive. And, it's not just thinking positive. It's really, really thinking it and trying things out even if you don't believe it. That's what's hard. I really have to work on that. Like, remembering my kids are one of the big things. They're great.

Interviewer: That's a big worthy part—you're a good mom.

Martha: I guess so. That's what they say. But I still have to remind myself. But they remind me, too. So does my sister. She's great, too. And I work now. I'm a radiology technician. That helps. It reminds me I'm being productive. I'm good at it. Actually, I enjoy it. If I start to think, "But I have all this education, I should be working as a veterinarian, I'm a failure," I have to catch my negative thinking. It's hard. I don't think I get up any day and not think about harming myself or suicide. It never goes away. Maybe it never will. But I know more what to do before things get so bad again.

Interviewer: So, you are back working at something that helps you believe you are worthy and productive, even though you still have to stay on top of negative thoughts and beliefs that creep back in. In closing, is there anything else about OT you'd like to share?

Martha: People need more OT. Crafts help. But they need help with ADLs like organizing and paying bills and grocery shopping, and with thoughts that get in the way. If you can't do those things, then you feel worse and think you can't do anything right. You actually have to do things to see you're not totally worthless or you'll still believe you are.

2007). Specifically, this theory posits that, when information is ambiguous, the worrier views the uncertainty as unacceptable (thoughts), which leads to anxiety and stress (feelings) and an inability to act (behavior). For example, a mother who is a chronic worrier is unable to stop thinking about the possibility that her son will get injured during a football game, until the game is over and her child is unhurt.

Obsessive compulsive disorder (OCD) is another anxiety disorder; it is characterized by intrusive thoughts and the engagement in rituals or compulsions to manage those thoughts. Cognitive theorists suggest that the distorted core beliefs in OCD include an inflated responsibility for negative events and a need for control and perfectionism (Abramowitz, Khandker, Nelson, Deacon, & Rygwall, 2006). This could help explain why a concern for contamination from germs leads to an overzealous need for cleanliness and rituals related to hand washing. In posttraumatic stress disorder (PTSD), individuals often describe cognitive distortions related to self-blame. For example, individuals who develop PTSD after childhood sexual abuse may report beliefs that they are the cause of the abuse (Feiring & Cleland, 2007).

Eating Disorders

Cognitive theories related to eating disorders include assumptions about the self and distortions related to eating (Cooper, 2005). Individuals with eating disorders tend to place much emphasis on self-worth in relation to appearance. Distortions such as "Nobody will like me if I am overweight" or "I'm unacceptable if I don't maintain a certain shape" are the types of thoughts associated with eating disorders. In addition, there are cognitions that are specific to anorexia and bulimia. Individuals with anorexia may avoid eating as a strategy to prevent other distressing thoughts from coming to the forefront, whereas individuals with bulimia may believe that they have no control (which results in bingeing) or have overly permissive thoughts that contribute to impulsive eating.

Conduct Disorders

Children with conduct disorders engage in antisocial behaviors that are beyond the typical realm of acting out and involve violating the basic rights of others (e.g., bullying, stealing, physical assault). Cognitive theory indicates that children with conduct disorders are more likely to interpret the social environment as hostile (van de Wiel, Matthys, Cohen-Kettenis, & van Engeland, 2002). Consequently, a child with conduct disorder may interpret a bump from another child during recess as an antagonistic action. In addition, children with conduct disorders tend to have fewer solutions to managing confrontation and are more likely to choose an aggressive response, believing that the aggression will result in positive outcomes.

Other Disorders

Other psychiatric disorders for which cognitive theorists have identified associated dysfunctional beliefs include substance abuse (A. Beck, Wright, Newman, & Liese, 2001; Ellis & Velten, 1992; Terjesen, DiGiuseppe, & Gruner, 2000), personality disorders (A. Beck, Freeman, Davis, & Associates, 2003; Ellis, 1994b; Linehan, 1993), and schizophrenia (Cather, 2005; Davis, Lysaker, Lancaster, & Bryson, 2005; Lysaker, Bond, Davis, Bryson, & Bell, 2005; Pfammatter, Junghan, & Brenner, 2006).

In addition, the impact of distorted cognitions on emotions, mood, and performance has been reported for a variety of nonpsychiatric conditions and intervention contexts. Examples include brain injury and stroke (Khan-Bourne & Brown, 2003); dementia (Kasl-Godley & Gatz, 2000); chronic fatigue syndrome (Price, Mitchell, Tidy, & Hunot, 2008); Parkinson's disease (Cole & Vaughan, 2005; Lyons, 2003); chronic pain (Molton, Graham, Stoelb, & Jensen, 2007; Strong, 1998; Thorn, 2004); persons with disabilities in vocational programs (Davis, Lysaker, Lancaster, & Bryson, 2005; Lustig & Strauser, 2003); health behaviors such as weight loss (Cooper, Fairburn, & Hawkes, 2003; Liao, 2000), smoking cessation (Perkins, Conklin, & Levine, 2008), and exercise adherence (Schneider, Mercer, Herning, Smith, & Davis, 2004); students in educational settings (Pajares, 1992); and work with children and adolescents in school, community, and therapy contexts (Bailey, 2001; Braswell & Kendall, 2001; Vernon, 2006; Vernon & Bernard, 2006).

Cognitive Behavioral Theory and Therapy

A number of models are included under the umbrella of **cognitive behavioral therapy (CBT)**, an intervention approach that is recognized as an evidence-based approach for the treatment of many psychiatric conditions (Butler, Chapman, Forman, & Beck, 2006). This chapter discusses four prominent models that have influenced the development and practice of CBT and that are also most often discussed as relevant to belief-oriented occupational therapy: learning theory and behaviorism, social learning theory and social cognitive theory, and behaviorally oriented CBT models, and cognitively oriented CBT models (Bruce & Borg, 2002; Duncombe, 2005).

Learning Theory and Behaviorism

Beginning in the late 1950s, clinical psychologists began applying experimentally based principles of behavior known as **classical (or respondent) conditioning** and **operant conditioning** to the modification of maladaptive human behavior (Eysenck, 1966; Wolpe, 1958). At that time, classical conditioning theory, with systematic desensitization as its major clinical application, and operant conditioning, with behavior modification and systematic use of rewards as its major clinical application, focused on producing changes in overt, observable, measurable behavior. A number of intervention strategies evolved as these theories were applied to the treatment of psychological and behavioral conditions, some of which include targeting specific behaviors for change; setting observable, measurable outcome goals; analyzing behaviors to be learned, breaking them down into smaller "chunks," and grading them from less difficult to more difficult; and using various skill-oriented teaching-learning strategies such as shaping and chaining; monitoring behavior and changes over time; and rewarding desired adaptive behaviors. In its classic form, behavioral learning theory (Skinner, 1953) focused on the use of external reinforcement to increase the likelihood that a desired behavior would be learned. Behaviorism sometimes acknowledged beliefs and thoughts, but they were excluded from scientific study and intervention because they could not be directly observed, manipulated, and measured. However, this approach was increasingly seen as inadequate for explaining not only psychopathology, but also all human behavior (Mahoney, 1974, 1977). Thus, interest in the role of a person's internal beliefs, thoughts, and feelings, which could be inferred or reported by the person, but not directly observed, spurred further theoretical and research developments.

Social Learning Theory and Social Cognitive Theory

Albert Bandura (1977, 1986) is one of the most prominent representatives of **social learning theory**, or **social cognitive theory**, the name he adopted to emphasize the critical role of both social and cognitive factors in his theory of human learning and behavior change. Four fundamental constructs characterize social cognitive theory and are particularly relevant to belief-oriented occupational therapy practice:

1. Observational Learning, Vicarious Reinforcement, and Modeling—learning can occur from watching and listening to other people without any external reinforcement of the behavior to be learned.
2. Reciprocal Causation—personal factors, environmental factors, and behavior operate dynamically and influence one another.
3. View of Human Functioning as Proactive, Self-Regulating, and Self-Reflective—individuals can reflect on their thoughts, feelings, and actions, as well as assert self-control over them as opposed to reacting solely to environmental forces.
4. Self-Efficacy Beliefs and Outcome Expectancies—belief that the persons have the capability to successfully set and pursue their desired goals.

Self-efficacy beliefs are particularly relevant to occupational therapy practice with its emphasis on occupations and performance (Gage & Polatajko, 1994). An individuals' self-efficacy beliefs are instrumental in whether they "will attempt certain behaviors, how much effort they will expend, and how long they will stick with the behavior, particularly if problems or obstacles arise" (Bandura, 1981, p. 215). They also influence "how persons will feel about what they are doing and ultimately whether or not they will succeed" (p. 215). According to Bandura (1986, p. 399), performance failures tend to lower efficacy beliefs, whereas interventions that help create performance successes in a particular situation typically raise efficacy beliefs.

Listed in the order of their hypothesized power and influence, Bandura (1986) hypothesized that four types of experiences are basic to the development and enhancement of self-efficacy beliefs: actual performance accomplishments, vicarious experience and modeling, verbal persuasion, and physiological and affective states (learning coping skills to minimize stressors). This social learning model also provides the basis for many performance skill- and occupation-based interventions used by occupational therapists. For example, two self-management occupational therapy programs for older adults that draw extensively on Bandura's work are described in the occupational therapy literature. Cook (2004) describes a self-management occupational therapy program for arthritis joint protection. Lyons (2003) describes a self-management occupational therapy program for persons with Parkinson's disease.

Behaviorally Oriented CBT Models

Throughout the 1970s, a group of behaviorally trained psychologists and educators began to develop new approaches that focus on acquisition of cognitive and behavioral skills for self-managing psychological and behavior problems. Donald Meichenbaum (1977), a behaviorally trained psychologist, focused his early career work on what he called **cognitive behavior modification**, a prototype of behaviorally oriented CBT. With his colleagues, he developed a program of "self-instruction training" for children with impulsive behavior problems that used cognitive and behavioral strategies to teach them how to replace thoughts or "self-talk" that were not instructive or helpful for managing their own behavior with conscious thoughts or "self-talk" that were instructive and helpful (Meichenbaum & Goodman, 1971).

Encouraged by the promising results from these studies, other investigators applied this "self-instruction training" approach with individuals diagnosed with schizophrenia, speech and test anxiety, and phobias (Mahoney, 1974). Cognitive Orientation to Occupational Performance (CO-OP; Polatajko & Mandich, 2004) is an example of an occupational therapy children's program that builds on Meichenbaum and Goodman's work. This program is further described in Chapter 18.

Another behaviorally oriented CBT program developed by Meichenbaum and Cameron (1973), known as **stress inoculation training**, incorporates education about stress and its relationship to beliefs, emotions, and behavior; self-instruction training; cognitive restructuring; and training in the use of cognitive and behavioral coping skills for managing one's own behavior when exposed to various stressors that interfere with performance in daily life. For more discussion of coping skill theories, interventions, applications, and supporting evidence, the reader is referred to Chapter 22.

It is important to clarify that the primary emphasis of these behaviorally oriented CBT approaches is not on *directly* changing a person's existing idiosyncratic, dysfunctional beliefs and thoughts (which is the primary focus of this chapter), but rather on *indirectly* influencing a person's beliefs and thoughts through the acquisition and use of generalizable cognitive and behavioral skills for coping with real life challenges that cause emotional distress and interfere with achieving desired goals.

Cognitively Oriented CBT models

In a context quite removed from learning theory and behaviorism, several psychoanalytically trained psychotherapists began to doubt the efficacy and effectiveness of the Freudian psychodynamic therapies for helping persons with emotional and psychological disturbance. Albert Ellis (1962), a psychologist, and somewhat later, Aaron Beck (1976), a psychiatrist, began to independently explore **information processing theory** as a framework for understanding the impact of beliefs and thoughts on emotion and psychopathology. Their approaches are the prototypes of the cognitively oriented CBTs that focus on identifying and *directly* changing beliefs and thoughts using **cognitive restructuring** strategies.

Rational Emotive Behavior Therapy

Ellis' (1962, 1993) **rational emotive behavior therapy (REBT)** was the first of the modern cognitively oriented theories to gain widespread clinical acceptance. The REBT model is based on Ellis' cognitive model of emotional response. The core tenet of this model is that irrational beliefs about how things "must" and "should" be for persons to be happy actually lead them to make themselves miserable.

In the early 1970s, Ellis identified a number of basic irrational beliefs (Dryden & Ellis, 2001, p. 304) that take the form of absolute "musts" (e.g., "I must be loved by everyone to be happy") and "shoulds" (e.g., "I should be respected and looked up to by others"). According to Ellis, these irrational expectations of the self and others do not cause emotional disturbance and behavior problems; rather, they are key features of emotional disturbance. In addition, most people with emotional problems tend to have a low frustration tolerance; tend to deprecate themselves and others; and tend to overgeneralize, catastrophize, and "awfulize" about their failures, rejections, poor treatment by others, and life's frustrations and losses.

Ellis (1962, 1994a) devised the "ABC model" as an acronym to explain this view of emotional disturbance. He theorized that people typically think that the unfortunate **activating events (A)** in their lives are the cause of the disturbing behavioral and emotional **consequences (C)** that they experience. However, from Ellis' perspective, these consequences are actually caused by people's irrational **belief system (B)**. For example, imagine a young woman who feels terrible and depressed as a result of being rejected by the college of her choice. She assumes that feeling terrible and depressed is the emotional consequence (C) of the activating event (A), rejection by the college of her choice. However, from the REBT perspective, it is her core belief (B), "Rejection means I am incompetent and worthless," that is the real cause of her emotional distress.

In REBT, clients are taught to use the ABC model to identify and actively challenge the irrational beliefs that are at the core of their emotional problems. Then they are encouraged to replace "shoulds" and "mustabatory" beliefs with a more stoic, rational belief system and philosophy of life (Ellis, 1962, 1994a). Therefore, if the young woman in the example disputed her irrational belief and revised it to something more rational (e.g., "I am competent. Rejection is just something unfortunate that happens. I can find another college to attend.") this more rational view would help her feel better and seek out other options rather than being stuck as a depressed victim of rejection.

Cognitive Therapy

In 1976, Aaron Beck introduced his cognitive model of psychopathology based on information processing theory. Initially, his early research focused on the psychopathology of depression. His identification of the "cognitive triad" of distorted thoughts present in persons with depression is explained previously in this chapter. Over time, however, A. Beck and his colleagues proposed that his cognitive model

is applicable to the understanding of many psychological disturbances (A. Beck, 2005; J. Beck, 1995). A. Beck (1976) theorizes that the symptoms and cognitive content associated with various disorders reflect the systematic dysfunctional thoughts, information processing biases, and distorted interpretations of environmental experiences that result from the activation of underlying unrealistic or distorted core beliefs and from fairly enduring cognitive schemas and structures. Based on his early research, Beck identified a number of core cognitive distortions that reflect the processing and interpretation errors typically present in persons who experience emotional problems. Examples include emotionalizing or emotional reasoning (e.g., presuming that feelings are facts and reflect the real situation as in "I feel desperate; thus, the situation I'm in must be a desperate one"); jumping to conclusions (e.g., focusing on one part of a situation as the only way to understand it as in "Because they haven't called me about the job, they must have decided not to hire me"); and all-or-nothing thinking (e.g., perceiving events or people in absolute, polarized terms as in "Something is either perfect or completely wrong"). The goal of A. Beck's cognitive therapy (CT) is to collaborate with clients in identifying, reframing, and replacing these cognitive distortions or appraisals of life events with more realistic and adaptive appraisals, thoughts, and core beliefs under the assumption that this will also support changes in a person's emotional distress and behavioral problems.

Although the terms *cognitive therapy* (CT) and *cognitive behavioral therapy* (CBT) are often used as synonyms, A. Beck's CT is based specifically on his cognitively oriented and evidence-based theory of psychopathology. CBT typically incorporates CT, but it is also the "umbrella" term for all cognitive behavioral approaches (A. Beck, 2005).

From an overall perspective, the various models included under the CBT umbrella are some of the most widely adopted and empirically supported forms of psychotherapeutic intervention in Western culture. In an extensive and widely acknowledged review of 16 published meta-analyses on the treatment outcomes of CBT for a wide range of psychiatric disorders, Butler et al (2006) concluded that they provide support for the efficacy of CBT. Butler and his colleagues also concluded that the findings of these meta-analyses are consistent with other reviewed methodologies that support CBT for many psychiatric disorders.

Use of CBT Models in Occupational Therapy

Although the compatibility between CBT and occupational therapy models has been identified throughout this chapter, it is important to also clarify their differences in purpose and intent. The cognitive behavioral models that focus *directly* on changing beliefs, such as REBT and CT, are based on theories of psychopathology for persons experiencing symptoms of emotional distress related to psychiatric and medical illness. The purpose of therapy is to address these emotional and behavioral problems by addressing the dysfunctional or distorted cognitions that mediate them. Focus on deeper level core beliefs or schema is considered the central focus of intervention. This approach is most realistically provided in outpatient psychotherapy with therapists who have specialized training and certification in CBT (A. Beck, 2005).

Occupational therapy's primary domain of concern focuses on enabling occupational performance in a client's current daily life (AOTA, 2008). Changing a person's beliefs for the purpose of facilitating changes in the emotional and behavioral symptoms of various psychiatric diagnoses is not the primary purpose of occupational therapy, although it may indirectly contribute to changes in these areas. Typically, occupational therapists focus on changing beliefs and thoughts only if they are interfering with desired occupational performance, referred to as a "top-down" approach. Therefore, an emphasis on more surface-level automatic thoughts, intermediate assumptions and "rules for living," and specific aspects of fairly accessible core beliefs related to occupational performance is most compatible with occupational therapy's philosophy, assessment, and intervention process. This focus on surface or peripheral change is not superficial in the sense of being less important than deep change in a person's core beliefs. It simply serves a different therapeutic purpose and goal.

Assessment of Beliefs in Occupational Therapy Practice

As with other client factors, a client's beliefs and how they facilitate or hinder desired occupational performance is an important aspect of a client's occupational profile (AOTA, 2008). When assessing and evaluating beliefs, occupational therapists are concerned with the following:

- Understanding how a person's beliefs and thoughts limit or facilitate desired occupational performance goals
- Establishing basic client capacities related to targeted beliefs that interfere with desired occupational performance
- Identifying possible beliefs and thoughts that need to be addressed to support occupational performance interventions and desired outcomes
- Identifying environmental and performance factors that may be contributing to distorted beliefs and occupational performance problems

The following general questions are offered as suggestions for assessing the impact of a person's beliefs on occupational performance, as well as for identifying possible goals and outcome expectations for therapy.

1. What does the person identify as his or her occupational performance strengths and limitations? How are these strengths and limitations related to intervention priorities?
2. What beliefs or thoughts does the person have that facilitate or hinder occupational performance in general, as well as specific intervention priorities?
3. What are the client's beliefs about his or her ability to successfully address these intervention priorities, including the challenges that might occur?
4. What are the person's beliefs and expectations about intervention outcomes? Are they realistic or unrealistic?

5. What environmental and performance factors facilitate or hinder a client's desired occupational performance? Confirm or disconfirm dysfunctional or distorted beliefs?
6. What physiological and emotional reactions trigger dysfunctional beliefs that affect occupational performance?

Formal Assessments

There are a number of formal, structured, assessment instruments for evaluating beliefs and belief systems that have been developed in the fields of education, psychology, mental health, and preventive health care (Blankstein & Segal, 2001; Pajares, 1992). Researchers in these fields, more than practitioners, have led the way in developing and using assessment instruments to validate theoretical constructs, establish accurate diagnoses, and evaluate outcomes of cognitive behavioral interventions.

In the occupational therapy literature, there are no psychometrically supported formal tests that have been developed for the specific purpose of assessing the content of a client's beliefs and their impact on occupational performance. Based on their review of the occupational therapy literature, Bruce and Borg (2002) and Duncombe (2005) identified several assessments proposed by occupational therapists as part of specific CBT-oriented treatment programs, but none of these measures has been psychometrically evaluated or adopted for use on a larger scale in occupational therapy practice. One exception is a test developed to measure self-efficacy, the Self Efficacy Gauge (Gage, Noh, Polatajko, & Kaspar, 1994). This measure, specifically designed for occupational therapists, examines self-efficacy in the context of occupational performance.

Several occupational performance outcome measures, particularly those that are client centered and include a structured or semistructured interview component, either formally or informally, provide an opportunity for exploration of a client's beliefs as part of the assessment of occupational performance. For example, see the Canadian Occupational Performance Measure (Law et al, 2005); the Occupational Self Assessment (OSA), Version 2.0 (Baron, Keilhofner, Iyenger, Goldhammer, & Wolenski, 2002), and the Child Occupational Self Assessment (COSA), Version 1.0 (Federico & Kielhofner, 2002); the Assessment of Occupational Functioning—Collaborative Version (ASOF-CV) (Watts, Hinson, Madigan, McGuigan, & Newman, 1999); and the Occupational Performance History Interview, Second Version (OPHI-II) (Keilhofner et al, 1997).

Informal or Semistructured Assessments

Informal and semistructured assessments offer valuable methods for identifying beliefs that contribute to occupational performance problems, as well as to emotional distress and behavior problems. Structured or semistructured initial interviews provide a more informal collaborative interaction with clients (J. Beck, 1995; Dryden & Ellis, 2001). For occupational therapists, this process might be guided by questions like those suggested previously for assessing the impact of a person's beliefs on occupational performance and for determining intervention priorities and goals.

Another approach is to embed assessment in the ongoing intervention process. The advantage of this approach is that it focuses on what clients view as their idiosyncratic, problematic beliefs and lends itself to addressing dysfunctional beliefs and thoughts as they "naturally" arise by evaluating them in the context of what the client is feeling and doing in "real time" (J. Beck, 1995; Dryden & Ellis, 2001). Thus, clients are actively engaged in a process of identifying and addressing problematic behaviors that mirrors the same self-management process they might use in "real life." This less structured, more informal, embedded, and flexible approach is illustrated at the beginning of this chapter in the description of the woman receiving occupational therapy following hip replacement surgery.

Structured Task Assessments

There are a number of more structured, but informal cognitive and behavioral methods for assessment of beliefs and their impact on emotions and behavior as part of initial, ongoing, and outcome assessment and intervention planning. Because these methods, such as use of Socratic questioning and guided discovery, Beck's dysfunctional thought record, Burn's TIC/TOC technique, and Ellis's ABC model are also important intervention strategies, they are described in more detail in the next section.

Intervention

The overarching CBT intervention principles and the specific intervention strategies and techniques that follow are selected for their applicability in belief-oriented occupational therapy intervention. The specific cognitive and behavioral strategies and techniques are grouped separately to emphasize the important contribution of each perspective to the intervention and ongoing assessment process, as well as the importance of incorporating both cognitive and behavioral strategies for effective belief-oriented interventions. Those specific strategies and techniques preceded by an asterisk are particularly useful for initial, ongoing, and outcome assessment, as well as for intervention.

Client-Centered, Collaborative, Educational, Empirical Approach

For both CBT and occupational therapy interventions, effectiveness relies on a client-centered, collaborative relationship. The therapist's role is to actively listen, teach, role-model, encourage, and give feedback. The client's role is to express concerns related to occupational performance strengths and limitations; to identify beliefs and thoughts that interfere with desired occupational performance; to learn new beliefs and ways of thinking, feeling, and behaving; and to test and apply that learning with problems that arise in their day-to-day lives. Therapists do not tell their clients *what* to do; rather, they collaborate with their clients in learning *how* to think and talk to themselves in ways that support them doing what they want and need to do (J. Beck, 1995). In addition, CBT interventions incorporate many teaching-learning strategies to encourage learning and self-discovery (e.g., use of didactic materials, handouts, workbooks; modeling and experiential learning methods; homework assignments).

Another characteristic of CBT is the use of scientific or empirical methods. Intervention is designed as a systematic, logical process that not only involves gaining new insights, but also actively experimenting and applying insights in the client's daily life. This approach is reflected in the use of a structured agenda and format for belief-oriented interventions (J. Beck, 1995). Typically, therapists have a specific agenda for each session that is collaboratively determined with the client. A common format for addressing this agenda, whether as part of an individual or group intervention, includes the following steps: review of homework; didactic education related to the agenda; modeling and demonstration of a technique or skill; practice using or applying the technique or skill; feedback from self-reflection, therapist, and/or peers; and the assignment of collaboratively determined homework to be reviewed in the next session.

Cognitive Strategies and Techniques

Cognitive strategies and techniques *directly* target beliefs and thoughts with an emphasis on "**cognitive restructuring**." They can be used to modify existing beliefs or to construct entirely new beliefs that a person aspires to embrace (Mooney & Padesky, 2000). For each strategy to be optimally effective, the responses or outcomes need to be reflected on by client and therapist and used to revise or create new beliefs, new hypotheses to test, etc, as part of the ongoing assessment, intervention, and goal attainment process.

*Socratic Questioning and Guided Discovery

Socratic questioning and **guided discovery** are hallmarks of CBT's overall client-centered, collaborative, educational, and empirical approach. When used appropriately, these open-ended, guiding questions avoid interpretation and ultimately lead both client and therapist to discover problems and alternative options for solving them. In addition, therapists often use these questions to guide the review and evaluation of responses to the other cognitive intervention strategies and techniques that we discuss here. For occupational therapists, use of Socratic questioning facilitates client-centered "discovery" and clarification of beliefs and thoughts that may support or hinder occupational performance and goal attainment.

Padesky (1993) identifies four phases of questioning that may proceed in a stepwise fashion and may shift from one to another depending on how the dialogue unfolds. Table 19-2 outlines each phase with examples of relevant questions that a therapist might ask.

Table 19-3 illustrates the use of three Socratic questions to facilitate guided discovery as part of what is sometimes formalized as the "Three Question Technique" (J. Beck, 1995). In this example, the Socratic questions guide the client to reframe his situation and, in so doing, "discover" how helpful or not his belief is for meeting his needs and goals. This opens up new options and the possibility of revising or creating new beliefs that are more realistically oriented toward addressing the problematic situation and related emotions.

Table 19-2 ● **Four Phases of Socratic Questioning**

Phase	Examples of Questions
1. Asking **informational questions** that the client can answer to help make concerns explicit and for the client to feel heard.	*What are you thinking or feeling when you do _____ ?* *Could you give me an example?* *Could you elaborate on that?* *What do you mean when you say _____ ?* *How long have you felt or believed this way?*
2. Asking **questions that reflect empathic listening** and summarize issues related to the problem.	*Let me see if I understand; do you mean _____ ?* *You seem to be assuming __? Do I understand you correctly?* *When you say _____ , are you implying _____ ?* *Let me summarize: are you thinking ____ ? or feeling ____ ?* *Are you saying you believe _____ when you do _____ ?* *I'm not sure I understand. Why is _____ ?*
3. Asking **questions that draw the client's attention to information relevant** to the issue being discussed, but which may be outside the client's current focus.	*What evidence do you have to support or refute that view?* *Have you ever been in a similar situation? What did you do? How did that turn out?* *What would you advise a friend who said something similar?* *Has something happened to lead you to this conclusion?* *What might someone who disagrees say?*
4. **Asking analytic or synthesizing questions** that guide the client toward new information to reevaluate a previous conclusion or construct a new idea.	*How could you find out whether that is true?* *How does _____ relate to _____ ?* *By what reasoning did you come to that conclusion?* *How does this information fit with _____ ?* *What are the advantages and disadvantages of _____ ?* *What are the implications or consequences of that belief?* *Are there alternative explanations of the situation or event?* *What do you know now that you didn't know before?*

Table 19-3 ● **Example Illustrating Use of Socratic Questions and Guided Discovery**

Situation: A man has recently lost his job.

Belief: *I will never work again.*

Socratic, Guiding Questions	Example
What is the **evidence** for and against the belief?	**For:** *I was fired from my job. I won't be able to get a reference from my boss.* **Against:** *I've found work in the past. There are others I can use as a reference. I have received positive work evaluations in the past. My resume will help me.*
What are the **alternative explanations** of the event or situation?	*My boss and I got off to a bad start and were never able to develop a good working relationship. It was time for me to find a new job anyway.*
What are the real **implications** or consequences if the belief is correct?	*It's possible that I won't get work in my field, but I could always do something else.*

*Dysfunctional Thought Record

Introduced by A. Beck, Rush, Shaw, and Emery (1979), the **Dysfunctional Thought Record** (DTR) is integral to CT. Comprised of three to five columns, a DTR usually includes the date and columns for describing a distressing situation (e.g., where, what, when), related emotional responses (e.g., what, intensity rating), and automatic thoughts (e.g., what, strength of belief rating). Additional columns may be included for identifying thought distortions (e.g., all-or-nothing thinking, overgeneralizing, jumping to conclusions, overpersonalizing, inappropriate blaming, magnifying/minimizing), an alternative response (e.g., other views, explanations, positive reframe of distortion), and outcomes (e.g., follow-up rating of emotional intensity and belief strength) (J. Beck, 1995). In its simplest form, a thought record might be set up as illustrated in Table 19-4 with additional rows for subsequent situations.

*TIC TOC Technique

The **TIC TOC Technique**, developed by Burns (1993), is particularly appropriate for occupational therapy interventions because it focuses on identifying and reframing thoughts or cognitions that interfere with undertaking and accomplishing desired tasks. First, the client identifies a task that he or she wants or needs to do, but is avoiding or resisting. Then the client completes a three-column worksheet that includes identification of TICs (task interfering cognitions), related thought distortions (e.g., emotional reasoning, all-or-nothing thinking, minimization, mind-reading, overgeneralization), and a reframed TOC (task-oriented cognition) related to the problematic task. As with similar techniques, this worksheet is used to "discover" new options for achieving desired goals. Table 19-5 outlines this technique.

Table 19-4 ● Sample Dysfunctional Thought Record

Date/Time	Situation	Emotion	Automatic Thoughts	Thought Distortions	Alternative Thought/View	Outcome
7/13/XX 7AM	Forget to set alarm. Oversleep and end up late for work.	Anger, anxious; Emotional intensity: 90%	I'll be fired. I always mess up. I'm an idiot. Belief strength: 90%	Fortune-telling, magnifying	Late once before, and I wasn't fired. I can offer to stay late to make up time. I need to be sure to set my alarm.	Emotional intensity: 40% Belief strength: 20%

Table 19-5 ● Sample TIC TOC Chart

Task-Interfering Cognitions (TICs)	Thought Distortions	Task-Oriented Cognitions (TOCs)
I'll never be able to live in my own apartment. Why bother trying?	All-or-nothing thinking	I'm not ready yet to live on my own, but if I take little steps, like learning to take the bus, I can work toward doing so.

*Identifying ABCs

Identifying ABCs makes use of Ellis' (1962, 1994b) ABC model of emotional distress. It provides a framework to identify the activating events (A), irrational beliefs (B), and emotional and behavioral consequences (C) related to specific situations, beliefs and thoughts, or emotions that are interfering with a person's well-being. This method highlights the irrational beliefs that are the real source of emotional distress and behavior problems. When identified, a person can then evaluate, dispute, and reframe these irrational beliefs to be more realistic or rational, initially with a therapist's guidance and, eventually, on one's own.

Acquiring Knowledge

Educational or psychoeducational sessions for individuals or groups may be designed to impart knowledge about a CBT concept, method, or skill as a way to help clients **acquire knowledge** for understanding the CBT approach. Knowledge about psychiatric conditions, medications, stigma, etc, that provides accurate and appropriate information is also important for assessing the validity of a person's beliefs. Homework assignments for acquiring knowledge are sometimes referred to as *bibliotherapy*. In its broadest sense, this approach also includes the use of audiotapes, videotapes, and computer programs (Cather, 2005). For useful examples of various books and workbooks, see the Resources section.

In the occupational therapy literature, psychoeducational groups are the most prevalent application of CBT's educational philosophy and method (Bruce & Borg, 2002; Duncombe, 2005). Typically, these groups address topics such as stress management, life skills, and social skills. They focus on imparting knowledge about the topic and teaching topic-related cognitive and behavioral skills (see, e.g., Crist, 1986; Johnson, 1987; Stein & Smith, 1989).

Behavioral Strategies and Techniques

Behavioral strategies and techniques focus on activating or monitoring overt observable behaviors, such as "doing" an action, activity, or behavioral experiment, or on covert behaviors, such as self-reported thoughts and feelings, and may be used to directly or indirectly affect beliefs.

Behavioral Experiments

Behavioral experiments are the most important behavioral strategy that is incorporated into CBT's empirical methodology (DeRubeis, Tang, & Beck, 2001; Dryden & Ellis, 2001). Working collaboratively, therapist and client create opportunities for the client to test thoughts, beliefs, and related behaviors as part of discovering their relative utility or validity (Beck et al, 1979). The typical behavioral experiment involves creating a hypothesis to test, predicting the outcome, undertaking the test or "experiment," evaluating the result, and then using this feedback to revise or create new perspectives. This powerful process is critical to belief change, particularly when used in combination with cognitive strategies. For example, a student might have the belief that his classmates will think he is stupid if he asks for help on an exam. He might test this belief in a behavioral experiment by actually asking classmates if they would think he is stupid if he asked for help. The outcome of this experiment provides feedback on the validity of his belief, an important aspect of the cognitive restructuring process.

*Assigning Homework

Assigning homework requires clients, as part of their daily lives outside therapy sessions, to experiment with, apply, practice, or supplement what is addressed in a therapy. The assigning of homework supports the assumption in CBT that the outcome is not just a change in beliefs. Rather, the expected outcome is a change in people's abilities to function and self-manage their emotions, thoughts, and behavior in their daily lives (Padesky & Greenberger, 1995). Most of the strategies and techniques presented in this chapter could be assigned as homework.

*Self-Monitoring

Self-monitoring is a self-regulatory or self-management process that involves paying deliberate attention to some aspect of one's behavior. Typically, it includes recording and

Both Automatic Thought Records (ATRs) and Behavioral Experiments (BEs) are important components of CBT interventions. Evidence suggests that BEs are perceived as more powerful and compelling than ATRs for actual changes in beliefs and behavior. Based on these findings, the researchers hypothesized that ATRs may be more useful for providing clarity and understanding of thoughts and beliefs along with new options and perspectives, whereas BEs may be more powerful for actual belief and behavior change. The implications of this evidence are relevant to occupational therapists' expertise and practice.

➤ Occupational therapists have expertise in analyzing and grading tasks, an essential aspect of planning and evaluating behavioral experiments.

➤ Occupational therapy provides a social and performance context for clients to carry out behavioral experiments while engaged in meaningful occupations such as work, leisure, and ADLs.

➤ Occupational therapists can provide detailed information on functional capacity and abilities to help determine whether a client's beliefs are valid or a mixture of performance deficits and cognitive distortions about abilities. This information is helpful for verifying the validity of ATRs and in designing appropriate behavioral experiments.

➤ Psychoeducational groups led by occupational therapists that include both acquisition of knowledge and its application through behavioral experimentation may be more powerful for creating change in beliefs and behavior.

Bennett-Levy, J. (2003). Mechanisms of change in cognitive therapy: The case for automatic thought records and behavioural experiments. *Behavioural and Cognitive Psychotherapy, 31*, 261–277.

tallying the frequency of behavior with associated thoughts and feelings for a designated period of time (e.g., on an hour-by-hour basis for 1 week). It may also involve monitoring and rating one's thoughts and feelings, or the degree of mastery or pleasure associated with each action or activity performed (e.g., on a scale from 0 to 100, where 0 is the worst one has ever felt or the most negative and 100 is the best or most positive) (Beck et al, 1979; DeRubeis et al, 2001). For example, if someone believes that they do nothing all day long, as homework they might self-monitor their behavior by keeping a record of what they are doing every half hour for several days to evaluate if, in fact, they do nothing 24 hours a day. This concrete feedback would provide evidence to dispute the person's beliefs.

Scheduling Activities

Making a list or calendar of daily and weekly activities and committing to engage in them can be another useful strategy. The behavioral activation component of CT suggests that individuals need to engage in positive and successful experiences to change negative thinking (Hopko, Lejuez, Ruggiero, & Eifert, 2003). A successful experience provides contradictory evidence to the belief that one is incompetent or worthless. Follow-through or failure to follow-through also provides a basis to discuss the beliefs and thoughts that

may be interfering with performance. Scheduling activities is frequently combined with self-monitoring as homework.

Other Assessment and Intervention Considerations

Thus far, the focus of assessment and intervention related to beliefs has focused primarily on approaches for *directly* assessing and intervening with beliefs as part of a person's internal processes. There are several other considerations that are important to this approach, as well as to the indirect approaches for belief change, and to the overall process of assessment and intervention. This section addresses four considerations that are particularly relevant: metacognitive demands of CBT, culture and beliefs, and interventions focused on environmental solutions or on occupation and performance skill training and participation.

Metacognitive Demands of CBT

Use of CBT—in particular, of cognitive restructuring strategies and techniques—as primary methods for belief-oriented intervention requires various metacognitive conceptual reasoning abilities (e.g., the ability to "reflect about one's thinking," to identify and evaluate the validity of one's own beliefs, to differentiate between beliefs and "reality," and to grasp the critical meditational role of beliefs related to feelings and behavior). When children and adults have cognitive limitations or impairments due to developmental ability, disease, illness, or incompatible learning style preferences, they may find the cognitive restructuring methods overwhelming and excessively demanding of time and effort (Bailey, 2001; Braswell & Kendall, 2001; Dagnan, Chadwick, & Proudlove, 2000; Lysaker et al, 2005).

Occupational therapists Duncombe (2005) and McCraith (1998) suggest use of the Allen Cognitive Levels, part of the Allen Cognitive Disabilities Model (Allen, Earhart, & Blue, 1992; Allen et al, 2007), as a helpful guideline for assessment and intervention that takes the metacognitive demands of

Activity scheduling is often incorporated as a component of cognitive behavioral therapy, but the efficacy of activity schedule alone has also been studied. A meta-analysis of 16 studies found a large effect size for activity scheduling in treating individuals with depression (d = 0.87). These results promote interventions that are highly compatible with occupational therapy and include the following:

➤ Helping individuals with depression monitor the relationship between daily activities, their moods, and beliefs by keeping an activity schedule and encouraging them to participate in activities that are associated with a better mood.

➤ Helping individuals with depression create a plan to increase the number of pleasant activities and the number of positive interactions with other people.

Cuijpers, P., van Straten, A., & Warmerdam, C. (2007). Behavioral activation treatment of depression: A meta-analysis. *Clinical Psychology Review, 27*, 318–326.

CBT into account. They propose that these demands be viewed along a continuum from more behavioral (concrete) to more cognitive (abstract). For persons with the capacity to use higher-level executive functions for new learning, conceptual reasoning, and generalization to various situations (Allen Cognitive Levels 5 and 6), they recommend selection of more cognitive strategies along with behavioral experimentation. In contrast, more behavioral CBT models and "uncomplicated" cognitive strategies and techniques may be more suitable for persons who learn best using concrete, repetitive, situation-specific strategies (Allen Cognitive Levels 3 and 4). In addition, interventions focused on cognitive and behavioral skill acquisition and on seeking environmental solutions or engagement in meaningful occupation as an indirect approach to modifying a person's beliefs may be more appropriate for this latter group of learners. As a general guideline, this perspective is also supported by educators and psychologists working with children (e.g., Bailey, 2001; Braswell & Kendall, 2001) and adults with cognitive limitations (e.g., Dagnan et al, 2000; Lysaker et al, 2005).

Culture and Beliefs

Hays and Iwamasa (2006), the editors of *Culturally Responsive Cognitive Behavioral Therapy*, point out that CBT research and clinical applications have focused primarily on European American perspectives and assumptions. They recognize that CBT's nonjudgmental focus on client strengths and an educational approach, as well as awareness of the importance of social context, support the appropriateness of CBT for people of diverse cultural identities. They have brought together a well-informed group of authors who focus on the applicability, limitations, and "use of CBT with ethnic cultures, including people of Native, Latino, Asian, and African American heritage, as well as people of Arab and Orthodox Jewish heritage." In this valuable resource, they also "address the use of CBT with people of non-ethnic minority groups: older adults, people with disabilities, and sexual minorities" (p. 13).

Acculturation, in particular, is an essential construct to consider with regard to the psychological functioning of immigrants and ethnic minorities (Tanaka-Matsumi, Higginbotham, & Chang, 2002). Information about the person's language(s), social supports, and participation in ethnic and cultural activities provides important data regarding the possible relationship between cultural adjustment difficulties and presenting problems and beliefs. A clients' "acculturation status can shape not only behavior, affect, and cognitions, but also responses to various assessment tools" (p. 250) and intervention approaches. Although there are few cognitive assessments that have been developed for diverse populations, the Culturally Informed Functional Assessment (CIFA) interview (Tanaka-Matsumi, Seiden, & Lam, 1996) "was designed to facilitate the integration of cultural observations into cognitive-behavioral assessment and treatment planning" (p. 256). Pride in one's cultural identify, culture-specific beliefs that help one cope, such as healing rituals, and cultural icons that can serve as role models may offer important perspective and support for reframing beliefs to be more adaptive. Ultimately, the greater the therapist's knowledge of the client's cultural definitions of beliefs, emotions, and behavior and what makes a belief irrational or unrealistic, appropriate or inappropriate, as well as cultural norms regarding change strategies and the change agents, the more accurate and useful assessment and intervention will be (Okazaki & Tanaka-Matsumi, 2006).

Environment-Focused Interventions

Environment-focused interventions address environmental solutions that have the potential to *indirectly* influence a person's thoughts and beliefs. For example, to address beliefs such as "My furniture has been stolen" or "This isn't my room," which are often expressed by persons with dementia who have recently moved into a new supervised living situation, family members may bring in familiar furniture, bedding, and wall décor to make the new room more familiar.

In addition, an individual's dysfunctional beliefs may reflect an accurate cognitive appraisal of environmental factors and contexts that account for those beliefs. In circumstances in which a person's negative or dysfunctional beliefs are actually supported by realistic environmental problems, it is appropriate to *indirectly* address dysfunctional beliefs by *directly* working toward environmental solutions for those problems (e.g., resolving a stressful living situation, revising inappropriate social expectations, expanding limited social supports, clarifying conflicting cultural values and norms, leaving an abusive spouse or a racist boss, replacing inadequate housing) (Hays & Iwamasa, 2006).

For example, a **supportive social environment** is critical for effective belief and performance changes. Stigma, cognitive biases, and negative beliefs about mental illness, disability, and cultural differences, or simply inadequate information can have a profound impact on a person's self-efficacy beliefs and recovery. Educating family, friends, caregivers, and health-care professionals using the same teaching-learning and CBT strategies and techniques used with clients is an environmentally focused intervention that can indirectly have a profound impact on modifying a person's dysfunctional beliefs.

Pat Deegan (1994) credits the positive social supports in her life as a major force in helping her move from believing her situation was hopeless to believing that she could recover. She explained that the people who "loved her and did not give up" (p. 153) and who "remained optimistic despite the odds" provided a "constant invitation . . . calling [her] forth . . . to be more than [she] was" (p. 154). Ultimately, Pat Deegan earned a PhD in psychology; she now works as an empowerment advocate for persons with psychiatric and physical disabilities, and is a well-known national and international speaker and author on recovery and empowerment. A number of research studies also support the presence of positive social supports as an essential factor in a client's ability to change dysfunctional beliefs and to develop more adaptive beliefs as part of psychosocial recovery (Landeen, Seeman, Goering, & Streiner, 2007; Sullivan, 1994).

Occupation and Performance Skill Interventions

As with environmental problems, cognitive and behavioral skill deficits (e.g., coping, problem-solving, assertiveness, social and time management skills), and occupational performance deficits related to work, leisure, and social participation may realistically contribute to the dysfunctional beliefs and

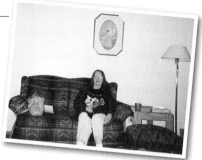

PhotoVoice

This is Pat. She's a good Christian and a good worker. I don't think she does anything wrong ever. She is a hard worker even though she has arthritis. She is always good. Pat lives with a mental illness. I see only her strengths.

thoughts that a person has about his or her abilities or situation (J. Beck, 1995; Dryden & Ellis, 2001; Meichenbaum, 1977). Clarifying performance skill strengths and deficits helps the therapist and client evaluate whether there is a realistic basis for the client's negative beliefs and what skill training may be important to incorporate into an intervention plan. For example, if a client believes that he is unable to assert himself and is therefore always taken advantage of by peers and coworkers, this belief may be realistically supported

by the fact that he has limited knowledge and skills for behaving in an assertive manner when appropriate. Assertiveness training may be a valuable component of his intervention plan. The occupational therapist's expertise in contributing assessment information related to occupational and skill performance strengths and deficits, as well as providing occupational and skill training as part of a treatment team in CBT-oriented intervention programs has been acknowledged by Wright, Thase, Ludgate, and Beck (1993).

Summary

Cognitive beliefs about oneself, other people, the world, and the future are part of the content of a person's internal cognitive processes. These beliefs are dynamically interrelated with emotions, physiological reactions, behavior, and the environment that comprise human functioning. Distorted cognitions and dysfunctional beliefs have been shown to be associated with a number of medical and psychiatric conditions. Cognitive behavioral theory and therapy offer a number of evidence-based approaches that are compatible with occupational therapy practice in mental health and can be used to address individuals' beliefs that interfere with achieving desired occupational performance outcomes.

Active Learning Strategies

1. Reflection

Reflect on a situation in which empowering thoughts and beliefs have given you the strength and courage to accomplish an important task or goal. Then, reflect again, this time selecting a situation when worry, procrastination, self-criticism, or other negative self-talk affected your mood and derailed you from achieving your goal.

Reflective Questions
● Describe the thoughts that were associated with each situation. What thoughts supported or interfered with working toward and achieving your goal?
● What environmental or performance factors helped or hindered you? What people and skills supported you or interfered with the process? Were there other environmental supports or barriers, such as finances, scheduling, or geography?

Reflective Journal

 Describe the experience in your **Reflective Journal**.

2. Practice Techniques

Based on the problematic situation you reflected on previously or another situation of your choosing, try out several of the cognitive and behavioral strategies and techniques described in the Intervention section for addressing dysfunctional beliefs (e.g., Thought Record, ABC method, TIC-TOC technique, behavioral experiments).

Reflective Questions
● How did the technique(s) facilitate or hinder your understanding of the beliefs and thoughts that affect your feelings and behavior related to the situation?
● What do you think it would take for you to change your problematic belief? What are the challenges involved?

Reflective Journal

 Describe the experience in your **Reflective Journal**.

3. Practical Application

Select a client in your fieldwork who is diagnosed with depression, anxiety, or another DSM-IV-TR condition for which there is evidence that supports use of CBT interventions. Read about this condition and how cognitive behavioral theory and therapy have been applied to the understanding of the condition and for intervention.

Reflective Questions
● What insights have you gained about this person as a result of your reading?
● How would you enhance or alter your occupational therapy interventions using CBT based on this information?

4. Justifying CBT by Occupational Therapists

An occupational therapist contacted me because her hospital had just been refused payment by Medicare for her services in a partial hospital day program for individuals with persistent mental illness. She explained that the program is based on CBT principles. As an occupational therapist, she leads a CBT group focused on teaching the ABC method to people with depression, a coping skills group focused on stress management, and a mindfulness group focused on meditation and related techniques. In refusing payment for her services, Medicare explained that occupational therapists are qualified to address functional skills, but are not qualified to provide cognitive behavioral group therapy.

Based on reading this chapter,

● What information and evidence might you give Medicare to educate them about occupational therapy and occupational therapists' qualifications to use CBT interventions?
● How might you redesign the title, purpose, and outcomes for these groups so that the occupational therapist could be reimbursed?
● Write a group protocol for one of the groups that this occupational therapist leads, applying what you have learned about belief-oriented occupational therapy.

Resources

Websites
● The Albert Ellis Institute: www.rebt.org
● The Beck Institute for Cognitive Therapy and Research—includes CBT information and Beck Scales such as the Beck Depression Inventory and Beck Youth Inventories: www.beckinstitute.org
● British Association for Behavioural and Cognitive Psychotherapies: www.babcp.com
● "Overview of Social Cognitive Theory and of Self-Efficacy," 2002, by F. Pajares. Available at: www.emory.edu/EDUCATION/mfp/eff .html (December 7, 2009)—a extensive overview of Albert Bandura, social cognitive theory, and self-efficacy
● New York Institute for Cognitive and Behavioral Therapies—includes useful resources and online continuing education courses on CBT: www.nyicbt.org

Workbooks
There are numerous workbooks available with cognitive behavior exercises that can be adapted for belief-oriented occupational therapy interventions. Following is a sampling of these resources:
● Addis, M. E., & Martell, C. R. (2004). *Overcoming Depression One Step at a Time: The New Behavioral Activation Approach to Getting Your Life Back*. Oakland, CA: New Harbinger.
● Beck, J. S. (2005). *Cognitive Therapy for Challenging Problems: What To Do When the Basics Don't Work*. New York: Guilford Press.
● Bourne, E. J. (2005). *The Anxiety and Phobia Workbook*. Oakland, CA: New Harbinger.
● Burns, D. B. (1993). *Ten Days to Self-Esteem*. New York: HarperCollins.
● Greenberger, D., & Padesky, C. A. (1995). *Mind Over Mood: Change How You Feel by Changing the Way You Think*. New York: Guilford Press.
● Knaus, W. J., & Ellis, A. (2006). *The Cognitive Behavioral Workbook for Depression: A Step by Step Program*. Oakland, CA: New Harbinger.
● McKay, M., Davis, M., & Fanning, P. (2007). *Thoughts and Feelings: Taking Control of Your Moods and Your Life*. Oakland, CA: New Harbinger.
● Stallard, P. (2002). *Think Good and Feel Good: A Cognitive Behavioral Therapy Workbook for Children*. West Sussex, UK: John Wiley & Sons.

References

Abramowitz, J. S., Khandker, M., Nelson, C. A., Deacon, B. J., & Rygwall R. (2006). The role of cognitive factors in the pathogenesis of obsessive-compulsive symptoms: A prospective study. *Behavioral Research, 44*, 1361–1374.

Allen, C. K., Austin, S. L., David, S. K., Earhart, C. A., McCraith, D. B., & Riska-Williams, L. (2007). *Manual for the Allen Cognitive Level Screen-5 (ACLS-5) and Large Allen Cognitive Level Screen-5 (LACLS-5)*. Camarillo, CA: ACLS and LACLS Committee.

Allen, C. K., Earhart, C. A., & Blue, T. (1992). *Occupational Therapy Treatment Goals for the Physically and Cognitively Disabled*. Bethesda, MD: American Occupational Therapy Association.

American Occupational Therapy Association (AOTA). (2008). Occupational therapy practice framework: Domain and process. *American Journal of Occupational Therapy, 62*(6), 625–683.

Anthony, W. (1993). Recovery from mental illness: The guiding vision of the mental health system in the 1990's. *Psychosocial Rehabilitation Journal, 16*(4), 11–23.

Bailey, V. (2001). Cognitive-behavioural therapies for children and adolescents. *Advances in Psychiatric Treatment, 7*, 224–232.

Bandura, A. (1977). Self-efficacy: Toward a unifying theory of behavioral change. *Psychological Review, 84*, 191–215.

Bandura, A. (1981). Self-referent thought: A developmental analysis of self-efficacy. In J. H. Flavell & L. Ross (Eds.), *Social Cognitive Development: Frontiers and Possible Futures* (pp. 200–239). New York: Cambridge University Press.

Bandura, A. (1986). *Social Foundations of Thought and Action: A Social Cognitive Theory*. Englewood Cliffs, NJ: Prentice Hall.

Bandura, A. (1997). *Self-Efficacy: The Exercise of Control*. New York: W.H. Freeman.

Baron, K., Kielhofner, G., Iyenger, A., Goldhammer, V., & Wolenski, J. (2002). *The Occupational Self Assessment* (ASA) (Version 2.0). Chicago: Model of Human Occupation Clearing House, Department of Occupational Therapy, College of Applied Health Sciences, University of Illinois at Chicago.

Baum, C., & Christensen, C. (2005). Person-environment-occupation performance: An occupation based framework for practice. In C. Christensen & C. Baum (Eds.), *Occupational Therapy: Performance, Participation and Well-Being* (pp. 243–266). Thorofare, NJ: Slack, Inc.

Beck, A. T. (1976). *Cognitive Therapy and the Emotional Disorders* (4th ed.). Madison, CT: International University Press.

Beck, A. T. (2005). The current state of cognitive therapy: A 40-year retrospective. *Archives of General Psychiatry, 62*, 953–959.

Beck, A. T., Freeman, A. M., Davis, D. D., & Associates. (2003). *Cognitive Therapy of Personality Disorders* (2nd ed.). New York: Guilford Press.

Beck, A. T., Rush, A. J., Shaw, B. F., & Emery, G. (1979). *Cognitive Therapy of Depression*. New York: Guilford Press.

Beck, A. T., Wright, F. D., Newman, C. F., & Liese, B. S. (2001). *Cognitive Therapy of Substance Abuse*. New York: Guilford Press.

Beck, J. S. (1995). *Cognitive Therapy: Basics and Beyond*. New York: Guilford Press.

Bennett-Levy, J. (2003). Mechanisms of change in cognitive therapy: The case of automatic thought records and behavioural experiments. *Behavioural and Cognitive Psychotherapy, 31*, 261–277.

Blankstein, K. R., & Segal, Z. V. (2001). Cognitive assessment: Issues and methods. In K. S. Dobson (Ed.), *Handbook of Cognitive Behavioral Therapies* (2nd ed., pp. 40–85). New York: Guilford Press.

Braswell, L., & Kendall, P. C. (2001). Cognitive-behavioral therapy with youth. In K. S. Dobson (Ed.), *Handbook of Cognitive-Behavioral Therapies* (2nd ed., pp. 246–294). New York: Guilford Press.

Bruce, M. A., & Borg, B. (2002). Cognitive-behavioral frame of reference—Thought and knowledge influence performance. In M. A. Bruce & B. Borg (Eds.), *Psychosocial Frames of Reference: Core for Occupation-Based Practice* (3rd ed., pp. 162–208). Thorofare, NJ: Slack.

Burns, D. D. (1993). *Ten Days to Self-Esteem.* New York: Harper-Collins.

Butler, A. C., Chapman, J. E., Forman, E. M., & Beck, A. T. (2006). The empirical status of cognitive-behavioral therapy: A review of meta-analyses. *Clinical Psychology Review, 26,* 17–31.

Cather, C. (2005). Functional cognitive-behavioural therapy: A brief, individual treatment for functional impairments resulting from psychotic symptoms in schizophrenia. *Canadian Journal of Psychiatry, 50*(5), 258–263.

Cole, K., & Vaughan, F. (2005). The feasibility of using cognitive behavior therapy for depression associated with Parkinson's disease: A literature review. *Parkinsonism & Related Disorders, (11),* 269–276.

Cook, A. (2004). Health education programming for older adults based on social cognitive theory. *Gerontology: Special Interest Section Quarterly, 27,* 1–3.

Cooper, M. J. (2005). Cognitive theory in anorexia nervosa and bulimia nervosa: Progress, development and future directions. *Clinical Psychology Review, 25,* 511–531.

Cooper, Z., Fairburn, C. G., & Hawkes, D. M. (2003). *Cognitive-Behavioral Treatment of Obesity: A Clinician's Guide.* New York: Guilford Press.

Crist, P. H. (1986). Community living skills: A psychoeducational community-based program. *Occupational Therapy in Mental Health, 6,* 51–64.

Cuijpers, P., van Straten, A., & Warmerdam, C. (2007). Behavioral activation treatment of depression: A meta-analysis. *Clinical Psychology Review, 27,* 318–326.

Dagnan, D., Chadwick, P., & Proudlove, J. (2000). Toward an assessment of suitability of people with mental retardation for cognitive therapy. *Cognitive Therapy and Research, 24*(6), 627–636.

Davis, L. W., Lysaker, P. H., Lancaster, R. S., Bryson, G. J., & Bell, H. D. (2005). The Indianapolis Vocational Intervention Program: A cognitive behavioral approach to addressing rehabilitation issues in schizophrenia. *Journal of Rehabilitation Research & Development, 42*(1), 35–46.

Deegan, P. E. (1994). Recovery: The lived experience of rehabilitation. In W. A. Anthony & L. Spaniol (Eds.), *Readings in Psychiatric Rehabilitation* (pp. 149–160). Boston: Boston University Centre for Psychiatric Rehabilitation.

DeRubeis, R. J., Tang, T. Z., & Beck, A. T. (2001). Cognitive therapy. In K. S. Dobson (Ed.), *Handbook of Cognitive Behavioral Therapies* (2nd ed., pp. 349–392). New York: Guilford Press.

Dryden, W., & Ellis, A. (2001). Rational emotive therapy. In K. S. Dobson (Ed.), *Handbook of Cognitive Behavioral Therapy* (2nd ed., pp. 295–348). New York: Guilford Press.

Dugas, M. J., & Robichaud, M. (2007). *Cognitive-Behavioral Treatment for Generalized Anxiety Disorder: From Science to Practice.* New York: Routledge.

Duncombe, L. (2005). The cognitive-behavioral model in mental health. In N. Katz (Ed.), *Cognition and Occupation Across the Life Span: Models for Intervention in Occupational Therapy* (2nd ed., pp. 187–210). Bethesda, MD: American Occupational Therapy Association Press.

Ellis, A. (1962). *Reason and Emotion in Psychotherapy.* New York: Lyle Stuart.

Ellis, A. (1993). Changing rational-emotive therapy (RET) to rational emotive behavior therapy (REBT). *Behavior Therapist, 16,* 257–258.

Ellis, A. (1994a). *Reason and Emotion in Psychotherapy, Revised and Updated.* Secaucus, NJ: Carol Publishing Group.

Ellis, A. (1994b). The treatment of borderline personalities with rational emotive behavior therapy. *Journal of Rationale-Emotive and Cognitive-Behavior Therapy, 12,* 101–119.

Ellis, A., & Vetten, E. (1992). *When AA Doesn't Work for You: Rational Separator Writing Alcohol.* New York: Barricade Books.

Eysenck, H. J. (1966). *The Effects of Psychotherapy.* New York: International Science Press.

Federico, J., & Kielhofner, G. (2002). *The Child Occupational Self Assessment (COSA) (Version 1.0).* Chicago: Model of Human Occupation Clearing House, Department of Occupational Therapy, College of Applied Health Sciences, University of Illinois at Chicago.

Feiring, C., & Cleland, C. (2007). Childhood sexual abuse and abuse-specific attributions of blame over 6 years following discovery. *Child Abuse and Neglect, 31,* 1169–1186.

Gage, M., Noh, S., Polatajko, H. J., & Kaspar, B. (1994). Measuring perceived self efficacy in occupational therapy. *American Journal of Occupational Therapy, 48,* 783–790.

Gage, M., & Polatajko, H. (1994). Enhancing occupational performance through an understanding of perceived self-efficacy. *American Journal of Occupational Therapy, 48,* 452–461.

Goldfried, M. R., & Davison, G. C. (1994). *Clinical Behavior Therapy* (2nd ed.). New York: John Wiley & Sons.

Harris, M. J., & Rosenthal, R. (1985). Mediation of interpersonal expectancy effects: 31 Meta-analyses. *Psychological Bulletin, 97,* 363–386.

Hays, P. A., & Iwamasa, G. Y. (Eds.). (2006). *Culturally Responsive Cognitive-Behavioral Therapy: Assessment, Practice, and Supervision.* Washington, DC: American Psychological Association.

Hopko, D. R., Lejuez, C. W., Ruggiero, K. J., & Eifert, G. H. (2003). Contemporary behavioral activation treatments for depression: Procedures, principles, and progress. *Clinical Psychology Review, 23,* 699–717.

Johnson, M. T. (1987). Occupational therapists and the teaching of cognitive behavioral skills. *Occupational Therapy in Mental Health, 7*(3), 69–81.

Kasl-Godley, J., & Gatz, M. (2000). Psychosocial interventions for individuals with dementia: An integration of theory, therapy, and a clinical understanding of dementia. *Clinical Psychology Review, 20*(6), 755–782.

Keilhofner, G. (2002). *Model of Human Occupation* (3rd ed.). Baltimore: Lippincott Williams & Wilkins.

Keilhofner, G., Mallinson, T., Crawford, C., Nowak, M., Rigby, M., Henry, A., & Walens, D. (1997). *A User's Guide to the Occupation Performance History Interview-II (OPHI-II) (Version 2.0).* Chicago: Model of Human Occupation Clearing House, Department of Occupational Therapy, College of Applied Health Sciences, University of Illinois at Chicago.

Khan-Bourne, N., & Brown, R. G. (2003). Cognitive behaviour therapy for the treatment of depression in individuals with brain injury. *Neuropsychological Rehabilitation, 13*(1–2), 89–107.

Landeen, J. L., Seeman, M. V., Goering, P., & Streiner, D. (2007). Schizophrenia: Effect of perceived stigma on two dimensions of recovery. *Clinical Schizophrenia & Related Psychoses, April,* 64–68.

Law, M., Baptiste, S., Carswell, A., McColl, M. A., Polatajko, H., & Pollock, N. (2005). *Canadian Occupational Performance Measure* (4th ed.). Ottawa, Ontario: Canadian Association of Occupational Therapists.

Law, M., Cooper, B., Strong, S., Stewart, D., Rigby, P., & Letts, L. (1996). The person-environment-occupational model: A transactive approach to occupational performance. *Canadian Journal of Occupational Therapy, 63,* 9–27.

Liao, K. L. (2000). Cognitive-behavioural approaches and weight management: An overview. *Journal of the Royal Society of Health, 120*(1), 27–30.

Linehan, M. M. (1993). *Cognitive-Behavioral Treatment of Borderline Personality Disorder.* New York. Guilford Press.

Lustig, D. C., & Strauser, D. R. (2003). An empirical typology of career thoughts of individuals with disabilities. *Rehabilitation Counseling Bulletin, 46*(2), 98–107.

Lyons, K. D. (2003). Self-management of Parkinson's disease: Guidelines for program development and evaluation. *Physical & Occupation Therapy in Geriatrics, 21*(3), 17–31.

Lysaker, P. H., Bond, G., Davis, L. W., Bryson, G. J., & Bell, M. D. (2005). Enhanced cognitive-behavioral therapy for vocational rehabilitation in schizophrenia: Effects on hope and work. *Journal of Rehabilitation Research and Development, 42*(5), 673–682.

Madon, S., Guyll, M., Spoth, R. L., Cross, S .E., & Hilber, S. (2003). The self-fulfilling influence of mother expectations on children's underage drinking. *Journal of Personality and Social Psychology, 84,* 1188–1205.

Mahoney, M. J. (1974). *Cognition and Behavior Modification.* Cambridge, MA: Ballinger.

Mahoney, M. J. (1977). Reflections on the cognitive learning trend in psychotherapy. *American Psychologist, 32,* 5–13.

McCraith, D. B. (1998). "Occupational Therapy Mental Health Practice Using a Cognitive-Behavioral Model." Handout presented at the World Federation of Occupational Therapists (WFOT) International Congress, June 1, Montreal, Canada.

Meichenbaum, D. (1977). *Cognitive-Behavior Modification: An Integrative Approach.* New York: Plenum Press.

Meichenbaum, D. (1992). Evolution of cognitive behavior therapy: Origins, tenets, and clinical examples. In J. K. Zeig (Ed.), *The Evolution of Psychotherapy—2nd Conference* (pp. 114–122). New York: Brunner/Mazel.

Meichenbaum, D., & Cameron, R. (1973). Training schizophrenics to talk to themselves: A means of developing attentional controls. *Behavior Therapy, 4,* 515–534.

Meichenbaum, D., & Goodwin, J. (1971). Training impulsive children to talk to themselves: A means of developing self-control. *Journal of Abnormal Psychology, 77,* 115–126.

Meyer, A. (1977). Philosophy of occupational therapy. *American Journal of Occupational Therapy, 31*(10). [Reprinted from A. Meyer. (1922). *Archives of Occupational Therapy, 1,* 1–10.]

Molton, I. R., Graham, C., Stoelb, B. C., & Jensen, M. P. (2007). Current psychological approaches to the management of chronic pain. *Current Opinion in Anaesthesiology, 20,* 485–489.

Mooney, K. A., & Padesky, C. A. (2000). Applying client creativity to recurrent problems: Constructing possibilities and tolerating doubt. *Journal of Cognitive Psychotherapy: An International Quarterly, 14*(2), 149–161.

Okazaki, S., & Tanaka-Matsumi, J. (2006). Cultural considerations in cognitive-behavioral assessment. In P. A. Hays & G. Y. Iwamasa (Eds.), *Culturally Responsive Cognitive-Behavioral Therapy: Assessment, Practice, and Supervision* (pp. 247–266). Washington, DC: American Psychological Association.

Padesky, C. (1993). "Socratic Questioning: Changing Minds or Guided Discovery?" Keynote address delivered at the European Congress of Behavioural and Cognitive Therapies, September 24, London. Available at: http://www.padesky.com/clinicalcorner/pdf/socquest.pdf. (accessed February 25, 2010).

Padesky, C. A., & Greenberger, D. (1995). *Clinician's Guide to Mind Over Mood.* New York: Guilford Press.

Pajares, M. F. (1992). Teachers' beliefs and educational research: Cleaning up a messy construct. *Review of Educational Research, 62*(3), 307–332.

Perkins, K. A., Conklin, C. A., & Levine, M. D. (2008). *Cognitive-Behavioral Therapy for Smoking Cessation: A Practical Guidebook to the Most Effective Treatments.* New York: Routledge.

Pfammatter, M., Junghan, U. M., & Brenner, H. D. (2006). Efficacy of psychological therapy in schizophrenia: Conclusions from meta-analyses. *Schizophrenia Bulletin, 32*(S1), S64–S80.

Polatajko, H. J., & Mandich, A. (2004). *Enabling Occupation in Children: The Cognitive Orientation to Daily Occupational Performance (CO-OP) Approach.* Ottawa, Ontario: Canadian Association of Occupational Therapists.

Price, J. R., Mitchell, E., Tidy, E., & Hunot, V. (2008). Cognitive behaviour therapy for chronic fatigue syndrome in adults. *Cochrane Database of Systematic Reviews, (3).* Art. No.: CD001027. DOI: 10.1002/14651858.CD001027.pub2.

Ridgeway, P. (2001). Restorying psychiatric disability learning from first person recovery narratives. *Psychiatric Rehabiliation Journal, 24,* 335–343.

Rosenfeld, M. A. (Ed.). (1997). *Motivational Strategies in Geriatric Rehabilitation.* Bethesda, MD: American Occupational Therapy Association.

Schneider, J. K., Mercer, G., Herning, M., Smith, C., & Davis, M. (2004). Promoting exercise behavior in older adults: Using a cognitive behavioral intervention. *Journal of Gerontological Nursing, 30,* 45–53.

Skinner, B. F. (1953). *Science and Human Behavior.* New York: Macmillan.

Snyder, M., & Stukas, A. A. (1999). Interpersonal processes: The interplay of cognitive, motivational, and behavioral activities in social interaction. *Annual Review of Psychology, 50,* 273–303.

Stein, F., & Smith, J. (1989). Short-term stress management programme with acutely depressed in-patients. *Canadian Journal of Occupational Therapy, 56,* 185–191.

Strong, J. (1998). Incorporating cognitive-behavioral therapy with occupational therapy: A comparative study with patients with low back pain. *Journal of Occupational Rehabilitation, 8*(1), 61–71.

Sullivan, W. M. (1994). A long and winding road: The process of recovery from severe mental illness. *Innovations and Research, 3*(3), 19–27.

Tanaka-Matsumi, J., Higginbotham, H. N., & Chang, R. (2002). Cognitive-behavioral approaches to counseling across cultures: A functional analytic approach for clinical applications. In P. B. Pedersen, W. J. Lonner, J. G. Draguns, & J. E. Trimble (Eds.), *Counseling Across Cultures* (5th ed., pp. 337–354). Thousand Oaks, CA: Sage.

Tanaka-Matsumi, J., Seiden, D., & Lam, K. (1996). The Culturally Informed Functional Assessment (CIFA) interview: A strategy for cross-cultural behavioral practice. *Cognitive and Behavioral Practice, 3,* 215–233.

Terjesen, M. D., DiGiuseppe, R., & Gruner, P. (2000). A review of REBT research in alcohol abuse treatment. *Journal of Rationale-Emotive and Cognitive-Behavior Therapy, 18*(3), 165–179.

Thorn, B. E. (2004). *Cognitive Therapy for Chronic Pain: A Step-By-Step Guide.* New York: Guilford Press.

van de Wiel, N., Matthys, W., Cohen-Kettenis, P. C., & van Engeland, H. (2002). Effective treatments of school-aged conduct disordered children: Recommendations for changing clinical and research practices. *European Child and Adolescent Psychiatry, 11,* 79–84.

Vernon, A. (2006). Depression in children and adolescents: REBT approaches to assessment and treatment. In A. Ellis & M. E. Bernard (Eds.), *Rational Emotive Behavioral Approaches to Childhood Disorders: Theory, Practice and Research* (pp. 212–231). New York: SpringerLink.

Vernon, A., & Bernard, M. E. (2006). Applications of REBT in schools: Prevention, promotion, intervention. In A. Ellis & M. E. Bernard (Eds.), *Rational Emotive Behavioral Approaches to Childhood Disorders: Theory, Practice and Research* (pp. 415–460). New York: SpringerLink.

Watts, J. H., Hinson, R., Madigan, M. J., McGuigan, P. M., & Newman, S. M. (1999). The Assessment of Occupational Functioning–Collaborative Version. In B. J. Hempill-Pearson (Ed.), *Assessments in Occupational Therapy in Mental Health* (pp. 239–248). Thorofare, NJ: Slack.

Wolpe, J. (1958). *Psychotherapy by Reciprocal Inhibition.* Stanford, CA: Stanford University Press.

World Health Organization (WHO). (2001). *International Classification of Functioning, Disability and Health (ICF).* Geneva, Switzerland: Author.

Wright, J., Thase, M., Ludgate, J., & Beck, A. T. (1993). The cognitive milieu: Structure and process. In J. Wright, M. Thase, J. Ludgate, & A. T. Beck, *Cognitive Therapy With Inpatients: Developing a Cognitive Milieu* (pp. 61–87). New York: Guilford Press.

CHAPTER 20

Sensory Skills

Catana Brown and Rebecca Nicholson

> "Not the senses I have but what I do with them is my kingdom.

—Helen Keller

Introduction

Barb and Joan are friends who like to go to the same exercise class; however, when they get to the gym they position themselves in different corners of the room. Barb likes to be in a spot where a large fan blows directly on her, whereas Joan is strategically located so that she can't feel the wind from any of the fans in the room.

Two children, Joshua and Aaron, attend the same preschool. Joshua digs right into the finger paints, play dough, and mud pile outside, whereas Aaron dislikes getting his hands dirty. He really enjoys the building blocks and puzzles at the school.

Allison and Sarah are college roommates. Allison likes to stay in the busy dormitory and study in the room with the radio playing or the TV turned on. Sarah finds this too distracting and has found a quiet study room in the library.

These individuals are successfully engaging in important occupations, but their preferences and ways of going about these occupations differ. These individuals have different reactions to sensation. Without even thinking about it, most people make choices about activities and create an environment that supports their own sensory preferences. However, sometimes we are unable to make adjustments to an environment, we lack self-awareness about our sensory preferences, or our sensory preferences are so constricting that they interfere with daily life. In these situations, occupational therapists can use their knowledge about sensory processing to design interventions that allow individuals to engage in important occupations, regardless of their particular sensory preferences.

Sensory Processing

Sensory processing is the means by which we obtain information about the world and our own bodies. In occupational therapy, the term *sensory integration* is often used broadly to refer to the same construct. However, drawing on the consensus work published in the *Sensory Integration Special Interest Section Quarterly* (Lane, Miller, & Hanft, 2000; Miller & Lane, 2000), the terms *sensory processing* and *sensory integration* are distinguished in this chapter. Sensory processing is the larger construct that encompasses sensory integration.

Sensory processing involves multiple steps at both the neural and behavioral levels. It includes noticing a stimulus, recognizing or classifying the stimulus, and then understanding or giving meaning to the stimulus. After the stimulus is processed, a behavioral response can occur. For example, when driving, you may startle when hearing a loud and unexpected noise, look in your rearview mirror, and determine that the noise is an ambulance siren coming from behind. You then decide that you should move out of the way and react by pulling over to the side of the road to let the ambulance pass.

Sensory integration, in contrast, is limited to the processes involved in organizing multiple sensations from the environment and the person's own body. According to Ayres (1979), sensory integration is followed by an adaptive response, which involves "a purposeful, goal directed response to a sensory experience" (p. 6). When playing tennis, you bring together the visual input of the ball, the tactile input of the racket in your hand, and the vestibular and proprioceptive input to position yourself to return the ball.

Sensory processing begins with the nervous system noticing or detecting sensory stimuli. Our nervous system relies on the peripheral ends of sensory neurons, or receptors, to detect sensory stimuli. There are different types of receptors for different types of sensory information. For example, chemoreceptors detect chemicals in the environment and are used in taste and smell, whereas mechanoreceptors detect changes in pressure, position, and acceleration, and are important in vestibular and proprioceptive perception. The receptors are concentrated on sensory organs such as the taste buds of the tongue, which act as the chemoreceptors for taste.

Stimulation of a neural receptor results in an action potential. When the stimulus is strong (e.g., the noise is loud, the lights are bright, the taste is intense), the neurons fire more rapidly, or more receptors respond, or for a longer period of time. In other words, the person is more likely to notice the stimulus because of the neuronal response. A weak stimulus results in impulses that are slower, shorter in duration, or involve fewer receptors. There is individual variability in receptor sensitivity based on the individual's threshold for detecting a particular stimulus. Many people have experienced a situation in which one person notices a smell, sound, or visual stimulus that another person missed. Within this continuum of receptor sensitivity, there can be great variability among individuals who remain functional. However, some individuals may be so **hyperresponsive** or so **hyporesponsive** that their conditions interfere with daily life.

After receptor stimulation, the second step of sensory processing involves the brain recognizing or classifying a stimulus. For example, the pitch and volume of a sound are deciphered into human speech, or a chemical in the environment is translated by the olfactory bulb as the smell of coffee brewing. Once a stimulus is identified, we typically attribute meaning to that information (e.g., words are not just sounds but can tell a story or provide a warning) and assimilate that information into what we are doing at the time.

Finally, the behavioral response to the stimulus is a complex reaction that can occur at the level of conscious or unconscious awareness and usually includes cognitive and motor processing. For example, after smelling the coffee, you may get out a mug and pour yourself a cup. Then again, you may decide that you have already had too much caffeine for the day and go on to something else.

Occupational therapists are concerned with all steps of sensory processing. Although most of the activity involved in sensory processing occurs at the neuronal level, occupational therapists may infer what is happening in the nervous system based on behavioral observation (Miller & Lane, 2000). It is important to recognize this distinction because our inferences may be incorrect at times. For example, an individual receiving a hug stiffens and makes a face that suggests displeasure. The therapist may interpret this response as tactile defensiveness, indicating the stimuli are too intense for this person. However, this assumption may be incorrect; the individual could be responding this way because he or she does not like the person doing the hugging. A simple solution in this case would be to ask the person about the reaction. Understanding the neurological systems involved provides important information to guide occupational therapy assessment and intervention. Questions the occupational therapist might ask when making an observation include the following:

- Does the person notice relevant stimuli, and can he or she screen out or habituate to irrelevant information?
- Can the person identify the sensory stimulus correctly?
- Does the person use the information effectively to better understand the environment or his or her own body?
- Does the person respond in a way that is productive or adaptive?

Sensory Processing Disorders

Recently, several experts in sensory processing disorders developed a nosology of sensory processing disorders to clarify different conditions (Miller, Anzalone, Lane, Cermak, & Osten, 2007). There are three classic patterns: sensory modulation disorders, sensory-based motor disorders, and sensory discrimination disorders. Each pattern includes subtypes.

The modulation disorders exist when behavioral responses are inconsistent with the available sensory stimuli such that some individuals underrespond, some overrespond, and others have an insatiable desire for a particular sensation. The sensory-based motor disorders include postural problems or difficulty stabilizing the body when moving and dyspraxia, which appears as poor motor planning or uncoordinated movement. Sensory discrimination disorders occur when the individual has difficulty processing sensory stimuli. This can be present in any of the sensory modalities. The role of the occupational therapist in assessment is to determine the particular area of sensory processing difficulty. Later in the chapter, particular assessment approaches are discussed. As an initial proposal, it is expected that this nosology will change with additional research.

Sensory Modalities

When asked to identify **sensory modalities**, people generally think of the five senses: vision, hearing, touch, taste and smell. However, there are two additional senses that are important. The proprioceptive and vestibular senses provide information that is essential to effective movement. The next section briefly describes each of the sensory modalities.

Visual System

Humans rely heavily on the visual system. The visual system provides information about the properties of an object, such as shape, size and color, and can tell us how close or far away something is. The lens of the eye is involved in focusing and, therefore, is connected with visual acuity (the ability to see things clearly). The visual field is the area in which an individual can see. In humans, the visual field of each eye overlaps, which creates our ability to perceive depth.

Photoreceptors are the receptors for the visual system, and there are two types: cones and rods. Rods are best at detecting motion and are more prominent on the periphery of the retina. Cones allow for the perception of color and produce sharp images in bright light. Schneider (1969) was one of the first to describe "two visual systems," with one system for movement (where something is) and the other for form (what something is). Parallel processing of form and movement is supported by clinical evidence (Kandel, Schwartz, & Jessell, 2000). For example, a lesion of the cerebral cortex can result in loss of vision for movement, yet the individual may still have adequate vision for form.

Auditory System

Like the visual system, the auditory system is important in the location of objects in the environment. In addition, the auditory system provides us with information about sounds, one of the most important being information about speech. Humans have an amazing ability to selectively attend to auditory input. Unlike visual stimuli, to which it is difficult to selectively attend (i.e., look in a particular direction and determine what you will and will not notice), with auditory input we frequently decide to listen to one conversation over another or ignore ambient sounds in the background.

Auditory input comes in the form of waves that can be measured in terms of amplitude and frequency. When the amplitude and frequency falls within our range, we can detect the sound. Amplitude refers to the number of vibrating particles, which accounts for its loudness. The frequency of sound is the rate at which the waves pass a given point. Frequency is roughly related to the pitch of a sound.

The detection of a sound begins when sound waves produce a vibration of the eardrum. This vibration is transmitted through the fluids of the inner ear and then hair cells, which results in the firing of nerve fibers. We can also hear through bone conduction, such as when we hear ourselves speak or chew. The reason that we sound different to ourselves (were you surprised the first time you heard yourself on a recording?) is because we hear ourselves through both bone and air conduction, whereas others hear our voice only through air conduction.

Tactile System

The tactile system works through a variety of sensory receptors found in the skin. Some of the receptors lie close to the surface of the skin, whereas others are found in the deeper subcutaneous tissue. Some of the receptors respond to light touch, which is an arousing sensation that causes us to pay attention and notice something in our environment. Another type of receptor responds to pressure and is the discriminative element of the tactile system. Discriminative touch tells us where and what we are feeling. In addition, the skin contains thermoreceptors that recognize hot and cold, and nociceptors that detect pain.

Our ability to localize and discriminate touch depends on several factors. First, the concentration of tactile receptors is not consistent over the body. Generally, the skin is more sensitive distally (e.g., fingers, toes) than proximally (e.g., shoulders, trunk), and the face is particularly sensitive to pressure. The adaptive state of the skin also influences the detection of tactile stimuli. For example, if a steady pressure is applied to the skin, we are likely to habituate to it and lose awareness of the stimuli. We are less likely to habituate to weaker stimuli that are presented intermittently. This explains why generally people are not constantly aware of the feel of their clothing unless they move and the site and type of touch changes as the clothing moves against the skin. It also explains why deep pressure is comforting, and light touch is arousing.

It is important to note that tactile sensitivity is an important component of food preferences. In addition to the taste of a food, we are very aware of the texture or feel of the foods we eat. Often, dislike for a particular food can be attributed exclusively to its tactile characteristics rather than taste—such as the sliminess associated with raw oysters or the fuzzy texture of a peach skin.

Taste (Gustatory) and Smell (Olfactory) Systems

Taste and smell are primitive senses. Smell is the only sense that connects directly to the amygdala and hippocampus before going to the thalamus. The amygdala and hippocampus have functions that are associated with emotional responses and the consolidation of memories. This connection may explain why smell is so strongly associated with feelings and memories (Herz & Engen, 1996). Undoubtedly, you have had the experience when a smell "takes you back" to a specific place and point in time.

The **gustatory** and **olfactory systems** are chemical sensory systems that are highly connected. In the case of smell, airborne molecules enter the nasal cavity and are detected by olfactory receptors that extend into the nostril as cilia or hair. With taste, a chemical (typically in the form of food) is placed directly on the tongue to activate the receptors in the taste buds. However, many of the nuances associated with taste are actually attributed to olfaction because when we taste a food we almost always smell it. Taste and smell are very important in food selection and food avoidance. These senses can help us identify unsafe or unpleasant foods. Human are able to detect the presence of an odor with relatively low levels of a stimulus; however, our ability to recognize odors (i.e., name the smell) is poor.

Proprioceptive System

Proprioception is the awareness of the body's position in space. Although you are not aware of it, proprioception is required for even automatic activities such as walking. Walking requires awareness throughout the body to maintain an upright posture and to strike your foot in a manner that moves you forward. Proprioceptive receptors detect changes in the position of muscles and joints, which provides us with information about the relative position of our body in space. This sense does not provide us with information about the outside environment; rather, it gives us important information about our own body. All movement results in proprioceptive input, but this sense becomes particularly important when movements are conducted without visual input (e.g., touch typing).

Muscle spindles act as receptors, providing information about muscle length and velocity of stretch. Golgi tendon organs provide information at the site where the tendon meets muscle. Therefore, without looking, we know when we have raised our arm and can approximate where our arm is in relation to the rest of our body.

Vestibular System

Of all the senses, we are typically the least conscious of the vestibular system—unless it becomes dysfunctional, and we experience the unpleasant sensations of dizziness and nausea. The **vestibular system** is responsible for balance through detection of the position and movement of the head in space. Receptors located in the semicircular canals of the inner ear lie in three different planes; thus, they are able to detect movement of the head in any direction. In addition to keeping the body balanced, the vestibular system allows us to keep our eyes fixed on a particular point in space even when our body is moving around.

Rarely do the sensory systems work independently. The simple act of taking notes in class provides a good example. The vestibular system keeps you balanced in your chair and helps you move your eyes from the instructor to your paper. In addition, there is the sensation of hearing the lecture, the use of visual input to keep your writing on the lines, and a great deal of tactile and proprioceptive sense to hold the pen and form the letters. Imagine how difficult the task would become without the input of just one of the sensory modalities. What would your notes look like if you could not see the page? How would you form the letters if you cannot sense the small movement of your hand?

We often take our senses for granted unless there is a problem. Children and adults with psychiatric disabilities can have sensory processing impairments that interfere with their daily life. The next section describes sensory processing impairments that are associated with particular psychiatric diagnoses.

Sensory Processing and Children With Psychiatric Disabilities

Working with children provides opportunities to observe the influence of sensory issues in their purest form. Walk into any preschool, and you can observe children reveling in the opportunity to create an artistic masterpiece using finger paints or diving into the sand or water tables. There will also be those children who are cautiously observing these activities at an arm's length.

Other children are unaware that certain sensory experiences are creating feelings of anxiety, distractibility, and even anger. Children are often unable to articulate or understand what is upsetting to them. For example, at the most primitive levels, a baby cries when it is hungry or wet, and a toddler throws a temper tantrum when splashed by a peer in the wading pool. However, in some cases, reactions to sensory experiences can result in behaviors that are disruptive to the child's daily life and sometimes to those around them. Teachers and parents are often unaware that there may be underlying sensory issues and may attempt to alleviate the problem through a strictly behavioral approach. Although behavioral strategies can be helpful when used in conjunction with sensory interventions, ignoring the sensory influences will not alleviate the problem and may make it worse.

The following sections explain sensory processing impairments that are associated with attention deficit-hyperactivity disorder (ADHD), autism spectrum disorder, and learning disabilities.

Attention Deficit-Hyperactivity Disorder

Children diagnosed with ADHD have patterns of sensory processing that are different from the typical child (Dunn, 1999). It is important to understand that children with ADHD do not simply have the inability to attend to information; rather, they have difficulty attending to relevant information in combination with filtering out extraneous stimulation.

This inability to process sensory information in their daily lives often leads to behavioral and social emotional problems. In one study, researchers examined health problems associated with ADHD, using the health-related quality of life questionnaires (Klassen, Miller, & Fine, 2004). Participants reported clinically important problems in psychosocial areas such as self-esteem, involvement in family activities, and emotional behavioral problems. In addition, the study explored the effects of this diagnosis on parents' emotional health and the negative effects on the function of the family in general daily life activities.

Vignette: ADHD — Tyler

An occupational therapist was providing services to Tyler, a first-grader with ADHD who was placed in a highly structured classroom. The teacher had a strict behavioral program in place that significantly limited movement in the classroom. The first-graders had individual trash receptacles placed at their desks, and there were no out-of-seat activities for a large portion of the morning. Even activities such as pencil sharpening occurred only at designated times. The team believed that this type of structure would be the answer for Tyler, who seemed to be in constant motion. Although the program was successful in limiting Tyler's out-of-seat behavior, he grew more anxious each day in the classroom.

After a few days in the classroom, the OT went to check with the teacher to see how things were going. This visit occurred during one of the designated movement times. The teacher reported successfully eliminating unnecessary movement, although task completion was still an issue. The children filed off to the restroom. As Tyler began walking down the hall, pieces of his clothing fell to the floor. By the time he had reached the restroom, most of his jeans and a large portion of his shirt were missing. Although Tyler had not been out of his seat all morning, he had been cutting his clothing rather than completing the group art project.

Although this vignette represents an extreme case of ADHD, it illustrates the fact that behavioral approaches can be ineffective in extinguishing sensory processing difficulties. Using a sensory frame of reference, the occupational therapist can provide insight to the types of sensory problems that interfere with daily performance and offer strategies to reduce the negative reactions to the sensory experiences. For Tyler, allowing periods of movement was critical to his ability to concentrate on the task at hand. When he was required to sit for long periods of time, he was less likely to attend to classroom tasks. In his case, the team reconvened, and a different classroom was selected that gave Tyler increased opportunities for movement throughout his day and a vestibular disk placed on his chair for in-seat activities. When movement strategies were incorporated into his classroom routine, his productivity increased. It is important to note that, in addition to sensory issues that interfered with performance, Tyler had cognitive challenges as well. It was the combination of adaptations in the cognitive demands, such as removing distractors and creating the optimal sensory environment, that led to more success in academic performance.

Allowing movement within the classroom is sometimes considered unacceptable to classroom teachers, but some of the literature suggests otherwise. In one study, the use of therapy balls for seating in classrooms during language arts activities was examined (Schilling, Washington, Billingsley, & Deitz, 2003). This study, completed on a group of 30 fourth-grade students, 3 of whom had been diagnosed with ADHD, found improvements in seated behaviors as well as increased legibility on writing tasks when seated on the therapy balls. All 3 of the subjects with ADHD reported that they found the use of therapy balls to be helpful in respect to comfort and ability to complete assignments in the classroom.

Children with ADHD often present patterns of sensory processing related to movement that are different from the typical child (Dunn,1999); however, it is important to recognize that patterns of sensory processing for children with ADHD are highly variable (Mangeot et al, 2001). Therefore, educational teams should resist the temptation to prescribe any sensory intervention based on diagnosis alone. For example, the use of weighted vests has been demonstrated to increase on-task behavior for children with ADHD (Vandenberg, 2001). Although this study provides support for deep pressure input for children with ADHD, it cannot be assumed that all children with ADHD would benefit from the use of a weighted vest. The child, the environment, and the demands of the activity are all important considerations in designing sensory interventions.

See Chapter 8 for more information on ADHD.

Autism Spectrum Disorder

It is important to note that the current accepted diagnostic criteria for pervasive developmental disorders, which include autism and Asperger's disorder, do not include difficulties with sensory processing. However, first-hand accounts of adults with autism include descriptions of sensory experiences such as an aversion to touch and a hypersensitivity to auditory stimuli. In an article by O'Neill and Jones (1997), possible problems with accepting these accounts as accurate are explored. Difficulties such as influence by coauthors, the respondents lack of understanding regarding what is "typical," and the fact that these accounts are from individuals on the high end of the functional continuum of autism warrant caution when interpreting these accounts. Therefore, making generalizations about what all children with autism experience in day-to-day sensory experiences is not advisable. In addition, the research may not always clearly describe the complexity of their responses in terms of cognitive, behavioral, and sensory influences. However, the authors acknowledge that, despite problems with overgeneralization of these accounts, there is adequate evidence to support the idea that abnormalities in sensory processing are often associated with diagnoses on the autism spectrum.

Although current criteria for diagnosis of autism and Asperger's disorder do not include impaired sensory processing, studies suggest that further investigation into sensory processing is warranted. Researchers such as Blakemore et al (2006) found evidence of hypersensitivity to certain tactile stimuli. In their study, they were able to demonstrate that children with Asperger's disorder had hypersensitive reactions to stimulation that was imposed on them from an outside source, but had a normal response to tactile stimulation they controlled. Hypersensitivity to touch in autism was also supported by research in the development of the Sensory Profile Questionnaire (Dunn, 1999; Kientz & Dunn, 1997). Lepisto et al (2005) examined the auditory processing of children with autism and found enhanced sound discrimination related to pitch. From this research study, the authors proposed a possible link between the hypersensitivity to low-level pitch and inability to comprehend higher-level language function. In these subjects, their comprehension of the meaning of speech decreased when they demonstrated superior skills in pitch processing; that is, the authors proposed that the hypersensitivity in these discrete areas of speech possibly interfered with their ability to derive meaning from speech.

In a study by Pierce, Glad, and Schreibman (1997), social perception by children with autism was examined. In this study, the investigators found that children with autism performed significantly poorer on tasks requiring visual recognition and processing of multiple social cues presented in short video vignettes. An interesting finding of this study was that it was only when the children were required to process multiple social cues that there were significant differences from typical children. These authors propose that it is possible that children with autism are not as impaired in visual recognition of social cues as is generally accepted; rather, it is when confronted with processing multiple environmental cues in combination that the interpretation of social experiences breaks down.

Children with disorders on the autism spectrum often have reactions to certain sensory experiences that interfere with their ability to perform daily life tasks. Children with autism sometimes have a heightened awareness of sensory stimulation and may even have unusual abilities related to sensory experiences.

Evidence-Based Practice

Deep pressure touch can have a calming influence. One way of providing a constant source of deep pressure is through the use of weighted vests. There is evidence that the use of weighted vests can increase on-task behavior for children with ADHD.

➤ Occupational therapists can consider weighted vests or other methods of deep pressure input for children with ADHD.

Vandenberg, D. L. (2001). The use of a weighted vest to increase on-task behavior in children with attention difficulties. *American Journal of Occupational Therapy*, 55(6), 621–628.

Vignette: Autism—Shawn

Shawn was an 8-year-old child with autism who had a heightened response to auditory stimulation. Often, she would be observed talking in her classroom at what appeared to be inappropriate times. The topics would be unrelated to what was happening in class, and it was difficult to refocus her attention on the subject at hand. On further examination of the verbalizations, the paraprofessional realized that Shawn was repeating exact phrases that were being spoken across the hall in another classroom.

In addition, Shawn would frequently come to school in the morning and begin reciting entire conversations between members of her family. After observing this child for some time, the educational team determined that when Shawn was provided with visual cues, she was able to concentrate on the relevant auditory stimulation in the environment. Working on a computer with head phones was a particularly successful activity.

Shawn's situation illustrates the extreme impact that a sensory processing issue can have on classroom participation. Although all children with sensory processing disorders have unique sensory needs, children with autism have different levels of need. Their seeking behaviors and avoidance behaviors go beyond just interfering with their ability to function. The child with autism is often dominated by the fear of certain stimuli or driven to the point of obsession to seek the stimulation they crave. Temple Grandin (2000), an adult with Asperger's disorder, describes her experiences as a child in a paper entitled, "My Experiences with Visual Thinking Sensory Problems and Communication Difficulties." Temple had an extreme hypersensitivity to touch and auditory stimulation. She described the following account from her childhood:

> When I was a child, I feared the ferry boat that took us to our summer vacation home. When the boat's horn blew, I threw myself on the floor and screamed. Autistic children and adults may fear dogs or babies because barking dogs or crying babies may hurt their ears. Dogs and babies are unpredictable, and they can make a hurtful noise without warning. . . . (p. 1)

When we accept the idea that stimulation for some children is not just upsetting, but even painful, it becomes clear that identifying the processing patterns is critical in the process of helping the child participate in daily activities. One of the challenges in working with children with autism is that it is difficult to release our own ideas about how we perceive stimulation from the environment; that is, we often make assumptions about how a child with autism is interpreting information based on how we would interpret it. A classical example of this is the general assumption that, when a child is not visually attending to a person or an activity, he or she is not engaged in the task.

Brockmeyer and Bundy (2001) describe the experiences of four adults with Asperger's disorder when questioned about the topic of eye contact during conversation. These individuals indicated that comprehending the verbal portion of the interaction was more difficult if they engaged in eye contact. In addition, the individuals with autism explained that the act of providing eye contact lacked social meaning.

We know that poor understanding of social cues is one of the criteria for the diagnosis of autism. Visual attention and, specifically, eye contact is one of the component skills of social interaction that is socially valued. However, we should consider the possibility that eye contact is an expectation of the person without autism who is engaging in the conversation, not the individual with autism. People with autism have identified strategies such as looking at the person's eyebrows or ears in an effort to concentrate on the conversation and still provide cues that they were in fact engaged in the interaction.

When we set expectations for certain skills to be in place in order for a child with autism to participate, we may, in fact, be interfering with strategies that the child has in place for coping with differences in his or her ability to process sensory information. For example, the child may be better equipped to attend to a classroom task if he or she were allowed to move to another part of the room when noise levels increase. We take for granted how few opportunities children in educational settings have to make decisions about the amount and type of stimulation they can handle in a given situation. When confronted with a situation that they may find overwhelming, children with autism may resort to behavioral outbursts because of lack of control of implementing coping strategies that are available to adults in the same situation.

Dunn, Myles, and Orr (2002) studied the sensory processing patterns of children with Asperger's disorder and found evidence of problems with sensory modulation, suggesting a fluctuating response that is both hypersensitive and hyposensitive. For example, a child may have extreme reactions to certain types of loud, unpredictable noises, such as when peers in the classroom become upset and yell or scream. Yet, surprisingly, the same child is not bothered by the loud ringing of the monthly fire drill alarm.

Pfeiffer, Kinnealey, Reed, and Herzberg (2005) examined the relationships between dysfunctions in sensory modulation, affective disorders, and adaptive behaviors in children and adolescents with Asperger's disorder. These researchers found significant relationships between hypersensitivity to sensory stimulation and negative impacts on community use and social skills. For example, hypersensitivity may prevent a child from play that involves physical contact or make it difficult to stand in line or attend community events that involve crowds. One explanation for the negative effects is that children and adolescents with Asperger's disorder do not have effective coping methods for dealing with the hypersensitivity, unlike adults, who are capable of recognizing their limitations and planning their lives accordingly. When a child is hypersensitive to certain types of sensory stimulation, he or she has little control in the educational setting. A child who cannot handle the noise and activity level of the gymnasium will not be excused from gym class. However, if the child's behavior disrupts the class or he or she becomes aggressive toward another student, the child is usually removed from the situation.

Occupational therapists are often asked to assist in developing interventions when children are unable to participate in educational activities. Too often, the referral is made based on a performance outcome, which may only be a small piece of the puzzle.

Evidence-Based Practice

Educational strategies such as reducing task difficulty and using small interactive groups and direct response questions are effective classroom techniques for children with learning disabilities.

➤ Occupational therapists should combine educational and sensory strategies when developing interventions for children with learning disabilities.

Vaughn, S., Gersten, R., & Chard, D. (2000). The underlying message in LD intervention research: Findings from research syntheses. *Exceptional Children*, 67(1), 99–114.

Vignette: Asperger's Disorder — David

David is an 11-year-old boy with Asperger's disorder who has been placed in a self-contained behavior disorder classroom for most of his academic instruction. He was removed from his classroom because of a biting incident on the playground and then referred to occupational therapy following an outside evaluation that revealed a significant delay on a standardized motor assessment. In addition, the classroom teacher indicated that he was unable to complete written work in the classroom.

The occupational therapist went into the classroom to observe his performance and carefully explained that she was there to help him improve his handwriting in class. He glanced at her, carefully took his pencil and scribbled out: "I hate you. This is irrelevant." After watching him for a short time, the therapist agreed completely. Although it was true that David had limited ability to produce written work in the classroom, he was able to provide great detail about topics he was reading and could verbally respond to any content question. Although the teachers reported that David was not interested or able to use a word processor to complete his work, he had never received consistent instruction in keyboarding because his behavior prevented him from participating in computer lab. The noise, the close contact with others, and even the tactile experience of the keyboard was problematic for him.

If the therapist had continued to look at David from a developmental frame of reference and failed to recognize his difficulties with sensory modulation, she would have constructed a handwriting program in which he would be in daily conflict with his teachers, paraprofessionals, and parents. David was exactly on target. His handwriting was irrelevant. The amount of time, effort, and cooperation required on his part would never have justified the end result.

To provide David with a method to complete written work, the Dragon Naturally Speaking software program was installed on the computer in the library, where David could go to complete assignments in a quiet setting. This program typed whatever David spoke into the computer. The team still believed that it would be useful for David to learn to type, so he was given an AlphaSmart Neo equipped with a typing tutorial and Co-writer word prediction software package. This portable word processing device was with him both at home and at school, and provided an effective method of storing assignments throughout the day so his parents were able to easily see what needed to be completed. As David became more efficient with typing, Inspiration software was also loaded on the computer in the library to use David's strengths in visual processing. This software allowed David to create visual concepts maps when learning new material. The Inspiration software was also useful when organizing group projects in his gifted class.

See Chapter 7 for more information on pervasive developmental disorders.

Evidence-Based Practice

Research on children with autism indicates a hypersensitivity to touch when the stimuli is imposed on the child, but a normal response when the child is able to control the stimuli. Children with autism also have difficulty processing multiple visual social cues, but perform well when presented with only one cue at a time.

➤ Occupational therapists can develop interventions that allow children with autism to have control over available sensory input (particularly tactile input).

➤ Occupational therapists can help individuals with autism to interpret social cues by creating situations in which the amount of visual stimuli is reduced.

Blakemore, S. J., Tavassoli, T., Calo, S., Thomas, R. M., Catmur, C., Frith, U., & Haggard, P. (2006). Tactile sensitivity in Asperger syndrome. *Brain and Cognition, 61*, 5–13.

Pierce, K., Glad, K. S., & Schreibman, L. (1997). Social perception in children with autism: An attentional deficit. *Journal of Autism and Developmental Disorders, 27*(3), 265–282.

Learning Disabilities

In the *Diagnostic and Statistical Manual of Mental Disorders, Fourth Edition, Text Revision* (DSM-IV-TR) (American Psychiatric Association, 2000), learning disorders are described as performance in academic achievement that is significantly lower than would be expected based on IQ, age, and schooling. In some cases, sensory processing problems may contribute to the learning difficulty, but there is great diversity in the type of sensory issues found in children with learning disabilities. For example, one child may have difficulty processing auditory information, while for another visual processing is difficult. It is important to note that a large percentage of children with ADHD have a learning disability with one study finding rates as high as 70% (Mayes, Calhoun, & Crowell, 2000). Therefore, many of the sensory strategies that are effective for children with ADHD are applicable to children with learning disabilities. The following vignettes illustrate different sensory processing concerns for two children with learning disabilities and examples of how an occupational therapist might approach these concerns.

Vignette: Learning Disability — Jacob

Jacob was a first-grader with a learning disability who was also diagnosed with ADHD. Jacob had tremendous difficulty focusing on important information in the classroom. One day, when asked to recount what he had been working on during his morning academics, he replied, "Oh, a whole GLOB of things." It was the perfect metaphor to how he saw the world—as a "glob" of things with indistinguishable features.

Jacob drew a picture of his creative writing story that was impossible to interpret. Whereas most children can isolate one important event, Jacob tried to draw a pictorial representation of the entire story. At first glance, his picture appeared to be meaningless and disorganized. However, with a more careful review, it revealed amazing detail and insight. Still, even Jacob could not fully describe each detail because, once completed, it was so visually challenging that he could not decipher what had been drawn.

This was often the case with his written work as well. On the days he was highly motivated to complete a story, he would go into too much detail and sometimes meander around to different topics. Eventually, he would get lost in the descriptions, and his handwriting would deteriorate so profoundly that, much to his frustration, little of the story could be salvaged when it came time for the final draft.

Many children with learning disabilities learn quickly to edit their work down to the bare bones as a survival skill in the area of written language. Thus, a paragraph once rich with detail becomes a two-sentence description that is not representative of the child's true cognitive potential.

Evaluating the sensory processing skills for children with learning disabilities can provide the team with important information that may be beneficial to the design of interventions. With learning disabilities, it is also important for occupational therapists to examine educational strategies that are supported in the literature and provide the team with information regarding both sensory and educational strategies. In a meta-analysis summarizing research in the field of learning disabilities, Vaughn, Gersten, and Chard (2000) found that control of task difficulty (e.g., sequencing of examples, small amounts of instruction at one time), use of small interactive groups, and direct response questioning ("thinking aloud") were critical components to the most successful educational strategies.

For Jacob, his diagnosis of ADHD adds an additional dimension to these strategies. Jacob was able to successfully process visual information, but had significant difficulties processing auditory information. Therefore, when implementing strategies for Jacob to effectively control task difficulty, it would be important to use visual cues, demonstration, or modeling, rather than a more verbal approach. In implementing small group strategies, it would be important to consider the environment in which the small group would convene, with a focus on the possible auditory distractions that could interfere with the intervention. In addition, although much evidence exists to support the use of the direct response strategy, perhaps for Jacob this strategy would be more effectively implemented when he receives instruction in the resource room rather than in a large class setting, where he might have more difficulty processing the auditory information.

Vignette: Learning Disability— Robert

Robert was a bright child with incredible verbal abilities who was unable to master the most basic prereading skill of letter recognition. His mother worked with him on his handwriting program on a daily basis, and Robert was highly motivated to complete the assigned home program in order to receive his reward. He had amazing recall for details of stories that had been read to him and had a well-developed vocabulary. He could also perform advanced math functions. However, Robert was well aware of his shortcomings and frequently resorted to manipulative behaviors to draw attention away from the skills he lacked. He had exceptional motor skills, but initially was not able to write a single letter after a full year of kindergarten.

One day when working with Robert, the occupational therapist began to discover the breadth of Robert's disability. He was pushing the limits at every turn. The therapist engaged in a discussion that would have been beyond the understanding of the average kindergartner, but in using a metaphor Robert was able to start talking about his problems. The occupational therapist described an angry meter explaining that everyone has an angry meter, and different things can make the angry meter have a high reading. The therapist informed Robert that his behavior had indeed activated her angry meter, and it was almost at the highest limit. This little description of a concrete representation of anger really hit home with Robert. He immediately started to tell the therapist about some of the things that activated his meter. Not the least of which was performing the daily letter recognition and phonics exercises in class. From that day forward, Robert never failed to ask the occupational therapist how her meter was doing and how his was measuring as well.

In contrast to Jacob, Robert's auditory processing was effective; however, his visual processing was not as strong. Robert was able to learn to write letters most effectively by coupling concrete verbal directions with the letter models. Although he was able to write every letter given a model, he was only able to accurately name about 25% of the letters. Robert was overwhelmed when presented with too much visual information at once. In addition, his emotional/behavioral response to frustration was problematic in the classroom. Because Robert had above average cognitive abilities, the therapist was able to help him recognize when he was reaching the limits of frustration. The classroom teacher was also more aware of the signs and could intervene before problems occurred. By providing additional verbal cues and limiting visual distractions, Robert was much more successful with daily classroom assignments.

Sensory Processing and Adults With Psychiatric Disabilities

Several psychiatric disabilities that are prevalent in adults also present with sensory processing difficulties.

Schizophrenia

The majority of this limited but growing area of research is focused on schizophrenia. There is a great deal of variability in schizophrenia; however, individuals with schizophrenia

The Lived Experience

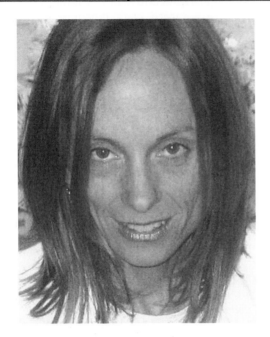

I am an occupational therapist who has struggled with sensory integrative dysfunction since childhood. Being an OT hasn't given me the magical ability to "cure" myself, but it has provided many tools that make what I experience manageable so that I can live a full life, experiencing ability instead of disability.

I was in my mid-30s before receiving a diagnosis on the autism spectrum. At that point, I had been diagnosed with a myriad of other things, including a generalized anxiety disorder, major depression, schizoaffective disorder, anorexia nervosa, and complex partial seizures. For me, these diagnoses bear dysfunctional sensory elements (although this may not be true for others), and I have grown to look at diagnoses more like stepping stones along a pathway of discovery.

At the time I received the autism diagnosis, life had been filled with challenges. I'd come to believe most were "emotionally based" and that I'd done something spiritually wrong. I spent much of my childhood and young adult years feeling frightened and overwhelmed—even within the safety of my home. I quickly felt dizzy, off-balance, and anxious, and this affected nearly everything I did. When I was at school, in crowds, on the playground, at a medical appointment, on family vacations, sleeping over at a friend's, riding horses, grocery shopping, playing my cello—I was prone to episodes where my equilibrium was challenged . . . and disrupted. Things that others don't seem to notice could make it impossible for me to concentrate or remain in a room—I felt tossed about and overstimulated so much of the time that I'd often leave a class early (causing me to get in trouble) or stay home from school entirely (causing missed assignments and social isolation). From an early age, I dreaded going to school but couldn't vocalize why—I knew it sounded "crazy" so I worked to keep the sensations I experienced quiet. I loved the "thinking" part of school, but the sensory overwhelm I experienced frequently ruined the adventure.

From early on, I couldn't eat foods with chunks or strange textures in them. I had episodes where parts of my body felt too big,

and I felt frightened and hypervigilant, worrying about when it might happen again. I was extremely introverted, seeming to lack the inner initiative to interact with others, although hanging out with one friend at a time was perfect. I preferred being in quiet places (or outside) to avoid feeling anxious and overwhelmed. Although most kids love breaks from school, I found the change in routine very difficult. I had a good childhood—but it was a constant effort to try and fit into the "mold" of a world that created so much disharmony for me. I developed intricate routines to follow to maintain inner order and stability—routines that later transformed into a serious eating disorder and other obsessive compulsive behaviors that have taken years to overcome. The rigid routines and beliefs helped me feel in control in a body and world that felt out of control, but they interfered deeply with developmental milestones and just being able to do the "normal" things in life.

Almost every day presented challenges—but I didn't necessarily realize it wasn't that way for others. You have to take life where it's at for you—finding ways to remain hope filled and grateful, and to reach the goals you set for yourself. My parents have always been huge encouragers—without them I would never have gone as far as I have. Strength does come from the support and love of others—those who help you face challenges with determination and an attitude of success. Another tool I've always used is my spiritual life and the inspiration of people I admire. Helen Keller's quote, "Keep your face to the sun and you will not see the shadows" is one of my personal mottos!

I grew from being a child with a dysregulated nervous system into an adult with a dysregulated nervous system. It seemed as if the wrong things got in, and in return, the wrong things resulted. I am proof that children with sensory integrative dysfunctions can become adults with them. Some of the behaviors and life concerns might change, but the core issues remain pretty steady.

It is through my personal journey of discovery that I stumbled on the field of occupational therapy. I was enthralled by the things OTs did to help people with sensory challenges, and was amazed at their approach to people who had autism, traumatic brain injuries, learning disabilities, cerebral palsy, and Parkinson's disease. I wanted to be part of this world! An OT worked with me during one of my hospitalizations, and we looked at the impact my health was having on a "circle of life domains" chart. It was the first time I realized there was a profession that took a whole-person, whole-life approach when treating people like me. OTs were always looking beyond the clinical environment (or taking treatment right into real life environments), examining how someone's challenges affected the quality of life in all life's domains. I began to understand what purposeful living meant and to learn new personal tools toward obtaining this.

I rejoiced when I was accepted to Colorado State University's Occupational Therapy Program, and graduated from it in 1994. School was difficult for me for the reasons I've already described. I underachieved at the goals I'd set, but in the midst of feeling discouraged, I began learning about accommodations and the Americans with Disabilities Act. I was blessed to receive accommodations that allowed me the chance to complete some assignments alternatively, as well as to succeed at all my fieldwork placements. In classes, these included taking tests alone,

The Lived Experience—cont'd

being allowed to sit in the back, having note takers, and presenting work to smaller groups. In fieldwork, these included working fewer hours and drawing the experiences out for longer time periods, getting frequent breaks, doing some of my paperwork in a quiet environment, and doing local placements so I didn't have to travel far or relocate. At this time, I was still mostly carrying the stigma of having many psychiatric diagnoses. It was embarrassing to tell others why I needed accommodations, and I didn't have the vocabulary to fully explain what I needed. I was determined to become an occupational therapist—but my inability to self-advocate often got in the way.

In 2000, an astute doctor gave me the autism diagnosis and helped me better understand what I experience as a syndrome that begins in my nervous system. This was a huge turning point for me. He was the one who really helped me understand the strong interplay among genetics, environment, and the neurophysical and neurochemical pieces when it comes to sensory disorders. For once, I stopped blaming myself and began to find new ways to engage in the life I desired—adopting a lifestyle that didn't include so many self-defeating challenges and negative inner voices.

I haven't grown far from the field of occupational therapy. I contribute to the psychosocial realm when the opportunity presents, finding new ways to use my skills (e.g., through writing and providing phone support on a warm line). I have learned that the core of healthy living is to find the ability to truly live it purposefully—in a way that causes one's soul to sing and dance. I have learned that hope and encouraging words are vital ingredients in the fuel that sustains courage and strength for clients who share their journeys with us. I have learned that labels can stigmatize, and that we owe it to others to listen with open minds and attitudes, forever seeing ourselves as students with so much more to learn.

Remember that within our uniqueness, we share a common space and thread—one that probably makes us more alike than different. My hope is that my dream to make the world a better place becomes part of yours, and that the special dreams you dream, become part of mine . . . and that we accept the challenges we encounter with an attitude of "YES!" . . . knowing we can—and do—make a difference.

---

generally seem to miss sensory input and yet, at the same time, are bothered by sensations. For example, a person with schizophrenia who is riding a public bus may not only miss the cues for the stop, but also find the visual and auditory stimuli in the bus overwhelming. For this reason, the person may choose not to use public transportation because it is too challenging.

In a study using the Adolescent/Adult Sensory Profile (A/ASP), individuals with schizophrenia, bipolar disorder, and no mental illness were compared (Brown, Cromwell, Filion, Dunn, & Tollefson, 2002). Individuals with schizophrenia had higher scores on low registration and sensation avoiding, and lower scores on sensation seeking than people without mental illness. This suggests that individuals with schizophrenia are not receiving adequate information about their environment and their own bodies. Not only do people with schizophrenia miss input, but also when they do detect sensory stimuli, they often find it unpleasant and engage in behaviors to avoid the sensation. In this study, individuals with bipolar disorder also had high scores on sensation avoiding, but were similar to people without mental illness on the low registration subscale. It may be that people with bipolar disorder are especially prone to avoiding behaviors when depressed, or that they may generally be more likely to actively control the sensory input they do receive.

Several laboratory studies indicate sensory processing differences in people with schizophrenia. Most of the research has focused on auditory and visual processing. In the area of auditory processing, one area of impairment has to do with selective attention. Individuals with schizophrenia have difficulty screening out irrelevant information (Mathalon, Heinks, & Ford, 2004), with some indication that selective auditory attention becomes more challenging for people with schizophrenia the longer they are required to attend. Leitman et al (2005) conducted a study that suggests that impairments in auditory sensory processing may contribute to social skill deficits. This study found that individuals with schizophrenia were less able to detect the vocal cues found in the intonation of language and were less able to use this information to determine the emotion being expressed by the speaker.

In a review of studies examining visual processing and schizophrenia, Butler and Javitt (2005) indicate that there is strong support from both electrophysiological and behavioral studies for a deficit in early stage visual processing. This review included many studies that contrasted magnocellular (motion detection) versus parvocellular (form detection) function in people with schizophrenia. Although deficits were found in form detection, there were more consistent and stronger findings of motion detection impairment in schizophrenia. In addition, these deficits are related to social and community functioning. For example, Sergi, Rassovsky, Nuechterlein, and Green (2006) found that early visual processing was related to social perception in schizophrenia, but social perception—not visual processing—accounted for more general impairments in functional status.

See Chapter 14 for more information on schizophrenia.

Other Psychiatric Diagnoses

There is less research on sensory processing and other psychiatric diagnoses in adults, although a few studies indicate sensory processing differences in borderline personality disorder and mood disorders. In a study using the Highly Sensitive Person Scale, individuals with borderline personality disorder with more symptoms tended to have higher levels of sensory sensitivity to aversive stimuli (Meyer, Ajchenbrenner, & Bowles, 2005). However, this finding deviates from the research that suggests that individuals with borderline personality disorder have reduced perception of pain (Bohus et al,

2000). Self-mutilation is a common symptom of borderline personality disorder, and many individuals report that they do not feel pain when they cut or burn themselves intentionally. This behavior is described as a coping mechanism to alleviate feelings of numbness or stun oneself out of negative emotions. The conflicting findings in borderline personality disorder could be related to the general instability and dysregulation of mood that are key features of the illness.

Two studies examining sensory sensitivity (using the Highly Sensitive Person Scale) and mood found that sensory sensitivity was associated with anxiety (Liss, Timmel, Baxley, & Killingsworth, 2005; Neal, Edelmann, & Glachan, 2002). Another study found an association with depression (Liss et al, 2005). This finding is consistent with a study comparing responses on the A/ASP and the New York Longitudinal Scales Adult Temperament Questionnaire, which found that sensory sensitivity was associated with serious or negative mood (Brown, Tollefson, Dunn, Cromwell, & Filion, 2001). Likewise, using a sensory history interview, Kinnealey and Fuiek (1999) found that sensory defensive adults had higher levels of depression and anxiety. These studies relied on self-reports of sensory sensitivity to environmental stimuli.

The processing of pain in people with depression is complicated. On the one hand, there is considerable evidence that people with depression experience higher levels of chronic pain (Aaron & Buchwald, 2001; Stahl & Briley, 2004). Physical pain is considered a common component of depressive symptomatology and may be related to dysfunction in the neurotransmitter systems of serotonin and norepinephrine. On the other hand, a systematic review of laboratory studies for pain tolerance and depression found that the pain perception threshold was higher in people with depression, meaning that individuals with depression did not register pain until the sensory stimulus was intense (Dickens, McGowan, & Dale, 2003). It may be that pain experienced in an acute laboratory condition is different from how an individual with depression experiences chronic clinical pain.

For more information, see Chapter 12 on mood disorders and Chapter 25 on pain regulation.

Models of Sensory Processing

Based on the pioneering work of Jean Ayres (1972a) on sensory integration, this domain of concern has evolved such that there are several different practice models or theoretical bases from which a therapist can practice. This section presents the different models of sensory processing in occupational therapy, including the theoretical base of each model and, when available, the associated assessments and intervention approaches.

Jean Ayres and Sensory Integration

A. Jean Ayers (1972a) developed the theory of **sensory integration** as a result of studying motor dysfunctions in children with mild to moderate learning problems. Although these children did not display any discernible central nervous system dysfunction, Ayres believed that the explanation for their problems was neurologically based. Ayers' theory proposed that interventions focused on improving responses to sensory stimulation could affect academic performance. Ayres examined the effects of sensory integration interventions on the academic skills of 148 children with learning disabilities. In this study, Ayres demonstrated a significant improvement in reading scores and concluded that the improvement was most likely the result of sensory integrative interventions.

Bundy and Murray (2002) describe the components of **sensory integrative theory** in terms of normal sensory function, sensory dysfunction, and possible interventions. In **normal sensory function**, learning occurs when an individual is able to effectively process the sensory information, and the result is an appropriate adaptive response. When this process is disrupted and **sensory dysfunction** occurs, the individual has difficulty performing physical and mental actions. The interventions recommended by the theory are based on the premise that the integration of the tactile, vestibular, and proprioceptive systems is not adequate to develop organization of the nervous system, which can result in postural instability, gravitational insecurity, occulomotor dysfunction, and oral motor difficulties. Subsequent levels of intervention involve the development of body perception, bilateral coordination, motor planning, activity level, attention to task, emotional responses, and visual motor integration.

The Southern California Sensory Integration Test (SCSIT; Ayers, 1972b) is the culmination of six-factor analysis studies by Ayres and the Goleta Union School District. The intent of this assessment was not only to identify those children whose sensory integrative abilities fell below the typical range based on normative data, but also to delineate the type of dysfunction associated with a particular aspect of sensory development. Ayres identified the four types of sensory integrative dysfunction categories as follows:

1. Form and space perception
2. Praxis
3. Postural and bilateral integration
4. Tactile defensiveness

The development of this assessment had a tremendous impact on pediatric practice in occupational therapy. Outlining normative data to describe underlying dysfunctions based on neuroscience theories provided legitimacy to sensory interventions that affected a child's development. To administer the assessment, therapists were required to complete a certification course, perform multiple practice administrations, and demonstrate competency to another person already certified in its use. Therapists in pediatric practice at that time who became certified in the SCSIT were considered on the cutting edge of professional development.

The theory of sensory integration continued to evolve, and eventually, the Sensory Integration Praxis Test (SIPT) was published (Ayres, 1989). The SIPT was developed as a result of the examination of practice abilities of adults with adult-onset brain damage. The dysfunctions associated with motor impairments in these adults were used to develop assessment of practice functions in children with normal intelligence and no known explanation of neurological injury. In addition, portions of the SCSIT that had failed to provide useful information were eliminated. The focus on examination of praxis was based on the trend in research at that time, which emphasized the interdependence of the brain's structures.

Recent critical analyses of the effectiveness of sensory integration intervention have brought into question some of the findings in Ayres' earlier work (Baranek, 2002). Criticism has focused on flaws in design, limited sample size, and lack of replication of the early studies. Although the impact on academic performance has not proven to be influenced by the sensory integrative approach, examining performance issues based on underlying neuroscience theories continues to be an impetus for current research in pediatric practice.

Georgia DeGangi

Georgia DeGangi is considered one of the leading experts in the field of sensory processing in infants and toddlers. Her work focuses on the importance of early intervention, as well as the influence of the family and environment in the child's development. Much of her research examines the significance of regulatory disorders and how these disorders affect development. Children with regulatory disorders respond to sensory stimuli with dysfunctional behaviors and emotions. They may cry easily and be difficult to soothe, or they may respond aggressively by biting or kicking. DeGangi, Breinbauer, Roosevelt, Porges, and Greenspan (2000) conducted a study to determine whether infants with regulatory disorders were a reliable predictor of future clinical diagnosis. Researchers found that children with moderate regulatory disorders in infancy were found to have a high incidence of developmental delays and parent–child relationship difficulties at age 3. DeGangi's (2000) *Pediatric Disorders of Regulation in Affect and Behavior* details normal regulatory functions in infants and toddlers, and suggests how to assess and treat regulatory problems in children.

DeGangi, Poisson, Sickel, and Wiener (1995) have developed a measure to assess regulatory disorders in infants and toddlers. The Infant/Toddler Symptom Checklist is a screening tool designed for young children who present difficult behaviors that interfere with daily activities such as eating, and sleeping. The screening identifies children who are at risk for regulatory disorders and may be in need of further diagnostic testing. Parents complete a questionnaire that examines self-regulation, attention, sleep patterns, eating, dressing, bathing and touch, movement, listening and language, looking and sight, and attachment or emotional functioning. The criterion-referenced checklist is available in a general screening version appropriate for ages 7 to 30 months, as well as five age-specific versions within that range. The authors of this assessment recommend that it be used in conjunction with other measures to provide a comprehensive understanding of the child's developmental level and sensory processing patterns. Developmental assessments and instruments that focus on underlying sensory functions are suggested.

DeGangi's approach to intervention places emphasis on the parent–child interaction. DeGangi offers descriptions of interventions to guide the parents in managing difficult behaviors associated with eating, sleeping, and emotional responses. In this approach, the activities are child centered, and the therapist provides sensory integrative techniques to elicit the desired response. The approach described in *Pediatric Disorders of Regulation in Affect and Behavior* (DeGangi, 2000) is a clinically based model in which the parent brings the child to a clinical setting for interventions sessions, with an emphasis on parent collaboration to carry over techniques in the home setting. For example, a therapist working with a mother who is constantly holding and rocking an irritable toddler can provide strategies for the mother to use to help the child learn to self-soothe. The therapist could demonstrate activities that involve tactile and movement stimuli to meet the child's sensory needs.

Wilbarger Approach

Patricia Wilbarger and Julia Wilbarger (2002) have developed a supplemental sensory intervention directed at treating sensory defensiveness. This intervention is widely recognized as the Wilbarger protocol. It is also commonly referred to as the "brushing technique," although the brushing procedure is only a part of the intervention approach. The Wilbarger approach to sensory defensiveness involves education of the caregivers and the client regarding the extent of sensory defensiveness and the impact on daily life experiences. The client is exposed to a sensory "diet" that provides a variety of sensory experiences embedded within daily activities. In combination with education and sensory diet, at frequent intervals throughout the day, the client undergoes an intensive treatment involving the application of deep pressure using a surgical brush. These intervals range from every 90 minutes to every 2 hours. The deep pressure brushing is applied to the hands, arms, back, legs, and feet. The brushing procedure is followed by joint compression in the legs, arms, and trunk. This procedure was developed specifically for clients with sensory defensiveness and is not recommended for individuals with medical or behavioral diagnoses for which deep pressure interventions might be contraindicated.

Dunn's Model of Sensory Processing

Dunn's (1997) Model of Sensory Processing provides a theoretical framework for understanding how individuals respond to sensory stimuli. This data-driven model was based on a factor analysis of 1,037 Sensory Profiles (SPs) of typically developing children. The factor analysis revealed that the items on the SP were best grouped according to particular patterns of sensory processing (e.g., visual or auditory) rather than sensory modalities. Dunn's model is comprised of four quadrants that are formed by the intersection of a neurological threshold continuum and a behavioral response/self-regulation continuum.

The neurological threshold continuum runs from low (sensitization) to high (habituation). A low threshold indicates that it takes less sensory stimuli or less intense stimuli for the nervous system to fire and take notice of the sensory stimuli, whereas a high threshold requires more or an increased intensity of the sensory stimuli. A very low threshold is equated with hypersensitivity, and a very high threshold with hyposensitivity.

The other continuum, behavioral response/self-regulation, moves from passive to active. A passive response is one in which the individual responds in accordance with his or her threshold, whereas an active response involves intentionally controlling, choosing, or changing environments to manage sensory input. The intersection of the two continua results in the four quadrants of Dunn's model.

Four Quadrants

The four quadrants of Dunn's model and their correspon-ding processing preferences include the following:

1. Low threshold and passive response = Sensory Sensitivity
2. Low threshold and active response = Sensation Avoiding
3. High threshold and passive response = Low Registration
4. High threshold and active response = Sensation Seeking

With a sensory processing preference of **sensory sensitiv-ity**, the person notices things that others do not notice. This can lead to a heightened awareness of the environment and more information with which to make decisions. In contrast, people who are sensory sensitive can be highly distractible and more likely to experience discomfort in high-intensity environments.

The individual with a processing preference of **sensation avoiding** creates or chooses environments that reduce sen-sory input. This individual can do well in low stimulus situ-ations or settings that others find dull. In addition, sensation avoiders tend to be skilled at adapting environments to meet their needs. Conversely, these individuals may miss impor-tant information and become distressed in situations in which they cannot control the environment.

People with **low registration** tend to miss input that oth-ers take in. They may be slow to respond or require repetition and cues. Yet, these individuals are highly flexible because they are not bothered by sensory stimuli and can typically manage distracting environments quite well.

Like the sensation avoiders, **sensation seeking** individu-als actively engage with their environment to meet their sen-sory needs. However, unlike the avoiders, they change the environment or select environments to obtain higher levels of sensory input. Sensation seekers are easily bored or frus-trated in environments that do not meet their elevated needs for sensation.

Sensory Profiles

The SPs are assessments specifically designed for use with Dunn's (1997) Model of Sensory Processing. There are several versions of the sensory profile that are intended for particular age groups. The Infant/Toddler Sensory Profile (I/TSP; Dunn, 2002) is designed for children ages birth to 3; the SP (Dunn, 1999) is designed for children ages 3 to 10; and the A/ASP (Brown & Dunn, 2002) is appropriate for ages 11 and older. The A/ASP is a self-report measure, whereas the SP and I/TSP are completed by a parent or caregiver. Each measure is a sur-vey with questions focused on sensory responses to everyday life activities. Subscale scores for each of the four quadrants: low registration, sensation seeking, sensory sensitivity, and sensation avoiding can be calculated from the measure. An important distinction exists for scoring the adolescent/adult versus the child versions. A high score on the A/ASP indicates more of a particular attribute (e.g., sensory sensitivity), whereas a low score in the SP or I/TSP indicates more of an attribute.

The Sensory Profile School Companion Manual (Dunn, 2006) provides a measure to be completed by school person-nel rather than the child's caregiver. This measure evaluates sensory processing related to performance within the school setting. This measure is to be completed by school personnel who know the child well and have observed his or her performance in a variety of school settings. Performance is based on typical performance during the school day. Al-though this assessment provides the opportunity for school personnel to contribute to information about sensory influ-ences, it is important that sensory information from the care-giver be given equal importance in the evaluation process. Using sensory information from the school setting alone will not provide the most complete picture of the child's sensory processing patterns. In addition, comparing performance in the two different settings may yield important information regarding possible interventions and help identify environ-mental influences.

Intervention in Dunn's Model

The primary intervention approach using Dunn's (1997) Model of Sensory Processing involves designing environments to meet an individual's sensory processing preferences. Con-sequently, the approach to intervention involves understand-ing the environmental features that match the sensory pro-cessing preference. Particular guidelines are associated with each sensory processing quadrant.

A person with sensory sensitivity will generally benefit from greater organization of stimuli and elimination of ir-relevant input. The environment should be adjusted to de-crease the intensity of the available sensations, with particu-lar attention given to the reduction of competing stimuli. Simple interventions might include having a student sit at the front of the class or having a distracted driver turn off the radio.

Interventions for sensation avoiding involve reducing the amount and intensity of sensation and increasing pre-dictability and familiarity. Established routines are generally helpful for the sensation avoider. In addition, allowing for breaks or providing a quiet space can be helpful, as well as giving the individual more control over sensory input.

For individuals with low registration, it is important to enhance relevant sensory stimuli so that the individual no-tices what he or she needs to notice. This might include in-creasing the intensity or amount of sensory input or reduc-ing the speed at which information is presented so the person has time to take in the information. Cues such as signs or a beeping alarm can be helpful for a person with low registration. It is also helpful to reduce the predictabil-ity or familiarity of the input, so signs may need to be changed regularly, and the individual may benefit from a change in setting.

The sensation seeker desires variety, intensity, and unpre-dictability in his or her environment, and he or she will ben-efit from opportunities to explore and take control of the en-vironment to create sensation. Sensations that may be distracting to others might be helpful for the sensation seeker to maintain arousal and focus. If the sensation seeker is required to be in a low stimulus environment, he or she may need breaks to get up and move around, talk, or spend time engaged in a higher level of activity.

Highly Sensitive Person Scale

Another measure that is similar to the sensory sensitivity subscale of Dunn's A/ASP is the Highly Sensitive Person Scale. This measure, developed by psychologists (Aron &

Evidence-Based Practice

Individuals with schizophrenia are more likely than individuals without mental illness to have sensory processing patterns characterized by low registration and sensation avoiding.

➤ Occupational therapists can create interventions that support occupational performance for people with schizophrenia by enhancing important sensory cues and reducing or eliminating excess or irrelevant sensory information.

Brown, C., Cromwell, R. L., Filion, C., Dunn, W., & Tollefson, N. (2002). Sensory processing in schizophrenia: Missing and avoiding information. *Schizophrenia Research, 55,* 187–195.

Aron, 1997), is a 27-item self-reported Likert scale assessment that asks respondents how they relate to environmental features such as noise, taste, and other people's moods. Unlike the A/ASP, the Highly Sensitive Person Scale contains several items that reflect greater interest and sensitivity to creative stimuli such as music and art.

Sensory Assessment in the Context of Occupational Performance

In addition to the use of assessments to detail sensory information regarding preferences, strengths, and concerns, it is important to examine sensory processing within the context of the demands of tasks. For the experienced therapist, structured observations in a variety of settings may be effective in providing supplemental information when designing a sensory program. However, for the novice therapist, it may be challenging to extract important information from observations. Videotaping may be helpful in analyzing observation information and is useful when discussing cases with experienced therapists. In addition, formal assessments that examine occupational performance may provide additional clues to sensory influences. Assessments such as the School Function Assessment (Coster, 2000), the Assessment of Motor and Process Skills (Fisher, 2001), and the Performance Assessment of Self Care Skills (Holm & Rogers, 1999) may help identify sensory influences in daily activities by examining patterns of performance.

Vignette: Sensitivity to Auditory Stimulation

A child with mental retardation who had been independent in toileting at school had a sudden decrease in performance with frequent accidents in the classroom. Based on information from the SP in combination with analyzing performance on the School Function assessment, a pattern of sensitivity to auditory stimulation was identified. In addition, he sometimes displayed hypersensitivity to tactile experiences. At first glance, this did not explain the decrease in independence in toileting tasks. However, on presenting this information to the team, the teacher was able to identify the source of the problem. Over the summer, all restrooms in the building had been renovated to include automatic toilets and faucets. As is often the case with automated flushing, the timing and frequency of flushes are not always predictable. The lack of control over the number of flushes was upsetting to the student, so he would either not use the restroom at all or would not complete the process, resulting in accidents in the classroom. Because of the child's cognitive level, he was not able to articulate his sensory needs. The only way to identify sensory influences was to use a sensory measure in combination with an assessment that examined performance in daily routines.

In another example, a therapist was called on to evaluate John, an adult with schizophrenia, who was having difficulty with his janitorial job. The A/ASP was administered, and there were clear patterns of sensory sensitivity and sensation avoiding. However, the relationship between these sensory processing patterns and problems at work were not apparent until the therapist observed John at work. John was not completing a major part of his job–vacuuming. When asked why he was avoiding this task, John explained that the sounds of the vacuum cleaner were overwhelming and also triggered auditory hallucinations. Once this was known, job reassignments were made, and John was once again successful at work.

Developmental Assessments in Combination With Sensory Measures

Depending on the requirements within a particular setting and the level of experience of the therapist, developmental assessments can provide supplemental information regarding sensory performance. Measures such as the Peabody Developmental Motor Scales (Folio & Fewell, 2000) and the Hawaii Early Learning Profile (Furuno et al, 1997) are commonly used in the field of pediatrics. These measures can help identify how a child compares to children of the same age on specific motor tasks. Strengths and weakness on specific motor tasks can be analyzed in conjunction with sensory assessments to try to identify patterns that may be interfering with performance.

It is important to consider additional influences in performance, even when sensory issues have been identified. Visual motor assessments and visual perceptual assessments such as the Beery Test of Visual Motor Integration (Beery, 2004), the Motor Free Visual Perceptual Test (Colarusso, Hammill, & Mercier, 1995), and the Test of Visual Motor Integration (nonmotor; Gardner, 1996) are measures that yield specific information that may provide guidance in terms of fine motor performance in the classroom. Difficulties with sensory processing may be complicated by underlying visual motor and perceptual problems. The Beery Test of Visual Motor Integration has been a reliable predictor of learning problems in the classroom. When coupled with classroom observations in daily tasks, these assessments can provide helpful information regarding areas of strength and weakness in classroom performance. When sensory information yields results that appear to be contradictory, underlying problems in visual motor or visual perceptual skills may provide possible explanations for these inconsistencies.

Snoezelen Environments

The Snoezelen environment was first developed by Jan Hulsegge and Ad Verheul (1987) in Holland. The term comes from the Dutch verbs "snuffelen," which means to seek, and "doezelen," which means to relax. Unlike other sensory approaches, the intent of the Snoezelen environment is not to develop specific skills per se but to promote restoration. In some literature, the Snoezelen environment is presented as an opportunity for leisure for individuals with severe disabilities (Haggar & Hutchinson, 1991). There are two critical variables for Snoezelen: the environment, which provides sensory stimulation that the person can explore and control, and the staff members who take part in the Snoezelen experience (Lancioni, Cuvo, & O'Reilly, 2002). The staff members act as enablers who guide the person to experience the available stimuli.

There are no specific assessments associated with the Snoezelen environment; however, the environment has been used most frequently with individuals who have severe impairments that limit communication and result in disruptive behaviors (e.g., severe mental retardation, dementia). Therefore, individuals who have a limited ability to communicate with others and are challenged to engage in any form of purposeful activity would be the best candidates for this intervention approach.

The Snoezelen environment is now commercially available and consists of a multimedia space of sensory experiences. The environment includes different areas to address the sensory modalities and objects, such as headphones for music, comfortable cushions, vibrating pads, mirror balls, and bubble machines. The therapist is expected to be in close contact with the client in the Snoezelen environment and promote exploration and enrichment.

Most of the research with the Snoezelen environment has been conducted with people with dementia or developmental disabilities. Occupational therapists studying the physiological and behavioral effects of Snoezelen (van Diepen et al, 2001) found positive short-term effects, including a reduction in agitation, but these improvements were short lived. A larger study found similar positive effects on agitation, as well as short-term improvements in mood and communication (van Weert, van Dulman, Spreeuwenberg, Ribbe, & Bensing, 2005). In a systematic review of 14 studies of people with developmental disabilities and 7 with people with dementia, the most consistent findings were related to positive effects while the person was in the Snoezelen environment (Lancioni et al, 2002). These positive effects were typically related to improved social engagement and reduced disruptive behavior. Long-term effects appear to be weaker and less consistent. Staff members are typically positive about using the Snoezelen

environment and find the experience pleasurable and humane (Lancioni et al, 2002).

Sensory Approaches to Reduce Seclusion and Restraint in Psychiatric Settings

The Massachusetts Department of Mental Health established a task force to reduce the use of restraints and seclusion (Carmen et al, 1996). Tina Champagne (an occupational therapist) and Nan Stromberg (a nurse) (2004) worked on the task force and incorporated sensory approaches as one of the strategies. Champagne and Stromberg use a combination of sensory models, including Dunn's (1997) Model of Sensory Processing and Wilbarger and Wilbarger's (2002) sensory diet. The use of restraints and seclusion for a person who is already overwhelmed with sensory stimuli will only magnify the difficult inner experience. Also, the lack of control further intensifies the feelings of being engulfed in a sensory inferno.

Champagne and Stromberg's (2004) work posits that meeting sensory needs can serve as an effective strategy to help the out-of-control individual regain control, and allows the staff to avoid the use of restraints and seclusion, which can have long-lasting negative effects on the individual. In general, the recommended approaches rely on activities that provide the appropriate type of sensory input for both the individual and the situation. In some situations, calming activities such as exercise against resistance, rocking, being wrapped up in a weighted blanket, deep breathing, and chewing gum may be helpful. In other situations, such as the anxiety associated with self-harm, orienting activities such as snapping a rubber band on the wrist or biting into a lemon are recommended. Champagne also advocates for the development of an individual crisis prevention plan before a crisis occurs. This way the staff members know what strategies have worked in the past and can honor the individual's request, which is more likely to prevent a crisis from occurring. A major component of this approach involves the training of staff in sensory processing theory and sensory approaches. Psychiatric units may need to develop more flexibility to allow individuals to engage in sensory activities that may "go against the rules" of the unit.

Summary

Occupational therapists have a long history of expertise related to understanding and providing interventions for sensory processing disorders, particularly for children. Newer models have expanded applications to adults with psychiatric disabilities. From a mental health context, this chapter provides information that can increase the opportunities for occupational therapists to use sensory processing theories for enhancing occupational performance in people of all ages.

Active Learning Strategies

1. Self-Inventory

Administer the A/ASP on yourself and score it.

Reflective Questions

- Are your scores and the patterns of sensory processing consistent with your view of your personal sensory processing preferences?
- Are there situations or behaviors not included on the measure that better represent your sensory processing preferences?
- Think about an important occupation. Are there ways in which you have constructed the environment in which you perform the occupation that assist in meeting your sensory needs?

2. Designing Environments

Select one of the occupations from the following list:

Studying

Cooking

Shopping for clothes

Watching a movie

Next, design an environment and adapt the task so that it would best meet the needs of a (1) sensory sensitive person, (2) sensation avoider, (3) low registration person, and (4) sensation seeker. What features of the environment or task did you consider most important when completing this exercise? Was it easier to create situations for particular preference (e.g., the one that you most relate to)?

Resources

- Assistive devices
- Nuance, the Nuance logo, Dragon, the Dragon logo, DragonBar, NaturallySpeaking, and RealSpeak are trademarks or registered trademarks of Nuance Communications, Inc. or its affiliates in the United States and/or other countries. All other trademarks are the property of their respective owners. ©2008, Nuance Communications, Inc. All rights reserved. http://www.nuance.com/naturallyspeaking/
- Inspiration Software, Inc. Copyright 2009
  9400 SW Beaverton-Hillsdale Hwy
  Suite 300
  Beaverton, OR 97005-3300
  http://www.inspiration.com/
- Infant/Toddler Symptom Checklist—a screening tool for parents developed by DeGangi, Poisson, Sickel, and Weinger: www.harcourtassessments.com
  http://www.pearsonassessments.com/HAIWEB/Cultures/en-us/Productdetail.htm?Pid=076-1643-559&Mode=summary
- OT Innovations—Web site describing Tina Champagne's sensory program: www.ot-innovations.com
- *Sensory Integration and the Child* by A. J. Ayres (Los Angeles: Western Psychological Services, 1979)—a classic text written for parents
- Sensory Integration and Praxis Test: www.wpspublishing.com
  http://portal.wpspublish.com/portal/page?_pageid=53,114668&_dad=portal&_schema=PORTAL
- Sensory Processing Disorder Foundation: http://www.spdfoundation.net
- Sensory Profile measures: www.sensoryprofile.com
- Snoezelen equipment: www.flaghouse.com/SnoezelenAL.asp
- Wilbarger protocol: http://www.sensory-processing-disorder.com/index.html

References

Aaron, L. A., & Buchwald, D. (2001). A review of the evidence for overlap among unexplained clinical conditions. *Annals of Internal Medicine, 134,* 868–881.

American Psychiatric Association. (2000). *Diagnostic and Statistical Manual of Mental Disorders* (4th ed., text revision). Washington, DC: Author.

Aron, E., & Aron, A. (1997). Sensory processing sensitivity and its relation to introversion and emotionality. *Journal of Personality and Social Psychology, 73,* 345–368.

Ayres A. J. (1972a). Improving academic scores through sensory integration. *Journal of Learning Disabilities, 5,* 338–343.

Ayres A. J. (1972b). *The Southern California Sensory Integration Test Manual.* Los Angeles: Western Psychological Services.

Ayres, A. J. (1979). *Sensory Integration and the Child.* Los Angeles: Western Psychological Services.

Ayres, A. J. (1989). *Sensory Integration and Praxis Tests Manual.* Los Angeles: Western Psychological Services.

Baranek, G. T. (2002). Efficacy of sensory and motor interventions for children with autism. *Journal of Learning Disabilities, 32*(5), 397–422.

Beery, K. E. (2004). *Developmental Test of Visual Motor Integration: Administration, Scoring, and Teaching Manual* (5th ed.). Minneapolis: NCS Pearson.

Blakemore, S. J., Tavassoli, T., Calo, S., Thomas, R. M., Catmur, C., Frith, U., & Haggard, P. (2006). Tactile sensitivity in Asperger syndrome. *Brain and Cognition, 61,* 5–13.

Bohus, M., Limberger, M., Ebner, U., Glocker, F. X., Schwarz, B., Wernz, M., & Lieb, K. (2000). Pain perception during self-reported distress and calmness in patients with borderline personality disorder and self-mutilating behavior. *Psychiatry Research, 95,* 251–260.

Brockmeyer, R. D., & Bundy, M. B. (2001). The effects of autism experience on life view and philosophy: A glimpse from one side of the looking glass. In R. A. Huebner (Ed.), *Autism: A Sensorimotor Approach to Management* (pp. 443–467). Gaithersburg, MD: Aspen.

Brown, C., Cromwell, R. L., Filion, C., Dunn, W., & Tollefson, N. (2002). Sensory processing in schizophrenia: Missing and avoiding information. *Schizophrenia Research, 55,* 187–195.

Brown, C., & Dunn, W. (2002). *Adolescent/Adult Sensory Profile.* San Antonio, TX: Psychological Corp.

Brown, C., Tollefson, N., Dunn, W., Cromwell, R., & Filion, D. (2001). The Adult Sensory Profile: Measuring patterns of sensory processing. *American Journal of Occupational Therapy, 55,* 75–82.

Bundy, A. C., & Murray, E. A. (2002). Sensory integration: A. Jean Ayres' theory revisited. In A. Bundy, S. J. Lane, & E. A. Murray (Eds.), *Sensory Integration Theory and Practice* (pp. 3–33). Philadelphia: F.A. Davis.

Butler, P. D., & Javitt, D. C. (2005). Early-stage visual processing deficits in schizophrenia. *Current Opinion in Psychiatry, 18,* 151–157.

Carmen, E., Crane, B., Dunnicliff, M., Holochuck, S., Prescott, L., & Reiker, P. (1996). *Massachusetts Department of Mental Health task force on the restraint and seclusion of persons who have been physically or sexually abused: Report and recommendations.* Boston: Massachusetts Department of Mental Health.

Colarusso, R. P., Hammill, D. D., & Mercier, L. (1995). *Motor Free Visual Perceptual Test-Revised (MVPT-R).* Novato, CA: Academic Therapy.

Champagne, T., & Stromberg, N. (2004). Sensory approaches in inpatient psychiatric settings: Innovative alternatives to seclusion and restraint. *Journal of Psychosocial Nursing and Mental Health Services, 42,* 34–45.

Coster, W. (2000). *The School Function Assessment Manual.* San Antonio, TX: Psychological Corp.

DeGangi, G. A. (2000). *Pediatric Disorders of Regulation in Affect and Behavior: A Therapist's Guide to Assessment and Treatment.* San Diego: Academic Press.

DeGangi, G. A., Breinbauer, C., Roosevelt, J. D., Porges, S., & Greenspan, S. (2000). Prediction of childhood problems at three years in children experiencing disorders of regulation during infancy. *Infant Mental Health Journal, 21*(3), 156–175.

DeGangi, G. A., Poisson, S., Sickel, R. Z., & Wiener, A. S. (1995). *Infant Toddler Symptom Checklist.* San Antonio, TX: Psychological Corp.

Dickens, C., McGowan, L., & Dale, S. (2003). Impact of depression on experimental pain perception: A systematic review of the literature with meta-analysis. *Psychosomatic Medicine, 65,* 369–375.

Dunn, W. (1997). The impact of sensory processing abilities on the daily lives of young children and their families: A conceptual model. *Infants and Young Children, 9*(4), 23–35.

Dunn, W. (1999). *Sensory Profile: User's Manual.* San Antonio, TX: Psychological Corp.

Dunn, W. (2002). *The Infant/Toddler Sensory Profile Manual.* San Antonio, TX: Psychological Corp.

Dunn, W. (2006). *The Sensory Profile School Companion Manual.* San Antonio, TX: Psychological Corp.

Dunn, W., Myles, B. S., & Orr, S. (2002). Sensory-processing issues associated with Asperger syndrome. *56,* 97–102.

Fisher, A. G. (2001). *Assessment of Motor and Process Skills, Vol. 2: User Manual* (4th ed.). Fort Collins, CO: Three Star Press.

Folio, M. R., & Fewell, R. R. (2000). *Peabody Developmental Motor Scales* (2nd ed.). San Antonio, TX: Psychological Corp.

Furuno, S., O'Reilly, K. A., Hosaka, C. M., Inatsuka, T. T., Allman, T. L., & Zeisloft, B. (1997). *The Hawaii Early Learning Profile.* Palo Alto, CA: Vort.

Gardner, M. (1996). *Test of Visual-Perceptual Skills (non-motor) Revised.* Burlington, CA: Psychological and Educational Publications.

Grandin, T. (2000). "My Experiences With Visual Thinking Sensory Problems and Communication Difficulties." Available at: http://www.autism.com/families/therapy/visual.htm (accessed February 15, 2010)

Haggar, L. E., & Hutchinson, R. B. (1991). Snoezelen: An approach to the provision of a leisure resource for people with profound and multiple handicaps. *Mental Handicap, 19,* 51–55.

Herz, R. S., & Engen, T. (1996). Odor memory: Review and analysis. *Psychonomic Bulletin and Review, 3*(3), 300–313.

Holm, M. B., & Rogers, J. C. (1999). Performance assessment of self care skills. In B. J. Hemphill-Pearson (Ed.), *Assessments in Occupational Therapy Mental Health* (pp. 117–124). Thorofare, NJ: Slack.

Hulsegge, J., & Verheul, A. (1987). *Snoezelen: Another World.* Chesterfield, UK: ROMPA.

Kandel, E. R., Schwartz, J. H., & Jessell, T. M. (2000). *Principles of Neural Science* (4th ed.). New York: McGraw-Hill.

Kientz, M. A., & Dunn, W. (1997). A comparison of the performance of children with and without autism on the Sensory Profile. *American Journal of Occupational Therapy, 51*(7), 530–537.

Kinnealey, M., & Fuiek, M. (1999). The relationship between sensory defensiveness, anxiety, depression and perception of pain in adults. *Occupational Therapy International, 6*(3), 195–207.

Klassen, A. F., Miller, A., & Fine, S. (2004). Health related quality of life in children and adolescents who have a diagnosis of attention-deficit/hyperactivity disorder. *Pediatrics, 114*(5), 541–547.

Lancioni, G. E., Cuvo, A. J., & O'Reilly, M. F. (2002). Snoezelen: An overview of research with people with developmental disabilities and dementia. *Disability and Rehabilitation, 24,* 175–184.

Lane, S. J., Miller, L. J., & Hanft, B. E. (2000). Toward a consensus in terminology in sensory integration theory and practice: Part 2: Sensory integration patterns of function and dysfunction. *Sensory Integration Special Interest Section Quarterly, 23*(2), 1–3.

Leitman, D. I., Foxe, J. J., Butler, P. D., Saperstein, A., Revheim, N., & Javitt, D. C. (2005). Sensory contributions to impaired prosodic processing in schizophrenia. *Biological Psychiatry, 58,* 56–61.

Lepisto, T., Kujala, T., Vanhala, R., Alku, P., Huotilainen, M., & Naatanen, R. (2005). The discrimination of and orienting to speech and non-speech sounds in children with autism. *Brain Research, 1066,* 147–157.

Liss, M., Timmel, L., Baxley, K., & Killingsworth, P. (2005). Sensory processing sensitivity and its relation to parental bonding, anxiety and depression. *Personality and Individual Differences, 39,* 1429–1439.

Mangeot, S. D., Miller, L. J., McIntosh, D. N., McGrath-Clarke, J., Simon, J., Hagerman, R. J., & Goldson, E. (2001). Sensory modulation dysfunction in children with attention-deficit-hyperactivity disorder. *Developmental Medicine & Child Neurology, 43,* 399–406.

Mathalon, D. H., Heinks, T., & Ford, J. M. (2004). Selective attention in schizophrenia: Sparing and loss of executive control. *American Journal of Psychiatry, 161,* 872–881.

Mayes, S. D., Calhoun, S. L., & Crowell, E. W. (2000). Learning disability and ADHD: Overlapping spectrum disorders. *Journal of Learning Disabilities, 33,* 417–424.

Meyer, B., Ajchenbrenner, M., & Bowles, D. P. (2005). Sensory sensitivity, attachment experiences, and rejection responses among adults with borderline and avoidant features. *Journal of Personality Disorders, 19,* 641–658.

Miller, L. J., Anzalone, M. E., Lane, S. J., Cermak, S. A., & Osten, E. T. (2007). Concept evolution in sensory integration: A proposed nosology for diagnosis. *American Journal of Occupational Therapy, 61,* 135–140.

Miller, L. J., & Lane, S. J. (2000). Toward a consensus in terminology in sensory integration theory and practice: Part 1: Taxonomy of neurophysiological processes. *Sensory Integration Special Interest Section Quarterly, 23*(1), 1–4.

Neal, J. A., Edelmann, R. J., & Glachan, M. (2002). Behavioural inhibition and symptoms of anxiety and depression: Is there a specific relationship with social phobia? *British Journal of Clinical Psychology, 41,* 361–374.

O'Neill, M., & Jones, R. S. P. (1997). Sensory-perceptual abnormalities in autism: A case for more research? *Journal of Autism and Developmental Disorders, 27*(3), 283–293.

Pfeiffer, B., Kinnealey, M., Reed, C., & Herzberg, G. (2005). Sensory modulation and affective disorders in children and adolescents with Asperger's disorder. *American Journal of Occupational Therapy, 59*(3), 335–345.

Pierce, K., Glad, K. S., & Schreibman, L. (1997). Social perception in children with autism: An attentional deficit. *Journal of Autism and Developmental Disorders, 27*(3), 265–282.

Schilling, D. L., Washington, K., Billingsley, F. F., & Deitz, J. (2003). Classroom seating for children with attention deficit hyperactivity disorder. *American Journal of Occupational Therapy, 57,* 534–541.

Schneider, G. E. (1969). Two visual systems. *Science, 163,* 895–902.

Sergi, M. J., Rassovsky, Y., Nuechterlein, K. H., & Green, M. F. (2006). Social perception as a mediator of the influence of early visual processing on functional status in schizophrenia. *American Journal of Psychiatry, 163,* 448–454.

Stahl, S., & Briley, M. (2004). Understanding pain in depression. *Human Psychopharmacology, 19,* S9–S13.

van Diepen, E., Baillon, S. F., Redman, J., Rooke, N., Spencer, D. A., & Prettyman, R. (2002). A pilot study of the physiological and behavioural effects of Snoezelen in dementia. *British Journal of Occupational Therapy, 65*(2), 61–66.

van Weert, J. C. M., van Dulman, A. M., Spreeuwenberg, P. M. M., Ribbe, M. W., & Bensing, J. M. (2005). Behavioral and mood effects of Snoezelen integrated into 24-hour dementia care. *Journal of the American Geriatric Society, 53,* 24–33.

Vandenberg, D. L. (2001).The use of a weighted vest to increase on-task behavior in children with attention difficulties. *American Journal of Occupational Therapy, 55*(6), 621–628.

Vaughn, S., Gersten, R., & Chard, D. (2000). The underlying message in LD intervention research: Findings from research syntheses. *Exceptional Children, 67*(1), 99–114.

Wilbarger, P., & Wilbarger, J. (2002). The Wilbarger approach to treating sensory defensiveness. In A. Bundy, S. Lane, & E. Murray (Eds.), *Sensory Integration Theory and Practice* (pp. 335–339). Philadelphia: F.A. Davis.

Communication and Social Skills

Virginia Carroll Stoffel and Jeffrey Tomlinson

> We can achieve high-quality lives of inner harmony by meeting our expectations, realizing our goals, and focusing on our ideals. Warm human contact and companionship, as well as general social recognition, can contribute to our success in these endeavors.
>
> —Esso Leete, 1993

Introduction

Across the life span, a person's ability to communicate and interact is at the heart of his or her social relationships and social participation. Nearly every occupational role (e.g., parenting, friend, student, employee) relies on the person's ability to communicate and interact. For persons who live with mental illness, the ability to engage in social relationships and respond to social demands can be affected by their condition. For example, a person with schizophrenia may initiate a conversation that is challenging to follow because of changing content that does not seem to be connected. Or a child with Asperger disorder may not show nonverbal responses to interaction initiated by others, despite intact verbal social skills.

Occupational therapy practitioners recognize the importance that communication and social skills play in carrying out numerous occupational roles, and they design therapeutic interventions and environments to facilitate communication for optimal occupational performance.

Successes associated with communication and social skills often lay in the person-to-person process, especially when, through careful listening, observation, and familiarity, the person receiving the message makes sense of what is meant to be communicated. Occupational therapy practitioners are committed to facilitating communication and interaction skills as part of the skill repertoire that supports successful occupational role participation.

This chapter provides foundational information that will prepare the practitioner to recognize and address communication and interaction challenges that can arise while working with individuals, families, and other relevant people with whom a person who has a serious mental illness interacts. Theories underlying communication and interaction are reviewed, as well as some of the common and unique communication challenges faced by persons with serious mental illness. Assessments and interventions for facilitating communication and social interaction are also offered. A first-person narrative from the perspective of a mother with a child who has autism offers insights into the importance of communication not only in the lives of people who live with a communication disability, but also the family members who work diligently to coordinate care and play a role in their everyday lives.

Communication and Social Skills as Performance Skills

The American Occupational Therapy Association's (AOTA's) *Occupational Therapy Practice Framework: Domain and Process, 2nd Edition* (2008) includes communication and social skills as one of the performance skills within the occupational therapy domain. Examples of communication and social skills include verbal and nonverbal capacities, such as initiating and answering questions; using eye contact, facial expressions, and gestures to convey intentions; acknowledging another person's perspective; and taking turns while interacting (AOTA, 2008). The ability to perform in any occupation requires the ability to communicate and interact effectively with others, whether in the context of work, education, home, or other community settings.

The Occupational Therapy Practice Framework notes that performance skills are interrelated; therefore, although this chapter focuses on communication and social skills, these skills are interrelated with **cognitive skills, emotion regulation skills, sensory-perceptual skills**, and **motor and praxis skills**. For example, a person who is less able to attend to the subtle, nonverbal cues exhibited by a person with whom they are communicating (e.g., a quick frown or hesitation that might convey discomfort) may be completely unaware of such discomfort unless the person expresses that in a manner that is understood by the other person. To fully understand what contributes to an individual's communication or social skill deficit, consider the impact of cognitive and emotion regulation skills (also see Chapters 18 and 24).

When considering an individual's communication and social skills, the occupational therapy practitioner may consider how they are linked to the following areas:

- Instrumental activities of daily living, such as care of others, child rearing, making arrangements for home maintenance (e.g., selecting and hiring a plumber or electrician)
- Educational activities, such as being a student from kindergarten through higher education
- Pursuit of work and volunteer roles

- Play and leisure activities
- Social participation, such as peer, friendship, and intimate relationships, as well as in family and community activities

Both communication and social skills are best practiced while engaged in a person's natural environments and typical occupations. Thus, skill building and training others in effective communication strategies might be the focus of individual and family interventions.

In some cases, the level of communication disability is such that a person requires the services of professionals who specialize in language and communication disorders, such as speech and language pathologists or augmentative communication specialists, such as for a child with autism. Persons with brain trauma, stroke, or dementia might also work closely with speech language pathologists as part of an overall interdisciplinary rehabilitation program. They might receive occupational therapy to address the sensory, motor, and cognitive limitations associated with these conditions, as well as the co-occurring depression, emotional lability, and overall stress that are associated with a challenging recovery process. Regardless of whether the occupational therapy practitioner is formally focused on communication skill building with the person who has a disability or involving the family in training to enhance his or her return to social roles in the home and community, a deep understanding of how communication and social skills can be used in the overall intervention plan is warranted.

Because communication is also one of the elements of therapeutic use of self that contributes to the effectiveness of an occupational therapy intervention, being an excellent communicator and careful listener, as well as providing clear information verbally and in writing, are all important tools of the practitioner.

Theories Underlying Communication and Social Interaction

An overview of the theories and principles that contribute to an understanding of communication and social interaction follows, including the Model of Human Occupation (MOHO;

Kielhofner, 2008), social learning theory, social cognition, and the social skills model, which is based on cognitive behavioral principles. These theories contribute important concepts for understanding the importance of communication and social interaction to the everyday lives of persons with serious mental illness. Given that social skills training is often carried out in groups, group therapeutic factors are also described.

Model of Human Occupation

Gary Kielhofner (2008), an occupational therapy researcher and theorist best known for his collaborative work on refining the MOHO, notes that the model was developed to focus theory, research, and practice on occupation. MOHO explains how occupation is motivated, patterned, and performed as individuals carry out their occupations in the three broad areas of activities of daily living, play, and productivity within various environments. Skills are discrete, purposeful actions that constitute occupational performance, comprised of motor skills, process skills, and communication and social interaction skills (Kielhofner, 2008).

MOHO provides a perspective on communication and social interaction skills that emphasizes the impact of the absence or presence of such skills on important, everyday occupations carried out by persons with mental illness as they engage in varied environments (home, community, work, school, or the treatment environment). A MOHO-based assessment, the Assessment of Communication and Interaction Skills (ACIS; Forsyth, Salamy, Simon, & Kielhofner, 1998), is an observational tool that is described later in the chapter.

Social Learning Theory

Social learning theory (Bandura, 1969) is based on the natural development and learning of social behavior. This theory postulates that the combination of observation and feedback in the form of natural consequences (positive and negative) shapes subsequent behavior. In other words, observing the actions of others is one way a person socially learns. Therapists often use explicit and frequent modeling of social skills as a means to facilitate social learning. When the social interaction is met with a desired or valued outcome (e.g., a smile or a warm welcome), the natural consequence is positively reinforcing to the individual. Frequent use of positive responses to the efforts of a person who is learning new expressive skills (e.g., making eye contact while greeting a person or initiating a conversation) will help positively reinforce that skill, whereas being put down or criticized will likely decrease that skill.

Successively shaping new skills, beginning with simple and successful steps, and working toward more complex skills over time, is recommended when designing social skills training for persons with serious mental illness. Bellack, Mueser, Gingerich, and Agresta (2004) suggest that overlearning skills by having a person repeatedly practice a skill to the point at which it becomes automatic can be facilitated by repeated practice in training sessions by using role-plays, planning homework assignments outside the group, and continued focus until the skill becomes second nature.

Generalizing use of the skills to naturally occurring interactions is the final piece of social learning theory that allows an individual to skillfully use new behaviors at home, on the job, and in the community. For some individuals, this best occurs in the community with case managers or peers who recognize and supply the needed coaching and reinforcement at the time, place, and natural space where the skill is needed.

Social Cognition

Social cognition is defined as "the processes and functions that allow a person to understand, act on, and benefit from the interpersonal world" (Corrigan & Penn, 2001, p. 3). When applied to schizophrenia, this theory proposes that, in addition to ameliorating the biological effect of the disorder with medications to improve the symptoms and resultant disabilities, social cognition offers a person the opportunity to "act on social information that reciprocally acts on the person" (p. 4), thereby addressing the interpersonal disabilities associated with the disorder. In other words, helping a person with schizophrenia to attend to and understand how nonverbal facial expression might convey interest in the form of eye contact, raised eyebrows, and a smile might facilitate a social response that builds a relationship based on shared interests. Application of social cognition to describing disorders and developing interventions has also occurred with depression and anxiety disorders (Abramson, 1988; Dobson & Kendall, 1993). Brothers (1990) links social cognition with behavior by describing social cognition as "the mental operations underlying social interactions, which include the human ability to perceive the intentions and dispositions of others" (p. 28).

Social cognitive deficits of persons with schizophrenia include difficulty communicating thoughts and feelings, as well as conveying and reading feelings nonverbally, resulting in a lack of empathy and difficulty assuming roles to help one's family or social group function more effectively. Social stimuli such as facial affect perception may not be perceived by people with schizophrenia, which is linked with poorer social functioning (Corrigan & Penn, 2001; Couture, Penn, & Roberts, 2006).

It is important to recognize that social cognition allows us to understand the limitations experienced by persons with serious mental illness, as well as the powerful impact that successful social interactions have on social participation.

Social Skills Model

Social skills must be considered in the social context within which they are used; there is considerable variance in what is expected in one social situation as compared with the next,

reflecting cultural and socioeconomic expectations and leading to varying reinforcement (Hersen & Bellack, 1976). Discerning the most appropriate method of requesting a dining table at a five-star restaurant versus a coffee shop, how to greet an elder within a specific culture, and asking about a person's marital status are all examples of social situations in which the context dictates the types of interactions that are considered socially appropriate. Social competence is considered to be an important part of what contributes to successfully finding a partner in marriage, establishing trusting relationships, finding employment well matched to one's capacities, and getting a respectful level of service (Bellack et al, 2004). Persons with serious mental illness may find social competence to be challenging and benefit from a **social skills training** program. It should be noted that these programs tend to be based on cognitive behavioral approaches where the person becomes highly aware of how faulty thoughts might lead to actions that might be less effective in developing strong and healthy relationships (Beck, Rush, Shaw, & Emery, 1979).

Social skills training has become one of the central approaches for developing communication and interaction skills with mental health clients. Social functioning and well-being are important outcomes for persons with psychiatric disability, and their social skills directly affect these important outcomes.

Tenhula and Bellack (2008) suggest that there are three component skills of social competence: social perception (receiving skills), social cognition (processing skills), and behavioral response (expressive skills). Deficits in any of these component skills can affect social functioning. These researchers suggest that the use of the term "skill" emphasizes that they are "learnable" and can be modified by training, practice, and use in everyday life. Table 21-1 outlines important skills for each component.

Of interest in considering occupational context is the distinction that Liberman, DeRisi, and Mueser (1989) make between instrumental social skills and affiliative social skills.

Social skills can be functionally separated into those that have value in instrumental roles and situations and those that are helpful in mediating affiliative relationships. Instrumental skills enable a person to attain independence and material benefits, such as money, residence, goods, and services. Affiliative skills make it possible for an individual to make friends, enjoy intimacy, obtain emotional support, exhibit warmth, and engage in reciprocity with friends and relatives. (p. 33)

Table 21-1 ● **Components of Social Skills**

Component	Skills
Social perception (receiving skills)	• Accurate detection of affect cues (e.g., facial and vocal expression), conveying feelings • Ability to perceive physical responses (e.g., gestures and body posture) • Ability to listen and clarify to promote accurate understanding of verbal message being conveyed and contextual information
Social cognition (processing skills)	• Effective analysis of social stimulus • Integration of current information and historical information • Ability to plan an effective response
Behavioral response (expressive skills)	• Ability to generate effective verbal content • Ability to speak with suitable nonverbal behaviors (e.g., facial gestures and posture) • Ability to maintain eye contact • Understanding of proxemics (physical distance between people while interacting)

Source: Data from Tenhula, W. N., & Bellack, A. S. (2008). Social skills training. In K. T. Mueser & D. V. Jeste (Eds.), Clinical Handbook of Schizophrenia (pp. 240–241). New York: Guilford Press.

When working on communication skills with individuals with serious mental illness, occupational therapy practitioners address the occupational roles that are important to the person, which guides the intervention as to which social skills are targeted and in specific contexts that match those valued by the client.

Group Therapeutic Factors

Groups provide a treatment medium for practicing communication and interaction skills. The **group** is a social microcosm, sometimes under the direction of a therapist, in which members have the opportunity to interact with each other. Yalom (2005) describes 11 primary therapeutic factors in groups, three of which specifically address the development of enhanced communication and interaction skills: socializing techniques, imitative behavior, and interpersonal learning.

Socializing techniques might be explicit (i.e., direct attention to the development of communication and interaction skills) or indirect (i.e., simply facilitating social interaction as part of the group process). **Imitative behavior** allows group members to observe the interactions and behaviors of the group leaders and other group members, and then experiment with applying these interactions themselves. **Interpersonal learning** occurs when the therapy group looks at the interpersonal distortions or misperceptions of others that impair social interaction. Through repeated opportunities for members to develop misperceptions of each other and then later correct those misperceptions, skills are gained as to how to correct or check their thoughts about one another (Yalom, 2005). Such interpersonal learning in groups can provide a rich opportunity to develop more accurate relations with others, greater interaction abilities, and more effective occupational performance.

Mosey (1986) describes group interaction skill as

> . . . the ability to be a productive member of a variety of primary groups. Through acquisition of the various group interaction subskills, the individual learns to take appropriate group membership roles, engage in decision making, communicate effectively, recognize group norms and interact in accordance with these norms, contribute to goal attainment, work toward group cohesiveness and assist in resolving group conflict. (p. 435)

Mosey further describes subskills of group interaction by developmental levels, including the age at which these group interaction skills are expected to emerge depicted in Table 21-2. This hierarchy of developmental groups allows a therapist to promote growth and learning through carefully designed groups that match the person's capacity and moves them toward higher levels of development.

Clients who receive interventions may present with group interaction abilities that match one of these levels. The therapist should consider each individual's ability when developing groups and take into account the developmental processes that can influence acquisition of social skills.

Occupation as a treatment medium provides excellent opportunities for exploring and practicing communication and interaction skills. Carefully planned activities can be designed to elicit different amounts and types of interaction. Mosey (1986) states,

> When people do not know each other, when they are somewhat uncomfortable with each other, a shared purposeful activity frequently allows them to become acquainted and more relaxed. Participation in an activity allows people to have something in common to discuss and serves as a bridge for more intimate communication. (p. 237)

Activity can be the context in which interaction begins. Therapists providing group counseling to very withdrawn clients have found that a group activity prior to the discussion period of the group provides an effective warm-up for group members to then interact.

Activities can also provide a natural environment for interaction when steps in the activity require the sharing of materials or the collaboration between individuals for successful completion of the task. For example, in a day program for individuals with serious and disabling mental illness, the therapist implements a prevocational group to develop work-related skills, such as attendance, punctuality, ability to accept directions from a supervisor, and ability to work with others. The primary gains made by many of the clients in the prevocational group are the development of social skills, with the clients using the context of the work setting as an opportunity to explore social connections with each other.

Table 21-2 ● **Subskills of Group Interactions by Developmental Levels**

Developmental Level	Typical Age When Skill Emerges	Description of Subskill
Parallel group	18 months–2 years	Individuals work or play in the presence of each other. There is an awareness of the others in the group, but not much interaction or sharing.
Project group	2–4 years	Interaction primarily involves the task of the group, with some sharing, cooperation, and competition.
Egocentric-cooperative group	5–7 years	Individuals are actively involved in selecting and jointly engaging in long-term tasks. Participation remains based on self-interest, but also involves recognition that their needs will be met through meeting the needs of others.
Cooperative group	9–12 years	Task is considered secondary to mutual need fulfillment; group membership is homogenous and compatible. Group leader is a consultant rather than an active authority figure.
Mature group	15–18 years	Membership can be heterogenous. Members participate flexibly in both task completion and the gratification of member needs. Members can assume a variety of roles, including leadership.

Source: Data from Mosey, A. C. (1986). Psychosocial Components of Occupational Therapy. New York: Raven Press.

The Lived Experience

From a Parent's Perspective: Ryan

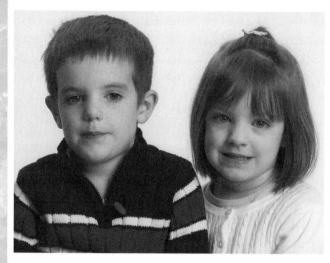

I am a single mom and have 5-year-old twins, Ryan and Tara. Although both children have special needs requiring the attention of a team of rehabilitation professionals, Ryan has a more severe social and communication disability because of his autism.

One of the recent areas where communication became a problem was with a new school bus driver who wrote up a disciplinary notice on Ryan. He was hitting himself and the window because he felt frustrated and wasn't able to communicate with her. He was extremely frustrated, and after using his typical signals to communicate—and because she didn't understand him—he simply regressed to moaning and hitting. That was frustrating for me as a mother because the bus ride is the only part of the day when my kids are in the care of someone who doesn't have any background except a valid driver's license, a clean drug test, and no relevant criminal background. In addition, even though I have tried to communicate clearly with the school bus service, my kids are the first ones picked up and the last to be returned home, which increases the amount of time they spend on the bus, which can be as long as an hour each day. Although his sister sometimes tries to communicate, and the others kids on the bus have special needs like Asperger's, Ryan can't directly ask for what he wants, and it's pretty scary when I think about it, really scary.

I have found a number of workshops to be helpful in learning all that I can about how to communicate with Ryan. In most cases, family members such as my mom and sisters attend with me because they all help out with and include my twins in family events and activities. First, we learned how to use WHO (Watch, Hear, and Observe), so that we watch Ryan and observe how he approaches everyday activities and what signals he gives in trying to communicate. We also learned how to use pictures with simple words, and he did really well with that. After a while, he started using single words and now that he is 5, he is able to initiate specific words to let us know what he wants (e.g., "drink") or what he would like to do (e.g., "Shrek"). He is not able to point, but looks at specific items to communicate what he wants, such as looking at the refrigerator, the TV, or the DVD player. If that

doesn't work, he takes my hand and leads me to where he wants to do something. If I still don't get it, he guides my hand to exactly what he wants to do because he knows sometimes he needs my permission to do something, like watch a DVD.

One of the other challenges when thinking about communication is that it takes a fair amount of time for someone to get to know Ryan, what he likes, and how he communicates, so if people change, there can be another period of time when he will be frustrated while people are learning. I know I can't form his world around him, so I just try to help him learn and adapt, too. When I'm at school or therapy, it can be helpful to see how other parents do that with their kids who are older and who are doing more.

When Ryan and his sister, Tara, try to communicate with each other, there's often a lot of yelling on both parts. Usually, she has a toy that he wants to play with (or vice versa), and they try to take them away from each other. We try to work on "Ryan share" and "Tara share," and what they do is yell that to get my attention while they hold onto the guitar that they don't want to share! Sometimes Ryan will say "Hi Tara" or "Hi Princess" when she is wearing her dress-ups. I think they probably communicate in other ways, more than I am even aware. Tara talks more with her cousins when they play together; however, her and her brother both watch out for each other and pay attention to what is happening with each other, especially at school. Sometimes Tara will say, "Where's my brother? Oh, okay, there he is," and then go on to her own activities.

Some of the things I see people do who are among the most effective communicators with Ryan include not using a lot of words, so the communication style is very simple—one-word questions, one-word responses. Not asking questions for which you would expect a verbal response, because he won't be able to give one, unless it's something like, "Do you want Cheetos or do you want Goldfish?" and no open-ended questions like, "How was your day?" The people who he gets along best with are not his peers, but are his therapists, his teachers, and his aides, along with his aunts, uncles, and Grandma. But he does really enjoy going to loud gatherings and events where he can enjoy and watch everyone, and simply be included in the gathering. He gets so excited when he knows he's going to a family party. And he really enjoys going to school and being with his peers. When you look at him, you can see he just enjoys being around others despite the absence of verbal communication or interactive play. He's playing by himself, but he enjoys being with others.

Ryan has started using the computer and seems to enjoy it. He uses the touch screen a lot, and his speech therapist seems to believe that he could really benefit from an augmentative communication tool (Tango). She's brought it over to our house for him to play with, and after he touches something on the screen, there is a little boy's voice that you hear. It's pretty pricey, but we hope to find ways to see if we can get this for him. It could really make a difference and reduce his frustrations each day.

Pictures, as a communication tool, really work well as a way to help Ryan get ready to go to see a dentist or any health professional. For example, when we have to go to the dentist, just having pictures of kids sitting on the dental chair and a picture of the dentist doing his or her work help prepare him to go there.

The Lived Experience—cont'd

I appreciate when I can get feedback from health professionals in written form because usually I am not always able to pay full attention and might be tired or forgetful, especially when the kids are screaming. Having it in writing also allows me to share it with others who can't be there. If it's easier to send an e-mail, that works well, too. As far as I am concerned, privacy doesn't really matter to me because I need to involve as many people as possible to make things work.

One final suggestion I have is from a workshop that I attended 4 months ago, where a set of parents who have two children with autism presented on their everyday living tips. They created a list of tips to share with others who might be involved in working with their children or who live in their neighborhood. When a new neighbor moved in, they made a picture of each child and provided them with information on the back, like, "This is my son John. If you see him in the neighborhood you may not be able to communicate with him because of his severe autism. Please contact me at (cell phone number), and our home is at (address)." Also, contacting the local police department when you move in to let them know you have children with special needs and the nature of those needs, how to get in contact with parents, what the best methods of communication might be, etc. Sometimes it's just the simplest way to include others so that they understand. Yesterday at day care, I said to one of the children in Ryan's classroom who had a Batman book, "Ryan likes Batman and Shrek, too," and the little guy went running up to Ryan and said, "Batman" and high fived him. Ryan smiled and felt included. That makes a world of difference to Ryan. They find what they have in common. That's the kind of communication that I plan to do next year when he goes to a special education kindergarten, where he'll be with a new group of kids who he'll likely spend time with over the years, so they can get to know each other.

The first word that Ryan said was when he was about 3.5 years old was "Shrek," and he started to say it while we were attending mass at our local church. I thought to myself, "Wait, not here," but at the same time was so excited to hear him say a word. So I figured out that he really didn't want to be in church, and he said "Shrek" out loud as many times as he could. Finally, I really knew what he wanted!

Communication and Social Skills in Persons With Psychiatric Disabilities

A number of common challenges in communication and social interaction skills faced by persons with psychiatric disabilities are summarized in this section, and the reader is also encouraged to review the chapters elsewhere in this text related to each psychiatric condition to more deeply understand these challenges.

Schizophrenia

The following set of instructions for family members, written by a person who lives with schizophrenia, offers the reader a sense of the challenges experienced by people who live with mental illness and provides the reader with straightforward suggestions that can lead to clear communication (Leete, 1993):

Recognize both our idiosyncratic thinking and the fact that we may not have the same communication style or skill as you do. First of all, try to minimize distractions during conversations. Be aware of surrounding stimuli and move to a different area if necessary. Communicate clearly and concisely. Speak slowly, in short sentences, if necessary. Give the information in small portions. Begin your answers with either "yes" or "no," then elaborate; otherwise your point may be missed. When we are speaking, try not to interrupt. This can be very confusing and frustrating. We're fighting hard enough to speak without being forced to stop and begin again, often on a tenuously held train of thought. (p. 124)

For individuals with serious mental health disorders, communication and interaction skills can be severely impaired. This is especially true for people with schizophrenia (Bellack et al, 2004; Corrigan & Penn, 2001; Tenhula & Bellack, 2008). People with schizophrenia experience positive symptoms (i.e., aberrations in behavior or behavior that is not typically present in other individuals) during the active phase of psychosis that interfere with communication and interaction, such as delusions, hallucinations, disorganized speech, and grossly disorganized or catatonic behavior (American Psychiatric Association [APA], 2000).

During periods of active positive symptoms, interactions with people in the community can be difficult and at times deleterious. People in the community may be uncomfortable or even frightened by the content of a client's communications, the disorganized speech, and the behavioral changes. Relationships in occupational and social contexts may be seriously strained during the active phase of schizophrenia. To allow the individual to develop successful occupational and social roles, relapse prevention and effective management of the illness is critical.

Individuals with schizophrenia experience challenges in social competence and may risk relapse associated with the anxiety, frustration, and isolation caused by poor social skills (Bellack et al, 2004). Although social skills are believed to be learned throughout development, researchers have postulated that certain aspects of social skills, such as facial expression showing feelings, might be genetically determined (Bellack et al, 2004). Psychotic symptoms such as intrusive verbal hallucinations can affect a person with schizophrenia's ability to attend to others, while interacting socially, thereby missing significant social information.

Because of social rejection and stigma, the person with schizophrenia might be less than motivated to seek out social contacts and avoid closer relationships. Social anxiety can result in avoidance and hesitation in engaging in social interactions. Due to attentional difficulties associated with schizophrenia, the information processing system related to memory, thinking, and learning affects social behavior in persons with schizophrenia (Green, Kern, Braff, & Mintz, 2000). Being able to discern what to attend to (e.g., when a person is talking at the same time a TV is on), focusing and sustaining attention, dealing with distractions, and tracking complex verbal and nonverbal messages associated with emotionally laden conversation can all present challenges to the person with schizophrenia.

Andreasen (1982) noted that the negative symptoms (i.e., the absence of typical function) associated with schizophrenia affect social skills; these can include an overall lack of motivation (avolition), low energy to participate in social situations (anergia), an inability to find pleasure in activities (anhedonia), and being challenged to initiate conversations (alogia).

Anxiety and Mood Disorders

Individuals with anxiety and mood disorders can also have a severe impairment in communication and interaction performance. In depressive disorders, the depressed mood, anhedonia, feelings of worthlessness, and diminished ability to concentrate are all symptoms that affect interactions with others (APA, 2000). Depressive disorders often lead to the extensive expression of negative thought content toward others, which people have great difficulty tolerating. Depression also results in extensive social withdrawal.

Individuals with bipolar disorder or manic episodes may have additional symptoms that affect interaction. The grandiosity, flight of ideas, pressured speech, distractibility, or excessive impulsive involvement in pleasurable activities have a negative impact on other people and can result in other people withdrawing from the client (APA, 2000).

Persons with anxiety disorder might convey a lack of interest in others due to heightened awareness of their own nervousness, lacking social attentiveness such as eye contact, and verbal tracking. Other symptoms such as intense fear also inhibit social interactions (APA, 2000).

Personality Disorders

Central to most personality disorders is some impairment in social interaction. These personality disorders include paranoid, schizoid, schizotypal, antisocial, borderline, histrionic, narcissistic, avoidant, dependent, and obsessive-compulsive disorders. People with these disorders may be experienced by others as odd and eccentric, or volatile and erratic. Individuals with these disorders usually have great difficulty sustaining positive relations with others (APA, 2000).

Substance Use Disorders

Although communication and interaction challenges are not specifically associated with the diagnosis of a substance use disorder, persons recovering from substance use disorders may find communication and social interaction to be a challenge in their recovery process. Finding new ways of being with others apart from a drinking or using environment, being able to assertively refuse offers of alcohol or other drugs, and using communication skills to build healthy relationships are all examples of the kinds of challenges frequently encountered by persons working on their recovery from substance abuse (Liberman, DeRisi, & Mueser, 1989; Stoffel & Moyers, 2004). For a person whose substance abuse developed during adolescence or early adulthood, recovery might also include learning to develop coping strategies for dealing with everyday anxieties and establishing friendships built on trust.

Pervasive Developmental Disorders

Children with autism spectrum disorders, including Asperger's disorder, tend to experience significant challenges with communication and social interaction, although individuals with Asperger's disorder do not often have delayed or impaired language (APA, 2000). Common communication and social deficits of persons with pervasive developmental disorders include difficulty attending to others' speech, difficulty attending to other's facial expressions, failure to vocalize, limited ability to shift gaze between people and objects, limited use of gestures, unusual speech tone and rhythm, and limited use of words (Audet, 2004).

Communication challenges for adults with Asperger's have been described as having monotone facial expressions and vocal intonation, yet they have highly sophisticated content of verbal expression with narration that depicts great attention to detail (Roy, Dillo, Emrich, & Ohlmeier, 2009). Eye contact tends to be avoided, and jokes and smiles often elicit no response. Adults with Asperger's syndrome tend to live a withdrawn life and have difficulties in partnering, appearing to be self-centered or "cold" toward others (Roy et al, 2009).

Dementia and Cognitive Disorders in Older Adults

Depending on the severity of the dementia or cognitive disorder, the individual may experience problems in language, such as rambling, disjointed, pressured, or incoherent speech that jumps from one topic to another. Such difficulty may also include writing or naming things. As the dementia progresses, the person may become more withdrawn and use language less often (APA, 2000).

Impact on Social Development

As part of this overview of psychopathology and its impact on communication and interaction, these disorders also affect social development. The onset of many of these disorders first occurs during adolescence or early adulthood, developmental periods that are critical for the acquisition of communication and interaction skills that are essential to occupational and social functioning. The marked disruption of development in adolescence and early adulthood by these disorders can have a profound and long-standing effect on the individual. For example, the repeated hospitalizations and chronic disability characteristics of schizophrenia can result in a separation from environments in which adolescents and young adults would typically develop socially. In addition, intolerance and judgment from others in the family and community can lead to further withdrawal from natural social settings.

In all diagnostic categories discussed in this chapter, individuals can be vulnerable to cognitive behavioral patterns that include faulty information processing and automatic thoughts that are dysfunctional. Automatic negative thoughts can have a destructive impact on communication and interaction with others. Automatic thoughts are evaluative thoughts that we all have about events around us. They may be preconscious (i.e., thoughts that we are not completely aware of), and they do not come from careful reasoning. Underlying these automatic thoughts are core beliefs developed early in life that are central to how individuals perceives themselves and events around them. These beliefs are held as absolute truths and overgeneralized; however, at the same time, they are usually not subject to self-awareness. For example, a client who has developed beliefs that he or she is not competent will then, when faced with new social situations, experience automatic thoughts that they cannot socialize, have nothing worth saying, and most likely will be rejected if they attempt to talk to others. The negative thoughts may either be expressed to others overtly in communications or may affect the individual's sense of self-efficacy and confidence in social situations (Beck et al, 1979).

Assessments

Both formal and informal assessment of communication and social interaction skills are commonly used by occupational therapy practitioners. The occupational profile (AOTA, 2008) may include observations of social interaction and communication in response to questions asked about one's typical day and valued occupational roles, such as questions about one's social network, relationships, and preferred communication modes. Social participation may be reviewed by asking questions about how the individual interacts with and engages in conversations with siblings, family members, and peers at home, in school, on the playground, and in other community settings (Frolek Clark, Miller-Kuhaneck, & Watling, 2004).

Formal assessments of communication and social skills have been developed by occupational therapists as well as speech language pathologists and psychologists. The tools reviewed here were selected based on a review of the occupational therapy literature.

Assessment of Communication and Interaction Skills

The ACIS is a formal observational assessment based on the MOHO, which measures a person's performance within a social context (Forsyth et al, 1998). This tool provides information about the individual's strengths and weaknesses related to interaction and communication while carrying out daily occupations that are meaningful and relevant to the client's life.

The optimum context for carrying out the ACIS is the client's actual environment (home, school, work, community) as he or she is engaged in dyadic interactions (1:1 contacts) and larger group contexts. The three domains of physicality, information exchange, and relations are assessed through a total of 20 items, rated on a 4-point scale. The scale was developed to use with a population of clients with psychiatric impairments and has been used with a wide range of children, adolescents, and adults who self-report difficulty in communication and interaction as young as age 3 to 4 (Kielhofner et al, 2008).

PhotoVoice

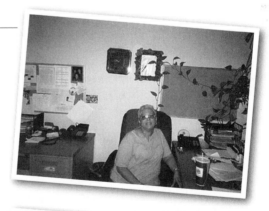

People are very important to my well-being. Going through rough times or just venting, it's good to have someone to talk to. Even though some move on, it's nice to know they were there when I needed them.

—Helen

The ACIS begins with an interview of the client or a significant other to determine the appropriate contexts for observation, and can be administered during a therapeutic group or in the client's natural environment. Observation time ranges from 15 to 45 minutes and rating time from 15 to 20 minutes, depending on the amount of qualitative information recorded by the therapist. Based on the strengths and weaknesses noted, targeted skills for the focus of intervention are identified. Social environments that may have a positive impact on the client's communication and interaction are identified, and can be used to determine group assignment or living placement.

Social Skills in the Workplace

Tsang, an occupational therapist, and Pearson, a social worker, developed this two-part measure of social competence in the workplace for people with schizophrenia, based on their model for assessing social skills (Tsang & Pearson, 1996, 2000).

Part one consists of a 10-item, self-administered checklist that measures perceived competence in handling work-related social situations, such as making an appointment for a job interview, requesting an urgent leave from a supervisor, or helping instruct a task for a new colleague. A 6-point scale is used to identify the level of difficulty experienced by the individual in carrying out the task.

Part two consists of a role-play of two simulated situations, a job interview and a request for an urgent leave from a supervisor. The role-play is rated by using a 5-point scale, with 4 representing normal performance and 0 representing poor performance, with either excesses or deficiencies in the desirable behaviors. Basic social survival skills, voice quality, nonverbal components, and verbal components, as well as situation-specific ratings, are analyzed after viewing the role-plays. Internal consistency of the self-administered checklist and role-play test (Cronbach alpha coefficients of 0.80 and 0.96, respectively), as well as test–retest reliability (0.35–0.78 for checklist) and interrater reliability (0.77–0.90 for role-play), have been established. The whole measure can be completed within 30 minutes and can be used to monitor baseline and progress over time.

Social Interaction Scale

The Social Interaction Scale (SIS) is one of two parts of the Bay Area Functional Performance Evaluation; the second part is the Task Oriented Assessment (Williams & Bloomer, 1987), a tool developed by two occupational therapists. The SIS is an observational assessment of seven verbal and nonverbal behaviors in five different settings: a 1:1 interview, mealtime, an unstructured group, a structured activity group, and a structured verbal group (Klyczek & Stanton, 2008). Ratings for the seven parameters of social interaction include verbal communication, psychomotor behavior, socially appropriate behavior, response to authority figures, independence/dependence, ability to work with others, and participation in group or program activities. A minimum of 10 minutes in each social setting within a 1- to 2-day period is recommended for completion of the SIS.

Comprehensive Occupational Therapy Evaluation

The Comprehensive Occupational Therapy Evaluation (COTE) was developed in 1975 by five occupational therapists, a psychiatrist and a psychologist, working together in Greenville, South Carolina (Brayman, 2008). The COTE ratings provide an overview of a person's occupational performance in three areas: general behaviors, interpersonal/communication skills, and task behaviors. The section on interpersonal/communication skills includes the following six behaviors, which are observed while the client is engaged in an occupational therapy environment: independence, cooperation, self-assertion, sociability, attention-getting behavior, and negative response from others.

Relevant Assessments Developed Outside Occupational Therapy

Several tools have been developed to assess various social and communication skills and may be used by occupational therapists and other mental health professionals in clinical and research programs to measure the effectiveness of social skills training and other programs. Most of the tools are interviews, self-report checklists (some confirmed by others such as family members), observational tools, and role-play with rating scales.

Social Functioning Interview

The Social Functioning Interview (Bellack et al, 2004) provides information about an individual's past and present role functioning (e.g., daily routines at home; as a student, worker, or volunteer; leisure activities; significant relationships; spiritual supports). It also explores social situations that the person sees as problematic, such as starting and holding conversations; managing conflicts; asserting self; living with others; having good relationships with family, partner, and friends; talking with treatment staff; and working or volunteering. This tool records the personal goals, as well as social skill strengths and weaknesses observed by the clinician during the interview.

Evidence-Based Practice

The question as to whether self-assessments are accurate in populations with serious and disabling mental illness was addressed in a study of 67 older adults with schizophrenia in whom self-assessment of social function was found to be inconsistent with actual performance of functional tasks. Clients with cognitive and functional impairment consistently overestimated their performance.

➤ Occupational therapy practitioners can use multiple methods to assess client social functioning, including naturalistic observation in settings typical for the person being assessed, self-report measures, role-play tests, and input from family and caregivers.

Bowie., C. R., Twamley, E. W., Anderson, H., Halpern, B., Patterson, T. L., & Harvey, P. D. (2007). Self-assessment of functional status in schizophrenia. *Journal of Psychiatric Research, 41,* 1012–1018.

Social Functioning Scale

The Social Functioning Scale (Birchwood, Smith, Cochrane, Wetton, & Copestake, 1990) was constructed to evaluate areas crucial to community living for persons with schizophrenia, such as social engagement or withdrawal (e.g., time spent alone, initiation of conversations, social avoidance), interpersonal behaviors (e.g., number of friends, heterosexual contact, quality of communication), prosocial activities (e.g., engagement in a range of common social activities), recreation (e.g., engagement in common hobbies, interests), independence-competence (e.g., ability to perform skills for independent living), independence-performance (e.g., performance of skills for independent living), and employment/occupation (e.g., engagement in productive employment or structured programs of daily activity). The tool identifies the client's strengths and weaknesses, and has been used to track the efficacy of family interventions.

Communication Skills Questionnaire

The Communication Skills Questionnaire (CSQ; Takahashi, Tanaka, & Miyaoka, 2006) was developed as a tool for evaluating the communication skills of persons with schizophrenia, mood disorders, and eating disorders. It can be administered as a self-report or by family or medical staff. The 29 items of the CSQ include 17 items concerning cooperative skills, 6 items addressing assertiveness skills, and 6 items concerning general communication skills, primarily nonverbal skills.

Independent Living Skills Survey

The Independent Living Skills Survey (Wallace, Liberman, Tauber, & Wallace, 2000) is described as a "comprehensive, objective, performance-focused, easy-to-administer measure of the basic functional living skills of individuals with severe and persistent mental illness" (p. 631). Two versions of the tool have been developed, one for informants and one for self-report. Of the 103 items on the scale, 9 are related to social skills, rated on a 6-point frequency scale from "always" to "never or no opportunity."

Maryland Assessment of Social Competence

The Maryland Assessment of Social Competence (MASC; Bellack, Brown, & Thomas-Lohrman, 2006) uses role-play procedures to evaluate social competence, that is, the ability to resolve interpersonal problems through conversation. Each of the four to six role-plays takes place in a 3-minute time period with a partner and is designed to capture the ability to think on one's feet and respond to the changing social cues or problems. The Social Skills Performance Assessment (Patterson, Moscona, McKibbin, Davidson, & Jeste, 2001) is abbreviated and adapted from the MASC and includes two role-plays, a social interaction (meeting a new neighbor), and an instrumental interaction (requesting attention from a landlord about a previously reported problem).

Social-Adaptive Functioning Evaluation

The Social-Adaptive Functioning Evaluation (SAFE; Harvey et al, 1997) was developed for geriatric clients with psychiatric disabilities to measure social-interpersonal, instrumental, and life skills functioning. It is designed to be rated by observation, caregiver contact, and interaction with the subject. Each of the 17 items is rated on a 5-point scale, where higher scores indicate more severe impairment in social-adaptive functioning. Ratings were found to be internally consistent and reliable across raters and across time. Seven of the 17 items were analyzed to be factors of the social functions component, including conversational skills, instrumental social skills, social appropriateness/politeness, social engagement, friendships, recreation/leisure, and participation in hospital programs (Harvey et al, 1997).

Social Occupational Functioning Scale

The Social Occupational Functioning Scale (SOFS; Saraswat, Rao, Subbakrishna, & Gangadhar, 2006) was developed as a "brief, yet comprehensive, easy to administer measure of social functioning for use in busy clinical settings" (p. 301). The 14 items measure adaptive living skills (bathing and grooming, neatness and maintenance activities, money management, orientation/mobility, instrumental social skills), social appropriateness (clothing and dressing, eating and diet, respect for property, independence/responsibility), and interpersonal skills (conversation skills, social appropriateness/politeness, social engagement, recreation/leisure) using a 5-point rating scale similar to the SAFE, which accounted for 59% variance in the total SOFS score (Saraswat et al, 2006).

A combination of naturalistic observation of the person in varied social contexts and systematic assessment of social and interaction skills will likely yield data that will allow the clinician to track progress and changes in social and interaction skills necessary for mental health recovery and living in the community.

Interventions

Once the occupational therapist and the person with a psychiatric disability have identified communication and social interaction as an important area for intervention, determination of the best intervention(s) for that person needs to take place. Building on the individual's strengths and intact skills and resources in his or her environment, intervention might include social skills training, problem-solving training, responsive social skills training, and generalization of social skills training.

Social Skills Training

Social skills training (SST) is an intervention that has been structured to target deficits in social problem-solving skills, with the overall goal of enhancing social functioning for persons with psychiatric disabilities (Bellack, 2004; Bellack et al, 2004; Kopelowicz, Liberman, & Zarate, 2006; Liberman et al, 1989; Tenhula & Bellack, 2008). Once the individual has established the social and interactional challenges and obstacles they encounter in their everyday lives, a focus on personal skill development is built into their treatment or wellness recovery plan.

Based on the Social Skills Model, social skills training emphasizes the development of learned skills that can be practiced and integrated into everyday occupational routines and situations related to establishing affiliative relationships and independent living. This highly structured approach to teaching skills involves breaking skills into discrete steps, rehearsing the behaviors through role-plays, and providing feedback and reinforcement to participants regarding their effectiveness (Tenhula & Bellack, 2008).

Peer support and role modeling are provided by the therapist and group participants, with an emphasis on tailoring the skills training toward problems identified by the person, based on personal goals (Kopelowicz et al, 2006). Typically, practice in natural environments is encouraged through homework assignments, which might be structured (e.g., "Find two to three opportunities each day to practice these skills when you go into the community") so that, at the start of the next group session, participants can report on their experiences with the targeted skills.

Skills training can be conducted individually, in groups, and with families. Group methods are the most common, consisting of 4 to 12 participants with 1 to 2 therapists for sessions that are conducted for 45 to 90 minutes, meeting 1 to 5 times per week (Kopelowicz et al, 2006). SST is conducted by diverse practitioners, including occupational therapists, nurses, social workers, psychologists, and paraprofessionals.

Each new skill begins with identifying a rationale for the skill (e.g., generated by the participants in response to a reflection exercise, such as "Why is this important to your mental health recovery?"), with instruction about the steps involved in the skill. This example is offered by Tenhula and Bellack (2008):

> For example, initiating conversations requires first gaining the other person's attention via introductory remarks ("Hi, is this seat taken?"; "Excuse me, does the number 2 bus stop here?"), asking general questions (e.g., How have you been?"; "Do you come here often?"), following up with specific questions (e.g., "Did you see the game last night?"), and sharing information with I statements (e.g., "I think . . .," "I feel . . ., "I like . . ."). Nonverbal and paralinguistic behaviors are similarly segmented (e.g., making eye contact, shaking hands, nodding one's head). Participants are first taught to perform the elements of the skill, then gradually learn to combine them smoothly through repeated practice, shaping, and reinforcement of successive approximations. (p. 242)

Role-playing simulated conversations and using behavioral demonstrations assist the person in identifying the most relevant social situations based on what would be most useful in his or her everyday life. Regardless of the level of skill demonstrated in the role-play, the therapist provides positive feedback about the role-play and offers suggestions about trying something different or adding something that was missing in the role-play (Tenhula & Bellack, 2008). Handouts and written prompts provide the participant with concrete reminders of each skill so that practicing the skills in everyday life can be completed more easily. Subsequent sessions always start with a review of the experiences between sessions associated with how the individual carried out that skill, including successes and challenges (Tenhula & Bellack, 2008).

SST curricula have been developed to support the domains of starting and maintaining conversations, assertiveness, friendship and dating, medication management, HIV prevention, job interviewing, and drug refusal skills, with the generic SST model used to teach any social skill identified by the participant (Bellack et al, 2004; Liberman et al, 1989; Tenhula & Bellack, 2008). Occupational therapy practitioners may find that they can aide generalization of skills by following group skills training with coaching and reinforcement in the actual occupational environments, such as community case management at the workplace, in the supported living apartment, or whatever the natural contexts are for the individual.

As in any therapy intervention, the treating therapists should always be sensitive to the clients' experiences of frustration, as well as their concerns about self-efficacy and the risk of failure. Liberman et al (1989) offer three important points in regard to preventing or reducing client frustration during social skills training:

1. "Remember the shaping principle. Like everything else in social skills training, you should start with easier assignments and gradually increase the difficulty and complexity as the patient's skill and confidence increase." (p. 118)
2. "The importance of setting the level of difficulty to maximize the probability of success can't be overemphasized." (p. 118)
3. "Always prepare the patients in advance for the real possibility of failure; in fact, patients should expect to succeed only some of the time with their assignments and not take failure personally." (p. 119)

The therapist may choose to reframe the experience of failure for the client by offering an alternative perception, such as an opportunity for learning, exploring, or evaluating one's current strengths and weaknesses.

An additional concern that the therapist must consider during social skills training is the difficulty some clients may have with attention. The therapist should monitor the clients' level of attention during the session. Are participants maintaining eye contact with the other participants in the session? Are they actively listening? Repetition of information, such as paraphrasing, summarizing information, and other techniques, can be helpful for clients who are having difficulty with attention. To keep everyone's attention on the social skills training group, Liberman et al (1989) recommend, "Stay on your feet! Most mental health professionals are used to conducting therapy sessions from a chair. . . . A blackboard or easel with newsprint pads should be available, since you will want to document the specific behavioral targets for training through the visual as well as audiochannel" (p. 75).

Problem-Solving Training

During social skills training, it usually becomes evident that many of the social situations in which clients experience difficulty involve something more than rote employment of specific interaction skills. Many social situations involve some assessment and problem-solving abilities to address the situation. What exactly is the other person saying? What does it mean to me? Am I interpreting the situation accurately? What is the best way to respond? Clients often demonstrate deficits in this assessment and problem-solving

The Lived Experience

Jose

Jose, a 48-year-old man with a diagnosis of schizophrenia, has now been working for 18 years. Jose recalls his treatment in the day program: "The role-play group really helped me at work and at home. It helped me to organize my thoughts, to know what to say. Things I learned how to do, I use at work when I have problems with my supervisor or with my coworkers. I feel I can talk for myself when I have to."

Evidence-Based Practice

Social skills training results in the acquisition of social skills through the use of instructions, modeling, role-play, reinforcement, corrective feedback, and in vivo exercises by homework assignments. A meta-analysis of social skills training efficacy studies confirms that acquired social skills are confirmed by changes as measured in role-play tests demonstrating enhancement of their assertiveness. In addition, social skills training consistently leads to a moderate but significant and stable improvement in social functioning, slightly reduces general psychopathology, and considerably decreases the hospitalization rate at follow-up.

➤ Occupational therapy practitioners should examine their social skills protocols to be sure that all aspects of best practice (instructions, modeling, role-play, reinforcement, corrective feedback, and homework) are included in their interventions.

Pfammatter, M., Junghan, U. M., & Brenner, H. D. (2006). Efficacy of psychological therapy in schizophrenia: Conclusions from meta-analyses. *Schizophrenia Bulletin, 32*(S1), S64–S80.

process. To address this problem and enhance further social functioning, many therapists have included problem-solving with social skills training. Bellack et al (2004) describe six steps to problem-solving:

1. Define the problem.
2. Use brainstorming to generate possible solutions.
3. Identify the advantages and disadvantages of each possible solution.
4. Select the best solution or combination of solutions.
5. Plan how to carry out the solution(s).
6. Follow-up on the plan at a later time.

Responsive Social Skills Training

Responsive social skills training combines problem-solving with social skills training in a group setting. For example, in long-term rehabilitation settings, a structured, preprogrammed social skills training sequence can be quickly exhausted, leaving the clients with incomplete acquisition of interaction skills. Clients often present with new and novel social situations with which they have had difficulty. In a **responsive social skills training** group, the clients are invited to report any recent events that have occurred in their lives that they would like to work on with the group. In addition, clients are invited to identify any anticipated social situations that may occur in the future. For example, the client may have an appointment at the Social Security office later in the week and have many concerns about what to say.

In a responsive social skills training group, the following sequence is followed:

1. Client(s) who were the focus of role-plays or who were given homework during the previous session are asked to report on their progress since that session.
2. Clients are invited to describe any social situations that they have experienced or that they anticipate occurring. If the clients cannot offer a situation, the group leaders may choose to introduce a situation or a choice of situations.
3. The group makes a decision about which situation to focus on.
4. Start the problem-solving sequence:
   - Define the problem.
   - Generate possible solutions for the problem.
   - Identify the pros and cons of each possible solution.
   - Select the best solution or combination of solutions.
   - Discuss how to carry out the solution in a social interaction.
5. Start the social skills training sequence:
   - Set up an interpersonal situation for a dry run role-play (i.e., the individual whose situation is being enacted runs it as it most recently occurred, without trying to use the most effective social skills).
   - Give instructions for the role-play.
   - Run the scene as a dry run.
   - Give positive and constructive feedback.
   - Use a model (another group member who can demonstrate more effective social skills) for another role-play of the same situation.
   - Verify that the client understands what has transpired in the second role-play, and identify the skills demonstrated by the model.
   - Give instructions to the client for a rerun of the role-play.
   - Rerun the role-play.
   - Give positive and constructive feedback.
   - Give a real life homework assignment.
   - Summarize skills covered in the session.

The added amount of information covered by a responsive social skills training group puts a heavy demand on the group. The group leaders may have to consider scheduling the group for a slightly extended time. The group leaders will need to move the group process along or risk running out of time. Liberman et al (1989) warn that

> Very early we found that people—both patients and therapists—had a tendency to talk a lot about the whys and wherefores of the problems, symptoms, and complexities present in any situation. Speculation on psychodynamics and motives, 'war stories' of various kinds, rationalizations, alibis, and other irrelevancies kept intruding and getting in the way of actually doing something. We found that such talk reduced the number of times a person could practice and get feedback. Be wary of this trap. (p. 74)

Generalization of Social Skills Training

Therapists often clearly describe progress observed in therapy sessions. However, one of the greatest concerns about social skills training is whether the client truly applies the techniques or skills learned in therapy sessions or groups to their actual life situations, that is, the generalization of skills learned in treatment. Bellack et al (2004) suggest a number of techniques that can be used to enhance generalization:

- Homework assignments
- Multiple exemplars and trainers
- Problem-solving strategy
- In vivo practice (meaning in the real life/world of the person)
- Fading of training structure, frequency, and supervision and reinforcement
- Treatment settings that approximate or simulate the "real world"

- Natural reinforcers to support acquired skills
- Skills that are "marketable" and self-sustaining in the community
- Client's use of self-reinforcement
- Repeated practice and overlearning
- Functional and attainable goals in training skills

In addition to these strategies, Kopelowicz et al (2006) suggest that promoting peer support specialists as part of community support programs could enhance the environmental supports for generalizing social skills in natural environments. Use of technology through social networking tools available on the Internet also allows for people with serious mental illness to select the method by which they are most comfortable in using their social interaction skills.

Summary

Occupational therapy practitioners play an important role in helping facilitate the communication and interaction skills necessary for individuals with mental illness to be full participants in everyday life in the community. Building on strengths, focusing on those skills that a person is able to do, coaching to enhance performance, and offering opportunities to use social and communication skills in everyday life are the building blocks that occupational therapy practitioners can use to enhance social competence. Working with families and promoting clear and open communication with all clients, families and community participants are key tools to affecting this important area of occupational performance.

Active Learning Strategies

1. Self-Assessment

Therapeutic use of self is a basic approach to social skills training. When the therapist is able to effectively model good communication in a variety of social settings, clients actively learn. Begin by assessing your own communication and social interaction skills.

Reflective Questions

- What are your strengths and weaknesses as a communicator? Comfort in social situations? Comfort leading groups? Comfort meeting new people?
- What interpersonal skills do you believe that you need to further develop? How do you plan to do so?
- How comfortable are you with collaborating with a client who is angry or agitated? Depressed?
- How will these communication skills be important in your future practice as an occupational therapist?

2. Role-Playing

Using either Liberman et al (1989) or Bellack et al (2004), practice role-playing a social skills training group session with

OT student peers. Trade roles (leader, participant, observer) during the role-play. Select either real life situations or hypothetical situations, such as a client talking to a doctor or a client asserting him- or herself in a difficult social situation. Develop a realistic homework assignment for each scenario.

3. Interview

Interview the family member of a person with a disability about his or her view of communication with health professionals. Ask for any suggestions he or she might have for improving communication with doctors, therapists, and other health professionals. Sample questions could include: What are the ways that you find most useful to communicate with your son's therapist? How do you think your communication could be improved?

Reflective Journal

Using your Reflective Journal, write about what you learned that will influence your communication as an occupational therapist in future practice.

Resources

- The National Association of School Psychologists (NASP) website provides many links to resources supporting social skill development and are noted as "Examples of evidence-based social skills programs": www.nasponline.org/resources/factsheets/socialskills_fs.aspx
- The "Free Social Skills Advice From a Former Shy, Awkward Guy" website offers information on social skills and how to get along with others: http://www.succeedsocially.com/
- The ACIS can be ordered via the MOHO Clearinghouse E-Store: http://ascendant.cas.uic.edu/retail/product.asp?catalog_name=MOHO&category_name=Assessments&product_id=0001301

References

Abramson, L. Y. (1988). *Social Cognition and Clinical Psychology*. New York: Guilford Press.

American Occupational Therapy Association (AOTA). (2008). Occupational therapy practice framework: Domain and process (2nd ed.). *American Journal of Occupational Therapy, 62*, 625–683.

American Psychiatric Association (APA). (2000). *Diagnostic and Statistical Manual of Mental Disorders* (4th ed., text revision). Washington, DC: Author.

Andreasen, N. C. (1982). Negative symptoms in schizophrenia: Definition and reliability. *Archives of General Psychiatry, 39*, 784–788.

Audet, L. R. (2004). The pervasive developmental disorders: A holistic view. In H. Miller-Kuhaneck (Ed.), *Autism: A Comprehensive Occupational Therapy Approach* (2nd ed., pp. 41–66). Bethesda, MD: AOTA Press.

Bandura, A. (1969). *Principles of Behavior Modification*. New York: Holt, Rinehart and Winston.

Beck, A. T., Rush, A. J., Shaw, B. F., & Emery, G. (1979). *Cognitive Therapy of Depression*. New York: Guilford Press.

Bellack, A. S. (2004). Skills training for people with severe mental illness. *Psychiatric Rehabilitation Journal, 27*, 375–391.

Bellack, A. S., Brown, C. H., & Thomas-Lohrman, S. (2006). Psychometric characteristics of role-play assessments of social skill in schizophrenia. *Behavior Therapy, 37*, 339–352.

Bellack, A. S., Mueser, K. T., Gingerich, S., & Agresta, J. (2004). *Social Skills Training for Schizophrenia: A Step-by-Step Guide* (2nd ed.). New York: Guilford Press.

Birchwood, M., Smith, J., Cochrane, R., Wetton, S., & Copestake, S. (1990). The Social Functioning Scale: The development and validation of a new scale of social adjustment for use in family intervention programmes with schizophrenic patients. *British Journal of Psychiatry, 157*, 853–859.

Bowie., C. R., Twamley, E. W., Anderson, H., Halpern, B., Patterson, T. L., & Harvey, P. D. (2007). Self-assessment of functional status in schizophrenia. *Journal of Psychiatric Research, 41*, 1012–1018.

Brayman, S. J. (2008). The Comprehensive Occupational Therapy Evaluation (COTE). In B. J. Hemphill-Pearson (Ed.), *Assessments in Occupational Therapy Mental Health: An Integrative Approach* (pp. 113–126). Thorofare, NJ: Slack.

Brothers, L. (1990). The social brain: A project for integrating primate behavior and neurophysiology in a new domain. *Concepts in Neuroscience, 1*, 27–61.

Corrigan, P. W., & Penn, D. L. (2001). *Social Cognition and Schizophrenia*. Washington, DC: American Psychological Association.

Couture, S. M., Penn, D. L., & Roberts, D. L. (2006). The functional significance of social cognition in schizophrenia: A review. *Schizophrenia Bulletin, 32*(S1), S44–S63.

Dickinson, D., Bellack, A. S., & Gold, J. M. (2007). Social/communication skills, cognition, and vocational functioning in schizophrenia. *Schizophrenia Bulletin, 33*, 1213–1220.

Dobson, K. S., & Kendall, P. C. (Eds.). (1993). *Psychopathology and Cognition*. San Diego, CA: Academic Press.

Forsyth, K., Salamy, M., Simon, S., & Kielhofner, G. (1998). *The Assessment of Communication and Interaction Skills (Version 4.0)*. Chicago: Department of Occupational Therapy, University of Illinois at Chicago.

Frolek Clark, G., Miller-Kuhaneck, H., & Watling, R. (2004). Evaluation of the child with an autism spectrum disorder. In H. Miller-Kuhaneck (Ed.), *Autism: A Comprehensive Occupational Therapy Approach* (2nd ed., pp. 107–153). Bethesda, MD: AOTA Press.

Green, M. F., Kern, R. S., Braff, D. L., & Mintz, J. (2000). Neurocognitive deficits and functional outcome in schizophrenia: Are we measuring the "right stuff"? *Schizophrenia Bulletin, 26*, 119–136.

Harvey, P. D., Davidson, M., Mueser, K. T., Parrella, M., White, L., & Powchik, P. (1997). Social-Adaptive Functioning Evaluation (SAFE): A rating scale for geriatric psychiatric patients. *Schizophrenia Bulletin, 23*, 131–145.

Hersen, M., & Bellack, A. S. (1976). Social skills training for chronic psychiatric patients: Rationale, research findings, and future directions. *Comprehensive Psychiatry, 17*, 559–580.

Kielhofner, G. (2008). *Model of Human Occupation: Theory and Application* (4th ed.). Philadelphia: Lippincott Williams & Wilkins.

Kielhofner, G., Cahill, S. M., Forsyth, K., de las Heras, C. G., Melton, J., Raber, C., & Prior, S. (2008). Observational assessments. In G. Kielhofner (Ed.), *Model of Human Occupation: Theory and Application* (4th ed.). Philadelphia: Lippincott Williams & Wilkins.

Klyczek, J. P., & Stanton, E. (2008). The Bay Area Functional Performance Evaluation. In B. J. Hemphill-Pearson (Ed.), *Assessments in Occupational Therapy Mental Health: An Integrative Approach* (2nd ed., pp. 217–237). Thorofare, NJ: Slack.

Kopelowicz, A., Liberman, R. P., & Zarate, R. (2006). Recent advances in social skills training for schizophrenia. *Schizophrenia Bulletin, 32*(S1), S12–S23.

Leete, E. (1993). The interpersonal environment: A consumer's personal recollection. In A. B. Hatfield & H. P. Lefley (Eds.), *Surviving Mental Illness: Stress, Coping, and Adaptation* (pp. 114–128). New York: Guilford Press.

Liberman, R. P., DeRisi, W. J., & Mueser, K. T. (1989). *Social Skills Training for Psychiatric Patients*. New York: Pergamon Press.

Mosey, A. C. (1986). *Psychosocial Components of Occupational Therapy*. New York: Raven Press.

Patterson, T. L., Moscona, S., McKibbin, C. L., Davidson, K., & Jeste, D. V. (2001). Social skills performance assessment among older patients with schizophrenia. *Schizophrenia Research, 482*, 351–360.

Pfammatter, M., Junghan, U. M., & Brenner, H. D. (2006). Efficacy of psychological therapy in schizophrenia: Conclusions from meta-analyses. *Schizophrenia Bulletin, 32*(S1), S64–S80.

Roy, M., Dillo, W., Emrich, H. M., & Ohlmeier, M. D. (2009). Asperger's syndrome in adulthood. *Duetsches Aerzteblatt International, 106*(5), 59(64. Available at: www.aerzteblatt.de/int/article.asp?id=63236 (December 8, 2009).

Saraswat, N., Rao, K., Subbakrishna, D. K., & Gangadhar, B. N. (2006). The Social Occupational Functioning Scale (SOFS): A brief measure of functional status in persons with schizophrenia. *Schizophrenia Research, 81*, 301–309.

Stoffel, V. C., & Moyers, P. A. (2004). An evidence-based and occupational perspective of interventions for persons with substance-use disorders. *American Journal of Occupational Therapy, 58*, 570–586.

Takahashi, M., Tanaka, K., & Miyaoka, H. (2006). Reliability and validity of Communication Skills Questionnaire (CSQ). *Psychiatry and Clinic Neuroscience, 60*, 211–218.

Tenhula, W. N., & Bellack, A. S. (2008). Social skills training. In K. T. Mueser & D. V. Jeste (Eds.), *Clinical Handbook of Schizophrenia* (pp. 240–248). New York: Guilford Press.

Tsang, H. W. H., & Pearson, V. (1996). A conceptual framework for work-related social skills in psychiatric rehabilitation. *Journal of Rehabilitation, July/August/September*, 61–66.

Tsang, H. W. H., & Pearson, V. (2000). Reliability and validity of a simple measure for assessing the social skills of people with schizophrenia necessary for seeking and securing a job. *Canadian Journal of Occupational Therapy, 67,* 250–259.

Wallace, C. J., Liberman, R. P., Tauber, R., & Wallace, J. (2000). The Independent Living Skills Survey: A comprehensive measure of the community functioning of severely and persistently mentally ill individuals. *Schizophrenia Bulletin, 26,* 631–658.

Williams, S., & Bloomer, J. (1987). *The Bay Area Functional Performance Evaluation.* (2nd ed.). Palo Alto, CA: Consulting Psychologists Press.

Yalom, I. D. (2005). *The Theory and Practice of Group Psychotherapy* (5th ed.). New York: Basic Books.

Coping Skills

Kristine Haertl and Charles Christiansen

> "*P*roblems are not the problem; coping is the problem.
>
> —Virginia Satir

Introduction

Coping is the process through which we adjust to the stressful demands of daily life. Through its emphasis on helping people address the performance demands of their life tasks, occupational therapy intervention can be described as therapy for coping. Little has been written in the occupational therapy literature about coping with stress or developing skills for coping, despite the reality that daily demands are often stressful. To the extent that some people have limitations related to moving, thinking, sensing, and/or feeling, they are faced with additional burdens and challenges in their everyday lives. Successful and satisfying occupational performance is the goal of occupational therapy intervention. Occupational therapists can be more effective when they include coping skills as one means of enhancing performance of life tasks. This chapter provides an overview of concepts pertinent to stress and coping, and describes the relationships between mental illness and coping.

Stress and Coping

It is interesting to note that the father of American psychiatry, Adolf Meyer, a Johns Hopkins Professor of Psychiatry, was the first influential leader in the United States to draw a link between stress and mental illness. In his work on the theory of psychobiology, Meyer observed that many of the patients he treated had conditions progressing from circumstances that overwhelmed their ability to cope with the demands of daily life (Meyer, 1921). Meyer, himself an immigrant from Switzerland, observed that the demands of a new culture during an era when technology was creating many changes in the way people lived their lives could easily overwhelm people and their ability to cope with these changes (Christiansen, 2007).

In today's fast-paced world, in which people in developed countries are quite accustomed to new technologies such as laptop computers, the Internet, and wireless phones, it is difficult to imagine what it must have been like when technology moved people from horse-drawn carriages to automobiles, or changed their circumstances from working on a farm in a rural community to working in a factory with assembly lines in a crowded urban setting. Yet, these were precisely the kinds of changes that affected people during the time when Dr. Meyer was helping establish the specialty of psychiatry in the early 19th century. Although many physicians tried to explain mental illness in terms of biological causes, Meyer was convinced that the stressful demands of living and the personal and social resources that people had available to assist them with coping were key factors in understanding most mental illness.

Meyer's model was perhaps the first **diathesis stress model**. The term *diathesis* refers to a predisposition, perhaps created by genetics or other background factors, that makes a person more vulnerable to the challenges of living.

Coping and Adaptation

Situations that require coping are often stressful. The risk of harm or loss is a natural part of everyday life, whether a person is crossing the street, driving on the freeway, doing a job interview, or taking an examination. Such stressful experiences, and the manner in which one copes with them, are viewed as important because of their relationship to a person's physical and mental well-being.

Some people use the terms *coping* and *adaptation* interchangeably. This chapter uses **adaptation** as a general term for human change based on challenges in the environment. For example, over extended periods, genetic changes in a species help assure survival as the environment creates demands that require such changes. Adaptation can thus be gradual and biological, or it can be more immediate and behavioral.

In contrast, the term **coping** is used more specifically to describe the explicit actions taken by individuals as they encounter difficult conditions in their daily lives. Coping takes place in response to situations that may be perceived as relevant or vital to an individual's well-being. The **coping process** involves information processing, emotions, and behavioral response (White, 1974). A person encounters a situation, appraises the situation as a potential threat, and then assumes a course of action to address the situation.

This process occurs repeatedly throughout life when people encounter unusual or novel situations that they perceive as relevant to their well-being. Consider encountering a stranger at the door who asks to use your telephone. At the point of the request, it is typical for a quick appraisal to be made of whether the stranger poses a danger. If so, our method of coping with that situation may be to politely deny the request, particularly if we are alone. However, if the person presents as well intentioned, well groomed, and polite, and we have friends in the house and have just completed a self-defense course, we might be more inclined to grant the request. The presence of friends and the ability to use self-defense are resources that are employed as part of our coping strategy.

Stress as a Mind-Body Connection

A Canadian physician-scientist, Dr. Hans Selye is now known as the father of modern stress theory. Selye identified a group of common symptoms during illness that he characterized as representing the body's ordinary physiological reaction to unfavorable conditions. He called this the **generalized adaptation syndrome** (Selye, 1946). Selye's work followed research by Walter Cannon, who established the concept of **homeostasis**, or the principle that the body works hard to maintain a favorable physiological balance and adjusts when external circumstances create abnormal circumstances (Cannon, 1929).

Holmes and Rahe (1967) published a landmark article in the 1960s that was the first to draw an association between abnormal life circumstances and illness. They hypothesized that, if people experience too much adversity in their lives, it will overwhelm their ability to cope, and illness will result. Their work used a now well-known scale of life events (the Schedule of Recent Experiences) to demonstrate a significant association between unfavorable life events and illness. It is important to remember that the link between the body and adverse events is the mind, that is, how we process and respond emotionally to information. Unless a person is physically assaulted or deprived of nutrients or shelter, the major consequences of adverse events are emotional. Emotions trigger the bodily mechanisms that create physiological consequences following stress.

Over the past two decades, scientists have begun unraveling the mechanisms that explain this connection. Psychoneuroimmunology is the specific area of study that explains this connection. Emotions resulting from events create changes in the endocrine system that prepare the body to respond to threats. Typically, the hormones involved in such readiness reactions (e.g., epinephrine, cortisol) are useful. However, over time, they can be harmful and create circumstances that damage the body's natural defensive (or immune) systems. The term given for the physiological changes that accompany the body's readiness activities is **allostasis**. The cumulative result of allostasis can be measured using physiological indicators that describe "allostatic load" (McEwen, 2002).

Hormones that trigger the body's physiological reactions to stressful circumstances are released after a person encounters and appraises a life situation. Such appraisals are accompanied by emotions that start the hormonal releases of allostasis. In his book *Why Zebras Don't Get Ulcers*, Sapolsky (2003) explains that the immune systems of animals are less prone to the ravages of stress because animals do not dwell on the past or future. When a zebra is directly threatened by a lion, it responds by running away. If it escapes, it does not spend time worrying about when and if a lion will reappear. Such thoughts themselves create the emotional responses

(e.g., fear, anxiety) that trigger the release of hormones that activate the immune system responses. Just as a fire department crew gets worn out over time with countless false alarms, so, too, does the immune system wear down with repeated activation from anxiety and worry about threats, both real and imagined.

Coping Theory and Research

The likelihood that an event will be perceived as a threat depends on a person's experiences, resources, and coping strategies. Therefore, people will respond differently to the same situation. Lazarus and Folkman (1984) were among the first researchers to propose a **transactional model** of the coping process that involves a series of appraisals, or situational assessments. In the initial appraisal, the situation or event is seen as irrelevant, benign, positive, or stressful. A stressful event is one with potential harm or loss, threat, or challenge that warrants a coping response. The secondary appraisal considers available options and likely outcomes of choosing those options. Once a coping or behavioral response to the stressful circumstance is selected and applied, the situation is reappraised, and the appraisal process begins again. If the threat is still present, other options must be considered until the situation is resolved.

Certain stressful situations are short term and acute (e.g., a flat tire), whereas others are persistent and chronic (e.g., a supervisor or coworker who has annoying habits). Elliott and Eisdorfer (1982) identified four major types of stressors. **Acute stressors** are short-term events that go away quickly. **Stressor sequences** represent a cascade of adversity, often resulting from a single event, such as loss of a job. There are also **chronic, intermittent stressors** (e.g., a car that breaks down frequently or regular visits by unwelcome in-laws), and finally there are **chronic, permanent stressors**, which are continuous. Chronic illness and disability is an example of a chronic permanent stressor that occupational therapists encounter regularly. Recent research in occupational science has identified chronic permanent stressors caused by the environment that restricts participation based on isolation (either because of incarceration or by geographic location). Situations that limit access to people and services are likely to represent conditions that lead to chronic stress.

Types of Coping

People cope in different ways. The particular coping strategy selected by an individual depends on that person's unique situation, background, and available resources. Resources may consist of personal skills and abilities, friends and relatives, beliefs, and personality characteristics, such as a sense of efficacy or optimism. Coping efforts tend be classified in three major categories: **behavioral strategies, avoidance**, and **cognitive strategies**.

Behavioral strategies involve some type of action to manage stress, such as confronting a person about a conflict or engaging in physical activity to manage the feelings. Avoidance can involve withdrawal, distraction, use of substances, or other methods of staying away from the stressor. Cognitive strategies typically include efforts to analyze the situation to fully understand the nature of the threat or challenge. Sometimes, people try to see the positive side of a difficult situation and, in so doing, manage their appraisal of the stressor. It is important to realize that how people perceive and interpret a situation influences the nature of their response. Often, during cognitive appraisal, the situation may be compared to similar experiences a person has encountered in the past.

Folkman and Lazarus (1984) noted that coping can be emotion focused or problem focused. That is, people can concentrate on reducing the sense of anxiety they feel, or they can address the sources of fear and anxiety directly. Problem-focused coping strategies are directed at solving a problem directly, through active efforts. Clearly, not all problems can be solved, but active efforts can be beneficial because they may divert attention away from the source of stress or provide a release of energy to help dissipate the arousal state that, when persistent, fosters the unnecessary release of hormones that stimulate the sympathetic nervous system.

Felton, Revenson, and Henrichsen (1984) found that, in groups of adults with chronic medical conditions, coping strategies tended to cluster within six major groupings, including

1. Cognitive restructuring—Efforts to find and embrace the positive aspects of a situation
2. Emotional expression—Directing anger or humor at the situation
3. Wish-fulfilling fantasy—Spending time imagining an improved situation
4. Self-blame—Refocusing attention as a part of avoidance
5. Information seeking—Seeking information and advice about the situation and active coping strategies used by others
6. Threat minimization—Putting distressing thoughts out of one's mind as a type of denial or avoidance

The research by Felton and colleagues corroborated the model by Folkman and Lazarus in that these efforts grouped readily within the categories of cognitive strategies, behavioral strategies, and avoidance.

Coping Resources and Resilience

A great deal has been written in the literature about those resources that are deemed essential for success in coping with the stressful situations of life. Early research directed at understanding the effect of major life events on stress was followed by recognition that people differed in their levels of activity, intensity, and competitiveness. The terms "type A personality" and "type B personality" were coined to describe the distinction between people whose lifestyles and personal attributes foster more stressful circumstances and those whose attitudes and pace of life are such that their emotional responses to circumstances are less likely to evoke physiological stress responses. Research has shown that personality type and attitude are related to the perception of stress, as well as to its physiological consequences, such as hypertension and heart disease (Myrtek, 2001).

Suzanne Kobasa (Kobasa, Maddi, & Kahn, 1981) pursued a line of research that attempted to identify the characteristics of those who were more successful at coping with life stressors. She described this constellation of traits as a type of stress resilience she called "hardiness." People with hardiness tended to have several characteristics in common,

which Kobasa summarized in three words: control, commitment, and challenge. Because of these characteristics, hardy people

- Believe that they can influence their life situations and act according to that belief.
- Consistently consider how they can change situations for personal advantage and seldom accept events at face value.
- Regard change as part of the normal course of events and see it as an opportunity for positive growth and development.
- Remain committed to learning and self-development.

Today, the notion of hardiness has given way to the concept of **resilience**, a general term that signifies a person is able to endure stressful situations without suffering the physiological or psychological consequences, such as illness or disease, typically associated with such adversity.

Aaron Antonovsky (1979), an Israeli sociologist, spent years studying the factors that distinguished individuals who were able to thrive despite lives filled with apparent stress and adversity. His research yielded a model of health, or **salutogenesis**, which he described as the sense of coherence. Sense of coherence, in Antonovsky's framework, described people for whom life was viewed as manageable, meaningful, and comprehensible. That is, they had the skills or resources necessary for managing their problems, a sense of meaning and life purpose that gave them a strong will to live, and a mental picture of their lives that made sense in the form of an understandable or coherent story.

More recently, psychologist Carol Ryff of Wisconsin worked with physiologists interested in the concept of allostasis to identify the resources and attributes that contribute to successful aging (Ryff & Singer, 2003). Ryff concluded that these factors group into six major categories: autonomy, environmental mastery, personal growth, positive relations with others, purpose in life, and self-acceptance.

The research of Kobasa (Kobasa et al, 1981), Antonovsky (1979), and Ryff and Singer (2003) provides a useful way of summarizing the resources and attributes necessary for successful coping. On careful examination, it is apparent that the personal factors that distinguish people who cope most successfully with life's challenges include the following:

- A sense of confidence or belief in one's ability to successfully deal with adversity and challenge
- A sense of personal commitment that provides the drive to keep going when things get tough
- An orientation toward continuous growth and self-development

Beyond these personal characteristics, having defined skills (e.g., problem-solving, influencing, organizing, or managing resources) and a network of friends and associates who can provide advice and assistance also seem to be valuable assets in helping people cope successfully with adversity. The following sections focus on the relationship between coping and mental illness, paying particular attention to the assessment of coping skills and approaches to intervention that can be useful to occupational therapists working in the area of mental health.

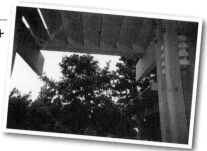

I see a place to sit down at a park shelter with a circular ray of light. There are also trees all around the shelter. I am searching for peace, and I found it in myself while sitting at this particular shelter. For those who have not experienced this peace, they too may benefit from the shelter within themselves.

—Grady

Mental Illness and Coping

There appears to be a dynamic link between mental illness and stress that is not dissimilar to the traditional contemplation, "Which comes first, the chicken or the egg?" Whereas the symptoms of mental illness cause additional stress, those individuals who have difficulty coping appear predisposed to developing mental health problems (Chapman, Chapman, Kwapil, Eckblad, & Zinser, 1994).

Diathesis stress models posit that individuals with a predisposition to psychiatric disorders are more prone to development of the illness in the presence of stress (Dangelmaier, Docherty, & Akamatsu, 2006). For example, if Mary, a woman with a genetic predisposition toward major depression, experiences the death of an immediate family member, it puts her at greater risk for the onset of depression. Yet, in the presence of adaptive coping skills, social support, and adequate resources, personal resilience may develop and protect individuals from the negative effects of stress. The means by which people cope with daily life stressors can serve either to buffer or exacerbate stressors. In the latter case, the exacerbation can trigger the onset of mental health symptoms such as psychosis (Dangelmaier et al, 2006).

Personal and contextual factors influence an individual's ability to cope with stress. A shopping trip to purchase food items may seem like a simple task, yet for individuals struggling with major mental illness, everyday tasks often pose challenges and bring about anxiety. The interaction between the individual, his or her view of the situation, personal stress and vulnerability factors, and the context and duration of the stressor affect an individual's ability to cope (Snyder & Pulvers, 2001; Wong, 2006).

Major mental illnesses such as schizophrenia often involve disturbances in self-identity, cognition, and relationships, all of which can negatively influence personal coping (Hatfield & Lefley, 1993). A client who actively hears voices, is overcome with depression, or has problems with attention and problem-solving may view the daily routine of getting up and preparing for school or work as overwhelming. A simple trip to the grocery store could be unmanageable for someone who has a fear of open spaces or who is actively hearing voices to engage in self-harm. A change in work schedule may become overwhelming for an individual who

has difficulty with transitions or is unable to figure out the change in bus schedule. Therapists must be empathic toward the challenges facing people with serious and persistent mental illness, and work to provide a "supportive, tolerant, and safe therapeutic environment" that facilitates client growth (Ghanstrom-Stranqvist, Josephsson, & Thom, 2004).

Personal narratives of individuals living with mental illness depict the shock, frustration, change in relationships, and altered identity that often emerge when diagnosed with a major mental illness. Chovil (2005) wrote, "I had an insidious onset of schizophrenia beginning in high school and gradually lost my human relationships over a 9-year period without anyone realizing I was completely alone by the time I was homeless . . . (I was) untreated for the next 10 years" (p. 407). Another author wrote, "Once a mishap or mistake occurred, a critical inner voice would berate me in a punishing way and send me into a tailspin and often into depression" (Weingarten, 2005, p. 77). Not only do the symptoms add to difficulty in coping with everyday stressors, but also individuals affected by mental illness must cope with the personal and societal stigma that often accompanies mental illness. Although mental illness often poses stress and barriers to successful coping, with adequate supports, interventions, and resources, individuals with psychiatric disorders can lead productive, healthy, enriching lives.

Family Coping

There is a significant amount of research on the impact of mental illness on the family (e.g., Fortune, Smith, & Garvey, 2005; Nehra, Chakrabarti, Kulhara, & Sharma, 2005; Tennakoon et al, 2000). Initial research focused heavily on a dysfunctional pattern of interaction between family members and individuals with mental illness. This pattern, termed "expressed emotion," was used to denote a pattern of hostility, criticism, and overinvolvement in relatives of those people with psychiatric conditions, particularly schizophrenia. Early studies (Brown, Birley, & Wing, 1972; Leff, Kuipers, Berkowitz, Eberlin-Vries, & Sturgeon, 1982) found that individuals with mental illness from families with high levels of expressed emotion were more likely to experience psychiatric relapse. Recent research questions whether the presence of mental illness in the family may actually contribute to the dynamics of the family dysfunction and abnormal interaction patterns (Weardon, Tarrier, Barrowclough, Zastowny, & Rawhill, 2000).

The stress, time, and energy required to care for a family member with a mental illness often disrupts daily activities. A mother coping with a teenage son who struggles with depression and suicidal tendencies may find the need to alternate her work schedule or secure community supports to ensure his safety during the day. A husband of a wife struggling with newly diagnosed schizophrenia faces major decisions regarding their relationship, supports needed, and parenting of the children. When family relationships break down and mental illness is perceived as overwhelming, caregivers often resort to both problem-based and emotional-based coping and use not only adaptive techniques, but also maladaptive strategies, such as avoidance, collusion, and coercion (Nehra et al, 2005).

Often stress buffers, such as seeking social support and using available resources, are helpful in ameliorating the anxiety caused by the mental illness (Nehra et al, 2000; Wong, 2006). Research suggests a dynamic interplay between the individual with the mental illness, the family's response to the mental illness, and services available to facilitate personal and familial coping.

Studies of caregiver burden suggest that familial social relationships, leisure time, daily routines, and personal health are altered as a result of caring for someone with mental illness (Ivarsson, Sidenvall, & Carlsson, 2004; Ostman, 2004). Family burdens as described by Wong (2006) include subjective burdens (social and psychological costs related to the care of individuals with mental illness) and objective burdens (practical difficulties encountered in the day-to-day interaction and care of relatives with mental illness). Although studies of caregiver burden are plentiful within the literature, one must be cautious because the use of the term "burden" often implicates the person with mental illness as the focus of the stress, a position that may be difficult for the client to accept (Abelenda & Helfrich, 2004). Furthermore, such conceptualizations may influence client identity and family relationships. A dynamic, competency-based approach to understanding family strengths and concerns allows for a balanced approach to family intervention.

Three areas of practical difficulties encountered by families affected by mental illness include understanding the disease, managing the symptoms, and coordinating therapy services (Wong, 2006). Additional subjective burdens cause emotional anxiety, frustration, guilt, and worry (Hatfield & Lefley, 1993). Including the family in evaluation and intervention helps mediate the difficulties often associated with caregiving. Evaluation methods using interviews and occupational history-taking provide a means to understand the daily routines and occupational patterns of the family (Chaffey & Fossey, 2004). Care must be taken to acknowledge patient privacy rights, and therefore, efforts should be made to determine the client's wishes related to the amount of information shared with the family. Efforts to facilitate open communication and collaboration between the therapist, client, and family often aid in transitions out of the hospital, particularly if the client will be returning home to live with the family. Areas to address with the family include the home environment, relational patterns, and resources used and needed, and existing family knowledge about the illness. A comprehensive, client/family-based approach to evaluation facilitates holistic intervention planning.

For information related to family assessment and interventions, see Chapter 29.

Client Evaluation

With the emergence of the recovery movement in psychiatric rehabilitation (Anthony, 1993), individuals with mental disorders are viewed as key informants related to intervention planning. Certainly, the course of the illness affects personal judgment, the capacity for insight, and the ability to actively engage in self-assessment and intervention (Cowls & Hale, 2005; Ivarsson et al, 2004). A recovery-oriented approach involves working collaboratively with the client and family to identify appropriate assessment tools. Several measurements

use self-assessment methods, yet retrospective self-reports of stress and coping may not always be accurate (Stone et al, 1998). Pairing personal assessment tools with additional objective and subjective measures can facilitate a more holistic approach to addressing the impact of stress and coping on personal occupational performance.

Occupational therapists work with clients to explore areas of current stress and personal coping methods in the context of their impact on quality of life and occupational performance. Measures of personal stress, trauma, and coping include checklists, self-appraisal instruments, physiological measures, observations, and interviews. Factors to consider when selecting a measure include the individual's cognitive level, potential for insight, motivation, and fit with the purpose of the tool.

Stress and Coping Measures

Whereas some events are considered inherently stressful and traumatic, such as war, natural disaster, and unexpected childhood death, others are deemed stressful based on the context and personal meaning assigned to the situation. Often events are not inherently bad or good, yet personal appraisal and perceived meaning of the occurrence has a bearing on well-being, equilibrium, and the need to cope (Zakowski, Hall, Klein, & Baum, 2001). Measures used to assess stress and its relationship to health are derived from three traditions (Stewart, 1999):

1. Environmental tradition—focused on events and experiences as they are objectively associated with adaptation and daily life demands
2. Psychological tradition—emphasizing individual (subjective) evaluation of coping abilities to meet life demands
3. Biological tradition—aimed at measuring the activation of physiological systems during times of stress

There are distinct pros and cons to each approach; therefore, selecting a measure is based on the purpose of the assessment and the client's condition. Stress and trauma-related measures tend to focus on three areas: life events, physiological responses to stress, and the subjective appraisal of stress through self-assessment. Additional assessment methods consider personal coping in response to life stress and the impact of stress and coping on health and wellness.

Self-Report Instruments

Self-report instruments are those in which the client provides his or her own perspective. They are the most commonly used method. Most measures assess the stressors that the individual is experiencing, some evaluate the type of coping method used, and others assess both stressors and coping methods.

Stress Measurement

Despite criticism within the literature, Holmes and Rahe's (1967) Social Readjustment Rating Scale (SRRS), remains one of the most frequently used tools to measure stress (Scully & Tossi, 2000). The scale was formulated based on research suggesting that stressful life events correlated with the onset of illness (Rahe, Meyer, Smith, Kjaer, & Holmes, 1964).

The SSRS consists of 43 life events in two categories: events that relate to the individual's lifestyle, and events that occur and include the individual. Items are ranked on a scale of 100 and include events such as (a) death of a spouse = 100, (b) marriage = 50, (c) retirement = 45, (d) change in sleeping habits = 16, and (e) vacation = 13. Respondents are asked to complete the checklist, based on the number of listed life events that have occurred within the past year. Total scores are compared to a scale that suggests the potential for developing a significant illness. A limitation of the measure is that it does not differentiate the reaction to positive and negative stress events.

In addition to the SSRS, examples of checklist and self-assessment tools used to rate personal stress include the Psychiatric Epidemiology Interview Life Events Scale (PERI) (Dohrenwend, Krasnoff, Askenasy, & Dohrenwend, 1978), the Recent Life Changes Questionnaire (Rahe, 1975), the Life Experiences Survey (Sarason, Johnson, & Siegel, 1978), and the Elder Life Stress Inventory (Aldwin, 1990). The PERI and Recent Life Changes Questionnaire are similar to the SSRS in assessing individual stress through use of an objective checklist of events encountered. The Life Experiences Survey seeks to broaden and differentiate stressors by identifying both positive and negative events. Additional instruments, such as the Occupational Stress Inventory–Revised (Osipow & Spokane, 1998) and Stress Symptom Checklist (Schlebusch, 2004), expand the measurement of stress beyond event occurrences through measurement of individual responses and coping in relation to stressors.

In addition to stress measurement tools derived from the field of psychology, a comprehensive occupation-based approach to measuring stress, the Stress Management Questionnaire (SMQ) provides a holistic view of stress and coping through self-assessment of problems and symptoms caused by stress, stressors eliciting the response, and coping activities that are currently used to manage stress (Stein & Cutler, 2002). The SMQ was developed from two descriptive studies in order to evaluate personal improved stress response following biofeedback and relaxation interventions. One advantage the SMQ offers over many of the other stress and coping tools is that it explores dimensions of both stress and coping responses. Stein reported the SMQ to be useful for facilitating therapist and patient collaboration in developing an individualized stress management program and tracking personal progress within therapy.

Coping Assessment

Coping measures are derived from theoretical frameworks and classifications of the coping process. Readers will recall that Lazarus and Folkman (1984) distinguished between problem-focused coping and emotion-based coping. Problem-focused coping is generally considered healthier (Schwarzer, Starke, & Buchwald, 2003) because it is directly focused on working through problems caused by the stress. Additional conceptualizations of coping classification identify active and avoidant styles of coping (Snyder & Pulvers, 2001; Suls & Fletcher, 1985). Active strategies are regarded as more adaptive and involve active means to change the stressor or emotional view of the situation in order to address it directly. Avoidant strategies use other means (e.g., alcohol, cigarettes, withdrawal) to avoid addressing the source of stress.

Traditionally, Folkman and Lazarus' (1988) Ways of Coping Checklist–Revised was the instrument of choice used to assess coping; however, newer measures have been developed in an attempt to improve psychometric rigor (Gol & Cook, 2004). Despite development and expansion of coping measures in recent years, the Ways of Coping Checklist–Revised continues to be used heavily in research and assessment within a variety of fields (Penley, Tomaka, & Wiebe, 2002). The checklist consists of 66 items rated on a 4-point Likert scale. Respondents are asked to identify strategies used to deal with life demands. The scale is easy to administer and results in a representation of the client's style of coping, including (a) problem focused, (b) wishful thinking, (c) distancing, (e) seeking social support, (f) emphasizing the positive, (g) self-blame, (h) tension reduction, and (i), self-isolation.

In addition, an abundance of coping self-assessment tools exist within the human service, health, and business fields. Three popular measures, the Coping Responses Inventory (Moos, 1990), the COPE scale (Carver, Scheier, & Weintraub, 1989), and the Coping Strategies Indicator (Amirkhan, 1990), all measure coping responses to daily stressors. The instruments are fairly easy to administer in both clinical and academic settings, yet as is often the case with coping measures, conceptual problems arise when separating out coping strategies from resources available (Schwarzer & Schwarzer, 1996). Given the limitations of such measures, additional evaluation techniques using observation, interview, history-taking, and formal task assessment provide a more holistic picture of the client's coping strategies and skills.

Children, Adolescents, and Parents

Based on age, context. and developmental stage, children's experience of stress and coping may differ from that of adults. Life event checklists for adults often include items that are not relevant for pediatric populations, and personal stressors differ based on age and development. Studies with children (Ayres, Sandler, West, & Roosa, 1996) suggest that a four-factor model of coping—active, distraction, avoidant, and support seeking—may fit better with childhood situational coping than the original coping theories developed by Lazarus and Folkman. Given the differences between children and adults, stress and coping evaluations for younger populations should include client and contextual factors such as the chronological and developmental age of the child.

Inventory tools available for coping assessment include the Life Events Coping Inventory for Children (Dise-Lewis, 1988), the Children's Coping Strategies Checklist (Ayres et al, 1996), the Adolescent Coping Scale (Frydenberg & Lewis, 1993), the Life Events Checklist (Johnson & McCutcheon, 1980), the Adolescent Perceived Events Scale (Compas, Davis, Forsythe, & Wagner, 1987), and the Parenting Stress Index (Abidin, 1990).

Additional Stress and Coping Measures

The limitations of self-appraisal instruments can be addressed with complementary assessment techniques that incorporate additional means of data gathering. These include interviews, stress diaries, physiological measures, observation, and resilience.

Interviews

Interviews serve to expand on information gained from inventories and allow the therapist to use clinical reasoning in the selection of areas for further inquiry. Interviews may be conducted on a formal or informal basis and may include the use of structured interview guides (Patton, 2002), an open-ended interview, or specific interview tools such as the Family Stress and Coping Interview (Nachshen, Woodford, & Minnes, 2003) or Interview for Recent Life Events (Paykel, 1997). Occupation-based tools such as the Canadian Occupational Performance Measure (Law et al, 1998) and the Occupational Case Analysis Interview and Rating Scale (Kaplan & Kielhofner, 1989) are helpful to provide a client-centered focus on perceptions of occupational performance as related to stress, coping, and quality of life.

Although these instruments do not expressly focus on stress and coping, responses to questions within the interview provide the therapist with relevant information related to the client's perception of function, life satisfaction, and goal areas. As with inventory measures, interviews do have limitations of self-report, yet they have advantages in their ability to expand and explore personal appraisal of stress and perceived efficacy of coping to a deeper level than traditional checklists.

Stress Diaries

Another approach to measuring stress and coping, the stress diary (Linehan, 1993), provides a means for clients and therapists to track stress and coping over time. Various forms of stress diaries exist; they generally involve a journal or recording of the times and events surrounding stress, personal reactions to events, and coping strategies used. One common form of the stress diary, Linehan's (1993) diary card, is used with dialectical behavioral therapy. This is a cognitive behavioral treatment that was originally designed for persons with borderline personality disorder, but has since been applied to a variety of populations, including persons with chemical dependency, eating disorders, depression, and anxiety. The diary card may be used to derive an initial baseline on maladaptive coping strategies used (e.g., alcohol, self-harm), as well as track the use of adaptive coping skills. The diary card serves as a means to provide feedback, increase insight into stressors that evoke maladaptive coping, and records skills that may be used to more positively work through the stress.

Physiological Measures

Whereas sophisticated physiological methods of measuring stress (e.g., cortisol levels) are often used for research purposes, the physiological measures of assessment in healthcare settings may include heart rate and skin temperature. Through the use of instrumentation such as biofeedback, clients work with the therapist to identify baseline physiological measures, experiment with various interventions (e.g., relaxation, meditation) in order to explore which stress-relieving activities are most effective and teach the client to self-regulate physiological responses to stress.

Additional physiological measures of stress include the use of heart rate, blood pressure, and galvanic skin response. The galvanic skin response uses surface electrodes on the fingers and can detect anxiety and skin resistance in response to an individual's emotional state (Storm, Shafiei, Myre, &

Raeder, 2005). Some programs use more basic measures, such as the use of stress patches or small thermometers that measure skin temperature (Needham, 1996) before and after intervention. With time, the aim of therapy is to teach clients to take control of their personal response to stress through adaptive techniques such as the use of deep breathing and relaxation.

Observation

Client observation in both natural and structured settings provides the therapist with insights into occupational performance. Although general observation is not included in many of the widely used stress and coping assessments, given the focus on task performance within therapy, occupational therapists are uniquely suited to make observations regarding a client's problem-solving capabilities, adaptive skills, and ability to cope with stress. As task-based assessments are performed, the therapist records observations of how the client responds to unexpected difficulties (or stress) within an assessment. For instance, if a client being assessed with the Kohlman Evaluation of Living Skills (Thomson, 1993) reacts to difficulty during the money management section by shouting at the therapist and stomping out of the room, the therapist gains valuable information about the client's current frustration level and reaction to the request to perform a task that may be beyond his or her current skill level.

A comprehensive assessment of the response behavior should include the client's perception of the situation, the therapist's view of the behavior, perceived and actual skill regarding the test, and antecedents and reasons for coping behaviors. Appraisal of the client and therapist interchange, as well as opportunities to reestablish rapport and develop positive coping skills, should be considered. A number of variables, including client factors such as emotional state, status of the psychiatric disorder, current medications, and rapport with the therapist, may all affect the client's ability to react to stressful situations. In addition, task demands and environmental factors affect the testing situation. A noisy, high-stimulus room may be perceived as far more stressful than a calm, quiet setting. Careful attention should be paid to the testing and intervention environment. Regardless of the task assessment tool, observations of the client's response to task demands provide valuable information regarding the client's occupational performance.

In addition to direct observation, several tools assess coping behaviors through interviews or questionnaires of caregivers based on client observation. These tools may be especially helpful with children, individuals with developmental disabilities, and clients with poor insight. Examples of assessments used to evaluate adaptive behavior include the AAMR Adaptive Behavioral Scale (Nihira, Leland, & Lambert, 1993), the Coping Inventory (Zeitlin, 1985), the Early Coping Inventory (Zeitlin, Williamson, & Szczepanski, 1988), and the Scales of Independent Behavior–Revised (Bruininks, Woodcock, Weatherman, & Hill, 1996). When selecting observation tools that are completed by the caregiver, careful consideration should be given as to who fills out the assessment, their level of involvement and scope of observation opportunities, and if they can accurately complete the form. At times, it is helpful to encourage the respondent to consult additional caregivers if the information is unknown (e.g., if completed by a teacher). Inclusion of direct observation is often helpful in order to assess current function and compare task performance in the testing situation to the trends reported over time.

Resilience

A final area of emphasis is the measurement and development of resilience or hardiness, which have been identified as the process and resources that allow people to competently and successfully deal with day-to-day challenges (Brooks & Goldstein, 2001). Similar to stress and coping, measures of resilience often include personal checklists (Hardy, Concato, & Gill, 2004; Reivich & Shatte, 2002) to self-assess resilience, identify controllable and uncontrollable factors related to resilience, and develop personal skills that will improve resilience. An example of a resilience measure, the Resilience Quotient (Reivich & Shatte, 2002), measures seven areas: (a) emotional regulation, (b) impulse control, (c) optimism, (d) causal analysis, (e) empathy, (f) self-efficacy, and (g) reaching out. In addition, the measure results in an overall resilient quotient. Based on research of the instrumentation and follow-up intervention techniques, the authors contend that resilience may be positively affected through mindfulness techniques aimed at transforming the thought process, an approach that is in line with cognitive behavioral therapy, an integral part of stress and coping intervention.

Intervention

Occupational therapists who work with clients to improve their performance skills are better equipping them to contend with the various problems and situations in their lives. In addition, through their contributions to their client's feelings of self-efficacy, they provide an important psychological element in an individual's coping toolkit; in so doing, it makes them more resilient to the consequences of stress over time. This section addresses how interventions relate to specific frames of reference and individual client needs.

Theoretical Frameworks for Intervention

Theoretical frameworks guide the selection of techniques used for intervention. Several frame of references used within occupational therapy are relevant to addressing stress and coping. For the purposes of this chapter, four are discussed: (a) psychodynamic/object relations (b) behavioral, and (c) cognitive behavioral.

Psychodynamic-Object Relations Approaches

The psychodynamic frame of reference draws on the work of theorists such as Freud, Jung, Rodgers, and Maslow. Occupational therapists are not trained in psychodynamic theory to the same extent as many psychologists and physicians; yet, the foundational knowledge of the theory provides a framework by which therapists can use expressive techniques in collaboration with the client to develop insights and understanding, and facilitate adaptive behaviors to meet goals. Mosey (1970) outlined major principles within this frame of reference and stressed the importance of the client's mental state, unconscious, utility of symbols, and creative expression to promote insight into the self. Mosey emphasized the significance of the therapist–client relationship and conscious use of self in order to develop rapport and foster a therapeutic environment conducive to intervention (Mosey, 1986). Empathy, compassion, humility, and unconditional positive regard were all considered by Mosey as foundations of the development of a positive therapeutic relationship between the therapist and the client in order to develop a collaborative partnership and foster goal attainment.

Key assumptions within the psychodynamic frame of reference emphasize that clients are personal experts on their lives and are capable of increased understanding of the self and others (Bruce & Borg, 2002). Some of the assumptions are as follows:

- Human behavior is influenced by the conscious and unconscious.
- Activities provide a means of personal exploration and feelings expression.

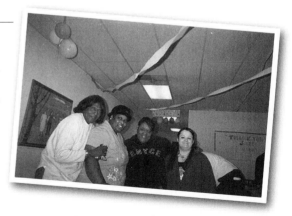

PhotoVoice

This is a group of successful women I know. These are the words they use to explain what makes their lives successful.

Jennifer—"My life is a success because I believe more in myself, and I have a lot more support."

Elise—"My life is a success because of God and because I pray all of the time."

Darlene—"I feel like I am very persistent, and I usually don't stop until I succeed."

Viola—"What has made me a successful life is, I started getting out of the house. This got rid of the depression. The sky is the limit of things I can do and accomplish. Also, my spiritual belief, there is a God of heaven. When I pray that will make everything better. That's called faith."

Knowing these women makes me have a successful life, and I am one of the women in the picture.

—Viola

- Structured activities provide improved functional performance, self-control, and personal safety.
- The client–therapist relationship is of distinct significance.
- The creation of an atmosphere of mutual respect contributes to personal safety and optimal group milieu.

Within this approach, interventions aimed at stress and coping often include creative media designed to provide a means for the client to express feelings and come to self-realization through the use of writing and creative expression such as art and dramatic play.

Writing

The use of therapeutic writing within the psychodynamic frame of reference incorporates open-ended, exploratory writing activities. Expressive techniques are helpful to facilitate understanding of the conscious and unconscious, which can lead to increased personal insight and goal attainment (Progoff, 1992). Studies demonstrate the effectiveness of therapeutic writing techniques, suggesting that personal expression in response to stress and trauma improve overall health and well-being (Esterling, L'Abate, Murray, & Pennebaker, 1999; Smyth, 1998). Expressive writing techniques may include the use of free writing and flow writing, stream of consciousness, journal writing, and expressive creative writing. Following completion of open-ended writing techniques, the client works with the therapist to explore themes within the writing and come to a new understanding.

Creative Expression

Another psychodynamic approach includes free-form art, sculpture, and improvisational drama or play. Media such as clay, finger paint, and watercolor are used because of their abstract properties and potential for free expression. The use of expressive media seeks to free underlying emotions and conflicts in order to heal the psyche (Samuels, 1995).

Some clients are more amenable to expressive techniques than others, and often children are more willing to engage in techniques such as finger painting or use of media that is harder to control because they may be less likely to personally judge the perceived quality of their work. Once expressive media creations are complete, the therapist and client work together to understand the underlying themes within the creation. Therapists must be cautioned not to overinterpret symbolism brought forth in the media, and should always consider the client as the expert related to the creation and the self. Given the emphasis on client insight, the cognitive capacity and ability to self-reflect should be considered. An example of creative expression as a psychodynamic approach to intervention is shown in Box 22-1.

Behavioral Frame of Reference

The use of behavioral approaches are often helpful with clients who need structure and an external locus of control. Behaviorism comes from the work of theorists such as Pavlov, Watson, and Skinner, and focuses on the study of the interactions between people and their environment. Behavioral perspectives emphasize objective behaviors with little focus on the emotions related to such behaviors.

Individuals with developmental cognitive deficits, those with low motivation, and children may respond to behavioral techniques. The use of structured reinforcement systems, such

---

BOX 22-1 ■ Client Example of Psychodynamic Intervention

Mary, a 15-year-old adolescent with a long history of abuse, depression, and conduct disorder, has difficulty communicating with others, isolates herself, and engages in maladaptive coping behaviors such as cutting her arms and abusing alcohol. During the initial interview and in the occupational therapy clinic, the therapist notices that Mary expresses feelings through the writing of poetry and painting of pictures. As rapport develops between the therapist and Mary, she becomes increasingly trusting of the therapist and willing to discuss her underlying fears of failure and rejection. The therapist and Mary work together to gain new insights from her creations, establish goals related to developing positive coping skills, and use media as an outlet when she is angry or frustrated.

Evidence-Based Practice

The use of expressive writing has been effective in improving physiological measures in response to stress and trauma, resulting in improved health and well-being (Esterling, L'Abate, Murray, & Pennebaker, 1999; Smyth, 1998).

➤ Regardless of the practice setting, occupational therapists are typically working with individuals that have or are currently experiencing stress and trauma. Occupational therapists can provide opportunities for expressive writing as an outlet to process and express emotions related to personal experiences.

➤ Occupational therapists might also consider using physiological measures of stress such as heart rate, blood pressure, or skin temperature to determine if the writing exercises are resulting in positive outcomes.

Esterling, B. A., L'Abate, L., Murray, E. J., & Pennebaker, J. W. (1999). Empirical foundations for writing in prevention and psychotherapy: Mental and physical health outcomes. *Clinical Psychology Review, 19,* 79–96.
Smyth, J. M. (1998). Written emotional expression: Effect sizes, outcome types, and moderating variables. *Journal of Consulting and Clinical Psychology, 66,* 174–184.

---

as token economies, is found in several areas of psychosocial practice. A token economy involves a reinforcement system, often unified for an entire group of clients (e.g., on a behavioral unit at the hospital). In simplified token economies, clients may be given a direct reinforcement following positive behavior or may be given a tangible symbol (e.g., a star) that counts toward the purchase of some larger reinforcement. In more sophisticated token economies, clients earn tokens and spend them, similar to spending money at a store. These systems may be used as an incentive for adaptive behaviors, and to teach skills surrounding money management and budgeting.

Despite a decline of research in token economies over the past two decades, studies suggest they are effective in decreasing maladaptive behaviors and violence within psychiatric settings (Le Page, 1999). Within occupational therapy, the pairing of behavioral techniques is often used with other approaches. For instance, clients may be given tokens or points for attending a therapy session focused on skill training. The use of the token economy is designed to promote and facilitate adaptive behaviors. One must be cautious, however, because the removal of the reinforcement can serve to decrease the desired behavior. An example of a behavioral approach to intervention is shown in Box 22-2.

In planning behavioral interventions, the therapist identifies behavioral patterns and the desired change in behavior, and then develops strategies to achieve the desired behaviors. Reinforcements may be tangible (e.g., material goods) or intangible (e.g., personal praise). Careful consideration of the client's motivation and ability to understand the program should be taken into account. Clients with low cognitive levels and poor impulse control may need immediate reinforcement, whereas those with higher levels of understanding are often able to engage in programs that implement delayed gratification.

Cognitive Behavioral Interventions

Cognitive behavioral interventions stem from social learning theory and the work of theorists such as Bandura, Ellis, and Beck. Rather than the reflexive, responsive focus of behaviorism, cognitive behavioral therapy stresses the role of our thought process in influencing emotions and behaviors. The emphasis within this intervention approach is to identify maladaptive behaviors and thinking patterns, and restructure these patterns with adaptive thoughts and actions. Kendall and Panichelli-Mindel (1995) provided a comprehensive definition, stating that cognitive behavioral therapy ". . . focuses on how people respond to their cognitive interpretations of experiences rather than the environment or experience itself, and how their thoughts and behaviors are related. It combines cognition change procedures with behavioral contingency management and learning experiences designed to help change distorted or deficient information processing" (p. 108).

Occupational therapists are often part of a multidisciplinary team approach that uses cognitive behavioral therapy to address stress, trauma, maladaptive behaviors, and coping skills. For more information on cognitive behavioral therapy, see Chapter 19.

Psychoeducation

As is true for family coping, psychoeducation emphasizes a multifaceted intervention approach to provide resources and education surrounding the client's illness. Research suggests the efficacy of using psychoeducational models to decrease stress and increase educational knowledge in individuals and families of those affected by mental illness (Pollio, North, Reid, Miletic, & McClendon, 2006; Pratt et al, 2005; Rotondi et al, 2005). When designing psychoeducation groups to address stress, trauma, and coping, there is often a dual emphasis on education and feelings expression; therefore, a group may take on a support emphasis in conjunction with serving the goal of delivering information. Depending on the type and severity of the illness, consideration should be given as to whether psychoeducation is performed individually or within a group. When determining the structure and content of the group, Knight (2006) stressed that clients new to therapy and those with PTSD may be more amenable to a time-limited, structured educational approach. Those who have been part of a group for a period of time may be suitable for a group focused on both the feelings and emotions related to stressors, as well as the skills necessary for successful adaptation to daily events.

The use of psychoeducation is suggested as evidenced-based practice in mental health occupational therapy (Tse, Lloyd, Penman, King, & Basset, 2004). Therapists often use an education approach along with experiential activities to provide opportunities to practice skills. Psychoeducation groups within occupational therapy are often used in conjunction with skill training and a holistic, client-centered approach.

BOX 22-2 ■ Client Example of Behavioral Intervention

Harry, a client with depression and schizophrenia, had difficulty coping with daily expectations, performing chores, and maintaining his hygiene routine. The therapist implemented a reinforcement program whereby Harry earned a coffee and donut every time he completed his morning routine. In time, the reinforcement was removed, in the hope that Harry would continue his routine without the reinforcement. Unfortunately, without an incentive, Harry fell back to his former pattern of behavior.

Unlike Harry, Mary, a 55-year-old woman with major depression and mild mental retardation, had difficulty with motivation and coming to her daily skill training group. Initially, she was placed on a token economy; every time she attended group, she earned points toward the purchase of items in the token store. As therapy continued, Mary made friends with other group members and began coming on her own. Mary informed the therapist that she no longer "needed those points" because she was satisfied with the group itself.

In these examples, Harry had no incentive to continue with his hygiene routine; he appeared to alter his behaviors for the sole purpose of the reinforcement. Mary, in contrast, needed the initial reinforcement as motivation, but later found that the group itself gave her enough intrinsic satisfaction that she no longer required an incentive to attend.

Evidence-Based Practice

The restructuring of thoughts and emphasis on the benefits of stressors and challenges has been shown in a meta-analysis to result in improved psychological and physical health and well-being (Helgeson, Reynolds, & Tomich, 2006). A meta-analysis of intervention strategies for persons with panic disorder suggests relaxation therapy, cognitive restructuring, and exposure as beneficial, and resulted in the most consistent effect sizes (Clum, Clum, & Surls, 1993).

➤ Occupational therapists can help individuals identify stressors and then rethink the meaning of the stressor. In many cases, although challenging, stressors create opportunities for growth and positive life changes.

➤ During the process of challenging thoughts, it is useful to provide the individual with evidence of self-efficacy (that he or she is capable of handling the challenge).

Clum, G. A., Clum, G. A., & Surls, R. (1993). A meta-analysis of treatments for panic disorder. *Journal of Consulting and Clinical Psychology, 61*, 317–326.

Helgeson, V. S., Reynolds, K. A., & Tomich, P. L. (2006). A meta-analytic review of benefit finding and growth. *Journal of Consulting and Clinical Psychology, 5*, 797–816.

Stein and Cutler (2002) presented a psychoeducational model in a cognitive behavioral framework that incorporates lecture, role-plays, behavioral rehearsal, and homework. Clients are presented with a variety of topics, including relaxation skills, stress management, self-regulation, and the use of humor. The use of worksheets provides a means for clients to work with the therapist to identify goals and track progress on goal attainment. Given the occupational nature of the profession, meaningful activity is integral to the delivery of psychoeducational groups in occupational therapy. Opportunities for experiential activities are key to provide the opportunity to practice skills necessary for stress and coping.

Relaxation and Meditation

The use of deep breathing and relaxation methods can decrease the stress response and facilitate adaptive coping (Janowiak & Hackman, 1994; Rausch, Gramling, & Auerbach, 2006). These techniques act on the autonomic nervous system to elicit a relaxation response. Davidson et al (2003) found a number of positive benefits of mindfulness meditation, including decreased anxiety and increased positive emotions. Meditation techniques may be used alone, or in conjunction with other practices such as Tai Chi, Qi Gong, and yoga. Some forms of meditation encourage the focus on an object or word/phrase (mantra), whereas others emphasize attention to the breath. With practice, individuals often become more focused and able to engage in the meditation process, as well as experience personal transformation and growth (Progoff, 1992; Uyterhoeven, 2006).

When used in therapy, training considerations should include the knowledge of the therapist on a given technique. Whereas basic breathing and muscle relaxation techniques are easy to learn and use in therapy, more sophisticated techniques involving practices such as yoga often involve certification from nationally recognized organizations.

Progressive muscle relaxation is a technique used to enhance personal self-control and reduce arousal levels (Lopata, Nida, & Marable, 2006). This technique encourages the individual to focus on specific muscle groups, tighten them, and slowly relax, thus affecting the autonomic nervous system and decreasing arousal. Within the progressive muscle relaxation training, clients are instructed to breathe slow and evenly. Whereas some meditation techniques place primary focus on the breath, progressive muscle relaxation emphasizes the contraction and subsequent relaxation and releasing of tension in the muscle groups throughout the body.

Although most individuals are able to learn relaxation techniques, some clients in acute phases of illness, particularly those with psychosis, may be less able to focus on the relaxation process. Caution should be used in selecting clients for group activities that involve quiet meditation and relaxation. In addition, clients with histories of sexual abuse and issues with body image may initially feel unsafe practicing relaxation in a group atmosphere. Therapeutic intervention should consider the client's need to practice the techniques alone and with the therapist prior to joining a group.

Relaxation and meditation methods may be used alone or in conjunction with other skills training techniques. Often the pairing of relaxation with an activity that may have some perceived stress (e.g., an agoraphobic attending a community outing to a mall) is useful to practice techniques as they are assimilated into everyday activities.

Health, Wellness, Nutrition, and Exercise

The incorporation of healthy life choices is effective in decreasing illnesses that lead to mortality and morbidity (Lloyd & Foster, 2006). Promotion of adequate nutrition, exercise, and healthy lifestyles not only decreases the incidence of major causes of death (Phillips, 2002), but may also serve to enhance personal well-being and decrease stress and depression (Ayse, Ardic, Ozgen, & Topuz, 2006; Ross & Hayes, 1988). A number of studies demonstrate a positive association between physical exercise and improved mood (e.g., Biddle, 1995; LaFontaine et al, 1992; Long & van Stavel, 1995). Persons with enhanced physical aerobic fitness appear to have more protection against stress than those who are less physically fit (Cox, 1998).

In designing health programs that include physical activity, Stein and Cutler (2002) emphasized the importance of considering the social and emotional requirements of the activities, purpose and achievability of goals, and frequency and duration of the program. Occupational therapists often work with other health professionals such as the physician, nurse, and dietician to develop health and wellness intervention. Programs designed for transferability and long-term health outcomes are necessary to enhance the continuing of physical activity and proper nutrition after discharge.

Interpersonal Skill Training

Interpersonal social and assertiveness skills may reduce anxiety in social situations and facilitate goal attainment in a socially acceptable manner (Rotheram-Borus, 1988). A major benefit of training is the provision for direct feedback, which can result in expectations of improvement in social and independent living and quality of life (Ikebuchi, Anzai, & Niwa, 1998). In conjunction with other techniques, cognitive behavioral therapy often includes social skills and assertiveness training through the use of role-plays, psychoeducation, and homework assignments.

Bruce and Borg (2002) identified three aspects of role-plays, including rehearsal, modeling, and coaching. In role-play, the client acts out social situations that have been set up. The therapist may take part in modeling the behavior, and then the client rehearses the social situation and receives coaching or feedback from the therapist and peers. Behaviors learned in the therapy situation are then practiced in real life situations. A fascinating example of the use of role-plays in a preventative stress atmosphere is that of training occupational therapists for military combat situations. Rice and Gerardi (1999) described a program that used education, training, and role-play practice to help military therapists learn to manage combat stress casualties.

Child and Adolescent Intervention

A challenge in the provision of services to address childhood stress and coping is the lack of well-developed theories for pediatric populations (Cohen & Park, 1992); therefore, many of the conceptual frameworks that guide assessment and intervention are based on studies of adult populations. Research demonstrates that the development of social skills and adaptive coping may buffer children from the negative effects of stress (Pincus & Friedman, 2004).

The Lived Experience

Bruce

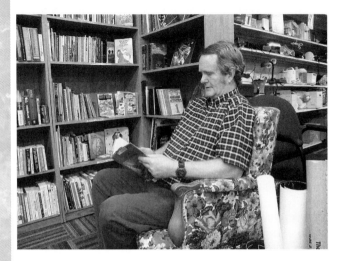

The following narrative communicates the difficulties of coping with a mental illness and the importance of meaningful occupation in the recovery process.

I first had mental illness in my life at age 24, and it seemed, in part, to be the result of a traumatic brain injury sustained in a car accident because of the proximity of the accident and my problems, and no history of mental illness in my family previously. However, I was treated for schizophrenia at least initially because medications worked.

My single biggest struggle was holding onto a sense of beauty in life with the illness bringing on much ugliness and uncomfortable feelings. I was blessed by an awareness of a divine angel, which to this day I believe was sent by God for my protection. For several months after the accident, and before I sought medical help, this angel was my only relief from feelings of pain, heightened awareness of violence in society, and deep grief.

When I did go for medical help finally, the meds were able to put me back into the mind-set I had before the accident, at least somewhat. However, I wanted to go forward with my life at age 24, seeing my future ahead of me. I wanted to explore spirituality, and specifically, this angel that had warmed my heart.

Some years later, 9 years to be exact, I found myself at Tasks Unlimited, a nonprofit mental health agency providing employment and housing for those with severe and persistent mental illness. After a 3-month training program I moved to a lodge, which was a peer-supported house in the community where clients of Tasks lived. I learned how to handle my mental illness socially in this setting. As a boy, I always had lots of friends and was quite active socially, so a big need of mine was to be social in my present situation with the added facet of having a mental illness. I spent 5 years at a lodge.

In this period, I developed a relationship at church with a woman who was a good influence in my life, and I was able to share some things with her. Nevertheless, I found it difficult to imagine how I could explain my illness to her, and we parted.

Since then, I've been able to feel more and more comfortable sharing my illness with others, particularly my family, and especially my parents. I've had great support from them. They are interested in my progress, and I've made significant achievements in this area.

If I allow the illness to take over, I get in serious trouble, so I must progress——always moving forward. To this end, I've made goals for myself.

I ran seven marathon races primarily to stay in shape, but also to provide a sense of achievement. I could get quite down on myself if I wasn't achieving in life. My goal was to run marathons the rest of my life, but I became sidelined with an injury. For my physical outlet, I've turned to karate. My goal, of course, is to get a black belt, but karate is demanding for anyone, and I find it especially so. I'm content to be making progress.

Another goal of mine was to buy my own place, which I've done. I own a condominium in downtown Minneapolis. I've had to work three jobs to accomplish this, but I'm very pleased with my living situation for now.

I alluded to work. If there's one single aspect of my life that makes me healthy, it's work. I've needed support in this area to build my confidence and not bring symptoms of mental illness to the workplace. I rely on a job coach in my job as a supervisor, although I feel my dependence is less and less. With my two other jobs, I work independently of the mental health system with good success. Work occupies my time, gives me income, contributes to self-esteem, and offers the chance to make and accomplish goals. Without work, I'd be in difficulty.

I mentioned the flagging sense of beauty brought on by the illness. More than anything else, I require beauty in my life. Because of my illness, I've had to work hard at this. I maintain good hygiene, eat healthy, and get a good night of sleep, although at this time I use a sleep aide, something I'd like to do away with eventually.

The biggest provider of beauty for me has been my church. I've had my struggles with organized religion, but I can't argue with the comfort I've felt there and the unconditional love of the parishioners and God. I'm looking for a woman friend in my life, but at this point I've been unable to find someone who can replace God in my life, and the answer, of course, is that maybe I can have both.

Interventions used with children often parallel adult techniques; yet, it is important to consider the developmental age of the child within the contextual framework. Similar to therapeutic approaches with adults, research demonstrates the efficacy of using a variety of methods for children and adolescents, including the use of relaxation, social skills, and interpersonal effectiveness training; cognitive behavioral techniques; behavioral reinforcement programs; and skills to promote self-control (Forman, 1993).

The use of play and media are often included to work on the expression of feelings and development of social skills, as well as to enhance physical, cognitive, and emotional development. Intervention approaches are aimed at facilitating adaptive coping through building stable coping resources and styles, and assisting the child in coping with specific stressors (e.g., divorce, abuse) (Sandler, Wolchik, MacKinnon, Ayers, & Roosa, 1997). Therapeutic goals include increasing the child's ability to discuss emotions, problem-solve, use adaptive coping techniques, and improve self-efficacy.

Research demonstrates that a child's self-esteem affects personal resilience and ability to cope (Brooks & Goldstein, 2001). Personal perception is affected by success and failure experiences. Children may experience barriers to success in school, daily life, and at home. Such barriers are often greater for those with mental health challenges. Many of the children seen within psychiatric settings have encountered abuse situations, trauma, and difficult home experiences. The incorporation of opportunities for success within the therapy environment may include the use of simple goal attainment strategies and reinforcements through positive feedback and behavioral programs such as token economies. Brooks and Goldstein (2001) identified the following principles to facilitate personal success in the promotion of self-esteem in children:

- Enjoy and celebrate the child's accomplishments.
- Emphasize the child's input in creating success.
- Reinforce the child's competence by "engaging in environmental engineering."
- Give strengths time to develop.
- Accept the unique strengths of each child.

As the therapist works with the child, emphasis is placed on helping the child realize his or her success experiences, thereby working to improve self-esteem and self-efficacy.

A key area of importance in the self-perception of children is that of peer relationships and the development of friendships. Children with mental health difficulties often have problems developing healthy peer interactions. Psychological conditions such as depression create problems in relationship formation (Panek & Garber, 1992) and develop a vicious circle, whereby the child may withdraw from others and thus feel isolated. His or her friends then respond with anger or by pulling away, reinforcing the child's self-perception of failure. Along with opportunities for success in therapeutic intervention, Seligman (1995) stressed the importance of developing social skills within a child. The ability to interact facilitates the development of friendships and positive peer interactions. The use of role-plays, cooperative peer environments, and storytelling is effective in teaching social skills (Gilbert & Mirawski, 2005). The use of popular movies, books, puppet shows, or drama may also be used to discuss social situations, morals, and values with children. The reinforcement of healthy lifestyles and personal choices through modeling, discussion, and opportunity for practice facilitates skill development. An example of coping intervention with a child is shown in Box 22-3.

In the previous client example, a transitional object was used to facilitate skill development and work with Jeremy to develop adaptive coping methods. Lifestyle patterns, behaviors, thoughts, and cognitions influence how adaptively individuals react to stress and function in society (Gilbert &

BOX 22-3 ■ **Client Example of Pediatric Coping Intervention**

Jeremy, an 8-year-old boy with fetal alcohol syndrome and conduct disorder, had a history of aggression, poor social skills, and low self-esteem. His mother complained that he did not have any friends and that all he ever wanted to do was play video games. On admission, the therapist conducted a comprehensive evaluation, including assessment of his developmental level, sensory processing, and perceived stress. A home observation and interview of the parents was also completed. Results indicated that Jeremy had difficulty not only with coping, but also with poor sensory processing, emotional dysregulation, and ineffective social skills.

In addition to play therapy and sensory-based approaches, the therapist used expressive media, storytelling, and role-play in order to teach Jeremy about social situations. Jeremy was initially resistant to engaging in therapy and discussing social scenarios, but this changed when the therapist incorporated a puppet of one of Jeremy's favorite cartoon characters. Through the use of puppetry, Jeremy projected onto the character his own feelings in situations and was able to learn basic coping techniques, such as deep breathing, to deal with stressful situations.

Mirawski, 2005). Because a child's patterns are often most influenced by his or her parents, the evaluation and intervention of children should include a comprehensive assessment of personal and environmental factors, including the child's home, school, and community life. Interventions are greatly affected by the social environment in which the child lives; therefore, occupational therapists are encouraged to involve the parents, school professionals, and other key individuals (e.g., grandparents, caregivers, siblings) in the provision of therapy services. Often, intervention with pediatric populations includes the use of family psychoeducation, an assessment of the home and school environment, and skill training for parents (Kumfer & Tait, 2000).

For those children who are recovering from trauma and disaster situations, Saylor, Belter, and Stokes (1997) emphasize the importance of restoring a sense of normalcy. Therapists can facilitate such normalcy through the use of predictable routines, consistent feedback, and the development of internal skills in conjunction with external supports. Consideration of follow-up should include home- and school-based programs designed to transfer the skills learned in therapy. Education of the family and school professionals is imperative in order to reinforce learning.

Summary

The process of coping is required to meet the demands of everyday life circumstances. An individual's personal appraisal of the situation, along with environmental and person factors, affect the ability to cope. Although mental illness may be triggered by life stressors, the symptoms of the illness itself cause additional stress and burdens in the process of coping. Through careful client-centered practice, occupational therapy can facilitate skill development to better equip clients to face everyday stressors, thus leading to increased productivity, self-efficacy, and life satisfaction.

Active Learning Strategies

1. Personal Assessment of Coping

Select and complete a self-assessment stress inventory and coping tool (either online or available from your instructor).

Reflective Questions

Following completion of the self-assessment tools, answer the following:

- What areas of your life currently cause you the most stress?
- What means of coping do you use to deal with stressors (e.g., avoidant coping, problem-focused coping)?
- If you were a therapist designing an intervention for yourself, what approaches would you take and why? (*Hint:* Think of the psychodynamic, behavioral, cognitive behavioral, and occupation-based approaches.)
- Write three realistic goals for yourself.
- What barriers do you anticipate in achieving your goals? How could you be proactive in addressing these barriers?
- Summarize your experience related to your self-assessment (i.e., how did it feel?, was it difficult?, what did you learn?)

2. Coping and Mental Illness

For each of the following scenarios, briefly describe how you would approach the client for evaluation and intervention as related to coping skills. (*Hint:* Your analysis will also need to identify areas for further information.)

- Mary is a 45-year-old woman with posttraumatic stress disorder following a severe car accident in which she lost her 8-year-old daughter and 49-year-old husband. She has a college degree, but has not worked for several years. She presents to you as depressed, anxious, and hopeless. Her self-described interests are crafts, aerobics, and gardening, yet she has no energy or drive to engage in anything except sleep and watching TV.
- Brian is a 24-year-old male with a newly diagnosed schizophrenia. He has been living at home, and his parents complain he became increasingly delusional and unable to meet his basic ADL needs. Both Brian and his parents are having considerable difficulty understanding his illness. Brian has also complained of the inability to cope with the "voices in his head."

Resources

Websites

- Scoring for the Holmes-Rahe Social Readjustment Scale: www.cop.ufl.edu/safezone/doty/dotyhome/wellness/HolRah.htm
- Ways of Coping Questionnaire, by Susan Folkman and Richard S. Lazarus (Menlo Park, CA: Mind Garden, Inc.): http://www.mindgarden.com/products/wayss.htm
- Psychological Assessment Resources, Inc. (PAR, Inc.)—several stress coping measures, including Coping Responses Inventory, Parenting Stress Inventory, and Occupational Stress Inventory: www3.parinc.com

Books

Diary Cards and Dialectical Behavior Therapy Skills Training

- Linehan, M. (1993). *Skills Training Manual for Treating Borderline Personality Disorder.* New York: Guilford Press.

Mindfulness Meditation

- Kabat-Zinn, J. (1994). *Wherever You Go There You Are: Mindfulness Meditation in Everyday Life.* New York: Hyperion.

Progressive Muscle Relaxation

- Jacobson, E. (1938). *Progressive Relaxation: A Physiological and Clinical Investigation of Muscle States and Their Significance in Psychology and Medical Practice* (2nd ed.). Chicago: The University of Chicago Press.
- Jacobson, E. (1942). *You Must Relax: A Practical Method of Reducing the Strains of Modern Living.* New York: McGraw-Hill.

Writing Techniques in Occupational Therapy

- Haertl, K. H. (2007). Journaling as an assessment tool in mental health occupational therapy. In B. Hemphill (Ed.), *Assessment in Occupational Therapy Mental Health* (2nd ed.) (pp. 61–80). Thorofare NJ: Slack.

References

Abelenda, J., & Helfrich, C. A. (2004). Family resilience and mental illness: The role of occupational therapy. *Occupational Therapy in Mental Health, 19,* 25–39.

Abidin, R. R. (1990). *Parenting Stress Index Manual* (3rd ed.). Charlottesville VA: Pediatric Psychology Press.

Aldwin, C. M. (1990). The Elders Life Stress Inventory: Egocentric and non-egocentric stress. In A. M. Stephens, J. H. Crowther, S. E. Hobfoll, & D. L. Tennenbaum (Eds.), *Stress and Coping in Late Life Families* (pp. 49–69). New York: Hemisphere.

Amirkhan, J. H. (1990). A factor analytically derived measure of coping: The Coping Strategy Indicator. *Journal of Personality and Social Psychology, 59,* 1066–1074.

Anthony, W. A. (1993). Recovery from mental illness: The guiding vision of the mental health service system in the 1990's. *Psychiatric Rehabilitation Journal, 16,* 11–23.

Antonovsky, A. (1979). *Health, Stress, and Coping: New Perspectives on Mental and Physical Well-Being.* San Francisco: Jossey-Bass.

Ayres, T. S., Sandler, I. N., West, S. G., & Roosa, M. W. (1996). A dispositional and situational assessment of children's coping: Testing alternative models of coping. *Journal of Personality, 64,* 923–958.

Ayse, S., Ardic, F., Ozgen, M., & Topuz, O. (2006). The effects of aerobics and resistance exercise in obese women. *Clinical Rehabilitation, 20,* 773–782.

Biddle, S. J. (1995). Exercise and psychosocial health. *Research Quarterly for Exercise and Sport, 66,* 292–297.

Brooks, R., & Goldstein, S. (2001). *Fostering Strength, Hope, and Optimism in Your Child: Raising Resilient Children.* Chicago: Contemporary Publishing Group.

Brown, G. W., Birley, J. L., & Wing, J. K. (1972). Influence of family life on the course of schizophrenic disorder: A replication: *British Journal of Psychiatry, 121,* 241–258.

Bruce, M. A., & Borg, B. (2002). *Psychosocial Frames of Reference: Core for Occupation-Based Practice* (3rd ed.). Thorofare, NJ: Slack.

Bruininks, R. H., Woodcock, R. W., Weatherman, R. F., & Hill, B. K. (1996). *SIB-R: Scales of Independent Behavior–Revised.* Itasca, IL: Riverside.

Cannon, W. B. (1929). *An Account of Recent Researches into the Function of Bodily Changes in Pain, Hunger, Fear, and Rage.* New York: Appleton and Co.

Carver, C. S., Scheier, M. F., & Weintraub, J. K. (1989). Assessing coping strategies: A theoretically based approach. *Journal of Personality and Social Psychology, 56,* 267–283.

Chaffey, L., & Fossey, E. (2004). Caring and daily life: Occupational experiences of women living with sons diagnosed with schizophrenia. *Australian Occupational Therapy Journal, 51,* 199–207.

Chapman, L. J., Chapman, J. P., Kwapil, T. R., Eckblad, M., & Zinser, M. C. (1994). Putatively psychosis-prone subjects 10 years later. *Journal of Abnormal Psychology, 87,* 399–407.

Chovil, I. (2005). First psychosis prodrome: Rehabilitation and recovery. *Psychiatric Rehabilitation Journal, 28,* 407–410.

Christiansen, C. H. (2007). Adolf Meyer revisited: Empirical thoughts on occupation and resilience. *Journal of Occupational Science, 14*(2), 63–76.

Cohen, L. H., & Park, C. (1992). Life stress in children and adolescents: An overview of conceptual and methodological issues. In A. M. LaGreca, L. J. Siegal, J. L. Wallander, & C. E. Walker (Eds.), *Stress and Coping in Child Health* (pp. 25–43). New York: Guilford Press.

Compas, B. E., Davis, G. E., Forsythe, J., & Wagner, B. M. (1987). Assessment of major and daily stressful events during adolescence: The Adolescent Perceived Events Scale. *Journal of Consulting and Clinical Psychology, 4,* 534–541.

Cowls, J., & Hale, S. (2005). It's the activity that counts: What clients value in psychoeducation groups. *Canadian Journal of Occupational Therapy, 72,* 176–182.

Cox, R. H. (1998). *Sport Psychology: Concepts and Applications* (4th ed.). Boston: McGraw-Hill.

Dangelmaier, R. E., Docherty, N. M., & Akamatsu, T. J. (2006). Psychosis proneness, coping, and perceptions of social support. *American Journal of Orthopsychiatry, 76,* 13–17.

Davidson, R. J., Kabat-Zinn, J., Schumacher, J., Rosenkranz, M., Muller, D., Santorelli, S. F., Urbanowski, R., Harrington, A., Bonus, K., & Sheridan, J. F. (2003). Alterations in brain and immune function produced by mindfulness meditation. *Psychosomatic Medicine, 65,* 564–570.

Dise-Lewis, J. E. (1988). The life events and coping inventory: An assessment of stress in children. *Psychosomatic Medicine, 50,* 484–499.

Dohrenwend, B. S., Krasnoff, L., Askenasy, A. R., & Dohrenwend, B. P. (1978). Exemplification of a method for scaling life events: The PERI Life Events Scale. *Journal of Health and Social Behavior, 19,* 205–229.

Elliott, G. R., & Eisdorfer, C. (Eds.). (1982). *Stress and Human Health.* New York: Springer.

Esterling, B. A., L'Abate, L., Murray, E. J., & Pennebaker, J. W. (1999). Empirical foundations for writing in prevention and psychotherapy: Mental and physical health outcomes. *Clinical Psychology Review, 19,* 79–96.

Felton, B. J., Revenson, T. A., & Henrichsen, G. A. (1984). Stress and coping in the explanation of psychological adjustment among chronically ill adults. *Social Science and Medicine, 18,* 889–898.

Folkman, S., & Lazarus, R. S. (1988). *Manual for the Ways of Coping.* Palo Alto, CA: Consulting Psychology Press.

Forman, S. G. (1993). *Coping Skills Interventions for Children and Adolescents.* San-Francisco: Jossey-Bass.

Fortune, D. G., Smith, J. V., & Garvey, K. (2005). Perceptions of psychosis, coping, appraisals, and psychological distress in the relatives of patients with schizophrenia: An exploration using self regulation theory. *British Journal of Clinical Psychology, 44,* 319–331.

Frydenberg, E., & Lewis, R. (1993). *Adolescent Coping Scale: Administrator's Manual.* Hawthorne: The Australian Council for Educational Research.

Ghanstrom-Stranqvist, K., Josephsson, H., & Thom, K. (2004). Stories of clients with mental illness: The structure of occupational therapists' interactions. *OTJR: Occupation, Participation, and Health, 24,* 134–143.

Gilbert, J. N., & Mirawski, C. (2005). Stress coping for elementary school children: A case for including lifestyle. *Journal of Individual Psychology, 61,* 314–328.

Gol, A. R., & Cook, S. W. (2004). Exploring the underlying dimensions of coping: A concept mapping approach. *Journal of Social and Clinical Psychology, 23,* 155–171.

Hardy, S. E., Concato, J., & Gill, T. M. (2004). Resilience of community dwelling older persons. *Journal of the American Geriatrics Society, 52,* 258–262.

Hatfield, A. B., & Lefley, H. P. (1993). *Surviving Mental Illness: Stress, Coping and Adaptation.* New York: Guilford Press.

Holmes, T. H., & Rahe, R. H. (1967). The social readjustment rating scale. *Journal of Psychosomatic Research, 11,* 213–218.

Ikebuchi, E., Anzai, N., & Niwa, S. (1998). Adoption and dissemination of social skills training in Japan: A decade of experience. *International Review of Psychiatry, 10,* 71–75.

Ivarsson, A., Sidenvall, B., & Carlsson, M. (2004). Performance of occupations in daily life among individuals with severe mental disorders. *Occupational Therapy in Mental Health, 20,* 33–50.

Janowiak, J. J., & Hackman, R. (1994). Meditation and college students self actualization and rated stress. *Psychological Reports, 75,* 1007–1010.

Johnson, J. H., & McCutcheon, S. (1980). Assessing life events in older children and adolescents: Preliminary findings with the life events checklist. In I. G. Sarason & C. D. Spielberger (Eds.), *Stress and Anxiety* (Vol. 7, pp. 111–125). Washington, DC: Hemisphere.

Kaplan, K., & Kielhofner, G. (1989). *Occupational Case Analysis Interview and Rating Scale.* Thorofare, NJ: Slack, Inc.

Kendall, P. C., & Panichelli-Mindel, S. M. (1995). Cognitive-behavioral treatments. *Journal of Abnormal Psychology, 61,* 235–247.

Knight, C. (2006). Groups for individuals with traumatic histories: Practice considerations for social workers. *Social Work, 51,* 20–30.

Kobasa, S. C., Maddi, S. R., & Kahn, S. (1981). Hardiness and health: A prospective study. *Journal of Personality and Social Psychology, 42,* 168–177.

Kumfer, K. L., & Tait, C. M. (2000). Family skills training for parents and children. *Juvenile Justice Bulletin, April,* 1–10.

LaFontaine, T. P., DiLorenzo, T. M., Frensch, P. A., Stucky-Ropp, R. C., Bargman, E. P., & McDonald, D. G. (1992). Aerobic exercise and mood: A brief review, 1985–1990. *Sports Medicine, 13,* 160–170.

Law, M., Baptiste, S., Carswell, A., McColl, M., Polatajko, H., & Pollock, N. (1998). *Canadian Occupational Performance Measure* (3rd ed.). Ottawa, Ontario: Canadian Association of Occupational Therapy.

Lazarus, R. S., & Folkman, S. (1984). *Stress, Appraisal, and Coping.* New York: Springer.

Le Page, J. P. (1999). The impact of a token economy on injuries and negative events on an acute psychiatric unit. *Psychiatric Services, 50,* 941–944.

Leff, J. P., Kuipers, L., Berkowitz, R., Eberlin-Vries, R., & Sturgeon, D. (1982). A controlled trial of social intervention in the families of schizophrenic patients. *British Journal of Psychiatry, 141,* 121–134.

Linehan, M. (1993). *Skills Training Manual for Treating Borderline Personality Disorder.* New York: Guilford Press.

Lloyd, P. J., & Foster, S. L. (2006). Creating healthy, high performance workplaces: Strategies from health and sports psychology. *Consulting Psychology Journal: Practice and Research, 58,* 23–39.

Long, B. C., & van Stavel, R. (1995). Effects of exercise training on anxiety: A meta-analysis. *Journal of Applied Sport Psychology, 7,* 167–189.

Lopata, C., Nida, R. E., & Marable, M. A. (2006). Progressive muscle relaxation: Preventing aggression in children with EBD. *Teaching Exceptional Children, 38,* 20–25.

McEwen, B. S. (2002). Sex, stress and the hippocampus: Allostasis, allostatic load and the aging process. *Neurobiology of Aging, 23,* 921–939.

Meyer, A. (1921). The contributions of psychiatry to the understanding of life's problems. In E. E. Winters (Ed.), *The Collected Papers of Adolf Meyer* (pp. 1–16). Baltimore: The Johns Hopkins University Press.

Moos, R. H. (1990). *Coping Responses Inventory Manual.* Palo Alto, CA: Center for Health Care Evaluation, Stanford University and Department of Veterans' Administration Medical Centers.

Mosey, A. C. (1970). *Three Frames of Reference for Mental Health.* Thorofare, NJ: Slack Inc.

Mosey, A. C. (1986). *Psychosocial Components of Occupational Therapy.* Philadelphia: Lippincott-Raven.

Myrtek, M. (2001). Meta-analyses of prospective studies on coronary heart disease, type A personality, and hostility. *International Journal of Cardiology, 79,* 245–251.

Nachshen, J. S., Woodford, L., & Minnes, P. (2003). The Family Stress and Coping Interview for families of individuals with developmental disabilities: A lifespan perspective on family adjustment. *Journal of Intellectual Disability Research, 47,* 285–290.

Needham, A. (1996). *The Stress Management Kit.* London: Connections.

Nehra, R., Chakrabati, S., Kulhara, P., & Sharma, R. (2005). Caregiver coping in bipolar disorder and schizophrenia: A re-examination. *Social Psychiatry and Psychiatry Epidemiology, 40,* 329–336.

Nihira, K., Leland, H., & Lambert, N. (1993). *AAMR Adaptive Behavior Scale—Residential and Community* (2nd ed.). Austin, TX: PRO-ED.

Osipow, S. H., & Spokane, A. R. (1998). *Occupational Stress Inventory Manual (Professional Version).* Odessa FL: Psychological Assessment Resources.

Ostman, M. (2004). Family burden and participation in care: differences between relatives of patients admitted to psychiatric care for the first time and relatives of re-admitted patients. *Journal of Psychiatric and Mental Health Nursing, 11,* 608–613.

Panek, W. F., & Garber, J. (1992). Role of aggression, rejection, and attributions in the prediction of depression in children. *Development and Psychopathology, 4,* 145–165.

Patton, M. Q. (2002). *Qualitative Research and Evaluation Methods* (3rd ed.). Thousand Oaks, CA: Sage.

Paykel, S. (1997). The interview for recent life events. *Psychological Medicine, 27,* 301–310.

Penley, J. A., Tomaka, J., & Wiebe, J. S. (2002). The association of coping to physical and psychological health outcomes: A metaanalytic review. *Journal of Behavioral Medicine, 25,* 551–603.

Phillips, P. (2002). The rising cost of health care: Can demand be reduced through more effective health promotion? *Journal of Evaluation in Clinical Practice, 8,* 415–419.

Pincus, D. B., & Friedman, A. G. (2004). Improving children's coping with everyday stress: Transporting treatment interventions to the school setting. *Clinical Child and Family Psychology Review, 7,* 223–240.

Pollio, D. E., North, C. S., Reid, D. L, Miletic, M. M., & McClendon, J. R. (2006). Living with severe mental illness—What families and friends must know: Evaluation of a one-day psychoeducation workshop. *Social Work, 51,* 31–38.

Pratt, S. I., Rosenberg, S., Mueser, K., Brancato, J., Salyers, M., Jankowski, M. K., & Descamps, M. (2005). Evaluation of a PTSD psychoeducation program for psychiatric inpatients. *Journal of Mental Health, 14,* 121–127.

Progoff, I. (1992). *At a Journal Workshop: Writing to Access the Power of the Unconscious and Evoke Creative Ability.* New York: Penguin Putnam Books.

Rahe, R. H. (1975). Epidemiological studies of life changes and illness. *International Journal of Psychiatry in Medicine, 6,* 133–146.

Rahe, R. H., Meyer, M., Smith, M., Kjaer, G., & Holmes, T. H. (1964). Social stress and illness onset. *Journal of Psychosomatic Research, 8,* 35–44.

Rausch, S. M., Gramling, S. E., & Auerbach, S. M. (2006). Effects of a single session of large group meditation and progressive muscle relaxation training on stress reduction, relaxation, and recovery. *International Journal of Stress Management, 13,* 273–290.

Reivich, K., & Shatte, A. (2002). *The Resilience Factor: 7 Essential Skills for Overcoming Life's Inevitable Obstacles.* New York: Broadway Books.

Rice, V., & Gerardi, S. M. (1999). Part II: Work hardening for warriors: Training military occupational therapy professionals in the management of combat stress casualties. *Work, 13,* 197–209.

Ross, C. E., & Hayes, D. (1988). Exercise and psychological wellbeing in the community. *American Journal of Epidemiology, 127,* 762–771.

Rotheram-Borus, M. J. (1988). Assertiveness training with children. In R. H. Price, E. L. Cowen, R. P. Lorion, & J. Ramos-McKay (Eds.), *Fourteen Ounces of Prevention* (pp. 83–97). Washington, DC: American Psychological Association.

Rotondi, A. J., Haas, G. L., Anderson, C. M., Newhill, C. E., Spring, M. B., Ganguli, R., Gardner, W. B., & Rosenstock, J. B. (2005). A clinical trial to test the feasibility of a tele-health psychoeducation intervention for persons with schizophrenia and their families: Intervention and three month findings. *Rehabilitation Psychology, 50,* 325–336.

Ryff, C., & Singer, B. (2003). Thriving in the face of challenge: The integrative science of human resilience. In F. Kessel, P. Rosenfield, & N. Andeson (Eds.), *Expanding the Boundaries of Health and Social Science* (pp. 181–205). New York: Oxford University Press.

Samuels, M. (1995). Art as a healing force. *Alternative Therapies in Health and Medicine, 5,* 38–40.

Sandler, I. N., Wolchik, S. A., MacKinnon, D., Ayers, T. S., & Roosa, M. W. (1997). Developing linkages between theory and intervention in stress and coping process. In S. A. Wolchik & I. N. Sandler (Eds.), *Handbook of Children's Coping: Linking Theory and Intervention* (pp. 3–39). New York: Plenum.

Sapolsky, R. (2003). *Why Zebras Don't Get Ulcers* (3rd ed.). New York: W. H. Freeman.

Sarason, I. G., Johnson, J. H., & Siegel, J. M. (1978). Assessing the impact of life changes: Development of the Life Experiences Survey. *Journal of Consulting and Clinical Psychology, 46,* 932–946.

Saylor, C. F., Belter, R., & Stokes, S. J. (1997). Coping with stress: The roles of regulation and development. In S. A. Wolchik & I. N. Sandler (Eds.), *Handbook of Children's Coping: Linking Theory and Intervention* (pp. 361–383). New York: Plenum.

Schlebusch, L. (2004). The development of a stress symptom checklist. *South African Journal of Psychology, 34,* 327–349.

Schwarzer, R., & Schwarzer, C. (1996). A critical survey of coping instruments. In M. Zeidner & N. S. Endler (Eds.), *Handbook of Coping: Theory, Research and Applications* (pp. 107–132). New York: Wiley.

Schwarzer, C., Starke, D., & Buchwald, P. (2003). Towards a theory based assessment of coping: The German adaptation of the Strategic Approach to Coping Scale. *Anxiety, Stress and Coping, 16,* 271–280.

Scully, J. A., & Tosi, H. (2000). Life events checklists: Revisiting the Social Readjustment Rating Scale after 30 years. *Educational and Psychological Measurement, 60,* 864–876.

Seligman, M. E. (1995). *The Optimistic Child.* Boston: Houghton Mifflin.

Selye, H. (1946). The general adaptation syndrome and the diseases of adaptation. *Journal of Clinical Endocrinology, 6,* 117–230.

Smyth, J. M. (1998). Written emotional expression: Effect sizes, outcome types, and moderating variables. *Journal of Consulting and Clinical Psychology, 66,* 174–184.

Snyder, C. R., & Pulvers, K. M. (2001). Dr. Seuss, the coping machine, and "oh the places you'll go." In C. R. Snyder (Ed.), *Coping With Stress: Effective People and Processes* (pp. 3–27). New York: Oxford University Press.

Stein, F., & Cutler, S. (2002). *Psychosocial Occupational Therapy: A Holistic Approach* (2nd ed.). San Diego: Singular Publishing Group.

Stewart, J. (1999). "Measures of Psychological Stress." John D. & Catherine T. MacArthur Research Network on Socioeconomic Status and Health. Revised February 9, 2000. Available at: www.macses.ucsf.edu/Research/Psychosocial/notebook/stress .html (accessed December 8, 2009).

Stone, A. A., Schwartz, J. E., Neale, J. M., Schiffman, S., Marc, C. A., Hickcox, M., Paty, J., Porter, L. S., & Cruise, L. J. (1998). A comparison of coping assessed by ecological momentary assessment and retrospective recall. *Journal of Personality and Social Psychology, 6,* 1670–1680.

Storm, H., Shafiei, M., Myre, K., & Raeder, J. (2005). Palmar skin conductance compared to a developed stress score and to noxious and awakening stimuli on patients in anesthesia. *Acta Anaesthesiologica Scandinavica, 49,* 798–803.

Suls, J., & Fletcher, B. (1985). The relative efficacy of avoidance and non-avoidant a coping strategies: A meta-analysis. *Health Psychology, 4,* 249–288.

Tennakoon, L., Fannon, D., Doku, V., O'Ceallaigh, S., Soni, W., Santamaria, M., Kuipers, E., & Sharma, T. (2000). Experience of caregiving: Relatives of people experiencing a first episode of psychosis. *British Journal of Psychiatry, 177,* 529–533.

Thomson, L. K. (1993). *The Kohlman Evaluation of Living Skills* (3rd ed.). Rockville, MD: American Occupational Therapy Association.

Tse, S., Lloyd, C., Penman, M., King, R. & Bassett, H. (2004). Evidence based practice and rehabilitation: Occupational therapy in Australia and New Zealand experiences. *International Journal of Rehabilitation, 27,* 269–274.

Uyterhoeven, S. (2006). Yoga and the autonomic nervous system: Re-educating the mind. *Yoga Therapy in Practice, August,* 23–25.

Weardon, A. J., Tarrier, A., Barrowclough, C., Zastowny, T. R., & Rawhill, A. A. (2000). A review of expressed emotion research in health care. *Clinical Psychology Review, 20,* 633–666.

Weingarten, R. (2005). Calculated risk-taking and other recovery processes for my psychiatric disability. *Psychiatric Rehabilitation Journal, 29,* 77-80.

White, R. W. (1974). Strategies for adaptation: An attempt at systematic description. In G. V. Coehlo, D. A. Hamburg, & J. E. Adams (Eds.), *Coping and Adaptation* (pp. 47–68). New York: Basic Books.

Wong, D. F. (2006). *Clinical Case Management for People With Mental Illness: A Biopsychosocial Vulnerability-Stress Model.* New York: Haworth Press.

Zakowski, S. G., Hall, M. H., Klein, L. C., & Baum, A. (2001). Appraised control, coping, and stress, in a community sample: A test of goodness-of-fit hypothesis. *Annals of Behavioral Medicine, 23*(3), 158–165.

Zeitlin, S. (1985). *Coping Inventory.* Bensenville, IL: Scholastic Testing Service.

Zeitlin, S., Williamson, G. G., & Szczepanski, M. (1988). *Early Coping Inventory.* Bensenville, IL: Scholastic Testing Service.

chapter 23

Motivation

Catana Brown

> "I think a lot of people around me had low, somewhat low expectations of me, and this especially includes family members. . . . I was so used to low expectations that I learned to expect nothing else. . . . I was barely hanging onto the concept of life at that time.
> —Person with schizophrenia, from Boydell, Gladstone, and Volpe, 2003

Introduction

Do you know the story of Oseolo McCarty? At the age of 87, Oseolo donated $150,000 to the University of Southern Mississippi—the largest gift ever received by the university from an African American donor (Bragg, 1995). However, this is not the amazing part of the story; many people donate large amounts of money to universities and other worthy causes. It is the source of the money that makes this story so remarkable.

Oseolo lived in a small frame house in Hattiesburg, Mississippi. When she was in elementary school, Oseolo started a savings account using the money she earned from odd jobs. In the sixth grade, she dropped out of school to take care of her aunt. Eventually, she started a small business out of her home, washing and ironing clothes. She did this for 70 years. It was her frugal living and value of saving that allowed Oseolo to save more money than most people who earn several times her income. Oseolo rarely spent money on herself, never owned a car, and, despite living in Mississippi, lived without air conditioning until her later years when others procured it for her. Oseolo's choice of lifestyle and the intentional efforts she made to save money meant that she was able to accumulate an impressive savings, most of which she donated to the University of Southern Mississippi.

As a culture, Americans are not ones to save money. So, what led this woman of meager means to save so much? And

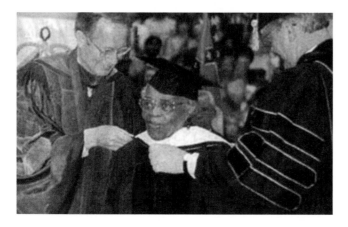

why did she decide to donate a large portion of this money to an institution that she never attended and that had never approached her about making a gift? In fact, for much of her lifetime, the university would have barred Oseolo and her family from attending because of their race. What motivated Oseolo to do the things she did? Those questions can never be answered completely; however, this chapter will help you think about Oseolo's motivations as it endeavors to explain what is it that moves people to do the things they do.

By nature, humans are curious and active beings who are naturally interested in acquiring new skills and connecting with others and the environment. Occupational therapy practice embodies this belief. As so eloquently stated by Suzanne Peloquin (2005), "Our ethos, in part, is this: Occupational therapy is a personal engagement—a mutual commitment to involve and occupy the self and be bound by promise. Guided by this belief, occupational therapy practitioners cocreate daily lives." (p. 615)

Our view of occupation as both a means and an end recognizes the inherent therapeutic value of participation. However, all participation is not healthy, and not all individuals find it easy to engage in life. The human condition is complex and variable. People can be highly motivated to engage in behaviors that are self-destructive, such as substance abuse, bulimia, and spending beyond one's means. Other times, people can find it difficult to be motivated to pursue activities that are life sustaining, as in the case of an individual who is grieving the loss of a loved one and stops eating or sleeping.

One concern of occupational therapy is the drifting toward passivity and withdrawal, in other words, a disengagement from participation. As an occupational therapy student or just as a concerned human, you have certainly observed variability in the degree to which people engage in their world. You have also noticed that some individuals seem destined to make harmful life choices. However, you may not have spent a lot of time thinking about what you can do as an occupational therapist to address these issues. By understanding motivation, occupational therapists are better positioned to assist individuals to engage or reengage in life, make life-sustaining and life-fulfilling choices, and participate in valued occupations.

This chapter presents several different perspectives on motivation through a review of major motivational theories. It also includes information on specific motivational impairments in psychiatric disabilities. Although motivation underlies everything people do, it often receives limited attention in occupational therapy practice. However, this chapter provides pragmatic information on assessing motivation and providing interventions to address motivation.

Theories of Motivation

Why are you reading this chapter? Are you driven by a personal interest in the topic? Possibly, but in all likelihood there are other factors at play. Is it a class assignment? Will there be a test on the material? Think about the factors that led to your decision to read the chapter. Once you get into it, how much energy will you devote to reading and understanding the concepts explained in the chapter? If you find the reading boring or difficult, will you persist?

There are many different explanations for what drives people to act, and some may explain your motivations for reading this chapter. The next section explores a variety of theories of motivation, including the following:

■ Maslow's hierarchy of needs
■ Approach/avoidance models
■ Self-efficacy
■ Self-determination theory
■ Flow theory
■ Transtheoretical model
■ Model of human occupation

As you read about these theories, reflect on which theories speak most to you and which explain what drives people to act, what causes people to give up, and what keeps people going, even when they experience challenges.

Maslow's Hierarchy of Needs

Abraham Maslow (1943) developed one of the earliest and most enduring models of motivation. Maslow asserted that people are motivated to act based on their most pressing need. Human needs are categorized and organized in a hierarchy, with basic needs at the bottom and higher-level needs at the top (Fig. 23-1). According to Maslow's hierarchy, the lowest-level need that has not been met must be addressed or satisfied before the individual can move onto higher-level needs.

The most basic needs are physiological such as hunger, thirst, and sleep. The next level of needs are safety and security needs, which involve feeling protected or out of danger. Once safety needs are met, the individual is focused on meeting affiliation, or belonging, needs. This means feeling connected to others, having friends, a supportive family, and belonging to groups. The next level of need is related to self-esteem; people are driven to achieve and want to be recognized or gain approval from others. Ultimately, according to Maslow, people are driven by the need for self-actualization. This concept is harder to define, but involves self-fulfillment and realizing one's potential and personal growth.

As a student, you know how difficult it is to study when you have just ended a relationship (affiliation needs) or your stomach is growling out of hunger (physiological needs).

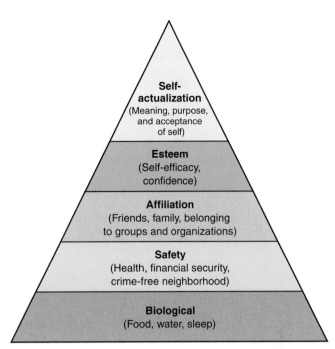

FIGURE 23-1. Maslow's hierarchy of needs. Lower-level needs must be met before higher-level needs can be addressed.

Likewise, occupational therapy clients may find it difficult to participate in a therapy session when they feel threatened (safety needs) or are dealing with other basic physiological needs such as lack of sleep or pain. Consider the child or adult who is homeless and the basic needs that this person must address each day. As an occupational therapist, it is important to consider the hierarchy of needs when providing services. For example, for a child to become motivated to participate in school work, he or she may need to feel safe from bullying, be a friend to other children, and be accepted by the teacher.

Approach/Avoidance Models

Approach/avoidance models provide one way of thinking about motivation. Individuals are driven to participate in activities (approach) when they will result in rewards, positive experiences, or pleasant emotions. In contrast, individuals may be reluctant to engage in goal-directed behaviors (avoid) if they anticipate that negative experiences or unpleasant emotions will result.

Gray (1991) postulates that these two dimensions of personality are biologically driven and regulated by two separate neurological systems. Gray refers to the approach dimension as the behavioral activation system (BAS) and the avoidance dimension as the behavioral inhibition system (BIS). The BAS is responsible for positive emotions, such as hope and happiness. Other characteristics associated with BAS include extraversion (Elliot & Thrash, 2002) and impulsivity (Diaz & Pickering, 1993). The BAS drives the person toward active engagement. The BIS, in contrast, alerts the individual to possible threats, danger, or punishment, which cause the individual to slow down and survey the situation. Inaction is often the result. In addition, the BIS is associated with negative emotions, particularly anxiety, but also depression.

According to Gray's (1991) model, individuals can be more or less sensitive to the BAS or BIS. The BAS-sensitive individual has a greater propensity for goal-directed activity and positive emotion, whereas the BIS-sensitive individual is more anxious and tentative.

Studies indicate that extreme sensitivity to either motivational system is associated with psychiatric disabilities. For example, one study found that individuals who were more sensitive to BIS were also more likely to be anxious or depressed, whereas substance abuse was associated with BAS sensitivity (Johnson, Turner, & Iwata, 2003). Another study found that high sensitivity to BAS is associated with manic symptoms (Bjorn, Rahman, & Shepherd, 2007).

An appreciation for approach/avoidance motivation theory can help occupational therapists better understand and provide interventions for their clients. For example, in a fearful client, the occupational therapist may need to employ interventions to reduce anxiety before a goal-oriented activity. An impulsive client may benefit from interventions aimed at slowing down and assessing the environment.

Self-Efficacy

Bandura (1999) identifies self-efficacy as the primary driver of humans. Self-efficacy is a belief in your own capability, which motivates you to act. People with high self-efficacy are more likely to set goals for themselves, persist longer when challenged, and remain resilient to failures.

Bandura identifies four sources of self-efficacy: mastery, modeling, social persuasion, and somatic/emotional states. **Mastery** is the strongest and most enduring source of self-efficacy. When individuals experience success, this leads to a positive belief about one's own skills and abilities. In contrast, failure can undermine self-efficacy. **Modeling** is another source of self-efficacy; however, all role models are not equally influential. People are more likely to be motivated by other individuals who are seen as similar to oneself. For example, a new mom who expresses a desire to exercise is less likely to be inspired by an elite athlete describing the joys of long-distance running, but might respond to a neighbor with young children who asks the new mom to join her morning walks.

Social persuasion refers to verbal encouragement. Although social persuasion tends to be a weaker source of self-efficacy, negative feedback in the form of harsh criticism or disapproval can serve to break down a person's beliefs in capability. Finally, **somatic/emotional states**, or the physical and emotional response to an activity, can either encourage or dishearten an individual. For example, extreme anxiety related to speaking in front of a group may cause even a strong public speaker to avoid this situation. One reason some people shun exercise is because they dislike the feelings of physical exertion and sweating, but the person who feels exhilarated when exercising is more likely to continue the activity.

Addressing Self-Efficacy

When individuals are reluctant to try a new task or give up easily when challenged, they may lack self-efficacy. Occupational therapists can promote self-efficacy by using the four sources and creating situations that promote beliefs related to capability. Table 23-1 provides specific examples.

Table 23-1 ● Examples of Addressing Sources of Self-Efficacy

Source of Self-Efficacy	Examples of Intervention
Mastery	• Create opportunities for successful experiences. • Break down tasks into achievable components.
Modeling	• Identify role models who are similar to the person. • Make available opportunities for modeling to occur.
Social persuasion	• Provide strong encouragement. • Impart feedback that is specific and genuine. • Withhold harsh criticism.
Somatic/emotional states	• Reduce anxiety. • Teach relaxation techniques. • Assist with reinterpretation of negative emotional states (e.g., soreness that comes from exercise can be interpreted as progress).

Culture and Self-Efficacy

Self-efficacy is not solely an individualistic notion. Bandura (2002) discusses three types of agency, or ways in which people meet goals: personal agency, proxy agency, and collective agency. **Personal agency** is exercised individually, as when a person joins a gym after making a New Year's resolution to lose weight and designs a schedule to exercise independently three times a week. **Proxy agency** is when the individual influences others to act on his or her behalf. Hiring a personal trainer would be an example of proxy agency because the individual is using the trainer for motivation. **Collective agency** is when people work together to shape their future. For example, everyone in a work site might agree to go for a walk together over the lunch hour three times a week. Self-efficacy is required for both personal and collective agencies. In collective agency, the individual must believe that he or she can work with others and contribute to the collective. People often use proxy agency when concerned about their own self-efficacy.

The pursuit of goals and the type of agency exercised occurs within a cultural context (Bandura, 2002). Very generally speaking, Western cultures are more individualistic, and Eastern cultures are more collective. However, much heterogeneity exists; some individuals from Western cultures have collective natures, whereas some individuals in Asian cultures are more individualistic. Therefore, it is important to avoid stereotyping individuals and to, instead, assess the unique nature of each person.

Furthermore, there are differences in collectivism, for example, in China and India, and even regional differences in individualism in the Northeast and Midwest regions of the United States. Nevertheless, occupational therapists can provide more effective interventions when they consider the propensity of the individual, that is, identifying whether the person has a cultural value for personal or collective agency.

Self-Determination Theory

Self-determination theory describes the dimensions of extrinsic and intrinsic motivation, as well as the conditions that support the more adaptive intrinsic motivation (Ryan & Deci, 2000). **Intrinsic motivation** is an innate tendency to seek novelty and strive for challenge and mastery. For example, the enjoyment that is derived from participating in a desired leisure activity is fueled by intrinsic motivation. **Extrinsic motivation** involves performance to obtain some outcome that is separate from the inherent satisfaction of the activity itself. A person who dislikes his or her work may only be motivated to stay at the job because of the extrinsic reward of good pay.

Ryan and Deci (2000) assert that intrinsic motivation is an innate human characteristic, however, maintaining and enhancing intrinsic motivation requires supportive conditions. These conditions are based on three fundamental psychological needs: competence, autonomy, and relatedness. Feelings of **competence** regarding a particular activity can enhance intrinsic motivation for that activity. Competence is analogous to self-efficacy, which is described previously. Positive feedback, the absence of criticism, and optimal challenge are all conducive to the development of feelings of competence.

Autonomy involves circumstances that promote individual action and decision. Autonomy, and thereby intrinsic motivation, is supported when there are opportunities for choice and self-direction. Furthermore, the acknowledgment of feelings reinforces autonomy. Controlling environments with deadlines, threats, and pressure is the antithesis of autonomy.

Finally, **relatedness** facilitates intrinsic motivation. When individuals feel secure in their relationships and connected to others, intrinsic motivation can flourish. It is important to note that, although competence, autonomy, and relatedness create supportive environments, the activity itself must be inherently enjoyable for intrinsic motivation to exist at all.

Although intrinsic motivation is desirable, most of what we do (particularly as adults) is motivated, at least to some extent, by extrinsic factors. One purpose of self-determination theory is to describe the differing degrees to which an extrinsically motivated activity can be autonomous because autonomous regulation leads to better performance and greater levels of persistence, creativity, self-esteem, and general well-being. **Self-regulation** is the mechanism that affects the degree of autonomy. There are four levels of self-regulation, from least to most autonomous (Table 23-2):

1. External regulation
2. Introjected regulation
3. Regulation through identification
4. Integrated regulation

The absence or lack of self-regulation can be manifested as procrastination. Procrastination is characterized by discounting the value of the long-term rewards and paying attention to the more immediately available rewards. One review of procrastination found that individuals are more likely to procrastinate when they find the task aversive or when they lack self-efficacy regarding the task (Steel, 2007). Personality characteristics are associated with procrastination, with impulsiveness leading to more procrastination and conscientiousness leading to less.

Occupational therapists are often interested in helping individuals become more motivated to engage in occupation. Everything we do requires some level of motivation. As therapists, we can promote self-regulation using the same factors that support intrinsic motivation: competence, autonomy, and relatedness. Poulson, Rodger, and Ziviani (2006) described how self-determination theory could be applied to a specific occupational therapy intervention for children, cognitive orientation to daily occupational performance (CO-OP). The child sets the goals (autonomy), the process of checking is used to promote successful performance of an activity (competence), and the intervention uses socializing agents, such as parents, teachers, and peers to enhance motivation (relatedness). Table 23-3 shows ways in which occupational therapists can create autonomy, competence, and relatedness.

Table 23-2 ● **Self-Regulation of Motivation**

	Type of Regulation	Source of Motivation	Examples
Most to least autonomous	External regulation	External rewards and punishment	• Doing a job just for the paycheck. • Driving the speed limit.
	Introjected regulation	Avoidance of guilt and anxiety or to enhance self-esteem	• Flossing your teeth regularly for 1 week before a scheduled dental check-up. • Wearing uncomfortable but attractive clothing for an important presentation.
	Regulation through identification	Activity is consciously and personally valued	• Attending your child's college graduation ceremony.
	Integrated regulation	Fully internalized to the self, but done for reasons outside inherent enjoyment	• Studying for the National Board for Certification in Occupational Therapy (NBCOT) exam to become a registered occupational therapist.

Table 23-3 ● **Strategies for Enhancing Self-Regulation**

Conditions That Support Intrinsic Motivation	Examples of Occupational Therapy Strategies
Competence	• Create opportunities for mastery. • Provide positive feedback that matches the accomplishment.
Autonomy	• Give choices. • Use client-centered practices so that the client is the primary decision maker and participates in all phases of the therapy process.
Relatedness	• Use group interventions. • Engage family members and friends in the therapy process.

Flow Theory

The concept of "flow" as a subjective experience was coined by the psychologist Csikszentmihalyi (2000). **Flow** is the experience of participation in an activity that is so intrinsically rewarding that the person loses him- or herself in the process. A basketball player having an incredible game, a day of practice when the pianist finds the piece coming together, and the occupational therapist connecting deeply with a client—all of these examples might be experienced as flow. Nakamura and Csikszentmihalyi (2002) describe the characteristics of flow as follows:

- State of intense and focused concentration on the activity
- Merging of action and awareness (i.e., the person does not have to think about what he or she is doing, but at the same time the person is intensely alert to what he or she is doing)
- Loss of self-consciousness (i.e., the person does not worry about being watched or judged by others)
- Deep sense of control
- Distortion in time (i.e., the individual loses all track of time, and hours seem like minutes)
- Absence of anxiety
- Activity is fully perceived as motivating in and of itself

Although the flow experience is intensely intrinsic, all intrinsically motivating activities do not result in flow. For example, a mother may be intrinsically motivated to feed her picky and trying toddler, and although the experience includes rewards and pleasures, it is not one in which the mother feels a great deal of control, she does not lose herself in the task, and minutes seem like hours instead of vice versa.

In flow theory, a particular compatibility must exist between the person and the activity; the activity must be challenging enough to illicit an internal feeling of satisfaction, but not so challenging that the individual fails. It requires just the right fit of skills from the person and challenge of the activity and the environment. It is very much a person-environment-occupation theory.

Occupational therapists can help promote flow for our clients. By knowing the skills of the person and applying the process of task analysis, an occupational therapist can find that "just right" challenge. In many cases, occupational therapists work with individuals who, because of a disability or illness, have lost the opportunity to engage in occupations that previously provided the feeling of flow. By completing an occupational profile, the occupational therapist can identify those valued occupations and then work to enhance the person's abilities, adapt the task, or modify the environment so that the individual can once again return to that occupation.

In other cases, the individual may need to identify alternative activities to meet that need. For example, a previous scratch golfer may be able to return to the activity, but no longer experiences flow because of a loss of sensorimotor abilities. An alternate leisure activity may need to be substituted.

Transtheoretical Model

The transtheoretical model (Prochaska, DiClemente, & Norcross, 1992) is a widely used theory of behavioral change. A major concept of the model is a description of the stages of change, which can be used to explain how people can begin a new behavior, such as exercising, and end an undesirable behavior, such as cigarette smoking. The five stages are precontemplation, contemplation, preparation, action, and maintenance. Instead of a linear model, the transtheoretical model is cyclical, recognizing that relapse can occur, but the person can then reengage in the change process (Fig. 23-2).

In **precontemplation**, the individual is not thinking about or intending to make a change in the near future. **Contemplation** is when the person starts thinking about the problem or concern, weighing the pros and cons of changing. Ambivalence toward change is a primary characteristic of this stage. The next stage is **preparation**, during which the person recognizes that the pros outweigh the cons in terms of changing. This stage involves planning for the change. In most cases, one can take multiple paths, so this phase involves the person weighing the options but not necessarily committing to the plan. The **action** phase is when the person actually makes the change. Action is still a fragile phase, and relapse is likely to occur. **Maintenance** comes into play when the person has maintained the behavioral change for at least 6 months. Generally, at this point, the behavior is easier to manage; although relapse can occur, it is less likely than in the action phase.

Attention to relapse is an important component of the transtheoretical model. Relapse is not seen as a failure, but a common part of the process. However, the person can more quickly reengage in the change process if he or she has already been through it before. Many changes in behavior take more than one trial. For example, people who successfully quit smoking usually attempt to quit several times before they are successful. In addition, the model is not meant to be unidirectional; that is, people generally move back and forth, perhaps contemplating a change, making a plan, and then going back to not thinking about the issue at all.

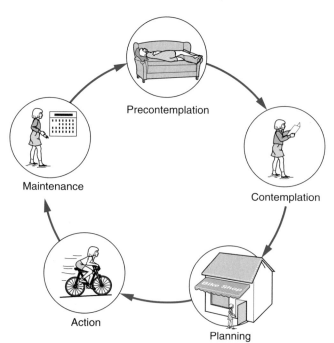

FIGURE 23-2. Stages of change process applied to increasing physical activity.

Some evidence suggests that the stages of change model does not adequately explain the complexity of the change process (Migneault, Adams, & Read, 2005; Spencer, Adams, Malone, Roy, & Yost, 2006). Research thus far indicates better evidence for the descriptive validity of the model, meaning that it can be helpful in describing the current stage of a person. There is less evidence to support the predictive ability of the model (e.g., whether the person will respond to an intervention, or which stage he or she will enter next). However, the model has been extremely useful in designing interventions to promote behavioral changes, particularly in helping people progress through the earlier stages of change. The old wisdom that a person will not change until he or she is ready to change is challenged by this model.

Most occupational therapy intervention targets people at the action stage. However, the stages of change model is useful in guiding occupational therapists and other practitioners to find strategies to help people move toward change, regardless of where they are in the stage process. Perhaps the strongest and most compelling argument of the model is that practitioners should not give up on people who have yet to make it to the action level. Table 23-4 identifies intervention strategies that target each stage of change.

Model of Human Occupation

The Model of Human Occupation (Kielhofner, 2008) is an occupational therapy model that explicitly addresses motivation. The model uses **dynamic systems theory** to explain the relationships between major concepts in the theory. In a dynamic system, all components are interrelated; if there is a change in one aspect of the system, the other components are affected.

Kielhofner (2008) identifies three person elements, or subsystems, that are interrelated: performance habituation, and volition. The **performance** comprises the mental and physical constituents (e.g., bones, muscles, nervous ystem) that provide the capacity for the person to engage in occupational performance. The **habituation subsystem** gives structure and routine to daily life. The habituation system comes into play during most activities of daily living. The execution of the activity, such as toothbrushing, is so familiar and practiced that the individual engages in the activity with little conscious effort. It is the **volitional subsystem** that is most relevant to this chapter. Volition provides motivation for occupation. Volition influences both our choice of occupation and our persistence when engaging in that occupation.

The volitional system is further divided into three components that affect motivation: interest, values, and personal causation (Kielhofner, 2008). **Interests** are those things that give pleasure and satisfaction. Certainly you have noticed that some activities have appeal to you, whereas others do not. In addition, there is individual variation in terms of how you perform these activities. For example, two people may enjoy eating out, but have very different ideas about the type of restaurant they prefer.

Values shape beliefs about what is important and worthy. There are many different sources of motivation, such as the opportunity to be with others you like, the creation of an end product, and the positive feelings associated with achievement. Interests are not the only factor that affects motivation. There are many activities that you may not find particularly pleasurable, but you still engage in them because of your values. Values are derived from the social and cultural environment, and represent what you think is important and meaningful. Doing the laundry could be an example for many. The activity is not pleasurable, but you value cleanliness of appearance.

Finally, **personal causation** as a contributor to motivation is closely linked to self-efficacy. You may have noticed by now that many of the motivation theories incorporate self-efficacy. Personal causation involves your personal assessment of abilities. You are more likely to engage in activities in which you expect success and avoid those in which you expect failure. Personal causation is also increased when you feel in control of the situation.

The Model of Human Occupation could be applied to an employment situation. Individuals with serious mental illness have high rates of unemployment, and the volitional subsystem should be addressed when supporting an

Table 23-4 ● Stages of Change Strategies to Promote Change	
Stage of Change	**Strategy**
Precontemplation	• Provide gentle encouragement and information. • Avoid lecturing and intensive approaches. • Express belief in the person's ability to make a change.
Contemplation	• Help person weigh the pros and cons for changing and elicit reasons that promote change (decisional balance). • Provide feedback to resolve person's ambivalence.
Preparation	• Help person make a realistic assessment of the difficulties related to making a change. • Provide options for ways to go about change. • Help person think creatively about the most effective plan.
Action	• Provide support for behavior. • Listen and affirm that person is doing the right thing. • Help person make changes in plan if having difficulties (i.e., build self-efficacy).
Maintenance	• Continue to provide support. • Recognize that people need time to make long-term changes. • Be prepared for the possibility of relapse. • If relapse occurs, help person reenter the change process.

Adapted with permission from Miller, W. R., & Rollnick, S. (2002). Motivational Interviewing: Preparing People for Change (2nd ed.). New York: Guilford Press.

individual to enter the workforce. Finding a job that matches the individual's interests is more likely to lead to success than one in which the individual is bored or detached. Values surrounding work should be explored so that the work situation is one that promotes those values. Different values surrounding work might include being productive, having a place to belong, contributing to others, developing an identity as a worker, and achieving financial independence. Finally, the person will need to believe that he or she can be successful. Creating a supportive work environment with reasonable accommodations can increase the likelihood that the individual will feel competent at work.

Motivation and Psychiatric Disabilities

Impairments in motivation or drives that are directed at self-destructive behaviors are common in many psychiatric disabilities. This section reviews those psychiatric disabilities in which a disturbance in motivation is a common characteristic, including schizophrenia, attention deficit-hyperactivity disorder, mood disorders, substance abuse, and developmental disabilities.

Occupational therapists need to be aware of the motivation dysfunction component of these particular psychiatric disabilities so that challenges in occupational performance are not misinterpreted. Much of the research into motivation and psychiatric disabilities has focused on reward sensitivity, with some literature examining success experiences and environmental factors. Although the research is just beginning, there appears to be a complex relationship between biological vulnerabilities and environmental influences that contributes to motivational dysfunction.

Schizophrenia

Impairment in volition is a core feature of schizophrenia. The Scale for the Assessment of Negative Symptoms, which is a measure used for determining degree of symptomatology in schizophrenia, lists **avolition** as one of five negative symptoms (Andreasen, 1984). On this particular scale, avolition includes lack of attention to grooming and hygiene, difficulty persisting at work or school activities, and physical inertia.

From a biological perspective, a disturbance in drive may be associated with the dysfunctional dopamine system in schizophrenia (Barch, 2005). The dopamine system is important in terms of "wanting" and working toward a desired goal. Furthermore, the dopamine system may be necessary for predicting rewards and learning from mistakes, a weakness that is common in schizophrenia.

A qualitative study (Boydell, Gladstone, & Volpe, 2003) involving interviews of six individuals with schizophrenia suggested other causes for motivational impairments. Five underlying causes were identified from these narratives. First, the experience of having a disabling condition made it difficult to be motivated. Specifically, hallucinations and delusions interfered with concentration, and secondary depression led to withdrawal. The sedating effects of medications were another cause of motivational issues. Spirit breaking by others was also associated with poor motivation.

Participants reported specific situations in which other people told them they would not be able to do something or made general comments about people with schizophrenia being limited in their capabilities. Similarly, stigma contributed to social isolation and negative feelings about the self. Finally, participants indicated that their social withdrawal or shutting down can be a defense mechanism to deal with the challenges of daily life. The combined biological vulnerability and multiple environmental factors challenge people with schizophrenia to participate in daily life. See Chapter 14 for more information on schizophrenia.

Attention Deficit-Hyperactivity Disorder

The motivational issue in attention deficit-hyperactivity disorder (ADHD) has also been associated with a dysfunctional dopamine system, but the manifestation of the impairment is very different than in schizophrenia. Whereas people with schizophrenia are less likely to initiate action to receive rewards, children with ADHD are compelled to seek out rewards (Holroyd, Baker, Kerns, & Muller, 2008). In addition, a diminished sensitivity to reinforcement often leads children with ADHD to become dissatisfied or frustrated when engaged in an activity because they do not anticipate the reward. As a result, impulsive acts are initiated in an attempt to obtain reinforcement, but there is a lack of persistence because rewards are not received. Occupational therapists can address these concerns by creating environments that provide stronger and more salient reinforcement to children with ADHD. See Chapter 8 for more information on attention deficit-hyperactivity disorder.

Mood Disorders

As explained in the description of the approach/avoidance theory of motivation, certain tendencies are associated with particular mood disorders. Those mood disorders that are characterized as dysphoric, or negative, are linked to a higher sensitivity to avoidance (Johnson et al, 2003). Fearfulness can also prevent an individual from engaging in activities. In contrast, mania is associated with a high sensitivity to approach behaviors (Bjorn, Rahman, & Shepherd, 2007), which may account for the impulsiveness and engagement in high-risk activities (e.g., substance use, excessive spending, promiscuity) that often accompany manic episodes.

Anhedonia, the inability to experience pleasure, is a core symptom of depression. Studies of anhedonia in depression suggest that these individuals are less responsive to pleasurable stimuli and have difficulty integrating rewards (Pizzagalli, Iosifescu, Hallet, Ratner, & Fava, 2008). As a result, individuals who are depressed lack the responses that lead to intrinsic motivation and, consequently, find it difficult to engage and persist in goal-directed activity. See Chapter 12 for more information on mood disorders.

Substance Abuse

The motivation to use substances in a self-destructive manner is also associated with reward sensitivities. In a study of adolescents, there was an association between high reward sensitivity, low punishment sensitivity, and substance abuse (Genovese & Wallace, 2007). This suggests that adolescents

The Lived Experience

Lee Beers

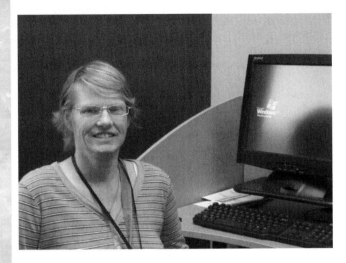

Lee describes the motivations and experiences associated with trying to lose weight. When reading this piece, attend to the internal, interpersonal, and spiritual motivators that contributed to her success story.

I was healthy as a child. I went to the Junior Olympics in the 600-yard dash and got a bronze medal. When I got older and almost died, I said, "This is for the birds and wanted to be healthy again." I had never been so heavy and sick. The grossness of it motivated me to get rid of my extra weight.

In 2007, at the Wyandot Mental Health Center, I worked for the diet-exercise (RENEW: Recovering Energy through Nutrition and Exercise for Weight Loss) program of Kansas University. Five years before, I was in the same program and, because of my success, I was asked to work as a peer mentor in the RENEW program. When I started the program, I weighed 289 pounds, had diabetes, and ended up with congestive heart failure. On the program, I lost 125 pounds. Over the past 5 years, I maintained at about 170 pounds. I hit a plateau at 170 when I went into the program again this time.

It took determination and dedication and help from the program with the diet (eating right and the right foods) and exercise. This time, while working as a peer mentor, I lost 22 pounds, now weighing 148. My doctor's recommendation was 146 pounds. I'm only 2 pounds away from my ideal weight. With the help of this program, my life was saved. Free food, great advice, great teaching, in-depth material, and humor, all this came from the program. I am grateful to Jesus for the program leaders, and I hope they will continue to help others for a long time.

I believe in the *Bible*; it is my greatest possession. I wanted to find a *Bible* verse that would say what the program is about: "Bear one another's burdens and so fulfill the law of Christ. Therefore as we have the opportunity, let us do good to all, especially to those who are of the household of faith" (Galatians 6:2).

Personally, I have made two good friends out of this program, and we help each other and support each other. We bear each other's burdens.

---

who are more susceptible to substance abuse have a greater response to the reward or pleasure of substance abuse and are less fearful or concerned about the negative consequences of substance use. Intervention models that promote natural and severe consequences for substance abuse are consistent with these findings.

A conventional wisdom regarding substance abuse is that the person must "hit bottom" before successfully engaging in treatment, the theory being that the person must be in an intolerable situation before he or she will be motivated enough to really make a change. However, this premise has been challenged by research. In fact, extreme depression, anger, and anxiety in people who abuse substances seem to interfere with engagement in treatment (Field, Duncan, Washington, & Adinoff, 2007). The transtheoretical model (Prochaska & DiClemente, 1982), including the stages of change, as discussed previously, provides guidance for occupational therapists to elicit the behavioral change for substance abusers. See Chapter 15 for more information on substance abuse.

Intellectual Disabilities

Self-efficacy, as a core element of motivation, has been studied in children with intellectual disabilities. Infants and very young children with intellectual disabilities appear to pursue

activities with the same sense of mastery motivation (Nichols, Atkinson, & Pepler, 2003). However, as children with these disabilities get older, there is a greater difference in their level of mastery motivation and the mastery of peers the same age. As the tasks become more complex, children with developmental disabilities are likely to have more and more

---

Evidence-Based Practice

A review of evidence-based interventions for substance abuse and the implications for occupational therapy indicates that strategies used to support an individual who is progressing through the stages of change may be most effective at the early stages. Individuals may need a combined approach at later stages, such as the addition of cognitive behavioral therapy.

➤ Occupational therapists should evaluate the individual's readiness to change to identify motivational change strategies.

➤ Occupational therapists should consider the addition of cognitive behavioral approaches to augment motivational interviewing during later stages of change.

Stoffel, V. C., & Moyers, P. A. (2004). An evidence based and occupational perspective of intervention for persons with substance-use disorders. *American Journal of Occupational Therapy, 58*, 570–586.

failure experiences. As children with intellectual disabilities get older, they express more frustration and less persistence in goal-oriented activity. Occupational therapists can help reduce the deficits in mastery motivation by modifying tasks so that children with disabilities can experience success and competence. See Chapter 9 for more information on intellectual disabilities.

Assessments

Even though motivation can seem like a fairly intangible concept, several standardized measures have been developed to assess motivation. Many of the measures are associated with a particular motivational theory.

BIS/BAS Scales

Carver and White (1994) developed the BIS/BAS scales to measure the two motivational systems described in Gray's (1991) theory of motivation. This brief self-reported measure uses a 4-point Likert scale, with 1 indicating *very true for me* and 4 indicating *very false for me*. The measure includes one BIS scale, which is described as a measure of punishment sensitivity. There are three BAS subscales: drive, fun seeking, and reward responsiveness. In validity studies, the measure tended to be better at discriminating BIS/BAS behaviors than alternative personality measures (Carver & White, 1994).

Goal Attainment Scaling

A challenge for assessing occupational therapy outcomes is finding a measure that can capture the diverse nature of the targets of therapy and the intervention process itself. Goals provide a motivational target in occupational therapy intervention. Goal attainment scaling (GAS) allows for the assessment of individualized progress, regardless of the outcome. Originally developed by Kiresuk and Sherman (1968) to assess adults in community mental health, the GAS method uses a 5-point scale (−2 to +2) to assess progress toward goal attainment. Zero is the expected level of performance, with the negative numbers indicating less than expected, and the positive numbers indicating higher than expected outcomes.

GAS is consistent with client-centered practice because the therapist and client work together to identify the primary goal and then specifically identify the expected level of success. Better and worse than expected outcomes are also specified for each point on the 5-point scale. Psychometric evaluations suggest that GAS can effectively distinguish between individuals who have made progress and those who have not (Kiresuk, Smith, & Cardillo, 1994).

Interrater reliability is less than optimal when compared with standardized assessments, but the measure provides greater flexibility for measuring diverse outcomes. There is also evidence that the collaborative nature of the GAS enhances participation in the therapy process.

Recently, occupational therapists have suggested that GAS may be useful for measuring outcomes in children with sensory integration dysfunction (Mailloux et al, 2007). These therapists provide guidelines and described the particular benefits of GAS for occupational therapy when trying to capture change for outcomes that tend to be highly variable and individualized.

Leisure Motivation Scale

The Leisure Motivation scale (Beard & Ragheb, 1983) assesses motivation within an occupational performance context, which increases its relevance for occupational therapy practice. The 48-item Likert scale is composed of four subscales: Intellectual, Social, Competence Mastery, and Stimulus Avoidance. The Intellectual subscale involves motivation to participate in thinking activities. The Social subscale is focused on the drive to engage in leisure activities with others, and the Competence Mastery subscale involves those activities that provide the individual with a sense of accomplishment. The Stimulus Avoidance subscale assesses the extent to which the individual is motivated to participate in activities that allow for escape from daily stress.

Occupational therapists used the Leisure Motivation scale within a clubhouse setting to determine the relationship between leisure motivation and recovery (Lloyd, King, McCarthy, & Scanlan, 2007). The study found that individuals with higher scores on the Leisure Motivation scale had more traits associated with recovery. The researchers suggest that occupational therapists should help individuals with serious mental illness reintegrate into leisure activities, particularly those that support socialization within the community.

University of Rhode Island Change Assessment

The University of Rhode Island Change Assessment (URICA) is frequently used as a measure of an individual's readiness to change (McConnaughy, Prochaska, & Velicer, 1983). Although most often used in substance abuse research, the general nature of the questions makes it more broadly applicable. In fact, it has been used to assess change across several different psychiatric disabilities, including obsessive compulsive disorder (Pinto, Pinto, Neziroglu, & Yaryura-Tobias, 2007), schizophrenia (Kinnaman, Bellack, Brown, & Yang, 2007), posttraumatic stress disorder (Hunt, Kyle, Coffey, Stasiewicz, & Schumacher, 2006), pathological gambling (Petry, 2005), and eating disorders (Hasler, Delsignore, Milos, Buddeberg, & Schnyder, 2004).

This 32-item measure includes just four of the stages of change subscales: Precontemplation, Contemplation, Action, and Maintenance. Validity studies have not supported four separate factors, so often a single score is obtained and used as a general measure of readiness to change (Sutton, 2001). Occupational therapists can use this measure when applying the transtheoretical model of change and then target interventions based on level of readiness.

Volitional Questionnaire and Pediatric Volitional Questionnaire

The Volitional Questionnaire (Chern, Kielhofner, de las Heras, & Magalhaes, 1996) comes out of the Model of Human Occupation and assesses the person's inner motives and the environment's impact on motivation. This observational assessment for adolescents and adults rates the individual in terms of three stages of volitional development: exploration, competency, and achievement. For each item, the individual is rated as passive, hesitant, involved, or spontaneous. There is also an Environmental Form that assesses the effect of the environment on the person's motivation. There is evidence supporting the measure's interrater reliability (de las Heras, 1993) and internal consistency (Chern et al, 1996). The Pediatric Volitional Questionnaire (Andersen, Kielhofner, & Lai, 2005) is designed for children ages 2 to 7. The child is observed in several different environments. Using this measure, the occupational therapist can determine if the individual is in the exploration, competency, or achievement stage in relation to a particular occupation.

Intervention

Generally speaking, individuals are not referred for occupational therapy or other services to exclusively address motivation. However, in occupational therapy practice, motivation is often a factor that interferes with successful occupational performance. It can also interfere with engagement in the therapy process. Too often, occupational therapists stop working with a patient or client because the person refuses therapy. From a different perspective, the refusal can become the initial target of intervention. The person who refuses therapy can benefit from strategies specifically focused on enhancing motivation for therapy. Intervention strategies for motivation are typically not the sole focus of the occupational therapy process, but are used in concert with other interventions to promote some type of behavioral change or to engage the individual in therapy or a valued occupation.

Interventions Linked to Theories

Previously in the chapter, various theories of motivation were presented with their implications for occupational therapy intervention. Table 23-5 describes the relevant applications and implications for intervention associated with the particular theory.

The Remotivation Process

The remotivation process is an occupational therapy intervention that arises from the Model of Human Occupation (de las Heras, Llerena, & Kielhofner, 2003). Targeting the volitional system, it considers motivation as a continuum that moves from exploration to competency to achievement (Fig. 23-3). The Volitional Questionnaire (described in the Assessment

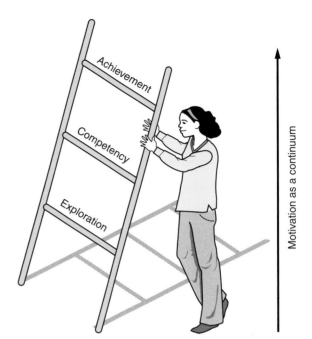

FIGURE 23-3. Remotivation process. The therapist provides activities to move the person through the different steps of the motivation process.

section) provides guidance for identifying where the individual falls on the continuum.

Once the developmental stage of motivation is identified, the therapist uses specific strategies to promote development to the next motivational level. For example, in the exploration stage, strategies include having the person engage in familiar activities in unfamiliar or new settings and exposing the individual to activities of interest. At the competency stage, the therapist helps the client identify goals, problem solve difficulties, and maintain engagement over time. To facilitate achievement, strategies include encouraging the individual to look for new challenges, take risks, and assume additional responsibilities. A manual is available from the Model of Human Occupation Clearinghouse (see the Resources section) that describes specific goals for the client at each stage and strategies for the therapist.

PhotoVoice

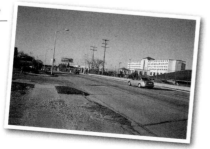

This is a picture of the West Allis skyline. The hustle and bustle of everyday life. Get out and get in the world. Being out stimulates and keeps our minds occupied so we don't focus on our mental illness so much. It's just one of the milestones in life, on our journey through life.

Evidence-Based Practice

In a study conducted by occupational therapists, individuals with serious mental illness who had a higher motivation for leisure activities (particularly social and intellectual leisure activities) also had higher scores on a measure of recovery. These results suggest that engagement in pleasurable leisure activities can enhance recovery.

➤ Occupational therapists can help people with psychiatric disabilities identify leisure interests and then create interventions to support participation in those activities.

Lloyd, C., King, R., McCarthy, M., & Scanlan, M. (2007). The association between leisure motivation and recovery: A pilot study. *Australian Occupational Therapy Journal, 54,* 33–41.

Table 23-5 ● **Motivation Theories and Intervention Approaches**

Theory	Relevant Application of Theory	Implications for Intervention
Maslow's hierarchy of needs	• Useful in all situations to help promote highest level of accomplishment • Neglecting to address lower-level needs can sabotage all progress	• Identify lowest level of unmet need, and address this need so that individual can work toward higher-level needs. • May need to establish rapport and demonstrate that person is safe before providing therapy.
Approach/avoidance models	• Applicable to situations in which individuals are avoiding necessary activities or approaching unhealthy ones, particularly when there tends to be an emotional component associated with the approach or avoidance	• Address emotions that might interfere with goal attainment, specifically anxiety and fear. • Address impulsiveness when there is little regard for danger or negative outcomes. • Support positive emotions that promote approach behaviors. • Change emotional associations (e.g., feelings of deprivation during dieting could be reframed as a demonstration of self-control). • Consider how to incorporate rewards or remove punishments associated with the activity.
Self-efficacy	• Appropriate for situations in which client expresses a lack of self-efficacy for a particular activity	• Break down activities so the individual can have multiple successful experiences that create sense of mastery. • Incorporate role models into occupational therapy intervention; role models should share important characteristics with client. • Provide positive, specific, and sincere feedback. • Avoid criticism.
Self-determination theory	• Helpful for all situations in which motivations is a limiting factor • Helpful for assessing environmental conditions that can be modified to promote intrinsic motivation	• Create conditions that support competence, autonomy, and relatedness. • Competence can be addressed in methods discussed previously related to self-efficacy. • Autonomy involves providing opportunities for choice and creating conditions in which the individual feels in control of the situation. • Relatedness is enhanced when the individual has positive interpersonal connections associated with the activity. • Consider group activities, mentorship, and role modeling.
Flow theory	• Relevant consideration for activities that already possess a strong intrinsic motivation for the person	• Identify activities of interest to client or activities that have the potential to be intensely interesting to the individual. • Create opportunities for the "just right" fit of challenge and competence. • Help individual identify lifestyle that supports more opportunities for flow experiences.
Transtheoretical model	• Focus is on situations in which person wants or needs to change a behavior—either to stop a negative behavior or begin a positive behavior	• Identify the current stage of change for the target behavior. • Use strategies that help person move to the next level.
Model of Human Occupation	• Applicable across all situations in which motivation is a barrier to performance	• Evaluate volitional system factors (interests, values, personal causation) that are associated with the activity in question. • Target intervention at the factor that is interfering with performance (e.g., consider how to increase interest, enhance value, or develop beliefs in ability to carry out the activity).

Motivational Interviewing

Motivational interviewing is a widely used approach that the developers describe as "a way of being with people" in the change process (Miller & Rollnick, 2002). It was initially applied to substance abuse intervention (Miller et al, 2006), but since then has been broadly adopted to address many types of change. The uses are too numerous to review here, but included are examples to demonstrate the wide-ranging applications. For example, motivational interviewing has been used for adopting healthier eating practices (Resnicow et al, 2008), increasing seat belt use (Fernandez et al, 2008), enhancing treatment for obsessive compulsive disorder (Simpson, Zuckoff, Page, Franklin, & Foa, 2008), and as a component of safe sex programs (Golin et al, 2007). Motivational interviewing is designed for people who are not ready to change or are ambivalent about changing.

The fundamental approaches of motivational interviewing are collaboration, evocation, and autonomy (Miller & Rollnick, 2002). These can be contrasted with opposing approaches that are also used in alternative counseling situations. **Collaboration** means that the therapist and client work together as partners. This is in contrast to confrontation (an approach frequently used in substance abuse treatment). Confrontation can lead to defensiveness, whereas collaboration supports engagement in therapy.

Evocation means drawing on the client to identify his or her own goals and values toward change. This is different from education that focuses on providing knowledge or skills to the client.

Finally, **autonomy** means that the client has the capacity for self-direction and makes his or her own choices, as opposed to authority, in which the therapist tells the client what to do.

The development of motivational interviewing was highly influenced by the transtheoretical model, particularly the stages of change (Miller & Rollnick, 2002). Motivational interviewing recognizes that people change gradually and that the intervention process can begin at any point in the change process.

General Principles

Along with the fundamental approaches to motivational interviewing, there are four general principles that guide the interaction:

- Express empathy
- Develop discrepancy
- Roll with resistance
- Support self-efficacy

Express Empathy

In motivational interviewing, it is important that the client knows that he or she is accepted. Often, the person has done things that are not valued by society, such as using illegal substances, inadequately parenting, unhealthy living, and trouble maintaining employment. Empathy does not mean approval; rather, it involves relating to the person without judgment, criticism or blame. Skills required for expressing empathy include reflective listening and the ability to convey respect and acceptance of the person. Expressing empathy often involves relating with the client that "change is hard" and that ambivalence to change is normal.

Develop Discrepancy

Although motivational interviewing relies heavily on reflective listening, it is also highly directive. This is where the principle of developing discrepancy fits in. The purpose is to call attention to the discrepancy between the present behavior and the person's goals and values. This is not done by having the therapist identify what is good and bad about a particular behavior, but comes from having the client elucidate his or her own perspective on the topic. One strategy used to develop discrepancy is a decisional balance exercise. In **decisional balance**, a grid is used to identify the pros of cons of both changing and not changing. Table 23-6 provides an example of a decisional balance exercise related to starting to exercise. People often consider the pros and cons of changing, but an important part of the decisional balance exercise is exploring the pros and cons of not changing (i.e., what makes the person want to keep things the way they are).

Roll With Resistance

When working toward change, clients often become resistant and sometimes even argumentative. This resistance undermines the change process and gives a cue that the therapist needs to be responding differently. It is important that the therapist avoid argument and not oppose the client's resistance. Instead, when the person begins expressing reluctance to change, it is helpful to acknowledge the ambivalence. Point out that you will not force the person to do anything; it is up to the client to decide what he or she will accept and reject. In rolling with resistance, it is also helpful to bring the problem back to the person in the form of a question. You might ask, "So how would you describe the problem, and how could you make things different?" These approaches can dispel defensiveness and reengage the person in the process.

Support Self-Efficacy

As identified in the Theories of Motivation section, self-efficacy is necessary for a person to believe that he or she can make a change. An individual can fully value the reasons for change, but if that person does not have self-efficacy, it is unlikely that a change will be attempted. One way to support self-efficacy as a therapist is to express your belief that the client can be successful. It is also important to explain to the client that he or she must make the change; the therapist cannot make the change for the client, but is there to help. The therapist can help the person identify past successes and individual strengths.

Application

There is extensive evidence indicating that motivational interviewing is effective for individuals with substance abuse (Miller & Rollnick, 1982). Stoffel and Moyers (2004) provide specific information on the role of occupational therapy and motivational interviewing with this population. However, motivational interviewing can be used across all occupational therapy practice settings and situations. It is a "way of being" with the person that addresses ambivalence toward change. Motivational interviewing is intended to be used alongside other intervention approaches. It is a tool the occupational therapist should consider whenever the client is reluctant to engage in the occupational therapy process or when the person has disengaged from life.

Summary

In occupational therapy practice, motivation is frequently talked about, but most often in terms of a client who is "unmotivated." In fact, lack of motivation, manifested as refusal of therapy, is a frequent cause for discharge from occupational therapy services. However, rarely is motivation evaluated, and seldom is motivation the target of occupational therapy intervention. This chapter attempts to alleviate this omission. The next time you find yourself describing a client as unmotivated, use the motivational theories in the chapter to help you better understand the underlying causes. Consider using the assessment tools and intervention approaches. By understanding and connecting with the client, you can increase the probability of engaging the person in occupational therapy and in life.

Table 23-6 ● **Decisional Balance Grid—Starting to Exercise**

	Changing	Not Changing
Pros	• Feel better • More energy • Lose weight • Good role model for children	• Have more time • Can keep my routine • Does not cost anything
Cons	• Worried that I cannot stick with it and will feel even worse • Family not interested in exercising with me	• Feel like a loser • May have long-term health problems • Gain more weight

Active Learning Strategies

1. Applying Motivation Theories

Identify an occupation that you engage in regularly and that gives you pleasure. Describe the activity. How often do you participate in it? How long have you been doing it? Is it something you do alone or with others?

Consider the different theories of motivation and how they might apply to your motivation to participate in this occupation.

Reflective Journal

Describe the exercise in your Reflective Journal.

Reflective Questions

- Maslow's hierarchy of needs—Which type of need is met by this occupation? Have there been occasions when you could not participate in the occupation because you had to meet lower-level needs?
- Approach/avoidance—What causes you to approach this occupation? What rewards, positive experiences, or pleasant emotions do you receive from participating in the occupation?
- Self-efficacy—Do you feel skillful/competent when performing this occupation? How did you learn to do this occupation?
- Self-determination—Does the occupation promote competence (self-efficacy), autonomy (you are in control), and relatedness (connection to others)?
- Flow—Is this a flow experience (i.e., do you lose yourself in the occupation?, lose track of time?, feel the "just right" challenge?)?

- Transtheoretical—Where are you in terms of your level of change, are their times when you have been less action oriented?
- Model of Human Occupation—Is this occupation a reflection of your interests, values, and competence?

2. Decisional Balance

Think of a behavior you would like to change, either something you want to stop doing (e.g., smoking, biting fingernails, gossiping) or something you want to start doing (e.g., exercise, getting more sleep, spending more time with family). Complete the decisional balance grid.

	Changing	Not Changing
Pros		
Cons		

Reflective Journal

Describe the exercise in your Reflective Journal.

Reflective Questions

- Which quadrants were the easiest to fill out?
- How could you enhance the pros of changing and cons of not changing?
- Can you use the motivational theories to help you make the change?
- What strategies could you use to get the change process going?

Resources

- BIS/BAS scales—The BIS/BAS scales are available online from the developer, Charles Carver, at the University of Miami website. The website also includes the items and instructions for scoring: www.psy.miami.edu/faculty/ccarver/
- Flow theory—Csikszentmihalyi, M. (2000). *Beyond Boredom and Anxiety: Experiencing Flow in Work and Play.* San Francisco, Jossey-Bass.
- Model of Human Occupation—Assessments (e.g., Volitional Assessments) and interventions associated with the Model of Human Occupation (e.g., Remotivation Process) can be obtained at the Model of Human Occupation Clearinghouse. The website also provides a reference list of publications: www.moho.uic.edu/
- Motivational interviewing—The Center on Alcoholism, Substance Abuse and Addictions includes information from William R. Miller on motivational interviewing and free downloads for many assessments: http://casaa.unm.edu/miller.html
Miller, W. R., & Rollnick, S. (2002). *Motivational Interviewing: Preparing People for Change* (2nd ed.). New York: Guilford Press.
- Self-efficacy theory—Website with Albert Bandura's biography and access to publications and videos: www.des.emory.edu/mfp/bandurabio.html
- Self-determination theory—Information, publications, and resources, including assessments related to self-determination theory: www.psych.rochester.edu/SDT/

- Transtheoretical stages of change model—The Health and Addictive Behaviors: Investigating Transtheoretical Solutions (HABITS) website includes information about the model and measures, including the University of Rhode Island Change Assessment (URICA) and the Decisional Balance scales: www.umbc.edu/psyc/habits/

References

Andersen, S., Kielhofner, G., & Lai, J. S. (2005). An examination of the measurement properties of the Pediatric Volitional Questionnaire. *Physical and Occupational Therapy in Pediatrics, 25,* 39–57.

Andreasen, N. C. (1984). *Scale for the Assessment of Negative Symptoms.* Iowa City: University of Iowa.

Bandura, A. (1999). Self-efficacy: Toward a unifying theory of behavioral change. In R. F. Baumeister (Ed.), *The Self in Social Psychology* (pp. 285–298). New York: Psychology Press.

Bandura, A. (2002). Social cognition theory in cultural context. *Applied Psychology: An International Review, 51,* 269–290.

Barch, D. M. (2005). The relationships among cognition, motivation, and emotion in schizophrenia: How much and how little we know. *Schizophrenia Bulletin, 31,* 875–881.

Beard, J., & Ragheb, M. (1983). Measuring leisure motivation. *Journal of Leisure Research, 15,* 219–228.

Bjorn, M., Rahman, R., & Shepherd, R. (2007). Hypomanic personality features and addictive tendencies. *Personality and Individual Differences, 42,* 801–810.

Boydell, K. M., Gladstone, B. M., & Volpe, T. (2003). Interpreting narratives of motivation and schizophrenia: A biopsychosocial perspective. *Psychiatric Rehabilitation Journal, 26,* 422–426.

Bragg, R. (1995). All she has, $150,000, is going to a university. *New York Times,* August 13.

Carver, C. S., & White, T. L. (1994). Behavioral inhibition, behavioral activation, and affective responses to impending reward and punishment: The BIS/BAS scales. *Journal of Personality and Social Psychology, 67,* 319–333.

Chern, J., Kielhofner, G., de las Heras, C., & Magalhaes, L. (1996). The volitional questionnaire: Psychometric development and practical use. *American Journal of Occupational Therapy, 50,* 516–525.

Csikszentmihalyi, M. (2000). *Beyond Boredom and Anxiety: Experiencing Flow in Work and Play.* San Francisco: Jossey-Bass.

de las Heras, C. G. (1993). *Validity and reliability of the Volitional Questionnaire.* Unpublished master's thesis. Tufts University: Boston, MA.

de las Heras, C. G., Llerena, V., & Kielhofner, G. (2003). *The Remotivation Process, Version 1.0.* Chicago: Model of Human Occupation Clearinghouse.

Diaz, A., & Pickering, A. D. (1993). The relationship between Gray's and Eysenck's personality spaces. *Personality and Individual Differences, 14,* 297–305.

Elliot, A. J., & Thrash, T. M. (2002). Approach-avoidance motivation in personality: Approach and avoidance temperaments and goals. *Journal of Personality and Social Psychology, 82,* 804–818.

Fernandez, W. G., Mitchell, P. M., Jamanka, A. S., Winter, M. R., Bullock, H., Donovan, J., George, J. S., Gallagher, S. S., McKay, M. P., Bernstein, E., & Colton, T. (2008). Brief motivational intervention to increase self-reported safety belt use among emergency department patients. *Academic and Emergency Medicine, 15,* 419–425.

Field, C. A., Duncan, J., Washington, K., & Adinoff, B. (2007). Association of baseline characteristics and motivation to change among patients seeking treatment for substance dependence. *Drug and Alcohol Dependence, 91,* 77–84.

Genovese, J. E., & Wallace, D. (2007). Reward sensitivity and substance abuse in middle school and high school students. *Journal of Genetic Psychology, 168,* 465–469.

Golin, C. E., Patel, S., Tiller, K., Quinlivan, E. B., Grodensky, C. A., & Boland, M. (2007). Start talking about risks: Development of a motivational interviewing–based safer sex program for people living with HIV. *AIDS Behavior, 11*(5 suppl), S72–S83.

Gray, J. A. (1991). The neuropsychology of temperament. In J. Strelau & A. Angleitner (Eds.), *Explorations in Temperament: International Perspectives on Theory and Measurement* (pp. 105–128). New York: Plenum Press.

Hasler, G., Delsignore, A., Milos, G., Buddeberg, C., & Schnyder, U. (2004). Application of Prochaska's transtheoretical model of change to patients with eating disorders. *Journal of Psychosomatic Research, 57,* 67–72.

Holroyd, C. B., Baker, T. E., Kerns, K. A., & Muller, U. (2008). Electrophysiological evidence of atypical motivation and reward processing in children with attention deficit hyperactivity disorder. *Neuropsychologia, 46,* 2234–2242.

Hunt, Y. M., Kyle, T. L., Coffey, S. F., Stasiewicz, P. R., & Schumacher, J. A. (2006). University of Rhode Island Change Assessment-Trauma: Preliminary psychometric properties in an alcohol-dependent PTSD sample. *Journal of Trauma and Stress, 19,* 915–921.

Johnson, S. L., Turner, R. J., & Iwata, N. (2003). BIS/BAS levels and psychiatric disorder: An epidemiological study. *Journal of Psychopathology and Behavior Assessment, 25,* 25–36.

Kielhofner, G. (2008). *Model of human occupation: Theory and application.* (4th ed). Baltimore, MD: Lippincott, William and Wilkins.

Kinnaman, J. E., Bellack, A. S., Brown, C. H., & Yang, Y. (2007). Assessment of motivation to change substance use in dually-diagnosed schizophrenia patients. *Addictive Behavior, 32,* 1798–1813.

Kiresuk, T. J., & Sherman, R. E. (1968). Goal attainment scaling: A general method for evaluating community mental health programs. *Community Mental Health Journal, 4,* 443–453.

Kiresuk, T. J., Smith, A., & Cardillo, J. E. (1994). *Goal Attainment Scaling: Applications, Theory and Measurement.* Hillsdale, NJ: Erlbaum.

Lloyd, C., King, R., McCarthy, M., & Scanlan, M. (2007). The association between leisure motivation and recovery: A pilot study. *Australian Occupational Therapy Journal, 54,* 33–41.

Mailloux, Z., May-Benson, T. A., Summers, C. A., Miller, L. J., Brett-Green, B., Burke, J. P., Cohn, E. S., Koomar, J. A., Parham, L. D., Roley, S. S., Schaaf, R. C., & Schoen, S. A. (2007). The issue is—Goal attainment scaling as a measure of meaningful outcomes for children with sensory integration disorders. *American Journal of Occupational Therapy, 61,* 254–259.

Maslow, A. H. (1943). A theory of human motivation. *Psychological Review, 50,* 370–396.

McConnaughy, E. A., Prochaska, J. O., & Velicer, W. F. (1983). Stages of change in psychotherapy: Measurement and sample profiles. *Psychotherapy: Theory Research, and Practice, 20,* 368–375.

Migneault, J. P., Adams, T. B., & Read, J. P. (2005). Application of the transtheoretical model to substance abuse: Historical development and future directions. *Drug and Alcohol Review, 24,* 437–448.

Miller, W. R., Baca, C., Compton, W. M., Ernst, D., Manuel, J. K., Pringle, B., Schermer, C. R., Weiss, R. D., Willenbring, M. L., & Zweben, A. (2006). Addressing substance abuse in health care settings. *Alcohol Clinical and Experimental Research, 30,* 292–302.

Miller, W. R., & Rollnick, S. (2002). *Motivational Interviewing: Preparing People for Change* (2nd ed.). New York: Guilford Press.

Nakamura, J., & Csikszentmihalyi, M. (2002). The concept of flow. In C. R. Snyder & S. J. Lopez (Eds.), *Handbook of Positive Psychology* (pp. 89–105). Oxford, UK: Oxford University Press.

Nichols, A., Atkinson, L., & Pepler, D. (2003). Mastery motivation in young children with Down's syndrome: Relations with cognitive and adaptive competence. *Journal of Intellectual Disability Research, 47,* 121–135.

Peloquin, S. M. (2005). The 2005 Eleanor Clarke Slagle Lecture—Embracing our ethos, reclaiming our heart. *American Journal of Occupational Therapy, 59,* 611–625.

Petry, N. M. (2005). Stages of change in treatment-seeking pathological gamblers. *Journal of Consulting and Clinical Psychology, 73,* 312–322.

Pinto, A., Pinto, A. M., Neziroglu, F., & Yaryura-Tobias, J. A. (2007). Motivation to change as a predictor of treatment response in obsessive compulsive disorder. *Annals of Clinical Psychiatry, 19*(2), 83–87.

Pizzagalli, D. A., Iosifescu, D., Hallet, L. A., Ratner, K. G., & Fava, M. (2008). Reduced hedonic capacity in major depressive disorder: Evidence from a probabilistic reward task. *Journal of Psychiatry Research, 43,* 76–87.

Poulson, A. A., Rodger, S., & Ziviani, J. M. (2006). Enhancing children's motivation from a self determination theoretical perspective: Implications for practice. *Australian Journal of Occupational Therapy, 53,* 78–86.

Prochaska, J. O., & DiClemente, C. C. (1982). Transtheoretical therapy: Toward a more integrative model of change. *Psychotherapy: Theory, Research, and Practice, 19,* 276–288.

Prochaska, J. O., DiClemente, C. C., & Norcross, J. C. (1992). In search of how people change: Applications to addictive behavior. *American Psychologist, 47,* 1102–1114.

Resnicow, K., Davis, R. E., Zhang, G., Konkel, J., Strecher, V. J., Saikh, A. R., Tolsma, D., Calvi, J., Alexander, G., Anderson, J. P., & Wiese, C. (2008). Tailoring a fruit and vegetable intervention on novel motivational constructs: Results of a randomized study. *Annals of Behavioral Medicine, 35,* 159–169.

Ryan, R. M., & Deci, E. L. (2000). Self determination theory and the facilitation of intrinsic motivation, social development and well-being. *American Psychologist, 55,* 68–78.

Simpson, H. B., Zuckoff, A., Page, J. R., Franklin, M. E., & Foa, E. B. (2008). Adding motivational interviewing to exposure and ritual prevention for obsessive-compulsive disorder: An open pilot trial. *Cognitive Behavior Therapy, 37*(1), 38–49.

Spencer, L., Adams, T. B., Malone, S., Roy, L., & Yost, E. (2006). Applying the transtheoretical model to exercise: A systematic and comprehensive review of the literature. *Health Promotion Practice, 7*(4), 428–443.

Steel, P. (2007). The nature of procrastination: A meta-analytic and theoretical review of the quintessential self-regulatory failure. *Psychological Bulletin, 133,* 65–95.

Stoffel, V. C., & Moyers, P. A. (2004). An evidence based and occupational perspective of intervention for persons with substance-use disorders. *American Journal of Occupational Therapy, 58,* 570–586.

Sutton, S. R. (2001). Back to the drawing board? A review of applications of the transtheoretical model to substance abuse. *Addiction, 96,* 175–186.

Emotion Regulation

Marian Scheinholz

> "*E*motions shape the landscape of our mental and social lives. Like the "geographical upheavals" a traveler might discover in a landscape where recently only a flat plain could be seen, they mark our lives as uneven, uncertain, and prone to reversal . . .
> —Martha Nussbaum, *Upheavals of Thought: The Intelligence of Emotions,* 2001

Introduction

Emotions are an ever present and essential facet of daily life. Our emotions help us interpret the world and guide us in our responses. However, emotions can also interfere with successful performance. A young child has a temper tantrum at the grocery store when the parent refuses to buy something the child wants. A college student cries uncontrollably after receiving a poor grade on an exam. A middle-age man gets in a fistfight over a minor argument at a bar. An older adult is completely unable to make a decision due to extreme feelings of anxiety. These are all examples of emotion dysregulation.

Although everyone experiences times when their emotions get in the way or result in a bad life decision, for some people emotion dysregulation is a constant problem that creates challenges for everyday life. Emotion dysregulation can be especially taxing for the maintenance of healthy interpersonal relationships. This chapter describes emotions, identifies psychiatric conditions in which emotion dysregulation is a primary concern, and describes assessment and intervention for emotion regulation.

Emotion

An **emotion** is an evaluative mental state produced by a neural impulse. Emotions include a combination of physiological arousal, subjective experience, and behavioral or affective expression (Western, 2003). Emotions have been characterized as the very essence of life—it is impossible to be alive without experiencing emotions (Curtis, 1986). Emotions are important to both the preservation of health and survival of organisms because they result in adaptive responses. Emotions enable communication; through the maturation of emotions, humans develop the ability to understand their own feelings and the feelings of others, resulting in the development of healthy relationships.

Emotions can be distinguished from **feelings**, which are considered to be an inner subjective sensation without a physiological response. However, often the terms "feeling" and "emotion" are used synonymously (Curtis, 1986). A persistent emotional state is called a mood. Individuals may experience contradictory emotions simultaneously, resulting in a state of ambivalence.

Physiology of Emotion

The nervous and endocrine systems provide most of the controlling functions of the body and are of great importance to the physiology of emotion. The limbic system and its connections to other parts of the brain play a central role in the origination and modulation of emotions. Receipt and interpretation of sensory input, memories of past experience (both conscious and unconscious), and the state of wakefulness or arousal of the brain can affect emotional and behavioral activity (Curtis, 1986).

The production and release of hormones by the endocrine system and the direct action of the autonomic nervous system also exert control over emotional responses. Because of the role emotions play in human physiology, emotional stress is a factor in the etiology of many physical and mental illnesses and disease (Lumley, Beyer, & Radcliffe, 2008; Taylor, 2007). **Emotional stress** can be defined as a sustained, damaging emotional response and the inability to control such responses. Psychosomatic disorders are considered to have emotional factors as their primary cause. In addition, there are emotional responses to any serious disease, with depression being the most prominent feature. The emotional response to diseases such as cancer has been reported to have significant impact on the patient's response to treatment and prognosis (Western, 2003).

Experience of Emotion

Psychologists define basic emotions as those that are common to the human species, having characteristic physiological, subjective, and expressive components (Ekman, 1999). Anger, fear, happiness, sadness, and disgust are generally accepted as basic emotions. These basic emotions are similar to primary colors in perception in that other emotions or emotional blends are derived from them, such as surprise, contempt, shame, guilt, joy, and anticipation (Western, 2003).

Culture, politics, and social structures appear to affect the subjective experience of emotions (Baerveldt & Voestermans,

2005). Social norms and individual history shape the way that humans experience emotions and how they respond, although certain human emotions appear to be universal. Fear, love, anger, and grief seem to be ubiquitous because they are based on the vulnerabilities and attachments that are common to all humans (Nussbaum, 2001). But emotional repertoires do differ, and the extent to which they differ may be related to culture or political structures. For example, one predictor of happiness is the extent to which a culture is individualistic, with a focus on the needs and desires of individuals, rather than the needs of the collective or group. Furthermore, a significant correlation (0.85) has been found between life satisfaction and the number of uninterrupted years of democracy in a country (Inglehart, 1990). In another example, the consequences associated with suppression of emotion may be culture specific. The suppression of emotions is generally associated with negative outcomes; however, this may be primarily a Western phenomenon (Butler, Lee, & Gross, 2007). It appears that there are fewer negative consequences associated with suppression in Asian cultures. A vast proportion of human behavior, including emotional responses, is conditioned based on social surroundings, developmental influences, and other environmental factors.

Individuals differ in the intensity of their emotional states. At the upper end of the continuum are individuals with certain types of severe personality disorders whose emotions are not well modulated, causing significant dysfunction in their daily lives (Linehan, 1993a, 1993b). In the middle of the continuum are well-adjusted individuals who experience a wide range of emotions, but are able to modulate and control their emotional experiences. Finally, some individuals may lack emotional experience and expression. For example, individuals with schizoid personality disorder often seem aloof with restricted emotional expression (American Psychiatric Association [APA], 2000). Emotions can be undesired to the individual feeling them, who wants to control them but cannot. Behavior, in response to emotions, also differs among individuals.

Cognition and Emotion

Emotions affect cognitive processes, in the same way that memory, judgment, and cognition influence emotions when people use situational cues to understand their physiological state of arousal. For example, an individual who was recently fired from a job may react with anger, depression, or anxiety, depending on the interpretation of the event. Someone who interprets the experience as unfair or as retribution is more likely to react with anger, whereas the individual who sees the loss of employment as a reflection of incompetence is more likely to feel depressed. Cognitive processes also influence one's interpretation of other people's emotions, particularly facial displays of emotions. The experience of emotions is more than the thought content, because it contains the "rich and dense perceptions of the object, which are highly concrete and replete with detail" (Nussbaum, 2001, p. 65). Therefore, the experience of an emotion, such as grief, brings with it "cognitively laden" memories, perceptions, and attitudes, in addition to the specific content. For example, memories of fighting with a loved one before an unexpected death can affect the grief process.

Emotions have a connection to the imagination and to creativity that is different from other abstract judgmental states. There is some evidence that negative emotions such as depression and anxiety are associated with higher levels of creativity (George & Zhou, 2002). There also appears to be a higher incidence of bipolar disorder among artists (Jamison, 1993). Bipolar disorder is characterized by extremes of emotions. Emotions also include sensory content that is inseparable from the experience of the emotion, such as the feeling of heaviness associated with depression or increased sensitivity to sound when anxious. The ability to imagine and to sense objects and situations that is derived from emotional experience is likely what explains emotion's contribution to survival (Nussbaum, 2001).

Emotional Function as a Client Factor

The Occupational Therapy Practice Framework (OTPF) defines **emotional functions** as a subset of specific mental functions, which are a body function category of client factors. Emotional functions are defined as "appropriate range and regulation of emotions, self-control" (American Occupational Therapy Association [AOTA], 2002, p. 625). The OTPF describes analysis of occupational performance as the consideration of "... the complex and dynamic interaction among performance skills, performance patterns, context or contexts, activity demands and *client factors* rather than any one factor alone" (p. 617, italics added). **Emotion regulation** refers to efforts to control emotional states. Regulation of emotional function is essential to successful occupational performance. Emotions can be regulated before or after they occur. One way that emotions are regulated is by reframing the meaning of events or putting perspective on events before they occur. For example, you may miss a party because you need to study for an important exam. Although you are disappointed, you also are proud of yourself for the self-discipline and recognize the potential rewards in the future.

Individuals can also suppress emotions after they occur. For example, you become angry at your boss for belittling you in front of others, but you decide not to say anything and try to ignore your angry feelings because you do not want to lose your job. However, this may interfere with the ability to engage in tasks (or, in the example, the ability to complete your work tasks successfully) because suppression often leads to increased sympathetic nervous system activity or arousal (Salters-Pedneault, Tull, & Roemer, 2004). In fact, trying not to think about something can have a paradoxical effect such that the individual actually thinks more about what he or she is trying to suppress.

Consequently, more recent conceptualizations of emotion regulation focus on the importance of experiencing all emotions, but in a way that allows the individual to control one's behavior and continue to engage in goal-directed activities. This conceptualization of emotion regulation includes the ability to

- Inhibit inappropriate behavior related to strong emotions.
- Accept and willingly experience negative emotions as part of a meaningful life.

■ Organize oneself independent of mood state to act to attain external goals.

■ Self-soothe physiological arousal when strong emotions occur.

■ Refocus attention in the face of strong emotions. (Gratz & Roemer, 2004)

Emotion dysregulation refers to emotional responses that are not adaptive to the particular situation (Schore, 2003). Dysregulated emotion does not always involve a negative emotion (although most frequently it does), but it involves an emotional experience that interferes with goal-oriented activity. For example, an individual may become bereft over losing a weekend tennis match and go home to fight with an unsuspecting spouse. Or, in another example, an individual is so excited about a new relationship that he or she is unable to concentrate at work and shares inappropriate information with coworkers and supervisors.

Another feature of emotion dysregulation is an impairment in modulation. Everyone has experiences of intense anger, sadness, or anxiety, but typically the intense feelings subside relatively soon. For people with emotion dysregulation, the intense feelings remain for a longer period of time, and the individual is unable to accept the experience and move on. Holding grudges, an inability to focus due to emotions, and lingering emotional reactivity are examples of problems with modulation.

Development of Emotion Regulation

Because emotions feel "good" or "bad" and lead to positive or negative responses, people learn to regulate their emotions early in life. Emotion regulation is a form of procedural knowledge that can be conscious or implicit. It is a skill that humans acquire as part of the developmental process. Infants and young children learn to regulate their emotions in the context of their primary relationships (Perry, 2006). Infants learn to regulate their emotional responses as they interact with caregivers and attend to the caregiver's emotional displays (Carver & Vaccaro, 2007). Adults help children meet their primary needs for sustenance and security and, in so doing, develop their emotional and stress response systems and the ability to self-regulate. When infants feel safe and know their needs will be met, they are able to self-soothe. Crying is a normal infant behavior, but excessive crying and lack of a response to soothing is an indication of emotion dysregulation in infants. Often called "colic," excessive infant crying has a complex and poorly understood etiology, but is mostly likely due to a combination of psychosocial factors (Akman et al, 2006). Most infants "grow out" of colic at 3 to 6 months of age, but decreasing negative emotional displays of parents and increasing routine are strategies that can help infants better regulate their emotions (St. James-Roberts, Sleep, Morris, Owen, & Gilham, 2001). Occupational therapists can teach parents how to apply these strategies.

Older children continue to learn how to tolerate distress based on the degree to which adults meet their needs, for example, thirst, hunger, and fear. Learning to tolerate distress, correctly label uncomfortable situations, and develop appropriate ways to respond to emotions is central to healthy development. However, as children get older, peers play a greater role in the development of healthy emotion regulation.

Some children demonstrate inherent difficulties with self-regulation due to poorly organized stress response systems and hyperreactivity. This could be due to a genetic predisposition, developmental issues, or exposure to chaos or violence early in life. These children may be impulsive, irritable, and require more structure, predictability, and repetition to learn and grow than other children of the same age (Perry, 2006).

A study of school-age children aged 5 to 12 examined the relationship of the child's predisposition to particular behavioral patterns and how these interacted with peer rejection (Ladd, 2006). The predispositions studied were aggression and withdrawal, which may be considered to be two different types of emotion dysregulation. Peer rejection had an additive effect on psychological maladjustment when combined with either aggression or withdrawal. Although the aggressive or withdrawn child may contribute to the peer rejection, Coie (2004) finds that once a child acquires a rejected status, that child tends to be treated more and more negatively.

Similarly, another study found that deficient emotion regulation skills mediated the relationship between peer group victimization and peer rejection (Kelly, Schwartz, Gorman, & Nakamoto, 2008). A role for occupational therapists is the creation of programs to increase peer acceptance and to help aggressive and withdrawn children develop more effective coping strategies.

Adolescence is a period of intense expression and great variability in moods (Silk, Steinberg, & Morris, 2003). Those adolescents who experience an intensity and lability (rapid change) that is beyond the typical adolescent experience are more likely to have behavioral problems and psychological disorders, particularly depression.

One study of the relationship of mood and activity in adolescents found that autonomy was an important feature for emotion regulation (Weinstein & Mermelstein, 2007). The type of activity was less important than the degree of personal choice and valuation that the individual associated with an activity. Increased autonomy was associated with more positive mood and greater emotional stability. Occupational therapists can help create situations in which adolescents have more choice in their selection of daily activities.

Neurophysiological Basis

Neuroscience research is revealing brain mechanisms that underlie the impulsivity, mood instability, aggression, anger, and negative emotion seen in emotion dysregulation. Studies suggest that people predisposed to impulsive aggression have impaired regulation of the neural circuits that modulate emotion (Davidson, Jackson, & Kalin, 2000). Brain imaging studies indicate possible involvement of the amygdala, the limbic system, and the prefrontal cortex in responding to perceived threats and negative emotions. In addition, it is believed that these neurophysiological responses might be more pronounced under the influence of drugs, such as alcohol, and with stress (Davidson, Putnam, & Larson, 2000).

Serotonin, norepinephrine, and acetylcholine are among the chemical messengers in these circuits that play a role in the regulation of emotions, including sadness, anger, anxiety, and irritability. Drugs that enhance brain serotonin function and mood-stabilizing drugs may help people with emotion dysregulation–related responses. Deficits in cognitive functioning, such as decision making (Bazanis et al, 2002), conflict resolution (Posner et al, 2002), and "effortful control" (Lenzenweger, Clarkin, Fertuck, & Kernberg, 2004; Posner et al, 2002) are reported. These deficits are believed to be mediated in the frontal lobe, although not all studies have found frontal lobe impairment related to cognitive functioning (Kunert, Druecke, Sass, & Herpertz, 2003).

Taken together, these studies suggest abnormalities in prefrontal, corticostriatal, and limbic networks, perhaps related to lowered serotonin neurotransmission and behavioral disinhibition (Johnson et al, 2003). In the future, such brain-based vulnerabilities may be managed with help from behavioral interventions and medications, much like people manage susceptibility to diabetes or high blood pressure (Siever & Koenigsberg, 2000).

Emotion Dysregulation and Psychiatric Disabilities

There are several diagnoses in which some impairment of emotion is a core symptom (mood and anxiety disorders being the most obvious); however, the particular symptom of emotion dysregulation is most often associated with borderline personality disorder (Reisch, Ebner-Priemer, Tshacher, Bohus, & Linehan, 2008). The following section focuses on borderline personality disorder, but also presents other psychiatric conditions in which emotion dysregulation is pertinent.

Borderline Personality Disorder

Borderline personality disorder (BPD) is a psychiatric diagnosis in which emotion dysregulation is identified as a core symptom. The DSM-IV-TR diagnosis of BPD includes symptoms of "affective instability due to a marked reactivity of mood," "chronic feelings of emptiness," and "inappropriate, intense anger or difficulty controlling anger" (APA, 2000, p. 689). Understanding emotion dysregulation in BPD has led to great advances, including an evidence-based intervention known as dialectical behavior therapy (DBT; Linehan, 1993a, 1993b). Marsha Linehan is responsible for much of this work and has developed a theory that describes the etiology of emotion dysregulation in BPD as the combination of emotional vulnerability and an "invalidating" environment.

A person with emotional vulnerability has an autonomic nervous system that reacts excessively to low levels of stress and/or has intense responses to emotional stimuli. In addition, their nervous system has a slow return to baseline after the emotional arousal. A person who is emotionally vulnerable tends to have quick, intense, and difficult-to-control emotional reactions that can affect performance of occupational roles. For example, the individual may get in physical or verbal fights or become tearful over minor incidents. However, emotional vulnerability is rarely the sole cause of psychological problems. Some people with emotional vulnerability are able to use effective coping strategies to modulate their emotions (see Chapter 22).

Consequently, Linehan (1993a, 1993b) hypothesizes that emotion dysregulation occurs when a child with high emotional vulnerability is exposed to an "invalidating" environment, that is, an environment in which the experiences and responses of the child are disqualified or "invalidated" by significant others. It is the combination of emotional vulnerability and the invalidating environment that leads to emotion dysregulation.

In an invalidating environment, the child's personal expressions of needs, fears, and desires are not accepted as an accurate description of true feelings. For example, if a child says, "I'm hurt," the parent might respond by saying, "Don't be a crybaby, just shake it off." Or a child might come home proud of a grade of 94%, but the parent only focuses on the questions that the child got wrong.

Extreme examples of invalidating environments include physical and sexual abuse, and indeed BPD is associated with high rates of abuse histories. Studies show that many, but not all, individuals with BPD report a history of abuse, neglect, or separation as young children (Zanarini & Frankenburg, 2001). Forty to 71% of BPD patients report having been sexually abused, usually by a noncaregiver (Zanarini, 2000).

Invalidating environments characteristically place a high value on self-control and self-reliance, and difficulties in these areas are not acknowledged. It is expected that the child will independently resolve problems easily, and failure to do so is ascribed to a lack of proper motivation or some other negative characteristic in the child. Emotionally vulnerable children in such an environment experience particular problems, including loss of the opportunity to label and understand their feelings and to learn to trust their own responses to events.

As a result, the child's behavior oscillates between emotional inhibition to gain acceptance and extreme displays of emotion in order to have feelings acknowledged. Erratic and inappropriate responses from the environment can result in intermittent reinforcement for these actions (e.g., giving in to a child's temper tantrum in a store by purchasing the item that was previously denied), resulting in a persistent behavior pattern that interferes with development of healthy habits and routines, and therefore the competent performance of occupational roles. In the extreme case, the ongoing erratic and inappropriate responses by significant others (parents and other adults) to the private experiences (beliefs, thoughts, and feelings) of an emotionally vulnerable child is believed to lead to emotion dysregulation and the development of BPD (Linehan, 1993a, 1993b).

One manifestation of emotion dysregulation that is highly associated with BPD is self-injury without suicide intent, as well as a significant rate of suicide attempts and completed suicide in severe cases (Gardner & Cowdry, 1985; Soloff, Lis, Kelly, Cornelius, & Ulrich, 1994). Patients often need extensive mental health services and account for 20% of psychiatric hospitalizations (Zanarini & Frankenburg, 2001).

Substance Abuse

Although not studied in as much depth as BPD, there is also evidence for emotion dysregulation in substance abuse. Impairment in impulse control is a type of emotion dysregulation that is common in substance abuse. Both neuropsychological and behavioral studies suggest that individuals with substance abuse problems are much more likely to make decisions based on immediate rewards as opposed to long-term consequences (Verdejo-Garcia, Perez-Garcia, & Bechara, 2006). This appears to be true, even when the decision will result in extremely negative outcomes. This helps explain why people that abuse substances will pursue and use substances even to the detriment of their work, children, and significant others.

Furthermore, triggers that elicit a craving, such as attending a celebration, anticipating a stressful event, driving by a liquor store, or meeting a friend who is also an abuser, are laden with emotional overtones (Quirk, 2001). Feelings that can be managed by someone with good coping skills become overwhelming for the person with emotion dysregulation.

More generally, there is evidence that people who abuse substances tend to experience more negative emotions such as depression and anxiety, greater variability in emotions, and more difficulty managing negative emotions (Bowen, Block, & Baetz, 2008; Dorard, Berthoz, Phan, Corcos, & Bungener, 2008; Fischer, Forthun, Pidcock, & Dowd, 2007).

Bipolar Disorder

Bipolar disorder is a mood disorder in which individuals must experience at least one manic episode at some point in the course of the illness, and most individuals also experience depressive episodes (APA, 2000). Bipolar disorder is characterized by both high levels of impairment and high levels of achievement (Nusslock, Ally, Abramson, Harmon-Jones, & Hogan, 2008). Emotion regulation involves the ability to manage emotions for goal-oriented activity; therefore, bipolar disorder presents an interesting question. Why is it that some individuals with bipolar disorder, who by definition experience extreme moods, are high achievers? Some great artists such as the composer Robert Schumann and the poet Lord Byron were most prolific during periods of mania (Jamison, 1993).

Some researchers attempt to explain bipolar disorder as a dysregulation of the behavioral approach system (BAS). (See Chapter 23 for a more thorough discussion of the BAS/BIS systems.) The BAS-sensitive individual is oriented toward receiving rewards and achieving goals (Gray, 1991). A person with low BAS would be characterized by anhedonia (the inability to experience pleasure) and low energy. Dysregulation of the BAS system could then explain both the mania and depression of bipolar disorder (Depue & Collins, 1999).

Urosevic, Abramson, Harmon-Jones, and Alloy (2009) provide a model of the course of bipolar disorder based on BAS dysregulation. The BAS system is activated when exposed to reward-inducing events, such as entering a contest, studying for an exam, or meeting an interesting person. The BAS system is deactivated when rewards are lost or there is an experience of failure (e.g., breaking up with a boyfriend, losing a job, failing an exam). BAS activation is associated with mania and deactivation with depression. Furthermore, individuals with bipolar disorder experience a greater magnitude of activation and deactivation than people without the disorder when exposed to these events.

Disruptive Behavior Disorders

Behavioral disorders in children and adolescents, such as conduct disorder, oppositional defiant disorder, and attention deficit-hyperactivity disorder, have been associated with emotion dysregulation (Beauchaine, Gatzke-Kopp, & Mead, 2007). Like bipolar disorder, some researchers suggest that behavioral disorders are related to an increased BAS activation and a decreased behavioral inhibition system (BIS) activation. BAS impairments are associated with externalized behaviors such as impulsivity and hostility. This BAS dysregulation causes children and adolescents to seek or approach larger and larger reinforcements. Therefore, they may engage in risk taking or other extreme activities to receive the rewards they are seeking. Furthermore, decreased BIS activity is linked to behavioral disinhibition (Beauchaine, 2001), such that these children and adolescents are less likely to avoid punishments or negative consequences.

Assessment for Emotion Dysregulation

Assessment instruments developed by Linehan and colleagues (Behavioral Research & Therapy Clinics, 2007a) are also available to collect clinical data for treatment purposes and outcome data for research or program evaluation purposes. The diary card is used as part of DBT skills training. It can be used by consumers for self-monitoring, as well as in interactions with therapists in both individual therapy and skills training groups. These cards help consumers keep track of their work on skills throughout the week, including a rating of 0 to 7 on how the skills are used each day. (The ratings correspond to whether the consumer tried to use the skills, was able to use the skills, and whether the skills helped.) The card keeps track of use of alcohol, medications (prescription and over the counter), and street/illicit drugs. In addition, suicidal ideation, self-harm, and misery ratings are included. It also tracks daily activities such as sleep, exercise, relaxation, social supports, and pleasure.

The social history interview is most applicable and useful to occupational therapy. It includes questions on various occupational roles (work, student, home management, family member, friend), as well as questions about housing, finances, and legal matters that are pertinent to daily living. It is completed based on an interview with the consumer.

The Difficulties in Emotion Regulation scale is a direct measure of emotion regulation (Gratz & Roemer, 2004). The 36-item scale measures six domains, including acceptance of negative emotions, engagement in goal-directed behavior, controlling impulsive behavior, emotion regulation strategies, emotional awareness, and emotional clarity. The items are written, and the scale is scored such that a higher score indicates more emotion dysregulation. Psychometric studies indicate the measure has high internal consistency and good test–retest reliability, and there is support for construct and predictive validity.

There are no specific occupational therapy assessments for emotion regulation. In contrast to the standard instruments used to assess personality structure, symptoms, and other traits, occupational therapy assessment focuses on the individual's occupational functioning in daily life. Individuals with emotion dysregulation have difficulties in many occupational performance areas, including instrumental activities of daily living, work, leisure pursuits, and social participation. The reader can refer to the chapters on occupation to identify specific assessments of occupational performance. Occupational therapy assessment can add valuable information to the treatment team in assessing behavior prior to beginning therapy and therapy progress.

Linehan (1993b) identifies specific areas of consideration that should be addressed in assessing consumers with emotion dysregulation. One area of difficulty in assessing the skills of individuals with emotion dysregulation is determining whether incapability is due to skill deficit, emotional inhibition, or environmental constraints. This is further complicated by the client's lack of self-knowledge. He or she may confuse being afraid of doing something with being able to do it, and thus, self-reporting assessment information may be flawed. Naturalistic observation of consumers can provide a means for assessing skill deficits that exist in specific environmental contexts.

Another factor to consider is that consumers may view their deficits as a result of lack of motivation on their part, rather than an actual lack of skill in that situation. This usually relates to the history of invalidation they have experienced with their family of origin or others, including treatment providers. To determine whether the consumer has a specific skill in his or her repertoire, the therapist may need to create the ideal circumstances under which the skill can be produced. For interpersonal skills, this may be accomplished through role playing with the therapist or another client. Coaching is permitted in order for the consumer to produce the behavior. This will also provide information to the therapist to counsel the consumer and the family or significant others on types of supports that may enable the consumer to act skillfully.

Interventions for Emotion Regulation

DBT is the first evidence-based approach with significant efficacy for individuals with BPD. Due to its strong evidence base and emphasis on emotion regulation issues, DBT will receive the most attention in this section. Other approaches occupational therapists might use to address emotion regulation are included, such as cognitive therapy, anger management, and a program to reduce excessive crying in infants.

Cognitive Therapy

Cognitive therapy, as defined by Beck (1993), is a mental health intervention that focuses on changing thinking patterns, especially automatic thoughts, to influence behavioral responses to situations in which emotions are evoked. Cognitive behavioral therapy has been widely used and described in the clinical literature to treat Axis I conditions (e.g., anxiety and depressive disorders) (APA, 2001). Cognitive behavioral therapy assumes that maladaptive, distorted beliefs and cognitive processes underlie symptoms and dysfunctional affect or behavior, and that these beliefs are behaviorally reinforced. It generally involves attention to a set of dysfunctional automatic thoughts or deeply ingrained belief systems (often referred to as schemas), along with learning and practicing new, nonmaladaptive behaviors.

Utilization of cognitive behavioral methods in the treatment of emotion dysregulation have been described (Beck & Freeman, 1990), but because persistent dysfunctional belief systems are usually "structuralized" (i.e., built into the patient's usual cognitive organization), substantial time and effort are required to produce lasting change. Modifications of standard approaches (e.g., schema-focused cognitive therapy, complex cognitive therapy, DBT) are often recommended in treating certain features that are typical of the persistent beliefs associated with emotion dysregulation. (See Chapter 19 for more information on cognitive behavioral therapy.)

Dialectical Behavior Therapy

Dialectical behavior therapy (DBT) is a comprehensive cognitive behavioral treatment protocol for complex and difficult-to-treat mental disorders that combines individual psychotherapy with psychosocial skills training (Linehan, 1993a, 1993b). DBT was originally designed to treat individuals who repeatedly engaged in suicidal or parasuicidal behaviors and had frequent hospitalizations. BPD is such a disorder, and DBT evolved into a treatment specifically for this illness. DBT has been adapted for other individuals with mental disorders involving emotion dysregulation, including those with co-occurring BPD and substance dependence (Bornovalova & Daughters, 2007), depressed elderly (Lynch, Morse, Mendelson, & Robins, 2003), suicidal adolescents (Paul, 2007), and binge eating (Telch, Agras, & Linehan, 2001). Applications of DBT tend to focus on populations in which impulse control and/or suicidal and self-harm behaviors are prevalent.

Designed as an outpatient therapy protocol, DBT has been applied in a variety of other settings, such as inpatient, partial hospitalization, and forensic settings (Dimeff & Linehan, 2001). Research has been conducted to determine efficacy in many of these populations and settings (Dimeff, Koerner, & Linehan, 2002).

In the classical sense, dialectical means the synthesis of opposites. In DBT, the primary dialectic is acceptance and change. The treatment program, the approach of the therapist, and the engagement of the consumer involves a process that validates the consumer's current emotional and functional state while promoting change in skills, behavior, and thinking. DBT is a modification of standard cognitive behavioral therapy (CBT), using standard CBT techniques, such as skills training, homework assignments, symptom rating scales, and behavioral analysis in addressing clients' problems. However, the standard overall approach of CBT was found by Linehan and colleagues (1993a, 1993b) to be ineffective with consumers with BPD. People with BPD were discouraged by the constant focus on change and believed that the degree of their suffering was underestimated and that their therapists were overestimating how helpful they were being. As a result, clients dropped out of treatment, became very frustrated, and/or shut down.

Linehan (1993a, 1993b) modified standard CBT by incorporating acceptance strategies and other "dialectics." The balance between acceptance and change strategies in therapy formed the fundamental "dialectic" that resulted in the treatment's name. "Dialectic" refers to considering and integrating seemingly contradictory facts or ideas in order to resolve the contradictions. There are four primary modes of treatment in DBT: individual psychotherapy, psychosocial skills training, telephone contact, and therapist consultation.

PhotoVoice

This is a picture of my DBT therapist. She is a person I can actually talk to about problems I may be having at that time. Sometimes she understands me better than I understand myself. She makes me feel comfortable about talking without making me feel ashamed to talk about my problems. Some of my problems are worrying about having a panic attack every time that I'm outside, physical pain and aches in my back. My DBT therapist is very friendly and very important to my recovery. Without her I don't know where I would be now.

—Sterling

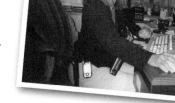

Psychotherapy

In DBT, the individual psychotherapist is the primary therapist. Unless the occupational therapist receives specialized training in this area, the psychotherapy is typically performed by someone from another discipline, such as psychology or social work. In individual psychotherapy, emotion regulation and other behavioral skills are acquired, strengthened, and generalized.

Because of the nature of BPD, consumers with this disorder often "burn out" therapists or drop out of therapy prematurely. DBT includes a therapist consultation team and specific procedures to address this challenge and to enhance the therapist's capabilities and motivation to treat clients effectively. Therapists receive support and consultation as an integral and essential part of the therapy.

To deliver DBT, therapists are asked to assume several working assumptions to establish the right attitude for the therapy, including (Linehan, 1993a)

- The consumer wants to change and is trying to do so, although at times it may not appear so.
- The consumer's behavior patterns are understandable in light of his or her history and present circumstances. Although it may be that the consumer's life is so terrible that it seems not worth living, the therapist never agrees that suicide is the appropriate solution. Rather, the therapist focuses on supporting the consumer to try to make life more satisfying and worthwhile.
- The consumer is not to blame for the ways things currently are in his or her life, but it is his or her personal responsibility to try to make them different.
- Consumers do not fail at DBT. If problems do not improve, it is the treatment that is failing and needs to be modified.
- Although the therapist may feel manipulated by the consumer, blaming or labeling the consumer as manipulative will not lead to successful therapeutic intervention.

In DBT, the therapist uses two dialectically opposed styles when interacting with the consumer. On the one hand, the therapist is warm, genuine, and responsive, and may appropriately self-disclose when it is beneficial to the consumer's interests. On the other hand, the therapist uses an "irreverent communication" style that is more confrontational and challenging, and that is directed at addressing situations in which the consumer is stuck or moving in the wrong direction. Overall, the therapist is accepting of the consumer, but encourages change and nurtures through benevolent demands.

Skills Training

DBT skills training is generally conducted in a group format (Linehan, 1993b). It is the skills training component of DBT that provides the natural role for occupational therapy leadership. The skills taught in DBT include mindfulness, interpersonal effectiveness, emotion regulation, and distress tolerance. As with all group formats, consumers benefit from the interpersonal interaction, support, and modeling of other consumers. The group format also supports the therapist staying with the skills training agenda and protocol even in the face of current problems or crises of the individual group members.

Linehan (1993b) provides an outline for the skills training group sessions in a training manual, and it is recommended that group leaders follow the manual closely, especially during the first few group meetings. Occupational therapy practitioners typically receive training during their educational preparation to lead skills and psychoeducational groups, and they may find the structure and content of the outlines and activities familiar and helpful in structuring groups.

The manual includes reproducible handouts and homework sheets, as well as content outlines of the skills in each of the four skills training modules. These outlines contain lecture and discussion points, practice exercises (activities), and notes to group leaders that provide advice on group process and on addressing common problems that may be encountered.

The four modules of skills training are mindfulness, interpersonal effectiveness, emotion modulation, and distress tolerance. Mindfulness has been defined as "awareness, without judgment, of life as it is, yourself as you are, other people as they are, in the here and now, via direct and immediate experience" (Sanderson, 2006, p. 1). The roots of mindfulness practice are in the contemplative practices common to both Eastern and Western spiritual disciplines and to the emerging scientific knowledge about the benefits of "allowing" experiences rather than suppressing or avoiding them. Mindfulness in its totality has to do with the quality of awareness that a person brings to everyday living; learning to control your mind, rather than letting your mind control you. Mindfulness as a practice directs a person's attention to only one thing, and that one thing is the moment in which one is living. Furthermore, mindfulness is the process of observing, describing, and participating in reality in a nonjudgmental manner, in the moment and with effectiveness.

The "interpersonal effectiveness skills" that are taught focus on effective ways of achieving one's objectives with other people: to ask for social relationships and to maintain self-esteem in interactions with other people. Interpersonal effectiveness training is designed to teach the application of specific interpersonal problem-solving, social, and assertiveness skills to enable participants to modify aversive environments and obtain their personal goals in interpersonal encounters. Skills are taught to accomplish this without damaging either relationships or the person's self-respect.

"Emotion modulation skills" are ways of changing emotional states, and "distress tolerance skills" include techniques for putting up with these emotional states if they can not be changed for the time being. The goals of this module are to enable participants to understand their emotions, reduce emotional vulnerability, and decrease emotional suffering. Specific skills that are taught to regulate emotions include identifying and labeling emotions, recognizing obstacles to changing emotions, and reducing vulnerability to being overly influenced by emotions.

Distress tolerance skills have to do with the ability to accept oneself and the current situation in a nonjudgmental and nonevaluative manner. Distress tolerance is the ability to experience an emotional state without attempting to change it and observing one's thoughts and actions without attempting to stop or control them. In essence, the current environment is observed and tolerated. This does not mean that the current reality is approved or cannot eventually be modified, rather that it is accepted at the present time. Distress tolerance skills are used to tolerate and survive the crises that are frequent occurrences in the life of many people with BPD. Crisis survival skills include distracting, self-soothing, improving the moment, and thinking of pros and cons.

Anger Management Programs

Anger is one of the most common and problematic disturbances associated with emotion dysregulation. Anger management programs are used for children, adolescents, and adults. One program with substantial research support is the Anger Coping program (Lochman, Barry, & Pardini, 2003). The program is designed for children and can be used in the school or clinic. Small groups of four to six students attend weekly meetings to improve perspective taking, problem-solving, recognizing emotions that lead to anger, and conflict resolution strategies. The program is based on cognitive behavioral principals, meaning that there is an emphasis on changing cognitive distortions or developing more accurate perspectives during social interactions. The training includes role-playing that is videotaped for feedback. Children also practice the skills in more natural settings. Throughout the program, children receive positive reinforcement whenever they demonstrate good anger management skills.

Evidence-Based Practice

Two early randomized controlled trials (RCTs) of dialectical behavior therapy (DBT) indicated that DBT is more effective than treatment-as-usual (TAU) in treatment of BPD and treatment of BPD and comorbid diagnosis of substance abuse (Linehan, Armstrong, Suarez, Allmon, & Heard, 1993; Linehan et al, 1999). Clients receiving DBT, compared with TAU, were significantly less likely to drop out of therapy and engage in parasuicide, and had significantly fewer parasuicidal behaviors. Furthermore, clients receiving DBT were less likely to be hospitalized, had fewer days in the hospital, and had higher scores on global and social adjustment. In the RCT conducted on DBT for women with comorbid substance abuse, in addition to similar findings to the original study, DBT was more effective than TAU at reducing drug abuse. Another RCT (Linehan et al, 2006) attempted to address some of the criticisms of previous studies (small number of subjects, lack of expertise in the TAU category therapists, unsustained gains after termination of treatment). This study of 101 participants contrasted 1 year of DBT with 1 year of therapy by experts in the community and 1 year of follow-up for both groups. The DBT participants had half the rate of suicide attempts, significantly decreased use of psychotropic medications, and significantly fewer emergency department visits and hospitalizations for psychiatric reasons.

➤ There is strong support for the efficacy of DBT with individuals with BPD. Occupational therapists that work with clients with BPD can use DBT as an intervention approach and are particularly well suited to providing the skills training component.

➤ The skills training component has been put into a manual. The manual is essential to ensure fidelity (meaning that the intervention provided is true to DBT principles).

Linehan, M. M., Armstrong, H. E., Suarez, A., Allmon, D., & Heard, H. L. (1993). Cognitive behavioral treatment of chronically parasuicidal borderline patients. *Archives of General Psychiatry, 50,* 157–158.

Linehan, M. M., Comtois, K. A., Murray, A. M., Brown, M. Z., Gallop, R. J., Heard, H. L., Korslund, K. E., Tutek, D. A., Reynolds, S. K., & Lindenboim, N. (2006). Two-year randomized controlled trial and follow-up of dialectical behavior therapy vs therapy by experts for suicidal behaviors and borderline personality disorder. *Archives of General Psychiatry, 63*(7), 757–766.

Linehan, M. M., Schmidt, H., Dimeff, L. A., Kanter, J. W., Craft, J. C., Comtois, K. A., & Recknor, K. L. (1999). Dialectical behavior therapy for patients with borderline personality disorder and drug-dependence. *American Journal on Addiction, 8,* 279–292.

Mary Tang (2001), an occupational therapist, described an anger management program for adults with mental health problems. This program was also based on cognitive behavioral therapy principles, with an emphasis on enhancing coping skills to address management of anger. Results from a pretest/posttest analysis revealed that participants had a significant reduction in the intensity of angry feelings and an improvement in anger coping strategies.

REST Program for Infant Irritability

Excessive crying, or colic, is the most common complaint among parents in the first year of life (Lindberg, 2000). The lack of response to soothing and difficulty modulating crying suggests emotion dysregulation of the infant. Although there is no universal agreement as to the definition

The Lived Experience

Marian Schienholz

Since the early years of adolescence, I have experienced symptoms of a mood disorder that affected my growth, development, and ability to function. One set of these symptoms with which I have struggled repeatedly over the years has been suicidal thoughts and ideas.

The first time I attempted suicide, I was 16. By then, I had been experiencing undiagnosed depression for several years. The incident that preceded my taking about 75 aspirin tablets involved a bell, a priest, and an adult religious education class—a very strange incident that retrospectively caused me shame and a deep sense of the worthlessness of my situation and my life. I awoke the next day and went to school without telling my family or friends. (My mother was very ill at that time.) I did confide what I had done to another priest, who served as a counselor at my school. He listened and sent me to the school nurse—when I told her I didn't feel well, she offered me, ironically, an aspirin! What he did not do was to refer me for further counseling or intervention, nor did he suggest I tell my family and ask for their help.

That incident occurred in 1970. I did not receive treatment for my symptoms until 1981 and, in the interim, experienced numerous episodes of depressed mood and suicidal thoughts and behaviors. I attempted to deal with the belief that I was a "bad, weak person" by intellectualization and engaging in erratic, self-destructive behaviors.

This story exemplifies how my emotional responses to situations were significantly colored by my predominantly depressive moods and beliefs about the world. My illness was complicated because I have bipolar II disorder, the milder form of bipolar disorder. This meant that I had fluctuating moods and functioning, so, for much of the time, I was able to hide my impairment. In fact, I excelled academically, but my self-esteem was severely impaired, and I experienced a sense of hopelessness and dread. I avoided many social situations and was fearful of opportunities that might result in failure. During adolescence, I spent a great deal of time isolated in my bedroom and secretly cried for no reason.

I now attribute the cause of this to genetic predisposition to clinical depression, a highly critical family, and a series of traumatic life events.

From my upbringing, I learned to suppress emotions, and I often turned anger and frustration inward and experienced them as depression. I did get help eventually for my illness when I entered graduate school at age 25 and experienced a severe depression after a painful breakup with a boyfriend. It has taken many years of therapy, medication, and using alternative methods for me to reach my current state of stability. I have been able to work for most of this time, although I was hospitalized for suicidal intentions several times. Due to ongoing issues, I allowed myself to be in dangerous situations and was victimized twice. I also experienced trauma during one of my psychiatric hospitalizations when I was admitted to a hospital of very poor quality. In addition, I have had some other serious medical problems (physical), and I lost my husband to cancer after only 6 years of marriage. But I have survived . . . and thrived thanks to the time, love, and patience of my family, friends, and mental health providers.

My Recovery

After nearly 35 years of living with a psychiatric disability, I have a regime that enables me to have a productive and satisfying life, and I do believe I am achieving my goal of contributing something worthwhile to others. I am recovering from my illness through personal exploration, coping mechanisms, a relationship with a supportive significant other and supportive friends, reasonable medical intervention, and ongoing therapy.

But I do still experience periods of increased symptoms—even occasional suicidal thoughts, to this day. This happens to me, especially during periods when my depressive symptoms are exacerbated due to external stress, anniversaries of difficult events, and hormonal fluctuations. Stressors include relationship issues, work pressures, and family difficulties.

I would like to share what has been important to my recovery and how I cope with the stress, and periodic occurrence of symptoms, in my daily life. I am sharing some of the things that have helped me, although I believe each *individual* must determine what works best for him- or herself. In my research into the theory and techniques of dialectical behavior therapy, I was struck with the similarity of much of the model to my own emotional "pain management" strategies.

These strategies are not listed in a particular order of importance; established external resources (mental health professionals and support groups) are at the end of the list, but not necessarily more or less helpful. The other ideas may help in the time between contact with these resources and as ongoing preventive/recovery strategies.

- Alternative Activities—Identify several activities that ease the feelings or provide distraction. These should range in degree of concentration and energy needed for engagement. These are very individual, but some of the ones that I use are taking a walk; having a bath; reading a magazine or an interesting, but not too complex book; calling or e-mail/instant messaging a friend/family member; going to a support group; visiting a bookstore or the library; gardening; crocheting; and playing with my cats. Outdoor activities have been particularly helpful to me, such as hiking in the woods, sitting by a lake or at the beach, or visiting a park. I think they bring a sense of peace and connection with nature. Activities should be meaningful to the person, productive if possible, and should be appropriate for the level of energy, concentration, and cognitive capacity of the individual.
- Rational Thoughts—I have a list of rational reasons why I feel depressed or think about suicide—things that challenge thinking "I'm an awful/bad/unlucky/stupid, etc. person" or "life is too much trouble, not worthwhile, too painful/difficult" or "no one really cares about me or loves me." This can include identifying the current stressors or anniversaries of stressful events. The list should include projections of how/when the stressor will abate.

I keep a list of the alternative activities and rational thoughts posted at home and/or carry it along with me when I am experiencing symptoms. Consulting the list when concentration or initiative is lacking is helpful.

The Lived Experience—cont'd

- Journaling—This is a special type of "alternative activity" that I find very helpful. It's a way to pour out negative thoughts and feelings, and then try to challenge them or reflect how they have diminished in the past. It is useful to journal the good times as well and reread these passages when one is feeling especially down.
- Relaxation—I find progressive relaxation and deep breathing helps ease the painful feelings. I sometimes use a guided relaxation tape if I am having more difficulty concentrating. Visualizing a peaceful place I have enjoyed during vacation enhances the effects for me. I am also now using a sound machine to relax. The sound of ocean surf, rain, and thunderstorms are relaxing to me. There are nine sound choices on the machine, and individuals may find one of them soothing.
- Creative Activities (Poetry/Dance/Art/Music, etc)—I find writing poetry to be helpful in expressing my feelings in a constructive way. I often do this as part of my journaling. I share some of my poetry with others, and some I don't. Dancing and doing crafts also relax and distract me. However, this can backfire if the level of the activity is too complex. It is important to identify and pursue an appropriate activity for one's state of mind.
- Identify a Reason to Go On!—Make it simple, if possible. It should be important and specific to the individual, and does not necessarily have to make sense or be important to others. For example, I have used the thought that I need to continue living to take care of and love my cats.
- Structure—During times of distress or symptom exacerbation, it is important to follow a normal daily schedule of structured activities, even if one is unable to engage in a normal daily routine (i.e., employment, school or volunteer job).
- Exercise—This is a critical part of my plan for recovery and can be very helpful in times of distress. Finding the motivation to exercise may be a problem, and I find that little tricks such as thinking "I will take a 5-minute walk" can often "get the sneakers on" and enable one to do more.

- Reward System—It is important to recognize and/or give oneself congratulations or praise for doing/getting through these simple daily tasks, such as personal hygiene, getting dressed, etc. They take energy and concentration, and, although they are simply part of one's day when a person is feeling well or does not suffer from depression or have suicidal thoughts, they are an accomplishment when a person does experience these things.
- Talk to Someone/Use Established Resources—For a very long time, I had difficulty calling my doctor or therapist in times of distress. I have kept fairly regular weekly appointments, but at times, I needed help in between. I am now better at this and have found the contact very helpful—it may mean "tweaking" medication or just getting support or suggestions for getting through the day. If a person is feeling suicidal, mental health professionals can assess the degree of danger of your thoughts and actions, as well as the need for immediate intervention.
- Self-Help or Support Groups—Such groups can provide persons who will listen, support, and share their experience in dealing with suicidal thoughts and urges. The National Depressive and Manic Depressive Association (www.ndmda.org) and the National Alliance for the Mentally Ill (www.nami.org) have established chapters and support groups in many areas of the United States. There is increasing evidence that people with long-standing mental illnesses will experience problems with substance misuse. I experienced this and have found Alcoholics Anonymous to be extremely helpful. The program, fellowship, and encouragement of seeing others who are living sober have been very helpful.

Finally, for all those who are experiencing symptoms of mental illness, have *hope.* Think about it, read about it, talk about it. Plan to do something that you want to do that is important to you and will make you happy. Believe it can and will happen. Keep a mental or written list of the times you hoped for something and it came true. This is what keeps us all alive after all—the hope for a better life, the continuation of current happiness, and the belief that things will turn around as the cycles of the seasons and all living things do.

---

of colic, a classic criteria is crying that occurs 3 or more hours per day, 3 or more days per week for at least 3 weeks (Zeskind & Barr, 1997). An intervention program developed by nurses, called the REST Routine program, is supported by randomized controlled trials (Keefe, Grose-Fretz, & Kotzer, 1997; Keefe, Karlsen, Dudley, Lobo, & Kotzer, 2006). It is presented here because the approach, either in its entirety or in components, would be appropriate for occupational therapists working with parents of infants. It includes the type of parent training that is common for occupational therapists working in birth to 3-year-old programs.

The program targets both the parent and the infant. For the infant, the REST intervention includes regulation (protection from overstimulation), entertainment, structure and repetition (to create routine and predictability for the infant), and touch (involving chest-to-chest contact). For parents, the intervention includes reassurance (that the child is not ill or in pain), empathy (listening and acknowledging the challenge), support, and time out (specifically, break time each day).

Summary

Emotions are embedded in everything people do, yet the impact of emotion regulation on occupational performance has received relatively little attention in the occupational therapy literature. This chapter provides occupational therapists with information to better understand emotion and provide interventions to address emotion regulation. More work is needed to develop specific occupational therapy assessments and additional interventions for emotion regulation. Occupational therapists have the potential to make a significant contribution to this area of practice by developing assessments and interventions that address emotion regulation in the context of occupational performance.

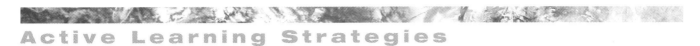

Active Learning Strategies

1. Mindfulness

Mindfulness is a core strategy taught in skills training in DBT. It comes from Asian meditative practice. Mindfulness involves being in the present moment. This is more difficult than it sounds because frequently we are either thinking about what we need to do next or reflecting on something that has happened in the past. Staying in the present moment is challenging. Mindfulness also involves noticing without judgment. It is about paying attention to the present without making an evaluation.

Try a mindfulness exercise: The next time you sit down for a meal, try to eat it mindfully. Turn off the television, music, or any other potential distractions. It is okay if you eat with others, but you may not interact while eating. To eat mindfully, you need to pay full attention to the experience of eating. Focus on the smells, tastes, and textures as you eat. Think about the feelings in your mouth, the sensation of chewing and swallowing. If other thoughts come into your head (e.g., the homework you need to do, an argument you had earlier in the day), do not criticize yourself, but just let go of those thoughts and refocus on the eating experience.

Reflective Questions
- How was the experience of eating mindfully different than your usual way of eating?

- Did you find your mind wandering away from the eating experience? How difficult was it to stay focused?
- After this experience, how do you think mindfulness could help a person with emotion dysregulation?

Reflective Journal

Describe the experience in your Reflective Journal.

2. Girl, Interrupted

Read the book *Girl, Interrupted* (or see the 1999 movie), an autobiography by Susanna Kaysen, who was diagnosed with BPD.

Reflective Questions
- What examples of emotion dysregulation do you see in the main character and in the character of Lisa?
- How does Lisa contribute to the emotion dysregulation of Susanna?
- What aspects of the hospitalization exacerbate Susanna's emotion dysregulation and what helps her?

Resources

- Anger Coping Program Manual:
  Larson, J., & Lochman, J. E. (2005). *Helping Schoolchildren With Anger: A Cognitive Behavioral Therapy Intervention.* New York: Guilford Press.
- Dialectical Behavior Therapy Manuals:
  Linehan, M. M. (1993a). *Cognitive Behavioral Treatment for Borderline Personality Disorder.* New York: Guilford Press.
  Linehan, M. M. (1993b). *Skills Training Manual for Treating Borderline Personality Disorders.* New York: Guilford Press.
- Dialectical Behavior Therapy Resources:
  Marsha Linehan's website includes assessments (diary cards and social history interview) as well as PowerPoint presentations on DBT and training resources: http://faculty.washington.edu/linehan/
  Kaysen, S. (1993). *Girl, Interrupted.* New York: Vintage Books. An autobiography of a girl with BPD.
- Mindfulness Meditation Resources:
  Books and practice CDs from Jon Kabat-Zinn: www.mindfulnesstapes.com
  Hanh, T. N. (1976). *The Miracle of Mindfulness: A Manual on Meditation.* Boston: Beacon Press.

References

Akman, I., Kusa, K., Ozdemir, N., Yurdakul, Z., Solakoglu, M., & Orham, L. (2006). Mothers' post partum psychological adjustment and infantile colic. *Archives of Diseases in Childhood, 91,* 417–419.

American Occupational Therapy Association (AOTA). (2002). Occupational therapy practice framework: Domain and process. *American Journal of Occupational Therapy, 56,* 609–639.

American Psychiatric Association (APA). (2000). *Diagnostic and Statistical Manual of Mental Disorders* (4th ed., text revision). Arlington, VA: Author.

American Psychiatric Association (APA). (2001). Practice guideline for the treatment of patients with borderline personality disorder. *American Journal of Psychiatry, 158,* 1–52.

Baerveldt, C., & Voestermans, P. (2005). Culture, emotion and the normative structure of reality. *Theory and Psychology, 15,* 449–473.

Bazanis, E., Rogers, R. D., Dowson, J. H., Taylor, P., Meux, C., Staley, C., Nevinson-Andrews, D., Taylor, C., Robbins, T. W., & Sahakian, B. J. (2002). Neurocognitive deficits in decision-making and planning of patients with DSM-III-R borderline personality disorder. *Psychological Medicine, 32,* 1395–1405.

Beauchaine, T. P. (2001). Vagal tone, development and Gray's motivational theory: Toward an integrated model of autonomic nervous system functioning in psychopathology. *Development and Psychopathology, 13,* 183–214.

Beauchaine, T. P., Gatzke-Kopp, L., & Mead, H. K. (2007). Polyvagal theory and developmental psychopathology: Emotion dysregulation and conduct problems from preschool to adolescence. *Biological Psychology, 74,* 174–184.

Beck, A. T. (1993). Cognitive therapy: Past, present and future. *Journal of Consulting and Clinical Psychology, 61,* 194–198.

Beck, A. T., & Freeman, A. M. (1990). *Cognitive Therapy of Personality Disorders.* New York: Guilford Press.

Behavioral Research & Therapy Clinics, University of Washington. (2006a). "Assessment Instruments." Available at: www.brtc.psych.washington.edu/pubs/instruments.html (accessed December 14, 2009).

Bornovalova, M. A., & Daughters, S. B. (2007). How does dialectical behavior therapy facilitate treatment retention among individuals with comorbid borderline personality disorder and substance use disorder? *Clinical Psychology Review, 27,* 923–943.

Bowen, R., Block, G., & Baetz, M. (2008). Mood and attention variability in women with alcohol dependence: A preliminary investigation. *American Journal of Addiction, 17,* 77–81.

Butler, E. A., Lee, T. L., & Gross, L. L. (2007). Emotion regulation and culture: Are the social consequences of emotional suppression culture specific? *Emotion, 7,* 30–48.

Carver, L. J., & Vaccaro, B. G. (2007). 12 Month infants allocate increased neural resources to stimuli associated with negative adult emotion. *Developmental Psychology, 43,* 54–69.

Coie, J. D. (2004). The impact of negative social experiences on the development of antisocial behavior. In J. B. Kupersmid & K. A. Dodge (Eds.), *Children's Peer Relations: From Development to Intervention* (pp. 243–267). Washington, DC: American Psychological Association.

Curtis, R. H. (1986). *Mind and Mood: Understanding and Controlling Your Emotions.* New York: Charles Scribner's Sons.

Davidson, R. J., Jackson, D. C., & Kalin, N. H. (2000). Emotion, plasticity, context and regulation: Perspectives from affective neuroscience. *Psychological Bulletin, 126*(6), 873–889.

Davidson, R. J., Putnam, K. M., & Larson, C. L. (2000). Dysfunction in the neural circuitry of emotion regulation—A possible prelude to violence. *Science, 289*(5479), 591–594.

Depue, R. A., & Collins, P. F. (1999). Neurobiology of the structure of personality: Dopamine, facilitation of incentive motivation, and extraversion. *Behavioral and Brain Sciences, 22,* 491–569.

Dimeff, L., Koerner, K., & Linehan, M. M. (2002). "Summary of Research on DBT." Behavioral Tech, LLC. Available at: http://www.behavioraltech.com/downloads/dbtSummaryOfData.pdf (accessed February 15, 2010).

Dimeff, L., & Linehan, M. M. (2001). Dialectical behavior therapy in a nutshell. *The California Psychologist, 34,* 10–13.

Dorard, G., Berthoz, S., Phan, O., Corcos, M., & Bungener, C. (2008). Affect dysregulation in cannabis abusers: A study in adolescents and young adults. *European Child and Adolescent Psychiatry, 17,* 274–282.

Ekman, P. (1999). Facial expressions. In T. Dalgleish & M. Power (Eds.), *The Handbook of Cognition and Emotion* (pp. 45–60). New York: John Wiley & Sons.

Fischer, J. L., Forthun, L. F., Pidcock, B. W., & Dowd, D. A. (2007). Parent relationships, emotion regulation, psychosocial maturity and college student alcohol use problems. *Journal of Youth and Adolescence, 36,* 912–926.

Gardner, D. L., & Cowdry, R. W. (1985). Suicidal and parasuicidal behavior in borderline personality disorder. *Psychiatric Clinics of North America, 8*(2), 389–403.

George, J. M., & Zhou, J. (2002). Understanding when bad moods foster creativity and good ones don't: The role of context and clarity of feelings. *Journal of Applied Psychology, 87,* 687–697.

Gratz, K. L., & Roemer, L. (2004). Multidimensional assessment of emotion regulation and dysregulation: Development, factor structure and initial validation of the Difficulties in Emotion Regulation scale. *Journal of Psychopathology and Behavioral Assessment, 26,* 41–54.

Gray, J. A. (1991). The neuropsychology of temperament. In J. Strelau & A. Angleitner (Eds.), *Explorations in Temperament: International Perspectives on Theory and Measurement* (pp. 105–128). New York: Plenum Press.

Inglehart, R. (1990). *Culture shift in advanced industrial society.* Princeton: Princeton University Press.

Jamison, K. R. (1993). *Touched With Fire: Mental Illness and Artistic Temperament.* New York: Free Press.

Johnson, P. A., Hurley, R. A., Benkelfat, C., Herpertz, S. C., & Taber, K. H. (2003). Understanding emotion regulation in borderline personality disorder: Contributions of neuroimaging. *Journal of Neuropsychiatry and Clinical Neuroscience, 15,* 397–402.

Keefe, M. R., Grose-Fretz, A., & Kotzer, A. M. (1997). The REST regimen: An individualized nursing intervention for infant irritability. *American Journal of Maternal Child Nursing, 22,* 16–20.

Keefe, M. R., Karlsen, K. A., Dudley, W. N., Lobo, M. L., & Kotzer, A. M. (2006). Reducing parenting stress in families with irritable infants. *Nursing Research, 55,* 198–205.

Kelly, B. M., Schwartz, D., Gorman, A. H., & Nakamoto, J. (2008). Violent victimization in the community and children's subsequent peer rejection: The mediating role of emotion dysregulation. *Journal of Abnormal Child Psychology, 3,* 175–185.

Kunert, H. J., Druecke, H. W., Sass, H., & Herpertz, S. C. (2003). Frontal lobe dysfunctions in borderline personality disorder? Neuropsychological findings. *Journal of Personality Disorders, 17,* 497–509.

Ladd, G. W. (2006). Peer rejection, aggressive or withdrawn behavior and psychological maladjustment from ages 5 to 12: An examination of four predictive models. *Child Development, 77,* 822–846.

Lenzenweger, M. F., Clarkin, J. F., Fertuck, E. A., & Kernberg, O. F. (2004). Executive neurocognitive functioning and neurobehavioral systems indicators in borderline personality disorder: A preliminary study. *Journal of Personality Disorders, 18,* 421–438.

Lindberg, T. (2000). Infantile colic: Aetiology and prognosis. *ACTA Paediatrica, 89,* 1– 2.

Linehan, M. M. (1993a). *Cognitive Behavioral Treatment for Borderline Personality Disorder.* New York: Guilford Press.

Linehan, M. M. (1993b). *Skills Training Manual for Treating Borderline Personality Disorders.* New York: Guilford Press.

Lochman, J. E., Barry, T. D., & Pardini, D. A. (2003). Anger control training for aggressive youth. In A. E. Kazdin & J. R. Weisz (Eds.), *Evidence Based Psychotherapies for Children and Adolescents* (pp. 263–281). New York: Guilford Press.

Lumley, M. A., Beyer, J., & Radcliffe, A. (2008). Alexithymia and physical health problems: A critique of potential pathways and a research agenda. In A. Vingerhoets, I. Nyklicek, & J. Donollet (Eds.), *Emotion Regulation: Conceptual and Clinical Issues* (pp. 43–68). New York: Springer Science.

Lynch, T. R., Morse, J. Q., Mendelson, T., & Robins, C. J. (2003). Dialectical behavior therapy for depressed older adults: A randomized pilot study. *American Journal of Geriatric Psychiatry, 11,* 33–45.

Nussbaum, M. C. (2001). *Upheavals of Thought: The Intelligence of Emotions.* Cambridge, UK: Cambridge University Press.

Nusslock, R., Ally, L. B., Abramson, L. Y., Harmon-Jones, E., & Hogan, M. E. (2008). Impairment in the achievement domain in bipolar spectrum disorders: Role of behavioral approach system hypersensitivity and impulsivity. *Minerva Pediatrica, 60,* 41–50.

Paul, A. (2007). Review of dialectical behavior therapy with suicidal adolescents. *Child and Family Behavior Therapy, 29,* 87–94.

Perry, B. D. (2006). "Developing Self-Regulation." Available at: http://content.scholastic.com/browse/article.jsp?id=1460 (accessed December 14, 2009).

Posner, M. I., Rothbart, M. K., Vizueta, N., Levy, K. N., Evans, D. E., Thomas, K. M., & Clarkin, J. F. (2002). Attentional mechanisms of borderline personality disorder. *Proceedings of National Academy of Science USA, 99,* 16366–16370.

Quirk, S. W. (2001). Emotion concepts in models of substance abuse. *Drug and Alcohol Review, 20,* 95–104.

Reisch, T., Ebner-Priemer, U. W., Tshacher, W., Bohus, M., & Linehan, M. (2008). Sequences of emotion in patients with borderline personality disorder. *Acta Psychiatrica, Scandinavia, 118,* 42–48.

Salters-Pedneault, K., Tull, M. T., & Roemer, L. (2004). The role of avoidance of emotional material in the anxiety disorders. *Applied and Preventive Psychology, 11,* 95–114.

Sanderson, C. (2006). "Mindfulness for Clients, Their Friends, and Family Members." Available at: http://behavioraltech.org/downloads/Mindfulness_for_clients_and_family_members.pdf (accessed December 14, 2009).

Schore, A. (2003). *Affect Dysregulation and Disorders of the Self.* New York: Norton.

Siever, L. J., & Koenigsberg, H. W. (2000). The frustrating no-man's-land of borderline personality disorder. *Cerebrum, The Dana Forum on Brain Science, 2*(4), 1–11.

Silk, J. S., Steinberg, L., & Morris, A. S. (2003). Adolescents emotion regulation in daily life: Links to depressive symptoms and problem behavior. *Child Development, 74,* 1869–1880.

Soloff, P. H., Lis, J. A., Kelly, T., Cornelius, J., & Ulrich, R. (1994). Self-mutilation and suicidal behavior in borderline personality disorder. *Journal of Personality Disorders, 8*(4), 257–267.

St. James-Roberts, I., Sleep, J., Morris, S., Owen, C., & Gilham, P. (2001). Use of a behavioural programme in the 1st 3 months to prevent infant crying and sleep problems. *Journal of Paediatrics and Child Health, 37,* 289–297.

Tang, M. (2001). Clinical outcome and client satisfaction of an anger management group program. *Canadian Journal of Occupational Therapy, 68,* 228–236.

Taylor, S. F. (2007). Neural correlates of emotion regulation in psychopathology. *Trends in Cognitive Sciences, 11,* 413–418.

Telch, C. F., Agras, W. S., & Linehan, M. M. (2001). Dialectical behavior therapy for binge eating disorders. *Journal of Consulting and Clinical Psychology, 69,* 1061–1065.

Urosevic, S., Abramson, L. Y., Harmon-Jones, E., & Alloy, L. B. (2009). Dysregulation of the behavioral approach system (BAS) in bipolar spectrum disorders: Review of theory and evidence. *Clinical Psychology Review, 118,* 459–471.

van den Bosch, L. M., Verheul, R., Schippers, G. M., & van den Brink, W. (2002). Dialectical behavior therapy of borderline patients with and without substance use problems: Implementation and longterm effects. *Addictive Behavior, 27,* 911–923.

Verdejo-Garcia, A., Perez-Garcia, M., & Bechara, A. (2006). Emotion, decision-making and substance dependence: A somatic-marker model of addiction. *Current Neuropharmacology, 4,* 17–31.

Weinstein, S. M., & Mermelstein, R. (2007). Relations between daily activities and adolescent mood: The role of autonomy. *Journal of Clinical Child and Adolescent Psychology, 36,* 182–194.

Western, D. (2003). *Psychology: Brain, Behavior, & Culture.* New York: John Wiley & Sons.

Zanarini, M. C. (2000). Childhood experiences associated with the development of borderline personality disorder. *Psychiatric Clinics of North America, 23*(1), 89–101.

Zanarini M. C., & Frankenburg, F. R. (2001). Treatment histories of borderline inpatients. *Comprehensive Psychiatry, 42*(2), 144–150.

Zeskind, P. S., & Barr, R. G. (1997). Acoustic characteristics of naturally occurring cries of infants with "colic." *Child Development, 68,* 394–403.

Pain Regulation

Joyce M. Engel

> "Pain has an element of blank;
> It cannot recollect
> When it began, or if there were
> A day when it was not.
> It has no future but itself,
> Its infinite realms contain
> Its past, enlightened to perceive
> New periods of pain.
>
> —Emily Dickinson

Introduction

Nearly everyone experiences pain at some point in his or her life: the sharp pain experienced after stubbing your toe, the dull pain in one's shoulders and neck after sitting in front of a computer too long, or intolerable pain after a severe injury. Pain can persist for a minute, a month, or for most of one's lifetime. Pain is a common occurrence. In 2006, an estimated one in four adult Americans reported that they experienced a day-long pain episode during the previous month, with 10% stating the pain lasted 1 year or more (National Center for Health Statistics, 2006). Back pain and headaches are the most common pain complaints (USDHHS–CDC, 2009) Pain is also often comorbid with psychiatric disorders, particularly mood and anxiety disorders (Bair, Robinson, Katon, & Kroenke, 2003). Despite people's use of pain medications, two-thirds of individuals experiencing chronic or persistent pain cannot perform routine occupations (American Pain Foundation, n.d.). The annual financial cost of all persistent pain syndromes, including direct medical expenses, lost income, and lost productivity, is at least $100 billion (American Pain Foundation, n.d.). Yet, the emotional and social costs of suffering cannot be estimated.

The obligation to manage pain and relieve suffering is now recognized by governing bodies as fundamental to health-care (Fishman, 2004; Hamdy, 2001). Pain may be a primary reason for seeking health-care (e.g., low back pain), coexist with a disease (e.g., arthritis, depression) or disability (e.g., spinal cord injury), or result from medical procedures (e.g., immunization). This chapter defines pain, describes the biopsychosocial model of pain, explains the relationship of pain to consumer factors and occupational performance, presents standardized assessments, interprets evidence-based practice interventions that are psychological in origin, and provides a first-person account of an individual with persistent pain, as well as self-reflection and experiential learning activities.

Defining Pain

The International Association for the Study of Pain (2007) defined **pain** as "an unpleasant sensory and emotional experience associated with actual or potential tissue damage or described in terms of such damage." This definition conveys that pain is primarily a subjective experience and that it is multifaceted. Individual variables, such as prior pain experiences, mood, cognition, sex, familial factors, and culture, are known to affect an individual's experience of pain (Baptiste, 1998; LeResche, 2001; Strong, Sturgess, Unruh, & Vicenzino, 2002).

Differentiating acute from chronic or persistent pain is critical to using the appropriate assessments and interventions. **Acute pain** and its associated physiological, psychological, and behavioral responses are almost always caused by tissue irritation or damage in relation to injury, disease, disability, or medical procedures. When pain persists beyond its typical course of recovery, it is classified as **chronic** or **persistent pain** (Turk & Melzack, 1992). Unlike acute pain, persistent pain does not appear to serve a biological purpose and is often experienced in the presence of minimal or no apparent tissue damage. Persistent pain may have an insidious onset or begin as acute pain. Persistent pain typically produces significant changes in mood, thoughts, attitudes, lifestyle, and environment (Unruh, Strong, & Wright, 2002).

Biopsychosocial Model of Pain

A dualistic model that suggests pain is either psychological or physical should be avoided. Conceptualizing pain using a **biopsychosocial model** can help clarify the complex, multifaceted nature of pain that is critical to accurate evaluation and effective intervention (Fordyce, 2001; Sullivan & Turk, 2001; Waddell & Burton, 2005). Loeser and Fordyce (1983) proposed the phenomenon of pain as divided into four distinct domains: nociception, pain, suffering, and pain behavior (Fig. 25-1).

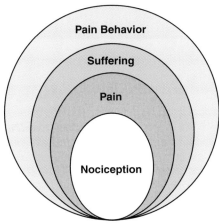

FIGURE 25-1. Loeser's model of pain. *Adapted from Loeser, J. D. (1982). Concepts of pain. In M. Stanton-Hicks & R. Boas (Eds.), Chronic Low Back Pain (p. 146). New York: Raven.*

Nociception is the perception of physical pain. Specialized sensory receptors in the skin and deeper structures detect current or impending tissue damage or irritation, and transmit this information by A-delta and C fibers in the peripheral nerves. Nociception is the body's message to do something or to stop doing something. For example, you are working at your desk and have ignored the tingling in your hand and wrist for weeks until today when you experience a sharp pain shooting through your wrist and up through your arm, signaling carpal tunnel syndrome. **Pain**, as stated previously, is an unpleasant sensory and emotional experience. In the previous example, it is the sharp pain that is likely signaling carpal tunnel syndrome. **Suffering** is the negative affective response to pain. For example, chronic pain is often associated with depression, dysthymic disorder, anxiety, substance abuse/dependence, and insomnia (Sullivan & Turk, 2001). Suffering can be manifest as fear, anxiety, or depression. Suffering is personal. The individual knows the impact of pain on his or her body, sense of self, social responsibilities, and daily occupations. **Pain behavior** is what a person says or does (e.g., moaning, taking pain medication) or does not do (e.g., job attendance), which communicates to others the presence of pain. Pain behaviors are observable and readily influenced by spiritual, cultural, familial, and environmental factors.

Loeser and Fordyce's (1983) biopsychosocial model purports that an individual can experience some domains of the model in the absence of others. In our carpal tunnel syndrome example, some of the initial tingling or numbness is ignored, and if the sharp pain is acute and subsides, the person may continue physical activity without any notable suffering or pain behavior. A biopsychosocial model of pain recognizes both biological and psychological features of pain. Occupational therapy has long embraced a biopsychosocial model in health-care for its emphasis on the interaction of the individual's body, mind, and social factors (Mosey, 1974).

Evaluation

An accurate and comprehensive evaluation of a client's pain is necessary in order to effectively manage the pain. Clinicians can consider pain to be the "fifth vital sign" (Fishman, 2004); if pain were assessed in a manner similar to other vital signs,

effective pain control would be more likely to result. Regular monitoring of pain can also be helpful in making a diagnosis and treating an illness. Consumers may need to be informed that they deserve to have their pain evaluated and treated.

A variety of standardized assessments are available to occupational therapists for pain evaluation, including the visual analogue scale (VAS), numerical rating scale, verbal rating scale, McGill Pain Questionnaire, Brief Pain Inventory, and the University of Alabama Pain Behavior Scale. Evaluation is facilitated by qualitative input such as interviews and observations using tools such as pain diaries, the Canadian Occupational Performance Measure, and motivational interviewing (MI), all of which can be used in conjunction with standardized assessments.

Visual Analogue Scale

The primary approach to pain assessment is the use of self-report measures (Turk et al, 2003). Single-item ratings of pain intensity are the most commonly used measure. A VAS (Fig. 25-2A) consists of a horizontal or vertical line, typically 100 mm long, with each end of the line labeled with descriptors representing the extremes of pain intensity (e.g., "no pain," "worst pain imaginable"). The consumer draws a mark on the line that represents his or her pain intensity, and the distance measured from the "no pain" anchor to the mark becomes that individual's VAS pain score.

Advantages of the VAS are that it has a high number of response categories, demonstrated sensitivity to changes in pain due to intervention or time, and high test–retest reliability. Some individuals, however, do experience difficulties with understanding and completing the measure (Bruera, Kuehn, Miller, Selmser, & MacMillan, 1991; Jensen, 2007.

Numerical Rating Scale

The numerical rating scale (NRS; Fig. 25-2B) is another measure of pain intensity. The NRS consists of a range of numbers, typically 0 to 10. Zero represents *no pain*, and 10 represents *extreme pain* (e.g., "worst pain possible"). The consumer indicates which number best represents his or her level of pain intensity, and that number becomes his or her pain intensity score.

The 0-to-10 NRS has been recommended as a useful measure of pain intensity because of (1) the strong evidence for its reliability and validity, as evidenced by its strong association with other measures of pain intensity and responsivity to analgesic treatment; (2) understandability and ease of use; and (3) ease of administration and scoring (Jensen & Karoly, 2001; Jensen, 2007). Farrar, Portenoy, Berlin, Kinman, and Strom (2000) suggest that a clinically significant change in pain intensity can be defined as an absolute change of 2 points on the NRS.

Verbal Rating Scale

The verbal rating scale (VRS; Fig. 25-2C) of pain intensity consists of a list of 4 to 15 descriptors and an associated number (e.g., 0 = *no pain*, 1 = *mild pain*, 2 = *moderate pain*, 3 = *severe pain*). The consumer selects the one word that best describes his or her pain intensity, and the corresponding number becomes the pain intensity score. Although the VRS

The Lived Experience

Viola Adkins

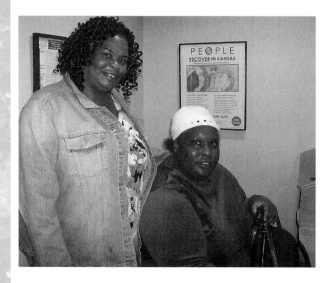

Viola experiences severe pain due to an accident she suffered many years ago. She shares a prayer that illustrates how spirituality provides her with a feeling of hope for the future. In addition, she finds that sharing her story and beliefs allows other people to better understand her situation. (Viola is shown on the right in the photo with her friend Cherie.)

When I was working at a nursing home, I slipped and fell and hurt my back and pelvis. Later, I was in a car accident that reinjured the pelvis. I experience pain unexpectedly. I take pain medicine, but the pain exceeds the medicine. A pain clinic helped me emotionally, but they were not able to get rid of the pain.

People see me everyday, but don't know what I'm going through. It's a challenge for me just to get up and leave my home to go to classes at the mental health center. I decided to write about this so others could understand. My spirituality gives me hope that the pain can go away through a miracle of God. I wrote this prayer in hope for the future. Even if the doctors can't fix you, it's important to know there is a higher power. Here is my prayer:

Dear Jesus, who is my rock, my salvation, my strength, my shield. My prayer is for a miracle to live. The mental and physical pain is too much to bear. I have tried everything I know to get rid of the pain. I tried medicine, diet, heating pads, exercise, talking to people, second opinions, walking, reading my Bible, going to church, laying on hands with prayer, and physical therapy. I tried concentrating only on the good things, not the bad.

Jesus, I still want the pain to go away and never come back. After all these things prayed and done, I still can tell I am only human. It is Jesus who gives hope, faith, blessing, peace, trust, and healing. All these things I learned from my Bible promise book. I learned you give these things freely when I accepted you as Lord and Savior of my life many years ago when I was just a little child, never knowing in the future I would need you so much. I thank you for your Holy Spirit that abides then and still now. I come to you with these prayers to the throne of grace and mercy, Lord. I pray that you hear this prayer for healing of my mind body and soul. Make me brand new. Lord, I know I have purpose here on earth and meaning. Lord, I know you have pain-free written just for me in the lamb book of life. All these words I have written as a prayer to you, Lord Jesus. Set me free from this pain, so I can enjoy life the way I know it can be. Through your son Jesus Christ the Savior, I pray. Amen

On a spirituality level, this prayer lets other people know what I'm going through. I've let others read the prayer, and they were more understanding of my situation, and it made me feel better. Saying the prayer gives me more faith that a miracle can happen. I feel more at ease. I hope the prayer will encourage others that are going through pain. It's something that needed to be told.

---

is easy to administer and score, consumers need to be cognizant of the possible lengthy list of verbal descriptors and may not find a descriptor on the list that is a match for his or her experiences (Jensen, 2007). VRSs are less reliable than other pain intensity measures (Ferraz et al, 1990).

McGill Pain Questionnaire

In addition to intensity, pain has many other dimensions. For example, pain can be described in terms of its temporal (e.g., flickering, throbbing), constrictive (e.g., pinching, pressing), or thermal (e.g., hot, scalding) dimensions, to name a few. The McGill Pain Questionnaire (MPQ; Melzack, 1975) or short-form MPQ (Melzack, 1987) consists of pain descriptors that are classified into 20 categories of pain that can be scored to assess a person's subjective experience of pain across three primary dimensions: sensory, affective, and evaluative, and one miscellaneous category of pain experiences. **Sensory dimensions** of pain include temporal, spatial, pressure, and thermal properties. **Affective dimensions** refer to fear, tension, and autonomic properties. **Evaluative dimensions** are the subjective overall intensity of the pain experience (e.g., annoying, miserable, unbearable).

The MPQ has four components. Part 1 consists of anterior and posterior drawings of the human body. The consumer marks on these drawings the area(s) where he or she feels pain. Part 2 consists of 20 sets of words describing pain. Consumers select one word from each of the sets that best describes his or her pain. These adjectives are ordered from least painful (e.g., "nagging") to most painful (e.g., "torturing"). Part 3 asks how pain has changed over time. Part 4 assesses pain intensity on a 5-point scale from mild to excruciating (Jensen, 2007).

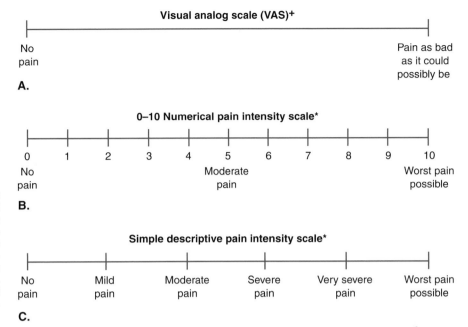

FIGURE 25-2. Examples of Pain Intensity scales. †A 10-cm baseline is recommended for Visual Analogue scales. *If used as a graphic rating scale, a 10-cm baseline is recommended. *From U.S. Department of Health and Human Services, Acute Pain Management Guideline Panel. (1995). Acute Pain Management in Adults: Operative Procedures. Quick Reference Guide for Clinicians. AHCPR Pub. No. 92-0019, Rockville, MD: U.S. Government Printing Office.*

The primary value of the MPQ for clinicians is to identify qualitative features of a consumer's pain experience and to detect subtle clinical changes (Strong et al, 2002). The MPQ has been criticized for its difficult vocabulary and lack of standard scoring format.

Pain Behaviors

Pain behaviors are frequently targeted in assessment. Pain behaviors include complaining about pain, guarded movement, bracing, posturing, limping, rubbing, facial expressions, health-care utilization, and receiving compensation (Fordyce, 2001). The University of Alabama Pain Behavior Scale (UAB; Richards, Nepomuceno, Riles, & Suer, 1982) is a standardized rating scale that is reliable, valid, and an easy method for documenting behaviors. This scale can be used to record the frequency of communication behaviors (verbal/nonverbal complaints, grimacing), mobility behaviors (postural adjustments, use of equipment), and the use of medications. Analysis of a consumer's pain behaviors before, during, and after intervention can provide valuable information about the role of environmental and learned factors in the individual's pain perception, as well as responses to intervention.

Brief Pain Inventory

The Brief Pain Inventory (BPI; Cleeland, 1991) is a reliable and valid instrument that is used to measure pain interference. Consumers rate on an ordinal scale of 0 (*no interference*) to 10 (*complete interference*) to indicate how much their pain has interfered with general activity, mood, mobility, work, interpersonal relationships, sleep, and enjoyment of life. This information can be helpful in determining baseline tolerance levels for specific occupations and participation that may be addressed in treatment as well as measuring change.

Pain Diaries

Paper and electronic pain diaries provide another means for the consumer to communicate his or her unique pain experiences to the health-care team. Because diaries can record pain triggers and temporal patterns, it is useful for the person to make regular entries (e.g., each morning or night or after an episode of pain). Typical entries should record rating of pain intensity, a list of medication taken and its effect, rest time, and satisfaction with pain control, activity level, mood, and recurrent thoughts (Partners Against Pain, n.d.; Turner & Romano, 2001a). Occupational therapists may also want the person to record what they were doing, where they were, and painfree activities throughout the day.

Canadian Occupational Performance Measure

The Canadian Occupational Performance Measure (COPM; Law, Baptiste, Carswell, McColl, Polatajko, & Pollock, 1998) is another valid and reliable measure that can be used in pain assessment. The COPM detects changes over time in the individual's perceptions of his or her occupational performance in the areas of self-care, productivity, and leisure, as well as the importance of being able to perform these occupations and the level of satisfaction with performance using 10-point scales. The COPM is especially helpful in collaborative functional goal setting (Rochman & Kennedy-Spaien, 2007).

Motivational Interviewing

Motivation appears to play an important role in whether people benefit from pain interventions, due to the consumer's need to acquire pain-related coping and self-management skills (Habib, Morrissey, & Helmes, 2005; Osborne, Raichle, & Jensen, 2006). Assessing readiness for change is critical for success. **Motivational interviewing** (MI) is a counseling approach that recognizes that consumers who need to make behavior changes approach intervention at different levels of readiness (Miller & Rollnick, 1991). This nonjudgmental approach attempts to increase the consumer's awareness of potential problems faced by the behavior and to engage them in identifying reasons (motivations) for change.

In MI, the person is challenged to envision how her life may improve by the behavior change. For example, an occupational therapist may ask, How important is it for you to complete (specific activity)? How confident do you feel about doing (activity)? In MI, the therapist provides a therapeutic environment that promotes behavior change through expressing empathy, develops discrepancy between the consumer's current behaviors and goals, avoids argumentation, rolls with resistance, and supports self-efficacy. In addition, the therapist helps the person consider behavior changes by helping him or her to examine the pros and cons of a particular line of action, by reviewing past efforts that have been successful, and by brainstorming and even fantasizing to identify creative solutions. The therapist develops interventions to address the challenges of the consumer's current stage of readiness to change. MI complements interventions used in persistent pain management (e.g., functional restoration) and addresses obstacles that can lead to relapse (Osborne et al, 2006). Information gathered from MI is then incorporated into a specific collaborative treatment plan. (Note that a more extensive discussion of MI is included in Chapter 23.)

Measuring Outcomes

Many of the assessments listed previously can be used to measure the efficacy of pain interventions. Clinical improvement can be measured as gains in occupational performance (as measured by standardized instruments), such as the BPI (Cleeland & Ryan, 1994) or COPM (Law et al, 1998), increased participation (e.g., as measured by increased percent of employment), reduction in pain intensity (e.g., as measured by a NRS or VAS), or elimination of pain behaviors (per UAB). Data from pain diaries could also be used to record increases in activities and social participation. The studies described later in the chapter report on one or more of these outcome measures.

Factors Influencing Pain

The outcome of an effective pain evaluation is a clear understanding of the person, his or her problem situation relative to pain, and the physical and social contexts that may be influencing the person's pain experience. The biopsychosocial model described previously reflects current theories of pain, which argue that pain is not simply the manifestation of an underlying injury or disease process. Contemporary theories of pain, like the biopsychosocial model, are useful for identifying factors that influence pain. For example, low activity levels, poor body mechanics, or inadequate pacing of physical activities can negatively influence the pain experience. Negative thoughts about one's pain experience (e.g., worrying,

ruminating on negative aspects of life, convincing self of worst possible outcome) and reactions to pain (e.g., depression, anger, hopelessness) can make adaptation to chronic pain more difficult. In contrast, increasing tolerance of activity, relaxation training, a positive attitude and focus on capabilities, and developing strategies to proactively manage one's pain are factors that support the adaptive management of pain. Gatchel (2004) suggests that as pain progresses from acute to chronic, factors other than tissue damage become more prominent.

Theoretical Approaches to Pain Management

Pain is a complex and multidimensional problem. The biopsychosocial model introduced previously postulates that the perception of pain is a function of the interplay of physical (e.g., disease, injury), psychological (e.g., anxiety, fear, control), and socioenvironmental (e.g., social supports, role obligations) factors. In the following section, several approaches that compliment a biopsychosocial model are presented. Many of these approaches directly address psychosocial factors that influence the pain experience. The primary goal of these approaches is to reestablish and increase the consumer's occupational roles, occupational performance, and participation *despite* pain.

Behavioral Approaches

Traditional medical and rehabilitative interventions have failed in reducing persistent pain, primarily because of their focus on impairments and body structures, rather than addressing the complexity of the problem (Meldrum, 2003). The behavioral approach to managing persistent pain does not emphasize treating an underlying organic etiology of the pain complaint; rather, it emphasizes involvement in activities and participation through cognitive changes, physical retraining, and environmental adaptations (Morley, Eccleston, & Williams, 1999). Multidisciplinary/interdisciplinary pain programs are goal oriented and integrated with an emphasis on activities and participation (Loeser & Turk, 2001). Because persistent pain is recognized as a multidimensional phenomenon, behavioral techniques are a critical component of comprehensive treatment. Behavioral approaches may involve three types of interventions: respondent or physiological (Fordyce, 1976), operant (Fordyce, 1976), and cognitive behavioral (Turner & Jensen, 1993) strategies.

Respondent or Physiological Strategies

According to Fordyce (1976), pain behavior can be classified as **respondent** if its onset and frequency of occurrence were due to preceding tissue damage. Respondent treatment approaches, therefore, strive to eliminate or reduce tissue irritation or damage. Intervention attempts to directly modify the physiological response system. For example, an individual with muscle contraction (tension) headaches uses biofeedback-assisted relaxation training to learn how to decrease scalp muscle tension, which is a presumed precipitating or exacerbating pain factor (Engel & Rapoff, 1990).

Occupational therapy practitioners can implement therapeutic exercise (Borelli & Warfield, 1986; Caruso, Chan, &

Chan, 1987; McCormack, 1988); relaxation training (Caruso et al, 1987; McCormack, 1988); physical agent modalities such as heat therapy (Breines, 2006; Rochman & Kennedy-Spaien, 2007); splinting (Davis, 1990); adaptive equipment (Borelli & Warfield, 1986; Tyson & Strong, 1990); consumer education in and the application of proper posture, body mechanics, and energy conservation principles for routine activities of daily living (Borelli & Warfield, 1986; Caruso et al, 1987; Rochman & Kennedy-Spaien, 2007); and environmental adaptations (MacRae & Riley, 1990) to eliminate or reduce tissue irritation or damage.

Respondent or physiological interventions may be most appropriate for acute pain conditions, but are not necessarily effective for persistent, nonmalignant painful conditions (Main, Sullivan, Watson, Greasley, & Sjolund, 2007). With acute pain, tissue irritation or damage is apparent, whereas the etiology of persistent nonmalignant pain is not clear.

Operant Strategies

Because pain is a subjective experience, there is no way to empirically measure an individual's pain. When pain occurs, a person's behavioral strategies may include analgesic use, avoidance of specific activities (Woby, Watson, Roach, & Urmston, 2004), and use of compensatory postures (e.g., hyperextend trunk when reaching overhead because of pain) in an attempt to reduce pain. **Operant conditioning** acknowledges that observable expressions of pain are not merely the consequence of impairments in body structure and body functions, but are influenced by the environment. Pain complaints are perpetuated

through increased attention, sympathy, pain medication use, financial compensation, reduced participation (e.g., release from work and social obligations), and other positive reinforcers that follow their occurrence (Main et al, 2007).

Operant intervention, therefore, incorporates learning theory principles with a focus on overt pain behaviors—not the subjective experience of pain (Fordyce, 1976). It is believed that pain interference will be reduced if the individual's well behaviors (e.g., health maintenance) are positively reinforced, especially by significant others, and observable pain behaviors no longer reinforced (Fordyce, 1990; Turner & Romano, 2001).

Outcome measures for operant programs have emphasized return to work, increased activity levels and participation, decreased pain-related health-care utilization, and restoration of well behaviors (Fordyce, 1976; Turk & Rhudy, 1990; Turner & Chapman, 1982b). Common treatment approaches used by occupational therapy practitioners include increasing physical activity through the use of graded activities, reinforcement of well behaviors, and ignoring overt expressions of pain (Fordyce, 1976). Merskey (1992), however, cautioned practitioners not to provide treatment for reducing pain behaviors in lieu of attempts at alleviating pain. Evaluation and intervention that focuses solely on observable pain behaviors can lead to the inaccurate conclusion that pain behaviors suggest malingering, lack of motivation, or hypochondriasis (Merskey, 1992).

Ideally, all members of the multidisciplinary/interdisciplinary pain management team use the same theoretical basis in a consistent manner. Strong (1996) pointed out that the use of operant principles might conflict with traditional occupational therapy interventions. For example, operant pain management programs aim to reduce and eliminate external approaches to pain control, such as adaptive equipment. In addition, the focus of occupational therapists on the meaning of pain in a person's life is not addressed in an operant approach.

Cognitive Behavioral Strategies

Cognitive interventions aim to identify and modify the consumer's thoughts, feelings, beliefs, and attitudes related to pain, disability, and quality of life. It is assumed that an individual's affect and behaviors are greatly influenced by cognitive appraisal, whereby the person interprets events in terms of his or her perceived significance. Cognitions emerge from attitudes and beliefs based on previous experiences (Turner & Chapman, 1982a; Turner & Romano, 2001b). Cognitive behavioral strategies typically aim to identify and change maladaptive cognitions, beliefs, and attitudes about pain and promote the use of adaptive behavioral coping skills training (e.g., cognitive restructuring), relaxation training (with or without biofeedback), imagery, distraction, and hypnosis (Turner & Jensen, 1993; Turner & Romano, 2001b). Cognitive behavioral principles integrate well with those of occupational therapy (see Chapter 19).

The outcome measures for **cognitive behavioral strategies** have emphasized subjective complaints of pain (Turner & Chapman, 1982b). In a variety of populations in which persistent pain is the primary disability (e.g., low back pain), cognitive behavioral interventions have been effective in improving function (Van Tulder et al, 2000).

It is difficult to compare the various behavioral intervention studies due to their different goals and subsequent outcome measures. Respondent or physiological interventions aim to normalize body functions and body structure. Operant interventions strive to increase work, other productive activity levels, and participation. Cognitive behavioral approaches focus on restructuring maladaptive cognitions, beliefs, and attitudes while improving mood (Turner & Chapman, 1982b).

Model of Human Occupation

The Model of Human Occupation (MOHO) conceptualizes the human as a dynamic complex organization of three subsystems: volition, habituation, and performance. According to Kielhofner (2002), these subsystems respectively motivate, organize, and make possible the performance of occupation. Occupational behavior results from the human's interactions with the environment.

Pain regulation strategies based on MOHO strive to improve occupational behavior. Gusich (1984) described in global terms the utility of MOHO in treating adults with persistent pain. Sample treatment goals include the reactivation of interests, the resumption of occupational roles, and the reestablishment of activities and participation (Strong, 1996).

Pain Management

The choice of intervention for pain control depends on objective findings (e.g., abnormal MRI), pain occurrence (e.g., frequency, duration, intensity), and the consumer's overt, covert, and physiological pain responses, in addition to the clinician's training and resources available. A variety of pain control options are available, including pharmacological interventions, surgical interventions, cutaneous stimulation, and occupational therapy interventions.

Pharmacological Interventions

Pharmacological interventions are typically the first pain intervention used due to their effectiveness and ease of use. Medications often provide partial, but not complete, pain relief and increase the individual's level of function. Short-term use of medications is usually safe, but prolonged use increases the likelihood of adverse reactions (American Chronic Pain Association, 2008). Because medications may have different effects on people, the individual should be closely monitored by his or her physician.

Three general categories of medications are used in the management of persistent pain: antidepressants, analgesics, and opioids/narcotics. **Antidepressants** (e.g., amitriptyline, Elavil) have been the most successful in reducing pain symptoms and depressive symptoms that are commonly experienced by individuals with persistent pain (Lynch, 2008).

Analgesics include acetaminophen (Tylenol), aspirin (Bayer), *nonsteroidal anti-inflammatory drugs (NSAIDs)*, ibuprofen (Motrin), and opioids, or narcotics. Acetaminophen is used when there is no inflammation at the pain site and the pain is of mild intensity. Aspirin may also be used in the treatment of mild intensity pain. Excessive use of acetaminophen or aspirin may result in kidney or liver damage. NSAIDs are typically used in acute pain or flare-ups of persistent pain (e.g., pain from osteoarthritis). Daily use of these drugs for an extended period of time can cause kidney damage or ulcers. COX-2

inhibitors (e.g., Celebrex) were developed to reduce those risks, but gastrointestinal bleeding or ulcers can result.

Opioids, or narcotics, are used when antidepressants and analgesics are insufficient. Long-acting opioids (e.g., Oxycodone [OxyContin], Methadone [Dolophine]) may afford better pain control for severe pain, but their long-term use is controversial (American Pain Society, n.d.). Potential side effects include nausea, hormonal effects, gastrointestinal upset, suppression of the immune system, depression, and addiction. Dependence occurs in approximately 5% to 15% of persons with persistent pain (Cluett, 2009). Treatment for substance abuse/dependence should precede rehabilitative chronic pain treatment (Sullivan & Turk, 2001).

The major and minor tranquilizers have been used to control anxiety, which is a precipitating pain factor. The use of marijuana for chronic pain relief is also controversial. Alcohol use is to be avoided. Consumers are encouraged to discuss openly their use of marijuana, alcohol, and other illicit drugs. It should be noted that a consumer's past history of substance abuse/dependence may lead to inadequate analgesia for current pain problems (Flugsrud-Breckenridge, Gevirtz, Paul, & Gould, 2007).

Medication for acute pain should be prescribed in anticipation of pain and to prevent its recurrence. When pain medication is administered regularly and prophylactically in a time contingent manner, the consumer need never experience pain, thereby preventing the occurrence of persistent pain and reducing the need for higher doses of opioids to relieve existing pain.

Surgical Interventions

Surgical pain relief procedures focus on interrupting pain pathways at the peripheral level (e.g., nerve block), spinal level (e.g., cordotomy), and brain level (e.g., stimulating electrodes in the thalamus). Surgical interventions are considered to be a last resort for persistent nonmalignant pain due to the resultant anatomical changes, possible iatrogenic difficulties (e.g., scar tissue with resultant decreased mobility), and the low success rate (Koestler & Meyers, 2002).

Cutaneous Stimulation

Transcutaneous electrical nerve stimulation (TENS), massage, thermotherapy (heat applications), and cryotherapy (cold applications) are often effective in remediating acute pain (Bracciano, 2000). Therapists use physical agent modalities as an adjunct to purposeful activity to promote performance (American Occupational Therapy Association, 2003).

Occupational Therapy Interventions

Occupational therapists provide interventions that address physical, psychosocial, and environmental factors that influence a person's experience of pain and interfere with occupational performance (Engel, 2006a). Because the etiology of pain is multifaceted, the approaches to pain management vary from person to person (Strong, 1996). Evidence-based interventions that address various occupational performance areas are listed here. (Note that the data are specific to the pain population identified for that intervention.)

A therapeutic focus on activity is the cornerstone of occupational therapy (Mosey, 1974). Persons with persistent pain often disengage from routine activities due to a fear of injury or of pain escalation (Strong, 1996; Woby et al, 2004). Therefore, increases in the consumer's activity levels and participation are common goals of chronic pain management programs. Occupational therapy interventions seek to increase the person's satisfaction with and performance of life tasks in multiple occupational roles.

Health maintenance is a primary focus of persistent pain interventions. All multidisciplinary/interdisciplinary team members emphasize functional restoration, psychological well-being, education about mind–body integration, and promotion of wellness, despite the pain (Loeser, 2001). Routines for health maintenance can include physical fitness, graded activities, quota programs, relaxation training, and biofeedback.

Physical Fitness

Exercise therapy is often prescribed for the relief of low back pain (LBP), one of the most frequent persistent pain complaints (Guisch, 1984). The landmark Nuprin Pain Report indicated that more than one half of the adult American population (56%) suffers from back pain each year (Sternberg, 1986). At least 26 million Americans between the ages of 20 and 64 experience recurrent back pain. Back pain is the leading cause of disability in persons younger than age 45 (American Pain Foundation, n.d.).

Frequently, the etiology of LBP is unclear. Trauma to the back, however, through a lifting, twisting, or falling injury is a common initial cause of LBP. Mechanical causes of LBP include poor muscle tone, curvature of the spine, and persistent strain from improper postures (Association for Advancement of Behavior Therapy, 1989). For many individuals who experience mild LBP, the pain typically resolves on its own. For those who seek health-care, most back pain complaints improve within a few months regardless of the treatment (Waddell, 1987). For those persons with persistent (i.e., 12 or more weeks) pain, interference with sleep, routine instrumental activities of daily living, work and other productive activities, and leisure may result and require rehabilitation (Association for Advancement of Behavior Therapy, 1989; Loeser, 2001).

Occupational therapy and physical therapy practitioners ideally collaborate with the consumer in the development and implementation of a reconditioning exercise program. Together, they treat the individual with deficits in neuromuscular performance components, such as range of motion, strength, endurance, and postural alignment. Occupational therapists use exercise to augment purposeful activity and prepare the consumer for performing occupations (Breines, 2006). Exercise, as part of an active rehabilitation program, is a common intervention used to resolve neuromuscular deficits in persons with LBP (Koes, Bouter, Beckerman, van der Heijden, & Knipschild, 1991).

Graded Activities

In conjunction with a physical therapist, an occupational therapist can facilitate increasing an individual's independence in occupational performance. Returning to the example of LBP, because it is conceptualized as a problem of activity intolerance, **graded activity programs** are used to restore function. Graded activities implement a biomechanical approach whereby purposeful activities are graded from low to high in demand with regard to performance components (e.g., range of motion, strength, endurance) (Strong, 1996).

When an individual is engaged in interesting and purposeful activity, he or she may be more relaxed, less preoccupied with the pain, and more fluid in movement. Task selection based on occupational roles, interests, and abilities is a unique contribution of occupational therapy in pain management (Breines, 2006; Heck, 1988; McCormack, 1988; Strong, 1996).

Quota Programs

Fordyce (1976) applied operant conditioning principles to a graded exercise program for persons with persistent pain. An individual's tolerance to activity can be achieved through the use of a **quota system**. Intervention begins with a series of baseline trials in which the individual is asked to perform a demonstrated exercise to tolerance. **Tolerance** is defined as the point at which an individual stops exercising due to pain or fatigue. Detailed baseline performances are recorded. The occupational or physical therapist then establishes a quota for each prescribed exercise to be performed daily. Initial quotas are slightly lower than baseline trials (e.g., approximately 75% of baseline mean) and are increased by predetermined small increments (e.g., about 10% every few days).

Unlike traditional graded activities in which the consumer exercises to tolerance, the individual achieves a quota. Rest breaks are scheduled. Resting at the time of the individual's reported pain onset or exacerbation is avoided because it may reinforce pain behaviors (Fordyce, 1976; Turner & Romano, 2001b). A gradual increase in activity and participation also lessens the likelihood of an exacerbation of pain.

Relaxation Training

Relaxation training is well recognized as a viable intervention for the alleviation of skeletal muscle tension, distraction

---

Evidence-Based Practice

Psychological interventions for chronic low back pain are effective. A meta-analysis of 22 randomized clinical trials (published between 1983 and 2003) evaluated the efficacy of psychological interventions in adults. Psychological interventions had a positive effect on pain intensity, quality of life, levels of depression, and pain-related interference with daily activity. The largest and most consistent effect of these interventions was on reducing pain intensity. Cognitive behavioral and self-regulatory interventions (e.g., biofeedback, relaxation) were found be particularly effective.

➤ Occupational therapists can incorporate psychological interventions in their treatment sessions, particularly cognitive behavioral and relaxation training approaches.

➤ Occupational therapists can share the results of this study with consumers, particularly to give hope that the person can not only learn to live more successfully with pain, but also can use these psychological approaches to reduce pain intensity.

Hoffman, B. M., Papas, R. K., Chatkoff, D. K., & Kerns, R. D. (2007). Meta-analysis of psychological interventions for chronic low back pain. *Health Psychology, 26*(1), 1–9.

from pain, reduction of fatigue, enhancement of additional pain relief measures, relief of anxiety, and elimination of insomnia (National Institutes of Health, 1995).

Many techniques are available for inducing relaxation. Abdominal breathing is the simplest way to encourage relaxation. The learning sequence involves (1) awareness of breathing pattern, (2) inhalation, and (3) slow exhalation (Engel, 2006b). Abdominal breathing is incorporated into the following relaxation techniques.

Progressive muscle relaxation (PMR) is used to relieve excess tension that can result in muscle spasms, pain, and fatigue. PMR involves (1) focusing attention on a muscle group, (2) systematic tensing and relaxing of major musculoskeletal groups for several seconds, (3) passive focusing of attention on how the tensed muscle feels, (4) release of the muscles, and (5) passive focusing on the sensations of relaxation (Bernstein & Borkovec, 1973).

Autogenic training (AT) involves the silent repetition of phrases about homeostasis. AT includes (1) scanning the mind and body for tension, (2) passively concentrating on physical and mental states, and (3) concentrating on cues for relaxation (Luthe, 1965). AT has proven effective in treating persons with tension headaches, substance abuse, and musculoskeletal disorders, in addition to promoting wellness (Payne, 2000).

Guided imagery is the purposeful use of images to reduce stress and distract attention away from intrusive thoughts. In this technique, the participant focuses on a relaxing environment (e.g., a peaceful garden) of his or her choice (Payne, 2000). Meditation (Payne, 2000), massage (De Domenico & Wood, 1997), yoga (Payne, 2000), and physical exercise (Rosch & Hendler, 1982) may also be used as relaxation approaches. Benson's (1975) relaxation response is another effective technique that involves the repetition of a word, prayer, or controlled muscular activity and a vigilant return to the repetition when everyday thoughts interfere with the relaxation process. The intent of this approach is to generate a physiological response characterized by decreased heart rate, metabolism, blood pressure, and rate of breathing (Benson, Beary, & Carol, 1974).

Biofeedback

Biofeedback refers to instrumentation used to provide consumers with feedback of electronically monitored physiological events (Rogers, Shuer, & Herzig, 1984). This intervention assumes a faulty body function is responsible for the pain; the impairment can be controlled when the individual with pain is provided with immediate feedback (Turner & Chapman, 1982a). Biofeedback is often used in conjunction with relaxation training. Skin temperature feedback to increase digital temperature in vascular conditions (e.g., migraine headaches) and electromyogram feedback to lessen muscle tension complaints (e.g., tension headaches) are standard treatments in multi- and interdisciplinary pain clinics.

Relapse Management

Consumers with persistent pain frequently experience an acute pain episode or flare-up that is not related to nociception, or a significant exacerbation of their pain that is activity related. Until the consumer has recovered from the acute episode, aerobic conditioning exercises (e.g., walking, stationary biking, swimming) should be performed on a daily basis to avoid dehabilitation. An incremental, gradual increase in activity should be implemented (Fordyce, 1995). The consumer should be encouraged to increase his or her use of coping and self-management strategies throughout the pain flare-up.

Summary

Evaluation and management of individuals with persistent pain is complex. Occupational therapists have a critical role in the prevention, evaluation, and treatment of persons experiencing persistent pain (International Association for the Study of Pain ad hoc Subcommittee for Occupational Therapy/Physical Therapy Curriculum, 1994). There are individual variances in the way people experience pain, feel about pain, and behaviorally respond to pain. There is not one treatment that works for every person, even for pain that is of the same type and etiology. Chronic pain challenges the mental health of people with physical dysfunction and adds a layer of complexity to interventions with people who have psychiatric illnesses. Use of a biopsychosocial model when evaluating and intervening with persons experiencing pain can help practitioners address pain management holistically. This chapter describes a variety of tools to evaluate a person's experience of pain and a range of treatment interventions that can be used to help people who experience pain continue to participate in productive and satisfying occupations.

Acknowledgment

Supported by grant PO1 ND/NS 33988, "Management of Persistent Pain in Rehabilitation," from the National Institute of Child Health and Human Development and the National Institute of Neurological Disorders and Stroke, National Institutes of Health.

Active Learning Strategies

1. Pain Narrative

Individually or with a partner, identify a person who is experiencing chronic pain or is a family member or primary caregiver for someone who is experiencing chronic pain. Set up a short interview, with the specific goal of eliciting the person's pain narrative. You might begin by asking the person to describe the pain and his or her beliefs about its origins. Specifically, ask how the person has dealt with his or her pain and any reductions in physical activities. Explore positive and negative aspects of the person's interactions and relationships with health-care professions who treat his or her pain symptoms. If your interviewee and you are both comfortable, you might also explore the following topics:

- Relationship between his or her pain experience and self-image
- Impact of his or her pain experience on relationships with family and friends
- Strategies that he or she uses to cope with pain

Share your interview experiences and stories with your peers. Look for similarities and differences between peoples' pain experiences.

Reflective Journal

In your Reflective Journal, consider the following questions: What did you learn about the pain experience and its impact on daily life? What strategies were most useful in managing pain? When comparing your interview with peers, what were common themes among the stories? What experiences were unique to your individual?

2. Pain Self-Assessment

Think back to your most recent pain experience. Rate your pain intensity using the VAS, NRS, and VRS.

Reflective Journal

In your Reflective Journal, identify which scale you prefer and why.

3. Using the COPM as a Pain Interview

Secure a copy of the Canadian Occupational Performance Measure (COPM). You will note that in this semistructured interview, there are no suggested questions that specifically focus on pain or pain management. With a peer, generate questions that could be incorporated into the COPM that would address pain management issues. Be sure to identify at least two questions in each component of the COPM (e.g., productivity, self-care, leisure).

4. Relaxation Techniques

Relaxation techniques are very helpful in controlling pain (Rochman & Kennedy-Spaien, 2007). The more one practices

a technique, the better pain relief is obtained. On a scale of 0 to 10, where 0 equals *completely relaxed* and 10 equals *as tense as can be*, what is your tension level? Go to a quiet dimly lit room to practice the following progressive relaxation exercise:

- Assume a comfortable body position, gently close your eyes, and listen to yourself breathe.
- Breathe in r-e-l-a-x-a-t-i-o-n and exhale t-e-n-s-i-o-n. Take about twice the time to exhale as to inhale.
- Allow your body to be supported.
- Feel your body sink.
- Scan your body for tension indicators.
- Feel the tension leaving your body as you become more r-e-l-a-x-e-d and c-o-m-f-o-r-t-a-b-l-e.
- Inhale and begin by tightening your arms and making fists.
- Study the tension.
- Now exhale, relax, and feel the tension leaving your arms.
- Next inhale and tighten your legs by pointing your toes.
- Now exhale and let your legs go limp with relaxation.
- Inhale and draw your abdominal muscles in, making the abdomen "hard."
- Release your breath and r-e-l-a-x.
- Inhale up into your chest.
- Hold your breath as you tighten your pectorals.
- Exhale, relax, and feel the tension leave your body.
- Inhale and tense your shoulders and back by shrugging.
- Breathe out as you let your shoulders and back relax.
- I-n-h-a-l-e and gently bring your chin toward your chest, hold it, and e-x-h-a-l-e as you relax.
- Breathe in and tense your face by squinting and pursing your lips.
- Exhale and let your face relax.
- Allow the relaxation to spread throughout your body.
- Be aware of how much more relaxed and comfortable you feel.
- As you return to your normal level of awareness, concentrate on bringing these feelings of deep relaxation and comfort back with you.
- Gradually open your eyes and stretch.

Using the 0-to-10 scale again, how tense do you feel now? What parts of your body feel more relaxed?

Reflective Journal

In your Reflective Journal, discuss your personal response to the exercise. Where you able to relax? Why or why not? What other methods/activities provide relaxation for you?

Resources

- The Psychological Management of Chronic Pain: www.continuingedcourses.net/active/courses/course016.php This is an online course approved for continuing education by the American Psychological Association, Association of Social Work Boards, and several other discipline-specific boards. It is designed for mental health professionals and provides a clear overview of contemporary theories of pain and pain management. It reviews evaluation and intervention planning with a clear focus on psychological interventions.
- National Center for Health Statistics. (2006). *Health, United States, 2006, With Chartbook on Trends in the Health of Americans.* DHHS Pub No. 2006-1232. Washington, DC: U.S. Government Printing Office. www.cdc.gov/nchs/data/hus/hus06.pdf This document represents the 30th report on the health status of the United States. The Secretary of the Department of Health and Human Services submits similar reports to the president and Congress regularly. This lengthy (559-page) report uses statistics from the National Center for Health Statistics (NCHS) and the Centers for Disease Control and Prevention (CDC) to provide a global picture of the health of the U.S. population. A 22-page special feature on pain provides a contemporary review of prevalence, a review of health-care treatment, and some discussion of effective interventions.
- International Association for the Study of Pain (IASP): www.iasp-pain.org/ The IASP is an international professional forum dedicated to advancing science, practice, and education in the field of pain. The IASP's official journal is *PAIN*, which is the premier journal on the subject of pain. You cannot access the journal from this site without a membership, but you do have access to *Pain: Clinical Updates*, which are short (4-page) briefs designed to disseminate contemporary information on therapeutic interventions for pain.
- The Oxford Pain Internet Site Pain Research at Oxford: www.medicine.ox.ac.uk/bandolier/booth/painpag/index2.html Based in Oxford, UK, this site disseminates evidence-based information on pain. The page includes many downloadable essays on a multitude of pain topics. The research group at Oxford has produced more than 100 systematic reviews on topics related to pain.

References

American Chronic Pain Association (ACPA). (2008). "ACPA Chronic Pain Medications Supplement 2008." Rockland, CA: Author. Available at: www.theacpa.org/documents/ACPA%20Chronic%20Pain%20Medications%20Supplement%202008.pdf (accessed December 16, 2009).

American Occupational Therapy Association (AOTA). (2003). Physical agent modalities: A position paper. *American Journal of Occupational Therapy, 57,* 650–651.

American Pain Foundation. (n.d.). "Pain Facts & Figures." Last updated July 8, 2009. Available at: www.painfoundation.org/newsroom/reporter-resources/pain-facts-figures.html (accessed December 16, 2009).

American Pain Society. (n.d.). "Advocacy—The Use of Opioids for the Treatment of Chronic Pain: A Consensus Statement from American Academy of Pain Medicine and American Pain Society." Available at: www.ampainsoc.org/advocacy/opioids.htm (accessed December 16, 2009).

Association for Advancement of Behavior Therapy (AABT). (1989, October). "Fact Sheet on Low Back Pain." New York: Author. Available at: http://horan.asu.edu/ced522readings/aabt/lowbackpain.htm (accessed December 16, 2009).

Bair, M. J., Robinson, R. L., Katon, W., & Kroenke, K. (2003). Depression and pain comorbidity: A literature review. *Archives of Internal Medicine, 163,* 2433–2445.

Baptiste, S. (1988). Persistent pain, activity, and culture. *Canadian Journal of Occupational Therapy, 55,* 179–184.

Benson, H. (1975). *The Relaxation Response.* New York: Avon Books.

Benson, H., Beary, J. F., & Carol, M. P. (1974). The relaxation response. *Psychiatry, 37,* 37–45.

Bernstein, D. A., & Borkovec, T. D. (1973). *Progressive Relaxation Training: A Manual for the Helping Professions.* Champaign, IL: Research Press.

Borelli, E. F., & Warfield, C. A. (1986). Occupational therapy for persistent pain. *Hospital Practice, 21*(8), 36–37.

Bracciano, A. G. (2000). *Physical Agent Modalities: Theory and Application for the Occupational Therapist.* Thorofare, NJ: Slack.

Breines, E. B. (2006). Therapeutic occupations and modalities. In H. M. Pendleton & W. Schultz-Krohn (Eds.), *Pedretti's Occupational Therapy: Practice Skills for Physical Dysfunction* (6th ed., pp. 658–679). St. Louis, MO: Mosby.

Bruera, E., Kuehn, N., Miller, M., Selmser, P., & MacMillan, K. (1991). The Edmonton Symptom Assessment System (ESAS): A simple method for the assessment of palliative care consumers. *Journal of Palliative Care, 1,* 6–9.

Caruso, L. A., Chan, D. E., & Chan, A. (1987). The management of work-related back pain. *American Journal of Occupational Therapy, 41,* 112–117.

Cleeland, C. S. (1991). Research in cancer pain: What we know and what we need to know. *Cancer, 67,* 823–827.

Cleeland, C. S., & Ryan, K. M. (1994). Pain assessment: Global use of the Brief Pain Inventory. *Annals of the Academy of Medicine, 23,* 129–138.

Cluett, J. (2009). "Types of Pain Medications." Available at: http://orthopedics.about.com/od/medicati3/p/medications.htm (accessed February 16, 2010).

Davis, J. (1990). The role of the occupational therapist in the treatment of shoulder-hand syndrome. *Occupational Therapy Practice, 1*(3), 30–38.

De Domenico, G., & Wood, E. C. (1997). *Beard's Massage* (4th ed.). Philadelphia: W.B. Saunders.

Engel, J. M. (2006a). Evaluation and pain management. In H. M. Pendleton & W. Schultz-Krohn (Eds.), *Pendretti's Occupational Therapy: Practice Skills for Physical Dysfunction* (6th ed., pp. 646–655). St. Louis, MO: Mosby Elsevier.

Engel, J. M. (2006b). Relaxation and related techniques. In D. Hertling & R. M. Kessler (Eds.), *Management of Common Musculoskeletal Disorders: Physical Therapy Principles and Methods* (4th ed., pp. 261–266). Philadelphia: Lippincott Williams & Wilkins.

Engel, J. M., & Rapoff, M. A. (1990). Biofeedback-assisted relaxation training for adult and pediatric headache disorders. *Occupational Therapy Journal of Research, 10,* 283–299.

Farrar, J. T., Portenoy, R. K., Berlin, J. A., Kinman, J. L., & Strom, B. L. (2000). Defining the clinically important difference in pain outcome measures. *Pain, 88,* 287–294.

Ferraz, M. B., Quaresma, M. R., Aquino, L. R., Atra, E., Tugwell, P., & Goldsmith, C. H. (1990). Reliability of pain scales in the assessment of literate and illiterate consumers with rheumatoid arthritis. *Journal of Rheumatology, 17,* 1022–1024.

Fishman, S. M. (2004, January). "Q&A About Pain: Fifth Vital Sign." Available at: www.painfoundation.org/learn/library/qa/fifth-vital-sign.html (accessed December 16, 2009).

Flugsrud-Breckenridge, M. R., Gevirtz, C., Paul, D., & Gould, H. J. III. (2007). Medications of abuse in pain management. *Current Opinion in Anaesthesiology, 20,* 319–324.

Fordyce, W. E. (1976). *Behavioral Methods for Persistent Pain and Illness.* St. Louis, MO: Mosby.

Fordyce, W. E. (1990). Contingency management. In J. J. Bonica (Ed.), *The Management of Pain* (2nd ed., pp. 1702–1710). Philadelphia: Lea & Febiger.

Fordyce, W. E. (1995). *Back Pain in the Workplace: Management of Disability in Nonspecific Conditions*. Seattle: IASP Press.

Fordyce, W. E. (2001). Learned pain: Pain as behavior. In J. D. Loeser, S. H. Butler, C. R. Chapman, & D. C. Turk (Eds.), *Bonica's Management of Pain* (3rd ed., pp. 478-482). Philadelphia: Lippincott Williams & Wilkins.

Gatchel, R.J. (2004). Comorbidity of chronic pain and mental health disorders. *American Psychologist, 59*, 795–805.

Gusich, R. L. (1984). Occupational therapy for persistent pain: A clinical application of the model of human occupation. *Occupational Therapy in Health Care, 1*, 59–73.

Habib, S., Morrissey, S., & Helmes, E. (2005). Preparing for pain management: A pilot study to enhance engagement. *Journal of Pain, 6*(1), 48–54.

Hamdy, R. C. (2001). The decade of pain control and research (editorial). *Southern Medical Journal, 94*(8), 753–754.

Heck, S. A. (1988). The effect of purposeful activity on pain tolerance. *American Journal of Occupational Therapy, 42*, 577–581.

International Association for the Study of Pain (IASP) (2007). IASP terminology. http://www.iasp-pain.org/AM/Template.cfm?Section=General_Resource_Links&Template=/CM/HTMLDisplay.cfm&ContentID=3058#Pain (retrieved February 16, 2010).

International Association for the Study of Pain ad hoc Subcommittee for Occupational Therapy/Physical Therapy Curriculum. (1994). Pain curriculum for students in occupational therapy or physical therapy. *IASP Newsletter, November/December*, 3–8.

Jensen, M. P. (2007). Pain assessment in clinical trials. In D. Carr & H. Wittink (Eds.), *Evidence Outcomes, and Quality of Life in Pain Treatment* (pp. 281–288). Amsterdam: Elsevier.

Jensen, M. P., & Karoly, P. (2001). Self-report scales and procedures for assessing pain in adults. In D. C. Turk & R. Melzack (Eds.), *Handbook of Pain Assessment* (2nd ed., pp. 15–34). New York: Guilford Press.

Kielhofner, G. (2002). *Model of Human Occupation: Theory and Application* (3rd ed.). Philadelphia: Lippincott Williams & Wilkins.

Koes, B. W., Bouter, L. M., Beckerman, H., van der Heijden, G. J. M. G., & Knipschild, P. G. (1991). Physiotherapy exercises and back pain: A blinded review. *British Medical Journal, 302*, 1572–1576.

Koestler, A. J., & Myers, A. (2002). *Understanding Chronic Pain*. Jackson: University Press of Mississippi.

Law, M., Baptiste, S., Carswell, A., McColl, M. A., Polatajko, H., & Pollock, N. (1998). *Canadian Occupational Performance Measure* (3rd ed.). Ottawa, Canada: CAOT Publications ACE.

LeResche, L. (2001). Gender, cultural, and environmental aspects of pain. In J. D. Loeser, S. H. Butler, C. R. Chapman, & D. C. Turk (Eds.), *Bonica's Management of Pain* (3rd ed., pp. 191–195). Philadelphia: Lippincott Williams & Wilkins.

Loeser, J. D. (2001). Multidisciplinary/interdisciplinary pain assessment. In J. D. Loeser, S. H. Butler, C. R. Chapman, & D. C. Turk (Eds.), *Bonica's Management of Pain* (3rd ed., pp. 363–367). Philadelphia: Lippincott Williams & Wilkins.

Loeser, J. D., & Fordyce, W. (1983). Chronic pain. In J. E. Carr & H. A. Dengerink (Eds.), *Behavioral Science in the Practice of Medicine* (pp. 331–345). New York: Elsevier.

Loeser, J. D., & Turk, D. C. (2001). Multidisciplinary/interdisciplinary pain management. In J. D. Loeser, S. H. Butler, C. R. Chapman, & D. C. Turk (Eds.), *Bonica's Management of Pain* (3rd ed., pp. 2069–2079). Philadelphia: Lippincott Williams & Wilkins.

Luthe, W. (1965). *Autogenic Training*. New York: Grune & Stratton.

Lynch, M. E. (2008). The pharmacotherapy of chronic pain. *Rheumatic Disease Clinics of North America, 34*(2), 369–385.

MacRae, A., & Riley, E. (1990). Home health occupational therapy for the management of pain: An environmental model. *Occupational Therapy Practice 1*(3), 69–76.

Main, C. J., Sullivan, M. J. L., Watson, P. J., Greasley, K., & Sjolund, B. H. (2007). *Pain Management: Practical Applications of the Biopsychosocial Perspective in Clinical and Occupational Settings*. Edinburgh: Elsevier Churchill Livingstone.

McCormack, G. L. (1988). Pain management by occupational therapists. *American Journal of Occupational Therapy, 42*, 582–590.

Meldrum, M. L. (2003). A capsule history of pain management. *Journal of the American Medical Association, 290*(18), 2470–2475.

Melzack, R. (1975). The McGill Pain Questionnaire: Major properties and scoring methods. *Pain, 1*, 277–299.

Melzack, R. (1987). The short-form McGill Pain Questionnaire. *Pain, 33*, 191–197.

Merskey, H. (1992). Limitations of pain behavior. *APS, 1*, 101–104.

Miller, W. R., & Rollnick, S. (1991). *Motivational Interviewing: Preparing People to Change Addictive Behavior*. New York: Guilford Press.

Morley, S., Eccleston, C., & Williams, A. (1999). Systematic review and meta-analysis of randomized controlled trials of cognitive behaviour therapy and behaviour therapy for persistent pain in adults, excluding headache. *Pain, 80*, 1–13.

Mosey, A. C. (1974). An alternative: The biopsychosocial model. *American Journal of Occupational Therapy, 28*, 137–140.

National Center for Health Statistics. (2006). *Health, United States, 2006, With Chartbook on Trends in the Health of Americans*. DHHS Pub No. 2006-1232. Washington, DC: U.S. Government Printing Office. Available at: www.cdc.gov/nchs/data/hus/hus06.pdf (accessed May 20, 2009).

National Institutes of Health. (1995, October 16). "Integration of Behavioral and Relaxation Approaches into the Treatment of Persistent Pain and Insomnia." NIH Technology Assessment Conference Statement..

Osborne, T. L., Raichle, K. A., & Jensen, M. P. (2006). Psychologic interventions for chronic pain. *Physical Medicine and Rehabilitation Clinics of North America, 17*, 415–433.

Partners Against Pain. (n.d.). Pain Management Kit. Available at: www.partnersagainstpain.com/professional-tools/pain-diaries.aspx?id=3 (accessed December 16, 2009).

Payne, R. A. (2000). *Relaxation Techniques: A Practical Handbook for the Health Care Professional* (2nd ed.). New York: Churchill Livingstone.

Richards, J. S., Nepomuceno, C., Riles, M., & Suer, Z. (1982). Assessing pain behavior: The UAB Pain Behavior Scale. *Pain, 14*(4), 393–398.

Rochman, D., & Kennedy-Spaien, E. (2007). Chronic pain management: Approaches and tools for occupational therapy (electronic version). *OT Practice, 12*(13), 9–15.

Rogers, S. R., Shuer, J., & Herzig, S. (1984). The use of biofeedback techniques in occupational therapy for persons with persistent pain. *Occupational Therapy in Health Care, 1*(3), 103–108.

Rosch, P. J., & Hendler, N. H. (1982). Stress management. In R. B. Taylor, J. R. Ureda, & J. W. Denham (Eds.), *Health Promotion: Principles and Clinical Applications* (pp. 339–371). Norwalk, CT: Appleton-Century-Crofts.

Sternberg, R. A. (1986). Survey of pain in the United States: The Nuprin Pain Report. *Clinical Journal of Pain, 2*, 49–53.

Strong, J. (1996). *Persistent Pain: The Occupational Therapist's Perspective*. New York: Churchill Livingstone.

Strong, J., Sturgess, J., Unruh, A. M., & Vicenzino, B. (2002). Pain assessment and measurement. In J. Strong, A. M. Unruh, A. Wright, & G. D. Baxter (Eds.), *Pain: A Textbook for Therapists* (pp. 123–147). New York: Churchill Livingstone.

Sullivan, M. D., & Turk, D. C. (2001). Psychiatric illness, depression, and psychogenic pain. In J. D. Loeser, S. H. Butler, C. R. Chapman, & D. C. Turk (Eds.), *Bonica's Management of Pain* (3rd ed., pp. 483–500). Philadelphia: Lippincott Williams & Wilkins.

Turk, D. C., Dworkin, R. H., Allen, R. R., Bellamy N., Brandenburg, N., Carr, D. B., Cleeland, C., Dionne, R., Farrar, J. T., Galer, B. S., Hewitt, D. J., Jadad, A. R., Katz, N. P., Kramer, L. D., Manning, D. C., McCormick, C. G., McDermott, M. P., McGrath, P., Quessy, S., Rappaport, B. A., Robinson, J. P., Royal, M. A., Simon, L., Stauffer, J. W., Stein, W., Tollett, J., & Witter. J. (2003). Core outcome domains for persistent pain clinical trials: IMMPACT recommendations. *Pain, 106*, 337–345.

Turk, D. C., & Melzack, R. (1992). The measurement of pain and the assessment of people experiencing pain. In D. C. Turk & R. Melzack (Eds.), *Handbook of Pain Assessment* (pp. 3–14). New York: Guilford Press.

Turk, D. C., & Rhudy, T. E. (1990). Neglected factors in persistent pain treatment outcomes studies—Referral patterns, failure to enter treatment and attrition. *Pain, 43*, 7–25.

Turner, J. A., & Chapman, C. R. (1982a). Psychological interventions for persistent pain: A critical review. I. Relaxation training and biofeedback. *Pain, 12*, 1–21.

Turner, J. A., & Chapman, C. R. (1982b). Psychological interventions for persistent pain: A critical review. II. Operant conditioning, hypnosis, and cognitive-behavioral therapy. *Pain, 12*, 23–46.

Turner, J. A., & Jensen, M. P. (1993). Efficacy of cognitive therapy for persistent low back pain. *Pain, 52*, 169–177.

Turner, J. A., & Romano, J. M. (2001a). Psychological and psychosocial evaluation. In J. D. Loeser, S. H. Butler, C. R. Chapman, & D. C. Turk (Eds.), *Bonica's Management of Pain* (3rd ed., pp. 329–341). Philadelphia: Lippincott Williams & Wilkins.

Turner, J. A., & Romano, J. M. (2001b). Cognitive behavioral therapy for chronic pain. In J. D. Loeser, S. H. Butler, C. R. Chapman, & D. C. Turk (Eds.), *Bonica's Management of Pain* (3rd ed., pp. 1751–1758). Philadelphia: Lippincott Williams & Wilkins

Tyson, R., & Strong, J. (1990). Adaptive equipment: Its effectiveness for people with persistent lower back pain. *Occupational Therapy Journal of Research, 10*, 111–121.

Unruh, A. M., Strong, J., & Wright, A. (2002). Introduction to pain. In J. Strong, A. M. Unruh, A. Wright, & G. D. Baxter (Eds.), *Pain: A Textbook for Therapists* (pp. 3–11). New York: Churchill Livingstone.

United States Department of Health and Human Services (USDHHS), Centers for Disease Control and Prevention (CDC). (2009). Summary health statistics for U.S. adults: National Health Interview Survey, 2008. DHHS Publication No. (PHS) 2010-157-. Hyattsville, MD: USDHHS.

Van Tulder, M. W., Jellema, P., van Poppel, M. N. M., et al. (2000). Lumbar supports for prevention and treatment of low back pain (Cochrane Review). In *The Cochrane Library*, Issue 4. Oxford: Update Software.

Waddell, G. (1987). A new clinical model for the treatment of low back pain. *Spine, 12*, 632–644.

Waddell, G., & Burton, A. K. (2005). Concepts of rehabilitation for the management of low back pain. *Best Practice & Research Clinical Rheumatology, 19*(4), 655–670.

Woby, S., Watson, P., Roach, N., & Urmston, M. (2004). Adjustment to chronic low back pain—The relative influence of fear-avoidance beliefs, catastrophizing, and appraisals of control. *Behavior Research and Therapy, 42*, 761–775.

Environment

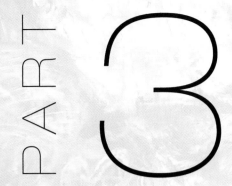

This part of the text is divided into two sections: the lived environment and practice settings. Although recognized as important by occupational therapists, the environmental component of the person-environment-occupation model has received the least attention. The lived environment section of the text aims to correct this neglect by providing the mental health practitioner with an explicit understanding of the environment and its impact on occupational performance, specific environmental assessments, and interventions aimed at creating a supportive environment. The setting section is devoted to the places that occupational therapists work, including settings with either a primary or secondary focus on mental health practice. Some of these settings are emerging areas of practice that have received little attention in previous texts. Each chapter includes a general description of the setting with information on the needs of the population served. The role of occupational therapy as well as assessment and interventions common to that setting are described.

CHAPTER

26

Introduction to the Environment

Catana Brown

> *You are a product of your environment. So choose the environment that will best develop you toward your objective. Analyze your life in terms of its environment. Are the things around you helping you toward success—or are they holding you back?*
>
> —Clement Stone

Introduction

Most people have experienced a situation in which lack of transportation hindered their activity. Perhaps their car was being repaired or someone had borrowed it. Maybe the weather prohibited them from driving or using public transportation. Such situations are temporary, but the same is not true for many people with serious mental illness. Lack of transportation is one of many environmental barriers that interfere with community participation.

Transportation is a common problem for people with mental illness. Most people with serious mental illness live in poverty (another environmental barrier) and are unable to pay for a car and the associated expenses. In addition, public transportation is limited or nonexistent in many communities. When it is available, public transportation may be expensive or difficult for someone with serious mental illness to manage.

Think about all of the trips you have taken from home in the past week. How would your activities have been different without a means of transportation? Would you have been able to get to work or school? Could you have gone to the grocery store and transported your groceries? What about visiting your friends, going to a movie, attending church, returning a book to the library, or getting to a doctor's appointment? Transportation, which most of us take for granted, can have a significant impact on the roles we assume, the social contacts we make, the places we go, and how we create our own personal routines of daily life.

It is common to think that the symptoms and impairments associated with mental illness are the reasons that many people with mental illness are restricted when it comes to participating in community life. Although depression, anxiety, psychosis, and cognitive deficits are certainly relevant for occupational performance, the environment has received very little attention as a component of the person-environment-occupation dynamic in understanding and providing interventions for people with serious mental illness. Cohen (2000) argues that psychiatry's emphasis on biological models has trivialized the importance of the social realm. Consequently, current methods for explaining and treating mental disorders are inadequate. People with serious mental illness have higher rates of unemployment, homelessness, poverty, and incarceration than the general population. Typically, mental illness is seen as the "cause" of these social conditions, but the relationship is not so simple; social factors can directly influence neurological functioning and impact the outcome and course of a mental disorder. More research that compares people with and without mental illness in similar social situations is warranted to better determine the impact of mental illness on community living.

This chapter introduces the environment as the context in which occupations are performed. It describes different components of the environment and explores environmental barriers that present common concerns for people with mental illness. The chapter also outlines environmental resources that support participation for people with serious mental illness. Part III, Section 2, includes chapters about environments and their impact on people with mental illness, and Section 3 contains chapters about practice settings in which occupational therapists work and address mental health issues.

Environment and Occupational Therapy

In occupational therapy and other disciplines, there is an increasing appreciation for the importance of the **environment**, and major conceptual models emphasize the importance of the environment in understanding occupational performance. For example, the Ecology of Human Performance model considers performance to be an outcome of the transactional process of the person, context (or environment), and task (Dunn, Brown, & McGuigan, 1994). One purpose for the model's development was to provide a framework by which occupational therapists and other members of disciplines could assess and design interventions that targeted the environment. In the Occupational Adaptation model, the environment demands mastery from the person, and the person's engagement with the environment results in an adaptive response (Schkade & Schultz, 1992). The Person-Environment-Occupation model (Law et al, 1996) views occupational performance as the convergence of the individual, the occupation and the environment. In this model, successful occupational performance is dependent on the fit of the person, occupation, and environment (see Chapter 3).

Components of the Environment

In 2002, the American Occupational Therapy Association published *Occupational Therapy Practice Framework: Domain and Process*, which describes seven environments, or contexts:

- Cultural
- Physical
- Social
- Spiritual
- Personal
- Temporal
- Virtual

The second edition of *Occupational Therapy Practice Framework* (AOTA, 2008) includes spirituality as a client factor and does not include a spiritual environment. This textbook discusses spirituality as both an occupation and an environment. The seven contexts are discussed in the following sections, and the different aspects of the environments are explained in greater detail in subsequent chapters.

Cultural Context

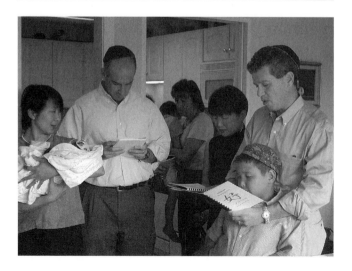

The **cultural context** includes the beliefs and behavioral expectations of the society. As occupational therapists, it is important to understand how the cultural environment influences the occupational performance of individual clients, appreciate how culture interacts with specific aspects of psychiatric disability, and recognize health care disparities that exist across cultures. For example, gender roles differ across cultures, as does the role of the family in caring for an ill individual. In addition, the incidence and manifestation of specific mental disorders can vary by culture; eating disorders are more common in Western cultures and in occupations where thinness is highly valued (e.g., modeling and ballet dancing) (APA, 2000). Finally, a significant disparity exists in access to and quality of mental health care for minority populations, which was described in an important Surgeon General's Report on mental health (USDHHS, 2001). The cultural context is more fully described in Chapter 30.

Physical Context

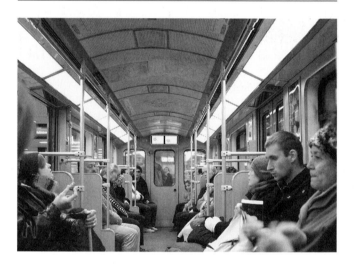

Both the manmade and the natural environments make up the **physical context**. The physical context includes large features, such as buildings and terrain, as well as smaller items, such as plants and tools. The impact of the physical environment is often ignored in psychiatric disabilities, but its influence should not be overlooked. The complexity of the modern world can create additional challenges for people with psychiatric disabilities, particularly those with cognitive impairments, such as dementia, attention deficit disorder, and schizophrenia. For example, a cluttered and noisy classroom can interfere with success in school for a child with attention deficit disorder, and an older adult with dementia is more likely to get lost and have difficulty engaging in activities of daily living when in an unfamiliar physical environment. Some evidence suggests that the physical environment can contribute to the etiology of mental illness; for example, a higher incidence of psychotic disorders occurs in urban settings, which may be attributed to the stress of city life (Eaton, Mortensen, & Frydenberg, 2000).

The physical environment is also of interest to occupational therapists because of its sensory qualities. An analysis

of the physical environment is therefore essential to the development of interventions focused on sensory processing concerns.

The physical environment is described more fully in Chapters 32 and 33.

Social Context

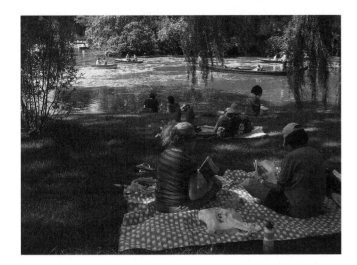

The **social context** is made up of relationships with individuals, groups, and organizations. Social support is crucial for good mental health, and several aspects of social support have been studied in relation to mental health. The size of an individual's social network is related to mental health. In a large study by Brugha et al (2005), a primary group (friends and family) size of three or fewer was predictive of diminished mental health.

However, it is not just the size of the social network but also the quality of the social support that is important. For example, Bertera (2005) found that negative relationships with family and friends are associated with an increase in anxiety and mood disorders. The extensive literature on expressed emotions in families finds that individuals with schizophrenia or mood disorders are two to three times more likely to relapse if they live in a family that is hostile, critical, and controlling (Hooley, 2004).

Equally important is what makes up a good social relationship. In a qualitative study by Rebeiro (2001), women with mental illness reported that an affirming social environment was important for occupational performance. The affirming environment was described as one in which sympathetic others are present and one is accepted, one's self-worth is acknowledged, and there is a safe place to belong.

The social environment is larger than friends and family. Groups and institutions can also provide either supports or barriers to people with mental illness. Some groups exclude people with mental illness and may engage in subtle or overt discriminatory practices. Other groups offer important services, a place to belong, or a sanctuary. Some of the relevant social groups to consider include schools, clubs and social centers, faith-based organizations, health care systems, and social service agencies. The social environment also includes the political world, such as legislative bodies

and court systems. Policies related to deinstitutionalization, psychiatric commitment, the Americans with Disabilities Act (ADA), and social security all have a great impact on people with mental illness in both negative and positive ways. For example, deinstitutionalization resulted in less unnecessary hospitalization but also contributed to higher rates of homelessness.

The social context is more fully described in Chapters 27, 28, and 29.

Spiritual Context

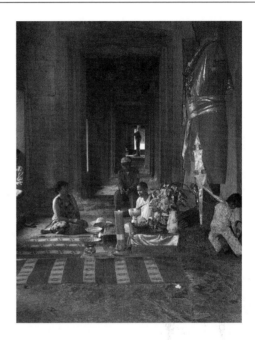

The **spiritual context** is a connection to the sacred that provides the underlying inspiration and motivation for one's life. An extensive literature review indicates that involvement in religious or spiritual practices is associated with better physical and mental health (George et al, 2002). Until recently, mental health practitioners often avoided and even discouraged discussion of spiritual topics with people with mental illness. In some cases, the practitioner was uncomfortable with the topic, and in others, there was a concern that religious ideations and delusions might be furthered. Although the spiritual context is still neglected, this view is changing.

The recovery model itself is recognized as a spiritual process, and recovery-oriented services are increasingly more likely to address the spiritual context. Even if service providers are slow to embrace spirituality, individuals with mental illness are not. One study found that the most common alternative health-care practices utilized by people with serious mental illness were religious/spiritual practices and meditation (Russinova, Wewiorski, & Cash, 2002). Furthermore, a central component of 12-step programs for addictions (e.g., Alcoholics Anonymous) is recognition that a higher power is essential to the recovery process. The spiritual context is more fully described in Chapter 31.

Studies have found that the most common alternative health care practices utilized by people with serious mental illness are religious/spiritual practices and meditation (Russinova, Wewioski & Cash, 2002). In addition, involvement in religious or spiritual practices is associated with better physical and mental health (George et al, 2002).

➤ Occupational therapists should evaluate the spiritual environment of their clients. Are spiritual practices important to the individual? Does the individual have the social and organizational/institutional supports he or she needs to engage in spiritual practices?

➤ Consider ways that you can promote spiritual environments for your client. Identify spiritual organizations in your community that are accepting and understanding of people with mental illness. Advocate for inclusive practices and/or provide the needed education at faith-based organizations.

George, L. K., Larson, D. B., Koenig, H. G., & McCullough, M. E. (2000). Spirituality and health: What we know, what we need to know. *Journal of Social and Clinical Psychology, 19*(1), 102–116.

Russinova, Z., Wewiorski, N. J., & Cash, D. (2002) Use of alternative health care practices by persons with serious mental illness: Perceived benefits. *American Journal of Public Health, 92,* 1600–1603.

Personal, Temporal, and Virtual Contexts

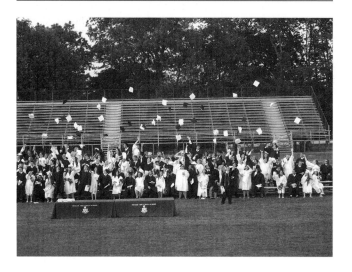

The *Occupational Therapy Practice Framework* (AOTA, 2008) includes three aspects of context that are not commonly discussed in descriptions of the environment: personal, temporal, and virtual. The **personal context** includes age, gender, socioeconomic and educational status, and the like. Although demographic characteristics are different from the health condition, they interact with mental health conditions. For example, the age of onset and course of particular mental disorders affect occupational performance. Attention deficit-hyperactivity disorder can be particularly challenging to successful school performance, and the onset of schizophrenia in early adulthood can interfere with establishing roles as a worker, spouse, and/or parent. Some disorders are more common in females (e.g., depression and borderline

personality disorder), and others are more common in males (e.g., autism and substance abuse). Socioeconomic status has a transactional relationship with serious mental illness in that people from lower socioeconomic groups are more likely to be diagnosed with a serious mental illness. Once diagnosed with a serious mental illness, an individual is more likely to experience a drop in socioeconomic status.

The **temporal context** refers to stage of life as well as time of day, year, and duration. Time of year is related to depression, as depression increases during the winter when there are fewer hours of sunshine. In bipolar disorder, some evidence suggests that disruptions in daily patterns, particularly morning routines, are associated with an increase in symptoms (Ashman et al, 1999).

The **virtual environment** is a new consideration for the environment. The Internet, chat rooms, text messaging, and other forms of virtual communication provide many opportunities for social connection, information gathering, and leisure pursuits. Yet some people with mental illness are often excluded from this environment due to limited access to electronic media.

The consumer movement and the resulting recognition of people with psychiatric disability as a minority group has revealed that people with psychiatric disability face discrimination in virtually all sectors of society.

Environmental Obstacles to Recovery and Empowerment

People with mental illness are frequently confronted with environmental barriers that may be less common or even nonexistent for the general population. In many cases, for people with mental illness, difficulty in successfully performing job tasks is related more to these environmental stumbling blocks than to the symptoms or deficits associated with the illness.

Attitudinal Barriers

One of the greatest environmental barriers that people with mental illness face is stigma and discrimination. The general public widely endorses stigmatizing attitudes toward people with mental illness, and stereotypes persist even in highly trained mental health professionals (Corrigan, 2000), such as occupational therapists. Although most of the literature related to stigma and psychiatric disability focuses on serious mental illness such as schizophrenia, there is also evidence of discrimination in other mental illnesses, such as depression (Kelly & Jorm, 2007) and anorexia nervosa (Mond, Robertson-Smith, & Vetere, 2006). Stigma can lead to discrimination at both the person and the public policy levels. For example, landlords are less likely to lease apartments to people with mental illness (Page, 1995), and the lack of parity between health-care coverage of physical and mental illnesses can be seen as a form of discrimination.

Individuals with "invisible disabilities" such as mental illness face unique challenges. For example, the stigma associated with mental illness can present a significant conundrum when it comes to disclosing the disability for employment accommodations. If the individual chooses to disclose a psychiatric disability, he or she risks alienation and questions of

The Lived Experience

Ron Nicholls

Ron describes his experiences with obsessive compulsive disorder. Notice how the environment influences his obsessions. Particular cues in the environment elicit the obsessions, and some environments are more challenging than others.

I am a 58-year-old American male in very good physical health. My education level I consider to be above average. As previously mentioned, my physical health is very good, but my mental health is not so lucky. In my studies of psychology I learned that I had OCD (obsessive compulsive disorder). After evaluating the situation, I was able to trace my OCD back at least twenty years (to age 20). I was at the time turning 40 years of age. What I am trying to stress is that I suffered OCD for at least twenty years without knowing that I had it. Until I studied about it in psychology, I had no idea what it even was. Even though there are a number of anti-OCD medications on the market in my case they have been very ineffective.

It is very important to understand that, to the uncontrolled OCD personality, the OCD controls the life of this person. Once the obsession enters their mind, it takes complete control over this person, often leading to obsessive compulsive rituals.

Let me describe some of my OCD traits, of which I have many. One of my earliest behaviors that I was able to trace back (and I still suffer this today) was the use of a blue ink, medium point, BIC pen. I began using such a pen in my early college days. To this day, this is the only kind of pen that I can use. I always carry such a pen with me because my OCD demands that I do it. If I ever need to sign my signature and another person hands me a pen to use, my obsessive compulsive mind says to me, "No, Ronald, you must use the blue ink, medium point BIC pen." On a few occasions when I did not have my BIC pen, I would become extremely anxiety ridden. My anxiety level became so bad that I could barely sign my signature.

Another OCD trait is what I call re-reading. I read part of a sentence and then my mind plays a trick on me. It tells me that I have to go back and re-read what I just read. The OCD cycle has gone into action, and I will have to go back and read the sentence over again. I might then read two or three sentences and again the OCD cycle will demand that I go back to begin reading at the beginning. It might take me four or five minutes to read a single paragraph. I do not understand how I made it through college. I rarely read anymore because this trait still exists, controlling my actions, and I have NO control over it. It controls me!

A related trait is when I go to a museum or a zoo, both of which I love to do. My OCD ruins these visits. My OCD demands that I read every sign, placard, or any other notes that describe the exhibit. Let me emphasize that my OCD demands that I read EVERY word of every sign. This is further complicated by the above mentioned re-reading. I discovered an interesting phenomenon the past year when I began traveling to foreign countries where the signs are in a different language. I found that I can go to a museum or a zoo and have a very enjoyable time. My mind knows that I am unable to understand the exhibit signs, so I just look at an exhibit and then continue on to the next exhibit.

Closely related to the above OCD experience is the reading of license plates, bumper stickers, and billboards. While I am driving my automobile around, my OCD mind might suddenly focus on a particular license plate, and my OCD mind says, "Let's play another trick on Ronald." I will be compelled to be sure that I have read all the numbers on the license plate, or all the words on the bumper sticker, or all the words on the billboard. If necessary I will drive around the block one, or two, or even three times to be sure that I have read all the words or all the numbers of the license plate.

When I leave for a vacation, I am sure that my water is turned off (which is not a bad idea); however, in my case my OCD mind compels me to check and recheck. I might check fifteen or twenty times. I know that it is turned off, but my OCD forces me to do this. Not only do I keep checking to be sure that the water is turned off, but I have gone beyond the typical OCD cycle and have developed what I will call an "OCD ritual." I not only check several times to be sure that the water is turned off, but I do it in a certain "ritualistic" pattern. I will put my hand on the valve and turn it a certain number of times to the right (clockwise). I will say to myself as I do it, "Right, right, right, clockwise, clockwise, clockwise, off, off, off." I will do this a specific number of times, and if I lose track of how many times I do this, I will start over.

Even though my obsessive compulsive disorder has not been controlled by medications, I did find a temporary relief for my OCD in something that was caused by my OCD. I have become a world traveler, having traveled to Europe seven times in the past year, South America three times, The Dominican Republic three times, to Mexico twice, to Puerto Rico twice, to another island in the Caribbean (Tobago), and I have no idea how many trips back and forth across the United States. I became this world traveler because of an obsessive compulsive desire to break *The Guinness Book of World Records* on how many trips a person could make traveling back and forth across the United States in a four-week period. I traveled to New York City, which was to be my home base. From NYC, I would fly to Seattle, only to return to NYC after being in Seattle for just a few hours. After arriving back in NYC, I would then be on another airplane to Los Angeles a few hours later. After arriving in Los Angeles, I would then be back on another airplane back to NYC after just a few hours in Los Angeles. I continued this for two weeks, but had to discontinue my endeavors because I became completely fatigued.

Although I did not complete my mission, I did discover something very interesting. During this two-week period I did not suffer from any symptoms of my OCD. I had become completely involved in what I was doing and somehow this "shorted out" in my mind the desire to do the obsessive compulsive things that I have described in the previous sections.

I found that I really enjoyed traveling, and it relieved to a large extent my obsessive compulsive habits. I found a way to travel inexpensively and I began traveling very extensively. I was seeing new things, doing things I had never done before, and for some unknown reason my OCD was pretty much under control. This, unfortunately, was not to last forever. After several months of traveling, I have found myself gradually beginning to do the obsessive compulsive things that I had done before my travel experiences began. The habits that I have listed are now haunting me even in my travels. I have no way to explain why they disappeared for a while and have now begun to reappear except that OCD seems to find a way to control my life.

Continued

The Lived Experience—cont'd

Airport monitor boards are a perfect example. After going through security, I go to the flight monitor board to check on my flight. I will look at my boarding pass to check the flight number and time, and then I will look at the monitor board to see if they are the same. I have now set myself up for an OCD ritual. I will check the pass against the board at least seven to ten times before I can convince my mind that they are the same. Often after doing this I will begin to walk away from the monitor board and have to turn around and go through the ritual again. I may do this two or three times. Unfortunately, this is not the end. When I get to the boarding gate, I will again check my boarding pass against the information posted at the boarding gate. I again will check

this seven to ten times before I can convince my mind that they are the same, another OCD ritual.

I feel that it is very important for the reader to understand that all people have some obsessive compulsive tendencies. Just because you (the reader) may undergo some type of patterned or ritualistic behavior, do not quickly conclude that you have OCD. It is important to understand the difference between obsessive compulsive behavior and obsessive compulsive DISORDER; only when the behaviors become so frequent and intense that they begin to interfere with your life can this be described as obsessive compulsive DISORDER. In more severe cases such as mine, these not only interfere with my life but they completely control it.

---

competency. On the other hand, without disclosure, the individual is not eligible for reasonable accommodations. Decisions related to when and how much to disclose can also be an issue in the formation of friendships and romantic relationships.

When stigma from the external environment becomes internalized, it is referred to as self-stigma. Cultural beliefs in Western society tend to include negative images of people with mental illness. Imagine the impact this has on a person who is recently diagnosed with a mental illness and who has grown up exposed to negative beliefs. This person is likely to assume that if others learn about the mental illness, they will reject or devalue him or her. A study of the consequence of stigma found that people with serious mental illness who held strong perceptions of devaluation had much lower self-esteem (Link et al, 2001).

Occupational therapists can address stigma by educating individuals or challenging institutions and policies that discriminate against people with mental illness. Occupational therapists can also support individuals with mental illness to

develop skills in self-advocacy so that they can become empowered to confront situations that are prejudicial or unjust. The topic of stigma is covered more thoroughly in Chapter 28.

Poverty

Where you live, what you eat, whom you interact with, and which leisure activities you engage in are greatly influenced by your financial resources. Many people with serious mental illness live in chronic poverty, which compromises their ability to fully participate in community life. Unemployment and underemployment, poor insurance coverage, high health-care costs, and financial disincentives all contribute to inadequate economic situations for people with serious mental illness. For people with schizophrenia unemployment rates have been reported at 85% in the United States (Rosenheck et al, 2006) and 80–90% in Europe (Marwaha & Johnson, 2004). These rates are likely higher given the current economic environment as employment rates for people with mental illness are affected by the general labor market in the United States (Becker, Xie, McHugo, Halliday, & Martinez, 2006), Europe (Marwaha et al, 2009) and Australia (Waghorn, Chant, Lloyd, & Harris, 2009). Furthermore, the majority of working people with serious mental illness are in part-time, low-paying, entry-level jobs. Therefore, even among the employed, people with mental illness have severely limited incomes.

Several factors, some of them interactive, explain the low employment rates (Cook, 2006). For example, although advanced education is increasingly important for well-paying jobs, many individuals with psychiatric disabilities have low levels of education. Poverty makes it challenging to seek advanced education. In addition, poverty may mean that individuals live in neighborhoods with few employment opportunities, lack access to transportation, and cannot consider employment that requires tools, uniforms, or other expenses.

Employment disincentives can also impact employment rates. For example, individuals who receive supplemental security benefits undergo a reduction in benefits of $1 for every $2 of earnings once their earnings reach $65 a month. Furthermore, other benefits, such as housing subsidies, food stamps, and transportation stipends, are often reduced or lost when an individual is working.

Evidence-Based Practice

The general public widely endorses stigmatizing attitudes toward people with mental illness, and stereotypes persist even in highly trained mental health professionals (Corrigan, 2000) such as occupational therapists.

➤ Explore your own biases and stigmatizing attitudes toward people with mental illness. Consider what you need to do to change these biases.

➤ Become an advocate for people with serious mental illness, both inside and outside your work setting. Provide educational opportunities to reduce stigma, talk to employers about reasonable accommodations, and challenge friends and family when they make discriminatory comments about people with mental illness.

Corrigan, P. W. (2000). Mental health stigma as social attribution: Implications for research methods and attitude change. *Clinical Psychology: Science and Practice, 7,* 48–67.

Currently, few occupational therapists work within supported employment programs, but this presents an opportunity for occupational therapists to contribute unique skills (such as activity analysis, environmental accommodation, skill training) to enhance the likelihood that individuals with mental illness may obtain and keep a job. Occupational therapists can also work within supported education settings so that individuals with mental illness can obtain additional skills and credentials necessary for better paying jobs.

Complex Physical Environments

With the ADA and other relevant legislation, the physical environment, particularly the manmade environment, is now recognized as a factor that can interfere with the life of a person with a physical disability (particularly wheelchair users). Curb cuts, enlarged bathroom stalls, and handicapped parking spaces are now expected in public places. Although the environment is not completely accessible for people with physical disabilities, there is at least some recognition that the physical environment presents barriers to wheelchair users and individuals with other physical disabilities. This is far less true for people with mental illness, who can also find aspects of the physical environment challenging.

Rapid advances in technology, the fast pace of society, and the demand for choice has resulted in a rich but complex physical world. Consider the large department stores or warehouse stores that offer items in bulk. Although these environments provide a lot of choice and convenience, it can be more challenging to sort through, screen out, and make decisions about products in this setting. The use of automated services such as electronic check-in at airports, ATM machines, self-checkout in grocery stores, online card catalogs at the library, and automated exercise machines at the gym can be especially intimidating to individuals with limited experience or exposure to technology.

Occupational therapists can provide skills training so that individuals with mental illness can learn to use everyday technologies. They may also provide supportive devices such as simple written directions or store maps to enhance performance in these challenging environments.

Lack of Choice

People with mental illness have far fewer choices for many aspects of community participation. Housing is a primary example. If you belong to the middle or upper class, you have many choices in terms of the neighborhood you want to live in and the type of apartment or house. However, the shortage of affordable housing means that people with serious mental illness have little to no choice regarding where they can live. Many people with serious mental illness live in congregate housing situations such as group homes, where choice is further restricted in terms of roommates, meals, and visitors.

Forchuk et al (2006) conducted a qualitative study on housing instability for people with serious mental illness. They reported that individuals with mental illness experience a turbulent pattern of losing, struggling, and gaining housing stability. The experience of losing housing can be particularly distressing, because the conditions under which many people lose their housing are often traumatic (e.g.,

fire, eviction, or condemned building). The individual often loses not only housing but also the possessions that were in the home. When individuals with mental illness are given more choice in programs like supported housing, they report greater satisfaction with their housing situation and an overall improvement in quality of life (Nelson et al, 2007).

Mental and physical health-care services are another area of narrow choice for people with mental illness. Private insurance provides limited coverage for mental health services. People with long-term mental illness typically receive services through the Medicaid/Medicare system, which restricts access to many providers and health-care systems. In addition, providers may lack training, and stigmatizing attitudes can interfere with health care provision.

Occupational therapists can work within supported housing programs to help individuals with mental illness develop the necessary skills to maintain an apartment. They may also provide education to health-care providers so that they may be more sensitive to the needs of people with mental illness.

Segregation and Isolation

Deinstitutionalization, which began in the 1960s and became the policy of most systems by 1980, was successful in creating policy that resulted in most people with psychiatric disabilities living outside of institutional settings. However, for some individuals, life in the community is characterized by loneliness and social isolation. A Department of Health Report from Australia revealed that among people with psychosis, 39% did not have a close friend and 45% wished they had a good friend (Jablensky, McGrath, & Herman, 1999).

In general, people with mental illness are lonelier than people without mental illness, although their particular housing situation does not seem to be related to the level of loneliness (Brown, 1996). It is likely a combination of factors, such as opportunities for socialization, level of acceptance by neighbors or roommates, comfort in social situations, and the social proficiency of the individual, that contribute to social connectedness. However, social support is an important factor in the quality of life of the general population and of people with mental illness.

Occupational therapists can refer individuals to consumer-operated programs or naturally occurring community organizations that might enhance the social network of the person with mental illness. Occupational therapists may also provide social skills training so that the individual with mental illness will be more accepted and feel more comfortable in social situations.

Criminal Justice System

The number of people with psychiatric disabilities in large mental hospitals has decreased dramatically, and some statistics suggest that jails are the new setting for institutionalization (Blumstein & Beck, 1999). Startling statistics indicate that up to 50% of people with serious mental illness may be arrested at some point in their lives. Several reasons beyond symptomatology could account for these rates. Draine et al (2002) argue that there are more powerful risk factors for crime than the illness itself. For example, unemployment, poverty, homelessness, and particularly substance abuse may play a greater role in the high rates of arrest and incarceration for people with serious mental illness.

The increase in arrest rates does not take into account that the arrest rates of the general U.S. population have increased dramatically. One study examining police reports found very few examples of offenses that could be attributed to mental illness, although approximately one quarter of the offenses were probably or definitely related to substance abuse (Junginger et al, 2006).

Some communities have developed programs that attempt to divert people with mental illness from the criminal justice system to community treatment (Munetz & Griffin, 2006); however, Draine et al (2002) argue that this approach may not be in the best interest of the offender. They suggest that an integrated approach that considers risk factors common to both mental illness and criminal behavior would more effectively address the problem.

Environmental Resources

Although the environment contains many barriers for people with psychiatric disabilities, the resources afforded by the environment are too often overlooked. Helping people with psychiatric disabilities access environmental resources is essential to effective occupational therapy practice. Key environmental resources include consumer-operated organizations, self-help and peer support, family and friends, and community resources.

Consumer-Operated Organizations and Self-Help/Peer Support

Self-help organizations are common in Western societies, particularly for addictions (e.g., Alcoholics Anonymous) and physical illnesses such as cancer. However, the use of peer support for mental illness is a more recent phenomenon. The consumer/survivor movement is responsible for the growing acceptance of mental health peer-support programs (Chamberlin, 1990) and the recognition that people who have experienced a mental illness have something unique to offer others who are going through a similar experience.

Consumer-run organizations and other peer-support services are increasing in numbers, and the mutual support they provide directly addresses the social environment of people with psychiatric disabilities. These programs help individuals develop social networks and create interpersonal connections and a sense of belonging. In describing a specific consumer-run organization, the Welcome Basket program, Chinman et al (2001) suggest that peers are particularly well equipped to create social supports and, in doing so, make a better "person–environment fit" than traditional mental health systems. The Welcome Basket program was effective in reducing the hospitalization rates of its participants. Although research into consumer-run organizations and peer-support programs is only beginning, there is some evidence that peer providers are able to more quickly form a strong working alliance, particularly with clients who have not responded to traditional care (Davidson et al, 2006). Consumer-operated organizations are more fully described in Chapter 35.

Family and Friends

For people with mental illness, a larger social network is associated with reduced symptoms, better quality of life, and higher self-esteem (Goldberg, Rollins, & Lehman, 2003). A social system that includes individuals from different groups (e.g., family, friends, and professionals) tends to be more beneficial. Corrigan and Phelan (2004) found that a larger social network was also associated swith greater levels of hope and a stronger orientation toward goals and success.

Consumer-run organizations and peer-support programs provide one resource for making social connections. Another model of programming is the clubhouse, a consumer-driven program that incorporates participation in work-oriented activities required to run the clubhouse. A central mission of the clubhouse is to develop an intentional community (Herman et al, 2005). Clubhouses can reduce social isolation and create a place of belonging. They are described in more detail in Chapter 39.

Mental health services directed by professionals can also contribute to the development of friendships. Catty et al (2005) found that social networks were increased in relation to the duration and attendance in a day center program. Individuals who attended the day center were more likely to confide in friends and neighbors than in professionals when compared with other individuals who received mental health services but did not attend the day program.

Families provide another source of social support. Although much of the research on families focuses on caregiver burden, there is also evidence that family members receive gratification from the caregiving relationship (Greenberg, Seltzer, & Judge, 2000). Programs such as Journey of Hope, in which families meet to learn about mental illness and develop strategies to better assist their family members, can help to develop positive family relationships. One study of the Journey of Hope program indicates improvements in caregiver satisfaction (Pickett-Schenk et al, 2006).

Community Resources

The community can provide a wealth of resources for people with mental illness. Therefore, it is important that occupational therapists learn what resources are available in the communities in which their clients live. Spend time

---

Evidence-Based Practice

A larger social network is associated with reduced symptoms, better quality of life, and higher self-esteem for people with mental illness (Goldberg, Rollins, & Lehman, 2003).

➤ Occupational therapists can make referrals to clubhouses, consumer-run organizations, and other groups that provide social opportunities for people with mental illness.

➤ Get involved with the family. Provide interventions that foster a more interdependent relationship between family members and the client.

Goldberg, R. W., Rollins, A. L., & Lehman, A. F. (2003). Social network correlates among people with psychiatric disabilities. *Psychiatric Rehabilitation Journal, 26*(4), 393–402.

driving around your clients' community, visit the businesses and services, look through the newspaper, and talk to other care providers such as social workers to learn about the community. For example, the local library can provide many resources. In addition to books, the library may also loan movies and music CDs and provide computer and Internet access. Food pantries and soup kitchens provide nutritional resources to individuals who have a limited income. Thrift stores and other discount retail outlets can make clothing, furniture, electronics, and other items more affordable.

The cooperative extension system is an educational network that provides free information on a variety of topics, such as nutrition and health, gardening and small business operation. Faith-based organizations address spiritual needs and can provide opportunities for socialization, education, and volunteering. These are just a few examples of common resources available in most communities. Viewing the community as a resource instead of a barrier and establishing alliances with these resources can enhance community participation for people with mental illness.

Summary

Although this chapter provides only an overview of information on the environment, this textbook includes seven chapters specifically devoted to the environment and its relationship to people with serious mental illness and 10 chapters describing practice settings. Environment is the most neglected component of the person-environment-occupation model. Occupational therapists can help rectify this omission by routinely considering the environment in their assessment and intervention planning and implementation.

Active Learning Strategies

1. Barriers

Think about an occupation you needed or wanted to do recently but either were unable to do it or were dissatisfied with the experience. List all of the factors that were barriers to performing this occupation.

Reflective Questions
- Were the barriers primarily environmental or personal?
- For you to succeed the next time, what would need to be different?
- Would you make a change in yourself, or would you change something about the environment?

 Describe the experience in your **Reflective Journal**.

2. Community Resources

Explore the environmental resources in your own community. Walk or drive through the neighborhood, look through the phone book and the newspaper. Identify low-cost and free services. Categorize these resources in terms of the areas of occupation they support (e.g., work, school, instrumental activities of daily living, activities of daily living, leisure, social participation). What are the strengths of your community? What is missing from your community?

References

American Occupational Therapy Association (AOTA). (2008). *Occupational Therapy Practice Framework: Domain and Process* (2nd ed.). Bethesda, MD: American Occupational Therapy Association.

American Psychiatric Association (2000). *Diagnostic and Statistical Manual of Mental Disorders: DSM-IV-TR* (4th ed., text rev.). Washington, DC: American Psychiatric Association.

Ashman, S. B., Monk, T. H., Kupfer, D. J., Clark, C. H., Myers, F. S., Frank, E., & Leibenluft, E. (1999). Relationship between social rhythms and mood in patients with rapid cycling bipolar disorder. *Psychiatry Research, 86*(1), 1–8.

Becker, D. R., Xie, H., McHugo, G. J., Halliday, J., & Martinez, R. A. (2006). What predicts supported employment program outcomes. *Community Mental Health Journal, 42,* 303–313.

Bertera, E. M. (2005). Mental health in U.S. adults: The role of positive social support and social negativity in personal relationships. *Journal of Social and Personal Relationships, 22*(1), 33–48.

Blumstein, A., & Beck, A. J. (1999). Population growth in U.S. prisons, 1980–1996. In M. Tonry & J. Petersilia (Eds.), *Crime and Justice: A Review of the Research, Vol. 26, Prisons* (pp. 17–61). Chicago: University of Chicago Press.

Brown, C. (1996). A comparison of living situation and loneliness for people with mental illness. *Psychiatric Rehabilitation Journal, 20*(2), 59–63.

Brugha, T. S., Weich, S., Singleton, N., Lewis, G., Bebbington, P. E., Jenkins, R., & Meltzer, H. (2005). Primary group size, social support, gender and future mental health status in a prospective study of people living in private households throughout Great Britain. *Psychological Medicine, 35*(5), 705–714.

Catty, J., Goddard, K., White, S., & Burns, T. (2005). Social networks among users of mental health day care: Predictors of social contacts and confiding relationships. *Social Psychiatry and Psychiatric Epidemiology, 40*(6), 467–474.

Chamberlin, J. (1990). The ex-patients' movement: Where we've been and where we're going. *Journal of Mind and Behavior, 11,* 323–336.

Chinman, M. J., Weingarten, R., Stayner, D., & Davidson, L. (2001). Chronicity reconsidered: Improving person-environment fit through a consumer-run service. *Community Mental Health Journal, 37,* 215–228.

Cohen, C. I. (2000). Overcoming social amnesia: The role for a social perspective in psychiatric research and practice. *Psychiatric Services, 51,* 72–78.

Cook, J. A. (2006). Employment barriers for persons with psychiatric disabilities: Update of a report for the president's commission. *Psychiatric Services, 57,* 1391–1405.

Corrigan, P. W. (2000). Mental health stigma as social attribution: Implications for research methods and attitude change. *Clinical Psychology: Science and Practice, 7,* 48–67.

Corrigan, P. W., & Phelan, S. M. (2004) Social support and recovery in people with serious mental illnesses. *Community Mental Health Journal, 40,* 513.

Davidson, L., Chinman, M., Sells, D., & Rowe, M. (2006). Peer support among adults with serious mental illness: A report from the field. *Schizophrenia Bulletin, 32,* 443–450.

Draine, J., Salzer, M. S., Culhane, D. P., & Hadley, T. R. (2002). Role of social disadvantage in crime, joblessness, and homelessness among persons with serious mental illness. *Psychiatric Services, 53,* 565–573.

Dunn, W., Brown, C., & McGuigan, A. (1994). The ecology of human performance: A framework for considering the impact of context. *American Journal of Occupational Therapy, 48,* 595–607.

Eaton, W. W., Mortensen, P. B., & Frydenberg, M. (2000). Obstetric factors, urbanization and psychosis. *Schizophrenia Research, 43,* 117–123.

Forchuk, C., Ward-Griffin, C., Csiernik, R., & Turner, K. (2006). Surviving the tornado of mental illness: Psychiatric survivors' experiences of getting, losing, and keeping housing. *Psychiatric Services, 57,* 558–562.

George, L. K., Larson, D. B., Koenig, H. G., McCullough, M. E. (2000). Spirituality and health: What we know, what we need to know. *Journal of Social and Clinical Psychology, 19*(1), 102–116.

Goldberg, R. W., Rollins, A. L., & Lehman, A. F. (2003). Social network correlates among people with psychiatric disabilities. *Psychiatric Rehabilitation Journal, 26*(4), 393–402.

Greenberg, J. S., Seltzer, M. M., & Judge, K. (2000). Another side of the family's experience: Learning and growing through the process of coping with mental illness. *Journal of the California Alliance for the Mentally Ill, 11,* 8–10.

Herman, S. E., Onaga, E., Pernice-Duca, F., Oh, S. M., & Ferguson, C. (2005). Sense of community in clubhouse programs: Member and staff concepts. *American Journal of Community Psychology, 36,* 343–356.

Hooley, J. M. (2004). Do psychiatric patients do better clinically if they live with certain kinds of families? *Current Directions in Psychological Science, 13,* 202–205.

Jablensky, A., McGrath, J., & Herman, H. (1999). *People Living with Psychotic Illness: An Australian Study 1997–1998.* Canberra: Australian Mental Health Branch, Commonwealth Department of Health and Aging.

Junginger, J., Claypoole, K., Laygo, R., & Crisanti, A. (2006). Effects of serious mental illness and substance abuse on criminal offenses. *Psychiatric Services, 47,* 879–882.

Kelly, C. M., & Jorm, A. F. (2007). Stigma and mood disorders. *Current Opinion in Psychiatry, 20,* 13–16.

Law, M., Cooper, B., Strong, S., Stewart, D., Rigby, P., & Letts, L. (1996). The person-environment-occupation model: A transactive approach to occupational performance. *Canadian Journal of Occupational Therapy, 63*(1), 9–23.

Link, B. G., Stuening, E. L., Neese-Todd, S., Asmussen, A., & Phelan, J. C. (2001). Stigma as a barrier to recovery: The consequences of stigma for the self-esteem of people with mental illness. *Psychiatric Services, 52,* 1621–1626.

Marwaha, S., & Johnson, S. (2004). Schizophrenia and employment—A review. *Social Psychiatry and Psychiatric Epidemiology, 39,* 337–349.

Marwaha, S., Johnson, S., Bebbington, P. E., Angermeyer, M. C., Brugha, T. S., Azorin, J. M., Killian, R., Hansen, K., & Tourni, M. (2009). Predictors of employment status change over 2 years in people with schizophrenia living in Europe. *Epemilogia e Psichiatria Sociale, 18,* 344–351.

Mond, J. M., Robertson-Smith, G., & Vetere, A. (2006). Stigma and eating disorders: Is there evidence of negative attitudes towards anorexia nervosa among women in the community? *Journal of Mental Health, 14,* 519–532.

Munetz, M. R., & Griffin, P. A. (2006). Use of the sequential intercept model as an approach to decriminalization of people with serious mental illness. *Psychiatric Services, 57,* 544–549.

Nelson, G., Sylvestre, J., Aubry, T., George, L., & Trainor, J. (2007). Housing choice and control, housing quality, and control over professional support as contributors to the subjective quality of life and community adaptation of people with severe mental illness. *Administration and Policy in Mental Health and Mental Health Services Research, 34,* 89–100.

Page, S. (1995) Effects of the mental illness label in 1993: Acceptance and rejection in the community. *Journal of Health and Social Policy, 7,* 61–68.

Pickett-Schenk, S. A., Bennett, C., Cook, J. A., Steigman, P., Lippincott, R., Villagracia, I., & Grey, D. (2006) Changes in caregiving satisfaction and information needs among relatives of adults with mental illness: Results of a randomized evaluation of a family-led education intervention. *American Journal of Orthopsychiatry, 76*(4), 545–553.

Rebeiro, K. L. (2001). Enabling occupation: The importance of an affirming environment. *Canadian Journal of Occupational Therapy, 68,* 80–90.

Rosenheck, R., Leslie, D., Keepfe, R., McEvoy, J., Swartz, M., Perkins, D., Stroup, S., Hsaia, J. K., Lieberman, J., & Catie Study Investigators Group. (2006). Barriers to employment for people with schizophrenia. *American Journal of Psychiatry, 163,* 411–417.

Russinova, Z., Wewiorski, N. J., & Cash, D. (2002) Use of alternative health care practices by persons with serious mental illness: Perceived benefits. *American Journal of Public Health, 92,* 1600–1603.

Schkade, J., & Schultz, S. (1992). Occupational adaptation: Toward a holistic approach for contemporary practice, part 1. *American Journal of Occupational Therapy, 46,* 829–837.

United States Department of Health and Human Services. (2001). *Mental Health: Culture, Race & Ethnicity. A Supplement to Mental Health: A Report of the Surgeon General.* Rockville, MD: US Department of Health and Human Services, Substance Abuse Mental Health Services Administration, Center for Mental Health Services.

Waghorn, G., Chant, D., Lloyd, C., & Harris, M. G. (2009). Labour market conditions, labour force activity and prevalence of psychiatric disorders. *Social Psychiatry and Psychiatric Epidemiology, 44,* 171–178.

CHAPTER
27

The Political and Public Policy Environment

M. Beth Merryman

> "He who influences the thought of his times influences the times that follow.
>
> —Elbert Hubbard

Introduction

Public policy can have a significant impact on the daily lives of people with mental illness. For example, social security disability insurance regulations influence their financial situations, the lack of affordable housing can lead to homelessness, and disincentives regarding employment often interfere with work.

Public policy impacts mental health specialty practice in occupational therapy. The Community Mental Health Centers Construction Act of 1963 led to a deinstitutionalization movement in the early 1960s that ultimately reduced the number of residents in state and county mental health hospitals from over a half million in 1956 to just over 60,000 in 1996 (Geller, 2000). Occupational therapy positions in institutions were reduced, but new practice opportunities for occupational therapists in community-based mental health services were created. In a similar vein, the New Freedom Commission on Mental Health (NFCMH) generated a 2003 report filled with policy recommendations that have implications for occupational therapy practice and advocacy (Cottrell, 2007). The Mental Health Parity Act, scheduled to take full effect in 2010, will create opportunities for occupational therapists to create new and expanded roles in mental health (Gallew, Haltiwanger, Sowers, & van der Heever, 2004).

Public policies generate shifts in the organization, financing, and delivery of services and can present opportunities for the profession, but we cannot realize them if we do not understand how policies are developed or how to shape them. Knowledge is power, and understanding the public policy environment enables professionals to advocate for access to occupational therapy services and foster full social participation for persons with mental illnesses.

This chapter describes the mental health public policy environment in the United States, with the goal of providing a broad understanding of the decision-making structure and major "players" in the mental health policymaking environment. The chapter begins by defining the values that frame current health and mental health policy in the United States, including the impact of deinstitutionalization, managed care, political issues, and funding challenges on a comprehensive, coherent policy. The current funding and administrative structures for public and private organizations are described, including information on funding sources, managed care principles, and administrative and legislative decision-making structures. The chapter explains how the policy agenda is established and how current mechanisms of influence on the local, state, and national levels are identified, including the impact of advocacy groups and inherent challenges of mental health policy to the policy agenda. Finally, a model for assessing policy issues relative to the profession is presented, and policy intervention in the form of individual, programmatic, and public policy advocacy is discussed, emphasizing the application of this information to concerns of occupational justice.

Influence of Values on Policies and Practices

Societal values influence public policy and mental health policy in the United States. The U.S. health care system has traditionally valued provider autonomy and consumer sovereignty over other values, such as social advocacy (Preister, 1992). That is, the provider, whether a physician or occupational therapist, can make his or her own decisions about the care provided. Consumer sovereignty means that the consumer can pick his or her health care provider, and decisions regarding treatment are made on an individual basis rather than categorically (i.e., everyone with a particular diagnosis receives exactly the same treatment). These values have contributed to both the strengths (e.g., technology and acute care) and limitations (e.g., access and community care) of the system. For example, in the United States, the technology available for health care is advanced, yet some people have limited access to even the most basic health care services.

Mechanic, Schlesinger, and McAlpine (1995) state that despite decades of growth and change, the core culture of U.S. medicine has remained stable and resilient. This culture involves an individual versus a community view, an emphasis on aggressive intervention and cure, and narrow biomedical measures of outcome. Consequently, health care in the United States focuses on the individual rather than on equal access, acute/short-term care rather than chronic/disability care, and hospital rather than community health. The mental health system struggles because the primary systems are not consistent with the needs of people with mental illness who lack access to care; have long-term, disabling illnesses; and need community care. In addition, the growth of managed care in the public sector may not adequately address important values such as consumer empowerment and cultural competence (Emery, Glover, & Mazade, 1998).

However, other systems do promote values that support the needs of people with mental illness. The World Health Organization (2001) embraces a universalist perspective relative to health and disability, emphasizing engagement in activity and social participation instead of symptoms. Occupational therapists have long embraced such measures of community participation as goals of health care intervention, a fact that was further supported in the *Occupational Therapy Practice Framework* (AOTA, 2008).

Impact of Policy Decisions on Practice

As a result of policy decisions such as deinstitutionalization and the development of various programs of social support, most mental health care occurs in the community (Scull, 1985). A review of key policy decisions over the past six decades highlights some of the current issues affecting both occupational therapists and the individuals they serve (Table 27-1).

The policy shift toward community-based mental health care emerged after World War II, with new federal monies increasing the role of the federal government in mental health services, policy, and research (Grob, 2001). The **Community Mental Health Centers Act** of 1963 was designed with the belief that changing the locus of care from hospital to community would in itself be therapeutic. However, a

Table 27-1 ● **Key Policy Actions Relative to Mental Health**

Decade	Major Mental Health Policy	Policy Impact	Impact on Occupational Therapy Practice
Post-WWII 1950s	Federal funds for services, policy, and research • National Institute of Mental Health (NIMH) • Hill-Burton Act • Mental Health Study Act (1955)	• Improved nation's hospital system; called for evaluation of the societal impact of mental illness • Increased federal role in mental health • Funding for mental health research (NIMH)	Increased opportunities for occupational therapists in hospital settings; some care for underserved
1960s	Federal legislation and funding • Community Mental Health Centers Act (1963) • Medicare (1965) • Medicaid (1965)	• Development of community philosophy and initial community legislation • Funds to construct but not staff community mental health centers • Reduction of state hospital populations • Increased coverage for treatment of psychiatric illnesses	Increased opportunities in community-based settings, halfway houses, partial hospitalization settings; Medicare and Medicaid funding for hospital-based care
1970s	Federal/state courts address civil rights • Social Security amendments (1972) • Right to treatment in least-restrictive environment Health Maintenance Organization Act (1973)	• Emerging civil rights issues relative to treatment and community living • Civil rights addressed in court • Funding for startup of HMO, including short-term mental health care	Court decisions influence practice environments, including physical setting, staffing levels, and individualized treatment plans
1980s	Federal monies reduced and shifted to block grants • State block grants • Decreased policy guidelines/requirements Managed care in public and private sector President Reagan repeals Mental Health Systems Act (1980)	• Attention to cost drives policy decisions • Decreased lengths of stay and increased alternatives to inpatient care • Issues of access, cost, and quality emerge • Advocacy more prominent	Managed care emphasizes lower levels of care and lower-cost professionals
1990s	Decade of the brain: increased neuroscience research • Report of the Surgeon General (1999) • Mental Health Parity Act (1996) Continued civil rights • Americans with Disabilities Act (1990) • Olmstead Act (1997) Expanded managed care • Medicaid waivers	Scientific evidence emerges as policy issue • Mental health as public health issue • Access to evidence-based practices • Antidiscrimination policies relative to care and community life • PL 104-21 prohibits SSDI or SSI disability benefits for addicts or alcoholics	Legal decisions supporting community-based placement creates potential for increased occupational therapy role in community-based settings

Table 27-1 ● **Key Policy Actions Relative to Mental Health—cont'd**

Decade	Major Mental Health Policy	Policy Impact	Impact on Occupational Therapy Practice
2000s	Consumer rights New Freedom Initiative (2001) • Transformation grant • Waivers	Consumer rights drive recovery orientation • Tension between safety and self-determination • Policy decision making shifts to states	Opportunities to develop independent living skills and vocational and transitional services for youth, adults, and elders with mental illnesses

negative outcome of this policy was fragmentation of services. A person with mental illness is now faced with negotiating separate complicated systems for financial, medical, employment, and housing services, which are often provided by different agencies in different parts of the community.

The enactment of Medicare and Medicaid in 1965 influenced both where services were delivered and how they were paid for. For example, many elderly individuals were transferred from state mental hospitals to nursing homes, most of which did not provide mental health services. As private third-party payers improved mental health coverage (a common trend is that private insurers follow the lead of Medicare), inpatient mental health care shifted to general hospitals. The increases in outpatient mental health insurance coverage and the policy shift to the community led to drastic reductions in state and county mental hospital populations and an increase in the numbers of episodes of care. By the late 1960s, state mental hospitals no longer provided long-term or custodial care but provided short- or intermediate-term care for persons with serious and persistent mental illness. The Social Security Act, as amended in 1972, enabled those individuals whose disability precluded them from working to receive federal income supports. This also made them eligible for Medicaid and other entitlements, further enabling community living for those with serious mental illness.

The 1980s brought policy shifts that greatly reduced the federal government's role in mental health. Federal funding for mental health was reduced, and grants to local communities to meet targeted needs of their mentally ill populations were converted to state block grants, with few policy guidelines or requirements (Grob, 1994; Sharfstein, 2000). The primary impact of public policies for mental health services in the 1980s was to reduce public funding for services and impose more stringent criteria for determining disability benefits (Geller, 2000). Although the service needs for persons with a serious mental illness (e.g., health care access, medications, housing, transportation, employment, and basic living expenses) were evident to mental health policymakers and providers, rising health care costs led to the development of various mechanisms to limit services and control costs.

Policies in the 1990s had two major foci: an emphasis on basic brain research and a renewed focus on creating opportunities for persons with mental illness in integrated community settings. Basic brain research centered on understanding the influence of biological and genetic factors on serious mental illnesses such as schizophrenia and bipolar disorder. The development of practice guidelines, treatment algorithms, and evidence-based practice for various mental disorders occurred as a result of this knowledge. In 1999, the Surgeon General of the United States issued a report on mental health, which encouraged a public health approach to mental health and illness, validated the biological evidence of mental disorders, articulated the value of using research evidence to determine interventions, and acknowledged the negative effects social stigma has on recovery from mental illness (U.S. Department of Health and Human Services [USDHHS], 1999).

The **Americans with Disabilities Act (ADA)** in 1990, the **Mental Health Parity Act (MHPA)** of 1996, and the ***Olmstead v. L.C. and E.W.*** decision of the U.S. Supreme Court (1999) all reflect policies aimed at addressing equality by eliminating discrimination against persons with disabilities (ADA); advocating that insurance plans provide equal coverage (MHPA) for mental and physical illnesses (Geller, 2000); and reducing community barriers to social participation in housing, employment, and transportation (*Olmstead*). On the reimbursement side, cost pressures continued, and managed care methodologies were introduced to reduce costs in both the private and public sectors. Payment became prospective, based on medical necessity, intensity of symptoms, and cost. Insurance providers were disinclined to pay for problems of daily life and a movement to pay for those illnesses that were shown to have a biological basis (e.g., mood disorders and schizophrenia). Overall, more individuals had some type of mental health insurance coverage, but the coverage they had was extremely limited.

In the early 21st century, the consumer rights movement led to the adoption of a belief that symptom relief was not enough and that individuals with mental illness should be fully involved in decisions about their care. The New Freedom Initiative of 2001 called for a transformation of the mental health delivery system to increase access to needed services and integrate Americans with disabilities into broad participation in community life (Cottrell, 2003). States are charged with addressing the goals and legislative mandates that focus on supporting full social participation in the least restrictive environment relative to mental health policies and administrative practices.

At the same time that states are adopting recovery-oriented services, some states are struggling with ways to offer mandated community treatment alternatives that do not interfere with civil rights, the most well known of which is New York's Kendra's Law (Monahan, Swartz, & Bonnie, 2003). Under Kendra's Law, judges have the authority to require an individual to receive involuntary outpatient treatment. Mental health advance directives also enable individuals to make decisions about their own treatment before any exacerbation occurs.

Individuals with mental illness can identify in writing what treatment they want to receive or may identify a proxy who can make such decisions on their behalf should they become mentally incapacitated.

In summary, the current mental health policy environment is based on a philosophy encompassing the following:

- Inclusion versus segregation.
- Modest support for parity in insurance coverage between biological and mental illnesses.
- Protection of the civil rights of the individual with mental illness in the form of laws and administrative rules relative to commitment, housing, and employment.
- Provision of a safety net through basic entitlements that, while enabling rudimentary community life, may not provide necessary funding to support individualized, recovery-oriented care delivery.

In this manner, the policy environment reflects American values, such as preserving the autonomy of individual consumers through privacy and civil rights actions; involving consumers in decisions about their care through the recovery philosophy; embracing private solutions to address public funding challenges, such as managed care adoption in both the private and public sectors, providing incentives for quality and access through state transformation grants and waivers; and maintaining provider autonomy by continuing to support a private system of health. It is important to note that the U.S. system is different from those in virtually all other developed countries, which utilize a government-run, single-payer system.

Administrative Structure and Funding

According to experts, there is no single mental health policy-making body in the United States. Regier et al (1993) referred to a de facto system of entities that deliver mental health services, including primary care, specialty care, human and social services, and voluntary sectors. The **primary care system** includes internists, pediatricians, and geriatricians. The **specialty care system** includes the traditional mental health continuum of specialty services, such as specialty inpatient units, partial hospitalization programs, and intensive outpatient programs. The **human and social services sector** is primarily involved with individuals who have serious and persistent mental illness and includes housing, employment, and income supports. The **voluntary sector** has grown tremendously as recovery has been embraced and includes support groups, advocacy, and self-help resources.

One of the greatest challenges to care delivery is the fragmented mental health system (NFCMH, 2003). Fragmentation and gaps in services exist for individuals with serious and persistent mental illness, leading to unnecessary costs and levels of disability, which contribute to school failure, homelessness, and incarceration (NFCMH, 2003). For example, an individual with severe and persistent mental illness may require services that include vocational rehabilitation, education, temporary financial assistance, services to ensure child welfare, and assistance with criminal or legal issues. Multiple programs exist to provide assistance, but Medicare, Medicaid, Social Security Income (SSI) or Social Security

Disability Insurance (SSDI), the Office of Vocational Rehabilitation, or Temporary Assistance for Needy Families (TANF) may variously finance these programs. In order to receive the needed services, the individual must negotiate this complex system and demonstrate that they meet the different requirements for receiving services from each program. The lack of a central agency or entity to coordinate mental health services dilutes influence in the policymaking arena as well, which creates a vicious cycle of underfunding and lack of influence in the policymaking process.

An adequate financing structure enables plans to be implemented; however, much of mental health planning is inadequately financed. According to the World Health Organization (2009), mental health policymakers must address three basic financial concerns: (1) developing and sustaining an adequate infrastructure to support service delivery, (2) allocation by need and priority, and (3) reasonable control of costs. Mental health financing in the United States is complex and compounded by numerous issues, not the least of which is that insurance plans have traditionally imposed greater restrictions on treatment for mental illness than for medical illnesses (NFCMH, 2003). The largest payer of mental health services in the United States is Medicaid. Medicaid and Medicare accounted for 33% of all public and private mental health spending in 1997 (Figure 27-1). Nearly a quarter (24%) of mental health spending was paid by state, local, and other federal sources. Another quarter (26%) were covered by private insurance, and the remaining 17% of services were paid for out of pocket (NFCMH, 2003).

Private, nonprofit general hospitals increasingly treat publicly financed patients who have more severe illnesses (Mechanic, McAlpine, & Olfson, 1998). Patients with private insurance are less likely to be admitted to inpatient beds than are individuals whose care is publicly funded. It is therefore critical for mental health advocates and policymakers to monitor Medicaid policy because Medicaid is the de facto long-term care policy for individuals with serious mental illness (Grob, 1994). Other critical funding policies that impact individuals with serious mental illness include those related to disability and income support. For example, a large and growing population of individuals comprise those receiving SSI and SSDI (Mechanic, 2008).

The Center for Mental Health Services (CMHS) is the federal agency that oversees state mental health plans. Each state develops its own plan for improving community-based services and reducing inpatient hospitalization. Since each state receives a block grant, and most care is delivered to

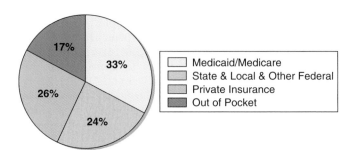

FIGURE 27-1. Sources of mental health expenditures. The greatest sources of funding for mental health services are public dollars. *Data from the New Freedom Commission on Mental Health Report (NFCMH, 2003, p. 22).*

The Lived Experience

Sarah

I have struggled with bipolar disorder since the age of 13 or so, but was diagnosed at the age of 18. Until that point I was characterized as "moody," "deep," and sometimes "self-absorbed" by those who knew me. I talked about God and death. I cried a lot. I isolated myself from friends and developed a paranoid outlook on life. It was only in 1996 after a complete departure from consensus reality that my treatment for mental illness began. Forced to leave a top-tier college due to a period of severe psychosis, I found myself bereft of any remaining social skills, unable to read and write due lack of concentration, and plagued by delusions that televisions were talking to me, and that an acquaintance was the incarnation of Jesus. I was brought to a hospital and stayed one and a half weeks in an inpatient psychiatric unit. Barely stabilized on medication, I was released.

My ten years in recovery from bipolar disorder have not been linear. Recovery from mental illness seldom is. It took me a long time to understand and accept that this illness is chronic, that it has a biological basis, and that I can't control its flare-ups. At times I have believed I can will myself to be better. This belief offers a sense of control—a last effort to maintain faith in my own sanity. Fueling this lack of acceptance is a society only beginning to acknowledge that mental illnesses are brain disorders. There were adult role models and friends who urged me to stop taking medication. There was a teacher who implied I was lazy, not ill. Who would say that a person with cancer is lazy? Who would say a person with cancer does not need some kind of treatment?

Some years after my first major episode in 1996 I found myself jobless after a period of sporadic part-time work. I called my local social security office to inquire about benefits, but was told I did not qualify to apply. This is what I would have believed to this day had my parents not known that I had been given false information. They contacted the National Alliance on Mental Illness (NAMI), a national, nonprofit organization that advocates, supports, and educates on behalf of people with mental illness. The local office supplied us with names of lawyers recommended by its members. These lawyers have expertise in navigating the social security system. How ironic that to get the help I desperately needed, I would have to pay out a percentage of any retroactive benefits to an expert on navigating bureaucracy.

Now equipped with the help of this expert I began a lengthy application for benefits. Already debilitated due to acute illness, I was forced to approach prior employers for written proof of my disability. The following is an excerpt from a letter written by a previous employer who took the time to help me apply for benefits:

We were struck with the realization that the bipolar disorder was permanent and that the severity of it was likely to be cyclical. Therefore, we could not rely on Sarah to perform the whole range of duties for which she was hired. We continued to see evidence of significant memory lapses. As we tried to give her more responsibilities again, we also found that she had great difficulty with relatively simple numerical calculations and with the accuracy of her

data entry. In short, we had to accept the fact that she was disabled to a degree that it made it impossible for us to assign her even the most basic tasks.

In addition to these disheartening proofs of my current disability, there were many painstaking details to uncover—dates of prior employment, periods of disability, accommodations made during employment, descriptions of work I was unable to do, past W2 forms, calculated percentages of my "net worth" as a disabled employee, records of my salary going back years, and finally, a detailed statement by my psychiatrist confirming my disability. According to my lawyer, all of this must be written in such a way that illustrated the chronicity of the illness, because when the illness was in remission I was much more capable and articulate.

It took months to fill out an application and to get signed documents from prior employers with busy schedules. With my parents' help I uncovered old records and filled out the necessary forms. I visited my doctor to get a statement from her confirming my disability. My lawyer then reviewed the documents with us and suggested some changes. Finally, I mailed in the application. During the lag time it took for the social security office to respond to my request, my parents absorbed the cost of my medical care. They saved me from destitution by putting a roof over my head, picking up my medication, driving me to and paying for appointments, and supplying me with a selfless stream of love and care.

Some months later I finally received a letter confirming I would receive some benefits. This was a surprisingly short timeframe within which to receive benefits, considering that so many others I know have waited up to two years for a similar outcome with appeals and visits to court in between. However, I did not qualify for Medicaid. The type of benefits I qualified for barred me from receiving immediate medical assistance, although they would supply me with Medicare after two years on benefits. The check I received monthly was not enough to live on and get medical care. Therefore, my parents continued to sink precious savings into my health care.

One of my greatest fears is that I will, without their support, one day end up on the streets—a victim of a malfunctioning system. I am, today, living proof that people can recover with proper care. I was privileged to receive such care during the time when I most acutely needed it. Without treatment would I still be walking the streets of the nation's capital blessing buildings, having conversations with imagined spirits, and approaching strangers? So many other people do not have the kind of support I have had. This keeps them from being able to pursue the type of recovery I have achieved.

Today I hold a full-time job with NAMI, the organization that helped me become an advocate, and I have the life every person deserves. I have a meaningful job, friends and family, my own apartment, a pet, music, books, poetry, and so much more. It shames me that our country does not adequately support individuals with mental illness and that our systems hold us back from the successes we truly can achieve.

individuals eligible for Medicaid, there are as many public mental health systems as there are states. Therefore, states differ in terms of availability, types of services, and quality of care. In addition, since so many recipients of public mental health services meet the eligibility requirements for Medicaid in terms of poverty and disability, Medicaid policy is closely tied to state mental health policy.

Another complexity of mental health financing is the emergence of managed care as the preferred cost-containment strategy in both the private and public sectors. Americans with private insurance generally have mental health and substance abuse coverage through employer-based managed care (Iglehart, 1996). Managed care is the predominant financing mechanism, with financial incentives aimed at controlling costs. Such measures include cost-sharing through copayments, deductibles, or co-insurance on the part of the policyholder (demand side) and **gatekeeping** (need for preauthorization of referrals to specialists), credentialing and provider panels, fee schedules, and capitation on the part of providers of services (supply side).

Capitation involves an insurer paying a fixed amount per enrollee in the plan; this system encourages the provider group to think about delivering care in the most efficient manner, because the group manages most of the economic risk. This often includes strategies such as hiring nonphysicians for lower-cost services, such as brief psychotherapy, and developing alternative delivery systems to inpatient care, such as intensive outpatient programs.

Private mental health insurance is typically provided through either a prepaid practice or a health maintenance organization (HMO), or it is contracted out and managed separately from other aspects of the insurance coverage, which is known as a "carve-out" contract. Carved-out plans enable access to specialists and services that are not common in HMOs, such as case management and psychosocial rehabilitation. Carve-out plans are most helpful for individuals with serious and persistent mental illness who benefit from a range of mental health services that would not likely meet the medical necessity criteria adhered to by HMOs (Goldman, McCulloch, & Sturm, 1998; Mechanic, 1998). The HMO structure, in contrast with the carve-out model, is more integrated between physical and mental health care, making access to general medical care and necessary prescriptions theoretically easier.

Some believe that the adoption of managed care in both the public and private sectors has created a crisis in financing and access to mental health care (Applebaum, 2003). For example, most acute inpatient mental health care occurs in the private sector despite an individual's insurance status. The financial risks of providing costly inpatient care are borne by the hospital, resulting in a serious impact on access and care delivery. Hospitals are seeing more acutely ill patients and discharging them more rapidly because of pressures of managed care (McKusick, Mark, King, Coffey, & Genuardi, 2002). Monitoring these strategies adds administrative costs to providers introduces potential issues of continuity of care for service recipients. Potential issues include whether an individual's mental health coverage includes access to levels of care other than inpatient or whether social issues such as transportation or ability to meet copayments impede access.

Every state has some type of Medicaid-managed mental health care program (Smith, Kennedy, Knipper, & O'Brien, 2005). Some of the benefits from a managed care structure include initial access to diagnosis and treatment, a flexible continuum of services designed to reduce unnecessary inpatient hospitalization, and cost savings associated with the ability to negotiate volume and reduced fees from providers (Mowbray, Grazier, & Holter, 2002). As a result, there may be reduced access to comprehensive care for individuals with more severe and persistent illnesses and incentives to cut costs at the expense of continuity of care. For example, managed care systems often use a "fail-first" policy, which restricts access to higher cost services unless the individual "fails" at a lower level of care.

Public sector–managed care often takes the form of statewide **waivers.** States are given the opportunity to apply for Medicaid waivers from the federal government to support innovation in care delivery without raising costs. States apply to waive either part of Medicaid requirements so that they can support novel programming or all Medicaid requirements in order to replace them with the state's proposed Medicaid plan. As the private sector learns to work with individuals with more complex mental health needs, the public sector increasingly finds itself competing for private funds.

Ongoing Policy Issues

Several ongoing policy issues affect occupational therapy practitioners and the individuals they serve:

- What will be covered?
- Who can provide services?
- How will care be funded and allotted?
- How will evidence-based practice be supported in routine practice?
- How can we deal with the challenges of stigma?

What Will Be Covered?

Regardless of the source of payment, decisions must be made regarding what conditions will be covered by insurance. There is disagreement on this issue among various stakeholder groups. Managed care organizations use the criteria of "medical necessity," which often covers initial access for evaluation and brief treatment and is less likely to cover long-term treatment, presenting challenges for individuals with serious and persistent mental illnesses.

There is ongoing tension about what mental health diagnoses will be covered by insurance. Some constituent groups advocate covering "biological illnesses" rather than "problems of daily living." This means that diagnoses determined to have a biological basis, such as mood disorders and schizophrenia, are covered, but other DSM-IV-TR diagnoses, such as a personality disorder, are not. This language was supported by advocates for mental health parity to counteract opposing arguments that mental health parity would have catastrophic economic consequences due to fears of extreme consumer demand for outpatient psychotherapy. A recent study found that the adoption of mental health parity along with managed care restrictions for federal employee health plans did not lead to catastrophic cost increases (Goldman et al, 2006). The study found that despite increased use of mental health services and increased costs, this effect was also seen in private sector insurance that had not adopted parity for mental health care and was primarily due to inflation and increases in health insurance premiums rather than to elimination of therapy caps.

Who Can Provide Services?

Another key policy decision involves who can provide service. One of the most challenging interprofessional issues to emerge includes direct access to nonphysician mental health providers for diagnosis, treatment, and medication. The medical profession has employed aggressive influence to prevent psychologists, nurses, and other licensed mental health providers from performing diagnostic and prescribing activities. Many states designate certain licensed disciplines (e.g., psychologists, social workers, marriage and family counselors) as Qualified Mental Health Providers (QMHPs). Designation as a QMHP allows a service provider to diagnose illnesses, provide interventions, request involuntary commitment, and so on. In practice, the designation also determines which disciplines will or will not get reimbursed. No state identifies occupational therapists as QMHPs, although in some states, such as Pennsylvania, they are considered "noncore" professionals who can provide mental health care and can be reimbursed for services. Exclusion from QMHP status restricts reimbursement, reduces access to occupational therapy services, and in some cases results in lower pay for occupational therapists, particularly in community-based settings. Occupational therapists have not been advocating for prescription writing or diagnostic ability but to provide mental health services according to state practice acts, typically in a community setting.

How Will Care Be Funded and Allotted?

Although most professionals agree that mental health care funding should follow individual clients and be allotted to community-based settings, there is often resistance to implementing such reforms. One challenge is mistrust in this policy area due to a history of underfunding. Mistrust may cause tension between hospital-based providers and community providers who fear that an increase in allotted community mental health funding will come at the expense of reduced state hospital funding. Economic and political concerns about hospital closings and job loss may emerge, including community concerns about housing and characteristics of the population joining the community. Some believe that further broadening the mental health service delivery system makes for more fragmentation and diffuse spending without a central accountable agency.

Different priorities among consumer and advocate groups also impact the policy agenda. For example, the National Alliance for Mental Illness, which primarily comprises family members, has supported initiatives such as the adoption of involuntary commitment laws to include conditions such as "gravely disabled" and the expansion of assertive community treatment programs, whereas consumer organizations such as the National Empowerment Center oppose these policies. Many of these conflicts are centered on the challenge of supporting the civil rights of individuals with serious mental illness while not denying needed care. As a result, states have grappled with various forms of outpatient commitment/ treatment protocols; the role of the criminal justice system; rights of the individual, families, and the community; and definitions of medical necessity that often preclude intervention until the individual is completely unable to function.

How Will Evidence-Based Practice Be Supported in Routine Practice?

A 2001 Institute of Medicine report stated that the time between research discoveries of treatment effectiveness and the incorporation of this evidence into routine care could sometimes take over a decade (Institute of Medicine, 2001). This issue was specifically addressed in the Surgeon General's report on mental health (USDHHS, 1999) and again by the NFCMH (2003). Both reports called for support for the dissemination of technologies that demonstrate positive research outcomes. States and accrediting agencies are invested in this issue. States are challenged to meet the demands of evidence-based practice fidelity due to funding and staffing issues, and accrediting agencies and payers are interested in whether programs are using best practices supported by research evidence and are applying pressure to do so. Nonetheless, to incorporate these effective services or treatments into practice, both public and private funders must constantly examine their coverage rules to support the adoption of new interventions. Presently, a practitioner seeking reimbursement for a new, effective treatment would have to work with the consumer to navigate the financing systems to get the appropriate permissions or waivers (NFCMH, 2003).

Additional challenges to implementing policies and administrative practices that support integration of evidence-based research into practice include funding problems, turnover of key state leaders, state bureaucracies, competing priorities, and lack of incentives (Goldman et al, 2001; Mechanic, 2002). This demonstrates that the historic fragmentation of the delivery system, lack of a policy champion, and divided responsibility of mental health service and delivery continues to negatively impact basic quality of and access to care.

How Can We Deal With Challenges of Stigma?

An inherent challenge to mental health policy is the stigma attached to mental illness. Mass media portrayals of individuals with mental illness often emphasize dangerousness and unpredictability. Research has shown that most individuals get information about mental illness from mass media sources despite statistics showing that one in four American adults experience a diagnosable mental disorder in any given year (Kessler, Chiu, Demler, & Walters, 2005). Studies indicate the American public increasingly believes in the biological basis of mental disorders and that most desire additional education and information about mental illness (Corrigan & Penn, 1999).

From a policymaking perspective, where competition for a place on the decision agenda and for limited funds is high, it is important that stigma be decreased. The population served by mental health policy is broad and heterogeneous and includes children, adults, and the elderly. The issues are just as complex and include oversight and approval of medications, education support, employment discrimination, mandatory outpatient interventions, civil rights, and fair and safe housing alternatives. It is challenging to advocate that additional public funds be allotted to a population that because of fear or misunderstanding is viewed by the public as undeserving. Nonetheless, to transform the mental health service delivery system, occupational therapists must play a leading role in helping people increase their understanding of mental illness and in decreasing the stigma toward both persons with mental illnesses and the act of seeking help to maintain one's mental health.

Basics of Policymaking

Policymaking is a decision-making process that includes three interdependent phases (Longest, 2002):

1. Policy formulation—problem definition and weighing alternatives.
2. Policy implementation—action and decisions in implementation process.
3. Policy modification—incrementalism.

Policy Formulation

The public policy agenda consists of issues that are commonly perceived by members of the political community as meriting attention (although not necessarily action) and falling within the community's legitimate domain or jurisdiction. Kingdon (1995) states that in order for an "issue" to become a policy problem that makes it onto the agenda, it must have the ability to evoke a relatively uniform public response and be "solvable." It also helps if there is someone, such as a policy entrepreneur, committed to its success.

Elected officials advocate for policy formation when they define problems by giving them a "human face" (Stone, 1989), such as by portraying "average citizens" struggling because of the policy problem or benefiting from the proposed policy solution. Examples could include senior citizens needing to choose between buying prescriptions or food and homeless persons with serious mental illness and/or addiction dying from hypothermia. One direct way occupational therapists can support policy formation is to provide their elected leaders with the personal stories that assist them in defining a policy problem and gaining public support for its placement on the policy agenda.

Schneider and Ingram (1993) discuss how the social construction of various populations determines success in getting on the policy agenda. They posit that some conditions are positively constructed, and the public feels these deserve policy attention, whereas some are negatively constructed and appear less deserving of policy benefits. In this typology, for example, conditions with known biological causes, such as Alzheimer disease, are more positively socially constructed, whereas a condition that is less understood and seen by some as being within the control of an individual, such as substance dependence, is more negatively socially constructed.

The second aspect of policy formulation includes identifying potential policy alternative solutions, which are based on the defined policy problem. Interest groups, or groups of individuals who are organized around a common interest and seek to influence public policy, are important participants because they often can present alternatives to current policies that reflect the needs of their constituencies (Weissert & Weissert, 1996). Three key strategies are employed by interest groups to influence policy:

- Lobbying for a particular policy alternative.
- Grassroots organizing to promote or block a particular policy alternative.
- Contributing to campaigns through political action committees (PACs).

Interest groups have grown exponentially in the past 30 years. Groups with interests in mental health include those seeking influence on the part of various provider groups, such as occupational therapists, states, private insurers, consumers of care, families, community activists, legal activists, hospitals, and employers. In general, interest groups are more successful with single, narrow issues rather than broad legislation. One recent trend is the development of temporary coalitions around issues such as fair and safe housing by groups with a single common interest. These collaborations typically do not last beyond the interest.

Policy alternatives are generated in a few ways, including examining the traditional types of alternatives (Table 27-3), adopting what has been successful elsewhere, and working with what is already the policy alternative by making incremental (small and politically possible) changes. Identifying multiple alternative policies for addressing an issue allows for some comparisons of both how the problem is perceived and what may be the best approaches to a solution to the problem. An example is pulling a medication from the market

Table 27-2 ● **Indicators That Determine the Policy Agenda**

Indicator	Example	One Policy Solution
Crisis/focusing event	Incident at Columbine led to increased interest in middle school–aged youth, alienation, and bullying	Direct service: Afterschool programs
Change in respected indicator	Relatively poor health outcomes for infants and children	Expanding current alternative: Children's Health Insurance Program (CHIP)
New technology and knowledge	Information on risk of self-harm and children and teens with depression on selective serotonin reuptake inhibitors (SSRIs)	Rule: Adopting a "black box" warning on SSRI prescriptions for children and adolescents
Public opinion	Rising drug costs to seniors	Direct service: A market-oriented Congress supported the current Medicare Part D prescription plan

Table 27-3 ▪ **Policy Alternatives**

Typical Alternative	Example
Subsidy	Provide additional funds to providers who treat underserved populations
Tax	Pay for expanded health coverage by tax on cigarettes
Incentive	Reward for adoption of desired policy, such as recruiting diverse student pool
Rule	Requirement to participate, such as license to provide care
Direct service	Demonstration project of new program

(preferred alternative of the Food and Drug Administration and some consumers and advocates) versus doing nothing and leaving the medication on the market (preferred alternative of the pharmaceutical industry and some professionals and consumers) versus permitting it to stay on the market with a "black box" warning label of potential risks and increased monitoring from psychiatrists (compromise based on scientific evidence). It is most common to choose the alternative that requires the least controversy and cost. Interest groups or their representatives compare alternatives in several ways, including identifying criteria by which they will be evaluated and examining positive and negative consequences (e.g., cost, morbidity, independence) to determine what is gained and lost.

Another consideration is whether the public can support the alternative. Community placement of drug treatment settings is an example of a fractious policy for which public support is challenging. This is the NIMBY (not in my back yard) phenomenon that often shows up when decisions about opening a substance abuse treatment center are discussed in a public venue. Geographic barriers relative to access are accentuated when such programs are concentrated in one area or neighborhood (Wolch, 1996). Another example was the compromise reached in the federal Mental Health Parity Act of 1996. It was found that the public would support aspects of parity for mental illness, but such support eroded when treatment for substance abuse was included in the plan. The final version that was enacted did not include substance abuse. Once a policy alternative is chosen, it proceeds to implementation.

Policy Implementation

The challenge of policy implementation is that it occurs with a different group of participants than those who defined the problem. On the federal level, this includes employees of government agencies that issue regulations for carrying out the law, such as the Centers for Medicare and Medicaid Services (CMS), Social Security Administration (SSA), and Occupational Safety and Health Administration (OSHA). This is the stage of policymaking during which interest groups, such as the American Occupational Therapy Political Action Committee (AOTPAC) or the National Alliance on Mental Illness (NAMI), are most active.

Policy implementation is not a systematic, linear process by which experts rationally define a problem, unanimously agree on the alternative solution, and assign it to a knowledgeable group of individuals with authority and accountability for its execution. There is rarely immediate and unified agreement among stakeholders; the participants come and go during the process; there is rarely a structured outline and timeline of decision point (rather, decisions evolve over time); and although the alternative may have improved some aspects of the issue, it likely does not fully "solve" the problem. An example is legislation that is the product of compromise, such as the Medicare Modernization Act, which includes the Medicare Prescription Drug Plan, or Medicare Part D. Legislation is passed, but the implementation involves assignment to an agency with oversight provided by another agency.

Events can change the implementation process; for example, election results that alter party control can dramatically change legislative and fiscal priorities as well as administrative leadership in agencies through political appointments. In addition, civil servants with technical expertise may transfer, be reassigned, retire, or impact implementation through funding shifts or other forms of political influence.

Policy implementation evolves, adapts, and comes with unintended consequences. Several authorities discuss the challenges of implementation. Kingdon (1995) states that fluid participation of participants and unclear technologies impede successful implementation. Hargrove (1981) identifies features that support implementation, including ensuring that the policy alternative has explicit boundaries, goals and objectives, and overtly defined trade-offs. He states that there are two phases of implementation: passing the law and making it happen. It is important to realize that policy implementation is not the end of the process. Opportunities arise to influence policy during and after implementation, and interest groups are very involved in policy modification.

Policy Modification

Inevitably, the implementation of a policy presents unintended consequences. Policies need to be modified. This modification process is parallel to a practitioner fine-tuning a treatment plan to address a person's problem of occupational functioning: an intervention plan to address the problem is generated through a collaborative process with the person (formulation), which is followed by a series of interventions (implementation) that help both the consumer and practitioner realize that the plan needs to be modified to ensure success (modification). One example of a policy modification is the decision to waive Medicare Part D late enrollment penalties for the first year for dually eligible individuals. As this policy was implemented, it became clear that there were unanticipated problems with consumers and their families understanding enrollment directives and accessing sign-up. No policy is 100% successful; errors and other challenges due to communication and access difficulties are common.

Policy Impact on Occupational Therapy: A Model for Analysis

One way to understand how policies influence occupational therapy practice is to apply a model that identifies and analyzes internal and external influences First, aspects of the issue relative to the profession of occupational therapy (internal influences related to practice, education, administration, and research) are examined. Then, outside influences (external issues including historical, political, economic, and social influences) are examined. This model assists in understanding the complexity of an issue beyond what may seem obvious (Morris, 2000). An example of application of the model is provided in Figure 27-2. The figure presents policy issues that affect occupational therapy's role in community based practice. By identifying and understanding the policy issues, occupational therapists can better work to influence policy.

In the example in Figure 27-2, the general **policy problem** is identified as "increased mental health costs and decreased access to mental health care," and the proposed alternative by the occupational therapy profession is to expand the role for occupational therapy in community mental health. On the professional level, then, an organized, multifaceted policy discussion would ensue. For example, a resolution might be proposed to the representative assembly to address the need to prepare occupational therapy students for roles in community mental health. A variety of policy alternatives might be generated:

- Direct service alternative—involve a task force to examine current practice influences.
- Rule alternative—involve curriculum mandates relative to mental health content and fieldwork.
- Incentive alternative—involve focused grant funding by the professional association for projects that lead to increased practice in community mental health that results in measurable outcomes.
- Subsidy alternative—involve the private or public employment sector in mental health, providing a stipend or tuition remission for graduates who work in community mental health.

Once a policy alternative is selected, the process moves to implementation. Implementation from this example would involve participants designing and following through with each action item. Then, reports and other data that were generated from the alternatives might be assembled into a position paper demonstrating benefits of occupational therapy in community mental health that could be presented by AOTA or AOTPAC representatives to key policymakers on the federal and/or state levels. Policy modification is often the point at which the profession is involved, because once policies are implemented, unintended consequences arise. For example, if the chosen alternative to improve access and reduce cost was unsuccessful or revealed complexities unanticipated in the original policy decision, there is another opportunity to propose the occupational therapy alternative. In this case, those who are prepared with brief, succinct data that demonstrates effectiveness can be successful over time. In other words, many changes emerge over time in the policy modification process, not just as the first chosen alternative.

If the issue example included an occupational therapist becoming aware of state funding for transforming the public mental health system due to a defined policy problem of not meeting state-mandated mental health **recovery standards** by developing a plan to apply for grant funds to improve the system, a programmatic effort of advocacy might include the following:

- Direct service alternative—providing key decision makers with a proposal for services or a state association position paper taking a stand on the issue.
- Incentive alternative—volunteering for a task force or board membership.
- Subsidy alternative—including in the proposal for services a fieldwork program model in which students serve to extend programmatic offerings in community mental health.
- Rule alternative—working, as a member of the state association and in conjunction with the national office, to advocate for the recognition of occupational therapists as QMHPs in the state.

Evidence-Based Practice

Advocacy interventions address issues at the individual, programmatic, and policy levels.

➤ Occupational therapists can advocate for clients at the individual level by providing client documentation to decision-making agencies in support of issues such as the following:
  - Additional intervention (third-party payer).
  - Housing decision (agency leadership).
  - Funding decision (disability determination).

➤ Occupational therapists can advocate for clients at the individual level by advising clients or family members of their rights, such as by providing information on the following:
  - Appealing decisions to policymakers (school system).
  - Contacting agencies for additional services (safety net).
  - Civil rights (ADA, Olmstead Act, Fair Housing Act).

➤ Occupational therapists can advocate for clients at the programmatic level by becoming involved in organizations and presenting information and advice on the benefits of policy change. This can be accomplished by occupational therapists volunteering, joining a board, and making a formal presentation (e.g., get invited to present to key groups; write focused letters to decision makers; solicit position papers from state organizations; solicit letters of support).

➤ Occupational therapists can advocate for clients at the policy level by getting involved with key decision makers and building relationships through:
  - Regular written contact with decision makers/legislators.
  - Staying abreast of professional issues on the federal and state levels.
  - Joining national and state occupational therapy associations.
  - Taking a leadership role or joining a task force.
  - Joining an advocacy group.
  - Joining the board of directors of an agency.
  - Volunteering on a key work group that determines policy.
  - Contributing funds.

Goodman-Lavey, M., & Dunbar, S. (2003). Federal legislative advocacy In G. McCormack, E. Jaffe, & M. Goodman-Lavey (Eds.) *The Occupational Therapy Manager* (4th ed.) (pp. 424–430). Bethesda, MD: AOTA Press.

Sandstrom, R. W., Lohman, H., & Bramble, J. D. (2009). Effecting policy change: Therapist as advocate. In *Health services: Policy and stems for therapists* (2nd ed.) (pp. 266–275). Upper Saddle River, NJ: Prentice Hall.

Policy Issue Analysis

Issue: Expanding the role for occupational therapy in community mental health practice

---

Internal Aspects:

Historical

Practice Trends
- Most U.S. mental health OT practice occurs in hospital-based settings
- Profession's adoption of OTPF encourages attention to community participation/recovery
- Managed care demands efficiency and attention to productivity

Education
- Entry-level focus on basic psychopathology and OTPF
- Continuing education focus on community practice, recovery model, and advanced skills/credentials
- Current standards do not prepare OTs to meet criteria as a qualified mental health practitioner (QMHP)

Administration
- "Manpower" issue — are there enough therapists? Do they want to practice in this area?
- Regulatory issues determine roles — can OT be recognized as a QMHP?
- Current reimbursement reinforces medical model
- Scope of practice supports broader role
- Supervision needs/mentoring for new roles — by whom?

Research
- Evidence-based research relative to profession and mental health — who is doing it? Findings?

External Influences:

Historical
- Alliance with moral treatment and mental hygiene movement to biological basis of illness and neuroscience and genetic findings of past decade
- Civil rights and individual self-determination drive policy shifts to community from institutional care
- Skyrocketing costs promote exploration of alternatives to inpatient care

Political
- Federal civil rights legislation and administrative actions support recovery philosophy, but not funding
- New Freedom Commission on Mental Health report lists multiple recommendations that are consistent with OTPF
- Potential to link with MH survivors and recovery-oriented grass roots organizations in strategic alliances to transform mental health service delivery systems

Economic
- Costs of care increase — desire for lower cost alternatives
- Cost shifting from payers to providers to individuals
- Chronic lack of funding for public mental health
- Increased attention to funding outcomes-based programs
- Consumer advocacy activities increase demand for quality
- Politics of the population — how perceived by the public?
- States have multiple competing health and social priorities to fund
- Organizational politics — state hospitals, community mental health at odds
- Provider conflicts divide potential coalitions and impact success

Social
- Increase in numbers of aging/disabled populations
- Increased diversity of population and mental health needs
- Increased involvement of adult/juvenile justice system
- Stigma of conditions/treatment impact?
- Effects of poverty, racism, and geography on access

FIGURE 27-2. Example of policy issue analysis. In the United States, occupational therapists have had limited visibility and influence in the area of community-based mental health. This figure identifies policies that have influenced community-based practice both within and outside of the profession.

Occupational Justice and Intervention in Public Policy

A discussion has emerged in the occupational therapy and occupational science literature regarding the political aspects of occupation. Townsend (2004) discussed the role of social justice in occupational therapy practice, and Townsend and Wilcock (2004) introduced the concept of **occupational justice**: "the equitable opportunity and resources to enable people's engagement in meaningful occupations (p. 85)." Watson and Swartz (2004) ask if we are ready to make occupation a political issue in terms of empowering others relative to sustainable livelihoods, service integration, and social inclusiveness.

Kronenberg, Algado, and Pollard (2005) identify "political activities of daily living" and state that the overarching aim of occupational therapy intervention is social integration. These political activities of daily living include advocacy activities on behalf of marginalized populations and empowering such individuals and communities to exercise agency on their own behalf. The authors challenge therapists to collaborate with those individuals who are powerful and those who are marginalized to promote social change. Certainly, understanding the policymaking process assists occupational therapy practitioners in advocating for access to needed services; adequate funding for safe, affordable housing; civil rights of individuals with mental illnesses relative to securing viable education and employment; and reducing social stigma to promote full participation in environments of choice. Terms relative to occupational justice are defined with examples in Box 27-1.

BOX 27-1 ■ Occupational Justice Terminology

Occupational alienation: When a person's need for meaningful and health-promoting occupations is unmet or systematically denied. Example: Do mental health policies support an individual's ability to find meaning in daily life? Do such policies deny opportunities for health promotion? Occupational alienation can occur as an unintended consequence, for example, when funds are cut or limits are set on which medications are available or when policies restrict employment by denying crucial benefits such as health care when an individual becomes employed, thereby denying a valued activity.

Occupational deprivation: When an individual experiences daily life as meaningless and purposeless. Example: As a result of organizational policies, are individuals able to exercise personal agency/self-determination in terms of valued activities and role development toward personally meaningful occupations, such as employee, parent, student, and home maintainer? Do such policies by design involve those individuals who are most affected (e.g., clients and families) in the design of intervention plans?

Occupational imbalance: When sufficient variations in daily occupations that are necessary to sustain well-being are rendered impossible due to personal or societal circumstances. Example: Do organizational policies support personal choice of activity? Is there too much of the same and too little variation for balance, due to funding challenges, staffing issues, or other organizational barriers?

Definitions adapted from Wood, W., Hooper, B., & Womack, J. (2005). Reflections on occupational justice as a sub-text of occupation-centered education. In F. Kronenberg, S. Algado, & N. Pollard (Eds.), *Occupational Therapy Without Borders* (p. 378–389). New York: Elsevier.

The person-environment-occupation model addresses the multiple aspects of the environment that impact social participation. Theorists discuss the multiple aspects of the environment that impact client performance and engagement in valued roles (Law et al, 2003). Five environmental domains have been described: physical, social, cultural, socioeconomic, and institutional/organizational. It is clear that public policy impacts the person and his or her environment in all five domains.

Assessment and Intervention of Client Needs: An Occupational Justice Perspective

Case Example

The following case example depicts the impact of public policy on the five environmental domains of physical, social, cultural, socioeconomic, and institutional/organizational.

Joe is a 23-year-old single male with a diagnosis of schizophrenia, paranoid type. Joe first became ill when he went away to college at age 18. He found the transition challenging and began isolating himself, drinking, and smoking marijuana to cope with the stresses of managing five classes and his life each week. He became increasingly paranoid and suspicious and began staying in his dorm room. His roommate eventually complained to the resident assistant that Joe was behaving and speaking bizarrely, claiming that the campus administration was tapping his phone and that he had to stay in bed to hide from the authorities.

Joe was hospitalized and left campus at that time. He has been in and out of inpatient, partial hospitalization, and community programs for the past five years. Inpatient hospitalization has typically been precipitated by Joe's return to drinking, smoking marijuana, and refusing to take his psychotropic medications. The longest that Joe has remained out of inpatient care over the past five years was 16 months. Joe was living with his mother until this last hospitalization. She has now decided that Joe needs to develop life skills and can best learn these in a supported housing environment and community rehabilitation program. Joe agrees but does not see the impact of substance use on his relapse history and overall illness management. Joe has recently been awarded SSI in the amount of $700 per month. He also has Medicaid coverage, and the state that he lives in provides pharmacy assistance that enables him to afford his medications.

To assist Joe in developing needed life skills and resuming valued roles as he recovers, the occupational therapist uses the person-environment-occupation framework to examine Joe's wants and needs. The *person* aspect includes Joe's wants, skills, and capacities relative to community living, which the occupational therapist addresses through assessment.

The *environment* aspect includes an examination of physical, social, cultural, socioeconomic, and institutional/organizational aspects of Joe's situation. Environmental knowledge relative to public policy includes the following:

■ Physical environment—What are Joe's housing options? What is the available housing market in Joe's community for someone with his income? What degree of involvement will Joe will have in determining his housing situation? This might include geographic location, which could impact continuity of care, transportation, and safety, as well as living arrangements, such as roommate(s), rules relative to taking medications and using substances, and amount of supervision.

■ Social environment—Is Joe aware of recovery-oriented consumer rights and support services? Are services coordinated in this state or fragmented and geographically dispersed? Are consumers involved in policymaking at the state and organizational/agency levels? Is there a NAMI affiliate or other venue for Joe's family to access for support and education? Is there a venue for Joe if he needs to advocate for assistance with living situation, legal needs, pharmacy assistance, or other need relative to successful community tenure?

■ Cultural environment—Does Joe's environment support the expression of his values and beliefs?

■ Socioeconomic environment—Can Joe live on his disability check? What resources are available to assist him?

■ Institutional/organizational/agency environment—What services are available in Joe's community relative to skill building and role performance? Are evidence-based practices, such as supported employment and family psychoeducation, available? If so, are they reimbursed by Medicaid? Do state policies support a recovery framework? Are there specialized and accessible services for individuals such as Joe who struggle with medication compliance and substance abuse, placing them in a higher risk category relative to criminal justice involvement or homelessness? Will Joe have access to occupational therapy after he leaves a hospital-based environment? Is the occupational therapist considered a mental health provider in this state?

The *occupation* aspect of the case refers to Joe's ability to engage in valued activities of daily life (occupations) based on the fit between his personal factors and what the environment provides and demands (Brown, 2009). When Joe's engagement in valued occupations is restricted, an occupational justice approach may be indicated.

From an occupational justice perspective, the occupational therapist working with Joe would be interested in the degree of self-determination that Joe is able to exercise relative to choice of housing and housing characteristics. Is Joe offered the opportunity to choose the activities that comprise his daily life? Simple daily choices, such as preferred foods, valued activities, and respect for religious and cultural practices impact quality of life and determine whether the organizations that serve Joe support a recovery framework or alienate, deprive, or marginalize service recipients. Social or community aspects reflecting issues of occupational justice include cost of housing and availability of safe, affordable housing and transportation. Institutional/system aspects include whether such policies support recovery or further marginalize recipients with restrictive barriers to employment participation, refusal to cover effective medications because of cost, or recommending discharge from all services once minimal function is demonstrated.

In terms of occupational justice, the occupational therapist is interested in whether Joe has access to needed services and resources to engage in valued activities in his community of choice. For example, the degree of self-determination in his living environment and skill-building program is significant, as is his ability to access social resources of interest. Attention to occupational issues will support Joe in rebuilding a life of meaning based on his valued interests and goals relative to recovery.

Summary

Occupational therapists who work in mental health must understand the structure and financing mechanisms of the mental health system as well as the social, legal, and other influences that affect the daily lives of individuals with mental illness. Necessary knowledge includes federal, state, and local laws, policies, and agencies that support the needs of individuals with mental illness living in the community. Such knowledge can be used to advocate for, develop, or provide access to occupational therapy services.

Active Learning Strategies

1. Educate Yourself About Current Policy Issues

● Go to the American Occupational Therapy Association website (www.aota.org). Click on the Legislative Action Center tab. Click on any of the Current Issues and learn more about current legislation that may impact the occupational therapy profession in mental health.

● Can you identify how the profession exercised influence in the design and/or modification of the selected policy? Who were our allies? What were the outcomes? Were there any unintended consequences? If the information is not clear, consider calling or writing the AOTA Federal Affairs Department at (301) 652-2682, extension 2010.

- Read the synopsis provided by AOTA, then go to one of the following sites to learn more and track the progress of the bill.
  - Thomas Library of Congress: http://thomas.loc.gov
  - GovTrack USA: http://www.govtrack.us
  - Open Congress: http://www.opencongress.org
- Note if a representative or senator from your state has signed on as a cosponsor. If not, consider calling or writing to your representative. There are links from the AOTA's Legislative Action Center to help you find your legislator and preformatted letters to get you started.

2. Bring a Bill to Class

- Go to the Library of Congress site (http://thomas.loc.gov) and type in the name of a bill. The AOTA Legislative Action Center can help you identify the specific name of the bill; for example, Medicare Home Health Flexibility Act of 2009 or the bill number (e.g., H.R. 1094).
- Enter the title or bill number and then follow the link to get the text of the legislation; print, read, and bring to class to share.
- Use the model for analysis of a practice issue to analyze this bill.

3. Find Out What National Mental Health Organization Are Focusing On

- Go to the National Alliance on Mental Illness (http://www.nami) or another organization that advocates for the rights of persons with mental illness. What are some initiatives that match interests of occupational therapy practitioners? How can occupational therapists get involved?
- Click on the link to Find Your Local NAMI to find organizations in your area.
- Look for a legislative link on your local NAMI's page and identify the key bills that this organization is tracking.
- Have peers do the same thing for various states in and out of your region of the country.
- Compare and contrast the key issues defined by these state organizations.
  - Do the legislative concerns of the NAMI members coincide or conflict with concerns of the occupational therapy profession?
  - Brainstorm ways to collaborate on advocacy campaigns.
  - Invite a member from NAMI to your class to discuss legislative issues and advocacy strategies.

4. Explore Your State's Mental Health Plan

- Go to the Substance Abuse and Mental Health Services Administration (SAMHSA) website (http://www.samhsa.org) and look up your state's mental health plan.
  - What information is available?
  - For example, is enrollment information available? Costs of mental health care? Eligibility criteria? Services offered? Evaluation measures and outcomes?
  - How does this information influence occupational therapy service delivery?

5. Explore Requirements for Being a Qualified Mental Health Practitioner in Your State

- Google "Qualified Mental Health Practitioner JOBS" and compare the variety of positions that come up. Discuss with peers whether occupational therapists have the skill set to compete for some of these jobs.
- Use your state's Department of Health and Human Services or State Licensure website to identify what disciplines have been designated QMHP in your state.
  - List the types of services QMHPs are able to perform in your state.
  - Compare the educational requirements of disciplines with QMHP status with your own mental health training in your occupational therapy curriculum.
  - Divide your class and debate whether occupational therapists should be identified as QMHPs in your state. Have half the students argue for and the other half argue against occupational therapists being designated as QMHPs.

6. Learn About Your Congressional Representatives

- Review and identify your federal and state House of Representative and Senate contacts.
  - What committees are they on?
  - Interview them about their positions on mental health issues, such as parity, seclusion and restraint, and Medicare (federal) and Medicaid (federal and state) funding initiatives.
  - Ask them about what is happening in your state relative to community-based mental health care.
  - Ask if there is occupational therapist representation on the state level for initiatives relative to housing, education, or employment supports for persons with mental illness.

7. Read Recent Governmental Reports

- Download the executive summary of the New Freedom Commission on Mental Health (http://www.mentalhealthcommission.gov/reports/reports.htm).
- Form six groups in your class and have each group examine one of the commission's six primary goals.
  - Have each group identify three to five talking points describing the key issues that will help colleagues understand the goal.
  - Have each group examine the NFCMH's recommendations for achieving the goal and identify three specific strategies that can be used to influence policies that could help implement these recommendations.

Resources

- National Alliance on Mental Illness: http://www.nami.org
- National Mental Health Association: http://www.nmha.org
- Bazelon Center for Mental Health Law: http://www.bazelon.org
- National Association of State Mental Health Program Directors: http://www.nasmhpd.org
- National Mental Health Information Center: http://www.mentalhealth.org
- Centers for Medicaid and Medicare Services: http://www.cms.gov
- Medicaid: http://www.cms.hhs.gov/home/Medicaid.asp. At this site are links for:
  - Medicaid Waiver and Demonstration Projects
  - Home and Community-Based Services
  - New Freedom Initiative
  - Medicaid Transformation Grants
  - Ticket to Work and Work Incentives Improvement Act (TWWIIA)
- Fair Housing Act: http://www.usdoj.gov/crt/housing/housing_coverage.htm
- National Center for Health Statistics: http://www.cdc.gov/nchs/hus.htm
- World Health Organization: http://www.who.int
- Institute of Medicine: http://www.iom.edu
- National Center for Education Statistics: http://www.nces.ed.gov
- National Council on Disability: http://www.ncd.gov
- Agency for Healthcare Research and Quality: http://www.ahrq.gov
- Robert Wood Johnson Foundation: http://www.rwjf.org
- National Empowerment Center: http://www.power2u.org
- Center for Reintegration: http://www.reintegration.com

References

American Occupational Therapy Association. (2008). Occupational therapy practice framework: Domain and process (2nd ed.). *American Journal of Occupational Therapy, 62,* 625–688.

Appelbaum, P. S. (2003). The "quiet" crisis in mental health services. *Health Affairs, 22*(5), 110–116.

Brown, C. (2009). Functional assessment and intervention in occupational therapy. *Psychiatric Rehabilitation Journal, 32,* 162–170.

Corrigan, P. W., & Penn, D. (1999). Lessons from social psychology on discrediting psychiatric stigma. *American Psychologist, 54,* 765–776.

Cottrell, R. P. (2003). The Olmstead decision: Fulfilling the promise of the ADA? *OT Practice, 8*(5), 17–21.

———. (2007). The New Freedom Initiative: Transforming mental health care: Will OT be at the table? *Occupational Therapy in Mental Health, 23,* 2, 1–25.

Emery, B. D., Glover, R.W., & Mazade, N. A. (1998). The environmental trends facing state mental health agencies. *Administration and Policy in Mental Health, 25,* 337–347.

Gallew, H. A., Haltiwanger, E., Sowers, J., & van der Heever, N. (2004). Political action and critical analysis: Mental health parity. *Occupational Therapy in Mental Health, 20,* 1, 1–25.

Geller, J. L. (2000). The last half century of psychiatric services as reflected in *Psychiatric Services. Psychiatric Services, 51,* 1, 41–67.

Goldman, H. H., Frank, R. G., Burnham, M. A., Huskamp, H. A., Ridgely, M. S., Normand, S. T., et al. (2006). Behavioral health insurance parity for federal employees. *New England Journal of Medicine, 354,* 1378–1386.

Goldman, H. H., Ganju, V., Drake, R., Gorman, P., Hogan, M., & Hyde, P. (2001). Policy implications for implementing evidence-based practices. *Psychiatric Services, 52,* 1591–1597.

Goldman, W., McCulloch, J., & Sturm, R. (1998). Costs and use of mental health services before and after managed care. *Health Affairs, 17*(2), 40–52.

Grob, G. N. (1994). Government and mental health policy: A structural analysis. *Milbank Quarterly, 72*(93), 471–500.

———. (2001). Mental health policy in 20th-century America. In R. W. Manderscheid, M. J. Henderson, (Eds.), Center for Mental Health Services, *Mental Health, United States 2000* (pp. 218–230). DHHS Pub. No (SMA) 01-3537 (Washington, DC: Government Printing Office).

Hargrove, E. C. (1981). The search for implementation theory. (ERIC Document Reproduction Service, No. ED207158).

Iglehart, J. K. (1996). Health policy report: Managed care and mental health. *New England Journal of Medicine, 334*(2), 131–135.

Institute of Medicine Committee on Quality of Health Care in America. (2001). *Crossing the Quality Chasm: A New Health System for the 21st Century.* Washington, DC: National Academies Press.

Kessler, R. C., Chiu, W. T., Demler, O., & Walters, E. E. (2005). Prevalence, severity, and comorbidity of twelve-month DSM-IV disorders in the National Comorbidity Survey Replication (NCS-R). *Archives of General Psychiatry, 62*(6), 617–627.

Kingdon, J. W. (1995). *Agendas, Alternatives and Public Policies* (2nd ed.). New York: HarperCollins.

Kronenberg, F., Algado, S. S., & Pollard, N. (Eds.). (2005). *Occupational Therapy Without Borders.* Philadelphia, PA: Elsevier.

Law, M., Cooper, C., Strong, S., Stewart, D., Rigby, P., & Letts, L. (1996). The person-environment-occupation model: A transactive approach to occupational therapy. *Canadian Journal of Occupational Therapy, 63,* 9–21.

Longest, B. B. (2002). *Health Policy Making in the United States* (3rd ed.). New York: Health Administration Press.

McKusick, D., Mark, T., King, E., Coffey, R., & Genuardi, J. (2002). Trends in mental health insurance benefits and out-of-pocket spending. *Journal of Mental Health Policy and Economics, 5,* 71–78.

———. (2002). Removing barriers to care among persons with psychiatric symptoms. *Health Affairs, 21*(3), 137–147.

———. (2008). Managed mental health care. In *Mental Health and Social Policy: Beyond Managed Care* (5th ed.). (pp. 185–221). Boston: Pearson Education.

Mechanic, D., McAlpine, D., & Olfson, M. (1998). Changing patterns of psychiatric inpatient care in the United States: 1988–1994. *Archives of General Psychiatry, 55*(9), 785–791.

Mechanic, D., Schlesinger, M., & McAlpine, D. D. (1995). Management of mental health and substance abuse services: State of the art and early results. *Milbank Quarterly, 73*(1), 19–55.

Monahan, J., Swartz, M., & Bonnie, R. J. (2003). Mandated treatment in the community for people with mental disorders. *Health Affairs, 22,* 28–38.

Morris, J. A. (2000). Playing policy pinball: Making policy analysis palatable. *Administration and Policy in Mental Health, 28,* 131–137.

Mowbray, C. T., Grazier, K. L. & Holter, M. (2002). Managed behavioral health care in the public sector: Will it become the third shame of the states? *Psychiatric Services, 53*(2), 157–170.

New Freedom Commission on Mental Health (NFCMH). (2003). *Achieving the promise: Transforming mental health care in America. Final report.* DHHS Pub. No. SMA-03-3832. Rockville, MD: author.

Olmstead v L.C. and E.W., 527 U.S. 581, 138 F.3d 893 (1999).

Priester, R. (1992). A values framework for health system reform. *Health Affairs, 11*(1), 85–107.

Regier, D. A., Narrow, W. E., Rae, D. S., Manderscheid, R.W., Locke, B. Z., & Goodwin, F. (1993). The de facto U.S. mental and addictive disorders service system: Epidemiologic and catchment area prospective one-year prevalence rates of disorders and services. *Archives of General Psychiatry, 50,* 85–94.

Schneider, A., & Ingram, H. (1993). Social construction of target populations: Implications for politics and policy. *American Political Science Review, 87*(2), 334–347.

Scull, A. (1985). Deinstitutionalization and public policy. *Social Science and Medicine, 20*(5), 545–552.

Sharfstein, S. (2000). Whatever happened to community mental health? *Psychiatric Services, 51*(5), 616–620.

Smith, G., Kennedy, C., Knipper, S., & O'Brien, J. (2005). *Using Medicaid to Support Working-Age Adults with Serious Mental Illness in the Community: A Handbook.* Rockville, MD: US Department of Health and Human Services, Office of the Assistant Secretary for Planning and Evaluation.

Stone, D. (1989). Causal stories and the formation of policy agendas. *Political Science Quarterly, 104*(1), 281–300.

Townsend, E. (2004). Occupational justice and client-centered practice: A dialogue in progress. *Canadian Journal of Occupational Therapy, 62*(5), 192–198.

Townsend, E., & Wilcock, A. (2004). Occupational justice. In C. Christiansen & E. Townsend (Eds.), *An Introduction to Occupation: The Art and Science of Living* (pp. 243–273). Upper Saddle River, NJ: Prentice Hall.

US Department of Health and Human Services (USDHHS). (1999). *Mental Health: A Report of the Surgeon General.* Rockville, MD: US Department of Health and Human Services, Substance Abuse and Mental Health Services Administration, Center for Mental Health Services, National Institutes of Health, National Institute of Mental Health.

Watson, R., & Swartz, L. (2004). *Transformation Through Occupation.* Philadelphia: Whurr.

Weissert, C. S., & Weissert, W. G. (1996). *Governing Health: The Politics of Health Policy.* Baltimore: Johns Hopkins University Press.

Wolch, J. R. (1996). Community-based human service delivery. *Housing Policy Debate, 7,* 649–671.

World Health Organization. (2001). *International Classification of Functioning, Disability and Health.* Geneva, Switzerland: Author.

———. (2009) Mental health financing. Available at: http://www.who.int/mental_health/resources/en/Financing.pdf (accessed September 27, 2006).

Attitudinal Environment and Stigma

M. Beth Merryman

> "The normal and the stigmatized are not persons but rather perspectives.
>
> —Erving Goffman, 1963 (p. 138)

Introduction

Imagine the challenge of an illness that derails your plans and dreams and robs you of the ability to think things through the way you are used to. Imagine being in your early 20s and experiencing mental confusion, extreme fatigue, and weight gain of 40 pounds as a result of medication compliance. Imagine that as you try to resume daily life with a serious mental illness, you are faced with questions such as whether or how much to disclose about your illness to family, friends, employers, teachers, and landlords.

Now imagine that instead of a serious mental illness, you experience a serious medical illness, such as multiple trauma from an automobile collision, which causes you to miss one semester of college. What would be different about your recovery? The physical fatigue and mental confusion may be similar, but would you have the additional stress of social integration? Would your recovery be complicated by issues of self-disclosure? According to the National Alliance for the Mentally Ill (NAMI), the recovery process from psychosis is physical and mental. Recovery is also a social process, and social support is a protective factor in recovery.

Both the recovery framework and the person-environment-occupation model value a collaborative approach in which the individual receiving care identifies the goals of intervention. Social and ecological models of care that enable us to view the person as "more than the illness" are being adopted. This shift in thinking moves us from an illness model that emphasizes a "problem" that resides solely within the person to a belief that many of the barriers to recovery reside in the environment. The role of the environment is examined in terms of supports and barriers to recovery. This perspective offers occupational therapists an opportunity to practice holistically (World Health Organization, 2001a). In holistic practice, the assessment process examines not only the individual and his or her wants and needs relative to occupation but also the supports and barriers in the environment.

According to the person-environment-occupation model, the environment is multifaceted and comprises five domains: the physical, social, cultural, socioeconomic, and institutional/organizational environments (Law et al, 1996). This chapter explores the role of the social environment, specifically social stigma, relative to mental health, occupational therapy practice, and the recovery process. It first describes stigma and theories about its origins, then discusses literature on the impact of stigma on those with mental illness and their families. Aspects of the social environment that support recovery are presented, and concerns regarding social stigma from an occupational justice perspective are explored. Finally, assessments and interventions relevant to stigma are addressed.

The Social Environment

The social environment includes aspects of daily life in which people interact with varying levels of intimacy. The social environment includes any type of interaction with another individual, such as family member, roommate, neighbor, coworker, and health care provider. According to the person-environment-occupation framework, the environment contains elements that either support or impede occupational performance. In the case of the social environment and recovery from serious mental illness, a support might involve the structured social opportunities offered through supported employment and assisted living environments. For example, does a person who lives in an assisted living environment and receives services have the opportunity to use community resources, such as an ATM machine or laundromat as needed, or is the use of community resources determined solely by staff? In a supported work setting, are a person's unique skills, education, and interests key components in determining the work setting, or is the person assigned to food service or janitorial services due to beliefs that individuals with mental illness are unable to work in other areas? A social barrier to recovery from serious mental illness involves social stigma.

Stigma

Stigma is "an attribute that is deeply discrediting," resulting in the marginalization of the stigmatized person in the eyes of others (Goffman, 1963). In the case of mental illness, stigma includes perceptions that the person with the illness may in some way be responsible for the illness or that the family is to blame (Smart, 2001). Although this chapter focuses on the stigma of mental illness, additional stigmatizing conditions such as homelessness, unemployment, poverty, substance abuse, and a record of incarceration are not uncommon for some people with serious and persistent mental illness. These social conditions are viewed quite negatively by the general public and may further compromise access to care, funding for services, and acceptance in the community. In fact, some believe that government underfunding for psychiatric disability in comparison to physical disability is in part due to the stigma attached to these conditions (Day, 2006). This lack of funding has contributed to the reduction in numbers of mental health occupational therapy practitioners in the United States because salaries (particularly in community-based practice) tend to be much lower when compared with opportunities in physical disabilities settings (AOTA, 2006).

The potential negative social environment for recovery due to public perception and stigma of mental illness is important for occupational therapy practitioners to consider. Practitioners may encounter these challenges more directly when working with people with serious mental illness in the community, where obtaining affordable and safe housing and adequate financial resources for the basic necessities of daily life are common challenges.

In addition to prejudice (a hostile attitude toward a person simply because she or he belongs to a group judged to have objectionable qualities), there is also the issue of "self-stigma," in which the person believes that he or she is deviant or shamefully different (Kleinman, 1988). Both internal and external stigmas are detrimental to recovery and full community participation for people with mental illness.

Negative consequences of social stigma may include marginalization, segregation, and restricted personal freedoms (Miller Polgar & Landry, 2004). An example is a person whose social invitations or opportunities at work are reduced following hospitalization for major depressive disorder.

Theories of Stigma

Goffman was the first to extensively discuss the negative effects of stigma on individuals with serious mental illness (1963). Initially, **labeling theory** and **normalization** were the predominant social science theories used to study stigma. Several other views have emerged over the past 30 years, including the minority group perspective and the rite of passage theory.

Labeling Theory

Labeling theory grew out of the sociological study of deviance. According to labeling theorists, certain groups have sanctioned power to define or "label" what is and is not socially deviant. Examples of such groups in power include government officials and medical professionals (Jones, 1998). For instance, police determine when an individual is demonstrating dangerous behavior and proceed according to their socially sanctioned role to maintain order. Mental health professionals determine if a person's self-report and observed behavior meet criteria for a *Diagnostic and Statistical Manual of Mental Disorders* Fourth Edition, Text Revision (DSM-IV-TR) diagnosis and proceed according to their socially sanctioned role to "label" someone with a mental illness and recommend treatment.

According to labeling theory, a person with a stigmatizing condition experiences three stages: (1) realization of stigma, (2) development of coping skills, and (3) learning to "pass" or cover their disability effectively to function in society (Taylor, 1991). Critics of labeling theory believe that this theory views those individuals with disability as passive recipients of discrimination. Challenging this view, these critics instead see disability as a sociopolitical construct impacted by broader social forces. They believe that labeling theorists focus too much on values of independence, self-reliance, beauty, and health (Hahn, 1985; Susman, 1994). For example, parents often experience ambivalence at having their child "labeled" with a learning disorder or psychiatric diagnosis. On the one hand, the parents recognize that the label is necessary for service delivery and insurance coverage, but they also wonder if the label will lead to a self-fulfilling prophecy in terms of how others will view the child. This could lead to lowered expectations and reduced social opportunities for the child.

Normalization Theory

Normalization theory is based on the work of labeling theorists and provides an alternative view that proposes how people who are typically disenfranchised in our society can be included (Jones, 1998). Normalization theorists believe that a label forces an individual into a deviant role, and subsequent behavior and response to others is determined by expectations surrounding the label. Normalization attempts to reduce elements that emphasize difference and develop social participation in the broader community. This theory is applied in the design of inclusive environments in education, reducing components that emphasize difference (e.g., "special" buses, camps, and congregate housing) and supporting interventions that emphasize social role development (e.g., friend, neighbor, student, and worker) rather than simple skill acquisition.

An example of "normalizing" behavior is providing an individual who is hearing voices with a headset and music to assist with reducing anxiety on an unfamiliar bus route. This adaptation enables the individual to use public transportation; without the adaptation, he or she would avoid riding the bus because of suspicion, anxiety, and paranoia. Another example is encouraging the parents of a child with social skills deficits and attention difficulties to join noncompetitive, age-appropriate social activities, such as Scouts, in which the child can develop skills with peers rather than focusing solely on a therapeutic social skills group.

Critics of normalization are concerned that normalization emphasizes the need of the person with the disability to change and "fit in" rather than requiring society to accept such differences as part of human diversity.

Minority Group Perspective

Some social scientists support a *minority group perspective* of disability. This view sees disablement as a consequence of oppression, demoralization, and marginalization of those individuals who deviate from the norm. Political activism is the primary intervention that has been used to combat stigma from this perspective. Stigma is seen as a civil rights issue; therefore, this view supports the consumer movement with the goal of expanding civil liberties (Susman, 1994; Vrkljan, 2005). An example is the political mobilization of

The Lived Experience

Grady Newton

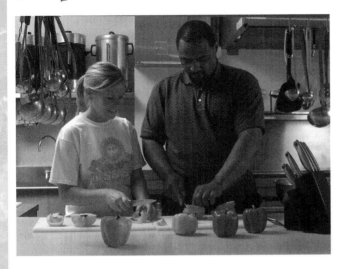

In 1990 I went through a two-hour psychodiagnostic test and verbal consultation with a psychiatrist, and he said I was sane. I then went for a second opinion with a different psychiatrist. Without any testing this psychiatrist called me a name, that I had a mental illness, and told me to go to the drop-in-center. That was the last time I saw that psychiatrist. I've seen four psychiatrists all together. Once you get diagnosed with mental illness, it's tough to get back into society without that name.

Writing this is one way for me to speak on my own behalf. When you are looked upon as mentally ill, you lose your voice. I want to give a general statement about what I live like. This is my viewpoint.

Wyandot Center is a place I attend that has a foundation, doctors, nurses, case management and staff. I respect the Wyandot Center with a good group of people that hear me. I feel like I've lost something in life by being called mentally ill; it is a personal loss. There are groups to attend, and I show up for my share of the program. When they have the groups and classes, I take in the information and enjoy it fully. In my everyday life, I know I am not alone or at least hope not. A goal of mine is persevering through this so-called mental illness. I don't believe the psychiatrist, I think I've been misjudged. My attitude and my behavior has to remain to the best of my ability even when relaxing.

I believe education is important. It helps you in the long run. I went to Kansas State University. I have 250 credits and a C average with a major in Social Sciences, with an emphasis in Criminology. I had a full football scholarship and I was a fifth-year senior. I red shirted myself, so I played for four of the five years. I was an outside linebacker, the most athletic position on the field. I was honorable mention, All-American even though I was on the losingest team in college football. I was team captain for the whole season. I was a free agent for the Washington Redskins. I signed the contract, I reported to training camp, but then I left. I looked at the situation and decided instead of seeking money I sought God. I got to keep the signing bonus.

I left the Redskins in 1988, and then I got a job as a detention officer in a correctional facility the same year. I worked there for two years. They terminated the whole job. Because I had this job, I now get an SSDI check—it is like workman's compensation. It shows that I have worked, but I'm disabled. I used to get the check myself in the mail, but I decided I wanted to have a payee. A payee is someone that takes the check, pays the rent and then gives me a disbursement check once a week. I get a little more than $100 a week. But once you have a payee it's hard to get it back. I have to decide what to do with the check, decide how to budget and what to eat.

When I have to see the psychiatrist, the nurse, OT students, take my medication, I feel like my life is the subject. I get fired up and empowered. I question why this is happening to me. So I go to the library to get books that help me learn. Checking those books out is my answer and antidote. I take my medication, but I have to find a way to heal myself, to be as healthy as I can. My reading consists of the Holy Bible King James Version, *Introduction to Criminology, Psychological Theories of Motivation, The 26 Letters, Evil the Shadow Side of Reality* and many more. These books help me gain strength during my life-long trial. Reading is like eating healthy food.

I watch what I say and I watch what I do for myself and the Wyandot Center Staff and business associates because sometimes people jump to conclusions or say things against me because of the stigma of this mental illness. For instance, one early mid-afternoon eating was on my mind. I decided to go to the cafeteria at KU Medical Center. I usually go there without incident. I was a few steps past the cafeteria when a policeman was standing in a door way on a cell phone talking to someone. I noticed him talking on the cell phone. He said "Hi" to me. I felt uncomfortable. I responded by saying, "Why are you saying hi to me?" He said "Hi" again, and I turned in the direction of peace toward him and repeated, "Why are you saying hi to me?" while he was still talking on his cell phone. The police officer then went screaming into hysterics. He disappeared through a door and alarmed the whole unit. They arrested me and handcuffed me from head to toe and gave me a ticket for resisting arrest. I believe this is associated with Wyandot Mental Health Center calling me mentally ill. I don't mean they know each other, but being called mentally ill and having this incident with the police officer reminds me of the same sort of stigma.

I didn't show up for my court date, but I turned myself in. They were not able to verify the arresting incident, but set another court date. I wrote a citizen's report explaining what had happened. I showed this to the prosecuting attorney and the attorney said the story coincides with the police report and dismissed the charges. This is unheard of. I have to say I won and I got my $100 back. I think the law should be respected because the law is there for a reason. Trying to figure out the problem personally on my own is my true nature. This is what I do to protect myself and my world. I have people telling me I'm mentally ill, but I tell myself I'm sane because that is my own interpretation of my past, present and future. Hopefully the interpretation of your own life story is protected, so you won't have to go through what I'm going through.

Continued

The Lived Experience—cont'd

I've developed a model to help me interpret my life. There are different elements that interact that form a variety of patterns that give the illusion of greater differences than really exist. When you are in a situation, this model helps explain how you look at the characters in the room, what is said, and how to pay attention to your surroundings. I call the model my PK matrix which can be viewed below:

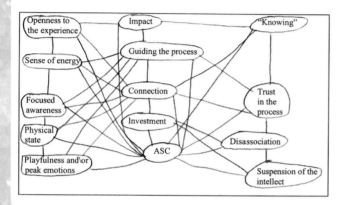

The Asbury Café is a place where I work. The café is held in a church every Wednesday. We fit into the church's schedule. The people that come to eat may go to the church but anybody who wants to get a meal can come to eat. I try to work harder when I'm there. I like the job. I've been there for seven years, and I've never had a job that long. I cook a little, I do clean up, take the money and am nice to the patrons that eat there and they are nice to me. I compare it to other restaurants in the area, and it is one of the best places that I've been to eat. I gave a speech during the church services to get more patrons to come to eat at the Asbury Café. I hoped that I could say something that would make them come and eat with us. Lately we have had new people coming to eat at the café, and we get compliments. They say the food is good every time. There is an incredible hospitality and respect that is shared at the Asbury Café.

mental health consumers and advocates to write letters to their congressperson or to hold a demonstration to voice concerns about the potential impact of Medicaid or Social Security funding cuts on their daily lives.

Rite of Passage Theory

Another theory that is relevant to stigma is based on Turner's (1969) *rite of passage theory.* According to this theory, life is a series of transitions, or rites of passage, each composed of three phases. The first phase is separation from the social structure. Following this separation, the individual loses prior social status and enters the second phase, or transition. This phase is also termed *liminal,* because it is exemplified by marginalized status while preparing for a new role or identity. The final phase is incorporation, in which the individual reenters society with a new identity. This theory has been applied to various disabling conditions, with the emphasis on the challenges of resolving the second, or liminal, stage, which is fraught with confusion and social isolation (Murphy, Scheer, Murphy, & Mack, 1988; Willett & Deegan, 2001).

In the first stage, the person is separated from his or her initial social status due to the disabling event. For example, a high-achieving graduate student experiences a psychotic break, and his status shifts from "promising college student" to "mental patient." During this stage, the person is afforded the sick role and is busy getting well. For individuals with somatic illnesses, the demarcation for this stage is clearer than for those with a mental illness, primarily because of the "invisibility" of mental illnesses.

During the second phase, the individual is no longer afforded the sick role by society, but he or she is still unable to fully perform valued social roles. The individual in the liminal stage typically struggles with self-identity and confusion due to feeling that he does not fit into valued roles, self-expectations, and the expectations of others. In addition, family and friends may be confused about the person's status, which can lead to even more isolation and loss of needed supports.

The individual may be attending a community program, working on skills, and transitioning to community life but is unsure of his capabilities and where he fits in terms of social roles. He is out of the hospital and wants to resume the role of promising graduate student, and he does not see himself as sick. Still, he is unsure where he fits in. Therapists who work with individuals in this stage should remember the value of focused goal setting in collaboration with the client and maintaining hope for the future.

The third stage, incorporation, involves resolution of liminal status and emergence of a new identity. This process is akin to recovery in that the individual acknowledges the illness as part of his or her identity but does not consider it the whole identity. Grady Newton (see this chapter's The Lived Experience) provides a good example. While he rebuffs the label "mentally ill," he acknowledges his illness by taking prescribed medications, attending a program at the Wyandot Mental Health Center, and assigning a payee who helps manage his money. He engages in daily life, using his "PK matrix" to help him cope with everyday situations, and he takes pride in his accomplishments and in his work at the Asbury Café.

Other Theories

Other theorists seek to understand the experience of the person who is the subject of stigmatizing attitudes. Kleinman (1988) discusses stigma in terms of both the person who devalues another individual and the internal feelings of the individual who is devalued. Kleinman studies this process through the construction of narratives or "mini-ethnographies" of individuals and families with chronic illness. These narratives provide stories that describe the social challenges of daily life.

The social environment of people with chronic illness is described as a series of exacerbations and remissions leading to numerous separations, transitions, and aggregations. The unpredictability of daily life produces stress on the individual and family, which compounds the stress caused by the symptoms of the illness.

Another theory examining the impact of stigma on the person is **modified labeling theory.** This theory argues that the act of labeling leads to negative outcomes (Link, Streuning, Cullen, Shrout, & Dohrenwend, 1989). Modified labeling theory was used to study the perception of social rejection by individuals seeking mental health treatment. Specifically, it was hypothesized that negative social consequences would result if people believed they would be devalued by others for seeking treatment. Link, Phelan, Bresnahan, Steuve, and Pescosolido (1999) found that if people felt threatened by devaluation from others if they sought mental health care, they were more likely to avoid social situations, engage in secretive behavior, and lose out on valuable coping and social supports. In this manner, perceived stigma negatively impacts successful recovery of those who seek mental health care.

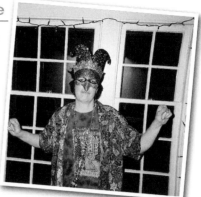

PhotoVoice

This is a picture of my older sister. Her name is Paula. This picture was taken at her Birthday and Mardi Gras party. She is wearing Mardi Gras clothes, beads, and a mask. This party reminds me of my high school parties and dances. That was the time when I started getting mental illness. This mask reminds me of mental illness because it covers up the real person inside. People may hide behind a mask because they fear mental illness.

Structural Stigma and Universalist Perspective

We often think of stigma in terms of individuals expressing a negative bias toward a particular person or group of persons. However, stigma can occur at the level of the institution or government. **Structural stigma** is described as a sociopolitical process in which the policies of private or governmental structures restrict the opportunities of stigmatized groups (Corrigan et al, 2005). Examples include states restricting the child custody rights of parents with mental illness and restrictions on the location of group homes that serve individuals who are recovering from mental illness or substance abuse. Of concern is the potential for discrimination, in which all members of a particular group are excluded from participation in social privileges simply because of membership in the group. This view of structural stigma is somewhat congruent with an emerging view of disability from a **universalist** perspective. The World Health Organization has shifted its description of disability to this social perspective, recognizing the need to examine the broader contexts beyond personal factors that impact the social participation of individuals with disabilities. The universalist view purports that policies are a reflection of the system in which they are decided and that change must occur at that level rather than at the individual level of intervention. This view reinforces the need for occupational therapy practitioners to be involved at the policy level to effect positive system change.

Social Environmental Barriers and Stigma

Much literature addresses the consequences of stigma for individuals with mental illness. For occupational therapists, it is important to recognize that stigma can present a major barrier toward participation in community life. The shift of mental illness care to the community from inpatient institutions moved opinions and views of individuals with mental illness into the public sphere.

A population survey focusing on seven conditions (depression, panic attacks, schizophrenia, dementia, eating disorder, alcoholism, and drug addiction) found that 77% of respondents knew someone with a mental illness (Crisp, Gelder, Goddard, & Meltzer, 2005). The most stigmatized conditions were schizophrenia and drug and alcohol addiction. People with schizophrenia were characterized as "unpredictable," "dangerous," and "hard to talk with." The same labels were applied to people with drug and alcohol addictions; in addition, these individuals were "to blame for their condition." Stigmatizing attitudes are not limited to the general public. Mental health professionals also hold stigmatizing views toward the very individuals they treat (Schulze, 2007).

In addition, there are specific issues surrounding stigmatizing attitudes toward children with mental illness. For example, children with depression may be seen as having a more serious illness, as more violent, and as more deserving of coerced care when compared with adults with depression (Perry, Pescosolido, Martin, McLeod, & Jenson, 2007). Adults with mental illness who received diagnoses as children believe that stigma began in treatment during childhood, which resulted in rejection at school (Pecosolida, Perry, Martin, McLeod, & Jenson, 2007). The National Stigma Study of Children (Pescosolido et al, 2008) found skepticism, misinformed beliefs, and a lack of knowledge about childhood mental illness. Such studies indicate that efforts aimed to reduce stigma must address the specific issues of childhood mental illness, such as acceptance at school, teacher education, and parenting.

Although negative attitudes about mental illness still exist, the general public has increased its level of understanding of mental illness (Sartorius, 2007), and people, particularly younger adults, are more accepting of seeking mental health treatment (Mojtabai, 2007). Other survey data reveal that most people obtain information about mental illness from mass media sources, such as television news and movies (Lopez, 1991; Wittman, 1994). Mental health advocates are greatly concerned about the source of information about mental illness because the content that "sells" media market share may not provide an accurate portrayal of daily life with a mental illness. For example, local news focuses on sensational news events such as a police standoff with a psychotic individual who threatens to take his or her life rather than on the less sensational, everyday lives of most individuals with mental illness. Sensationalist media coverage is not likely to engender support for vital community mental health services such as housing and employment.

Researchers indicate that persons with mental illness tend to be portrayed by mass media in one of three ways: (1) a person to be feared, (2) a person with special and marvelous powers, and (3) a rebellious free spirit (Corrigan & Penn, 1999). It is believed that such portrayals reinforce stereotypes of individuals with mental illness that negatively impact policy decisions. Both the World Health Organization (2001b) and the World Psychiatric Association (2002) have initiated campaigns to address the stigma of mental illness. Advocacy groups such as the National Alliance for Mental Illness (NAMI) launched antistigma campaigns in the 1990s to address stereotypic media portrayals through targeted protest and education methods aimed at key decision makers in the mass media. Research addressing attitudes toward individuals with mental illness has been important because of treatment, policy, and funding implications.

Stigma and Culture

Although some research suggests that mental illness stigma is more prevalent in the Western world and less so in Africa and Asia (Fabrega, 1991), more recent studies indicate stigma is a worldwide experience. A study of Nigerian university students found higher levels of desire for social distance toward individuals with mental illness when compared with those of Western cultures (Adewuya & Makanjuola, 2005).

A study of college students in the United States found stigmatizing attitudes among all groups, but African Americans and Asians considered people with mental illness to be more dangerous and wanted more social distance than did Caucasians (Rao, Feinglass, & Corrigan, 2007). Latinos had the least stigmatizing attitudes. Even finer distinctions may be made. For example, in comparing different Asian cultures, one study in Singapore suggested that Malaysians held more tolerant attitudes than the Chinese (Chong et al, 2007). A study comparing Caucasians and African Americans in the United States found that African Americans were more likely to view people with schizophrenia and major depression as violent, but they were less likely to believe that these people should be blamed or punished for their behavior (Anglin, Link, & Phelan, 2006). A study comparing Chinese and United States employers' concerns about hiring people with psychotic disorders found some similarities of stigma for both groups, but Chinese employers were more likely to see people with mental illness as having a weaker work ethic and less loyal to the company (Tsang et al, 2007).

Viewing stigma in light of cultural contexts requires a shift from an individual perspective to an understanding of the societal forces that shape discrimination. In order for stigma to be addressed in a culturally sensitive manner, it is important to understand how different cultures conceptualize mental illness. This research is only just beginning, but initial studies suggest there are important distinctions among cultures. For example, the extreme discrimination faced by individuals with mental illness in Chinese cultures may be related to the cultural norm of "face" (Yang, 2007). Chinese social interaction is based on a reciprocation of favors that is central to identity. Schizophrenia consequently results in a "loss of face" when the individual is unable to engage in this type of social interaction. The loss of face is experienced by the individual as well as strongly associated with the family.

Thus far, this section has discussed how different cultural groups view mental illness. Gary (2005) presents the concept of **double stigma**, which is the result of prejudice and discrimination that occurs when the individual both has a mental illness and belongs to an ethnic minority group. This double stigma can lead to increased isolation, limited access to services and health care, higher rates of incarceration, and greater levels of self-stigma. The New Freedom Commission on Mental Health (2003) identifies disparities in access to and quality of care for individuals of different cultural groups in the United States and sets a goal of equal access and culturally competent mental health care for all Americans.

Stigma and Community Integration

Social stigma impacts successful community integration. This occurs through both stigma perceived from the attitudes of others and self-directed stigma. According to Smart (2001), there is a hierarchy of stigma relative to the type of disability. In this hierarchy, which consists of physical disability, intellectual and cognitive disability, and psychiatric disability, individuals with a psychiatric disability experience the most stigma. Smart states that the individual with a disability must learn not only to manage the disability but also to recognize and manage the stigma of the disability.

Caltaux (2002) discussed self-stigma (in which individuals self-discriminate on the basis of their beliefs about their own limitations) and the negative impact it has on successful recovery. Examples include individuals who believe their illness leaves them socially undesirable, so they tolerate an abusive or exploitative relationship; individuals who believe their illness leaves them less competent, so they do not pursue employment opportunities; and individuals who believe their illness leaves them incapable of caring adequately for their children, so they do not seek social support to assist them with the challenges of parenting. In each of these examples, the individual self-imposes beliefs about his or her own competence or worth due to the illness. This lack of self-efficacy negatively impacts successful recovery and social role performance. It is critical to support the self-concept of the individual with mental illness through collaborative and client-centered interactions that promote self-determination.

Occupational therapists often address self-efficacy in their interventions. Because of the impact of self stigma, it is particularly important for occupational therapists to consider approaches that can improve an individual's sense of self-worth, which includes but is not limited to:

■ Providing "therapeutic use of self" strategies indicating you believe in the individual.

- Using cognitive behavior strategies to change distorted thinking.
- Providing activities in which the individual can have a mastery experience.

A study of individuals with serious mental illness who lived in the community examined consumer perspectives on community versus institutional life. Although most consumers (98%) preferred community life, one of the most frequently identified barriers to community integration was the stigma of mental illness (Davidson & Hoge, 1996). Consumers felt that stigma left them socially isolated and reduced their opportunities in the community. Prince and Prince (2002) examined the perceptions of individuals with mental illness and found that despite intensive structure and community support, clients receiving assertive community treatment believed that members of the community would reject them.

Other researchers studied quality of life from the perspective of individuals with serious mental illness and found that the most frequently unmet need was information and help related to stigma (Perese, 1997) and that a major factor related to quality of life was being perceived as "normal" by others (Laliberte-Rudman, Yu, Scott, & Pajouhandeh, 2000).

Lloyd, Sullivan, and Williams (2005) examined the interpersonal relationships of young males who experienced psychotic behavior. Participants revealed that their relationships had become more superficial, and they were less involved in terms of personal decision making, both of which they attributed to the stigma of mental illness.

Quinn, Kahng, and Crocker (2004) studied the effects of self-disclosure relative to mental illness on cognitive performance. They found that individuals with mental illness exhibited vigilance for cues in the environment that they would be devalued or marginalized and that hypervigilance resulted in subjective emotional stress and disrupted focused attention.

In each of these studies, the perception of individuals with mental illness was that they were judged negatively by others because of their illness. In some of the studies, the judgment was a result of the mental illness label; in others, it related to concerns that they were not perceived as "normal" because of a label or behavior. These results have implications for providers dedicated to supporting recovery and successful role performance. For example, an occupational therapist may confuse hypervigilance and the resulting disrupted attention as a symptom of the mental illness rather than as vigilance due to fear of judgment. The intervention would be different depending on the source of the vigilance or attention issue.

Social value is assigned to the work that an individual does, and dependence or the inability to work is viewed negatively. Research indicates that despite the desire to work, very few individuals with serious mental illnesses are gainfully employed (Anthony, Cohen, & Farkas, 1990). Attitudinal barriers are some of the most difficult to overcome for individuals with mental illness who want to work (Van Niekerk, 2004).

Both external stigma and self-stigma create barriers to successful work experiences for people with mental illness. Strong and Rebeiro (2003) discuss the self-stigma individuals experience in a system that focuses on their skill deficits. The social environment, including negative attitudes toward mental illness, was the greatest barrier to successful employment, according to participants in a study by Rebeiro (1999). Deegan (1992) described the barriers that the system of care places on users of services, stating that such attitudes lead to disempowerment and despair.

Barriers can be organizational in nature and often reflect attitudes and beliefs that are not consumer centered or supportive of resumption of valued roles in the community environment. Examples of such barriers include lengthy waiting lists for service, services that do not engage users in defining goals and preferences, messages that employment success is solely due to service user efforts, and a community view that individuals with mental illness are dangerous or unpredictable in the workplace. In addition, education within existing employment settings is made difficult because of the secrecy individuals with mental illnesses often adopt for fear of discrimination after self-disclosure.

Impact of Stigma on Mental Health Treatment

Stigma can impact treatment-seeking behavior. For example, even though most treatment for depression occurs in primary care settings, and medications are effective for up to 70% of individuals with depression, it is estimated that depression is seriously undertreated. Barriers include that patients are hesitant to discuss concerns; physicians are reluctant to ask; and the symptoms of depression, such as self-blame and cognitive distortion, make it difficult for accurate diagnosis to occur (Stimmel, 2001).

Mechanic (2002) believes the stigma toward serious mental illness, particularly psychosis, is detrimental to accessing both mental health and general health care. Of concern is the individual's ability to successfully navigate challenging bureaucracies. In environments such as health maintenance organizations, in which pressure is intense to see large numbers of patients, it may be challenging to get a timely appointment, and knowledge of specialized problems is questionable. Mechanic believes these organizational practices do not support the needs of the individual with serious mental illness.

> *The epidemic of mental illness in children is all around us, but it is not something we talk about easily. I didn't. In the days after Alex was admitted to the hospital, I told people that he had a bad case of the flu. "Don't tell anyone at school what's happening," I told Liz. "We don't want the other parents to be afraid to let their kids play with Alex."*
>
> *Paul Raeburn, 2004 (p. 9)*

Impact of Stigma on Families

Stigma also affects the families of individuals with mental illness. Family members have discussed feelings of "stigma by association" simply because their family member was known to have a mental illness (Friesen, 1996). In addition to studies that report on the challenges of illness management, families report disrupted household routines, neglect of other family needs, and reduced social contacts. Research indicates the most common behavior exhibited by families is concealing information about the family member's mental illness (Phelan, Bromet, & Link, 1998). This reduces opportunities for necessary social support and adds unneeded stress to the family system.

Other issues include disrupted individual and family roles, including decisions about financial and living arrangements that deviate from the norm (Teschinksy, 2000). For example, in a family in which the parent has a serious mental illness, adult children may assume a caretaking role, including long-term financial and health planning. In families in which a child has a serious mental illness, there may be financial strain and the need for comprehensive long-term care for the child, which impacts the retirement planning of the parents.

Family psychoeducation and support have been identified as evidence-based practices for individuals with serious mental illness (Lincoln, Wilhelm, & Nestoriuc, 2007). Occupational therapists can use psychoeducation approaches to address stigma as it relates to the family. The perceived social risks of self-disclosure may prevent family members from accessing such valuable services or advocating for such a service to be offered or covered by insurance.

Public Policy Impact of Stigma

Stigma impacts the types of public policy alternatives that are considered by the political system. The Surgeon General's report on mental health identified reduction of stigma as critical to addressing the mental health needs of the population (Tanaka, 2003; U.S. Department of Health and Human Services, 1999). Yet there are conflicting points of view as to how this should occur. In the 1960s and 1970s, policies were focused on equality for all. Some believe that there has been a shift away from egalitarianism toward a belief that individual success is possible, but not for all. This shift results in less tolerance for risk and less concern for the civil rights of others (Borinstein, 1992).

This conflict is played out in numerous policies regarding individuals with mental illness. For example, despite surveys showing that the public believes mental illnesses should be covered by insurance at the same rate as physical illnesses, there has been little public identification of this belief as an issue for aggressive action. Despite evidence of the cost of substance abuse to society in terms of lost productivity, physical illness, and social costs, little public outcry is made over the lack of treatment availability.

People with psychiatric disabilities are the only Americans who can have their freedom taken away and be institutionalized or incarcerated without being convicted of a crime (Cook & Jonikas, 2002). According to civil rights advocates, many laws affecting people with mental illness are designed on the basis of what a person *might* do rather than what they *have* done. On the other hand, some believe there is prejudice in denying disability status to those with mental illness. This is exemplified in policies that protect civil liberties at all costs, including treatment refusal to those who are severely psychotic. This view sees psychosis as a medical problem that is no more under the control of the individual than dementia is under the control of a person so afflicted.

A policy shift to a recovery framework, by design, must support self-determination and empower individuals to move beyond survival to recover and thrive in communities of choice. This is a challenge because of the need to address both self-determination and issues of safety.

Another policy impacted by stigma is parity, or equality of insurance coverage for mental and physical illnesses.

There is a long history of discriminatory insurance coverage for mental illnesses and addictive disorders (Hanson, 1998). Although the proportion of insured workers with mental health benefits actually increased between 1991 and 1995, mental health care, as defined by hospital care and physician visits, was covered less frequently than other conditions (Jensen, Rost, Burton, & Bulycheva, 1998). This study found that only 18% of individuals with mental health coverage had benefits for inpatient care similar to those with physical illnesses. Only 2% had outpatient mental health coverage that equaled their benefits for other physician visits. It was concluded that more individuals had mental health coverage, but the depth of benefits shrunk. It was also found that the percentage of insurance plans that limited inpatient psychiatric care increased from 38% to 57%.

Despite the presence of federal legislation passed in 1996 and enacted in 1998, states and private insurers found many loopholes to avoid full mental health parity. These include exclusions for the size of a workforce, "hardship" to the employer, and restricting coverage by diagnosis (Amaro, 1999). Despite fears that parity would exponentially increase costs of insurance, Goldman et al (2006) found that, combined with managed care strategies, mental health parity improved insurance coverage without increasing total costs.

Poverty is an additional social barrier for individuals with mental illness. The burden of mental illness and disability is higher among people with low income than among people of means. Generally, those with higher income and education are more likely to use mental health services. At the other end of the socioeconomic continuum, expanded Medicaid coverage led the poor to be almost as likely as the wealthy to use mental health services. The group with the lowest rates of mental health visits are the "near poor," because they are the least likely to have access to private, employment-based insurance or government entitlements designed for the poor (Mechanic, 1998).

Other social barriers to those with mental illness include inequitable housing, education, and income support. Many agree that housing, disability and welfare policies, and human services are vital components of the mental health system for individuals with serious and persistent mental illnesses (Goldman et al, 2006). Many individuals with serious mental illness live in high-crime areas with substandard housing (Carling, 1990). If there are large numbers of individuals with mental illness in a particular neighborhood, they may experience backlash from the community. This is referred to as NIMBYism (not in my backyard) and highlights the conflict between the policy (those in the neighborhood support community mental health) and the implementation of the policy (they just support it somewhere else).

Research shows that individuals with mental illness prefer community to institutional life and prefer to have a choice regarding their housing situation rather than being assigned to congregate arrangements such as group homes (Nelson, Sylvestre, Aubry, George, & Trainor, 2007). The recovery model supports the involvement of the individual in the housing process. Policies such as the Earned Income Tax Credit and Section 8 housing vouchers provide opportunities to reduce the impact of poverty on low-income families. Such policies are more critical in the current environment of community-based care and recovery (Cottrell, 2003). Such policies specifically support individuals with low income and enable community living. Chronic underfunding and unpredictable funding levels threaten the safety net that is critical for some of society's most marginalized citizens.

Social issues of race and class also impact recovery. In a study in which the authors viewed mental health beyond disorders to include other social problems, it was found that individuals of color were less likely to seek care unless severely ill and were less likely than the nonminority population to be insured (Alegria, Perez, & Williams, 2003). Research shows that lower education levels are also associated with poorer psychological functioning and higher risk for negative mental health outcomes. Those of low-income and minority status are more likely to be identified for special education and less likely to receive services, graduate, and work at gainful employment. Advocates are concerned that individuals with mental illness who are also poor, have lower education levels, and/or are members of minority groups are further marginalized in the current system.

Social Environmental Supports and Recovery

The effects of stigma can be buffered by positive social support. The literature emphasizes the value of social support, hope, and feedback from others in promoting successful recovery (Liberman & Kopelowicz, 2002; Noordsy et al, 2002; Pettie & Triolo, 1999). Health, mental health, and social services delivered by individuals who not only believe that persons with mental illness recover but provide those services in a system that is not encumbered with bureaucratic challenges appear to support recovery (Mancini, Hardiman, & Lawson, 2005; Rebeiro, 1999). First-person accounts detail the importance of engagement with a person or persons who "believed in" the individual or did not give up on him or her (Deegan, 1988). The value of an attitude that positive change is possible cannot be underestimated. However, this is not possible if the provider supports negative stereotypes of individuals with mental illness.

An affirming social environment is associated with successful recovery. This means that service systems need to develop environments in which the individual is empowered through collaborative decision making and self-determination, and families are provided with education and support regarding the illness (Jacobson & Greenly, 2001). Inadequate funding has made such services difficult to reliably implement (Spaniol, Wewiorski, Gagne, & Anthony, 2002).

Occupational therapists can address social issues by empowering individuals to act as community participants to support social inclusion (Kronenberg, Algado, & Pollard, 2005; Watson & Schwartz, 2004). Galheigo (2005) discusses the need to address the macrostructures of society by working on the local level to identify needs, develop supports, and empower individuals to take collective action to address social inequities.

Assessments of Stigma and Recovery

Assessments that examine stigmatizing attitudes can be useful for occupational therapists who are interested in better understanding the social environment of the people they serve. Stigma assessments can also be administered to staff in the mental health setting to identify and, if they exist, address negative stereotypes among mental health professionals. Recovery-oriented assessments help to determine the impact of the social environment on the individual with mental illness and the person's resilience.

Attitudinal Assessments Relative to Stigma

One method of attitudinal assessment uses a case study approach. Using Corrigan, Markowitz, Watson, Rowan, and Kubiak's attribution model (2003), case studies are developed and respondents answer questions about the person described in the vignette. Attribution theory posits that a person's beliefs about a condition are related to what he or she believes caused the condition. If the person is considered responsible for the condition, this belief can result in responses that reject the person. One study applied this model to vignettes describing an individual with one of three psychiatric diagnoses. Varied information was provided to participants in the following ways: type of illness, whether the vignette included a diagnostic label or simply a description of behavior, and whether situational information was provided. Questions related to the perceived cause, controllability, stability, and violence potential relative to the individual in the vignette. Results indicated that a diagnostic label affected perception of cause, controllability, and stability measures. Individuals with attention deficit-hyperactivity disorder were viewed more positively than were those with other mental illness diagnoses (Demaio, 2006).

Many researchers have studied attitudes toward individuals with mental illness (Keane, 1991; Singh, Baxter, Standen, & Duggan, 1998). Attitudes imply beliefs, and research has shown that negative attitudes among mental health professionals affect client outcome (Murray & Steffen, 1999). Several instruments measure attitude, but few specifically address attitude toward mental illness. One exception is the Opinions of Mental Illness (OMI) by Cohen and Streuning (1962). The OMI, developed in the early 1960s, measures attitude toward mentally ill individuals, etiology, and treatment. The instrument is a 51-item, five-factor scale in which each factor coincides with a belief about mental illness. The factors include authoritarianism (people with mental illness need to be controlled to behave), benevolence (people with mental illness need to be protected—paternalism), mental illness ideology (mental illness is a medical problem), social restrictiveness (people with mental illness are threatening), and interpersonal ideology (mental illness is caused by interpersonal deficits). This instrument has been widely used to assess professional students and staff attitudes in order to facilitate best practices in education.

Another instrument is the Attitudes toward Mental Illness Questionnaire (AMI) developed by Singh et al (1998). This 20-item questionnaire includes content relative to causes, treatment, and consequences of mental illness. Items are scored on a 5-point Likert scale with a higher score indicating a more favorable attitude toward mental illness.

Link et al (1989) developed the 12-item Devaluation-Discrimination Scale that measures stigma from the perspective of the individual who experiences it. This measure allows the individual with mental illness to rate his or her own experiences of discrimination. In studies of people with mental illness, discrimination is associated with rejection (Bjorkman, Svensson, & Lundberg, 2007) and low self-esteem (Berge & Ranney, 2005).

Occupational therapy researchers have studied student attitudes regarding mental illness and other conditions (Lyons & Hayes, 1993; Penny, 2001). Results indicate that occupational therapy students are no different from other students in their opinions. In both studies, students had significant differences in attitude between mental and physical illness and a desire for greater social distance from individuals with mental illness than from those with physical illness. Authors believe that the educational environment was in part to blame. For example, fieldwork often exposes students only to severely ill individuals, which reinforces a less hopeful attitude toward recovery. In addition, coursework focuses on pathology and the deficit approach at the expense of recovery. It is also believed that media sensationalism may further contribute to students' views of the dangerousness of mental illness (Lyons & Ziviani, 1995).

Recovery-Oriented Assessments

In addition to addressing professional staff attitudes related to stigma, it is important to address consumer/client self-stigma and degree of self-efficacy. These constructs are typically assessed using measures of recovery. One relevant instrument is the Recovery Assessment Scale (Corrigan, Giffort, Rashid, Leary, & Okeke, 1999). This consumer-developed instrument is a 41-item measure on which participants describe themselves using a 5-point scale (5, *strongly agree*; 1, *strongly disagree*). One sample item is, "I can handle it if I get sick again." The instrument has demonstrated adequate reliability and validity.

Another relevant instrument is the Empowerment Scale (Rogers, Chamberlin, Langer Ellison, & Crean, 1997). This consumer-developed scale includes 28-items about empowerment that participants respond to on a 4-point scale (4, *strongly disagree*). Analysis reveals five factors: self-efficacy–self-esteem, power–powerlessness, community activism, righteous anger, and optimism–control over the future. Additional testing to determine validity is ongoing. A sample item is, "I am often able to overcome barriers."

Other instruments relevant to measuring self-efficacy include those that assess quality of life (Lehman, 1988). For example, Lehman's Quality of Life Interview contains six items on various domains relevant to quality of life. Participants respond on a 7-point scale (7, *delighted*; 1, *terrible*). The instrument has demonstrated adequate reliability and validity.

Interventions to Address Stigma

As this chapter has explained, stigma is a major barrier toward successful occupational performance for people with serious mental illness; however, it is often overlooked in the intervention process. Occupational therapy practice that is recovery oriented and sensitive to environmental influences should adopt intervention approaches that target the reduction of stigma at the level of the social environment of the individual with mental illness, the larger society as a whole, and within the individual with mental illness who has adopted self-stigmatizing attitudes. Following is a discussion of potential interventions that address stigma.

Interventions to Address Public, Student, and Professional Attitudes

The literature on interventions to address professional attitudes toward mental illness includes education, protest, and contact (Corrigan & Gelb, 2006).

Educational interventions have been described with varying success. Crowe, Deane, Oades, Caputi, and Morland (2006) found that a brief staff recovery orientation addressing attitude and hopefulness was effective. Corrigan, Watson, Warpinski, and Gracia (2004) examined public education program effects on perception of individuals with mental illness. Those who completed a program that highlighted the association between mental illness and violence were more likely to support services that restricted autonomy, exercise avoidance behavior, and report fearful attitudes.

Interventions aimed at changing student attitudes typically include focused coursework, fieldwork reflective of community living and aftercare, and reflective journaling. Educational interventions that have been identified as successful varied between formal coursework (Penny, Kasar, & Sinay, 2001) and contact beyond the context of the caregiver role (Lyons, 1991). Penn et al (1994) found that, in general, increased knowledge about mental illness, specifically knowing someone with a mental illness, reduced negative judgment. However, knowledge of only the acute phase of serious mental illness actually increased stereotyped beliefs about mental illness. Professional education in which learners were exposed primarily to cases in which individuals were seriously ill without attention to the aftercare plan reinforced hopelessness and the deficit approach (i.e. "what was wrong" with the individual).

Protest methods include such activities as focused letter writing, boycotts, and public endorsement that draw attention to the injustice and ask for behavior to change. This form of attitude change is sometimes criticized because it addresses the behavior after it has been expressed. Studies have shown that this method may have little effect on attitude but does have some influence on behavior toward individuals with mental illness (Corrigan, 2004; Corrigan et al, 2001).

Methods that include contact with individuals with mental illness are often based on Allport's (1954) cognitive theory, which proposes that to change attitude between two groups, there needs to be contact between them. This theory identifies four critical factors to ensure a positive outcome of the contact: equal group member status, common goals, intergroup cooperation, and support of authorities. An alternative, recategorization theory, proposes that contact positively shifts the outsider's status (Couture & Penn, 2006).

Corrigan et al (2001) found that contact was more successful than both education and protest in producing targeted effects on attitude toward specific mental illnesses. Several researchers have found that contact with individuals who have mental illness in which the social status of both parties are similar reduces perception of mental illness as "dangerous" (Holmes, Corrigan, Williams, Canar, & Kubiak, 1990; Kolodziej & Johnson, 1996; Penn et al, 1994; Wittman, 1994). Contact has been proposed to impact attitude, but the type and frequency of contact seems to matter. This has implications for occupational therapy education and fieldwork experiences, meaning it is important for occupational therapy students to have positive contact with people with mental illness.

Interventions to Address Self-Stigma and Self-Efficacy

According to the literature, some individuals with mental illness are negatively affected by stigma. Others are mobilized by it to become socially active, and still others do not appear to be affected. Among the strategies to address self-stigma are those that support recovery principles. These include engaging in activities that are personally meaningful and empowering, such as peer support and consumer-operated services (Corrigan et al, 2001), and in activities that involve exercising self-determination and choice, as well as accepting both aspects of health and illness in daily life (Davidson & Strauss, 1995). These interventions are familiar to occupational therapy, which is based on client-centered intervention in which the first contact elicits the client's view of what he or she wants and needs to do. Engaging the client through exploration of personal interests, goals, and valued roles addresses the need that all individuals have for finding meaning in daily life. Occupational therapists address this need through intervention

---

Evidence-Based Practice

What does the evidence say creates a supportive environment?

Individual level:

➤ Hopeful, empowering professionals

➤ Accessible mental health and health-care network

➤ Basic necessities: shelter, food, and self-care items, including medications, clothing and hygiene

➤ Opportunities for self-determination and meaningful decision making in daily life

➤ Social support

➤ Information about illness and recovery

Family level:

➤ Psychoeducation

➤ Information about illness and recovery

➤ Social support

Community level:

➤ Public education about mental illness

➤ Client-centered services

➤ Policies that promote client centeredness

➤ Adequate funding to enable access and fidelity to evidence-based practice

Professional education and training:

➤ Knowledge about mental illness

➤ Hopeful attitude toward disability

➤ Classroom content beyond acute illness episode, including aftercare plan, understanding of person beyond the illness

➤ Contact with individuals with mental illness outside of the care provider relationship

➤ Attitudes of professional colleagues/mentors toward individuals with mental illness

➤ Collaborative style of intervention

Occupational therapy practice:

➤ Client-centered assessment and intervention

➤ Advocacy at the client, organization, and community levels

Cook, J. A., & Jonikas, J. A. (2002). Self-determination among mental health consumers/survivors: Using lessons from the past to guide the future. *Journal of Disability Policy Studies, 13*(2), 87–95.

Corrigan, P. W. (2004). Target-specific stigma chance: A strategy for impacting mental illness stigma. *Psychiatric Rehabilitation Journal, 28,* 113–121.

Crowe, T. P., Deane, F. P., Oades, L. G., Caputi, P., & Morland, K. G. (2006). Effectiveness of a collaborative recovery training program in Australia in promoting positive views about recovery. *Psychiatric Services, 57*(10), 1497–1500.

Corrigan, P. W., & Gelb, B. (2006). Three programs that use mass approaches to challenge the stigma of mental illness. *Psychiatric Services, 57,* 393–398.

Corrigan, P. W., & Penn, D. (1999). Lessons from social psychology on discrediting psychiatric stigma. *American Psychologist, 54*(9), 765–776.

Corrigan, P. W., River, L. P., Lundin, R. K., Penn, D. L., Uphoff-Wasowski, K., Campion, J., Mathisen, J., Gagnon, C., Bergman, M., Goldstein, H., & Kubiak, M. A. (2001). Three strategies for changing attributions about severe mental illness. *Schizophrenia Bulletin, 27*(2), 187–195.

Corrigan, P. W., Watson, A. C., Warpinski, A. C., & Gracia, G. (2004). Implications of educating the public on mental illness, violence, and stigma. *Psychiatric Services, 55,* 557–580.

Friesen, B. J. (1996). Family support in child and adult mental health. In G. H. S. Singer, L. E. Powers, & A. L. Olson (Eds.). *Redefining Family Support: Innovations in Public–Private Partnerships* (pp. 259–274). Baltimore: Brookes.

Lincoln, T. M., Wilhelm, K., & Nestoriuc, Y. (2007). Effect of psychoeduction for relationships, symptoms, knowledge, adherence and function in psychotic disorders: A meta-analysis. *Schizophrenia Research, 96,* 232–245.

Nelson, G., Sylvestre, J., Aubry, T., George, L., & Trainor, J. (2007). Housing choice and control, housing quality, and control over professional support as contributors to the subjective quality of life and community adaptation of people with serious mental illness. *Administration and Policy in Mental Health, 34,* 89–100.

Penn, D. L, Guynan, K., Daily, T., Spaulding, W., Garbin, C., & Sullivan, M. (1994). Dispelling the stigma of schizophrenia: What sort of information is best? *Schizophrenia Bulletin, 20*(3), 567–578.

Perese, E. F. (1997). Unmet needs of persons with chronic mental illnesses: Relationship to their adaptation to community living. *Issues in Mental Health Nursing, 18,* 19–34.

Singh, S. P., Baxter, H., Standen, P., & Duggan, C. (1998). Changing the attitudes of "tomorrow's doctors" towards mental illness and psychiatry: A comparison of two teaching methods. *Medical Education, 32,* 115–120.

Stimmel, G. L. (2001). Maximizing treatment outcome in depression: Strategies to overcome social stigma and noncompliance. *Disease Management Health Outcomes, 9*(4), 179–186.

Strong, S., & Rebeiro, K. (2003). Creating supportive work environments for people with mental illness. In L. Letts, P. Rigby, & D. Stewart (Eds.), *Using Environments to Enable Occupational Performance.* Thorofare, NJ: Slack.

with the client as well as in the multiple contexts in which they perform daily activity.

Interventions Supporting Occupational Justice

Research indicates there are negative consequences to social stigma, including the chronic stress of self-deprecation, which in turn reduces self-determination and full participation in community life (Wright, Gronfein, & Owens, 2000). Since one of the goals of the recovery movement is consumer-driven care and social participation in communities of choice, anything that impedes an individual from exercising self-determination is of concern to occupational therapy providers.

Some occupational therapists are beginning to embrace a model of universalism in which issues of access, equality, and inclusion are more relevant than concepts such as "functionality" (Galheigo, 2005). Galheigo identifies the three main social concepts of importance to occupational therapists as marginality, exclusion, and disaffiliation. **Marginality** refers to individuals experiencing a lack of integration with cultural experiences and norms. An example of marginality is a 42-year-old, single woman with serious mental illness who lives in supported housing and attends psychosocial rehabilitation. This person is marginalized in that she is not participating in typical occupations of a person of that age, such as employment, a home of her own, and an autonomous social network.

Exclusion, once defined in terms of banishment, confinement, or social control, now also includes those whose main occupation is daily survival due to social exclusion. An example of exclusion would be individuals who attend a psychosocial rehabilitation program (PRP) who wish to engage in a daily fitness regimen. However, due to poverty and marginal social status, they attend a daily group at the PRP rather than access the local health club. Another example is an individual with serious mental illness who is looking for an apartment in the community. Due to poverty and marginal social status, the only rental units available are in unsafe geographic locations or requires that the individual take three buses to get to the PRP. Despite the policy shifts away from institutional care, the daily reality for individuals with serious mental illness living in the community is social exclusion from participation with the exception of that structured by the PRP.

Disaffiliation refers to those whose circumstances have devolved to such a level of disruption that they are viewed as "other" (e.g., street people or the homeless). Miller Polgar and Landry (2004) discuss the notion of sanctioned and unsanctioned occupations. Sanctioned occupations are those that are socially accepted, whereas unsanctioned occupations are those that are considered socially deviant from the norm. An example of an unsanctioned occupation is living on the street, which is the case for some with serious and persistent mental illness. Homeless individuals are typically segregated and may have personal freedoms restricted. This is certainly the case in some jurisdictions that arrest individuals for loitering or panhandling under "nuisance" laws.

Some occupational therapists are calling for support of individual mental well-being by addressing social strategies beyond traditional occupational therapy intervention, particularly for individuals whose self-determination is impacted by poverty, unemployment, and/or unstable housing (Duncan, 2004). Such occupational therapy intervention includes occupational empowerment, enablement, and enrichment to address occupational risks associated with deprivation, alienation, and imbalance. These interventions occur not only at the individual level but also at the community and policymaking systems levels. Many of the individuals who are marginalized due to illness clearly have serious and persistent mental illness, and their issues with poverty, unemployment, and fair housing are well documented in the literature.

Other occupational therapists believe community practice demands that advocacy, knowledge of civil rights, and formation of strategic community alliances become part of everyday occupational therapy practice (Christiansen & Townsend, 2004; Strong & Rebeiro, 2003). In this manner, occupational therapists practice what has been called political activities of daily living. For example, Strong and Rebeiro (2003) advocate for a full range of employment-oriented services to meet the needs of a diverse population of individuals with mental illness who desire employment. The shift to a social model of disability and adoption of the person-environment-occupation framework support an individualized approach to employment based on the desires and needs of the consumer, intervention in the environment, and attention to work that is meaningful. Attention is given to the social environment, where hope, trust, and acceptance are critical to recovery.

Van Niekerk (2004) discusses several roles for occupational therapists to include working to remove attitudinal and other barriers in "regular" work environments, developing meaningful supported employment, and exploring volunteerism and consumer-run businesses. Again, these interventions occur on the individual, community, and policymaking systems levels.

Summary

Like other helping professionals, occupational therapists often provide services to people with mental illness with a focus on ameliorating impairments or acquiring community living skills. This focus can neglect the important role that the social environment, particularly stigma, can play in obstructing community participation. Occupational therapists may even contribute to stigma. Therefore, to realize the vision of full participation for all people, occupational therapists should become advocates for wiping out stigma and work with individuals with mental illness to develop their own self-advocacy skills.

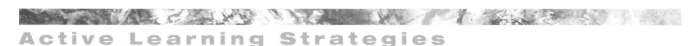

Active Learning Strategies

1. First-Person Accounts

Read a first-person account that describes the experiences of an individual with mental illness in a community social situation.

- Nonfiction examples: *Darkness Visible* (William Styron, Vintage Books, 1992); *An Unquiet Mind: A Memoir of Moods and Madness* (Kay Redfield Jamieson, Vintage Books, 1997); *The Noonday Demon: An Atlas of Depression* (Andrew Solomon, Scribner, 2001); *Crazy: A Father's Search Through America's Mental Health Madness* (Paul Earley, Putnam's Sons, 2006); *Acquainted with the Night* (Paul Raeburn, Broadway Books, 2004); *Smashed* (Koren Zailckas, Viking, 2005); *A Beautiful Mind* (Sylvia Nasar, Simon & Schuster, 1994).
- Fiction examples: *72-Hour Hold* (Bebe Moore Campbell, Alfred A. Knopf, 2005); *Stones from the River* (Ursula Hegi, Simon & Schuster, 1997).

Reflective Journal

In your Reflective Journal, describe your reactions to the writer's description of mental illness. How is the writer perceived by others, and how does that impact the writer's social experiences in the community?

2. Films

View a movie (nondocumentary) that depicts mental illness (examples: *Girl, Interrupted; Ordinary People; Silence of the Lambs; A Beautiful Mind; Shine; Benny & Joon; The Soloist*).

Reflective Questions

- How is the character portrayed?
- How are family members portrayed?
- How do other people respond to the person with mental illness?

- When was the film made, and what was the prevailing theory/belief about mental illness at the time?
- What has and has not changed since that time?

Reflective Journal

In your Reflective Journal, describe the view of mental illness as portrayed by the film.

3. Support Groups

Gather information about support groups in your community. Are there any differences between accessing support groups for individuals with mental illness and for those with physical illness? Reflect and comment.

4. Job Applications

Collect job applications from entry-level employers, such as discount stores, fast food restaurants, and other service-oriented businesses. What information is asked regarding health and mental health? Reflect on the challenges of an individual with mental illness relative to self-disclosure, stigma, and civil rights.

5. Public Transportation

Use public transportation and observe individuals who are also using it. How do you assess your own comfort? What does this say about your own biases?

6. Housing

Call a local housing agency and ask for information on finding supported housing for an individual with mental illness who is leaving the hospital. What did you learn about this process? Consider the challenges of obtaining safe, affordable, and appropriate housing of choice in your community.

Resources

- Breaking the Silence offers lessons on mental illness for children and adolescents: http://www.btslessonplans.org
- Chicago Consortium for Stigma Research includes publications on stigma and downloadable stigma measures: http://www.stigmaresearch.org
- Institute for the Study of Human Resiliency offers resources on recovery with programs and research to support resiliency for people with serious mental illness: http://www.bu.edu/resilience
- National Alliance for the Mentally Ill is a major advocacy organization with information on policy issues affecting people with mental illness and initiatives to fight stigma. Information on a public education program called "In Our Own Voice" is available at the website: http://www.nami.org
- New Freedom Commission on Mental Health presents a final report addressing issues of stigma and provides a vision of hope and recovery for people with serious mental illness: http://www.mentalhealthcommission.gov

- Substance Abuse and Mental Health Services Administration (SAMHSA) Resource Center to Address Discrimination & Stigma Associated with Mental Illness (ADS Center): http://www.adscenter.org

References

Adewuya, A. O., & Makanjuola, R. O. (2005). Social distance toward people with mental illness amongst Nigerian university students. *Social Psychiatry and Psychiatric Epidemiology, 40,* 865–868.

Alegria, M., Perez, D., & Williams, S. (2003). The role of public policies in reducing mental health status disparities for people of color. *Health Affairs, 22*(5), 51–64.

Allport, G. (1954). *The Nature of Prejudice.* Cambridge, MA: Addison-Wesley.

American Occupational Therapy Association (AOTA) (2006). 2006 AOTA workforce compensation survey: Occupational therapy salaries and job opportunities continue to improve.

http://www.aota.org/Pubs/OTP/1997-2007/Features/2006/f-091106
.aspx (accessed March 1, 2010).

Amaro, H. (1999). An expensive policy: The impact of inadequate funding for substance abuse treatment. *American Journal of Public Health, 89*(5), 657–659.

Anglin D. M., Link, B. G., & Phelan, J. C. (2006). Racial differences in stigmatizing attitudes about people with mental illness: Extending the literature. *Psychiatric Services, 57,* 857–862.

Anthony, W., Cohen, M., & Farkas, M. (1990). *Psychiatric Rehabilitation.* Boston: Center for Psychiatric Rehabilitation.

Berge, M., & Ranney, M. (2005). Self-esteem and stigma among persons with schizophrenia: Implications for mental health. *Care Management Journal, 6,* 139–144.

Bjorkman, T., Svensson, B., & Lundberg, B. (2007). Stigma among persons with serious mental illness. Reliability, acceptability and construct validity of the Swedish versions of two stigma scales measuring devaluation, discrimination and rejection experiences. *Nordic Journal of Psychiatry, 61,* 332–338.

Borinstein, A. B. (1992). Public attitudes towards persons with mental illness. *Health Affairs, 11*(3), 186–196.

Caltaux, D. (2002). Internalized stigma: A barrier to recovery. *New Zealand Journal of Occupational Therapy, 49*(1), 25–27.

Carling, P. (1990). Major mental illness, housing and supports: The promise of community integration. *American Psychologist, 45*(8), 969–975.

Chong, S. A., Verma, S., Vaingankar, J. A., Chan, Y. H., Wong, L. Y., & Heng, B. H. (2007). Perception of the public towards the mentally ill in developing Asian country. *Social Psychiatry and Psychiatric Epidemiology, 42,* 734–739.

Christiansen, C. H., & Townsend, E. A. (2004). *Introduction to Occupation: The Art and Science of Living.* Upper Saddle River, NJ: Prentice Hall.

Cohen, J., & Streuning, E. L. (1962). Opinions about mental illness in the personnel of two large mental hospitals. *Journal of Abnormal and Social Psychology, 64*(5), 349–360.

Cook, J. A., & Jonikas, J. A. (2002). Self-determination among mental health consumers/survivors: Using lessons from the past to guide the future. *Journal of Disability Policy Studies, 13*(2), 87–95.

Corrigan, P. W. (2004). Target-specific stigma chance: A strategy for impacting mental illness stigma. *Psychiatric Rehabilitation Journal, 28,* 113–121.

Corrigan, P. W., & Gelb, B. (2006). Three programs that use mass approaches to challenge the stigma of mental illness. *Psychiatric Services, 57,* 393–398.

Corrigan, P. W., Giffort, D., Rashid, F., Leary, M., & Okeke, I. (1999). Recovery as a psychological construct. *Community Mental Health Journal, 35*(3), 231–239.

Corrigan, P. W., Markowitz, F., Watson, A., Rowan, D., & Kubiak, M. A.(2003). An attribution model of public discrimination towards persons with mental illness. *Journal of Health and Social Behavior, 44*(2), 162–179.

Corrigan, P. W., & Penn, D. (1999). Lessons from social psychology on discrediting psychiatric stigma. *American Psychologist, 54*(9), 765–776.

Corrigan, P. W., River, L. P., Lundin, R. K., Penn, D. L., Uphoff-Wasowski, K., Campion, J., Mathisen, J., Gagnon, C., Bergman, M., Goldstein, H., & Kubiak, M. A. (2001). Three strategies for changing attributions about severe mental illness. *Schizophrenia Bulletin, 27*(2), 187–195.

Corrigan, P. W., Watson, A. C., Heyrman, M. L., Warpinski, A., Gracia, G., & Slopen, N. (2005). Structural stigma in state legislation. *Psychiatric Services, 56*(5), 557–563.

Corrigan, P. W., Watson, A. C., Warpinski, A. C., & Gracia, G. (2004). Implications of educating the public on mental illness, violence, and stigma. *Psychiatric Services, 55,* 557–580.

Cottrell, R. P. (2003). The Olmstead decision: Fulfilling the promise of the ADA? *OT Practice, 8*(5), 17–21.

Couture, S.M. & Penn, D.L. (2006). The effects of interpersonal contact on psychiatric stigma: A prospective approach utilizing volunteers from the community. *Journal of Community Psychology, 34,* 635–645.

Crisp, A., Gelder, M., Goddard, E., & Meltzer, H. (2005). Stigmatization of people with mental illnesses: A follow-up study within the Changing Minds campaign of the Royal College of Psychiatrists. *World Psychiatry, 4,* 106–113.

Crowe, T. P., Deane, F. P., Oades, L. G., Caputi, P., & Morland, K. G. (2006). Effectiveness of a collaborative recovery training program in Australia in promoting positive views about recovery. *Psychiatric Services, 57*(10), 1497–1500.

Davidson, L., & Hoge, M. A. (1996). Hospital or community living? Examining consumer perspectives on deinstitutionalization. *Psychiatric Rehabilitation Journal, 19*(3), 49–58.

Davidson, L., & Strauss, J. S. (1995). Beyond the biopsychosocial model: Integrating disorder, health, and recovery. *Psychiatry 58*(1):44–55.

Day, S. L. (2006). Issues in Medicaid policy and system transformation: Recommendations from the President's Commission. *Psychiatric Services, 57,* 1713–1718.

Deegan, P. E. (1988). The lived experience of rehabilitation. *Psychosocial Rehabilitation Journal, 11*(4), 11–19.

———. (1992). The independent living movement and people with psychiatric disabilities: Taking back control over our own lives. *Psychosocial Rehabilitation Journal, 15*(3), 3–19.

Demaio, C. (2006). Mental illness stigma as social attribution: How select signals of mental illness affect stigmatizing attitudes and behavior. *Dissertation Abstracts International, 66*(7-B), 3997.

Duncan, M. (2004). Promoting mental health through occupation. In R. Watson & L. Swartz (Eds.), *Transformation Through Occupation.* Philadelphia: Whurr.

Fabrega, H. (1991). Psychiatric stigma in non-Western societies. *Comprehensive Psychiatry, 32,* 534–551.

Friesen, B. J. (1996). Family support in child and adult mental health. In G. H. S. Singer, L. E. Powers, & A. L. Olson (Eds.), *Redefining Family Support: Innovations in Public–Private Partnerships* (pp. 259–274). Baltimore: Brookes.

Galheigo, S. M. (2005). Occupational therapy and the social field: Clarifying concepts and ideas. In F. Kronenberg, S. Algado, & N. Pollard (Eds.), *Occupational Therapy without Borders.* New York: Elsevier.

Gary, F. (2005). Stigma: Barriers to mental health care among ethnic minorities. *Issues in Mental Health Nursing, 26*(10), 979–999.

Goffman, E. (1963). *Stigma: Notes on the Management of Spoiled Identity.* Englewood Cliffs, NJ: Prentice-Hall.

Goldman, H. H., Frank, R. G., Burnham, M. A., Huskamp, H. A., Ridgely, M. S., Normand, S.T., et. al. (2006). Behavioral health insurance parity for federal employees. *New England Journal of Medicine, 354*(13), 1378–1386.

Hahn, H. (1985). Towards a politics of disability: Definitions, disciplines, and policies. *Social Science Journal, 22,* 87–105.

Hanson, K. W. (1998). Public opinion and the mental health parity debate: Lessons from the survey literature. *Psychiatric Services, 49*(8), 1059–1066.

Holmes, E. P., Corrigan, P. W., Williams, P., Canar, J., & Kubiak, M. A. (1999). Changing attitudes about schizophrenia. *Schizophrenia Bulletin, 25*(3), 447–456.

Jacobson, N., & Greenly, D. (2001). What is recovery? A conceptual model and explication. *Psychiatric Services, 52,* 482–485.

Jensen, G. A., Rost, K., Burton, R. P., & Bulycheva, M. (1998). Mental health insurance in the 1990s: Are employers offering less to more? *Health Affairs, 17*(3), 201–208.

Jones, D. (1998). Deviance. In D. Jones, S. Blair, T. Hartery, & R. K. Jones (Eds.), *Sociology and Occupational Therapy: An Integrated Approach* (pp. 93–104). Philadelphia: Churchill Livingstone.

Keane, M. (1991). Acceptance vs. rejection: Nursing students' attitudes about mental illness. *Perspectives in Psychiatric Care, 27*(3), 13–18.

Kleinman, A. (1988). *The Illness Narratives: Suffering, Healing and the Human Condition.* New York: Basic Books.

Kolodziej, M. E., & Johnson, B. T. (1996). Interpersonal contact and acceptance of persons with psychiatric disorders: A research synthesis. *Journal of Consulting and Clinical Psychology, 64,* 1387–1396.

Kronenberg, F., Algado, S. S., & Pollard, N. (2005). *Occupational Therapy without Borders: Learning from the Spirit of Survivors.* Philadelphia: Elsevier.

Laliberte-Rudman, D., Yu, B., Scott, E., & Pajouhandeh, P. (2000). Exploration of the perspectives of persons with schizophrenia regarding quality of life. *American Journal of Occupational Therapy, 54*(2), 137–147.

Law, M., Cooper, B., Strong, S., Stewart, D., Rigby, P., & Letts, L. (1996). The person-environment-occupation model: A transactive approach to occupational performance. *Canadian Journal of Occupational Therapy, 63,* 9–23.

Lehman, A. F. (1988). A Quality of Life Interview for the chronically mentally ill. *Evaluation and Program Planning, 11*(1), 51–62.

Liberman, R. P., & Kopelowicz, A. (2002). Recovery from schizophrenia: A challenge for the 21st century. *International Review of Psychiatry, 14,* 245–255.

Lincoln, T. M., Wilhelm, K., & Nestoriuc, Y. (2007). Effect of psychoeducation for relationships, symptoms, knowledge, adherence and function in psychotic disorders: A meta-analysis. *Schizophrenia Research, 96,* 232–245.

Link, B. G., Phelan, J. C., Bresnahan, M., Steuve, A., & Pescosolido, B. A. (1999). Public conceptions of mental illness: Labels, causes, dangerousness, and social distance. *American Journal of Public Health, 89,* 1328–1333.

Link, B. G., Streuning, E., Cullen, F. T., Shrout, P. E., & Dohrenwend, B. P. (1989). A modified labeling theory approach to mental disorders: An empirical assessment. *American Sociological Review, 54*(3), 400–423.

Lloyd, C., Sullivan, D., & Williams, P. L. (2005). Perceptions of social stigma and its effect on interpersonal relationships of young males who experience a psychotic disorder. *Australian Occupational Therapy Journal, 52,* 243–250.

Lopez, L. R. (1991). Adolescents' attitudes toward mental illness and perceived sources of their attitudes: An examination of pilot data. *Archives of Psychiatric Nursing, 5,* 271–280.

Lyons, M. (1991). Enabling or disabling? Students' attitudes towards persons with disabilities. *American Journal of Occupational Therapy, 45*(4), 311–316.

Lyons, M., & Hayes, R. (1993). Student perceptions of persons with psychiatric and other disorders. *American Journal of Occupational Therapy, 47,* 541–548.

Lyons, M., & Ziviani, J. (1995). Stereotypes, stigma, and mental illness: Learning from fieldwork experiences. *American Journal of Occupational Therapy, 49,* 1002–1008.

Mancini, M., Hardiman, E., & Lawson, H. (2005). Making sense of it all: Consumer providers' theories about factors facilitating and impeding recovery from psychiatric disabilities. *Psychiatric Rehabilitation Journal, 29*(1), 48–55.

Mechanic, D. (1998). *Mental Health and Social Policy: The Emergence of Managed Care* (4th ed.). Boston: Allyn & Bacon.

———. (2002). Removing barriers to care among persons with psychiatric symptoms. *Health Affairs, 21,* 137–147.

Miller Polgar, J., & Landry, J. E. (2004). Occupations as a means for individual and group participation in life. In C. H. Christiansen & E. A. Townsend (Eds.). *Introduction to Occupation: The Art and Science of Living* (pp. 197–220). Upper Saddle River, NJ: Prentice Hall.

Mojtabai, R. (2007). Americans' attitudes toward mental health treatment seeking: 1990–2003. *Psychiatric Services, 58,* 642–651.

Murphy, R. F., Scheer, J., Murphy, Y., & Mack, R. (1988). Physical disability and social liminality: A study in the rituals of adversity. *Social Science Medicine, 26,* 235–242.

Murray, M., & Steffen, J. (1999). Attitudes of case managers toward people with serious mental illness. *Community Mental Health Journal, 35*(6), 505–514.

Nelson, G., Sylvestre, J., Aubry, T., George, L., & Trainor, J. (2007). Housing choice and control, housing quality, and control over professional support as contributors to the subjective quality of life and community adaptation of people with serious mental illness. *Administration and Policy in Mental Health, 34,* 89–100.

New Freedom Commission on Mental Health. (2003). Transforming mental health care in America. Final Report. DHHS Pub. No. SMA-03-3832. Rockville, MD: U.S. Government Printing Office.

Noordsy, D., Torrey, W., Meuser, K., Mead, S., O'Keefe, C., & Fox, L. (2002). Recovery from severe mental illness: An interpersonal and functional outcome definition. *International Review of Psychiatry, 14,* 318–326.

Penn, D. L., Guynan, K., Daily, T., Spaulding, W., Garbin, C., & Sullivan, M. (1994). Dispelling the stigma of schizophrenia: What sort of information is best? *Schizophrenia Bulletin, 20*(3), 567–578.

Penny, N. H. (2001). Longitudinal study of student attitudes toward people with mental illness. *Occupational Therapy in Mental Health, 17*(2), 49–81.

Penny, N. H., Kasar, J., & Sinay, T. (2001). Brief report: Student attitudes towards persons with mental illness: The influence of course work and level I fieldwork. *American Journal of Occupational Therapy, 55*(2), 217–220.

Perese, E. F. (1997). Unmet needs of persons with chronic mental illnesses: Relationship to their adaptation to community living. *Issues in Mental Health Nursing, 18,* 19–34.

Perry, B. L., Pescosolido, B. A., Martin, J. K., McLeod, J. D., & Jenson, P. S. (2007). Comparison of public attributions, attitudes and stigma in regard to depression among children and adults. *Psychiatric Services, 58*(5), 632–635.

Pescosolido, B. A., Jensen, P. S., Martin, J. K., Perry, B. L., Olafsdottir, S., & Fettes, D. (2008). Public knowledge and assessment of child mental health problems: Findings from the National Stigma Study–Children. *Journal of the American Academy of Child and Adolescent Psychiatry, 47*(3), 339–349.

Pescosolido, B. A., Perry, B. L., Martin, J. K., McLeod, J. D., & Jenson, P. S. (2007). Stigmatizing attitudes and beliefs about treatment and psychiatric medications for children with mental illness. *Psychiatric Services, 58*(5), 613–618.

Pettie, D., & Triolo, A. (1999). Illness as evolution: The search for identity and meaning in the recovery process. *Psychiatric Rehabilitation Journal, 22,* 255–263.

Phelan, J. C., Bromet, E. J., & Link, B. G. (1998). Psychiatric illness and family stigma. *Schizophrenia Bulletin, 24,* 115–126.

Prince, P. N., & Prince, C. R. (2002). Perceived stigma and community integration among clients of assertive community treatment. *Psychiatric Rehabilitation Journal, 25*(4), 323–331.

Quinn, D. M., Kahng, S. K., & Crocker, J. (2004). Discreditable: Stigma effects of revealing a mental illness history on test performance. *Personality and Social Psychology Bulletin, 30*(7), 803–815.

Raeburn, P. (2004). *Acquainted with the Night: A Parent's Quest to Understand Depression and Bipolar Disorder in His Children.* New York: Broadway Books.

Rao, D., Feinglass, J., & Corrigan, P. (2007). Racial and ethnic disparities in mental illness stigma. *Journal of Nervous and Mental Diseases, 195,* 1020–1030.

Rebeiro, K. L. (1999). The labyrinth of community mental health: In search of meaningful occupation. *Psychiatric Rehabilitation Services, 23*(2), 143–152.

Rogers, E. S., Chamberlin, J., Langer Ellison, M., & Crean, T. (1997). A consumer-constructed scale to measure empowerment among users of mental health services. *Psychiatric Services, 48*(8), 1042–1047.

Sartorius, N. (2007). Stigma and mental health. *Lancet, 370,* 810–811.

Schulze, B. (2007). Stigma and mental health professionals: A review of the evidence on an intricate relationship. *International Review of Psychiatry, 19,* 137–155.

Singh, S. P., Baxter, H., Standen, P., & Duggan, C. (1998). Changing the attitudes of "tomorrow's doctors" towards mental illness and psychiatry: A comparison of two teaching methods. *Medical Education, 32,* 115–120.

Smart, J. (2001). *Disability, Society and the Individual.* Austin, TX: ProEd.

Spaniol, L., Wewiorski, N., Gagne, C., & Anthony, W. (2002). The process of recovery from schizophrenia. *International Journal of Psychiatry, 14,* 327–336.

Stimmel, G. L. (2001). Maximizing treatment outcome in depression: Strategies to overcome social stigma and noncompliance. *Disease Management Health Outcomes, 9*(4), 179–186.

Strong, S., & Rebeiro, K. (2003). Creating supportive work environments for people with mental illness. In L. Letts, P. Rigby, & D. Stewart (Eds.), *Using Environments to Enable Occupational Performance.* Thorofare, NJ: Slack.

Susman, J. (1994). Disability, stigma and deviance. *Social Science Medicine, 38*(1), 15–22.

Tanaka, G. (2003). Development of the Mental Illness and Disorder Understanding Scale. *International Journal of Japanese Sociology, 12,* 95–107.

Taylor, M. C. (1991). Stigma: Theoretical concept and actual experience. *British Journal of Occupational Therapy, 54*(11), 406–410.

Teschinsky, U. (2000). Living with schizophrenia: The family illness experience. *Issues in Mental Health Nursing, 21,* 387–396.

Tsang, H. W., Angell, B., Corrigan, P. W., Lee, Y. T., Shi, K., Lam, C. S., Jin, S., & Fung, K. M. (2007). A cross-cultural study of employers' concerns about hiring people with psychotic disorder: Implications for recovery. *Social Psychiatry and Psychiatric Epidemiology, 42,* 723–733.

Turner, V. (1969). *The Ritual Process: Structure and Anti-Structure.* Chicago: Aldine.

U.S. Department of Health and Human Services. (1999). *Mental Health: A Report of the Surgeon General.* Rockville, MD: U.S. Department of Health and Human Services, Substance Abuse and Mental Health Services Administration, Center for Mental Health Services, National Institutes of Health, National Institute of Mental Health.

Van Niekerk, L. (2004). Psychiatric disability in the world of work: Shifts in attitude and service models. In R. Watson & L. Swartz (Eds.), *Transformation through Occupation.* Philadelphia: Whurr.

Vrkljan, B. H. (2005). Reflections on dispelling the disability stereotype: Embracing a universalistic perspective of disablement. *Canadian Journal of Occupational Therapy, 72*(1), 57–59.

Watson, R., & Schwartz, L. (2004). *Transformation through Occupation.* Philadelphia: Whurr.

Willett, J., & Deegan, M. J. (2001). Liminality and disability: Rites of passage and community in hypermodern society. *Disability Studies Quarterly, 21*(3), 137–152.

Wittman, P. (1994). Social stigma: What it means to occupational therapy. *Mental Health Special Interest Section Newsletter, 17*(4), 1–4.

World Health Organization. (2001a). *International Classification of Functioning, Disability, and Health.* Geneva: Author.

———. (2001b). *Mental Health: New Understanding, New Hope.* Geneva: Author.

World Psychiatric Association. (2002). *Schizophrenia: Open the Doors Training Manual: Global Program against Stigma and Discrimination because of Schizophrenia.* Geneva: Author.

Wright, E. R., Gronfein, W. P., & Owens, T. J. (2000). Deinstitutionalization, social rejection, and the self-esteem of former mental patients. *Journal of Health and Social Behavior, 41*(1), 68–90.

Yang, L.H. (2007). Application of mental illness stigma theory to Chinese societies: Synthesis and new directions. *Singapore Medical Journal, 48,* 977–985.

Families Living With Mental Illness

Christine Urish and Barbara Jacobs

> "Call it a clan, call it a network, call it a tribe, call it a family. Whatever you call it, whoever you care, you need one.
>
> —Jane Howard, *Families*, 1980

Introduction

Mental illness impacts thousands of individuals and their families each year. In 2002, over one fourth of all adults (18 years and older) and one fifth of all youth (9–17 years) had at least one mental disorder (U.S. Department of Health and Human Services, 2007). Mental health treatment has increasingly shifted toward short hospital stays to manage acute symptoms and early discharge with medication management and outpatient follow-up (Sharfstein & Dickerson, 2009). Statistics from 2004 indicate that 74.9% of people with mental illness are discharged home and usually reside with their families (Center for Mental Health Services, 2004). Families seeking to understand their loved one's mental illness and the treatment options available to them often encounter a mental health service delivery system that is fragmented and confusing (New Freedom Commission on Mental Health, 2003).

Many of the chapters in this text describe the impact of mental illness on the occupational functioning of the individual, but illness and disability often negatively impact family functioning as well (Lawlor & Mattingly, 2009). Families often have little understanding of the symptoms or course of a mental disorder. Many are ill prepared to navigate the mental health system, address a family member's difficult behaviors, or cope with the isolation and stigma they may experience as a result of having a family member with a mental illness (Shankar & Muthuswany, 2007).

In past centuries, it was commonly believed that families were the cause of mental illness (Spaniol et al, 2004). Although we know families do not cause mental illness, many textbooks that are used to train professionals continue to perpetuate such misinformation regarding families and mental illness (Spaniol et al, 2004). "Best practices now require a professional re-education perspective to counter this persistent family-culpability bias" (Stuart, Burland, Ganju, Levounis, & Kiosk, 2002, p. 326). One goal of this chapter is to break this cycle of misinformation by providing insights into the challenges facing families coping with mental illness. Descriptions and definitions of family environment are presented for consideration in establishing family-centered services. The relationship between the environment and occupation are examined, and assessments and models of intervention that can be beneficial in working with families are presented.

Description of the Family Environment

A family is a social system composed of a group of individuals whose occupations are interrelated (Humphrey & Case-Smith, 2001). The term **family** includes "those who undertake the care and support of a person with severe mental illness, regardless of whether they are related or live in the same household" (Substance Abuse and Mental Health Services Administration [SAMHSA], 2003, p.3). SAMHSA's description of family is not limited to a specific family structure, the number or gender of the people in the family group, or the biological (genetic) relationships among family members. It is inclusive, defining family as people who voluntarily consider themselves to be family as a result of their interaction, situation, psychological attachment, or capacity to reciprocally satisfy social needs. Despite that some clients will claim they have "no family," all individuals survive within the social environment.

Family environment is a term used variously in the mental health literature; it often connotes family characteristics such as family communication patterns (e.g., conflict, caring), relationships and family processes (e.g., availability, instability), family functioning (e.g., economic, educational), and family stressors (e.g., unemployment, health crises) (Rangarajan & Kelly, 2006). When occupational therapy practitioners consider the family environment, several factors should be taken into account, including (Marsh 1998; Spaniol, Zipple, Marsh, & Finley, 2000):

- Family's emotional response (i.e., the subjective and objective burdens associated with mental illness in the family).
- Family culture as context.
- Family lifespan and developmental roles.

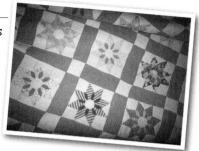

Who am I? Like this quilt sewn of scraps and pieces representative of my family life, I too am a product of my family life. A combination of nature and nurture. I am a crazy yet congruous mix of colors and patterns.

—Jill

Emotional Response

Burland (2001) identified three typical emotional responses that can occur when a family member is diagnosed with a mental illness:

1. Dealing with catastrophic events.
2. Learning to cope.
3. Moving into advocacy.

When mental illness is diagnosed in a family, the family often experiences feelings of crisis, chaos, and a world "turned upside-down" (Burland, 2001). A diagnosis to some may be an answer to prayer (e.g., "We finally have an answer as to why this has been happening"), whereas to others this news can evoke a state of shock. Family members may deny there is anything wrong with their loved one (e.g., "The diagnosis must be a mistake"). Others may hope that this is a phase or a stage and that things will return to "normal" once again.

Burland calls this emotional response "dealing with catastrophic events" (2001, p. 1). The powerful emotions that family members experience are often described as the **subjective burden** of family caregiving (Marsh, 1998). This subjective burden can include feelings of grief; symbolic loss of the hopes, dreams, and aspirations that were held for a loved one with mental illness; a sense of chronic sorrow; empathic pain; and the emotional "roller coaster" that individuals may feel they are riding during the relapse and remission their loved one experiences (Marsh, 1998). Another emotional response that family members often experience is anger (e.g., "Why is this happening to our family?"), guilt (e.g., "I must have done something wrong for this to be happening to my family"), and resentment (e.g., "Why do other families look so 'perfect,' yet my family is filled with turmoil?").

The burden of caring for a family member with mental illness is associated with higher levels of stress, lower levels of self-efficacy and personal sense of well-being, and adverse effects on physical health (Hirst, 2005; Treasure, 2004). Occupational therapists can address these aspects of burden by educating families about their family member's mental illness, teaching problem-solving methods for managing behavior, and helping the family identify resources and make plans for backup or emergency care as necessary.

The learning-to-cope response is manifest as families experience the **objective burden** of having a loved one diagnosed with a mental illness (Marsh, 1998). The objective burden of family caregiving refers to the challenges of addressing a myriad of practical problems associated with mental illness. These might include managing positive (e.g., hallucinations and delusions) and negative (e.g., lack of motivation, poor daily living skills and hygiene) symptoms and adapting to a family member's mood swings and socially inappropriate or self-destructive behaviors. The need to orchestrate family routines to provide the necessary care and supervision of the family member while minimizing family disruption and stress is also an example of objective burden (Marsh, 1998).

Occupational therapists working from a family-centered perspective can address these caregiver burdens by helping family members develop pragmatic strategies that compensate for an ill family member's decline in occupational role functioning while simultaneously providing opportunities to support the individual's recovery.

The third emotional response family members may experience is moving into advocacy (Burland, 2001, p. 1). Within this stage, families demonstrate a greater understanding of mental illness, share an acceptance of the impact of mental illness on their family and society, and move into an advocacy/action mode. For example, families can join their local National Alliance on Mental Illness (NAMI) affiliate or begin to advocate for family involvement in therapeutic interventions at the mental health agencies where their family member is receiving services.

These three emotional stages are not linear, and family members do not necessarily move through each stage in sequence or even fully experience each stage. A family member may spend a significant amount of time dealing with catastrophic events and move toward learning to cope when something drastic may happen, such as incarceration of their loved one or increased hospitalizations and severe decompensation of their loved one's level of function.

Family Culture as Context

In addition to the emotional responses of the family, it is important for occupational therapy practitioners to understand the particular family culture as an overarching context. Communication styles, problem solving, decision making, conflict resolution, family roles, and mental health–seeking attitudes and behaviors need to be examined in cultural context.

Cultural and ethnic barriers in the mental health system may be present and limit the family's and consumer's access to services (Spaniol et al, 2000). For example, in many Hispanic families, family unity is highly valued, and the network of social relationships often extends beyond marital or biological ties. Although this can be an important source of social support, it can also delay mental health treatment or even the recognition that professional help is needed (Garcia Preto, 2005).

Practitioners need to look at each family as a unique culture with an individual worldview and set of unique perceptions (Spaniol et al, 2000). It is useful for practitioners to be open regarding their own worldview and values and to share these directly and respectfully with family members.

Of significant importance is the ability for the practitioner to identify the family group's perception of mental illness, the cultural traditions in place with regard to seeking assistance, and preferred coping strategies. Occupational therapy practitioners can then work with family members to develop supports that are acceptable to the family from a cultural perspective.

For example, in some cultures, a frank discussion of mental health issues may be considered inappropriate and insensitive, whereas in other cultures emotional information may be reported as bodily symptoms (e.g., fatigue may mean despair in Chinese culture) or problems may be expressed in metaphoric terms or named in the language of a particular culture (e.g., *ataque de nervious* can be used to explain anxiety or dissociation in some Latino cultures). Chapter 30 describes a variety of strategies for demonstrating culturally responsive caring practices for individuals, which can also be applied to families.

Life Span and Occupational Roles

Occupational therapists are trained to evaluate normal development (e.g., physical, social, cognitive). A life-span perspective requires that the practitioner consider the life stage of the family member who has the illness and the occupational roles (e.g., child, sibling, parent, spouse) that may be associated with this life stage (Marsh, 1998). A family life-span perspective also necessitates that the life stage of all family members be considered.

Early family development theories proposed that the family unit could be viewed as a developing organism with a life cycle reflecting a distinct sequence of changes in family composition, roles, and relationships (Duvall, 1977). In nuclear families (husband, wife, and at least one child), Duvall proposed eight stages:

1. Married without children.
2. Childbearing family.
3. Family with preschooler.
4. Family with school-aged children.
5. Family with teenagers.
6. Family launching young adults.
7. The empty nest.
8. The aging family.

In this stage model, there are specific developmental tasks to be accomplished in each particular life stage. Disequilibrium is a hallmark of transition of one stage to the next, and failure to achieve the specific tasks of any stage can lead to distress in the family and influence the achievement of future life stages (Hill & Rodgers, 1964).

In any given stage of the family life cycle, individual family members occupy specific occupational roles. For example, school-aged children may possess several roles, including student, friend, and hobbyist, and each of these roles can be impacted when the family member with a mental illness is a parent who is frequently hospitalized or unable to function in the role as a parent. When a child's sibling has a mental illness, parents often need to spend a significant amount of time meeting the needs of the sibling and negotiating the mental health system to access effective services. The needs of the other siblings may be overlooked or viewed as less important during crisis times. Children and adolescents may not have developed resources or strategies for coping with the challenging issues they may be experiencing (Marsh, 1998).

Adults also participate in a variety of roles, including worker, caregiver, home maintainer, friend, and family member. How do these roles change due to mental illness? Are persons with mental illness able to fulfill these roles and the accompanying responsibilities? Do they turn to a spouse or life partner for assistance? Do they turn to their parents or siblings? Are there sources of reliable support outside the family? Family members often become the primary caregivers for their loved one, and this burden may be of specific concern to aging parents and spouses (e.g., "Who will care for my child or spouse when I am no longer here?") (Marsh, 1998).

Generally speaking, using a developmental perspective that considers the family life stage and the various roles of family members can be useful for anticipating the challenges that may exist and marshaling the family's strengths and resources to manage these challenges. On the other hand, this developmental approach uses a traditional nuclear family as the norm. Not all families reflect this nuclear family structure. Every family is unique in its composition. Nonetheless, when used as a general framework, a life-span, developmental perspective can help practitioners structure their clinical reasoning by asking questions such as, Where is this family on the continuum of family life-cycle stages? What occupational roles are associated with these stages? What life tasks are or are not being accomplished by the family or individuals in the family? Practitioners might help a family understand the developmental stages of individuals and the family as a unit, to recognize the disequilibrium that is normal during family life-cycle stages, and to proactively plan to meet the developmental challenges of each stage. Information specifically related to parenting is presented in Box 29-1.

BOX 29-1 ▪ Parenting *by Alexis D. Henry*

Making the decision to have a child is momentous. It is to decide forever to have your heart go walking around outside your body.

ELIZABETH STONE

The decision to become a parent is indeed momentous, and parenting is one of the most challenging, yet one of the most common, occupations that adults take on. Adults with mental illness have the same desires to be parents as those without mental illness, and research shows that even adults with serious disorders such as schizophrenia are just as likely as those without mental disorders to become parents (Nicholson, Biebel, Katz-Leavy, & Williams, 2004; Nicholson & Henry, 2003). There are millions of adults and children in the United States coping with parental mental illness.

Continued

BOX 29-1 ▓ **Parenting** *by Alexis D. Henry—cont'd*

Parenting as Occupation

Like other parents, adults with mental illness want to be the best parents they can be (Perkins, 2003). While parental mental illness can present challenges and risks for parents and their children, many adults with mental illness are parenting successfully. Being a parent can be an organizing life role, promoting recovery and sometimes providing the motivation a parent needs to stay in treatment (Mowbray, Oyserman, Bybee, MacFarlane, & Rueda-Riedle, 2001; Nicholson, Sweeney, & Geller, 1998).

Parents with mental illness face the same daily demands that all parents face (Henry & Nicholson, 2005; Nicholson & Henry, 2003; Nicholson et al, 1998). Typical daily demands faced by all parents can include finding safe and affordable housing for one's family; accessing childcare, health care, and transportation; and managing daily household responsibilities, such as cooking, shopping, cleaning, laundry, and family finances. Parents must provide hands-on caretaking for infants and toddlers; help older children with schoolwork; and provide their children with opportunities for play and recreation. In addition to these daily activities, parents need to teach their children social and self-management skills and to manage interpersonal relationships with their children and other family members. Many parents also need to balance their family demands with work responsibilities (Henry, 2005; Henry & Nicholson, 2005; Nicholson & Henry, 2003).

In addition to meeting the everyday demands faced by all parents, parents with mental illness face some unique challenges. Meeting one's own mental and physical health needs is crucial to being able to meet the needs of children and other family members. Psychiatric symptoms can make it difficult for a parent to meet the daily demands of parenting, but parents may also need to manage the impact of treatment on their ability to meet parenting responsibilities. For example, while psychiatric medications may be effective in controlling symptoms, medication side effects (e.g., fatigue) might make it difficult for a parent to be involved in a routine activity such as helping a child with homework. Single parents facing hospitalization will need to ensure that someone can care for their children while they are gone from home.

Parents with mental illness often worry about the impact of their illness on their children and may struggle to find ways to talk to and help their children understand about mental illness. Because children in families coping with parental mental illness may also have difficulties, many parents need to become skilled at advocating for school-based or mental health services for their children (Henry & Nicholson, 2005; Nicholson & Henry, 2003). The varied challenges that parents with mental illness can face point to multiple opportunities for providing services and supports to these families.

Assessment Considerations

Knowing that a parent has a mental illness says very little about his or her ability to meet the obligations of parenting, about the daily challenges that she or he might face, or about the supports that might best help that parent manage daily demands. Asking the right questions is key to conducting a family-centered and strengths-based assessment of parenting. A good place to begin is with an interview aimed at understanding the particular strengths, challenges, goals, resources, and needs of the parent and his or her family members.

An interview about parenting can begin with a discussion of a typical day in the family's life. What is the routine on a typical day, from the time everyone in the family wakes up until bedtime? Who does what and when? What things does the parent do well? What things do the children do well? What types of challenges make the family's daily routine break down? What resources and supports does the family have? What do they need? What are the parent's goals for himself or herself and for the family?

An interview can be followed by a discussion of priorities for change. A collaborative goal-setting tool specifically designed for use with parents with mental illness, the *ParentingWell Strengths and Goals* form (Figure 29-1), can be used by practitioners to help parents identify things they do well and areas for change.

Services for Parents

Until recently, the needs of parents with mental illness and their families have generally been overlooked by mental health service providers (Hinden, Biebel, Nicholson, Henry, & Katz-Leavy, 2006; Nicholson, Hinden, Biebel, Henry, & Katz-Leavy, 2007). However, there are many opportunities for occupational therapy practitioners to provide services to parents with mental illness and their families. Occupational therapy practitioners may encounter parents and/or children coping with parental mental illness across a variety of practice settings, including psychiatric hospitals, community mental health programs, early intervention programs, and school systems.

Practitioners working on inpatient psychiatric units may offer parent–child activity groups or other structured opportunities for children and parents to visit with each other on the unit or might otherwise help parents maintain communication with their children while in the hospital. Practitioners might help parents anticipate daily parenting challenges they are likely to face after discharge and help parents to identify ways to manage these challenges and to find parenting supports in their local communities. Practitioners working with adults in community mental health programs might offer parent support groups or skills training groups addressing daily tasks of parenting. Practitioners providing home-based services to families might offer similar parenting skills training interventions. Practitioners might also work with parents to help them develop natural supports for themselves and their families through schools, churches, or other community programs.

There are no evidence-based practices or programs for parents with mental illness and their families. However, recent efforts by Nicholson and colleagues (Hinden et al, 2006; Nicholson et al, 2007) have attempted to articulate the common philosophies and strategies used by several community-based programs across the country that have been developed specifically to address the needs of parents with mental illness and their families. These programs share several important assumptions, including the beliefs that:

- Adults with mental illness have strengths and can successfully parent.
- Adults with mental illness deserve the opportunity to parent and to receive the supports necessary to function as well as possible in the parenting role.
- Enhanced parenting is related to enhanced child development.
- Trusting relationships between practitioners and parents is central to successful interventions. (Nicholson et al, 2007, pp. 404–405)

Virtually all programs provide family-centered case management services, addressing needs of both parents and children, as well as parenting support, education, and skills training interventions. The common goals of these programs are to enhance quality of life for parents and their children by enhancing parenting self-efficacy, enhancing child development, strengthening parent–child relationships, decreasing family isolation, and stabilizing parents' mental health.

ParentingWell® Strengths & Goals

Here is a list of things you may need to do as a parent. For each one that applies to you, *circle* the answer that describes you best.	This is a strength of mine.	I do this okay.	I'd like to do this better.	Does not apply.	Check items to work on.
1. Manage everyday household tasks	Strength	Okay	Better	DNA	
2. Plan and make healthy meals	Strength	Okay	Better	DNA	
3. Understand the relationship between my feelings and my actions	Strength	Okay	Better	DNA	
4. Manage my family's money	Strength	Okay	Better	DNA	
5. Set limits with my child	Strength	Okay	Better	DNA	
6. Have positive interactions/visits with my child	Strength	Okay	Better	DNA	
7. Have a pleasant routine with my child	Strength	Okay	Better	DNA	
8. Find fun things to do with my child	Strength	Okay	Better	DNA	
9. Get adequate child care for my child	Strength	Okay	Better	DNA	
10. Balance work or school, and parenting	Strength	Okay	Better	DNA	
11. Know what to do when my child has problems	Strength	Okay	Better	DNA	
12. Identify my child's strengths	Strength	Okay	Better	DNA	
13. Have positive "family time"	Strength	Okay	Better	DNA	
14. Know my legal options as a parent	Strength	Okay	Better	DNA	
15. Get help for myself, if I need it	Strength	Okay	Better	DNA	
16. Talk with my child about my situation or worries	Strength	Okay	Better	DNA	
17. Keep in touch with my child who is not living with me	Strength	Okay	Better	DNA	
18. Live a substance-free lifestyle	Strength	Okay	Better	DNA	
19. Communicate well with my child	Strength	Okay	Better	DNA	
20. Have good relationships with my child's caregivers/helpers	Strength	Okay	Better	DNA	
21. Express anger without hurting anyone	Strength	Okay	Better	DNA	
22. Keep my child and myself safe	Strength	Okay	Better	DNA	
23. Make time to take care of myself	Strength	Okay	Better	DNA	
24. Manage stress and worries in healthy ways	Strength	Okay	Better	DNA	
25. Cope with bad things that have happened to me in my life	Strength	Okay	Better	DNA	
26. Get special services and supports for my child	Strength	Okay	Better	DNA	
27. Other:	Strength	Okay	Better	DNA	

FIGURE 29-1. ParentingWell® Strengths & Goals assessment form. A collaborative goal-setting tool specifically designed for use with parents with mental illness, this tool can be used by practitioners to help parents identify things they do well and areas for change. *Reprinted with permission from J. Nicholson & A. Henry. ©2003. ParentingWell® is a trademark of Strengths Based Solutions, LLC. www.parentingwell.org.*

Continued

BOX 29-1 ■ **Parenting** *by Alexis D. Henry—cont'd*

REFERENCES

Henry, A. D., & Nicholson, J. (2005). Helping mothers with serious mental illness. In Flach, F. E. (Ed.), *Directions in Rehabilitation Counseling*, Vol. 16, Lesson 3. (pp. 19–32). Long Island City, NY: Hatherleigh.

Hinden, B. R., Biebel, K., Nicholson, J., Henry, A., Katz-Leavy, J. (2006). A survey of programs for parents with mental illness and their families: Identifying common elements to build the evidence base. *Journal of Behavioral Health Services and Research, 33,* 21–38.

Mowbray, C. T., Oyserman, D., Bybee, D., MacFarlane, P., & Rueda-Riedle, A. (2001). Life circumstances of mothers with serious mental illness. *Psychiatric Rehabilitation Journal, 25*(2), 114–123.

Nicholson, J., Biebel, K., Katz-Leavy, J., & Williams, V. F. (2004). Prevalence of parenthood in adults with mental illness: Implications for state and federal policymakers, programs, and providers. In R. W. Manderscheid & J. J. Henderson (Eds.), *Mental Health, United States,*

2002. DHHS Pub No. (SMA) 3938 (pp. 12–137). Rockville, MD: Substance Abuse and Mental Health Services Administration.

Nicholson, J., & Henry, A. D. (2003). Achieving the goal of evidence-based psychiatric rehabilitation practices for mothers with mental illness. *Psychiatric Rehabilitation Journal, 27,* 122–130.

Nicholson, J., Hinden, B. R., Biebel, K., Henry A. D., & Katz-Leavy, J. (2007). A qualitative study of programs for parents with serious mental illness and their children: Building practice-based evidence. *Journal of Behavioral Health Services & Research, 34,* 395–413.

Nicholson, J., Sweeney, E. M., & Geller, J. L. (1998). Mothers with mental illness: I. The competing demands of parenting and living with mental illness. *Psychiatric Services, 49*(5), 635–642.

Perkins, L. (2003). Personal accounts: Mental illness, motherhood and me. *Psychiatric Services, 54,* 157–158.

Environmental Assessments

Occupational therapists can initially examine the family environment through observation and completion of an occupational profile. The occupational profile can provide information about the client's occupational history, experiences, daily living patterns, values, needs, interests, and current situation (American Occupational Therapy Association [AOTA], 2002). The occupational profile is designed to be used in a client-centered fashion to gather information about the client, from his or her perspective. It is important to note that, according to the *Occupational Therapy Practice Framework,* the client is defined as individual, caregiver, group, and population. A family member can be considered the client within the role as caregiver for the family member with mental illness (AOTA, 2002).

In considering the occupational profile of family members, the occupational therapist can elicit information on the impact of having a family member with a mental illness on their engagement in daily occupations as well as what problems they are experiencing. The therapist should consider the family members' priorities and outcomes as well as how these goals and priorities are similar to or different from the goals and outcomes desired by their loved one. Desired outcomes may be different for the individual diagnosed with mental illness than for the family member or caregiver. For example, a young adult with a serious mental illness may believe that a supportive education program can help him or her achieve a sense of normalcy and structure in his or her life, whereas the parents are convinced the family member is setting himself or herself up for failure and should be discouraged from pursuing higher education. Clarifying desired outcomes is very important to address early on to ensure that the occupational therapy practitioner has a clear perspective regarding the goals of all family members and where these goals may intersect or compete.

While completing the occupational profile, the occupational therapist must be sensitive to the values of the family, culture, family environment, and contextual factors that may impact family system functioning. Professionals also must acknowledge the strengths, resources, and expertise of families. Families may present with numerous challenges,

and family members are often doing the very best they can. Promoting a sense of control for the family and acknowledging strengths can assist families in development of the necessary skills to cope with mental illness and address the specific needs identified by the family. Establishing rapport is critical. "Rapport is enhanced when practitioners have an understanding of the family experience of mental illness, a respectful and humane attitude toward families and a commitment to family empowerment" (Marsh, 1998, p. 13). Listening in a nonjudgmental, responsive, and empathetic manner and using clear, direct, and supportive communication supports the maintenance of rapport and development of positive therapeutic relationships.

When a family member has a mental illness, individual family members can experience a disruption or discontinuation of a valued role or experience stress and strain related to the demands of caregiving. The role checklist (Oakley, 2006) can be used to ascertain current family roles and the value of the identified roles to the family member. A completed checklist offers a starting point for exploring how valued roles have been impacted by a family member's mental illness and for developing intervention strategies that can ensure the continuation of meaningful and productive role patterns. The Occupational Performance History Interview II is another assessment that can be considered for use with family members. This instrument provides information on participation in occupational choices, routines related to valued roles, life events, and environmental influences that can assist the occupational therapist in developing effective interventions (Chaffey & Fossey, 2004). Caregiver burden is complex and has been shown to include areas of activities of daily living, worry, and social strain (Ivarsson, Sidenvall, & Carlsson, 2004). A brief, reliable, and valid measure for assessing the family's level of burden is the Burden Assessment Scale (BAS) for Families of the Seriously Mentally Ill (Reinhard, Gubman, Horwitz, & Minsky, 1994). This 19-item scale can be self-administered or used as an interview. Practitioners working with families using an individual consultative or psychoeducational approach may consider using this assessment as a program evaluation measure by determining the level of burden at baseline and at the completion of their intervention program (Reinhard et al, 1994).

For example, Ivarsson et al (2004) found that caregivers needed more resources for managing burdensome situations related to daily activities than for managing issues related to their loved one's behavior. Assessing those aspects of daily life that a family experiences as adding to their caregiving burden can support intervention planning and referrals to other agencies or support groups. As of this writing, no study exists that addresses subjective or objective burdens for family members in the areas of activities of daily living and household routines. These are areas that occupational therapy practitioners are well equipped to address. When occupational therapists address the consumers' ability to establish routines, it can afford caregivers more time to engage in meaningful occupations unrelated to caregiving (Chaffey & Fossey, 2004).

Assistance for Families

Because many family members provide crisis intervention and serve as informal case managers for their loved ones, it is important for professionals to be able to clearly identify how they can effectively help family members perform the variety of roles they hold (National Alliance on Mental Illness New York State [NAMI NYS], 2006). Family members may find themselves responsible providing basic needs for their ill loved one, including housing, financial support, and socialization, as well as serving as his or her advocate. Often, families provide these services because there may be, or they may feel there are, few options available. Families need three specific types of assistance: collaboration, education, and support (NAMI NYS, 2006; Spaniol et al, 2000; Spaniol et al, 2004).

Collaboration

Collaboration is a partnership built on mutuality. Collaboration involves the development of mutually agreed-upon goals, shared decision making and planning, willingness to engage in a reciprocal relationship based on mutual respect, and honest and open dialogue and information sharing (Weist, Evans, & Lever, 2007). When family members learn a loved one has a mental illness, a major change often occurs within the family system and within family roles (Spaniol et al, 2004). During these initial stages of coping, many family members feel ill prepared to help their loved one and unsure of their role with health-care providers. Therefore, the professional should take the lead and clearly explain the collaboration process to the family (NAMI NYS, 2006; Spaniol et al, 2004).

Families should be included in treatment planning, and information should be sought from the family regarding the history of the client and the day-to-day wellbeing of their loved one (NAMI NYS, 2006). The Center for Psychiatric Rehabilitation reported that 80% of persons with mental illness who reported for a treatment appointment accompanied by a family member followed through with treatment, whereas only 55% of those who were unaccompanied followed through with treatment (Spaniol et al, 2004). The outcomes represented by these percentages emphasize the importance of family involvement in client care.

Open and reciprocal communication facilitates collaboration and results in families feeling respected and validated. The collaborative approach assumes that families are competent or potentially competent and focuses on the strengths rather than weaknesses within the family. This approach is a partnership in which the main goal is the utmost consideration of recovery for the loved one with a mental illness and the family as a whole.

Education

Families benefit from education about mental illness, diagnosis, and intervention (Bond & Campbell, 2008). The timing of family education should be carefully considered because it must be congruent with the family's emotional response stage (i.e., stage of dealing with catastrophic events versus moving into advocacy) (Burland, 2001, p. 1). Families can benefit from receiving printed information similar to that presented to their loved one upon admission into psychiatric treatment (NAMI NYS, 2006). Information on the role and responsibilities of occupational therapy professionals, the services provided by occupational therapists, and community support information and referral (i.e., NAMI support group) can also be provided. Education can assist the family in understanding the diagnosis, confronting stigma and negative attitudes, and advocating for their family and loved one. It can also decrease family stress and feelings of guilt and anxiety (Spaniol et al, 2004).

Support

Support, including emotional and practical support, is essential in helping families become successful in coping with the life changes they are experiencing (NAMI NYS, 2006). Support can come from professionally led support groups and **family respite**. Family respite care services provide brief periods of relief for families providing care to persons living in the community (Jeon, Brodaty, & Chesterson, 2005). Family-led support groups offer family members the opportunity to share stories and learn from one another (Spaniol et al, 2004). Within these groups, family members can develop helpful and supportive bonds and work collectively to advocate for positive changes within the mental health system that could benefit people with mental illness and families. Many families have experienced frustration with mental health providers. It is essential to utilize effective professional communication skills and actively listen without judging or becoming defensive when families express concern (Spaniol et al, 2004).

Barriers to family involvement include the consumer being disconnected from the family unit, increased stress within the family, and dissatisfaction with the family (Spaniol et al, 2004). Despite research that provides evidence of the needs of family members, very few families receive services (Sherman & Carothers, 2005). Dixon, McFarlane, et al (2001) note that few programs are available that specifically address family needs and suggest that problems with reimbursement and the logistical challenges of providing services at times that accommodate working families' schedules complicate the delivery of family services.

Prochaska and DiClemente (1983) developed the transtheoretical model (also called the stages of change model) to gain understanding of how individuals change behavior. The five stages of the transtheoretical model (precontemplation, contemplation, preparation, action, and maintenance) can be useful in considering issues presented by family members, clinicians, clients, and administrators of mental health services. This model is fully described in Chapter 23. When considering the potential for implementation of family services, it is important for the occupational therapist to assess the readiness to change of each group (family members, clinicians, clients, and administrators of mental health services) (Sherman & Carothers, 2005).

Table 29-1 provides information on issues families are experiencing at each stage of change and corresponding intervention approaches (Sherman & Carothers, 2005).

Family Participation in Mental Health Care

Family members have reported more adaptive coping when they possess a large social support system; have positive self-efficacy; belong to NAMI; and feel affirmed, valued, and respected for the information, knowledge, and abilities they possess (SAMHSA, 2003). Practitioners should work to create and maintain trusting environments that emphasize the strengths of the family.

Lakeman (2008) defined a set of family-centered practices that can support effective family participation in mental health care. Many of these expectations emphasize reciprocity and the family's right to give and receive information that supports the care of their family member and facilitates healthy family functioning. For example, family-centered practices respect the family's right to give and receive information about diagnosis, assessment, the strengths and limitations of their family member, and the goals and structure of the treatment plan. Further, family's have the right to expect to receive information, education, and support, including referrals to appropriate organizations and services that may benefit them or their loved one (Lakeman, 2008).

Family members provide many supports to their loved one. They are often the first responders when their loved one becomes ill or relapses (NAMI NYS, 2006). "Family connections are very powerful whether they are positive or negative" (Spaniol et al, 2004). As a result, occupational therapists should listen closely to family concerns. When family members call with a crisis at hand, practitioners should be prepared to offer concrete information and assistance.

The role of case management is one in which family members often find themselves by default. Family members often take responsibility to ensure that treatment plans are followed, medications and finances are managed, transportation is provided, and any number of daily stress situations are defused or resolved. Basic needs of consumers, such as housing, home maintenance, shopping, and cooking, often become the responsibility of the family (NAMI NYS, 2006). Although some family members do not wish to be responsible for these duties, they often have very limited alternatives (Spaniol et al, 2004). Occupational therapy practitioners can work collaboratively with the consumer and family to develop goals and interventions that work toward the functional independence of the consumer in these basic areas.

Family members are often responsible for providing opportunities for social participation (NAMI NYS, 2006). It is also important for the consumer to have outlets for communication and social interaction outside of the family system. Family members need to be encouraged to take advantage of family respite to strengthen their interactions with friends and others in the community. It is important for professionals to develop a positive relationship with the family because they know their loved one well and are often best suited to serve as the advocate with and for their family member (Spaniol et al, 2004). Family "case managers" need collaboration and support from mental health service providers. Family members can give service providers a great deal of information and insight into the history of their loved one's illness (NAMI NYS, 2006).

At times, family members may find themselves excluded from the therapeutic environment. Adults can refuse to allow family members access to records or refuse to participate in scheduled family meetings, and mental health professionals may operate in a way that excludes the family from assessment and treatment planning (Jakobsen & Severinson, 2006). This situation is not advised because the family often encourages attendance in community support programs, medication management, and other therapeutic activities (NAMI NYS, 2006). Family members should be actively involved in the treatment plan and have a clear understanding of the roles and responsibilities of the occupational therapists and all care providers.

Services to families should cover the spectrum from family psychoeducation to support groups, counseling, and informational materials. It is important that family members are not given false hope through this intervention. Although the goal of intervention is recovery, this does not mean

---

Table 29-1 ● **Transtheoretical Model Applied to Families That Include a Person With a Mental Illness**

Stage of Change	Possible Family Issues	Intervention Approach
Precontemplation	Feeling blamed for behavior of loved one	Display respect and empathy for family's experience
Contemplation	Considering treatment but may demonstrate ambivalence	Illicit pros and cons of participating in family members' treatment
Preparation	Evaluating benefits of treatment and possible options	Suggest support groups and other intervention options; help family make a commitment
Action	Involved in treatment	Remind family of long-term benefits and observe for potential obstacles to participation
Maintenance	Integrates new ways of coping and advocating	Provide flexible supports depending on family's changing needs

The Lived Experience

Jordan

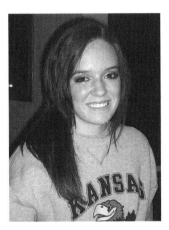

This narrative is shared by family member Jordan Hildebrand about her experience with the mental illness of her father, who has the diagnosis of bipolar disorder.

Everyone has hardships in their lives, but some are worse than others. Some people have lost a loved one or seen their house burn to the ground. No, no one extremely close to me has died, but I have lost the emotional connection to someone that I love very much. That may not seem like much, but for me it makes my world fall apart. It feels kind of as if you have been working on a puzzle for months and then your dog rips it to shreds.

Ever since I can remember, my dad has had bipolar disorder. Bipolar disorder is a disease that messes up your mind, and things happen like you think things that are not true, or you may hear voices in your head. Sure, there are medicines to treat it, but if you stop taking your medicine, or have to change your medicine, it can be disastrous. My dad has been in and out of psychiatric hospitals my whole life, and each time it doesn't get any easier. Usually I will just think, "Well, here we go again," but deep down it still hurts.

I remember one time that my dad's illness got really bad. My dad had been in the hospital for maybe three days, and my mom and I were going to the hospital to visit him. I guess he was just really angry because when we walked in what I never expected to happen did in fact happen. He started yelling at the top of his lungs and banging on the wall like it was a punching bag! My mom grabbed me. As we ran out, I remember looking back and seeing an attendant running back to help! I could hear the constant, "bam, bam, bam" sound of my dad letting loose a barrage of punches against the wall reverberating through the hallways! That was the day that my dad broke his hand. He was in the hospital for about a month longer after that—a very, very long month.

That may seem bad to you, but scarier than seeing the potential for physical harm is hearing the verbal harm that is committed. I remember one time when dad was yelling stuff to my mom like, "Get out of my house and don't come back." That was one of the scariest days of my life. Also, my dad becomes very "to himself," I guess you could say. Usually, when he is not sick, he will just sit upstairs and watch television anyway, but it gets a lot worse when he is sick. It feels like you are being rejected over and over again with each of his episodes. I just constantly remind myself that when he is sick it is not really my dad, but it is the illness.

Over the years I have learned just to love my dad and know that he loves me. Every time he gets admitted to the hospital it seems like you are getting whacked in the face. I have just learned that it is okay to be sad about it and that you just need to allow yourself time to heal. One of the most important things that I have learned is that you shouldn't dwell on the things that you can't control, but do treasure the moments that you have with loved ones because it could all change in a flash. I love my dad like any daughter would, but I just hope that maybe that emotional connection will be there again. Deep down, I know it will, and with that it will make this puzzle I call "My world" a little easier to put back together.

PhotoVoice

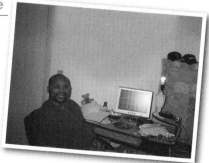

This is a picture of my brother. We have been friends all my life. My brother is my best friend—he is someone I can talk to as a great support system. Every time I need help he's always there for me. He provides a good sense of security for getting me out of the house. He is welcoming and friendly and we have a good, positive relationship as brother and as friends.

—Sterling

"cure" (NAMI NYS, 2006). Recovery is a process of living a full, meaningful, and productive life in spite of the illness and accompanying symptoms.

Professional Competencies in Working With Families

In considering the essential elements for any successful intervention with families, seven professional competencies must be considered in professionals who plan to offer services to families (Marsh, 1998):

1. Developing a collaborative relationship with the family.
2. Providing information on psychiatric disorders.
3. Enhancing coping and stress management skills of family members.
4. Assisting family members in navigating the mental health system.

Evidence-Based Practice

Compelling evidence shows that family psychoeducation as a systematic approach is an effective, evidence-based mental health practice (Dixon et al, 2004). When families are included as members of the treatment team, families report reduced burden, and the effectiveness of other intervention approaches is enhanced (Murray-Swank & Dixon, 2004). There is also strong evidence that family psychoeducation approaches result in reduced rates of relapse (McFarlane, Dixon, Lukens, & Lucksted, 2003). When creating psychoeducational groups, input from family members, persons with mental illness, and mental health providers should be considered in curriculum development. Curriculum should be flexible and able to accommodate varied individual needs of all groups (Pollio, North, & Foster, 1998).

➤ Occupational therapy practitioners are directed to consider family needs individually and suggest engagement in family psychoeducation or family education based on the individual needs of the family.

➤ Practitioners should provide families with information about a broad range of mental illnesses in a clear and concise manner and help families learn to access accurate facts about mental illness and effective interventions.

➤ Practitioners can integrate psychoeducational teaching approaches with traditional occupational therapy "doing" approaches to help families learn strategies to deal with mental illness and its effects.

➤ Practitioners can develop a psychoeducational curriculum for families or use programs readily available through NAMI. Useful objectives for psychoeducational programs may include but are not limited to the following:
  • Help families understand symptoms of mental disorders that affect mood, self-esteem, thinking, activity, sleeping and eating patterns, and occupational and social behavior.
  • Examine the changes that occur in occupational role functioning, including caregiving roles, that occur throughout the various stages of recovery.
  • Explain the range of interventions and the potential advantages of the various approaches.
  • Teach the family to identify and access community supports that can facilitate their family member's participation in a functional pattern of occupation.

Dixon, L., Lucksted, A., Stewart, B., Burland, J., Brown, C. H., Postrado, L., McGuire, C., & Hoffman, M. (2004). Outcomes of the peer taught 12 week family-to-family education program for severe mental illness. *Acta Psychiatrica Scandinavica, 109,* 207–215.

McFarlane, W. R., Dixon, L., Lukens, E. P., & Lucksted, A. (2003). Family psychoeducation and schizophrenia: A review of the literature. *Journal of Marital and Family Therapy, 29,* 223–245.

Murray-Swank, A. B., & Dixon, L. (2004). Family psychoeducation as an evidence-based practice. *CNS Spectrums, 9,* 905–912.

Pollio, D. E., North, C. S., & Foster, D. A. (1998). Content and curriculum in psychoeducation groups for families of persons with severe mental illness. *Psychiatric Services, 49,* 816–822.

5. Facilitating family members' ability to meet their own individual needs.
6. Assisting family members in understanding and dealing with the individual characteristics presented by their family member.
7. Successfully managing professional issues.

Occupational therapists who feel unprepared to work with consumers and families with mental illness can benefit from NAMI's Provider Education Program. This 10-week program is taught by a five-member team (a professional provider who is a family member, two family members, and two consumers) to employees of community mental health agencies. The program is taught in the true team spirit, as there is no leader, and the sessions are taught collaboratively by all team members (Mohr, Lafuze, & Mohr, 2000). Practitioners can contact their local NAMI affiliate to ascertain if the Provider Education Program is available in the area. Box 29-2 includes professional tips for working with families.

BOX 29-2 ■ Professional Tips for Working With Families

"What Hurts/What Helps: A Guide to What Families of Individuals with Serious Brain Disorders Need from Mental Health Professionals," a pamphlet published by the National Alliance on Mental Illness (2002) provides a basic reading list of books and resources that are helpful to professionals preparing to work with persons with mental illness and their families. Additional information essential to professional consideration includes the following tips:

What Helps
■ Practitioners must refrain from imposing their treatment agenda on families in crisis and pain. Working collaboratively and as a consultant will allow families to feel understood and assisted.
■ Professionals must critically examine their own beliefs regarding families "causing" mental illness.
■ Actively listen to the families' concerns and goals.
■ Recognize and value family strengths in dealing with stressful, life-changing situations.
■ Professionals who plan interventions after assessing the situation from a personal, social, and service support system perspective to reduce the strain on the family are helpful.
■ Family members benefit when professionals are compassionate and helpful in sharing information in a collaborative fashion.
■ Engaging in activities to lessen family burden (subjective and objective) and meet individualized family needs is essential.

What Hurts
■ Families complain when staff appears impatient, insensitive, unavailable, judgmental, or patronizing. It is important that staff not "talk down" to family members.
■ Families do not benefit from staff that blame or stigmatize them. Families do not cause mental illness.
■ Professionals who are insensitive to the needs of families add to the pain, grief, and anxiety that families experience. Insensitivity makes families feel isolated and rejected.
■ When families are left out of treatment planning and professionals do not communicate with them, a sense of frustration is heightened in families where frustration levels are most often already high.
■ Families complain when professionals fail to engage in collaborative efforts and are misinformed about the biological basis of mental illness.
■ Families worry if they express opinions or rejections and protest that they will be labeled as "troublemakers." Labeling behavior on the part of professionals does nothing to help the client.
■ Hurtful professionals only increase the pain family members are experiencing. These professionals add to the burden experienced by the family and cause increased stress and family burnout. Professionals should strive to engage in helpful rather than hurtful communication and behavior.

SAMHSA's poster illustrating core values of providing care to children with mental illness and their families (Figure 29-2) is consistent with the core values of occupational therapy.

Occupational Therapy Models and Frames of Reference

Several specific intervention approaches for families exist, and research demonstrates the efficacy of these approaches (Dixon, Stewart, et al, 2001; Solomon, 1996). However, these approaches often do not specify the role of the occupational therapist in providing services to the family. Two occupational therapy models and frames of reference are well suited for consideration in this area: the model of human occupation (Kielhofner, 2008) and Allen's cognitive disabilities frame of reference. (Allen & Blue, 1998).

Model of Human Occupation

The model of human occupation is considered an appropriate frame of reference to utilize with families because it addresses volition, habituation, and performance capacity (Abelenda & Helfrich, 2003). "**Volition** refers to the motivation for occupation. **Habituation** refers to the process by which occupation is organized into patterns or routines, and **performance capacity** refers to the mental and physical abilities that underlie skilled performance" (Kielhofner, 2008, p. 12). Volition is reflected in the family members' choices about what aspects of care are most important as well as in their perceptions of their personal capacities and effectiveness in these chosen tasks. The concept of habituation can be applied when the practitioner considers how different family members have internalized various family roles and how each organizes habits and daily routines to support individual and family functioning. It is important to consider the cognitive and physical performance capacities of each family member to understand areas where skill development may improve occupational functioning (Abelenda & Helfrich, 2003).

Within this frame of reference, the environment and individual work in cooperation to produce occupation. Individuals participate in a variety of activities of daily living within their social roles and develop occupational competence. As individuals examine their performance against societal expectations and demands, occupational identity is developed (Abelenda & Helfrich, 2003). Individuals identify their strengths and limitations and then develop plans for whom they want to be and what they would like to achieve in their lives. This newly developed identity facilitates engagement in occupations that are related to their competence. Through occupational adaptation, both competence and occupational identity are achieved.

The process of exploration, competence, and achievement occurs throughout an individual's occupational life when new roles are identified, new habits are developed, or occupational challenges are managed. For example, when a family member discovers a loved one has been diagnosed with mental illness, shock, disbelief, and feelings of helplessness may occur (Spaniol et al, 2000). Before family members can develop new methods for addressing their day-to-day lives, it is important for them to acknowledge that past habits, roles, and skills may be ineffective within the new situation they face (Abelenda & Helfrich, 2003).

To develop resilience, families often need to explore different methods of responding to new demands. This may involve modifying their daily routine to include and facilitate participation of their family member in daily occupations. Within the competency stage of the model, strategies that the family determines to be useful are organized into habits.

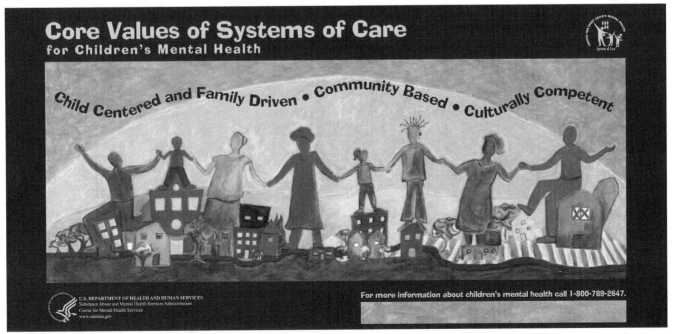

FIGURE 29-2. Core Values of Systems of Care for Children Mental Health poster. *Courtesy U.S. Department of Health and Human Services, Substance Abuse and Mental Health Services Administration, Center for Mental Health Services.*

As a result, the family may feel more in control of the new situations they find themselves in and better able to cope with the changing demands of their new environments and occupations (Abelenda & Helfrich, 2003).

In the achievement stage, a family member is able to integrate the newly developed habits into his or her ongoing lifestyle. This process assists families in being successful despite ongoing change and possible exposure to catastrophic events. Resilience is considered a dynamic process that changes over time and is contextual. Resilience exists when an effective match between family skills and resources and environmental challenges is present (Abelenda & Helfrich, 2003). Consider the following example of family resilience.

Case

When Joe experienced his first episode of mental illness, his wife, Mary, felt completely overwhelmed and panicky. She called her in-laws for help because they had experience in dealing with the mental illness of Joe's brother and had attended educational programs and support groups for several years. Her mother-in-law went to their house to assess the situation and offer any help and support she could. She told Mary not to try to take Joe to the hospital by herself.

Later that night, Mary called her in-laws and asked them to help her take Joe to the emergency room. He went without incident and was eventually hospitalized for 7 days. After being stabilized on medication, he was sent home with an aftercare program, which he closely followed. He also learned what he could about his illness.

A year later, Joe experienced a second episode. Mary again called her in-laws for support. Joe was not as sick as he had been the year before and was more aware of his symptoms than he had been during his first episode. He was also able to participate in the problem-solving related to the situation. Eventually, it was determined that he would go to his parents' home to spend the night, and Mary would take their son to her parents' home. By changing their environments, each of them was able to feel safe in the situation and get the help and support they needed. Joe called his doctor in the morning and made an appointment to see him later that week. Hospitalization was unnecessary this time.

Allen's Cognitive Disabilities Frame of Reference

One role that an occupational therapist can play is in helping families understand the cognitive function of their loved one and how cognition impacts one's ability to carry out everyday occupations in varied settings. Allen's cognitive disabilities frame of reference can be helpful in this regard. The Allen Cognitive Level Screen (ACLS) can be administered to ascertain the cognitive level of the individual diagnosed with mental illness. Standard practice when applying this model is to administer the ACLS and then verify the person's cognitive level of functioning by administering

the Routine Task Inventory or an Allen Diagnostic Module project (Allen, 1999; Allen, Kehrberg, & Burns, 1992). Other assessments that can be utilized to ascertain the client's cognitive level according to this frame of reference include the Cognitive Performance Test (Burns, 2002) and the Routine Task Inventory-Expanded (Katz, 2006).

Through understanding the client's cognitive level, the occupational therapist can assist the family in understanding what the client can do (realistic abilities that are biological in nature and may be limited by a disability); what the client will do (relevant abilities that are psychological in nature and can be limited by motivation); and what the client may do (abilities that are social in nature and can be limited by a caregiver or financial means).

In considering what the client may do, caregivers can be instructed in methods of structuring the environment for client success as well as what types of sensory cues (verbal or visual) are most effective for the client (Allen, 1999). Caregiver guidelines provide information for family members with regard to the level of supervision, environmental setup, structure, type of communication, and level of independence family members can anticipate in daily tasks such as medication management, nutrition, bathing, dressing, toileting, mobility and positioning, safety, and leisure for their loved one (Champagne, 2003).

SAMHSA-CMHS Family Psychoeducation Program Toolkit

Family **psychoeducation** is "a method of working with families, other caregivers and friends who are supportive of persons with mental illness" (SAMHSA, 2003). This model is based on a collaborative partnership and includes accurate information about mental illness, problem-solving, communication skills, coping, and the development of social support. The goals of this intervention are to improve consumer outcomes and quality of life while reducing family stress and strain. Psychoeducation is not a method specific to occupational therapy, but the philosophy of collaboration and active teaching and learning processes complement the occupational therapy model discussed earlier.

SAMHSA offers a free toolkit that can be obtained from its website. Occupational therapists are considered professionals who demonstrate capability in conducting this model of treatment. This intervention can be provided individually to family members or through multifamily groups. Family members may become coteachers in the multifamily group approach. Research indicates that 90% to 96% of family members considered the program's sources of help, lectures and books, classes and workshops, support groups, and friends to be valuable (SAMHSA, 2003).

Although the current toolkit was developed and found most effective for persons diagnosed with schizophrenia, modifications have been developed and tested for other mental illnesses, including bipolar disorder, depression, borderline personality disorder, and obsessive-compulsive disorder. Family psychoeducation is targeted to support both the consumer and family members. Research indicates that this model can provide the skills that family members need to contribute to the recovery of their loved one.

The model emphasizes basic communication skills and problem-solving, two areas in which occupational therapists have significant training. The core elements to all family psychoeducation programs are as follows:

- Joining (establishing a respectful, helpful relationship).
- Education (about mental illness).
- Problem-solving (identification of strategies for managing difficult situations).
- Structural change in treatment (focus on strengths-based environment aimed at recovery).
- Multifamily contact (encouragement of participation in family support groups to reduce social isolation).

Rather than working with consumers and family members individually, this model includes all parties for successful collaborative intervention in which practitioners work *with* rather than *on* the family and consumer (SAMHSA, 2003, p. 9). Family psychoeducation programs may vary in length from three to more than nine months. Outcomes from research indicate that longer programs yield better results. In fact, rehospitalization and relapse rates of consumers decreased by 40% to 70% over a 2-year period when compared to consumers who received individual therapy alone (Bond & Campbell, 2008).

A study conducted with parents of children diagnosed with a mood disorder who were involved in a **multifamily psychoeducation group** based on the model presented by Hatfield yielded positive outcomes according to parental reports (Goldberg-Arnold, Fristad, & Gavazzi, 1999). The intervention was conducted with parents and children who were diagnosed with mood disorder in an outpatient setting over a 6-week period. The program included parents and children at the start and end of each session, with groups conducted by trained facilitators for the parents and children in separate groups.

Parents in the study identified increased knowledge of the diagnosis of mood disorder and increased social support as a result of participating in the group intervention. On follow-up at 6 months, parents reported information and coping skills gained as a result of the intervention as important and reported attitude shifts as more significant. The attitudinal change included improved attitude when considering mental illness in their child, current family situation, and educational and mental health systems. The researchers identified that through participation in the intervention, parents gained knowledge related to mental illness, and moreover, their attitude toward their life and situation became more positive (Goldberg-Arnold, Fristad, & Gavazzi, 1999).

The multifamily psychoeducation group is viewed as effective and efficient because the therapist can work with many people at once, and families have the opportunity to learn from one another through observation and identification of situations with other families. When families participate in multifamily psychoeducation group interventions, the change of one member of the family can potentially impact all of the other family members and other group members as well. Group members may come to view their family situation differently upon listening to the stories and situations shared by other group members (Olson, 2006).

Despite research describing family intervention for children with mental illness, limited experimental studies are available for review to provide conclusive evidence that family-based services will improve mental health outcomes for children and adolescents (Hoagwood, 2005). As researchers identify needs, organizations such as SAMHSA and NAMI continue to

conduct research and publish information to benefit families. In May 2007, NAMI published "Choosing the Right Treatment: What Families Need to Know about Evidence-Based Practices." This guide can be ordered in printed format or is available in a PDF format at no charge from the NAMI website (Gruttadaro, Burns, Duckworth, & Crudo, 2007).

Resources and Programs

Occupational therapists who work with people with mental illness should be aware of resources and programs available to assist family members who have a loved one with a mental illness. Numerous programs and supports exist, including Operation Healthy Reunions, NAMI Family-to-Family Education Program, Visions for Tomorrow, Parents and Teachers as Allies, and the SAMHSA-CMHS Family Psychoeducation Program Toolkit.

Operation Healthy Reunions

Operation Healthy Reunions, a program sponsored by Mental Health America (formerly known as the National Mental Health Association, NMHA), was developed to combat stigma surrounding mental health issues and provide education to address the mental health issues of military families. Considering that mental disorders are being reported in 26% of soldiers returning from Iraq and Afghanistan, this program clearly meets a need in society at present (NMHA, 2006).

Best Practices in Family Intervention for Serious Mental Illness

The University of Oklahoma Health Science Center maintains a website with resources for practitioners who work with family members. Best Practices in Family Intervention for Serious Mental Illness (http://w3.ouhsc.edu/bpfamily) assists practitioners by providing titles of journals, contacts for training, relevant websites, information about a listserv hosted by Diane Marsh, PhD, as well as hot topics and recent advances in the area of family psychoeduation.

NAMI Family-to-Family Education Program

The NAMI Family-to Family-Education Program (FFEP) is a free, 12-week, evidence-based program that provides information on mental illness for family members who have an adult loved one with a mental illness (Dixon et al, 2004). FFEP was developed by Joyce Burland (2001), a psychologist who has experienced mental illness within her family. The FFEP program is delivered in the community and facilitated by two family members who receive extensive training. The facilitators present the program from a scripted manual that is updated annually.

The weekly program, 2 to 3 hours per session, includes information about mental illness, treatment, medication, and recovery. Through their attendance in the FFEP, family members gain information on self-care, communication skills, problem-solving, and advocacy. Participants can gain insight into their reaction toward mental illness within their family (Burland, 2001). FFEP is grounded in theory related to stress and coping, trauma recovery, adaptation, and support aimed at the family member's wellbeing.

The Lived Experience

Linda (A Mother's Narrative, as told to Barbara Jacobs)

"I didn't know." "I thought she was just shy. But she was so shy that she couldn't order her own food at McDonald's." In order to tell her own story, Linda had to talk about her daughter and how she learned that Kristen has a mental illness. Linda describes Kristen as shy, saying that she'd been shy and withdrawn since age 2. Kristen was 6 months old and her older brother was 3 when they came to their current suburban Midwestern home from Korea. They were adopted by a middle-class white family and raised in a community that was not racially diverse.

As Kristen grew older, she was aware that she was different, and her shyness worsened. She felt shunned by her peers at school. She was always very mature and a good student, and she began to realize that the differences she was feeling were more than skin deep. At age 14, after seeing a commercial on TV for Paxil, she decided to do some research on the Internet and found that she had a lot in common with the description there of social anxiety disorder. She went to her parents and asked for help.

Feeling like she was navigating totally unfamiliar territory, Linda immediately went to her pediatrician for guidance. The doctor recommended that Kristen see a psychiatrist, and Linda and her husband set about trying to find someone who would fit their daughter's needs. The "perfect" psychiatrist had a 3-month waiting list, so Kristen saw a therapist in the interim.

Kristen was initially treated for social anxiety disorder, but it wasn't too long before Linda noticed signs of depression and obsessive-compulsive disorder. Kristen became a "cutter" and was hospitalized six times during her sophomore year of high school. Linda and her husband got caught up in trying to control the situation by monitoring Kristen's computer use, locking up all the medications, and taking away access to large amounts of money. The family environment became one of mistrust and suspicion, with fear and anger just below the surface.

Linda quit her part-time job to accommodate Kristen's needs. She and her husband kept their problems with Kristen largely to themselves, not even telling their parents. They decided that they couldn't leave Kristen home alone, so they seldom went out together. Linda's outlets were playing tennis and taking the dog for walks.

On the recommendation of her therapist, Kristen began volunteering at the local NAMI office. It was through this connection that Linda became aware of NAMI's Family-to-Family program and joined the next class. Prior to this, Linda was more concerned about finding support for Kristen than for herself, although she now states, "I wish I would have known to reach out to other people sooner."

Since receiving some education and support through the Family-to-Family program, Linda reports having a better understanding of mental illness and a more realistic picture of what the future might hold. She's been able to accept some of Kristen's behaviors as being part of the illness and has let go of some of her expectations. She's more aware of the difficulties in finding appropriate medications and is appreciative of Kristen's willingness to comply with her medication regimen. She's learned that it's okay to talk about the mental illness with friends, family, and even acquaintances and has discovered that most of the people she's talked to are very supportive and compassionate. She realizes how important her tennis is to her own wellbeing and her ability to care for her family.

Linda finds that it's easier to talk openly with Kristen about what's going on, which helps to alleviate some of the anger. She's able to tell Kristen what she's learning at Family-to-Family, which lets Kristen know that she cares about her and wants what's best for her. She realizes that it's okay for Kristen to be angry at her because she knows not to take it personally.

Linda admits that she and her husband don't have much of a life—that it's still dominated by Kristen and her illness. But that seems to be okay for now. She states, "I know there's help out there if I need it in the future."

A study examining the efficacy of the FFEP found that participants experienced reduced subjective burden of worry and displeasure regarding the mental illness of their family member (Dixon et al, 2004). The participants' level of empowerment within the community, their family, and the mental health service system was increased. Participants in the FFEP also demonstrated increased knowledge of mental illness and the mental health system and demonstrated improved self-care. The positive benefits of an increased sense of empowerment and decreased subjective burden were maintained by study participants for 6 months beyond the end of the study. It is important to note that the FFEP did not change the level of objective burden of the family participants. The FFEP is not intended to directly change or alter the behavior and individual needs of a family member with a mental illness; rather, it builds capacity in the family to effectively support their family member's recovery using strategies that support overall family coping and functioning (Dixon et al, 2004).

Visions for Tomorrow

Visions for Tomorrow is a free course offered by several state and local NAMI affiliates around the United States (NAMI Iowa, 2005) This program was developed by NAMI Texas (Burland & Nemec, 2007). It is designed for parents and caregivers of children and adolescents with brain disorders (NAMI Iowa, 2005). Family members in this program learn about resources, find support, and examine strategies to cope with mental illness for their child or adolescent family member.

Through their participation in Visions for Tomorrow, family members have reported feeling understood and validated. Within the program, family members learn about a variety of disorders, including autism, attention deficit-hyperactivity disorder, bipolar disorder, depression, eating disorders, and anxiety disorders. Families and caregivers also learn about effective record keeping, coping, self-care, rehabilitation, recovery, transition, advocacy, and stigma (NAMI Iowa, 2005).

In Ohio, NAMI developed a program for young families called Hand to Hand, which presents content and focus similar to the Visions for Tomorrow program (Burland & Nemec, 2007).

Parents and Teachers as Allies

The Parents and Teachers as Allies program addresses mental illness in children through educating teachers via a 2-hour session on mental illness in children and adolescents. The information provided assists teachers in helping to recognize and identify early-onset mental illness in children and adolescents in their classrooms. The inservice is led by parents and mental health consumers who have worked to cope with mental illness while in school (Burland & Nemec, 2007).

In addition to this program, NAMI New York developed a curriculum for use by teachers at all academic levels. This curriculum, Breaking the Silence, is aimed at reducing the stigma that surrounds mental illness (Burland & Nemec, 2007).

Summary

Occupational therapy practitioners working with family members should view their roles as multifaceted. They may serve as direct care provider, consultant, advocate, and societal systems change agent. Occupational therapy practitioners, because of their education and holistic approach to individuals, are well suited to address the complex needs of families. Development of family-based intervention may be challenging because of reimbursement issues; however, research has shown family-based intervention is beneficial, and "everyone wins" in terms of positive outcomes. Occupational therapists should strongly consider the potential for family involvement within their service delivery setting.

Active Learning Strategies

1. Role Checklist

Complete the role checklist (Oakley, 2006). Consider all of the roles you are currently participating in (e.g., student, worker, volunteer, caregiver, home maintainer, friend, family member, religious participant, hobbyist/amateur, and participant in organizations). Reflect on how your identity roles would be impacted if a member of your family were diagnosed with a mental illness. The family member could be your son or daughter, spouse, parent, sibling, or grandparent.

Reflective Questions
- Would you continue to participate in these roles?
- If so, would your participation continue at the current level, or would it change? How?
- Would you find some roles less valuable than others and perhaps relinquish them due to family demands and time?
- How would you feel if your caregiver role was consuming 99.9% of your time?
- How would you work toward developing balance between the roles you feel you "must" fulfill and those in which you participate for the enjoyment and fulfillment they provide your life?
- How would the diagnosis of mental illness within your family impact the occupations you perform on a regular basis?
- How would you work with family members who are experiencing similar situations (change in roles and change in occupational participation)?
- How could you, as an occupational therapist, assist a family member who is experiencing significant role change as a result of his or her loved one's mental illness?

 Record your thoughts in your **Reflective Journal**.

2. Local Resources

Explore what resources exist for families in your community. Search the Internet for resources for family members who are looking for support in your community. Does your NAMI offer a Family-to-Family Education Program? At present, 45 states, Puerto Rico, and two Canadian provinces offer this course (Dixon et al, 2004). Develop a list of family resources, including support groups, family education programs, and current reading materials appropriate for families.

3. Collaboration

Identify specific benefits to working in a collaborative fashion with family members (Spaniol et al, 2000).

Reflective Questions
- What barriers do you think you might be faced with in trying to work collaboratively with family members?
- What specific things could you do to try to diminish these barriers?
- What types of environments, policies, and communication styles facilitate communication? How can you create these environments or policies if they do not exist where you are currently practicing or hope to practice?
- What might be specific issues of children diagnosed with mental illness? Conversely, what might be the needs of children who have a parent or parents diagnosed with a mental illness?

Record your thoughts in your **Reflective Journal**.

4. Professional Attitudes

NAMI has identified professional attitudes that are valued by families of individuals with serious brain disorders. These include compassion, respect, flexibility, accessibility, candor, hopefulness, and commitment (NAMI, 2002).

Reflective Questions
- Do you possess these qualities? If so, to what degree?
- Do you feel you could further develop any of these qualities? How?

- Identify from your experience what essential knowledge and skills an occupational therapy practitioner needs to possess to work effectively with family members.
- Identify specific steps you can take to gain knowledge and develop effective skills to provide services to family members.
- What materials, information, or resources do you feel you would need to obtain to be successful?
- Do you have access to these resources and supports? If not, could you gain access? How?

 Record your thoughts in your **Reflective Journal**.

Resources

Books
- Amador, X., & Johanson, A. (2007). *I Am Not Sick, I Don't Need Help: Helping the Seriously Mentally Ill Accept Treatment: A Practical Guide for Families and Therapists.* New York: Vida Press
- Andreasen, N. (1984). *The Broken Brain: The Biological Revolution in Psychiatry.* New York: Harper & Row.
- Hatfield, A. (1993). Dual diagnosis: substance abuse and mental illness. Available at: http://www.schizophrenia.com/family/dualdiag.html.
- Hatfield, A. (1983). What families want of family therapists. In W. R. McFarlane (Ed.), *Family Therapy in Schizophrenia.* New York: Guilford Press.
- Nathiel, S. (2007). *Daughters of Madness: Growing Up and Older with a Mentally Ill Mother.* Westport, CT: Praeger.
- Torrey, E. F. (2001). *Surviving Schizophrenia: A Manual for Families, Consumers and Providers* (4th ed.). New York: HarperCollins.
- Torrey, E., & Knable, M. (2002). *Surviving Manic Depression: A Manual on Bipolar Disorder for Patients, Families and Providers.* New York: Basic Books.
- Woolis, R. (1992). *When Someone You Love Has a Mental Illness: A Handbook for Family, Friends, and Caregivers.* New York: J.P. Tarcher/Perigree.

Organizations
- Alcoholics Anonymous
  940 Rockefeller Building
  614 Superior Avenue, N.W.
  Cleveland, OH 44113
  (216) 241-7387
- Children and Adults with ADHD (CHADD)
  http://www.chadd.org
  8181 Professional Place, Suite 150
  Landover, MD 20785
- Depression and Bipolar Support Alliance (DBSA)
  http://www.dbsalliance.org
  730 N. Franklin Street, Suite 501
  Chicago, Illinois 60610-7224
  (800) 826-3632
- Families Anonymous, Inc.
  P.O. Box 528
  Van Nuys, CA 91408
- Mental Health America (MHA)
  http://www.nmha.org
  Find an affiliate in your area:
  http://www.nmha.org/go/searchMHA
  2000 N. Beauregard Street, 6th Floor
  Alexandria, VA 22311
  (800) 969-6642

- National Alliance on Mental Illness
  http://www.nami.org
  2107 Wilson Boulevard, Suite 300
  Arlington, VA 22201-3042
- Obsessive Compulsive Foundation
  http://www.ocfoundation.org
  676 State Street
  New Haven, CT 06511
  (203) 401-2070

References

Abelenda, J., & Helfrich, C. A. (2003). Family resilience and mental illness: The role of occupational therapy. *Occupational Therapy and Mental Health, 19*(1), 25–39.

Allen, C. K. (1999). Stage one workshop Allen's cognitive levels: How to use the Allen's cognitive levels in daily practice. Allen Conferences, Inc: Ormond Beach, FL.

Allen, C. K., & Blue, T. (1998). Cognitive disabilities model: How to make clinical judgments. In N. Katz (Ed.), *Cognition and occupation in rehabilitation: Cognitive models for intervention in occupational therapy* (pp. 225–280). Bethesda, MD: American Occupational Therapy Association.

Allen, C. K., Kehrberg, K., & Burns, T. (1992). Evaluation instruments. In C. K. Allen, C. A. Earhart, & T. Blue (Eds.), *Occupational Therapy Treatment Goals for the Physically and Cognitively Disabled.* Bethesda, MD: American Occupational Therapy Association.

American Occupational Therapy Association (AOTA). (2002). Occupational therapy practice framework: Domain and process. *American Journal of Occupational Therapy, 56,* 609–639.

Bond, G. R., & Campbell, K. (2008). Evidence-based practices for individuals with severe mental illness. *Journal of Rehabilitation, 74,* 33–44.

Burland, J. (2001). *Family-to-Family Education Program Teaching Manual.* Arlington, VA: National Alliance on Mental Illness.

Burland, J., & Nemec, P. (2007). NAMI training programs. *Psychiatric Rehabilitation Journal, 31* (1), 80–82.

Burns, T. (2002) *Cognitive Performance Test 2002 Manual.* Minneapolis, MN: Department of Veterans Affairs.

Center for Mental Health Services. (2004). 2004 CMHS uniform reporting system output tables. Available at: http://www.mentalhealth.samhsa.gov/media/ken/pdf/URS_Data04/IA04.pdf (accessed July 18, 2006).

Chaffey, L., & Fossey, E. (2004). Caring and daily life: Occupational experiences of women living with sons diagnosed with schizophrenia. *Australian Occupational Therapy Journal, 51,* 199–207.

Champagne, T. (2003). Allen cognitive level caregiver guidelines. Available at: http://www.ot-innovations.com/content/view/21/28 (accessed July 18, 2006).

Cole, M. B., & McLean, V. (2003). Therapeutic relationships redefined. *Occupational Therapy in Mental Health, 19*(2), 33–56.

Crowley, K. (2000). *The Power of Procovery in Healing Mental Illness.* Los Angeles, CA: Kennedy Carlisle Publishing.

Dixon, L., Lucksted, A., Stewart, B., Burland, J., Brown, C. H., Postrado, L., McGuire, C., & Hoffman, M. (2004). Outcomes of the peer taught 12 week family-to-family education program for severe mental illness. *Acta Psychiatrica Scandinavica, 109,* 207–215.

Dixon, L., Lyles, A., Scott, J., Lehman, A., Postrado, L., Goldman, H., & McGlynn, E. (1999). Services to families of adults with schizophrenia: From treatment recommendations to dissemination. *Psychiatric Services, 50*(2), 233–238.

Dixon, L., McFarlane, W. R., Lefley, H., Lucksted, A., Cohn, M., Falloon, I., Mueser, K., Miklowitz, D., Solomon, P., & Sondheimer, D. (2001). Evidence-based practices for services to families of people with psychiatric disabilities. *Psychiatric Services, 52*(7), 903–910.

Dixon, L., Stewart, B., Burland, J., Delahanty, J., Lucksted, A., & Hoffman, M. (2001). Pilot study of the effectiveness of the family to family education program. *Psychiatric Services, 52*(7), 965–967.

Duvall, E. M. (1977). *Marriage and Family Development* (5th ed.). Philadelphia: J.B. Lippincott.

Eklund, M. (1997). Therapeutic factors in occupational therapy identified by patients discharged from a psychiatric day centre and their significant others. *Occupational Therapy International, 4,* 199–212.

Farhall, J., Webster, B., Hocking, B., Leggatt, M., Riess, C., & Young, J. (1998). Training to enhance partnerships between mental health professionals and family caregivers: A comparative study. *Psychiatric services, 49*(11), 1488–1490.

Friesen, B. (2007). Recovery and resilience in children's mental health: Views from the field. *Psychiatric Rehabilitation Journal, 31*(1), 38–48.

Garcia Preto, N. (2005). Latino families: An overview. In M. McGoldrick, J. Giordano, & N. Garcia Preto (Eds.), *Ethnicity and Family Therapy* (3rd ed.) (pp. 153–165). New York: Guilford Press.

Goldberg-Arnold, J. S., Fristad, M. A., & Gavazzi, S. M. (1999). Family psychoeducation: Giving caregivers what they want and need. *Family Relations, 48,* 411–417.

Gruttadaro, D., Burns, B. J., Duckworth, K., & Crudo, D. (2007). *Choosing the Right Treatment: What Families Need to Know about Evidence-Based Practices.* Arlington, VA: National Alliance on Mental Illness.

Hill, R., & Rodgers, R. H. (1964). The developmental approach. In H. Christensen (Ed.), *Handbook of Marriage and the Family* (pp. 171–211). Chicago: Rand-McNally.

Hirst, M. (2005). Carer distress: A prospective, population based study. *Social Science Medicine, 61,* 697–708.

Hoagwood, K. E. (2005). Family-based services in children's mental health: A research review and synthesis. *Journal of Child Psychology and Psychiatry, 46*(7), 690–713.

Hughes, I., & Hailwood, R. (1996). Developing a family intervention service for serious mental illness: Clinical observations and experiences. *Journal of Mental Health, 5*(2), 145–150.

Humphrey, R., & Case-Smith, J. (2001). Working with families. In J. Case-Smith (Ed.), *Occupational Therapy for Children* (pp. 95–135). St. Louis: Mosby.

Ivarsson, A., Sidenvall, B., & Carlsson, M. (2004). The factor structure of the Burden Assessment Scale and the perceived burden of caregivers for individuals with severe mental disorders. *Scandinavian Journal of Caring Science, 18,* 396–401.

Jakobsen, E. S., & Severinson, E. (2006). Parents' experiences of collaboration with community healthcare professionals. *Journal of Psychiatric and Mental Health Nursing, 13*(5), 498–505.

Jeon, Y. H., Brodaty, H., & Chesterson, J. (2005). Respite care for caregivers and people with severe mental illness: Literature review. *Journal of Advanced Nursing, 49*(3), 297–306.

Katz, N. (2006). Routine task inventory–Expanded. RTI-E manual, prepared and elaborated on the basis of C. K. Allen (1989, unpublished). Available at: http://www.allen-cognitive-network.org/pdf_files/RTIManual2006.pdf (Accessed July 18, 2006).

Keilhofner, G. (2008). *Model of Human Occupation: Theory and Application* (4th ed.). Philadelphia: Lippincott, Williams & Wilkins.

Lakeman, R. (2008). Practice standards to improve the quality of family and career participation in adult mental health care: An overview. *International Journal of Mental Health Nursing, 17,* 44–56.

Lawlor, M. C., & Mattingly, C. (2009). Understanding family perspectives on illness and disability experiences. In E. B. Crepeau, E. S. Cohn, & B. A. Boyt Schell (Eds.), *Willard and Spackman's Occupational Therapy* (11th ed.) (pp. 33–45). Philadelphia: Lippincott, Williams & Wilkins.

Looper, K., Fielding, A., Latimer, E., & Amir, E. (1998). Improving access to family support organizations: A member survey of the AMI-Quebec Alliance for the Mentally Ill. *Psychiatric Services, 49*(11), 1491–1492.

Marsh, D. T. (1998). *Serious Mental Illness and the Family: A Practitioner's Guide.* New York: Wiley.

McFarlane, W. R., Dixon, L., Lukens, E. P., & Lucksted, A. (2003). Family psychoeducation and schizophrenia: A review of the literature. *Journal of Marital and Family Therapy, 29,* 223–245.

Mohr, W., Lafuze, J., & Mohr, B. (2000). Opening caregiver minds: National Alliance for the Mentally Ill's provider education program. *Archives of Psychiatric Nursing, 14*(5), 235–243.

Murray-Swank, A. B., & Dixon, L. (2004). Family psychoeducation as an evidence-based practice. *CNS Spectrums, 9,* 905–912.

National Alliance on Mental Illness (NAMI). (2002). *What Hurts What Helps: A Guide to What Families of Individuals With Serious Brain Disorders Need From Mental Health Professionals* (5th ed). Arlington, VA: Author.

National Alliance on Mental Illness. (2007). "What Is Mental Illness: Mental Illness Facts." Available at: http://www.nami.org/Content/NavigationMenu/Inform_Yourself/About_Mental_Illness/About_Mental_Illness.htm (accessed July 7, 2007).

National Alliance on Mental Illness Iowa (2005). *The Handbook of Mental Illnesses* (2nd ed.). Des Moines: Author.

National Alliance on Mental Illness New York State (NAMI NYS). (2006). *Helping Families to Help Their Loved Ones With Serious Mental Illness.* New York: Author.

National Empowerment Center. (2006). "Hearing Voices That Are Distressing: A Simulated Training Experience and Self-Help Strategies." Available at: http://www.power2u.org/mm5/merchant.mvc?Screen=CTGY&Store_Code=NEC&Category_Code=workshops (accessed July 18, 2006).

National Mental Health Association. (2006). "Operation Healthy Reunions." Available at: http://www.nmha.org/reunions/index.cfm (accessed July 18, 2006).

New Freedom Commission on Mental Health. (2003). Achieving the promise: Transforming mental health care in America. DHHS Pub. No. SMA-03-3832. Rockville, MD: U.S. Department of Health and Human Services.

Oakley, F. (2006). Revised role checklist. Available via e-mail from FOakley@cc.nih.gov.

Olson, L. (2001). Child psychiatry in the USA. In L. Lougher (Ed.), *Occupational Therapy for Child and Adolescent Mental Health* (pp. 175–176). Edinburgh: Churchill-Livingstone.

Olson, L. (2006). What do we know about the daily interactions between children with mental illness and their parents? *Occupational Therapy in Mental Health, 22*(3/4), 11–22.

Perlick, D. A., Rosenheck, R. A., Clarkin, J. F., Maciejewski, P. K., Sirey, J., Struening, E., Link, B. G. (2004). Impact of family burden and affective response on clinical outcome among patients with bipolar disorder. *Psychiatric Services, 55*(9), 1029–1035.

Pollio, D. E., North, C. S., & Foster, D. A. (1998). Content and curriculum in psychoeducation groups for families of persons with severe mental illness. *Psychiatric Services, 49,* 816–822.

Prochaska, J. O., & DiClemente, C. C. (1983). Stages and processes of self-change of smoking: Toward an integrative model of change. *Journal of Consulting and Clinical Psychology, 51*, 390–395.

Rangarajan, S., & Kelly, L. (2006). Family communication patterns, family environment, and the impact of parental alcoholism on offspring self-esteem. *Journal of Social and Personal Relationships, 23*, 655–671.

Reinhard, S. C., Gubman, G. D., Horowitz, A. V., & Minsky, S. (1994). Burden assessment scale for families of the seriously mentally ill. *Evaluation and Program Planning, 17*(3), 261–269.

Schultz-Krohn, W. (2007). Assessments of occupational performance. In I. Asher (Ed.), *Occupational Therapy Assessment Tools: An Annotated Index* (3rd ed.) (pp. 53–54). Bethesda, MD: AOTA Press.

Shankar, J., & Muthuswamy, S. S. (2007). Support needs of family caregivers of people who experience mental illness and the role of mental health services. *Families in Society, 88*(2), 302–310.

Sharfstein, S. S., & Dickerson, F. B. (2009). Hospital psychiatry for the twenty-first century. *Health Affairs, 28*(3), 685–688.

Sherman, M. D., & Carothers, R. A. (2005). Applying the readiness to change model to implementation of family intervention for serious mental illness. *Community Mental Health Journal, 41*(2), 115–127.

Solomon, P. (1996). Moving from psychoeducation to family education for families of adults with serious mental illness. *Psychiatric Services, 47*(12), 1364–1370.

Spaniol, L., Pulliam, L., Gilman, S., Goldman, C., Harris, B., Husar, L., et al. (2004). *What Professionals Need to Know About Families.* Boston: Center for Psychiatric Rehabilitation.

Spaniol, L., Zipple, A. M., Marsh, D. T., & Finley, L. Y. (2000). *The Role of the Family in Psychiatric Rehabilitation: A Workbook.* Boston: Center for Psychiatric Rehabilitation.

Steele, D. (1998). *His Bright Light: The Story of Nick Traina.* New York: Random House.

Stuart, G. W., Burland, J., Ganju, V., Levounis, P., & Kiosk, S. (2002). Educational best practices. *Administration and Policy in Mental Health, 29*(4/5), 325–333.

Substance Abuse and Mental Health Services Administration (SAMHSA). (2003). *Family Psychoeducation Workbook.* Available at: http://www.mentalhealth.samhsa.gov/media/ken/pdf/toolkits/family/16.FamPsy_Workbook.pdf (accessed July 18, 2006).

———. (2006). "National consensus statement on mental health recovery." Available at: http://www.mentalhealth.samhsa.gov/media/ken/pdf/SMA05-4129/trifold.pdf (accessed July 18, 2006).

Treasure, J. (2004). Review: Exploration of psychological and physical health differences between caregivers and non-caregivers. *Evidence-Based Mental Health, 7*, 28–35.

U.S. Department of Health and Human Services. (1999). *Mental Health: A Report of the Surgeon General—Executive Summary.* Rockville, MD: U.S. Department of Health and Human Services Administration, Center for Mental Health Services, National Institutes of Health, National Institute of Mental Health.

Wang, P. S., Lane, M., Olfson, M., Pincus, H. A., Wells, K. B., & Kessler, R. C. (2005). Twelve-month use of mental health services in the United States: Results from the National Co-morbidity Survey replication. *Archives of General Psychiatry, 62*, 629–640.

Weist, M. D., Evans, S. W., & Lever, N. A. (2007). *Handbook of School Mental Health.* New York: Springer.

Mental Health Practice in a Multicultural Context

Jaime Phillip Muñoz

> "*It is what we think we already know that prevents us from learning.*
>
> —Claude Bernard (1949)

Introduction

Imagine that you are in the fourth week of a level II fieldwork rotation, working in the acute psychiatric unit of a general hospital located in an urban environment in a mid-sized city. Over the past few weeks, you have completed occupational histories with many different consumers: a Hispanic woman who told you she was seeking treatment because she was losing her soul; an American Indian woman who disclosed that she could not escape her spirit song; and an African American male who reported that the devil was sitting next to him as he was driving and warned him that his life's road was heading for some nasty turns. You have searched through the course notes from your mental health classes and found no references to soul loss, spirit songs, or conversations with the devil.

It is likely that much of your training has encouraged you to view abnormal behavior from a medical model perspective, which presumes a biological basis for behavior. Examined from this perspective, it would be understandable to conclude that each of these individuals was describing an experience consistent with a psychotic delusion. If these interactions are viewed from a multicultural perspective, however, you may arrive at a very different conclusion. **Multicultural context** refers to a person's family, community, and the effects of stigma associated with mental illness in society that influences their cultural identity (Cloutterbuck & Zahn, 2005). If occupational therapists are to provide culturally responsive care, they must understand multicultural context, including the social, cultural, political, and historical realities that impact the lives of the people they encounter in their practice.

This chapter frames mental health practice within a multicultural context. An understanding of the context begins with recognition that both the person with a mental illness and the occupational therapist possess cultural identities and worldviews that contribute to their explanations of the causes and treatments for mental illness. Multicultural context can influence how individuals explain the cause of their mental illness, how they exhibit its primary symptoms, how they interact with their family and community to manage their illness, and how or whether they use professional mental health services.

This chapter begins by outlining some arguments, grounded in the contemporary context of service delivery, U.S. demographics, and evidence for mental health care disparities, that support the need for culturally competent mental health care. Culture, models of cultural competency, and perspectives on culture-bound syndromes in mental health are discussed, and the chapter closes by addressing cultural assessment and intervention strategies. This chapter encourages you to consider mental illness from a multicultural viewpoint and to see and understand yourself and the people you work with as cultural beings.

Diversity Within the United States

The demographics of the United States indicate a shift in ethnic and racial populations, supporting the need to provide mental health care in a multicultural context. Ethnic and racial minorities are now numerical majorities in Texas, Hawaii, New Mexico, California, and the District of Columbia; in five other states (Maryland, Mississippi, Georgia, New York, and Arizona), ethnic and racial minorities exceed 40% of the population (U.S. Census Bureau, 2005). The United States is a multicultural, multiracial, and multilingual society, and it is important to consider some general trends that cross the various ethnic and racial minority groups.

General Trends

Although ethnic minority populations are generally younger than the non-Hispanic Caucasian majority, an increase in the ethnic elder population is on the horizon. In addition, much of the continuing diversification of U.S. society is the result of immigration (U.S. Department of Health and Human Services [USDHHS], 2001a). **Acculturation** is the processes that occur when people from different cultural groups have continuous contact, which results in changes in the cultural patterns of either group or both groups. Acculturative stress can result "when an individual's adaptive resources are insufficient to support adjustments to a new cultural environment" (Roysircai-Sodowsky & Maestas,

2000, p. 138). Immigration status, legal and illegal, is known to generate acculturation stress, as individuals are often coping with language barriers, unemployment, limited social and financial resources, and disorientation to an unfamiliar environment (Pumariega, Rothe, & Pumariega, 2005). This multicultural pluralism has a notable impact on mental health care.

Culture is known to influence communication in the therapeutic relationship, a person's conceptualization of mental health and illness, the manifestation of psychiatric symptoms, the timing and frequency of help-seeking behaviors, the experience of stress and behavioral coping styles, and the availability of family and community support systems (Institute of Medicine, 2003).

Language discrepancies among the consumer, family, and health care providers can be a critical barrier to culturally responsive caring. Consumers with limited English proficiency are less likely to have a regular source for health care, less likely to receive preventative services, and report being less satisfied with clinician communication (Green et al., 2005; Institute of Medicine, 2003). Although some studies show that interpreter services improve the health care experience and outcomes of consumers with limited English proficiency (Green, et al., 2006), others suggest poorer outcomes, particularly when children are used as interpreters and when interpreters are not experienced or well trained (Institute of Medicine, 2003; USDHHS, 2001b).

Culturally and linguistically appropriate services "are respectful and responsive to [the] cultural and linguistic needs [of consumers and their families]" (USDHHS, 2001b, p. 5). The publication *National Standards on Culturally and Linguistically Appropriate Services in Health Care* helps practitioners develop the knowledge and skills to make their services more culturally responsive (USDHHS, 2001b).

Practitioners should also consider their consumers' ability to understand and use written communication. **Health care literacy** refers to the consumers' ability to read, understand, and use health care information, including having the social skills and motivation to gain access to this information and the cognitive skills to process and use the information to make appropriate decisions about their health. An inability to receive effective and satisfying mental health services due to language discrepancies is a common issue for many racial and ethnic minorities.

Ethnic and Racial Minority Groups

The 2010 U.S. census has greatly expanded the categories for ethnicity and race. First the ethnicity categories—Hispanic orgin and Not of Hispanic origin—are distinguished. The 2010 census now further specifies Hispanic, Latino, or Spanish origin as Mexican, Mexican American, Chicano, Puerto Rican, Cuban, or another Hispanic, Latino, or Spanish American origin. Racial categories include White; Black, African American, or Negro; American Indian or Alaska Native (with space to identify tribe); and multiple categories of Asian (Asian Indian, Chinese, Filipino, Japanese, Korean, Vietnamese, Native Hawaiian Guamanian, Chamorro, Samoan other Asian and other Pacific Islander); However even these expanded. These designations are not without problems. The categories used by the U.S. government do not reflect allow the considerable variation within groups in each category. The designation White, used to classify the majority population in the United States, is an umbrella

term that could just as well apply to an American of Italian, Dutch, French, or German descent.

A definition of race focused on biology emphasizes biological distinctions among human populations based on physical characteristics. Yet most genetic researchers agree that biological arguments for dividing people into distinct racial categories are of limited use (Owens & King, 1999) and that race is a socially constructed, multidimensional construct (Ford & Kelly, 2005). **Ethnicity** designation suggests that a group, such as Cherokee Indians or Mexican Americans, share a common ancestry (Zenner, 1996), but this designation can also be confusing and is inconsistently applied (Cokley, 2005; Pahl & Way, 2006).

Limiting any discussion of culture to ethnicity and race is, at best, misguided; nonetheless, much of the research on culture and mental health uses this organizing framework, and race and ethnicity do provide a starting point for a broader consideration of culture and mental health. These ethnic and racial categories recognize the distinct histories and social treatment of ethnic and racial minorities in the United States. It is also clear that many, but not all, members of these groups share some common cultural beliefs, norms, and values, and these cultural characteristics impact mental health care.

Three major national studies provide insight into ethnic minority populations: the National Survey of American Life (Chernoff, 2002), the National Comorbidity Survey (USDHHS, 2001a), and the Epidemiologic Catchment Area Study (Robins & Reiger, 1991). Box 30-1 summarizes the findings from these studies along with findings from selected studies of mental health in ethnic and racial minority communities and data from the Institute of Medicine's report on health care disparities in mental health (2003).

As you read the information in Box 30-1, you are encouraged to reflect on three characteristics of a culturally competent provider described by Stanley Sue (2006). Sue argues that in order to ensure effective cross-cultural interactions, providers must demonstrate culture-specific expertise, scientific-mindedness, and dynamic sizing skills. **Culture-specific expertise** requires that the provider possess a strong base of cultural information for all groups, but especially for groups the therapist is likely to treat. Practitioners are **scientific-minded** when they draw on their knowledge about a cultural group yet approach each new person they treat without assumptions (scientifically), holding only hypotheses that can be tested and modified as more cultural information is collected. For example, a scientific-minded, culturally responsive practitioner would not let assumptions about a new client dictate the approach to therapy, (e.g., the client and family are speaking Spanish, so they must be Mexican). Rather, the practitioner would gather more information and test any hypotheses about culture by asking questions.

Finally, **dynamic sizing** refers to the practitioner's capacity to ask himself or herself whether what he or she knows about a person's cultural group fits the particular individual being treated. For example, a client who is of Mexican descent, but whose family has lived in the United States for five generations, will likely manifest culture differently than a client who is also Mexican but a recent immigrant. A therapist with dynamic sizing skills knows that "one size does *not* fit all" and consciously determines when to generalize cultural knowledge and when to elicit more specific cultural data. Keeping these characteristics in mind, therapists can increase their culture-specific

BOX 30-1 ■ Summary of National Studies on Ethnic Minority Populations

Hispanic Americans

■ It is estimated that in 2005, 14.2% of the U.S. population was Hispanic (U.S. Census Bureau, 2005). This population has now surpassed African Americans as the largest minority group in the United States, and some census estimates suggest that Hispanics will constitute 25% of the total U.S. population by 2050.

■ Compared with other ethnic and racial minority groups, Hispanics are more unified linguistically; however, they constitute a very heterogeneous cultural group, and there are cultural differences among people of Mexican, Cuban, Puerto Rican, South American, and Central American descent.

■ In general, Hispanics constitute a younger, poorer, and less-educated population that is twice as likely as non-Hispanic Caucasians to be uninsured (USDHHS, 2001a).

■ There is a high incidence of co-occurring disorders, especially with alcohol use (Beals, Novins, Mitchell, Shore, & Manson, 2001).

■ When considered as a group, the risk of anxiety and depression is higher for Hispanics than for non-Hispanic Caucasians (Manoleas, Organista, Negron-Velasquez, & McCormick, 2000).

■ Among Mexicans, overall rates for mental illness seem lower than among non-Hispanic Caucasians (Sue & Chu, 2003).

■ As a group, Hispanics are much less likely than Whites or Blacks/African Americans to receive specialty mental health care (USDHHS, 2001a).

■ Hispanic utilization of mental health services is very low, and language barriers are a key limiting factor (USDHHS, 2001a).

■ The expression of symptoms in Hispanic cultures often includes somatization to express distress (e.g., muscle, skeletal, stomach or chest pain, fatigue, dizziness) (Cloutterbuck & Zahn, 2005).

African Americans

■ The 2004 American Community Survey estimated that 12.8% of the U.S. population was African American (U.S. Census Bureau, 2005).

■ The majority of African Americans are native born, but people with ancestry in Africa, South America, or the Caribbean Islands are also considered African American.

■ African Americans are overrepresented in homeless shelters, correctional institutions, child welfare systems, and as victims of violence (USDHHS, 2001a).

■ This population is more likely to receive mental health care in an emergency room or from a primary care physician than from a mental health professional (Institute of Medicine, 2003).

■ In general, prevalence rates for mental illness in African Americans are comparable to rates in non-Hispanic Caucasians (USDHHS, 2001a).

■ Compared with non-Hispanic Caucasians, more African Americans are uninsured (Chernoff, 2002).

■ The percentage of African American psychiatrists, psychologists, social workers (and occupational therapists) is very low (Institute of Medicine, 2003).

Asian Americans

■ In 2004, it was estimated that 4.2% of the U.S. population was Asian American (U.S. Census Bureau, 2005).

■ The category of Asian American is exceptionally diverse, including over 40 distinct ethnic subgroups and more than 100 different languages. Chinese Americans make up the largest percentage of the Asian American population, followed by Asian Indians, Filipinos, Koreans, Vietnamese, and Japanese. Smaller populations of Hmong, Taiwanese, Cambodian, Sri Lankan, Samoan, and Laotian peoples are other examples of Asian Americans in the United States.

■ A clear picture of the mental health needs of Asian Americans is unclear secondary to their limited involvement in epidemiological studies (USDHHS, 2001a).

■ Some studies suggest higher levels of acculturation correlate with improved mental health, and rates of depression are lower compared with Non-Hispanic Caucasians (Takeuchi et al, 1998).

■ A primary reason the Asian American population does not access mental health services is because of language barriers (Phan, 2000).

■ Asian Americans seeking mental health care seek out practitioners fluent in their language, naturalists, spiritualists, and folk healers (Phan, 2000).

■ Compounding the problem of low utilization of mental health care is the timing of help seeking; that is, most seek help at a crisis stage (Sue & Chu, 2003).

■ Shame and stigma are strong cultural factors that further limit Asian Americans' use of mental health services (Sue & Chu, 2003).

American Indians and Alaska Natives

■ People of American Indian and Alaska Native (AIAN) descent made up 1.5% of the total U.S. population in 2005 (U.S. Census Bureau, 2006).

■ There are over 500 recognized tribes in the United States and another 100 tribes not formally recognized by the U.S. government. Approximately one in five American Indians lives on one of over 275 federally recognized reservations. The majority of this population is concentrated in four states: California, Alaska, Arizona, and Oklahoma.

■ Like Asian Americans, AIANs are a linguistically diverse group, having over 200 distinct languages.

■ As a group, AIANs are less likely than Non-Hispanic Caucasians to graduate from high school and twice as likely to be unemployed (U.S. Census Bureau, 2006).

■ AIANs are overrepresented in homeless facilities, correctional institutions, and drug and alcohol programs (U.S. Census Bureau, 2006).

■ Evidence suggests prevalence rates for many mental illnesses for AIAN groups are higher than in the general population (Sue & Chu, 2003).

■ The suicide rate for AIANs is 1.5 times the national rate, and people in this group are twice as likely to be victims of violence.

■ The AIAN rate of posttraumatic stress disorder is nearly three times the national average (Sue & Chu, 2003).

---

expertise and recognition that what you learn must be "sized" to fit each person you treat.

The growing diversification of the U.S. population, coupled with clear evidence of mental health care disparities for ethnic and minority populations, which is described in the next section, suggests that occupational therapists have a moral and ethical obligation to ensure culturally competent care.

Mental Health Care Disparities

Considerable evidence shows that disparities exist in the diagnosis and treatment of mental illness among various ethnic and racial minorities. Several recent national reports underscore the need to address these disparities. *Mental Health: A Report of the Surgeon General* (USDHHS, 1999) concludes that significant information on the prevalence and etiology of mental illness existed, that etiologic research was increasing, and that efficacious treatments are available for most mental illnesses. However, a 2001 supplement to the report, *Mental Health: Culture Race and Ethnicity* (USDHHS, 2001a), highlights substantial disparities for ethnic and racial minorities. Specifically, ethnic and racial minorities are more likely to be overdiagnosed, underdiagnosed, or misdiagnosed; have poorer access to mental health care in general and limited access to culturally competent services in particular; are less likely to receive evidence-based treatments; and are often overinstitutionalized in inpatient mental health facilities, correctional institutions, and child welfare or juvenile justice systems.

President Bush's New Freedom Commission on Mental Health, which was appointed to study the mental health service delivery system, not only confirms the existence of health care disparities but also recommend a fundamental transformation of the mental health system to eliminate these disparities and improve access to quality culturally competent care (USDHHS, 2003). The Institute of Medicine (2003) examined the research evidence that confirmed mental health care disparities in a document titled *Unequal Treatment: Confronting Racial and Ethnic Disparities in Healthcare*. This report details findings from a systematic examination of evidence substantiating health care disparities relative to quality of care, within patient provider interactions, and in decision making for mental health treatment.

For many ethnic and racial minorities, seeking mental health care is the result of a complex interaction among individual and family variables, cultural beliefs and practices, and issues of access to and trust of the mental health care delivery system (Cauce et al, 2002; Yeo, 2000). Yeo (2000) suggests that ethnic and racial minorities typically seek mental health care in the following ways:

1. No help seeking.
2. Using personal resources and family coping strategies.
3. Consulting with a trusted friend or extended family members.
4. Consulting with a traditional, spiritual, or faith-based healer.
5. Seeking help from a professional mental health care provider.

The national reports discussed previously enumerate multiple barriers that contribute to mental health care disparities. Some of these include the underrepresentation of minority health care professionals, failure to provide culturally and linguistically appropriate care, fear of discrimination, culturally insensitive mental health providers, and immigration or legal status (Clark, Anderson, Clark, & Williams, 1999; Sue & Sue, 2003; USDHHS, 2001a, 2003). Additional barriers are illustrated in Figure 30-1.

Occupational therapy mental health care is more likely to overcome these barriers and health care disparities when practitioners recognize that social, cultural, and environmental characteristics influence a person's perception of mental health and mental illness, access and health-seeking behaviors, the experience and expression of psychiatric symptoms, and the ease or difficulty of participating fully in psychiatric care and treatment.

Evidence-Based Practice

Significant findings from relevant research studies examining mental health care with ethnic and racial minorities identify disparities in mental health care. As you examine the evidence presented here, bear in mind that well-designed and well-executed studies of mental health outcomes for ethnic and racial minorities are very limited (Miranda et al, 2000; USDHHS, 2001).

➤ Among some African Americans, mental illness can be viewed as a punishment for wrongdoing. Women in particular can be stigmatized and disgraced partially as a result of being seen as incapable of handling the responsibilities of motherhood.

➤ Racism toward African Americans can create psychologically and physiologically unhealthy responses.

➤ Delays in seeking care and barriers to access often mean that problems reach an intense and chronic stage before help is sought, which in turn requires more costly health care services.

➤ Among unacculturated Mexican Americans, the term *nervios* refers to various types of psychiatric distress; however, the condition is not considered blameworthy.

➤ Ethnic and racial minorities are less likely than non-Hispanic Caucasians to seek out and access mental health services.

➤ Stigma related to mental illness can lead ethnic racial minorities to deny problems and can increase nondisclosure of symptoms, somatization, or delays in seeking professional help.

➤ Ethnic and racial minorities may initially or exclusively seek mental health care from a traditional healer and are more likely than non-Hispanic Caucasians to terminate therapy after one visit to a mental health professional.

➤ Cultural resources and collective resilience offered in ethnic and racial minority communities can serve as protective factors.

Miranda, J., Duan, N., Sherbourne, C., Schoenbaum, M., Lagomasino, I, & Wells, K.B. (2000). Can quality improvement interventions improve care and outcomes for depressed minorities? Results of a randomized controlled trial. *Health Services Research, 38*, 2, 613–630.

U.S. Department of Health and Human Services (USDHHS). (2001). *Mental Health: Culture, Race And Ethnicity – A Supplement To Mental Health: A Report Of The Surgeon General*. Rockville, MD: Author, Public Health Service, Office of the Surgeon General. Available at: http://www.surgeongeneral.gov/library (accessed January 26, 2007).

Culture

Most of the multiple definitions of **culture** suggest that it is a worldview learned and shared among members of a group and that it is cumulative and dynamic. Culture includes a system of shared meaning through language and nonverbal communication. It is value laden and defines norms for roles, relationships, obligations, beliefs, health practices, and behavior (Bonder, Martin, & Miracle, 2002). Metaphorically, culture is often described as a lens, suggesting that everyone interprets the world through his or her own particular cultural lens, which influences a person's thoughts and behaviors:

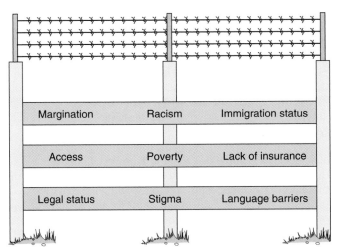

FIGURE 30-1. Barriers to utilization of mental health services.

Culture is a set of guidelines (both explicit and implicit) which individuals inherit as members of a particular society and which tells them how to view the world, how to experience it emotionally, and how to behave in it in relation to other people, to supernatural forces or gods, and to the natural environment. . . . To some extent, culture can be seen as an inherited "lens" through which the individual perceives and understands the world he inhabits and learns to live within it. Growing up within any society is a form of enculturation, whereby the individual slowly acquires the cultural lens of that society. Without such a shared perception of the world, both the cohesion and the continuity of any human group would be impossible (Helman, 1994, pp. 2–3).

Consider objects that have lenses, such as cameras, telescopes, glasses, binoculars, and microscopes. The lens can bring a subject into clearer focus but also limits the scope of what can be seen. In the same way, a cultural lens can influence a person's focus and how that person understands and categorizes what he or she observes. One aspect of the cultural lens is the division of the world and the people within it into different categories—for example, kinsfolk or strangers, normal or abnormal, mad or bad, healthy or ill. All cultures have elaborate ways of moving people from one social category into another (such as from "ill person" to "healthy person") and also of confining people—sometimes against their will—to the categories into which they have been put (such as "mad," "disabled," or "elderly") (Helman, 1994, p. 3).

Helman's description of an "inherited" lens could be interpreted to mean we are "stuck" with the lenses we are born with or socialized into, but more likely, the intent is to emphasize that when we look at the world and the people in it, we look first through the lenses that we know, value, and feel most comfortable with. Further, Helman's description seems to suggest that this act of looking through our own lenses in inevitable, but that does not preclude us from looking through other lenses as well.

In occupational therapy, as in many health professions, culture is often seen primarily through a lens of race or ethnicity. This is a very narrow lens that often puts some of the most obvious markers of culture, such as appearance, dress, and rituals or traditions of heritage, in the foreground while paying less attention to societal, organizational, and political characteristics of culture. Matsumoto (2006) provides a broader perspective that occupational therapists can appreciate when he says that culture "touches on all aspects of life, including general characteristics of food, clothing, housing, technology, economy, transportation, individual and family activities, community and governmental systems, welfare, religion, science, sex and reproduction, and the life cycle" (p. 35).

Describing culture solely through a lens of race and ethnicity is inadequate. Culture is broader and permeates multiple dimensions of occupation in everyday life. Many other lenses beyond race and ethnicity influence people's perception and daily occupations, including gender, age, cohort (e.g., Baby Boomer, Generation X), socioeconomic status, religious persuasion, professional or political affiliations, immigration status, sexual preference, physical ability, family structure, and geographic locale.

Occupational therapists, as person-centered professionals, are perhaps at their best when they intentionally look through multiple lenses in order to uncover the distinct ways in which people experience, understand, and organize their occupational behavior. From a mental health care perspective, this means seeking to understand how culture can influence the expression of emotion, the interpretation of objectionable symptoms, the manifestation of suffering or distress, and the selection of occupations a person may choose when recovering from a mental illness.

Cultural Definitions of Normal and Abnormal Behavior

Conceptually, culture is an abstraction that is most often used to examine how groups of people may be similar or different, but it also can be used to consider cultural worldviews and cultural practices. A person's worldview includes values, beliefs, and assumptions about the world that differ among individuals and are influenced by a person's cultural, social, religious/spiritual, and racial/ethnic background. A **cultural worldview** is the way in which a person or group looks at the world and their place in it. It is a belief system grounded in moral and ethical reasoning, magicoreligious beliefs, cosmology, values, social relationships, and connection to nature (Purnell & Paulanka, 2003).

Cultural practices can be thought of as the *doing* of culture, or the "discrete, observable, objective and behavioral aspects of human activities in which people engage related to culture" (Matsumoto, 2006, p. 35). Understanding a person's cultural practices is an important aspect of culturally responsive care precisely because these behaviors are embedded in a person's daily occupations. Cultural practices can be seen in the way individuals cook their food, care for their living space, engage in worship, work, play, and discipline their children.

Ethnocentrism is the universal tendency of humans to appraise ways of thinking, acting, and believing according to their own experience and cultural background—that is, to see the world and what passes for normal behavior through one's own cultural lens (Purnell & Paulanka, 2003).

In considering cultural practices, it is essential to apply a broad cultural lens because cultural practices that seem familiar and universal to you may seem strange and obscure to someone outside your cultural group. Wurzel (1988) quotes Aldous Huxley, who, upon returning from his first trip around the world, summarized his experiences with different cultures:

> So the journey is over and I am back again, richer by much experience and poorer by many exploded convictions, many perished certainties. For convictions and certainties are too often the concomitants of ignorance. . . . I set out on my travels knowing, or thinking I knew, how men should live, how be governed, how educated, what they should believe. I had my views on every activity of life. Now, on my return, I find myself without any of these pleasing certainties. . . . The better you understand the significance of any question, the more difficult it becomes to answer it. Those who attach a high importance to their own opinion should stay at home. When one is traveling, convictions are mislaid as easily as spectacles, but unlike spectacles, they are not easily replaced. (As quoted in Wurzel, 1988, p. 3.)

Huxley's comments reveal that what we consider the "right" or "normal" way to do things is heavily influenced by our worldview, or the cultural lens we use to see the world and the people in it. It is not hard to find examples throughout U.S. history of intelligent, clear-thinking individuals, convinced that their own worldview was accurate and "normal," using that perspective to define the cultural practices of others as abnormal. Consider the decimation of the American Indian people and their cultures in the United States. When viewed through the U.S. settlers' Christian-European worldview, American Indian culture was barbaric. Given this perspective, it seemed reasonable to forcibly remove American Indian children from their own culture and assimilate them into American culture by placing them in institutions where traditional cultural practices could be "replaced," a practice that began in the 1880s and continued through the 1920s (Wallace, 1995). Or consider the diagnosis of drapetomania, a so-called mental illness proposed by Samuel Cartwright (1851) to explain the tendency of black slaves to flee captivity. In his description of the diagnosis, Cartwright suggests that the practice of slavery was the natural execution of an owner's God-given right of power over others. Through this lens, the slaves' behavior was disordered.

These two examples reflect some extraordinary and tragic examples of ethnocentrism. One only needs to pick up the newspaper, watch television, or Google "hate groups" to recognize that some humans continue to label that which differs greatly from their own beliefs as strange, dangerous, unenlightened, or bizarre. Conceptualizations of what constitutes abnormal behavior inevitably are grounded in some notion of what is standard, normal, and proper behavior. The symptomatic expression of mental disorders varies across cultures (Guarnaccia & Rogler, 1999). The standard for defining normal and abnormal behavior in psychiatry is the *Diagnostic and Statistical Manual of Mental Disorders,* Fourth Edition, Text Revision (DSM-IV-TR).

Culture and the DSM-IV-TR

Throughout this text, and particularly in Part II, "The Person," you have read what constitutes normative behavior and personality development and how abnormal behavior is understood and treated. Diagnosing mental illness and designing interventions are, for the most part, based on a Western analytic scientific paradigm manifest in the DSM-IV-TR (APA, 2000).

One assumption of biomedical psychiatry is that psychiatric disorders can be described in a universal language without regard to cultural differences. "Genetic factors, molecular biological processes, and neurologically situated 'lesions,' processes and/or mechanisms account for the manifestations of behavior disturbances of 'mental illnesses' that the science of psychopathology describes and codifies" (Fabrega, 2004, p. 30). From a strict neurobiological perspective, disorders exist within the brain, and eventually laboratory science will evolve to the point that diagnosis is a matter of applying a proscribed set of tests and procedures.

The DSM-IV-TR is a product of this Western biomedical, psychiatric culture (Kress, Eriksen, Rayle, & Wood, 2005). From a cultural perspective, the disorders in the DSM-IV-TR center on psychopathology within the person, and the cultural, environmental, or situational context is of limited importance (Lopez et al, 2006). In fact, the term *culture* did not appear in the index of the DSM until 20 years ago (Paniagua, 2001). Further, acculturation is not defined in the DSM-IV-TR glossary of technical terms; only the following sentence suggests a link between psychiatric symptoms and acculturation processes: "[The category V62.4 Acculturation Problem] can be used when the focus of clinical attention is a problem involving adjustment to a different culture (e.g., following migration)" (APA, 2000, p. 741). Trauma related to migration or immigration is not specifically addressed. Disorders related to gender identity are included, but ethnic-racial identity confusion is not. There is also no discussion of adjustment issues related to the social environment, to housing or economic problems, or to racism or discrimination.

This said, the DSM-IV-TR is the primary diagnostic system that professionals use to communicate about individuals and their symptoms, to conceptualize a person's mental health issues, and to obtain reimbursement for mental health services. It is not likely to be replaced anytime soon, though some have proposed alternatives that give more attention to sociocultural and environmental problems and resources when determining diagnoses (Lopez et al, 2006). Occupational therapists do not make a psychiatric diagnosis; they are typically focused on how a person's psychiatric symptoms impact occupational functioning. Nonetheless, it is useful for practicing occupational therapists to understand the DSM-IV-TR's strengths and weaknesses as a culturally sensitive diagnostic system.

Diagnosis in Cultural Context

The DSM-IV-TR (APA, 2000) offers two resources that can help mental health practitioners, including occupational therapists, consider mental illness in cultural context: a cultural formulation outline and a glossary of culture-bound syndromes.

The Cultural Formulation Outline

The **cultural formulation outline** suggests that culturally responsive mental health evaluation and intervention practices consider and integrate the following five points (APA, 2000):

1. Establish the person's cultural identity.
2. Elicit cultural explanations for mental health issues.
3. Determine cultural factors related to the person's psychosocial environment.
4. Consider factors that might influence the relationship between the counselor and the client.
5. Make a global cultural assessment to determine how cultural considerations will influence mental health care.

The cultural formulation outline is intended as a resource to supplement the multiaxial diagnostic assessment process. Table 30-1 identifies the specific outcomes for each step in the cultural formulation process and suggests strategies that occupational therapists can apply to support culturally responsive mental health care.

Culture-Bound Syndromes

The DSM-IV-TR also provides a glossary of 25 **culture-bound syndromes**. "Culture-bound syndromes are generally limited to specific societies or culture areas and are localized, folk, diagnostic categories that frame coherent meanings for certain repetitive, patterned, and troubling sets of experiences and observations" (APA, 2000, p. 898). The syndromes included in the DSM-IV-TR do not generally have one-to-one correspondence with specific DSM diagnostic categories, nor do they constitute an exhaustive list, but these syndromes are important to consider because they demonstrate that expressions of mental distress reflect an individual's sociocultural context. The syndromes exemplify not only how different cultures establish and interpret behavior but also how groups label behavior with names that are then used to describe and understand these behaviors (Cloutterbuck & Zahn, 2005). It is important to recognize that although the belief systems that underlie these syndromes may differ, each approach to understanding the client's behavior is respected within its own culture. It is when these belief systems collide with

---

Table 30-1 ● **Strategies for Completing a Cultural Formulation**

Outcomes: Cultural Formulation	Strategies for the Occupational Therapist
Understand the cultural identity of the person	Hone your cultural curiosity • Determine the person's ethnic or cultural reference group • Identify the degree of involvement with the culture of origin and the host culture • Establish language abilities and preferences
Elicit the person's cultural explanation for his or her illness	Remember that all behaviors are learned and displayed in a cultural context • Seek to establish the person's description of physical or psychosocial symptoms • Compare the person's description of meaning/severity of symptoms with the norms of his or her cultural group • Determine preferred coping patterns • Explore past experiences with professional mental health care
Identify factors related to the sociocultural environment that support/impede the person's level of functioning	Consider person–environment interaction through a cultural lens • Understand the family's reaction to the person's illness • Discover the degree to which religion or kinship networks provide psychosocial, instrumental, or informational supports • Explore interactional patterns in the home and neighborhood • Recognize stresses in the local social environment • Identify socioeconomic resources or barriers • Determine if culturally relevant healers have been consulted
Appreciate the cultural elements of the person–practitioner relationship	Recognize that both the person and the practitioner come to the interaction with personal cultural worldviews • Identify your own unique cultural identity • Consider that differences in cultural and social status can exist and influence the therapeutic relationship • Ensure the person has the opportunity to communicate in his or her first language and offer interpreters if difficulties arise • Recognize that power differentials often exist between those providing and those receiving services
Intentionally address culture in the assessment process and intervention planning	Make your attention to cultural components a deliberate aspect of providing care • Determine if the assessment tools you employ integrate social and cultural components • Discuss the cultural relevance of assessment and intervention options with the person and his or her family • Identify and integrate culturally appropriate occupations in the occupational therapy intervention process

Western biomedical beliefs that the perspectives on mental illness are questioned.

Table 30-2 includes several culture-bound syndromes that are included in the DSM-IV-TR. Data has been expanded in this table to include both primary and associated features of these syndromes and to provide information on cultural explanations for the syndromes. Additionally, to challenge you to consider how the expression of mental distress reflects the individual's sociocultural context, anorexia nervosa and chronic fatigue syndrome, two entries that are not listed as culture-bound syndromes in the DSM-IV-TR, have been added to this table. These syndromes are diagnosed primarily in Non-Hispanic Caucasians in North America and Europe.

Culturally Responsive Caring in Mental Health Practice

Collectively, definitions of **cultural competence** suggest that it is a complex, multidimensional construct that integrates cognitive, affective, and behavioral components. In other words, cultural competency is manifest in what you know in your head, what you feel in your heart, and what you can demonstrate through your presence in the cross-cultural encounter.

Models of Cultural Competency

Models of cultural competency have been developed in many allied health fields, but they are particularly well developed in the counseling psychology and nursing disciplines.

Counseling Psychology Models

In counseling psychology Sue, Arredondo, and McDavis (1992) proposed a framework of cultural competency that is organized around three critical dimensions:

1. The capacity to be aware of one's own assumptions, values, and biases.
2. An understanding of the worldviews of culturally different clients.
3. The ability to develop appropriate intervention strategies.

The tripartite structure of this model established a framework for multicultural education and research within counseling psychology (APA, 2002). It also supported

---

Table 30-2 ● **Culture-Bound Syndromes**

Syndrome	Primary Population	Primary Features	Symptoms	Cultural Explanation
Amok	Males from Malaysia, Laos, Philippines, and Polynesia	Dissociation, paranoia, uncontrollable rage	• Withdrawal • Violent or aggressive behavior • Persecutory ideation	Perceived slight or insult to male honor
Ataque de nervios	Men and women in and from Latin American and Caribbean countries	Somatic complaints, anxiety, dissociation	• Uncontrolled shouting or crying • Convulsions, shaking • Verbal or physical aggression • Palpitations, dyspnea, dizziness • Tight chest, shortness of breath	Stressful event related to the family such as death or conflict; episodic expression of pent-up anger
Hwa-byung	Koreans and Korean Americans; more common in women	Somatic complaints, anxiety, depression, social distress	• Epigastric pain • Dysphoria • Panic, depression, tiredness • Insomnia, fatigue • Fear of death	Attributed to the suppression of anger and subsequent imbalance
Shin-byung	Korean and Korean American men and women	Somatic complaints, anxiety, dissociation	• Weakness, dizziness • Exploding sensation in the chest • Anorexia • Insomnia • Epigastric problems	Possession by ancestral spirits
Susto	Men and women in and from Latin American countries; more common in women	Somatic complaints, anxiety, dissociation, depression, anorexia	• Anorexia, vomiting, diarrhea • Muscle aches and pains • Troubled sleep • Avolition • Anxiety, depression, irritability	Soul loss brought on by a frightening event
Zar	Men and women in many North African and Middle Eastern countries	Dissociation, apathy, withdrawal	• Shouting, laughing, head banging • Singing or weeping • Refusal to eat • Ignoring daily activities	General term recognizing that a person has been possessed by spirits

The Lived Experience

Cynthia

There are many stories that could have been told here. There are many stories in which the main character is someone whose culture seems exotic, strange, or different. Cynthia is an African American woman in her mid-40s. She was chosen to write this narrative because she is not exotic; in fact, on the surface, she seems plainly American. In order to better understand her cultural identity, however, challenge yourself to move beyond a lens of race and explore how poverty, homelessness, and mental illness impact her lived experience. Does living in poverty have distinct cultural patterns that impact occupation? How does one become homeless? Can people with mental illness be said to have their own cultural group?

I was diagnosed with depression way back in 1996. But in reality, I've been depressed all my life. I can remember when I was in preschool. The teacher told my mother that I was an antisocial person. I wouldn't socialize with the other children. I had one friend, and if she wasn't there, then I had no friends and I kept to myself. I wasn't mean. I was doing my own thing. I was always real shy to where I was even scared to talk to my own mother. I'm just getting out of that within the last couple years. I've always been off by myself, not an antisocial person, but I function better by myself. Most of my friends also have a mental illness. My closest friend, she has a mental illness. I think sometimes that I can relate more to a person who has a mental illness because if a person doesn't understand mental illness, like if you tell them that you have a mental illness, they'll think that you're crazy. That's their automatic thought. It has to be something that you're off balance or crazy. That's the way they explain you. It gives people the excuse not to even try to know you.

Sometimes *I AM* off balance. At those times, I can relate to my friend because when I'm feeling down or some other kind of way, then I can talk to her because she can understand what I'm feeling because she's been there too. Sometimes other people don't get it; even my own sister. When I tell my sister, she's like, she says, "It's a mind thing and you can get out of it." My son's father is like that too, he's like, "It's just a will thing." That might be a general feeling within black communities; just be stronger, get faith. It's a weakness thing, something that you should be able to overcome. It's not something that requires medication and stuff like that. It's not a disease. It's just something that you can overcome if you want to overcome it. My sister is slowly coming around more to understand that I do have a mental illness and it's not something that I can just turn on and turn off. It's not something that I control, so she's coming around to that.

I don't tell certain people because, to me, I think people will judge you if you have a mental illness and I think it will hinder you in a lot of different things. Like I couldn't go to a job and say, "I have a mental illness." You know, I might not get that job because I told them. That is society in general. When people see homeless people on the street, they try to avoid them. They think that they are crazy, but that's not the case a lot of times. It's just that certain circumstances happen. Things happen. That's how I think people think about mental illness too. I think that if people knew you had a mental illness, they would walk around you to avoid you.

I was in a welfare office applying for housing once, and I decided I'm not going to tell them that I am mentally ill because it's a judging thing. In the welfare office they make it so hard for you to get benefits, and sometimes the workers act like they are paying you out of their own pocket. I feel like, OK, I have worked in my life too and I'm not planning on being on welfare all of my life. It is supposed to be there for people who need it when they need it. But they judge you. They judge you and they make you go through some pain. Especially when you get a worker who thinks that they are better than you are because you aren't working and they are. So you learn little tricks through experience and word of mouth. I'm not going to say that I work the system, but I've learned that there are certain things you have to do with the system because if you don't, you're not going to get any benefit. People with mental illness or who are homeless tell each other what we need to know, because the workers won't tell you nothing. You share information.

I graduated from the occupational therapy employment program and my intentions were to get a job. I did get a job last October, but I didn't keep it very long, and after awhile I decided I should apply for social security disability. That's my record; after a while I can't keep a job. I thought that a job would keep me sane, but it didn't. I felt that if I had a job, I would feel like I had a purpose in life because I felt useless when I wasn't working. I actually like to work, but I don't tend to stay on a job for a long time. I felt like I was getting worse instead of getting better, and I stopped taking my meds. So my depression came back. I was trying to change with the OT employment program, but it didn't work out. I'm to the point right now where I really want to work. I honestly do want to work, but with social security, you can only work so many hours before you lose your benefits. It's risky for me.

If I were to describe myself culturally, I would say I am middle-aged but I'm still young. I'm a person with a mental illness. I have been an addict. I consider myself as a mother; a mother of three. I'm not going to say lower class, but I live in poverty. I think I struggle a lot with identifying myself or who I am or my purpose, that's what I struggle a lot with. What is my purpose?

the continued refinement of a descriptive taxonomy of multicultural counseling proficiencies (Arredondo & Toporek, 2004) and provided the basis for the introduction and testing of several instruments designed to measure these competencies (Dunn, Smith, & Montoya, 2006). This research demonstrates that cultural knowledge is essential for effective and ethical health care service delivery and that it is influenced by education and training (Sue & Sue, 2003). Findings also suggest that cultural awareness is a key component of cultural competency but that practitioners and students may find it easier to learn about others than to reflect on their own attitudes or challenge how their personal biases may influence their practice behaviors (Arredondo & Toporek, 2004).

This model of multicultural counseling competencies may be useful for occupational therapy. Like occupational therapists, counseling psychologists take a life-span perspective in their work with people with mental illnesses. They specifically address personal and interpersonal functioning in a variety of areas, such as vocational, social, educational, and familial aspects of a person's life. Finally, counseling psychologists typically assume humanistic and holistic approaches and use methods that are problem oriented and goal directed.

Nursing Models

The nursing profession has developed multiple models of cultural competency. Madeleine Leininger pioneered the development of transcultural nursing nearly 60 years ago (Leininger, 2002). **Transcultural health care** is defined as "formal areas of study and practice in the cultural beliefs, values, and life ways of diverse cultures and in the use of knowledge to provide culture-specific or culture-universal care to individuals, families, and groups of particular cultures" (Leininger, 1997, p. 342). In the past few decades, others have continued to develop and synthesize transcultural nursing knowledge in novel ways, with some theorists suggesting that their models are designed to be used by health professionals from many disciplines (Campinha-Bacote, 2003; Giger & Davidhizar, 2004; Purnell, 2002). It is essential that occupational therapists are knowledgeable about these models and evaluate their usefulness for guiding occupational therapy practice.

Much of the research in nursing has focused on uncovering cultural universals that can be applied to transcultural health care. Transcultural nursing research has generally sought to closely examine nursing care with very specific ethnic and cultural groups. This literature is significant in the breadth of cultural groups that have been investigated, the depth of the research that has been completed, and the application of research results in the development and refinement of models of culturally competent care in nursing (Campinha-Bacote, 2003; Leininger, 2002; Purnell, 2002).

Leininger (2002) developed the sunrise model of culturally congruent care based on decades of clinical practice and research in transcultural nursing. A major assumption of Leininger's model is that culture care concepts vary transculturally but that diversities and universalities can be established across cultures. "The central purpose of the theory is to discover and explain diverse and universal culturally based care factors influencing the health and well-being, illness or death of individuals or groups" (Leininger, 2002, p. 190).

Leininger's sunrise model is simultaneously culture specific, broad, and holistic. Specific cultural and social dimensions of this model include educational and economic factors, political and legal factors, cultural values, beliefs and lifeways, kinship and social factors, religious and philosophical factors, and technological factors. From a broader contextual perspective, this model also encourages practitioners to examine a person's environmental context and linguistic and ethnic histories. This model assumes that every clinical encounter is cross-cultural. Opportunities for culturally competent care exist in the space created by the intersection of the cultural practices of the individual and the professional care practices of the health care provider. It is likely that assumptions inherent in this nursing model also apply in occupational therapy practice, but occupational therapists need to critically question whether theories of cultural competence imported from nursing fit the realities of occupational therapy practice.

Purnell (2002) defines cultural competence as "the adaptation of care in a manner that is consistent with the culture of the client and is therefore a conscious process and nonlinear" (p. 193). Purnell's framework for understanding culture includes 12 interrelated cultural domains:

- Overview/heritage
- Communication
- Family roles and organization
- Workforce issues
- Biocultural ecology
- High-risk behaviors
- Nutrition
- Pregnancy and childbearing practices, including fertility
- Death rituals
- Spirituality
- Health care practices
- Health care practitioners

Collectively, these domains provide an organizing framework for culturally competent assessment and intervention. For example, the new admission to your mental health center may be a 32-year-old migrant farm worker from the highlands of Guatemala (overview/heritage) who speaks an Indian dialect (communication), is undocumented, and has been unable to find any employment despite being healthy and willing to work (workforce issues). This individual involuntarily migrated to the United States to escape political persecution and torture (overview/heritage). He lives in a section of the city known as an ethnic enclave for immigrants from Central America (family roles and organization) and is distrustful of the professionals at the mental health center (health care practices), preferring instead to visit a *curandera* in his neighborhood (health care practitioners). As seen in this example, many of the domains in Purnell's framework may serve occupational therapists as they strive to provide culturally competent interventions. On the other hand, some of the domains, such as biocultural ecology, nutrition, pregnancy and childbearing practices, or death rituals, may be less consistently useful in occupational therapy practice.

Occupational Therapy Models

When compared with the efforts of the counseling psychology and nursing professions, the development of models of cultural competency that can guide practice within occupational therapy is a more recent occurrence. Two recent approaches include the culture-emergent model by Bonder, Martin, and Miracle (2002) and Iwama's *kawa* [river] model (2005).

Culture-Emergent Model

The **culture-emergent model** advocates an inquiry-centered approach to developing the knowledge, attitudes, and skills for culturally competent practice. In this process-oriented approach, the specific culture is irrelevant. The model stresses the development of skills for cross-cultural interactions—that is, learning to ask questions. Many of the approaches are grounded in classic anthropological and ethnographic methodologies, such as making skilled observations of objects, time use and socialization, paying close attention to interpersonal patterns, and intentionally studying culture. Practitioners applying a culture-emergent approach must develop the ability to skillfully manage an intercultural interaction, including learning how to directly elicit cultural information.

In the culture-emergent model, Bonder et al (2002) argue that culture is

- Learned
- Localized
- Patterned
- Evaluative
- Persistent but incorporates change

Practitioners can use these five primary assumptions to reflect on their own cultures and as a framework to understand the worldview of others. These assumptions can be observed in the following story:

When I was young, I read from the Bible and sang a solo during the church services for my eighth grade graduation ceremonies. I have over 60 first cousins on my mother's side of the family alone, so the church was full of family and it was a proud day. After mass had ended and we had all left the church, my Tio [Uncle] Ramón came over to me. He pinched my arm so hard I let out a surprised yelp, and then he hugged me. As he did, he spoke into my ear, saying, "Do not let your head grow too big. When you do good, you do good for the family, and when you do bad, it's the same. Today the family is proud, hijo [son]."

Let's examine how the assumptions of the emergent-culture model are expressed through this story.

- *Culture is learned* and transmitted in countless observations and interactions throughout a person's life. This learning can be referred to as **enculturation**, the process whereby an individual is taught the norms of the culture. In my family culture, my Tio Ramón and my mother's six other brothers all conveyed cultural lessons.,
- *Culture is localized* because it is situated in personally meaningful environments. In the story, the locale is the church, the scene of many events that shaped my cultural identity. My abuelita's [grandmother's] house was another meaningful locale, as it was the place where the family routinely gathered. Cultural practices for occasions that called for celebration, condolences, and every emotion in between were localized in that house.
- *Culture is patterned* in the rituals of the family life cycle. For example, weddings, baptisms, confirmations, and midnight mass on Christmas Eve followed by tamales and *menudo* at my abuelita's house were all events that established norms, customs, and expectations for behavior.
- *Culture is evaluative* because it structures and influences our choices. When my Tio Ramón pinched me, I focused on the pain, but the value orientation was his true message, and I have transmitted that same message to my own children. Cultural values are often not communicated so explicitly but are more often transmitted through action and example.

- Finally, *culture is persistent but incorporates change.* A person's core cultural identity is stable, but cross-cultural encounters lead to acculturation. Enculturation is described as the way we learn the norms of our own culture, but acculturation describes the way we borrow ideas, objects, and processes from other cultures and incorporate them into our own.

Kawa Model

Iwama (2005) introduced the *kawa* (river) model as a culturally relative approach to understanding a person in sociocultural context. The kawa model grew out of the clinical practice of Japanese occupational therapists who were struggling to explain occupational therapy to both consumers and colleagues from other disciplines. They were frequently frustrated by attempts to apply models of occupational therapy grounded in Western perspectives to Japanese practice. These practitioners recognized that models of occupational therapy based on Western cultural norms presented conceptualizations of occupation that did not always match the cultural realities of the people they treated. These practitioners were searching for a culturally relative and culturally safe model with which to describe their practice.

Cultural safety is a term that arose from an Aotearoan (New Zealand) perspective and was coined in response to the lived experience of health disparities realized by the Maori, the indigenous people of New Zealand (Jungerson, 1992). The concept of cultural safety extends notions of cultural sensitivity or cultural competency, which often ignore the power dynamics between those providing and those seeking services, particularly marginalized populations. In effect, this concept suggests that health care providers must recognize the broader sociopolitical aspects of providing care to marginalized persons. This includes understanding that health disparities are often perpetuated by historical, social, and political processes and that when consumers are being assessed and treated using standards grounded in a different context that these practices are, at best, culturally unsafe and, at worst, dangerous (Jungerson, 1992).

The kawa model is a culturally safe model grounded in an East Asian worldview. This model challenges occupational therapists to explore how concepts typically found in occupational therapy practice models, such as autonomy, independence, self, and temporality, translate when taken outside of middle-class, social, and cultural norms (Iwama, 2005).

Unlike Western-based models of practice, the individual is not the central feature in the kawa model. The self is decentralized in response to the assumption that harmony and balance in life are not individually determined but are dependent on the fluidity of all elements of the social, cultural, and environmental contexts. Imbalance, then, reflects a disruption of the collective synergy of these contextual elements rather than a disruption of the personal harmony within the self. Therefore, the central focus of occupational therapy intervention is to restore the harmony of the person within their surrounding contexts (Iwama, 2005).

The Japanese word *kawa* means river. The choice of a river, which conjures images embedded in nature, was intentionally selected as a means to convey the dynamics and structure of the model. The key elements of the kawa model extend the metaphor of a river:

- *Mizu* (water), the central concept in the metaphor, represents the life energy of the person; it both influences and is influenced by the surrounding context.
- *Kawa no suku heki* (river side wall) and *kawa no zoko* (river floor) are critical environmental elements that represent the social and physical context, which can impact the person's flow of life energy.
- *Iwa* (rocks) represent life circumstances that crop up in one's river of life. For a person with mental illness, the *iwa* in his or her life river can be manic symptoms or the experience of being stigmatized, either of which can impede the person's flow of life energy.
- *Ryuboku* (driftwood) in the river represents attributes of the person (e.g., values, character, personality traits, special aptitudes) and resources within his or her sociocultural context (e.g., relationships or material assets), which can both positively or negatively affect life flow.
- *Sukima* (the spaces between the obstacles) is where the promise of occupational therapy lies (Iwama, 2005). It is in these spaces that the person's life force still flows. These are often the occupations so meaningful and valuable that the person commits his or her life force to maintain engagement in these activities and roles. The astute practitioner will seek out these spaces, recognizing that the likelihood of success is highest in those areas where the person continues to commit his or her life energy.

The kawa model epitomizes a culturally relative approach that seeks to understand the person in context. The metaphor of the river and the natural context suggests that culturally competent practitioners recognize that the central measure of adaptation is not necessarily to control every circumstance of life but to find a way to keep one's life force flowing in harmony with them.

Assessment and Intervention

Muñoz (2002) elicited descriptions of care from 12 experienced practitioners who served culturally diverse populations and had the capacity to reflect on and describe their clinical encounters. His study sought to illuminate the basic social processes practitioners engaged in when providing care to culturally diverse populations. Findings revealed that practitioners who provide culturally responsive care achieve a synergistic mutuality with the people they work with and are actively engaged in the process of developing this synergy. These practitioners intentionally consider culture as a necessary variable to know and care for the person. Becoming a practitioner who provides culturally responsive care is an intentional endeavor. It is part of a personal quest not only to deliver the best possible service but also to personally become a more multicultural being.

Culturally responsive practitioners routinely inventory their own thinking and participate in social and educational activities that help them refine a personal database of cultural knowledge. Muñoz (2002) argued that occupational therapists provide culturally responsive caring when they (1) generate cultural knowledge, (2) build cultural awareness, (3) apply cultural skills, (4) engage others, and

(5) explore multiculturalism. These five components can be used to extend our discussion of culturally responsive assessment and interventions.

Generating Cultural Knowledge

Culturally responsive practitioners routinely consider the limits of their cultural knowledge. With each new person, practitioners asks themselves whether they are knowledgeable about the person's worldview and culture-bound illnesses within the person's cultural group (Campinha-Bacote, 2003). Practitioners who actively expand their knowledge base about different cultural groups are *generating cultural knowledge.* This requires a commitment to understand culturally based health practices of various groups. Practitioners with a strong foundation of cultural knowledge are more likely to intentionally seek to understand the cultural context of the person, their family, and the community; to know about and use culturally responsive intervention strategies; and to integrate the use of cultural resources when working with culturally different persons and their families.

For mental health practice, this also means exploring multicultural perspectives on mental health and illness, on stress and coping, and on cultural variations in the presentation of psychiatric symptoms. Culturally responsive practitioners intentionally study the cultures of people they are most likely to see in practice via continuing education and professional development activities, consultation with colleagues and key informants in the community, and reading and research. As already discussed, some of the transcultural nursing models present frameworks that delineate critical cultural characteristics that health care practitioners can target for their learning (Andrews & Boyle, 2003; Purnel & Paulanka, 2003).

Culture-specific knowledge is necessary to deliver culturally responsive care, but it is only a starting point. It is essential to recognize that considerable variability exists within cultures and that culture-specific information about any particular cultural group may or may not be relevant to a particular individual's care.

Building Cultural Awareness

Ask yourself toward which groups you hold the most bias. Chances are that this question makes you uncomfortable. It makes most people uncomfortable because no one wants to believe they hold any biases. When practitioners work toward *building cultural awareness*, they seek to recognize their own biases and prejudices toward people from other cultures and their own capacities and limitations in overcoming these biases when providing care. Practitioners can build cultural awareness through deliberative cognitive processes and reflection on their own prejudices and biases, values, beliefs, problem-solving strategies, and worldview.

Self-assessments can be useful tools to initiate critical reflection. Social attitude or bias scales, racial identity scales, assessment of spirituality, or tests to measure your level of cultural understanding relative to ethnic, racial, religious, or sexual preference minorities can be easily found online.

One basic tool, the Heritage Assessment Tool (Spector, 2004), is a 29-item self-assessment that therapists can use to explore their own heritage and also use with consumers to gain a deeper understanding of their heritage consistency. **Heritage consistency** is the degree to which a person's lifestyle reflects his or her traditional ethnic, religious, and cultural heritage. Heritage consistency is believed to exist on a continuum from more traditional to more acculturated. For example, a person of Italian descent who socialized in an Italian ethnic neighborhood where her grandparents, who lived with her family, spoke and expected her to speak Italian is likely to have a high level of heritage consistency. Someone without these experiences may have less. As practitioner, we can explore our client's heritage consistency by determining whether our client's lifestyle is consistent with a traditional ethnic, religious and cultural heritage. An understanding of a person's heritage and the potential strengths and supports within his or her family and community may help you more effectively plan interventions.

Other tools, such as the Inventory for Assessing the Process of Cultural Competence Among Health Care Professionals–Revised (IAPCC-R), encourage health professionals to examine their level of cultural competency. This 25-item, self-assessment tool is based on Campinha-Bacote's (2003) process model of cultural competency and measures the five cultural constructs of her model:

1. Cultural awareness: the limits of the respondent's competence when interacting with culturally diverse consumers.
2. Cultural knowledge: the respondent's understanding of the worldviews or health care practices of cultural groups.
3. Cultural skills: the respondent's ability to question a person about his or her ethnic or cultural background
4. Cultural encounters: direct engagement in cross-cultural interactions with persons from diverse backgrounds. Items on the IAPCC-R reflective of cultural encounter attempt to measure the respondent's habits of engaging others from diverse cultural backgrounds. A representative item is "I am involved with cultural/ethnic groups outside my healthcare setting role."
5. Cultural desire: the respondent's motivation to "want to" understand others. Cultural desire items on this self-assessment measure the degree to which the respondent has a genuine desire and motivation to work with culturally different consumers.

The IAPCC-R offers a scoring key that roughly places the respondent on a continuum from culturally proficient to culturally incompetent; however, rather than conceptualizing cultural competence as something you have more or less of, it is better to examine patterns in your responses as a way to consider next steps in your own cultural journey. For example, it may be that your results rate you high on cultural knowledge, awareness, and desire, but your lack of cultural encounters may have provided insufficient opportunities for you to test your knowledge and build your skills. Cultural awareness requires sensitivity and openness to understanding, valuing, and respecting the lifeways and cultural patterns of others and a willingness to explore the impact of prejudice and bias at personal, institutional, and societal levels. Building cultural awareness also requires practitioners

to appreciate their own cultural identity and how their cultural heritage impacts their beliefs and their clinical practices.

Applying Cultural Skills

Culturally responsive practitioners integrate their cultural knowledge and awareness into their clinical reasoning processes and intentionally make culture a central aspect of clinical assessment and intervention. Occupational therapy is a social process; thus, *applying cultural skills* requires practitioners to demonstrate the capacity to create an interpersonal connection with culturally diverse consumers that supports effective cultural assessment and interventions. This can be accomplished by maintaining an open and welcoming stance, by reading and responding to the dynamics of the clinical encounter, and by engaging each person with a purposeful intent to identify, explore, and honor their cultural lifeways. Cultural skills are also manifest when a practitioner selects occupations that are familiar and that hold cultural meaning for the persons they treat.

Models by Leininger (2002) and Purnell (2002) (discussed earlier) provide some useful assessment frameworks for occupational therapists to consider. Other nursing models (Andrews & Boyle, 2003; Giger & Davidhizar, 2004) go a step further and define very specific questions that can be used when completing a cultural assessment. For example, Giger and Davidhizar's (2004) approach to cultural assessment includes six cultural variables that may influence mental health and illness behaviors: communication, space, social organization, time, environmental control, and biological variations (Figure 30-2). In this model, each individual is seen as a culturally unique individual, and thus assessment begins with some understanding of the person's cultural identity. A useful starting point would be to understand the person's cultural heritage, educational and economic status, and acculturation level.

Level of acculturation can be determined by engaging the person in a discussion about his or her preferred language, educational background, religious beliefs, social relations, gender roles, cultural and racial identity, and use of folk healers. Occupational therapists often ask consumers about their current living situation, but asking where the consumer grew up may give insight about the cultural patterns of life into which the person was socialized and which may persist as important cultural factors than can support recovery. An approach that reflects genuine curiosity is often quite effective. A practitioner may ask, "I am interested in knowing about your family beliefs and traditions. Can you tell me a bit about your family's culture?"

In their model, Giger and Davidhizar advocate the use of specific interview questions during a cultural assessment of each variable. For example, Hispanic consumers who speak English can be asked what their preferred language is and, if appropriate, arrangements can be made for an interpreter. The authors also suggest asking directly about issues of touch and proximity and gathering clues for communication patterns by asking questions like, "If you have something important to discuss with your family, how would you approach them?" (2004, p. 10).

Andrews and Boyle (2003, p. 533–539) developed the Transcultural Nursing Assessment Guide, which offers a

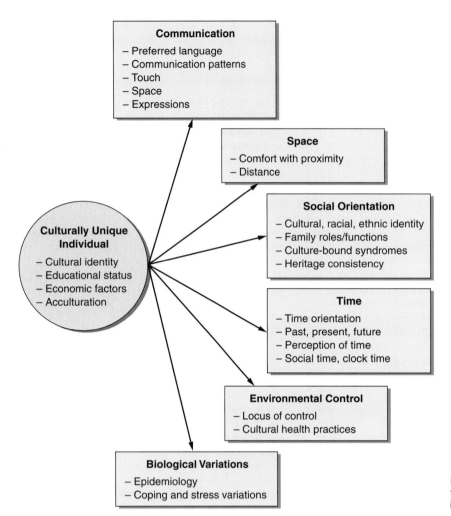

FIGURE 30-2. Giger and Davidhizar's transcultural assessment model in which each individual is seen as a culturally unique individual.

comprehensive approach to cultural assessment. It examines 13 cultural components, including cultural affiliations, values orientation, cultural sanctions and restrictions, communication, health-related beliefs and practices, nutrition, sociocultural considerations, organizations providing cultural support, educational background, religious affiliation, cultural aspects of disease incidence, biocultural variations, and developmental considerations. Andrews and Boyle propose that cultural assessment be integrated into a practitioner's overall assessment plan. Occupational therapists intending to apply this framework should examine where the components identified in Andrews and Boyle's transcultural assessment guide best fit their occupational therapy assessment process. Selected components from the assessment and potential questions for occupational therapists to employ are included in Table 30-3.

Kleinman (1988) suggests that a critical step for intervening in a culturally responsive manner is to assess the person's worldview and explanatory models for their illness. The basic question to consider is, how does the person see the world and his or her place in it? Explanatory models, or informal descriptions that consumers and their families have about an illness episode, can be helpful in answering this question and understanding the consumer's culture and life experiences.

Kleinman proposed three simple questions to elicit a consumer's explanatory model: "What do you think is wrong?

What caused it? What do you want me to do?" (1988, p. 239). Two follow-up questions include, "What is the chief way this illness (or treatment) has affected your life? What do you fear most about this illness (or treatment)?" (p. 239). Much of an occupational therapist's explanatory model for mental illness is based on his or her formal training. For example, consider a diagnosis of depression. What causes the disorder? What influences its onset? How is it experienced in a person's body? What is its course, and how do you predict the future course? What influences whether or not a person improves? How is it most likely to affect a person's life? If you reflect on your answers to these questions, you will undoubtedly find that your responses are informed by your education, life experiences, and Western biomedical perspectives. Now take these same questions and reword them using Kleinman's (1988) perspective on explanatory models. Hopefully, you will be able to understand how consumers' responses to such questions can provide a window into their lived experience of their mental illness and how their hopes, fears, and sense of control (or lack thereof) is embodied.

In order to take consumer's sociocultural context into consideration, it is essential to also assess the impact of the person's mental health problems on his or her family, work, and community. In some families, mental illness is perceived

Table 30-3 ● **Transcultural Assessment Components**

Component	Cultural Data to Collect	Sample Assessment Questions
Communication	• Preferred language • Need for interpreter • Styles of verbal/nonverbal communication	• What language do you speak at home? • What is a good distance when you are communicating with family or friends? Is this a comfortable distance between us now?
Cultural sanctions and restrictions	• Perspectives on the expression of emotions • Issues related to gender • Restrictions related to touch or specific topics	• Can you tell me about ways that people in your family talk about depression, anxiety, and so on? • In your culture, are their restrictions on topics we discuss or the ways we work together that I should know about?
Kinship and social networks	• Consumer's social network • Family influence on health behaviors • Roles in decision making	• How does your family respond when someone in the family is ill? • Are there people who help you cope when you are going through a difficult time? What do they do to help?
Health-related beliefs and practices	• Explanatory models of illness • Cultural group's view on mental disorders • Cultural healers or practices	• What do you think caused your illness? • When someone in your family has this illness, are there certain things you do, foods you eat, or healers you see to get better?

and addressed as the isolated illness state of the individual, but in many others, it is a social, family, and community matter. In a broader sociocultural context, the family's beliefs about emotional problems and mental illness, the way similar problems have been handled in the family, and the manner in which decisions about care are made and communicated within the family all become part of a comprehensive cultural assessment.

The need to use culturally responsive interaction skills in interview and intervention sessions has been suggested by several authors (Bonder, Martin, & Miracle, 2002; Ivey & Ivey, 2003; Sue & Sue, 2003). The goal is to solicit detailed information in a nonthreatening manner and with an intentional culturally relevant perspective. A practitioner can take a cue by approaching the person in an interpersonal style that is consistent with the client's own style and/or that is consistent with the interpersonal style of other people in the client's life.

One final perspective on applying cultural skills is the ETHNIC framework proposed by Levin, Like, and Gottlieb (2000). *ETHNIC* serves as a mnemonic device for critical questions to consider in the assessment process and specific culturally responsive strategies to integrate into the intervention process. Table 30-4 provides an overview of the ETHNIC framework.

Engaging Others

Engaging others who are culturally different is a process whereby practitioners actively seek to encounter consumers and other individuals who are culturally different from them. These encounters allow the practitioner to develop their cultural awareness, apply cultural skills, and generate cultural knowledge. By engaging others, practitioners ultimately increase their capacity to provide culturally responsive care. Critical self-evaluative questions that practitioners can ask themselves are, "How often do I engage consumers from diverse cultural backgrounds in face-to-face encounters? Do I put myself in environments where I am likely to encounter people who are culturally different than myself?" (Campinha-Bacote, 2003). It is often easier for practitioners to learn about other cultures through reading, watching films, or other passive means; however, actively engaging others provides substantial opportunities for multicultural learning.

Practitioners should recognize that encounters are not always harmonious. Engaging others can result in a clash

Table 30-4 ● **ETHNIC Framework for Culturally Competent Assessment and Intervention**

Framework	Strategies for Assessment and Intervention
Explanation	*Assess explanatory models:* Why do you think you might have this problem? Why do you think these problems started when they did? What do friends and family say about your symptoms?
Treatments	*Elicit person's beliefs about treatment:* Are there things you do to stay healthy (e.g., things you eat, drink, do or avoid doing)? What kinds of things have helped in the past? Are their medicines or home treatments your family or friends suggest?
Healers	*Determine use of cultural healers:* Are there healers that you or others in your family or neighborhood use when you become ill? Have you sought this person's advice? Are you comfortable telling me about these treatments? May I speak with this healer?
Negotiate	*Involve person in planning for assessment and intervention:* Make intervention planning an active, collaborative process; suggest and have the person suggest culturally relevant intervention options that incorporate the person's beliefs.
Intervention	*Incorporate culturally meaningful intervention activities:* Integrate culturally relevant occupations (e.g., cooking, dressing, leisure) and cultural healing activities and healers.
Collaboration	*Work in partnership with the person and his or her family:* Actively consider and integrate all cultural resources in the person's network (family, friends, spiritual leaders, cultural healers) and collaborate with other team members.

between the practitioner's and the consumer's cultural values or perceptions. In the study by Muñoz (2002), experienced practitioners shared incidents in which they failed to interpret or they misinterpreted cultural information about the consumer or they faced a difficult clinical choice due to differences in cultural perceptions, attitudes, or behaviors between them and the consumer or their families. Engaging others is a critical aspect of making connections. Practitioners in this study consistently sought opportunities outside their day-to-day clinical practices to engage others who were culturally different. These encounters supported them as they developed their capacity to become fully aware of themselves and others as cultural beings. It was through engaging others that a practitioner tested the depths and recognized the limits of his or her cultural knowledge and practiced and developed cultural skills for connecting and responding. Without engagement, a practitioner's journey toward multicultural understanding could be hampered.

Exploring Multiculturalism

Exploring multiculturalism is a reflective process whereby practitioners demonstrate a desire and intentional drive to broaden their cultural understanding and continue their own journey toward multiculturalism. In her model of cultural competence, Campinha-Bacote (2003) defines this intentional drive as "cultural desire," the practitioner "wanting to" go out and be curious about other people and other cultures. Your attitudes and actions relative to multiculturalism reflect your spirit of exploration: if you have a

tendency to be fascinated by cultural aspects of humanity and a passion for actively seeking knowledge about different cultures, then you have a strong drive to explore multiculturalism. Participation in the multicultural journey is motivated by a practitioner's cultural desire and commitment to learn about people from different cultures. As such, exploration is a purposeful act that is grounded in the practitioner's commitment to address culture in clinical practice as a means of providing the most efficacious service to clients. In many models of cultural competency, the ultimate manifestation of this spirit of exploration and cultural desire is to engage in social action that works to eliminate injustices such as racism, stigma, and poverty (Sue et al, 1992; Wurzel, 1998).

Summary

Culture is intimately intertwined with our identity, so much so that often we are unaware of our own cultural background, beliefs, rituals, and routines. This is particularly true of those who make up the dominant culture and/or when there is limited exposure to different cultures. Likewise, culture is embedded in occupational performance. Culture influences values and choice for particular occupations, the manner in which we participate, the people who share in our occupations, and the ways in which we evaluate our performance. Effective occupational therapy intervention requires a deep appreciation for culture and the unique nature of cultural expression for each individual.

Active Learning Strategies

1. The Culture of Occupational Therapy

Culture is a shared system of concepts and knowledge that influences our behavior. If you are an occupational therapy student, you are currently in a process of being socialized into the profession: you are learning the occupational therapy culture. You also are likely to come in contact with students from other disciplines. Consider the following questions:

Reflective Questions
- What are characteristics of the occupational therapy culture?
- How have you been enculturated?
- How is physical therapy culture like occupational therapy culture?
- Do pharmacy majors look at the world through a different lens than health science majors?

 Capture your responses to these questions in your **Reflective Journal**.

2. Examining Cultural Identity

Cultural identity refers to the culture you identify with and that you look to for standards for your behavior (Cooper &

Denner, 1998). Write a description of your cultural identity, then reflect on the following questions. After you have considered each question, pair up with a peer, share your description of your culture, and compare your responses.

Reflective Questions
- What was my first or most automatic thought when I started this task?
- How did I experience the task? How difficult did I find the task? Why was it simple or hard for me?
- What aspects of my identity did I automatically include in my description? What cultural lenses did I look through?
- What aspects of my identity took more reflection to include or were not included?
- What aspects of identity are the same as or different from those my peer chose to include in his or her description?

 Capture your responses to these questions in your **Reflective Journal**.

3. The Impact of Culture on Behavior

What if we used a multicultural lens to understand and situate behavior in multicultural context? Read and reflect on the following questions and write brief answers to each of them. These questions are designed to help you examine how you have come to think about what constitutes normal and abnormal behavior and to consider the impact of culture on behavior. For each question, try to provide an example that helps explain your response. When you have responded to each question, pair up with a peer and compare your responses.

Reflective Questions

- What constitutes abnormal behavior, and how have I learned to define what constitutes normality?
- What assumptions underlie the conceptual models I use to understand the behavior of others?
- How might contextual issues in contemporary U.S. society, such as racism, poverty, homophobia, or violence, influence human experience and behavior?
- Is it possible for a person's culture to affect his or her perception of reality?
- How might culture influence a person's experience of stress and the coping strategies he or she uses?
- In what ways might culture impact the duration, course, or outcome of mental illness?
- Can culture influence the kinds of problems a person reports or the meaning a person attaches to these problems?

 Capture your responses to these questions in your Reflective Journal.

4. Context and Mental Illness

Reread the definition of culture-bound syndromes and review the list of culture-bound syndromes in Table 30-2. Review the essential features of anorexia nervosa in the DSM-IV-TR or online. Google "chronic fatigue syndrome" and/or examine the definitions of this disorder in Wikipedia. Then, working with a peer, create two lists:

- List 1: Why anorexia nervosa and chronic fatigue syndrome *should be* considered culture-bound syndromes.
- List 2: Why anorexia nervosa and chronic fatigue syndrome *should not be* considered culture-bound syndromes.

Share your lists with your peers. What do you find are the most convincing arguments? Is one diagnosis easier than the other to define as a culture-bound syndrome?

5. Applying the Culture-Emergent Model

Reconsider the five assumptions of the culture-emergent model:
1. Culture is learned.
2. Culture is localized.
3. Culture is patterned.
4. Culture is evaluative.
5. Culture is persistent but incorporates change.

In your **Reflective Journal**, consider your own family culture:

- Think of, and write down, a story that reflects cultural learning (i.e., one that illustrates how you were socialized

to think about relationships, self-responsibility, motivation, how to handle disappointment or loss, or ways of coping and dealing with stressful situations).
- Provide an example of a personally meaningful environment where your family culture is localized.
- Identify a recurrent ritual in your family life cycle and consider the significance of this ritual in shaping your cultural identity.
- List the top three family values that you feel were communicated to you in the behavior of your family of origin.
- Identify what you feel may be the most significant changes that may have occurred in your cultural identity in the past 3 years (as a result of your cultural encounters).

6. Applying the Kawa Model

Consider the idea that life is a river:
- If life is like a river, what is a drought in one's life?
- If life is like a river, how can we think about the currents in river of life?
- If like is like a river, what is a flood in someone's life river?
- If your life is a river, would you rather be a meandering stream or a forceful rapid?

Now, create a drawing that depicts your current life situation as a river.
- Draw the floor and sidewalls of your life's river. In the floor and sidewalls, embed the names of
  - People who provide you with the most support—true friends.
  - People who provide you with material support and resources.
  - Places you frequent that build you up, refresh or replenish you, inspire or direct you.
- Somewhere along the bottom or the sides, draw the rocks. Label each rock as a problem or difficulty you are currently experiencing.
  - Draw as many or as few rocks as you like.
  - Make the size of each rock relative to the degree of impediment these problems create in your life.
- Draw driftwood in your river to represent your assets.
  - Label the driftwood with some of your best features or characteristics.
  - Label other driftwood as some of your most important skills/attributes.
- Now focus on the spaces between the floor, walls, rocks, and driftwood.
  - Label these spaces with the occupations in your life that hold the most meaning for you.
  - Be judicious and include only those things that are important for you to carry on no matter what life throws at you; these are things that are the essence of you.

Look at what you have created and, if you feel comfortable, share the picture with a peer. Do you think you could use the metaphor of life as a river as a way to help you consider a person in sociocultural context?

Resources

Books

- Gielen, U. P., Fish, J. M., & Draguns, J. G. (2004). *Handbook of Culture, Therapy and Healing.* Mahwah, NJ: Erlbaum. This informative collection of works written by authors from diverse fields such as psychology, anthropology, sociology, comparative religion, and nursing explores the convergence of culture, healing, and psychotherapy.
- Illovsky, M. E. (2003). *Mental Health Professionals, Minorities and the Poor.* New York: Brunner-Routledge. Illovsky defines this book as a "think about what you are doing" text that seeks to inform readers about issues in mental health specific to therapeutic interventions with minorities and people living in poverty. The book offers alternatives to standard care practices and sections devoted to sexual orientation minorities, minorities with disabilities, ethnic minority children, women and elders, and minorities in rural America.
- Murphy-Berman, V., & Berman, J. J. (2003). *Cross-Cultural Differences in Perspectives on the Self: Volume 49 of the Nebraska Symposium on Motivation.* Lincoln: University of Nebraska Press. This text examines cultural differences in models of psychological agency, motivations for self-improvement, choice, and intrinsic motivation and offers a cross-cultural perspective of Maslow's theory of self-actualization.
- Peacock, J. L. (1988). *The Anthropological Lens: Harsh Light, Soft Focus.* Cambridge: Cambridge University Press. This text on cultural anthropologies may help readers expand their use of multiple cultural lenses when examining culture and cultural identity. The author uses examples and storytelling to clearly describe concepts of race and culture while providing practical strategies that may help health professionals intentionally consider culture and cultural identity in all phases of their interventions.
- Royeen, A. M., & Crabtree, J. L. (2006). *Culture in Rehabilitation: From Competency to Proficiency.* Upper Saddle River, NJ: Pearson Education. This text covers a broad range of ethnic and cultural groups, including explorations of cultural issues related to poverty, gender, age, and sexual orientation. Multiple case stories help readers apply cultural considerations to rehabilitation practice.
- Wong, P. T., & Wong, L. C. (2006). *Handbook of Multicultural Perspectives on Stress and Coping.* New York: Springer Science and Business Media. This collection of works examines theoretical and methodological issues related to understanding stress and coping cross-culturally; it includes descriptive chapters on acculturative stress, coping and resilience, and work-related issues from a cross-cultural perspective.

Websites

- American Anthropology Association offers an excellent discussion of race, called *Race—Are We So Different?* http://www.understandingrace.com/home.html
- Diversity Rx provides models of practices that support culturally competent care and resources to help you understand policy and legal issues that impact the quality of health care for minority, immigrant, and ethnically diverse communities: http://www.diversityrx.org/HTML/DIVRX.htm
- Mind Freedom International is an organization advocating for the human rights of mental health consumers and promoting humane alternatives in mental health. Many of its members have personally experienced the mental health system: http://www.mindfreedom.org
- The National Center for Cultural Competence website provides a wealth of information about cultural and linguistic competence. Among other things, you will find information about conceptual frameworks for cultural competency, tools for assessing your own cultural competence, and practical resources to support cross cultural care for children, adults, and families: http://www11.georgetown.edu/research/gucchd/nccc
- The Office of Minority Health website is maintained by the U.S. Department of Health and Human Services and includes a wealth of information about minority health. The site includes newsletters, publications, statistics, and links to federal government clearinghouses and information centers and has a separate section addressing cultural competence: http://www.omhrc.gov
- The Stanford Geriatric Education Center has a unique site dedicated to multidisciplinary ethnogeriatric education. There are resources here for educators and practitioners, training and intervention materials, research findings, and policy analysis: http://sgec.stanford.edu

References

American Psychiatric Association. (2000). *Diagnostic and Statistical Manual of Mental Disorders: DSM-IV-TR* (4th ed., text rev.). Washington, DC: Author.

American Psychological Association. (2002). *Guidelines on Multicultural Education, Training, Research, Practice and Organizational Change for Psychologists.* Washington, DC: Author. Available at: http://www.apa.orgpi/multiculturalguidelines.pdf (accessed February 2, 2007).

Andrews, M., & Boyle, J. (2003). *Transcultural Concepts in Nursing Care* (3rd ed.). Philadelphia: Lippincott.

Arredondo, P., & Toporek, R. (2004). Multicultural counseling competencies = ethical practice. *Journal of Mental Health Counseling, 7,* 44–55.

Beals, J., Novins, D. K., Mitchell, C., Shore, J. H., & Manson, S. M. (2001). Comorbidity between alcohol abuse/dependence and psychiatric disorders: Prevalence, treatment implications and new directions among American Indian populations. In P. Mail (Ed.), *National Institute on Alcohol Abuse and Alcoholism Monograph.* Washington, DC: U.S. Government Printing Office.

Bonder, B., Martin, L., & Miracle, A. (2002). *Culture in CLINICAL CARE.* Thorofare, NJ: Slack.

Campinha-Bacote, J. (2003) *The Process of Cultural Competence in the Delivery of Healthcare Services,* 4th ed. Cincinnati: Transcultural C.A.R.E. Associates.

Cartwright, S. A. (1851). Report on the diseases and physical peculiarities of the Negro race. *New Orleans Medical and Surgical Journal,* 691–715. Reprinted in A. Caplan, T. Engelhardt, & J. McCartney (Eds.), *Concepts of Health and Disease in Medicine: Interdisciplinary Perspectives.* Boston: Addison-Wesley, 1980.

Cauce, A. M., Paradise, M., Domeneche-Rodriquez, M., Cochran, B. N., Shea, J. M., Srebnik, D., & Baydar, N. (2002). Cultural and contextual influences in mental health help seeking: A focus on ethnic minority youth. *Journal of Counseling and Clinical Psychology, 70*(1), 44–55.

Chernoff, N. N. (2002). NIMH study: Blacks mentally healthier. *American Psychological Society, 15,* 21–36.

Clark, R., Anderson, N. B., Clark, V. R., & Williams, D. R. (1999). Racism as a stressor for African Americans. *American Psychologist, 54,* 805–816.

Cloutterbuck, J., & Zhan, L. (2005). Ethnic elders. In K. D. Melillo & S. C. Houde (Eds.), *Geropsychiatric and Mental Health Nursing* (pp. 69–86). Sudbury, MA: Jones and Bartlett.

Cokley, K. O. (2005). Racial(ized) identity, ethnic identity, and Afrocentric values: Conceptual and methodological challenges in understanding African American identity. *Journal of Counseling Psychology, 52,* 4 517–526.

Cooper, C. R., & Denner, J. (1998). Theories linking culture and psychopathology: Universal and community-specific processes. *Annual Review of Psychology, 49,* 559–584.

Dunn, T. W., Smith, T. B., & Montoya, J. A. (2006). Multicultural competency instrumentation: A review and analysis of reliability generalization. *Journal of Counseling and Development, 84,* 471–482.

Fabrega, H. (2004). Culture and the origins of psychotherapy. In U. P. Gielen, J. M. Fish, & J. G. Draguns (Eds.), *Handbook of Culture, Therapy and Healing* (pp. 15 –35). Mahwah, NJ: Erlbaum.

Ford, M. E., & Kelly, P. A. (2005) Conceptualizing and categorizing race and ethnicity in health services research. *Health Services Research, 40,* 5, 1658–1675.

Giger, J., & Davidhizar, R. (2004). *Transcultural Nursing: Assessment and Intervention.* St. Louis: Mosley Year Book.

Green, A. R., Ngo-Metzger, Q., Legedza, A., Massagli, M. P., Phillips, R. S., & Iezzoni, L. I. (2005). Interpreter services, language concordance, and health care quality: Experiences of Asian Americans with limited English proficiency. *Journal of General Internal Medicine, 20,* 11, 1050–1056.

Guarnaccia, P. J., & Rogler, L. H. (1999). Research on culture-bound syndromes: New directions. *American Journal of Psychiatry, 156*(9), 1322–1327.

Helman, C. G. (1994). *Culture, Health and Illness: An Introduction for Health Professionals* (3rd ed.). Oxford, UK: Butterworth-Heinemann.

Institute of Medicine. (2003). *Unequal Treatment: Confronting Racial and Ethnic Disparities in Healthcare.* Washington, DC: National Academies Press.

Ivey, A. E., & Ivey, M. B. (2003). *Intentional Interviewing and Counseling: Facilitating Client Development in a Multicultural Society.* Pacific Grove, CA: Brooks/Cole.

Iwama, M. K. (2005). The kawa (river) model: Nature, life flow, and the power of culturally relevant occupational therapy. In F. Kronenberg, S. Algado, & N. Pollard (Eds.), *Occupational Therapy Without Borders: Learning from the Spirit of Survivors* (pp. 213–237). Edinburough: Elsevier Churchill Livingstone.

Jungerson, K. (1992). Culture, theory and the practice of occupational therapy in New Zealand/Aoteareo. *American Journal of Occupational Therapy, 46,* 745–750.

Kress, V. E., Eriksen, K. P., Rayle, A. D., & Wood, S. J. (2005). The DSM-IV-TR and culture: Considerations for counselors. *Journal of Counseling and Development, 83*(1), 97–104.

Kleinman A. (1988). *The Illness Narratives: Suffering, Healing and the Human Condition.* New York: Basic Books.

Leininger, M. (1997). Transcultural nursing research to nursing education and practice: 40 years. *Image Journal of Nursing Scholarship, 29*(4), 341–347.

———. (2002). Culture care theory: A major contribution to advance transcultural nursing knowledge and practices. *Journal of Transcultural Nursing, 13*(3), 189–192.

Levin, S. J., Like, R. C., & Gottlieb, J. E. (2000). ETHNIC: A framework for culturally competent clinical practice. *Patient Care, 34*(9), 188–189.

Lopez, S. J., Edwards, L. M., Pedrotti, J. T., Prosser, E. C., LaRue, S., Spalitto, S. V., & Ulven, J. C. (2006). Beyond the DSM-IV: Assumptions, alternatives and alterations. *Journal of Counseling & Development,84,* 259–267.

Manoleas, P., Organista, K., Negron-Velasquez, G., & McCormick, K. (2000). Characteristics of Latino mental health clinicians: A preliminary examination. *Community Mental Health Journal, 36,* 383–394.

Matsumoto, D. (2006). Culture and cultural worldviews: Do verbal descriptions about culture reflect anything other than verbal descriptions of culture? *Culture and Psychology, 12*(1), 33–62.

Muñoz, J. (2002). *Culturally responsive caring in occupational therapy: A grounded theory.* Unpublished doctoral dissertation, University of Pittsburgh, Pittsburgh.

Owens, K., & King, M. C. (1999). Genomic views of human history. *Science, 286,* 451–453.

Pahl, K., & Way, N. (2006). Longitudinal trajectories of ethnic identity among urban black and Latino adolescents. *Child Development, 77*(5), 1403–1415.

Paniagua, F. A. (2001). *Diagnosis in Multicultural Context: A Casebook for Mental Health Practitioners.* Thousand Oaks: Sage.

Phan, T. (2000). Investigating the use of services for Vietnamese with mental illness. *Journal of Community Health, 25*(5), 411–425.

Pumariega, A. J., Rothe, E., & Pumariega, J. B. (2005). Mental health of immigrants and refugees. *Community Mental Health Journal, 41*(5), 581–597.

Purnell, L. D. (2002). The Purnell model for cultural competence. *Journal of Transcultural Nursing, 13*(3), 193–196.

Purnell, L. D., & Paulanka, B. J. (2003). *Transcultural Health Care: A Culturally Competent Approach* (2nd ed.). Philadelphia: F. A. Davis.

Robins, L., & Reiger, D. A. (1991). *Psychiatric Disorders in America: The Epidemiologic Catchment Area Study.* New York: The Free Press.

Roysircai-Sodowsky, G. R., & Maestas, M. V. (2000). Acculturation, ethnic identity, and acculturative stress: Evidence and measurement. In R. H. Dana (Ed.), *Handbook of Cross-Cultural and Muticultural Assessment* (pp. 131–172). Mahwah, NJ: Erlbaum.

Spector, R. E. (2004). *Culture Care: Guide to Heritage Assessment and Health Traditions* (3rd ed.). Upper Saddle River, NJ: Prentice Hall.

Sue, D. W., Arredondo, P., & McDavis, R. J. (1992). Multicultural competencies/standards: A pressing need. *Journal of Counseling and Development, 70*(4), 477–486.

Sue, D. W, & Sue, D. (2003). *Counseling the Culturally Different* (4th ed.). New York: Wiley.

Sue, S. (2006). Cultural competency: From philosophy to research and practice. *Journal of Community Psychology, 34*(2), 237–245.

Sue, S., & Chu, J. Y. (2003). The mental health of ethnic minority groups: Challenges posed by the supplement to the surgeon general's report on mental health. *Culture, Medicine and Psychiatry, 27,* 447–465.

Takeuchi, D. T., Chung, R. C., Lin, K., Kuraski, S. K., Chun, C., & Sue, S. (1998). Lifetime and twelve-month prevalence rates of major depressive episodes and dysthymia among Chinese Americans in Los Angeles. *American Journal of Psychiatry, 155,* 1407–1414.

U.S. Census Bureau. (2005). Texas becomes nation's newest "majority-minority" state. *U.S. Census Bureau News,* U.S. Department of Commerce, August 11, 2005. Available at: http://www.census.gov/PressRelease/www/releases/archives/population/005514.html (accessed March 2, 2007).

———. (2006). *Nation's population one-third minority.* U.S. Census Bureau News, U.S. Department of Commerce, May 10, 2006. Available at: http://www.census.gov/Press-Release/www/releases/archives/population/006808.html (accessed March 2, 2007).

———. (2008). Race data. Available at: http://www.census.gov/population/www/socdemo/race/racefactcb.html (accessed December 22, 2009).

U.S. Department of Health and Human Services (USDHHS). (1999). *Mental health: A report of the surgeon general.* Rockville, MD: author, Public Health Service, Office of the Surgeon General. Available at: http://www.surgeongeneral.gov/library (accessed November 14, 2006).

———. (2001a). *Mental Health: Culture, Race and Ethnicity—A Supplement to Mental health: A Report of the Surgeon General.* Rockville, MD: Author, Public Health Service, Office of the Surgeon General. Available at: http://www.surgeongeneral.gov/library (accessed January 26, 2007).

———. (2001b). *National Standards for Culturally and Linguistically Appropriate Services in Health Care: Final Report.* Washington, DC: Author. Available at: http://www.omhrc.gov/assets/pdf/checked/finalreport.pdf (accessed April 5, 2009).

————. (2003). *Achieving the Promise: Transforming Mental Health Care in America, Final Report.* President's New Freedom Commission on Mental Health. Rockville, MD: Author, National Health Information Center. Available at: http://www.mentalhealthcommission.gov (accessed December 2, 2006).

Wallace, D. W. (1995). *Education for Extinction: American Indians and the Boarding School Experience 1875–1928.* Lawrence: University Press of Kansas.

Wurzel, J. (1988). The multicultural world. In J. S. Wurzel (Ed.), *Toward Multiculturalism: A Reader in Multicultural Education* (pp. 2–10). Yarmouth, ME: Intercultural Press.

Yeo, G. (Ed.). (2000). *Core Curriculum in Ethnogeriatrics* (2nd ed.). Palo Alto, CA: Stanford Geriatric Center.

Zenner, W. (1996). Ethnicity. In D. Levinson & M. Ember (Eds.), *Encyclopedia of Cultural Anthropology* (pp. 393–395). New York: Henry Holt and Company.

The Spiritual Environment

Mary Egan and Suzette Phillips

> "The best of modern therapy is much like a process of shared meditation. . . . In this joint meditation, the therapist joins in the listening, sensing, and feeling and may direct the client toward ways to pay a deeper attention to the roots of his or her suffering, entanglements, and difficulty.
>
> —Jack Kornfield, 1993, p. 245.

Introduction

The lived experience of mental illness often includes a crisis related to self-identity and meaning (Wisdom, Bruce, Saedi, Weis, & Green, 2008). It is through recovery that individuals can create a positive sense of self and find meaning for their lives. Marcia Murphy (1998) provides a poignant account of her own struggle, which includes the following:

> An integral part of my recovery has been my search and discovery of meaning for my life. This is a philosophical and psychological issue that goes beyond mere chemical imbalances in the brain. In this search I have developed a new worldview. (p. 188)

This emerging worldview points to the reality of a spiritual environment within the heart, mind, and experience of every person. Meaning in life, the core of an individual's sense of self and purpose, is to be found within this rich and mysterious environment.

The importance of spirituality in the recovery of those struggling with mental illness has been increasingly recognized. This is evidenced by the inclusion of spirituality in key occupational therapy documents such as the "Occupational Therapy Practice Framework" (American Occupational Therapy Association [AOTA], 2002) and the Canadian model of occupational performance (Law, Polatajko, Baptiste, & Townsend, 1997). Consideration of the client's spiritual environment as well as the incorporation of the spiritual domain into occupational therapy practice is therefore necessitated. Yet therapists are often unsure how to address this component of human experience and occupation.

Surveys of occupational therapists in the United States and Britain have demonstrated that although occupational therapists believe that spirituality is important to health and rehabilitation, few therapists were confident addressing this area in practice or were certain that spirituality was within their scope of practice (Belcham, 2004; Enquist, Short-DeGraff, Gliner, & Oltjenbruns, 1997; Rose, 1999; Udell & Chandler, 2000). One barrier to the inclusion of spirituality in practice is a lack of education and training (Belcham, 2004; Thompson & MacNeil, 2006). This chapter, along with Chapter 54, addresses the educational needs of occupational therapists.

This chapter heightens the awareness of occupational therapists to integral elements of the spiritual dimension, particularly as regards the individual struggling with mental illness, the person or the therapist working with the client, and the therapeutic environment in which therapy is offered. It is hoped that the information provided will equip occupational therapists with resources that support their inclusion of spiritual considerations as a component of their practice.

In this chapter, various aspects of the spiritual environment—that worldview and personal outlook held by each person that gives life a sense of meaning or meaninglessness—are considered. An occupational therapist might wish to consider these elements when attempting to explore and understand the client's worldview and identify interventions that may promote recovery. In addition, this chapter describes the importance of the therapist's awareness of his or her own spiritual context. Questions that the occupational therapist may use for self-reflection are offered.

To accomplish its aim, the chapter considers the place of spirituality in the process of recovery, presents a definition of the spiritual environment, reflects on ways in which recovery can be supported by the spiritual environment, identifies various components of the person's spiritual environment, describes influences on the spiritual context, explores ways in which an occupational therapist might explore the spiritual context with a client, suggests avenues through which a therapist might come to understand his or her own spiritual environment, describes practice structures that support recovery, and identifies ways in which the spiritual environment may be considered from an evidence-based perspective.

The Place of Spirituality in Recovery

Spirituality holds an important place in the process of recovery from a mental illness. In fact, spirituality is often recognized as a key component of recovery (Bussema & Bussema, 2007).

In a review of several first-person accounts, Andresen, Oades, and Caputi (2003) described the components of recovery as (1) finding hope, (2) reestablishing identity, (3) finding meaning in life, and (4) taking responsibility for recovery. For many individuals, both with and without mental illness, hope, meaning, and identity are derived from some spiritual source.

Spiritual practices are clearly associated with improved outcomes for people living with mental illness. Tepper, Rogers, Coleman, and Malony (2001) found that 80% of individuals with mental illness relied on religious coping methods and that these practices appeared to reduce symptoms. Another study found that individuals with a higher frequency of religious attendance demonstrated fewer suicide attempts (Rasic et al, 2009). In the general population, participation in spiritual practices is associated with a reduction in mortality even when behavioral factors such as smoking, drinking, and exercise are taken into consideration (Chida, Steptoe, & Powell, 2009).

Defining the Spiritual Environment

The environment in which a client finds himself or herself provides the context for everyday activity. In occupational therapy, we are very familiar with the physical context of occupation, particularly in terms of the impact of architectural barriers on participation in meaningful activities (Stark, 2004). Increasingly, we are learning to consider social, cultural, and political contexts and their effects on occupation (Letts, Rigby, & Stewart, 2003; Townsend, 1997). Close examination of these contexts reveals their interdependence. For example, the built physical environment is shaped by social, cultural, and political ideas. Likewise, the natural physical environment affects social relationships, molds cultural artifacts (e.g., art, sports, and folklore), and shapes all levels of political life.

But what is the **spiritual context** of daily activity? When spiritual terms are used in occupational therapy, they generally refer to something inside the person (as in spirituality) or to issues beyond the realm of material concerns (as in spiritual needs or issues) (Egan & Swedersky, 2003). Does a spiritual environment exist, though? If the term *spiritual* is used to refer to immaterial or abstract aspects of context, what would *not* be included? Clearly, we can acknowledge a spiritual environment only if we keep in mind the interdependence of all aspects of the environment and view it as the context that includes action, ideas, feelings, and beliefs.

Defining and addressing the **spiritual environment**, however, is challenging. As professionals who wish to provide the best care possible, occupational therapists have a tendency to look for definitions and guidelines that will help us understand what we are dealing with and master at least enough knowledge to allow us to competently and comfortably address various components of the person—including the spiritual context. When entering into the spiritual environment, however, definitions and guidelines are somewhat more difficult to articulate and delineate.

As described previously, the spiritual context includes action, ideas, feelings, and beliefs that affect a person's daily life and relationships. It consists of both the individual's internal world and his or her external practices that are revealed in word and action. Some aspects of the spiritual environment—behaviors and speech—can therefore be observed and measured, whereas other elements—feelings, thoughts, ideas—can only be subjectively related to the therapist by the client. This can make it difficult for the therapist, particularly when exploring the client's internal world. Despite the challenges, addressing the spiritual component as one of many important and interdependent aspects of the individual's context can contribute to practice that more fully addresses the needs of the individual.

In entering into the client's spiritual environment, occupational therapists are encouraged to reflect on the complexity of this dimension and on the fact that we are discussing realities that often defy language and will remain for us largely unknowable and incomprehensible. Perhaps the best we can do is listen and appreciate that there is an enormous diversity of contexts, shaped by many factors that we can at best only partially understand. Trying to comprehend it is nonetheless important if not critical when supporting someone in the process of recovery.

How can the spiritual environment be more clearly described? Sandra Schneiders (1998) proposed that spirituality as subject matter or a material object—we could say the spiritual environment—is "the experience of conscious involvement in the project of life-integration through self-transcendence toward the ultimate value one perceives" (pp. 2–3). The *Occupational Therapy Practice Framework* defines the spiritual context as "the fundamental orientation of a person's life; that which inspires and motivates that individual" (AOTA, 2002, p.11). Spirituality is seen as a source of meaning. It provides the individual with a sense of purpose and connectedness to the world and others. It has been noted that for individuals with mental illness, the recovery process often involves a connection to the spiritual (Bussema & Bussema, 2007).

Another way to define the spiritual context is to consider what this environment affords the individual. As spiritual beings, all people are considered to have a spiritual context, or environment, within which their meaning in life and perspective of life (their spiritual outlook, or "lens") is formulated (Figure 31-1). The spiritual environment provides a framework through which individuals attempt to do the following:

- Accept, make sense of, and find meaning in life.
- Resolve loss and grief issues.
- Understand and relate to oneself and others.
- Solve problems.
- Make life decisions.
- Cope with struggles.
- Embrace joys.
- Adjust to change.
- Find strength.
- Face fears.
- Become vulnerable.
- Dedicate oneself to something or someone beyond one's self.

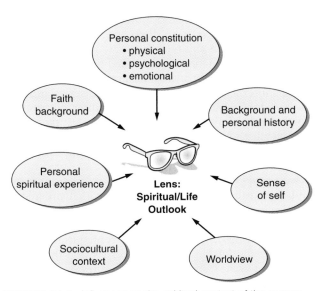

FIGURE 31-1. Influences on the spiritual context of the person.

Supporting Recovery Through Considering the Spiritual Environment

A goal of this textbook is to describe occupational therapy practice that best supports recovery. Recovery can be viewed as a lifelong process of learning, growth, and transcendence—a

process that occurs as much because of the presence of mental illness as it does in spite of it (Liebrich, 2002). Within supportive environments, people embrace their own strengths and weaknesses and, in doing so, accept who they are and realize their potential (Vanier, 1998). Ideally, occupational therapists are part of such a supportive environment.

Occupational therapists contribute to the formation of a supportive environment through three interrelated processes:

1. They listen for the uniqueness of the person.
2. They study their own contexts to ensure that their ideas, feelings, and beliefs do not become barriers to clearly understanding who the other person is and what he or she is experiencing.
3. They work to develop and maintain practice structures that allow and encourage recovery.

As you learn about these processes, we encourage you to use them as a springboard for your own exploration of the spiritual context of occupational therapy.

Listening for the Uniqueness of the Person

Within occupational therapy, every person is considered to be spiritual; that is, he or she is unique and truly human. The spirit is the deepest, most authentic component of the self, and it is expressed in actions and speech within relational and social contexts. Recognizing people as spiritual beings involves appreciating the intrinsic value of each person and respecting the other's life experiences, relationships, beliefs,

The Lived Experience

Jeff D.

Jeff experiences episodes of depression, anxiety, and agoraphobia. He shares how his lending a hand to others through volunteer work provides him with a sense of purpose, meaning, and hope. He finds that sharing his story allows other people to respect, understand, and accept him.

When I was young, I was bullied in schoolyards and laughed at by my schoolmates. My teachers and parents didn't do much to support me; they didn't know how to, I guess. I always felt like an outsider, never fitting in. I couldn't share my pain or my thoughts with anyone—no one knew me . . . no one understood the pain I felt inside.

I grew to fear being in crowds and felt different, unacceptable, and awkward. Anxiety would overcome me when I left the house, let alone if I had to talk with anyone. I felt this way despite my deep longing to be with people . . . to have real friends. And so I sat alone and in fear within the walls of my parents' home.

One day, a house build for Habitat for Humanity was advertised. A cousin of mine let me know about it and asked if I'd be up to going with him to check it out. I'd never done any carpentry work before, so I was uneasy—but somehow, nonetheless, mustered the courage to say yes. On the way to the building site, he told me about the family who had been selected to have the

house. It almost brought me to tears as the youngsters were just like me—bullied and ostracized. Something made me want to make a difference for them.

Arriving at the build site, anxiety started to rise, as there were many people around. One gentleman, the build captain, however, saw my cousin and me standing on the periphery of the group and personally approached us. He made me feel welcome and was grateful for my being there. He introduced us to the family—the youngsters. Though they were shy, I could tell that they too were grateful for us being there.

The captain gave my cousin and me each a carpenter's apron, a hard hat, some gloves, and a hammer. After showing us exactly what to do so that we couldn't help but do it right, we started framing walls and then, a few hours later, lifted them into place to the applause of the crowd. Watching the faces of the youngsters was incredible; feeling a tremendous sense of pride and contribution was amazing. All of a sudden I felt alive. I felt value, worth, and possibility. I touched hope.

Though it was difficult to face the anxiety and fear the next day, the feelings and experience of lending a hand moved me enough to push beyond it, and have each day since. That house was built with many hands—mine included. And so was the next, and the next. And each family, each kid, had a brighter future because of it . . . and so do I.

values, and goals—regardless of ability, age, or other characteristics (Townsend, 1997).

Within a therapeutic context, it is essential that the spiritual component of the person be respected, thereby validating the personhood of the client. "When our personhood is honored, we feel comfortable; when it is not taken into account by others, we feel 'depersonalized'" (Buzzell & Gibbon, 1991, p. 33). For individuals who struggle with mental illness, personhood and the spiritual have often been dishonored, which contributes to a compromised sense of self. For example, when an individual's personal views (perhaps his or her perception of the reasons for various difficulties or of actions that are most important for wellness) are disregarded, it impresses on the person that his or her thoughts and feelings have no value. Within the recovery context, honoring what has often been devalued is critical to the healing process.

Influences on the Spiritual Context

An individual's spiritual context is influenced by multiple elements, including personal constitution (physical, psychological, and emotional), background and personal history, faith background, personal spiritual experiences, and sociocultural context. Central to this spiritual environment is the person's relationship with self, others, the world, and for some, the Transcendent. These elements collectively contribute to a sense of self and a worldview or spiritual/life outlook.

Personal Constitution

An individual's **personal constitution** involves physical, psychological, and emotional factors that influence his or her spiritual context and outlook. Age, gender, physical and physiological status, and neurological and developmental state can all affect a person's outlook. Psychological factors, including cognitive abilities, thought processes, thinking style (e.g., concrete or abstract), personality, perceptual abilities, intuition, coping styles and skills, attitudes, thoughts, memory, motivational level, and goals, likewise affect the spiritual dimension of the person. Emotional factors are also noteworthy, as are feelings, desires, degree of self-control, emotional resilience, vulnerability, and impressionability. For example, a 45-year-old male who is cognitively astute, physically healthy, able to abstract, and possesses a significant degree of self-mastery will have a very different spiritual/life outlook than a highly impressionable 18-year-old woman with a diagnosis of schizophrenia, a history of sexual abuse, little emotional resilience and resources, and poor coping skills. Both will approach and handle the spiritual context and life itself very differently.

Background and Personal History

An individual's **background and personal history** further influences his or her spiritual context. Background includes life experiences within the family of origin, extended family, neighborhood(s), school(s), spiritual community, society, and world. Within each of these elements, individuals engage in numerous relationships—which can include the self, parents, family members, friends, teachers, authorities, strangers, society, creation, and, for many, the Transcendent. Each of these relationships has its own unique dynamics, which affect the spiritual environment.

Within these contexts and amidst these relationships, people either discover who they are; develop personal strengths, skills, and abilities; and grow to trust in themselves and others, or they are restricted by limitations and inabilities and grow distrusting. As a result, life experiences in these contexts leave a person with both positive and negative "residue." Healthy, uplifting, validating occurrences support the development of the self and give people a sense of self-worth and mastery, whereas wounding, invalidating, and hurtful experiences can leave behind many emotional scars.

One study examining spirituality and schizophrenia found that feeling connected to the spiritual provided a buffer against a poor social support system and also provided a sense of control in a world that often feels uncontrollable (Mohr, Brandt, Borras, Gilleron, & Huguelet, 2006).

Unresolved grief, family of origin issues, and trauma are often evident in the stories and feelings expressed by individuals living with mental illness who are in recovery. Trauma is a common feature of the lives of people with mental illness (Onken, Dumont, Ridgway, Dornan, & Ralph, 2002); in fact, trauma may have been a contributing factor in the development of mental illness, and/or the presence of mental illness may have increased the risk of or vulnerability to trauma. Consideration and appreciation of past trauma are essential to recovery of persons receiving mental health services (Onken et al, 2002).

Trauma is often considered a psychological event that happens to an individual. In a spiritual sense, however, it is important to recognize that trauma can be experienced by groups of persons and deeply affect the lives of the group members. For example, many aboriginal Canadians suffered trauma as a result of the residential school experience. During most of the 20th century, aboriginal children were taken from their communities to live at such schools, where they were isolated from family and often suffered abuse (Assembly of First Nations, n.d.). For individuals, affected by this experience (as well as their families and communities), a hospital ward room with multiple beds might trigger associations with this past trauma. Similarly, persons of Jewish descent, given the history of persecution and genocide of the Jewish people, may find it traumatizing to be brought to a strange place, have their possessions taken away, and be processed administratively (Lis-Turlejska, Luszczynska, Plichta, & Benight, 2008).

Faith Background

Another contributing factor that influences an individual's spiritual context is his or her **faith background**, or spiritual or religious experiences and beliefs. These beliefs are often adopted from communities that adhere to a particular spiritual tradition and are passed on to members through relationships, language, culture, symbols, teachings, rituals, and practices. In exploring a person's faith background, it is important to consider the individual's formative faith background (if the person has in fact been exposed to a particular faith tradition), present-day beliefs, and the relationship between the two. In struggling to make sense of life and experiences, individuals may cling to their belief systems or develop beliefs that differ significantly from the faith traditions to which they may have once belonged. Regardless of how conventional or informal their beliefs may be, individuals find acceptance of their particular beliefs to be important for recovery (Onken et al, 2002).

Personal Spiritual Experience

Although an individual's faith background is significant, his or her **personal spiritual experience** has an even greater impact on the spiritual context. An individual's personal spiritual experience often affects the degree to which he or she participates in spiritual practices and the value he or she places on the spiritual dimension of life. For example, Wilding, May, and Muir-Cochrane's (2005) qualitative study of the experience of spirituality among individuals diagnosed with mental health problems demonstrated that spirituality was literally "life-sustaining" for the six participants. The spirituality of these individuals infused their everyday lives, making their occupations more meaningful, achievable, and pleasant. In fact, all participants directly or indirectly stated that it was their spiritual beliefs that kept them from attempting suicide when the pain in their lives became overwhelming.

Although spirituality may be significant to some people, it does not hold a primary place in the lives of all persons. Individuals vary in their spiritual development and maturity, the types of spiritual experiences they have had, progress they have made along the spiritual path outlined in a particular tradition, and their understanding of a religious tradition, spiritual values, beliefs, attitudes, and commitment. Each of these aspects affects the individual's spiritual/life outlook, coloring the spiritual lens through which he or she looks at self, life, and relationships.

Sociocultural Context

People experience life and spirituality within particular **sociocultural contexts**. Sociocultural contexts are milieus shaped by the accepted norms, rules, assumptions and expectations governing what is understood to be significant within a particular community or social group, as well as what is taken to be appropriate or inappropriate. Such a context includes issues of geography, culture, ethnicity, gender, income, education, and capability. Symbols, rituals, language, music, literature, history, stories, art, dance, customs, and architecture are but a few of the many means by which a particular sociocultural context finds expression.

Given the pluralistic nature of society, any individual may be influenced by one or more sociocultural contexts simultaneously with differing perspectives and values. For example, a person might be a member of a group that adheres to strict norms regarding modest attire while also being a member of a society that encourages more provocative dress. Likewise, a person might live in a society in which mental health issues are accepted and treated just as would be any other medical condition. However, he or she might also be part of a group that both stigmatizes and ostracizes those who experience depression, mania, or delusions and regards such states as being unacceptable aberrations. Attempts to reconcile the two perspectives are often made by the person to varying degrees of success.

Views maintained within particular sociocultural contexts are produced not only through the values, beliefs, and practices that are passed on within an ethnic heritage but also through a unique blend of historical and present-day regional, economic, and educational influences (Krefting & Krefting, 1992). As a result, sociocultural contexts and the ideas they hold have a profound impact on people's lives, mental health, functional abilities, and the perceived meaning of different occupations. For example, a man living in a society and culture in which being a "good husband" means that he must provide financially for his family at all times may experience profound despair if he has difficulty maintaining employment. Given the profound ways in which the sociocultural context can affect a person's perceptions and life choices, it is essential that it be kept in mind when considering the spiritual environment of both the client and the therapist.

Sense of Self

A person's sense of self is colored by all of the aforementioned elements. This **sense of self** can be called the "anthropological view" of the person. The anthropological view includes the person's understanding of what it means to be human, the components that constitute the self (e.g., body, spirit, soul, feelings, will, mind, and heart), and how he or she perceives the self (e.g., lovable/unworthy, good/bad, or capable/incapable).

An individual's recovery is fundamentally linked to his or her sense of self. Distorted views of the self dishonor a person's self-image and identity, impairing the ability to believe in himself or herself and to develop to his or her full potential. For example, an individual with psychotic thinking and behaviors may be excluded from activities with the family that might result in embarrassment, such as eating out, family reunions, or vacations. This can result in self-stigmatization: the individual accepts that he or she is not welcome in typical occupations that involve interactions with the public (van Zelst, 2009). Conversely, the development of a healthy sense of self allows the person to fully accept himself or herself and to become as relational and functional as he or she is able to be. A new innovation in some community mental health centers is the use of a shared decision-making model for psychiatric medications (Deegan, Rapp, Holter, & Riefer, 2008). This type of program honors the expertise of the individual with mental illness and fosters participation and collaboration in the treatment process.

Worldview

A person's worldview, or ideological framework and outlook, is also influenced by all of the elements previously identified. The worldview a person upholds affects his or her perception of others, the world, creation, and the Transcendent. Influenced by social, cultural, political, spiritual, and familial contexts, the unique person assimilates and internalizes various aspects from each of these and many other sources. The development of an internal spiritual environment follows as he or she formulates beliefs, values, attitudes, relationships, expectations, choices, and a worldview amidst shifting life experiences. The person's outlook gradually takes shape, and he or she views and interacts accordingly with the world and relationships in it. For example, an individual's worldview regarding "free will" can impact that person's perspective as to how much influence he or she can actually have on the course that his or her life takes.

Exploration of the Individual's Spiritual Context

Throughout this chapter, we consciously avoided the terms *evaluation* and *assessment*. These two terms imply a standardized method of measurement as well as the sense that we can (and should) compare individuals in terms of quantity and quality, concepts we believe to be inappropriate in this context. We believe the terms *listen for* and *explore* better convey how we should consider the spiritual environment within occupational therapy practice. That is, through dialogue and observation, the occupational therapist learns about the spiritual environment of the client as well as about his or her own spiritual environment. This understanding unfolds gradually within a mutually trusting relationship.

To consider how occupational therapists can explore an individual's internal spiritual environment and its impact on the realization of meaningful occupation, it is necessary to examine some basic, yet often unrecognized, assumptions that underlie how we consider aspects of persons. As occupational therapists, we are accustomed to looking at people and their environments in terms of discreet component parts. For example, we may test cognition with mental status examinations or test strength through manual muscle testing. We understand that each component part contributes to a healthy whole, and addressing each part with standardized assessment methods is ultimately helpful. The pervasive underlying assumption is that it is possible (and desirable) to form a mental equation of how much of one thing and how much of another is required to obtain a specific goal, such as getting dressed in the morning or managing a household budget.

Such "equations" are sometimes applicable. For example, experience has demonstrated that specific degrees of pressure, shear forces, humidity, and temperature can lead to the development and worsening of pressure sores among individuals with mobility problems. A structured examination of the damaging forces and the amount of time over which they have been applied helps occupational therapists make changes that promote healing. In other words, application of principles of biology and physics can be used effectively to control pressure sores: x pounds over y minutes with z shear = pressure sore development. Lower the numbers through intervention, and the pressure sore will be prevented. This type of **logos reasoning** is extremely relevant in this kind of problem.

However, sometimes logos reasoning is not particularly helpful. For example, can you imagine a mathematical relationship between an individual's view of mankind, thinking style, history of trauma, and culture and his or her ability to carry out desired occupational goals? Although this type of question has been asked, and often underlies much of the research in mental health, it is helpful to step back and consider the assumptions for treatment. If we could classify and quantify the elements in this kind of equation, would it be helpful? Attempting to quantify, predict, and control complex human behavior that unfolds over time is generally done only with a fair bit of error. People with a wide range of incapacities are often able to accomplish much more than was ever considered "logically" possible. Reliance on such equations to make decisions about what people will or will not be able to do may negate such future possibilities.

When quantification, prediction, and control are not possible or desirable, but understanding and support are the goal, we are better served by **mythos reasoning** (Armstrong, 2001). In mythos reasoning, we think in images and stories

rather than in factors. Consider the PhotoVoice created by Viola. Using logos thinking, the therapist might determine that the kite making was obsessive and an indication of an exacerbation of symptoms. However, using mythos reasoning, Viola's story about the kites is one of hope and security. Given the mythos nature of the spiritual context, it is likely more appropriate to listen and reflect on the individual's story (Kirsh, 1996) rather than to question or listen in order to classify or "rate" the person on particular characteristics.

We listen and reflect to learn about the person's particular viewpoint. We also ask questions. For example, how does the person experience the world? Seen through this individual's lens, are people generally good and striving to be better? Or are they essentially evil and require saving from a deity to whom they must submit? Does this person believe that humans have a specific purpose on earth, and does he or she feel capable of fulfilling that purpose? What is the story of this person's life so far? What kind of trauma, if any, has been suffered? What has helped this person in the face of suffering?

Who and what has shaped his or her values and beliefs? How are these beliefs and values similar to and different from those of family members and friends? Which cultural groups does this individual feel most closely aligned to in beliefs and values? Has this changed over time? What events and stories have shaped the experiences of these groups (Martsolf, 1997)? Exploration questions such as these can help the occupational therapist develop an evolving understanding of the internal spiritual environment of the individual. This will help the occupational therapist appreciate the potential personal meaning of particular daily activities.

Studying One's Own Spiritual Context

The ability of the occupational therapist to appreciate his or her own spiritual environment is required before he or she can develop a meaningful understanding of another's (Moran, 2001). When an occupational therapist comes into

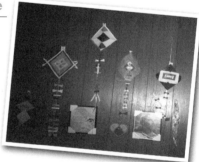

PhotoVoice

One day I made kites. Big kites, medium size kites, and very small kites. All kinds of kites I made. At church I learned, praise goes up and the blessings of God come down. To represent praises going up I use the kites. Then I receive blessings from the Lord by praising Him. I went into the hospital the day I made over 50 kites to praise God. I was afraid to leave my home. When I returned home from the hospital, I gave thanks to the Lord for an uplifting idea. The praise kites worked. When I walked into my home I was safe. Every now and then I still make a kite.
—Viola

the environment of a person receiving occupational therapy, his or her own spiritual environment becomes part of the other person's environment. The therapist's awareness of his or her own spiritual environment and appreciation of the distinctness of this environment from the client's environment can help ensure a supportive environment—a "safe space" where healing can occur (Wendler, 1996). This is an atmosphere in which the person feels that he or she will not be punished for viewing the world in a certain way or for living life as he or she has.

To be able to provide a safe space, an occupational therapist must have a clear understanding of his or her own beliefs and values so that these can be acknowledged as personal rather than part of a universal system that may exclude the individual receiving therapy services. Therefore, it is important for occupational therapists to regularly examine their spiritual environment. One way to do so is by directly reflecting on the aspects of the spiritual environment identified in the previous section. For example, how do we view human beings? How do events from our own lives shape our spirituality, and how do we relate to others? Which cultural groups do we most identify with, and what impact do the experiences of these groups have on our worldviews?

A helpful tool for students and therapists to use to examine their own spiritual context is Martsolf's (1997) Self-Assessment of Culture as Related to Spirituality (Table 31-1). When we work with people to support their participation in meaningful occupations, it is particularly important to understand our own viewpoints with regard to this concept. For example, given our own historical, cultural, and spiritual

lenses, what kinds of occupations do we particularly value? What kinds of occupations do we view as worthless, dangerous, or immoral?

Despite the pervasive view in occupational therapy that we support the autonomy of those individuals we serve (Townsend, 1997), differences in the way individuals and their occupational therapists interpret particular situations can lead therapists to override these dreams and goals. Speaking about their research on practice with seniors, Russell, Fitzgerald, Williamson, Manor, and Whybrow (2002) note a "safety clause." "People can be *allowed* to be independent (autonomous decision-makers) as long as they are safe to do so—in the opinion of the therapist" (p. 375). Given conflicting interpretations of a situation that is safe versus not safe, most of the therapists studied by these researchers had difficulty imagining that the client's interpretation could be the correct one. Further, therapists believed that safety issues (as they interpreted them) overruled any consideration of patient autonomy. Deegan (1996) provides a comical but instructive example of this kind of situation in mental health:

People who have not been psychiatrically labeled are allowed to make dumb, uninsightful decisions all the time in their lives. My favorite example is Elizabeth Taylor, who just got her eighth divorce. We might say, "She lacks insight! She is failing to learn from past experience!" However, when she embarks on marriage #9, no SWAT team of nurses with Prolixin injections will descend upon her "in her best interest." But just imagine if a person with a psychiatric disability were

---

Table 31-1 ● **Self-Assessment of Culture as Related to Spirituality**

Issue	Reflective Questions
Degree of cultural affiliation	• With what groups am I most closely affiliated now? • Has any change occurred in my group affiliation throughout my lifetime?
Life meaning in cultural context	• What do I believe is the meaning and purpose in life? • How did I obtain this belief? • Who in my life would readily understand my beliefs about the meaning of life? Who would least understand? • What words do I use to communicate this belief? • How does my sense of meaning in life affect the rules that I live by, the roles that I enact, and what I do each day?
Values in cultural context	• What do I value the most? • How did I obtain these values? • Who would readily understand my values? Who would least understand? • What words do I use to communicate these values? • How do my values affect the rules that I live by, the roles that I enact, and what I do each day?
Transcendence in cultural context	• What is my experience with a dimension beyond myself? • Who in my life would readily understand these experiences? Who would least understand? • What words do I use to communicate these experiences? • How do these experiences affect the rules that I live by, the roles that I enact, and what I do each day?
Connection in cultural context	• What are the characteristics of my relationship with myself? Others? God or a higher power? Nature? • Who in my life would readily understand my relationships? Who would least understand? • What words do I use to communicate the characteristics of these various relationships? • How do these relationships affect the rules that I live by, the roles that I enact, and what I do each day?
A sense of becoming in cultural context	• What is my life story? • How have I grown and developed as a person? • Where am I headed in life? • Is my life story, my development as a person, and my direction in life similar to that of any particular group of people?

Adapted with permission from Martsolf, D. S. (1997). Cultural aspects of spirituality in cancer care. Seminars in Oncology Nursing, 13, 231–236. St. Louis: Elsevier.

to announce to their treatment team that they were about to get married for the 9th time! People learn, and sometimes don't learn, from failures. We must be careful to distinguish between a person making (from our perspective) a dumb or self-defeating choice and a person who is truly at risk.

Therapists may be able to avoid the trap of labeling dreams and desires as too risky if we get in the habit of reviewing the context of our discomfort with certain goals. Following are reflective questions to consider:

- Does this discomfort come from a concern about safety?
- Is there concrete evidence that pursuit of the goal will result in an immediate, life-threatening situation for the individual?
- Is the goal illegal?
- If the answers to the above questions are no, why do we remain uncomfortable with the goal?
- What in our own spiritual context makes it impossible to view this goal as worthy?
- Do we feel that it is our responsibility to control every situation—to promote our vision of safety at any price?
- Are we adverse to some activities due to our own personal, spiritual, or cultural backgrounds?

Another issue that needs to be addressed in considering our own spiritual context is the impact of the therapist's personal beliefs on his or her ability to enable the occupations of others. Religious and/or cultural beliefs can greatly influence many therapists' perception of what constitutes a healthy individual and meaningful occupation.

Although it is rarely discussed, it is realistic to assume that some occupational therapists experience profound tension between a religiously mandated duty to live out and share their beliefs with others and a professional responsibility to unconditionally accept and support their clients regardless of how their perspectives may conflict with the therapist's own worldview. For example, a therapist whose belief system opposes sexual activity outside of marriage may have a strong reaction to unwed clients in a long-term care facility or group home engaging in sexual relations. Conversely, a therapist whose belief system is unconcerned with such activity may have greater ease accepting and working with it. When difficult moral or ethical situations arise, therapists are encouraged to be true to their own conscience regarding their person and practice while also maintaining professional boundaries and a client-centered focus that ensures that each client is both respected and receives the best care and services possible. Managing such situations is neither simple nor straightforward.

It is also important for the occupational therapist to be aware of power differentials with clients. When the client's beliefs are marginalized in a society and the therapist's belief system corresponds with the dominant belief system, the result may be a lack of "cultural safety" for the patient. Maori nursing scholar Irihapeti Ramsden (2000) developed the term **cultural safety** to describe a process of providing care that acknowledges power differentials and how they affect the ability of marginalized individuals to acquire health care services. Individuals tend to seek a "trust moment"— an instance in the therapeutic relationship that provides

evidence that they can be themselves without being criticized for their differences. There is evidence that occupational therapy clients who identify themselves as minority group members introduce hints about their life situations to see if it is safe to talk to the therapist (Kirsh, Trentham, & Cole, 2006).

What can we do to ensure a safe context for our clients whose lives and beliefs do not resemble those of our families and friends? Beagan (2003) proposes that health professionals reflect not only on differences (e.g., ethnic origin, gender, wealth) but also on the feelings that these differences evoke within the professionals themselves. Echoing Ramsden, Beagan states it is imperative for health professionals to acknowledge that power imbalances exist and are maintained through the ideas of the dominant culture.

It seems difficult but necessary to accept that no matter how open and welcoming we feel, our contexts ensure there will be things we do not understand or even feel comfortable with. It takes courage to move beyond our immediate circles and quietly listen as other people speak of their experiences. As occupational therapists, we may need to rephrase our routine questions in terms that are more likely to lead to a trust moment. For example, "Do you have a significant other?" rather than "Are you married?" "Would you like to rely on him or her to help you with some of your daily activities?" We cannot assume that all relationships conform to our ideas (Beagan, 2008).

Ensuring That Practice Structures Support Recovery

As Leibrich (2002, p. 150) states: "Health, literally means *being whole*. Health means *making whole*. . . . Any therapy that treats a person in a disintegrated way is not just ineffective, it is actually harmful because it can reinforce the disintegration of illness and erode a person's innate power to heal themselves." The third aspect of considering the spiritual environment involves continually ensuring that the way we work promotes wholeness and helps people to realize their full potential.

In her critique of occupational therapy mental health services, Townsend (1998) describes how occupational therapists often unwittingly further practices that foster disempowerment and chronic dependency. Although it appears evident that mental health systems naturally foster dependence through structures that control decision-making and minimize risk, occupational therapists tend to dismiss concerns that we operate in systems that do not allow health. For example, to save time or minimize perceived risks, we may use simulated occupations with our clients rather than work with them in their real environments. "We subjectively know how the routine organization of mental health services limits practice; but daily practice is conducted with an optimism and pride that renders practitioners unconscious of this organizational knowledge and the contradictions of trying to enable empowerment while perpetuating dependence" (p. 166). To help us understand the limitations of the present systems and move closer to a health-promoting way of working, Townsend contrasts occupational therapy practice that enables participation with practice that maintains dependence (Table 31-2).

Table 31-2 ● **Contrasting Practices That Enable Participation Versus Promote Dependency**

Enable Participation	Promote Dependency	Questions to Ask Ourselves
Inviting participation	Objectifying cases	Is participation in this program dependent on occupational issues rather than diagnostic criteria?
Facilitating individual and social action	Accounting for individual cases	Do program activities contribute to betterment of the life situations of participants and potential participants?
Encouraging collaborative decision-making	Controlling decisions hierarchically	Do people in this program have an opportunity to participate in decision-making regarding aspects of this program (including entry, activities, evaluation, and financing)?
Guiding critical reflection and experiential learning	Educating through standardized simulations	Do people in this program have an opportunity to reflect on their readiness for risk taking?
Supporting risk taking for transformative change	Managing safety and liability	Does intervention allow for supportive risk taking in the participant's actual environments?
Promoting inclusiveness	Preserving exclusion	Do program activities lead to the creation of a more inclusive environment?

Adapted with permission from Townsend, E. (1998). Good Intentions Overruled: A Critique of Empowerment in the Routine Organization of Mental Health Services. Toronto: University of Toronto Press.

Questions to consider when determining whether practice structures promote recovery include the following:

- Does the service allow people to be seen as whole beings who are, or strive to be, part of the larger community?
- Do assessment procedures allow for a deeper knowledge of the person, his or her context, and his or her dreams rather than reinforcing the idea that people are the sum of their parts and we must measure the degree of dysfunction of these parts?
- Do administrative structures allow and encourage participation in all levels of decision-making on the part of persons who receive services?
- Is risk taking within the context of real life (rather than simulations) supported and encouraged to allow transformative learning?
- Are there opportunities to work collectively for social change?

Borthwick et al (2001) make similar recommendations reflecting on how aspects of moral treatment, a philosophy that is considered fundamental to occupational therapy, can be applied to 21st-century mental health services. This includes respecting the human rights and personal integrity of persons in recovery; promoting the importance of real, useful occupation; emphasizing the social and physical environments; and appreciating the spiritual needs of the individual and the healing potential of human relationships.

In many countries, faith communities are an important part of the social environment; occupational therapists can work with faith communities to ensure that congregations are welcoming of persons in recovery. Foskett et al (2004) make recommendations for health-care workers who wish to promote such a linkage, suggesting that they learn how to refer for spiritual care and work with faith communities to ensure better inclusion of individuals in recovery. This would consist of a "deeper recognition of the fear engendered by mental health problems and encouragement of congregations to face their fears" (p. 45). Occupational therapists, with their knowledge of meaningful occupation and appreciation of spiritual issues, could provide an important

---

Evidence-Based Practice

Onken et al (2002) held 10 focus groups in nine states with the goal of determining what recovery meant to people diagnosed with mental health problems and what factors facilitated and hindered this recovery. Spirituality was seen as "a source of meaning that supports recovery," and individual and/or shared spiritual beliefs provided hope. In addition, spiritual communities provided both intangible and tangible support. However, the work of Foskett et al (2004) suggests that many community religious leaders lack good information about mental health issues and that their congregations may be fearful of including individuals in recovery in their communities.

➤ Occupational therapists can provide consultation or education to faith communities to promote successful integration or reintegration of people with mental illness.

➤ Identifying existing faith communities that are already supportive of individuals with mental illness provides a resource to clients who are searching for a spiritual home.

Foskett, J., Roberts, A., Mathews, R., Macmin, L., Cracknell, P., & Nicholls, V. (2004). From research to practice: The first tentative steps. *Mental Health, Religion & Culture, 7*, 41–58.

Onken, S. J., Dumont, J. M., Ridgway, P., Dornan, D. H., & Ralph, R. O. (2002). "Mental Health Recovery: What Helps and What Hinders?" Available at: http://www.nasmhpd.org/general_files_publications/ntac_pubs/reports/MHSIPReport.pdf (accessed September 19, 2006).

---

service in bridging the gap between people in recovery and faith communities.

Summary

Our reflection on the spiritual environment in occupational therapy leads us to see this context as something within the person receiving services, within the person providing services, and within the agency and the larger social environment, including faith communities. This information can provide a launching point for personal reflection and a more thorough discussion of the spiritual environment and its considerations for practice.

Active Learning Strategies

1. Self-Assessment

Complete Martsolf's Self-Assessment of Culture as Related to Spirituality (see Table 31-1). Compare your responses with those of a fellow student or friend, preferably someone you think may have responded to the questions quite differently.

Reflective Questions

● What did you learn about yourself and the other person who filled out the assessment?
● How were your responses similar or different?
● Now that you have this information, can you think of a situation in which your values and beliefs might conflict with a client's? How would you use this information to ensure that you are able to develop rapport with the client and respect the client's views, goals, and uniqueness?

 Capture your experience and thoughts in your **Reflective Journal**.

2. Revising Dialogue

Make a list of five questions that you routinely ask people during your work, writing each question in the way you tend to ask the question. Review your list and identify any underlying assumptions in the way you ask the questions. Next, rewrite the questions so they do not reflect any such assumptions. For example, perhaps you typically ask, "What kind of work do you do?" with the assumption that the person is working. Instead, you might start by saying "Tell me about a typical day."

3. Fieldwork Reflection

Think back to your clinical fieldwork experiences to date. Using the reflective questions in Table 31-2, determine whether the work of therapy in each organization tended to enable participation or promote dependency. Suggest one thing you could do to shift the balance toward enabling participation if you were acting in each of the following roles:

● Student
● Occupational therapist
● Manager

Resources

Books
● Peteet, J. (2007). Selected annotated bibliography on spirituality and mental health. *Southern Medical Journal, 100,* 654–659. Reviews 27 books and journal articles published since 1998.

Videos
● *Creating Caring Congregations,* produced by Mental Health Ministries: —http://www.mentalhealthministries.net
● *Fierce Goodbye: Living in the Shadow of Suicide* and *Shadow Voices: Finding Help in Mental Illness,* both produced by Mennonite Media: http://www.mennomedia.org

Websites
● Mental Health Ministries offers resources to help faith communities become caring and comfortable with people with mental illness: http://www.mentalhealthministries.net
● The National Alliance on Mental Illness website's mission is to create supportive faith communities and point out the value of spirituality in recovery. It offers newsletter with articles and many resources: http://www.nami.org/namifaithnet
● The report on "Mental Health Recovery: What Helps and What Hinders" includes sections on the importance of spirituality: http://www.nasmhpd.org/general_files_publications/ntac_pubs/reports/MHSIPReport.pdf
● The Pathways to Promise: Ministry and Mental Illness provides technical assistance and a resource center of liturgical and educational materials: http://www.pathways2promise.org

References

American Occupational Therapy Association. (2002). Occupational therapy practice framework: Domain and process. *American Journal of Occupational Therapy, 56,* 609–639.

Andresen, R., Oades, L., & Caputi, P. (2003). The experience of recovery from schizophrenia: Towards an empirically validated stage model. *Australian and New Zealand Journal of Psychiatry, 37,* 586–594.

Armstrong, K. (2001). The future of God. In D. A. Brown (Ed.), *Christianity in the 21st Century* (pp. 13–23). New York: Crossroad.

Beagan, B. L. (2003). Teaching social and cultural awareness to medical students: "It's all very nice to talk about it in theory, but ultimately it makes no difference." *Academic Medicine, 78,* 605–614.

———. (2008). "Cultural competence? A critical approach to working with diversity." Keynote address presented at OT Atlantic, October 3, Halifax, Nova Scotia.

Belcham, C. (2004). Spirituality in occupational therapy: Theory in practice? *British Journal of Occupational Therapy, 67,* 39–48.

Borthwick, A., Holman, C., Kennard, D., McFetridge, M., Messruther, K., & Wilkes, J. (2001). The relevance of moral treatment to contemporary mental health. *Journal of Mental Health, 10,* 427–439.

Bussema, E. F., & Bussema, K. E. (2007). Gilead revisited: Faith and recovery. *Psychiatric Rehabilitation Journal, 30,* 301–305.

Buzzell, M., & Gibbon, M. (1991). Personhood. *Canadian Nurse, 87*(6): 32–33.

Chida, Y., Steptoe, A., & Powell, L. H. (2009). Religiosity/spirituality and mortality: A systematic quantitative review. *Psychotherapy and Psychosomatics, 78,* 81–90.

Deegan, P. (1996). "Recovery and the conspiracy of hope." Paper presented at the Sixth Annual Mental Health Services Conference of Australia and New Zealand, Brisbane. http://www.bu.edu/resilience/examples/recovery-conspiracyofhope.txt (retrieved March 2, 2010).

Deegan, P. E., Rapp, C., Holter, M., & Riefer, M. (2008). Best practices: A program to support shared decision making in an outpatient psychiatric medication clinic. *Psychiatric Services, 59,* 603–605.

Egan, M., & Swedersky, J. (2003). The experience of occupational therapists who consider spirituality in practice. *American Journal of Occupational Therapy, 57,* 525–533.

Enquist, D. E., Short-DeGraff, M., Gliner, J., & Oltjenbruns, K. (1997). Occupational therapists' beliefs and practices with regard to spirituality and therapy. *American Journal of Occupational Therapy, 51,* 173–180.

Foskett, J., Roberts, A., Mathews, R., Macmin, L., Cracknell, P., & Nicholls, V. (2004). From research to practice: The first tentative steps. *Mental Health, Religion & Culture, 7,* 4–58.

Kirsh, B. (1996). A narrative approach to addressing spirituality in occupational therapy: Exploring meaning and purpose. *Canadian Journal of Occupational Therapy, 63,* 55–61.

Kirsh, B., Trentham, B., & Cole, S. (2006). Diversity in occupational therapy: Experiences of consumers who identify themselves as minority group members. *Australian Occupational Therapy Journal, 53,* 302–313.

Kornfield, J. (1993). *A Path with Heart—A Guide through the Perils and Promises of Spiritual Life.* New York: Bantam Books.

Krefting, L. H., & Krefting, D. (1992). Cultural influences on performance. In C. Christiansen & C. Baum (Eds.), *Occupational Therapy: Overcoming Human Performance Deficits* (pp. 100–122). Thorofare, NJ: Slack.

Law, M., Polatajko, H., Baptiste, S., & Townsend, E. (1997). Core concept of occupational therapy. In E. Townsend (Ed.), *Enabling Occupation: An Occupational Therapy Perspective* (pp. 29–56). Ottawa: CAOT.

Leibrich, J. (2002). Making space: Spirituality and mental health. *Mental Health, Religion and Culture, 5,* 143–162.

Letts, L., Rigby, P., & Stewart, D. (2003). *Using Environments to Enable Occupational Performance.* Thorofare, NJ: Slack.

Lis-Turlejska, M., Luszczynska, A., Plichta, A., & Benight, C. C. (2008). Jewish and non-Jewish World War II child and adolescent survivors at 60 years after war: Effects of parental loss and age at exposure on wellbeing. *American Journal of Orthopsychiatry, 78,* 369–377.

Martsolf, D. S. (1997). Cultural aspects of spirituality in cancer care. *Seminars in Oncology Nursing, 13,* 231–236.

Mohr, S., Brandt, P.-Y., Borras, L., Gilleron, C., & Huguelet, P. (2006). Toward an integration of spirituality and religiousness into the psychosocial dimension of schizophrenia. *American Journal of Psychiatry, 163,* 1952–1959.

Moran, F. M. (2001). *Listening—A Pastoral Style.* Victoria, Australia: David Lowell Publishing.

Murphy, M. A. (1998). Rejection, stigma and hope. *Psychiatric Rehabilitation Journal, 22,* 186–188.

Onken, S. J., Dumont, J. M., Ridgway, P., Dornan, D. H., & Ralph, R. O. (2002). "Mental Health Recovery: What Helps and What Hinders?" Available at: http://www.nasmhpd.org/general_files_publications/ntac_pubs/reports/MHSIPReport.pdf (accessed September 19, 2006).

Ramsden, I. (2000). Cultural safety/kawa whakaruruhau ten years on: A personal overview. *Nursing Praxis in New Zealand, 15*(1), 4–12.

Rasic, D. T., Belik, S. L., Elias, B., Katz, L. Y., Erins, M., Sareen, J., & Swampy Cree Suicide Prevention Team. (2009). Spirituality, religiosity and suicidal behavior in a nationally representative sample. *Journal of Affective Disorders, 114,* 32–40.

Rose, A. (1999). Spirituality and palliative care. *British Journal of Occupational Therapy, 62,* 307–311.

Russell, C., Fitzgerald, M. H., Williamson, P., Manor, D., & Whybrow, S. (2002). Independence as a practice issue in occupational therapy: The safety clause. *American Journal of Occupational Therapy, 56,* 369–379.

Schneiders, S. M. (1998). The study of Christian spirituality: Contours and dynamics of a discipline. *Christian Spirituality Bulletin, 6*(1), 2–3.

Stark, S. (2004). Removing environmental barriers in the homes of older adults with disabilities improves occupational performance. *OTJR: Occupation, Participation and Health, 24,* 32–39.

Tepper, L., Rogers, S. A., Coleman, E. M., & Malony, H. N. (2001). The prevalence of religious coping among persons with mental illness. *Psychiatric Services, 52,* 660–665.

Thompson, B. E., & MacNeil, C. (2006). A phenomenological study exploring the meaning of a seminar on spirituality for occupational therapy students. *American Journal of Occupational Therapy, 60,* 531–539.

Townsend, E. (Ed.). (1997). *Enabling Occupation: An Occupational Therapy Perspective.* Ottawa: CAOT.

———. (1998). *Good Intentions Overruled: A Critique of Empowerment in the Routine Organization of Mental Health Services.* Toronto: University of Toronto Press.

Udell, L., & Chandler, C. (2000). The role of the occupational therapist in addressing the spiritual needs of the client. *British Journal of Occupational Therapy, 63,* 489–495.

Vanier, J. (1998). *Becoming Human.* Toronto: Anansi.

van Zelst, C. (2009). Stigma as an environmental risk in schizophrenia: A user perspective. *Schizophrenia Bulletin, 35*(2), 293–296.

Wendler, M. C. (1996). Understanding healing: A conceptual analysis. *Journal of Advanced Nursing, 24,* 836–842.

Wilding, C., May, E., & Muir-Cochrane, E. (2005). Experience of spirituality, mental illness and occupation: A life-sustaining phenomenon. *Australian Journal of Occupational Therapy, 52,* 2–9.

Wisdom, J. P., Bruce, K., Saedi, G. A., Weis, T., & Green, C. A. (2008). "Stealing me from myself": Identity and recovery in personal accounts of mental illness. *Australian and New Zealand Journal of Psychiatry, 42,* 489–495.

The Neighborhood and Community

Terry Krupa

> "As I sobered up I realized I was in a genuine resort. Carpets, cable TV, three meals a day served by waitresses, people to talk to, and a view of 50 acres of partly forested grounds. I was discharged "involuntarily" to my usual accommodation, a small basement room, admittedly without the cockroaches, but I was the typical abandoned ex-patient. Some days I had to go buy a chocolate bar just to have a conversation with another human. "That will be $1.19 please. Thank you very much."
>
> —Jan Chovil (2000, p. 745)

Introduction

In recent years, increase attention has been directed toward understanding and capitalizing on the capacity of neighborhoods and communities to influence the mental health and wellbeing of citizens. This growing interest in neighborhoods and communities within the mental health field is good news for occupational therapists. The profession is defined by its focus on meaningful occupations, which naturally occur in neighborhood and community environments and are an integral part of all flourishing communities (Christiansen & Townsend, 2004). It is consistent with contemporary occupational therapy conceptual frameworks that an understanding of the performance and experience of occupation is determined by transactions among the person, environment, and occupation. Targeting the environment lends credibility to a broad range of occupational therapy approaches and interventions, including those directed at evaluating and changing the neighborhood and community to enable the occupational lives of people with mental illness.

This chapter focuses on a neglected but important environment, the neighborhood. People live, socialize, recreate, and conduct most of their instrumental activities of daily living within their neighborhood. This chapter describes the neighborhood and its associations with occupational performance and the particular challenges for people with mental illness. In addition, it provides strategies for assessing and providing interventions that target the neighborhood.

Current Interest in Neighborhoods and Communities

There are several reason for the increased interest in the impact of neighborhoods and communities on people with mental illness. First is the growing recognition that our understanding of mental health and mental illness has been overly focused on individual risk and that we need to develop a more balanced view that integrates social and ecological perspectives (Yen & Syme, 1999). Emerging research has begun to provide us with the evidence base we require to understand how neighborhoods and communities influence mental health and mental illness.

For example, a study by Xue, Leventhal, Brooks-Gunn, and Earls (2005) demonstrated that neighborhood disadvantage was associated with more mental health problems among children, and Kubzansky et al (2005) showed that poor neighborhoods were associated with higher levels of depressive symptoms among the elderly. A large epidemiological study (Silver, Mulvey, & Swanson, 2002) demonstrated an association between neighborhood and disadvantage and higher rates of mental disorder and suggested that particular features of the neighborhood environment can be associated with specific types of mental disorders.

A second reason for the increased attention to neighborhood and community relates to the outcomes of the policy of deinstitutionalization. Although the original intent of deinstitutionalization was to promote the community reintegration of people who experienced long stays in psychiatric hospitals, it has evolved to include the *prevention* of institutionalization of people living with mental illness in the community. The outcomes associated with the policy of deinstitutionalization have been mixed. Models of service delivery in community mental health have demonstrated the ability to decrease hospitalization, thereby locating people in community neighborhoods. They have, however, been less successful in demonstrating that they enable the people they serve to become established and active members of these communities.

For example, a participatory study of assertive community treatment, a best practice model in community mental health, found that people receiving the service experienced active support for managing symptoms of illness and crisis situations to keep them living in the community but less assertive support for ensuring their full community participation, personal growth, and development in the context of the broader community. (Krupa et al, 2005; also see Chapter 40.)

The failures of deinstitutionalization have shown us that people living with mental illness require more than stabilization of their mental illness and their housing situations to ensure that they become neighbors and community participants. They require complex skills of community living and the resources and supports that all citizens need to establish themselves in their communities. Policy failures have also shown us how our history of institutionalizing people with mental illness affected neighborhoods and communities. Simply put, it created a community culture of segregation. Structures, practices, rituals, and other symbols of community membership were developed without the need to consider institutionalized persons, and they were excluded from shared community routines, habits, and expectations. It also created a situation in which some community members perceive them as a threat to community wellbeing and order, which subsequently subjects individuals with mental illness to stigma and marginalization (Jenkins, 2004; Nelson, Lord, & Ochcocka, 2001).

A third reason for increased attention on neighborhoods and community in influencing the mental health and wellbeing of citizens is related to the current interest in enabling older people with dementia and other progressive health conditions associated with impaired cognitive and psychological function to remain in their homes and communities. The neighborhood has been identified as potentially supportive in enabling their supporting community living. For example, people in the neighborhood can perform surveillance functions that reduce the risks associated with wandering or vulnerability to crime that may be experienced by people living with dementia in the community (Gilmour, 2004). However, shifts in neighborhood communities, such as changes in the demographics and the transformation of aging neighborhoods, can be a barrier to community living when caregivers of persons with dementia depend on established neighborhood supports to assist them with caregiving in the community (Ortiz, Simmons, & Hinton, 1999).

Defining Neighborhoods and Communities

When we speak of our neighborhood and/or community, we are typically referring to a geographic location. Although the terms may be used interchangeably, neighborhoods often more specifically refer to the area in close vicinity to our place of residence, whereas the community may indicate a larger area. Our neighbors are the people with whom we share this defined, if loosely bound, locality. Neighbors can become friends, but even when they do not, we often consider our neighbors to be a potential source of informal support. They might, for example, take in our mail when we are away, lend us a rake, or perhaps send their children over to help with shoveling snow. At the very least, neighbors are people whom we might expect to share our interest in maintaining our community as a good place to live.

Services and resources that are nearby become part of our understanding of our neighborhoods. For example, we check the newspapers for local events, send children to the neighborhood school, enjoy neighborhood parks, and visit the neighborhood coffee shop. There are specific activities that we associate with participation in our neighborhoods, such as belonging to the Neighborhood Watch, planning a neighborhood garage sale, or attending a neighborhood block party.

Our neighborhoods also connect us to higher levels of social organization and governance. For example, attending a neighborhood church connects an individual to the larger structure of the religion, and local schools connect us to local educational governance structures and, ultimately, to government. Similarly, neighborhoods are represented at municipal and higher levels of government through elected representatives.

Neighborhoods have characteristics that allow us to identify them as distinct communities, even when we do not reside there. Efforts to promote tourism frequently focus on the allure of specific neighborhoods. Distinguishing neighborhood features can include the common types of residences, the ethnic composition and population mix, the way land is used, the way neighbors are organized, the activities that take place, and the types of businesses and services available.

PhotoVoice

This is a quiet suburban residential neighborhood. Although I cannot see the people, I know they are inside their homes, just going about their daily business. Being at home gives us a sense of security, which gives us peace of mind, especially those with mental illness. The neighborhood residents are somewhat of a close-knit community, and many of the people know each other, which provides them with a sense of comfort. It is good to know the people of the neighborhood live in peace with each other and that they care and look out for each other. I am a firm believer in the adage, no one is an island. Even though it is plain to see everyone does not have the gift of gab, we can nurture the willingness to communicate by at least greeting the people we see every day.

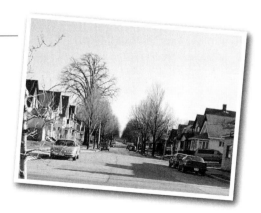

Relationship of Neighborhood Environment to Occupation

The literature and research base focused directly on the neighborhood environment and its relationship to occupation in the context of mental illness is relatively sparse. We can, however, use dimensions of neighborhoods that have been associated with mental health and mental illness to begin to build a framework for understanding how neighborhoods and communities enable or constrain the occupational lives of people and ultimately influence mental health and mental illness. These dimensions include the following:

- Organization and activism
- Socioeconomic status
- Safety
- Resident mobility
- Diversity
- Attitudes

Neighborhood Organization and Activism

Neighborhoods with social structures and interactions that are characterized by civic participation, a sense of identity and equality among members, and community responsibility and reciprocity are believed to promote mental health and prevent mental illness among community members (De Silva, McKenzie, Harpham, & Huttly, 2005). These characteristics, which engender cooperation among community members, have come to be known as **social capital**. With its focus on action and doing, social capital is a form of occupation that sustains both individuals and their communities (Christiansen & Townsend, 2004).

The mechanisms by which social capital influences the mental health of individuals are complex and not fully understood. There is, for example, reason to suspect that people who experience acute anxiety and depression will continue to have relatively low levels of activity participation despite being surrounded by a neighborhood characterized as high in social capital (De Silva et al, 2005). Yet it is fairly certain that any efforts made by these individuals to engage in community-based activities will be thwarted in neighborhoods that are low in social capital, both because of the general lack of community activities and because of the risks associated with social relationships that are not bound by trust, cooperation, and equality. Neighborhood relationships defined by cooperation and mutual respect are likely fundamental to building the personal sense of worth and legitimacy that is often missing in people with mental illness.

Neighborhood Socioeconomic Status

Neighborhood communities characterized by socioeconomic disadvantage have been associated with higher rates of mental illness among residents (Jarvis, 2007). The reasons for this are complex but likely include the threats to function and wellbeing that are associated with living in adverse neighborhood conditions, including high unemployment, financial hardship, and a general lack of material resources. Another potential reason is that once people experience mental illness, they are more likely to experience persistent poverty and subsequently be forced to live in disadvantaged neighborhoods (Silver et al, 2002).

Research indicating that people living with mental illness in nonindustrialized and developing countries may have better outcomes than those living in industrialized countries suggests that the relationship between socioeconomic status and mental health is complex (Fieldhouse, 2000; Warner, 1994). It suggests that other community structures may lessen the impact of socioeconomic disadvantage. For example, nonindustrialized communities may experience pressure to include all available human resources in an effort to sustain the community economy, or perhaps the nature of the occupations that sustain nonindustrialized communities are a good match for the capacities of people with mental illness.

Socioeconomic disadvantage is reflected in the neighborhood population in many ways, including high rates of unemployment and underemployment, lower educational performance among students of neighborhood schools, low rates of home ownership, and the disruption of families. It has been argued that the neighborhood environment provides opportunity structures that influence the occupational goals and expectations of residents (Furlong, Biggart, & Cartmel, 1996). For example, individuals are less likely to engage in meaningful work if unemployment in their neighborhood is high and if there is limited access to public transportation. However, a thriving economic environment can increase the likelihood that individuals will have good jobs, which also leads to better housing and educational opportunities.

Current conceptualizations of recovery from mental illness suggest that the same argument can be made for persons with mental illness. Neighborhoods constitute an important external condition for recovery by offering access to a range of work, education, self-care, social, and recreational opportunities that are consistent with basic human rights. These opportunities can create a positive culture of hope that can enable a full occupational life beyond the limits of mental illness (Jacobson & Greenley, 2001).

The relative social and economic disadvantage of neighborhood communities contributes to the pressure for local resources and services to address the specific needs of residents. For example, neighborhoods that include a large number of people with mental illness living at poverty levels will experience pressure to ensure a variety of services that support the daily occupations of these individuals, such as assistance to find and keep housing, food banks, access to public transportation, and community programs that provide social and recreational programming. There are many, many examples of communities that, despite being characterized by socioeconomic disadvantage, demonstrate a tremendous capacity to organize to ensure the wellbeing of residents.

Socioeconomic disadvantage within a neighborhood community may also be reflected in the presence of services associated with negative social behaviors or the exploitation of people with limited financial means (Kubzansky et al, 2005). For example, people with mental illness can often receive disability income as their means of financial support. As for many people who lived on fixed and limited incomes, banking services may be inaccessible or unhelpful. In response, these individuals come to depend on their neighborhood "cash-marts," which charge exceptionally high rates to cash disability pensions, pay bills, and borrow money. Situations such as this can further compromise an individual's already limited financial resources and compromise the ability to budget.

Socioeconomic disadvantage is also reflected in decrepit conditions that are uninviting to involvement and activity. A study by Boydell, Gladstone, Crawsford, and Trainor (1999) indicated that people with psychiatric disabilities living in an urban center tolerate exceptionally noxious conditions in their immediate neighborhood environments, perhaps due to lack of choice of living environments or prolonged desensitization to these environments. These conditions may be more than unpleasant—they can be harmful. A study by Krupa (2004) indicated that for some people living with serious mental illness, offensive community environments can provoke intense thoughts and feelings that aggravate the symptoms of their illness.

Neighborhood Safety

The relative prevalence of crime and violence is of particular concern in disadvantaged neighborhoods. Poor mental health and mental disorder have been linked to involvement in personally valued daily activities that are subject to uncontrollable negative events that affect personal safety and wellbeing (Dohrenwend, 2000; Whitley & Prince, 2005b). Individuals with mental illness living in urban environments feel more threats to safety than do individuals in rural environments (Schomerus et al, 2007), and one study found that individuals with psychosis who spent even short periods of time in a busy urban shopping environment had an increase in paranoid thinking (Ellet, Freeman, & Garety, 2008). Concerns about personal security and the presence of antisocial behaviors in the neighborhood, such as drug use and dealing, have been associated with psychological distress and poor levels of mental health. For people with mental illness, the experience of occupational inactivity and underachievement, coupled with the presence of an active drug culture in the neighborhood, may lead to increased participation in substance using occupations (Fieldhouse, 2000). This can result in a worsening psychiatric condition by creating co-occurring disorders of mental illness and substance abuse, which also leads to increasing vulnerability to victimization by drug dealers. A study by Whitely & Prince (2005b) found that neighborhood residents with mental health problems live with the fear of crime at a disproportionate rate, that fear is highest among women and older people, and that this fear causes them to restrict their activities.

The participants living with mental illness in Boydell et al's (1999) study described witnessing illegal and frightening events in their immediate neighborhood environments and being the target of abusive comments from community neighbors. The research indicated that participants actively used strategies to manage in such unpleasant environments and that some of these strategies, such as social distancing, could easily be interpreted as symptoms of mental illness rather then active efforts to adapt and cope. Any thorough explanation of decreased activity participation, withdrawal or isolation, and low levels of attendance at community mental health services by people living with mental illness must address the possibility that these are strategies implemented

to cope with fear for personal safety (Boydell et al, 1999; Holter & Mowbray, 2005; Whitely & Prince, 2005a, 2005b).

The common assumption that people with mental illness are prone to violence has been the subject of much debate, but research suggests that people with mental illness are not major contributors to community violence (Stuart & Arboleda-Florez, 2001). When they do participate in violent behaviors, the violence is more likely to occur in the context of socially disadvantaged communities where personal concerns about safety and security are heightened (Silver, 2000). People with mental illness experience higher rates of victimization in their community neighborhoods, likely due to a combination of the dimensions of social disadvantage of their neighborhoods and their personal vulnerabilities (Hiday, Swartz, Swanson, Borum, & Wagner, 1999; Teplin, McClelland, Abram, & Weiner, 2005).

Of particular relevance to occupational therapists are research findings indicating that lack of involvement in meaningful daily activity is a major predictor of victimization among community-dwelling people with serious mental illness (Fitzgerald et al, 2005). The researchers propose that involvement in activity can reduce exposure to threatening situations, and daily activity may also decrease personal vulnerability in a number of ways. For example, people involved in daily activities may move with an attitude of purpose in their neighborhoods that protects them from victimization, have somewhere to be where there are people who expect them, and be surrounded by a concerned social network, leaving them less vulnerable to harassment and victimization. In addition, the knowledge and skills acquired through involvement in occupations can potentially be generalized to successfully negotiate situations of neighborhood conflict. For example, social skills developed through regular interactions with neighbors may be used when a dispute occurs because of an overcharge at the grocery store.

Resident Mobility

Resident mobility is the movement of residents in and out of a neighborhood over time (Silver et al, 2002). In a neighborhood with high resident mobility, people do not stay very long, and there is a high rate of "turnover" in homes. High levels of resident mobility are believed to compromise the development and stability of social networks that could support occupation. For individuals living with mental illness, the combination of disruption of personal social abilities with high levels of residential mobility can seriously undermine social integration and leave individuals vulnerable to experiences of exploitation. For example, the mentally ill renter with impaired social skills and without stable neighbors who might act as advocates is in a more vulnerable position when it comes to dealing with an unscrupulous landlord.

Diversity

Some research supports the concept that some level of diversity and social disorganization (e.g., varied housing and landscape or mixed demographic structures such as young singles, families, and elders) in a neighborhood community can enable community mental health and support the community lives of persons with mental illness. Harkness, Newman, and Salkever (2004) propose that neighborhoods with "socioeconomically and demographically diverse populations, with a mix of commercial and residential land uses and not physically pristine" (p. 1344) should be linked to better community outcomes because they are more likely to support the anonymity of persons with mental illness and thereby reduce experiences of stigmatization and discrimination. Neighborhoods with greater variety in housing, people, and businesses should be associated with high levels of community tolerance.

Community Attitudes

Public stigma and the discrimination of people who experience mental illness is a well-known issue that is explored in Chapter 28. It is of particular importance when considering neighborhood because social proximity and social interactions characterize community environments. Stigma can enforce exclusion from relationships, activities, and physical spaces and places that constitute the neighborhood.

Interestingly, despite the high-profile resistance in some neighborhoods to community mental health residences or services, research has indicated that community members assume that their behaviors will be neighborly toward individuals with mental illness who live in their neighborhood (Aubry, Tefft, & Currie, 1995). These neighborly activities include offering information about home care services, offering information about professional services, offering a ride, and conversing on the street. Neighborhood residents may become more likely to accept

their neighbors with mental illnesses over time, with multiple contacts, and through the opportunity to interact collaboratively and as equals (Estroff, Penn, & Toporek, 2004).

Stigma or the perception of stigma in the neighborhood may affect an individual's willingness to accept treatment or rehabilitation services (Elbogen, Soriano, Van Dorn, Swartz, & Swanson, 2005; Lee, Chiu, Tsang, Chui, & Kleinman, 2006). In fact, people receiving community mental health services have indicated that these services can be delivered in a manner that compromises their status as neighbors. For example, participants in a study by Krupa et al (2005) described mental health professionals contributing to their experience of stigma by openly carrying medications into their homes and by arriving in cars for scheduled community appointments in a manner that would readily be identified by neighbors as treatment visits by mental health professionals.

Intervening to Develop Supportive Neighborhood Communities

Most mental health services are primarily directed at attending to the needs, limitations, and strengths of the individual with mental illness, with a view to enabling person-level changes that will lead to community integration. So, for example, occupational therapy practices have

The Lived Experience

Malcolm

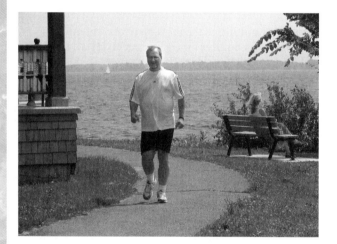

I'm a big believer in neighborhoods and community environments and their influence on recovery. When you experience a serious mental illness, like I have, your personality and coping can be fractured by the bomb that goes off in your brain. Recovery from this kind of trauma can be greatly enhanced by the environment around you. This is where neighborhoods and communities can have a positive influence as you relearn, develop new attitudes,

values, and beliefs. This helps with developing coping strategies and skills. It's invaluable to success.

When I think of neighborhoods, I think of a geographic location where people live, within fairly defined boundaries. I live in a nice enough neighborhood right now, but I don't socialize in my apartment building and I'm not really active in that neighborhood. The people in the building, they know my name and are friendly, but they are elderly. I like my building, it's in a mature area, quite green, and safe, and so it's a nice place to live.

My real community is my friends who live in other neighborhoods in the city and my activities outside of my local neighborhood. I participate in a power walking program through a local running store. Everyone in the running program is upbeat, positive, and supportive. The attitude is, "If the activity hurts, then you take a rest and look at why it's hurting." They don't try and push you through the pain, so they don't make the activity stressful. I've also started to get involved with golf and cross-training. I'm looking into some low-cost sailing courses or cycling for next year. I want to try and use my community to make some non–mental health contacts, to move beyond the illness and experience life from a different perspective. I'm looking for some new balance in my life.

A community might look different to different people. My city isn't a very big place, but I have a fairly active life. I do have

The Lived Experience—cont'd

schizophrenia, but I am involved. I know a fellow living with schizophrenia who basically lives in his apartment building, visits the psychiatric hospital and one local community organization. My friends and I find this distressing, and we are trying to encourage him to broaden his community. It's hard to say why he is so restricted. It may be his own outlook, it might be the opportunities available to him, or it might be the influence of his family.

I have always made my own community. Even if my local neighborhood doesn't have what I need, I can make my own personal community. I think of a personal community as being unique to an individual, not only how they interact in their local neighborhood, but also how they relate to a global village by making connections further afield. With the Internet, travel and relocation to various parts of a province, country, or internationally, a person can make many contacts and friends, and they all can have benefits to development and life.

I have found neighborhoods that are eclectic to be emotionally positive. By this I mean neighborhoods with a wide range of people from different backgrounds. The important thing is it can't be a ghetto, a place where people live because they are somehow disadvantaged. A ghetto isn't a healthy place. I live in a neighborhood where I feel safe and secure, that has some mature green space and isn't subject to stigma. These things can be hard to find in a ghetto environment. Unfortunately, social housing and poverty can be a barrier to where you live. If a person lives in a less desirable area, they can try to be a voice of change and development. Ultimately one has to stand up for their beliefs and goals regardless of influence. Not all of real life is going to be supportive. I have seen how communities can really be turned around even when they don't have a lot going for them. For example, I have seen how community centers can work as a place where people from the local neighborhoods get together to meet the needs of the people living there.

I also think that communities are enhanced when they have a range of resources available. I have really benefited from communities that have a nearby college or university. This has allowed me to meet people with different educational backgrounds and different interests. Colleges and universities encourage a willingness to learn that I think can bring out the best in people. They also offer opportunities like courses, access to technology, athletics, and the presence of the arts. I realize churches can be a touchy subject, but I must admit my experience with them is both positive and negative. I've always found the clergy to be excellent, but in some churches I've attended there can be an undercurrent in the congregation. Other churches I've experienced have been positive and helpful organizations in the community. Colorful local people also add a lot to a community. I remember back in Toronto we had a restaurateur who was a real character. People loved to congregate at his place.

For me, banks have been a very important part of my communities. They have had a tremendous influence on my financial security and self-esteem, and they have also caused me financial distress. Back in 1995 when I lived on the East Coast I was laid off from my job. It was a hard time. I had a farm and rental property as well as that small B&B, but I counted on the income from that job. I had very little debt, but my bank put a lot of pressure on me to sell my farm to one of their other customers. It was like all of a sudden I wasn't a worthy customer. I had always been good at managing my relationship with banks, but this was such a shaky time in my life and I decided to close the door on that community and leave because I was so worn out. In contrast, in another community my bank manager was willing to loan me money even though I didn't have a lot of collateral. He treated me like the good customer I had always been. He said, "You have a good history with me, I'll loan you the money." He gave me a good loan with a good interest rate and payback plan.

I've lived in several neighborhoods over the course of my recovery, and I've had my ups and downs in these neighborhoods. In the end, each one of these neighborhoods has contributed to my network of friends and contacts and the development of my interests and activities in some way. They have all been a piece of my many life adventures.

largely focused on the skills that people need to "fit in" and successfully participate in meaningful neighborhood community occupations.

Within in-patient and day program settings, occupational therapists are challenged in their efforts to address the occupational issues of their clients because they practice at a distance from the neighborhoods and community contexts within which these occupations occur. Today, people who are admitted to in-patient mental health settings are typically experiencing acute illness or their mental health has destabilized in the midst of a crisis in community life. Although the number of long-term in-patient rehabilitation patients has declined, there are still many individuals who have been long-term in-patients. It can be difficult in these circumstances for an occupational therapist to envision the individual making the transition back to neighborhood life. However, the occupational therapist role still must include integrating the neighborhood and community context into short- and long-term goals—and encouraging the health care team to do the same.

Likewise, adolescents with mental illness or developmental disabilities may benefit from services to assist with transition to independent community living.

In community-based settings, occupational therapists have the opportunity to practice directly in the individual's neighborhood and community environment. They also can develop community-based programs that offer individuals access to a range of self-care, productivity, and leisure interventions to address occupations experienced in daily life and to reduce their experiences of marginalization. If these programs are truly part of the neighborhood, they will be sensitive to the types and range of knowledge and skills that are expected of all community residents, including those with mental illness. These programs capitalize on the individual's personal abilities and potentials within communities. When the community is viewed as a resource and interventions are designed to assist individuals with mental illness to truly become members of their communities, the result can be a feeling of belonging instead of isolation.

The information provided in this chapter thus far has highlighted the profound influence that the neighborhood and community have on the occupational lives of people with mental illness. It suggests that in addition to our individual-level service approaches in community mental health, adequate attention must be given to approaches directed to the level of the neighborhood and community. Rather then focusing on the individual, these approaches focus on identifying the needs, limits, and capacities of the neighborhood and community, with a view toward facilitating the capacity of the neighborhood to enhance, and be enhanced by, the occupational lives of all their residents. These approaches can be conceptualized as **community development**, a process of building local communities to support the wellbeing of both individual community members and the community as a whole.

It is important to remember that occupational therapy values remain fundamental to community development approaches. Occupational therapy practice focused at the level of the neighborhood and community will still reflect the fundamental values of personal choice, empowerment, respect for basic human dignities, and respect for client knowledge and experience. A community development approach includes the values of equal access to meaningful occupations within the community and to the resources and supports that facilitate these occupations. The implementation of these values in practice will increase the likelihood of sustainability of positive change.

Assessing Neighborhoods and Developing a Neighborhood Profile

Despite their relatively small size, neighborhoods are complex entities. They have multiple structural and relational components, which can make assessment overwhelming. The dimensions of neighborhood communities described earlier provide a basic framework for community assessment and understanding the complex associations between occupation and the neighborhood environment. These dimensions can be used by occupational therapists to work collaboratively with persons with mental illness to create a **neighborhood profile**. The profile can include both a description of important neighborhood characteristics and a visual map locating important resources and activities.

The neighborhood profile gains meaning when it leads to a process of exploration and evaluation in relation to the individual's occupational performance and experience. For example, a community profile can identify specific resources in the community to support leisure interests. It can also lead to a discussion of neighborhood barriers that interfere with active participation in these community supports, such as the fear of encountering neighborhood drug dealers or difficulties accessing the resources because of limited transportation options. In this way, the neighborhood profile becomes personalized—that is, a vehicle for raising the individual's awareness of the context of his or her daily life and reflecting on himself or herself as a member of a community.

The neighborhood profile can lead to discussions about other potentially supportive neighborhoods. Individuals, for example, may continue to maintain social and occupational connections with their previous neighborhoods, and these may serve to counterbalance challenges arising in the present neighborhood. Similarly, extending the boundaries of the neighborhood can reveal opportunities that are aligned with the individual's values and interests and are still readily accessible. Community colleges, for example, often offer a wide range of courses and educational schedules that are accessible to the larger community.

Occupational therapists who work in programs that serve a large number of individuals from one or only a few neighborhood communities will benefit from developing **formal neighborhood profiles**. Formal neighborhood profiles create an accurate representation of a neighborhood community with regard to information about the population, employment rates, business and industry, land use, educational opportunities, housing, recreational resources, and health services. These profiles are developed both from spending time in and being immersed in the community and also from existing databases that can be accessed through Internet and library services. Figure 32-1 is a sample template for a neighborhood profile.

Beyond collaboration with individual clients, this type of neighborhood profile is essential for larger initiatives focused on assisting individuals with mental illness as a collective or social group to establish themselves in their communities. For example, occupational therapists who are interested in developing employment, occupational, and leadership opportunities for people living with mental illness in a particular neighborhood can initiate and support the development of affirmative or consumer-run businesses. This type of community economic development effort will depend on the resources and services available and the economic needs of the community to ensure viability of the business. The profile will also help reveal the potential for the credibility and recognition of the business, and subsequently the employees, in the community.

Dynamic Assessment of Neighborhood and Community Capacity

A second approach to neighborhood community assessment focuses on revealing the potential assets and capacities of communities. Community researchers Kretzman and McKnight (1993) argued that the traditional path to community development, overcome by the overwhelmingly negative influences that exist in neighborhoods in trouble, has centered on identifying needs, problems, and limitations. The result is that the interventions that follow are based on the view that the neighborhood is deficient and requires external resources to diagnose and correct the problems. This deficit-based approach can leave the community reliant on external expertise.

Kretzman and McKnight, and other community researchers, argue that all communities have the inherent capacity for sustained regeneration. To release this capacity, they highlight the importance of approaches that serve to identify and build on the community's own capacities. This community-building perspective has gained respect as the preferable approach to guide the development of occupational therapy practice in the area of community development (Fieldhouse, 2000).

Neighborhood Profile	
Considerations	
1. Demographics of individuals living in the neighborhood — age, family structure (single, couples, families with young children), ethnic/cultural groups, socioeconomic status	1. _____ _____ _____ _____

2. Housing
   a. Types of housing — single family, apartments, condos
   b. Availability
   c. Cost
	2. _____
	   a. _____
	   b. _____
	   c. _____

3. Safety
   a. Crime rates, types of crime
   b. Policing, neighborhood watch organizations
   c. Dangerous/safe areas
	3. _____
	   a. _____
	   b. _____
	   c. _____

4. Businesses
   a. Shopping (grocery stores, pharmacy, clothing, thrift stores)
   b. Banks and other financial services (money orders)
	4. _____
	   a. _____
	   b. _____

5. Leisure and recreational resources — parks, movie theatres, walking paths, coffee shops, museums	5. _____ _____ _____

6. Employment
   a. Types of employment in the neighborhood
   b. Unemployment rates
	6. _____
	   a. _____
	   b. _____

7. Public transportation
   a. Cost, availability of passes for people with mental illness
   b. Routes, access to important locations.
	7. _____
	   a. _____
	   b. _____

8. Social services — health services, food banks, housing assistance	8. _____
9. Educational resources — libraries, schools (K–12), community colleges	9. _____
10. Day care (child and elder); after-school programs	10. _____
11. Religious organizations	11. _____
12. Community clubs and organizations (e.g., scouting, recreational sports, political organizations, social clubs)	12. _____ _____
13. Neighborhood newspapers/newsletters, online resources	13. _____
14. Aesthetics — architecture, cleanliness, art, natural spaces, pollution	14. _____
15. Intangibles — friendliness, openness to outsiders, acceptance of nonconformity	15. _____

FIGURE 32-1. Sample template for a neighborhood profile.

Occupational therapists who assess a neighborhood from a capacity-building approach would focus their efforts on understanding how to release the assets of the community to successfully engage persons with mental illness in the occupations of the neighborhood. Using the framework proposed by Kretzman and McKnight (1993), the assessment would include the following steps (Figure 32-1):

1. Identify the skills and resources (e.g., time, skills from past education and work experiences, knowledge of music, family and friends with a range of skills and resources, computer experience, and previous experience in organizing or participating in communities) that people living with mental illness can contribute to their communities.

2. Identify community assets (e.g., local associations, community groups, churches, and public institutions such as schools, libraries, and local businesses) that could serve as potential partners for people with mental illness.

3. Determine how reciprocal and productive connections can be formed using the capacities of people

with mental illness and the assets of the community. For example, the local senior center may wish to hire individuals to assist with lawn mowing and landscaping; local public schools may be interested in developing opportunities for students to learn about diversity and acceptance, including gaining an understanding of mental illness; or a local committee focusing on accessibility issues may benefit from members who can help broaden their view beyond physical accessibility.

Practices to Support Change

Considering the neighborhood as the target of intervention requires practices that may be unfamiliar or uncomfortable to some occupational therapists. Following are suggestions for ways in which occupational therapists can become more involved in neighborhoods and creating environments that support community living for people with mental illness.

Promoting Neighborhood Regeneration

Occupational therapists who work in community mental health can make significant contributions by promoting initiatives to overcome the dimensions of neighborhood environments that are barriers to occupation. Typically, efforts to change the community include advocacy efforts directed at municipal or state governments to influence these structures to change community conditions. Although advocacy efforts will always be an integral part of community development, it is possible for occupational therapists, together with the individuals they serve, to identify and collaborate with local community networks to participate in the process of **neighborhood regeneration**, which involves eliminating barriers and creating supports that promote satisfying and productive daily life for people in that community.

Research has indicated that even small neighborhood regeneration efforts can have a significant impact on the activity and community participation of people with mental illness. For example, Whitley and Prince (2005a; 2005b) found that even small improvements to the physical condition and security of potentially high-traffic community areas and facilities could enable occupation and promote coping and function. They also found that eliminating the financial barriers to accessing public transportation by providing free bus passes gave people the opportunity to connect with activities and social networks within and beyond their neighborhoods, reducing their sense of alienation and providing some stress relief (Whitley & Prince, 2005b).

Supporting Neighborhood Partnerships

Building partnerships that connect the occupation-related assets of neighborhood communities and residents can require considerable attention and support. Therapists will need to apply their broad base of knowledge and critical reasoning skills to enable the growth of this partnership. Consider the example of a senior center that partners with individuals with mental illness to develop employment opportunities. The therapist may find that an individual expresses a desire for employment and a genuine interest in this employment opportunity but still experiences difficulty in carrying out the work. In this case, the therapist must work with the individual to identify and address the barriers

Evidence-Based Practice

Feeling safe in one's own neighborhood is important for positive occupational performance. One study of adults found that perceptions that a neighborhood was unsafe along with a negative reputation for the neighborhood contributed to social isolation and retreat into one's own living space (Rogers, Huxley, Evans, & Gately, 2008). A study of children found that feeling unsafe walking alone in one's neighborhood was associated with mental health diagnoses (Meltzer, Vostanis, Goodman, & Ford, 2007).

➤ Occupational therapists working in community regeneration can address safety by working with community leaders and agencies to increase the patrol of parks and play areas, increase lighting at night, develop Neighborhood Watch programs, and increase affordable public transportation.

➤ Occupational therapists can work with individuals and their families to develop strategies for increasing feelings of personal safety, such as providing information about where and when to travel outside the home, identifying others to walk with, and increasing social connections with neighbors.

Meltzer, H., Vostanis, P., Goodman, R., & Ford, T. (2007). Children's perceptions of neighborhood trustworthiness and safety and their mental health. *Journal of Child Psychology and Psychiatry, 48,* 1208–1213.
Rogers, A., Huxley, P., Evans, S., & Gately, C. (2008). More than jobs and houses: Mental health, quality of life and the perceptions of locality in an area undergoing urban regeneration. *Social Psychiatry and Psychiatric Epidemiology, 43,* 364–372.

to this partnership. Perhaps it is a person-level issue, such as physical conditioning or the lack of a specific task or social skill that is the issue. Perhaps the barrier is the occupation itself, such as a lack of adequate equipment to carry out the job. Or perhaps the problem rests in the environment, such as a disability pension system that presents the individual with a financial disincentive for paid work.

An important consideration in supporting neighborhood partnerships is the need to avoid the tendency to automatically explain partnership struggles as evidence of limitations and functional difficulties associated with mental illness. Building partnerships to enable occupation is a strategy based on developing new types of relations and interactions. In a situation in which there is limited experience with this type of partnership, and therefore few concrete examples to draw on, the automatic response can be to define the current struggles based on the old and familiar social relationships and labels.

PhotoVoice

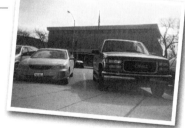

This is the library where I go on the first of the month to see if they have new magazines. They used to have groups play live music in the summer time to raise money. Children can watch videos. I used to work there vacuuming and putting books back on the shelves.

—Dennis

Empowering Peer Support

There is a high rate of mental illness in our neighborhood environments, and individuals living in the community with mental illness are not alone. Yet our communities and service systems have historically been constructed in a way that isolates them from the supportive structures of their neighborhood communities and the support and experiences of their peers. Engagement in peer support is not for everyone, but for many individuals with mental illness, their experiences with peer support can be transformative (Solomon, 2004). In addition to the enormous potential for benefits to the individual, peer initiatives are vehicles for individuals with mental illness, as a collective, to develop a shared legacy of support, skills, and experience.

Supporting the development of peer partnerships in neighborhood communities can be a distinct intervention of occupational therapy practice. This may include initiatives such as facilitating the development of self-help groups and consumer-run centers. Empowering peer support can also be an important underlying element of all occupational therapy intervention in neighborhoods. Emerging from our previous examples, we might see developing the employment opportunity through the senior center into a registered business, owned and operated by individuals with mental illness; evolving the partnership with the accessibility committee into a participatory research project that engages individuals in hosting focus groups to involve others in the community who live with mental illness; and displaying artwork at the public library as a vehicle for establishing an artist's cooperative.

Table 32-1 summarizes three potential areas of neighborhood intervention.

Summary

Although community-based mental health services are now practically universal, little attention is actually given to the neighborhoods and communities in which the clients of these services reside. Neighborhoods can present both opportunities and barriers to occupational performance for people with mental illness. A thorough knowledge of the neighborhood can lead to occupational therapy interventions that eliminate barriers or help individuals with mental illness take full advantage of existing opportunities.

Table 32-1 ● Example of Neighborhood Interventions

Category of Intervention	Examples
Neighborhood regeneration	• Establish Neighborhood Watch programs • Promote affordable child care • Work with local law enforcement on mental illness awareness • Start monthly neighborhood clean-up activities • Put on block parties or community fairs • Create a safe walking path • Develop an afterschool program • Establish reduced-cost bus passes for people with disabilities
Neighborhood partnerships	• Public library provides meeting space; people with mental illness create art displays • Senior center members have opportunities for employment (e.g., mowing lawns); people with mental illness have time and services to volunteer or provide for pay • Public schools and community colleges are interested in disability awareness; people with mental illness can provide educational programs • Accessibility committees need information to improve neighborhood accessibility; people with mental illness have real-life experiences
Peer support	• Develop a consumer-run organization • Create a consumer business • Connect consumers who live in the same apartment complex • Establish a mentorship program (e.g., one peer teaches others how to use public transportation)

Active Learning Strategies

1. Your Neighborhood

Think about your current neighborhood. Does it have characteristics that enable mental health and wellbeing? Are there aspects of your neighborhood that help you feel connected to others? What resources in the neighborhood support your physical or mental health? Are there characteristics of the neighborhood that make you anxious, frustrated, unhappy, and/or lonely? Do you feel at home in your neighborhood? Why or why not? Explain your answer and give examples.

2. The Mission of a Community

Jean Vanier, the founder of the L'Arche communities, once wrote, "The mission of a community is to give life to others, that is to say to transmit new hope and new meaning to them." Do you agree with this idea? Organize a group of four or five friends and discuss with them their views on this quote.

Describe what you learned from this discussion in your **Reflective Journal**.

3. Barriers to Activities

Choose an activity that you regularly engage in within your neighborhood. While you are participating in this activity, think about how a person experiencing mental illness might be included or excluded from participating. Consider how the activity might be changed to make it more inclusive. What barriers would you expect, and how might they be overcome?

References

Aubry, T. D., Tefft, B., & Currie, R. F. (1995). Public attitudes and intentions regarding tenants of community mental health residences who are neighbors. *Community Mental Health Journal, 31,* 39–52.

Boydell, K. M., Gladstone, B. M., Crawsford, E., & Trainor, J. (1999). Making do on the outside: Everyday life in the neighborhoods of people with psychiatric disabilities. *Psychiatric Rehabilitation Journal, 23,* 11–19.

Chovil, I. (2000). First person account: I and I, dancing fool, challenge you the world to a duel. *Schizophrenia Bulletin, 26,* 745.

Christiansen, C., & Townsend, E. (2004). The occupational nature of communities. In C. Christiansen & E. Townsend (Eds.), *Introduction to Occupation: The Art and Science of Living* (pp. 141–169). Upper Saddle River, NJ: Prentice-Hall.

De Silva, M. J., McKenzie, K., Harpham, T., & Huttly, S. R. (2005). Social capital and mental illness: A systematic review. *Journal of Epidemiology and Community Mental Health, 59,* 619–627.

Dohrenwend, B. P. (2000). The role of adversity and stress in psychopathology: Some evidence and its implications for theory and research. *Journal of Health and Social Behaviour, 41,* 1–19.

Elbogen, E. B., Soriano, C., Van Dorn, R., Swartz, M. S., & Swanson, J. W. (2005). Consumer views of representative payee use of disability funds to leverage treatment adherence. *Psychiatric Services, 56,* 45–59.

Ellet, L., Freeman, D., & Garety, P. A. (2008). The psychological effect of an urban environment on individuals with persecutory delusions: The Camberwell walk study. *Schizophrenia Research, 99,* 77–84.

Estroff, S. E., Penn, D. L., & Toporek, J. R. (2004). From stigma to discrimination: An analysis of community efforts to reduce the negative consequences of having a psychiatric disorder and label. *Schizophrenia Bulletin, 30,* 493–510.

Fieldhouse, J. (2000). Occupational science and community mental health: Using occupational risk factors as a framework for exploring chronicity. *British Journal of Occupational Therapy, 63*(5), 211–217.

Fitzgerald, P. B., de Castella, A. R., Filia, K. M., Filia, S. L., Benitez, J., & Kulkami, J. (2005). Victimization of patients with schizophrenia and related disorders. *Australian and New Zealand Journal of Psychiatry, 39,* 169–174.

Furlong, A., Biggart, A., & Cartmel, F. (1996). Neighborhoods, opportunity structures and occupational aspirations. *Sociology, 30,* 551–565.

Gilmour, H. (2004). Living alone with dementia: risk and the professional role. *Nursing Older People, 16*(9), 20–25.

Harkness, J., Newman, S. J., & Salkever, D. (2004). The cost-effectiveness of independent housing for the chronically mentally ill: Do housing and neighborhood features matter? *Health Services Research, 39,* 1341–1360.

Hiday, V. A., Swartz, M. S., Swanson, J. W., Borum, R., & Wagner, H. R. (1999). Criminal victimization of persons with severe mental illness. *Psychiatric Services, 50,* 62–68.

Holter, M. C., & Mowbray, C. T. (2005). Consumer-run drop-in centres: Program operations and costs. *Psychiatric Rehabilitation Journal, 28*(4), 323–331.

Jacobson, N., & Greenley, D. (2001). What is recovery? A conceptual model and explication. *Psychiatric Services, 42,* 482–485.

Jarvis, G. E. (2007). The social causes of psychosis in a North American Psychiatry: A review of a disappearing literature. *Canadian Journal of Psychiatry, 52,* 287–294.

Jenkins, R. (2004). *Social identity* (2nd ed.). London: Routledge.

Kretzman, J. P., & McKnight, J. L. (1993). *Building Communities From the Inside Out: A Path Toward Finding and Mobilizing a Community's Assets.* Chicago: ACTA Publications.

Krupa, T. (2004). Employment, recovery and schizophrenia: Integrating health and disorder at work. *Psychiatric Rehabilitation Journal, 28*(1), 8–15.

Krupa, T., Eastabrook, S., Hern, L., Lee, D., North, R., Percy, K., Von Briesen, B., & Wing, G. (2005). How do people who receive assertive community treatment experience this service? *Psychiatric Rehabilitation Journal, 29,* 18–24.

Kubzansky, L. D., Subramanian, S. V., Kawachi, I., Fay, M. E., Soobader J., & Berkman, L. F. (2005). Neighborhood contextual influences on depressive symptoms in the elderly. *American Journal of Epidemiology, 162*(3), 253–260.

Lee, S., Chiu, M. Y., Tsang, A., Chui, H., & Kleinman, A. (2006). Stigmatizing experiences and structural discrimination association with the treatment of schizophrenia in Hong Kong. *Social Science in Medicine, 62,* 1685–1696.

Nelson, G., Lord, J., & Ochocka, J. (2001). *Shifting the Paradigm in Community Mental Health.* Toronto: University of Toronto Press.

Ortiz, A., Simmons, J., & Hinton, W. L. (1999) Locations of remorse and homelands of resilience: Notes on grief and sense of loss of place of Latino and Irish-American caregivers of demented elders. *Culture, Medicine and Psychiatry, 23*(4), 477–500.

Schomerus, G., Heider, D., Angermeyer, M. C., Bebbington, P. E., Azorin, J. M., Brugha, T., & Toumi, M. (2007). Urban residence, victimhood and the appraisal of personal safety in people with schizophrenia: Results from the European Schizophrenia Cohort (EuroSC). *Psychological Medicine, 38,* 591–597.

Silver, E. (2000). Race, neighborhood disadvantage and violence among persons with mental disorders: The importance of contextual measurement. *Law and Human Behavior, 24,* 449–456.

Silver, E., Mulvey, E. P., & Swanson, J. W. (2002). Neighborhood structural characteristics and mental disorder: Faris and Dunham revisited. *Social Science and Medicine, 55,* 1457–1470.

Solomon, P. (2004). Peer support/peer provided services underlying processes, benefits, and critical ingredients. *Psychiatric Rehabilitation Journal, 27,* 392–402.

Stuart, H., & Arboleda-Florez, J. (2001). A public health perspective on violence among persons with mental illness. *Psychiatric Services, 52,* 654–659.

Teplin, L. A., McClelland, G. M., Abram, K. M., & Weiner, D. A. (2005). Crime victimization in adults with severe mental illness: Comparison with the National Crime Victimization Survey. *Archives of General Psychiatry, 62,* 911–921.

Warner, R. (1994). *Recovery from Schizophrenia: Psychiatry and Political Economy*. London: Routledge.

Whitley, R., & Prince, M. (2005a). Can urban regeneration programmes assist coping and recovery for people with mental illness? Suggestions from a qualitative case study. *Health Promotion International, 21,* 19–26.

———. (2005b) Fear of crime, mobility and mental health in inner-city London, UK. *Social Science and Medicine, 61,* 1678–1688.

Xue, Y., Leventhal, T., Brooks-Gunn, J., & Earls, F. J. (2005). Neighbourhood residence and mental health problems of 5-to 11-year olds. *Archives of General Psychiatry, 62,* 554–563.

Yen, I. H., & Syme, S. L. (1999). The social environment and health: A discussion of the epidemiologic literature. *Annual Review of Public Health, 20,* 287–308.

Supported Housing: Creating a Sense of Home

Deborah B. Pitts

> "There's no place like home. There's no place like home. There's no place like home.
>
> —Dorothy in *The Wizard of Oz*
>
> Every person with a psychiatric disability deserves a range of housing choices and to live in a home of his or her own. That includes the full rights of tenancy, including a lease, a key, privacy, and the choice of roommate, where relevant.
>
> —Center for Mental Health Services, 2006, p. 3

Introduction

Recovery for persons living with psychiatric disabilities involves a "reclaiming of the self" (Davidson & Strauss, 1992; Sells, Stayner, & Davidson, 2004), a self compromised by disruptions in engagement in occupational roles and social stigma attached to mental illness. This reclaiming of the self is best accomplished through "role recovery" processes that include access to opportunities for engagement in occupations within supportive contexts. Consistent with the "Occupational Therapy Practice Framework" (American Occupational Therapy Association [AOTA], 2008), supportive contexts help persons with mental illness to take the risks of engaging in occupation. Supported housing is one type of supportive context developed to promote recovery by providing persons with mental illness access to the role of "tenant." For persons seeking recovery, having a sense of home as a safe, supportive place to live, sleep, and carry out meaningful occupational roles can make the difference between full and limited participation in everyday life.

This chapter introduces the world of housing options that might be available to persons who are considered disabled on the basis of their psychiatric condition (those not considered disabled are unlikely to be able to access several of the options, given that they may not be eligible for publicly funded housing support). In addition to ensuring that there is a match between the person and the housing environment, the impact of varied neighborhoods and communities on the level of mental health recovery experienced by the person should be considered. The expertise of the occupational therapist provides this important interpretation from making the match to assessing and/or providing the ongoing support needed to increase the chances of success in community living for persons with serious mental illness.

Description of Supported Housing

Supported housing is described as "independent housing coupled with the provision of community-based mental

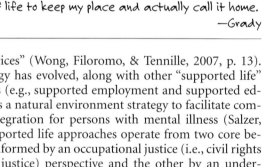

PhotoVoice

This is a picture of my building. I live in apartment # 200. This structure involves a transcendent level of interconnectedness.
This states I am in a safe place and on an ongoing way of life to keep my place and actually call it home.

—Grady

health services" (Wong, Filoromo, & Tennille, 2007, p. 13). This strategy has evolved, along with other "supported life" approaches (e.g., supported employment and supported education), as a natural environment strategy to facilitate community integration for persons with mental illness (Salzer, 2006). Supported life approaches operate from two core beliefs: one informed by an occupational justice (i.e., civil rights and social justice) perspective and the other by an understanding of the contextualized nature of learning and habit formation.

From an advocacy stance, supported life approaches claim that people with disabilities should have access to the same living, learning, and working environments as those individuals without disabilities; they should not be segregated in "specialized" settings such as congregate living, or group homes, and/or sheltered work situations (Salzer, 2006). These approaches acknowledge that persons with disabilities *may* need certain types and intensity of support beyond that typically accessed by persons without disabilities. However, supported life advocates emphasize the interdependent nature of human existence and remind us that everyone, even people without disabilities, need ongoing support to sustain participation in our living, learning, and working environments of choice.

Supported Housing Among Supported Life Approaches

Whatever the nature of supports, the supported life perspective emphasizes that the support should be provided in real-world contexts and only at a level preferred by the person with the disability to ensure that he or she can sustain successful and satisfying participation in that environment. For persons with psychiatric disabilities, this is particularly critical, as stigma and discrimination are significant barriers to recovery in general and access to safe and affordable housing in particular (Link, Struening, Neese-Todd, Asmussen, & Phelan, 2001; Perlick et al, 2001; Yanos, Rosenfield, & Horwitz, 2001). Community resistance (i.e., "Not in my back yard," or NIMBYism) to locating housing for different disability groups has been documented, and the reactions of communities toward integration of persons with psychiatric disabilities has been particularly harmful (Piat, 2000; Zippay, 2007).

Supported life approaches argue that the best way to learn to do "something" is to *do* that something. This is most commonly referred to in the community-integration literature as a paradigm shift from a "train-place" to a "place-train" perspective in psychiatric rehabilitation philosophy (Corrigan, 2001). The **place-train perspective** acknowledges the contextualized nature of learning and habit formation, particularly for major life roles, and eschews assumptions regarding the need for preparatory or transitional experiences (hence questioning the programs that train first in simulated environments) for persons with disabilities. In addition to the emphasis on placing a person in a housing situation first, and then offering the training and support to facilitate successful everyday living, an added emphasis is on helping the person to remain successfully housed (Yanos, Felton, Tsemberis, & Frye, 2007).

Although advocates of this approach acknowledge the developmental nature of skill building and habit formation across the life span, they remind us of how we all learned and established our self-care, domestic care, and work-related habits and routines. We did so by practicing them in those contexts in which they would be used with the specialized support of more skilled others and with the socioemotional support needed to take the risk of action. An example of the place-train approach is placing a person with a psychiatric disability in an apartment and offering occupational therapy and peer support to strengthen money management skills and communication skills with landlord and neighbors.

Federal Mental Health Policy Affecting Housing

In response to federal-level initiatives during the 1990s and early 2000s, specifically the Olmstead decision (Allen, 2004; *Olmstead v L.C. and E.W.,* 1999), the New Freedom Commission on Mental Health (2003), and the Substance Abuse and Mental Health Administration's Transformation Action Agenda (U.S. Department of Health and Human Services [USDHHS], 2005), supported housing has become one of several resources informed by a psychiatric rehabilitation perspective and adopted by state and local mental health authorities to promote recovery for persons with psychiatric disabilities. Although there were efforts by some institutions during the mid-1800s "moral treatment" and the early 1900s "mental hygiene" eras in the United States to help those individuals being discharged to resettle into the community following an extended hospitalization experience (Goldstein & Godemont, 2003; Meyer, 1916/1952; Tuntiya, 2006), these programs were never widespread.

Choice and Supports

Although it is acknowledged that there are conceptual problems in defining supported housing, given that the specific housing types and supports offered are not fully standardized across mental health programs and research (Fakhoury, Murray, Shepherd, & Priebe, 2002), Nelson and Peddle (2005) distinguished supported housing from other approaches to providing housing for persons with psychiatric disabilities, specifically supportive and custodial housing, because of its fundamental commitment to providing consumers with "choice/control over where they live, how they live, and the professional support that they receive" (p. 1573). They credit Paul Carling (1993; 1995) and Ridgway and Zipple (1990) with defining this key characteristic of supported housing and note that supportive housing grew out of the philosophical perspective of the independent living movement for persons with physical disabilities.

In supported housing, the tenant is the primary lesee or mortgage holder, not a mental health agency, and the housing is typical of that available in the community in which the person is living, such as an apartment, duplex, condominium, co-op, or single-family home. A critical aspect of supported housing is that it is a "home for life . . . [not a] treatment way-station" (Bigelow, 1998, p. 403) and is based solely on the person meeting his or her tenancy obligations, not on the individual's compliance with treatment. Common support services used by people with mental illness include financial support to pay for rent, professional support to assist with obtaining and maintaining the apartment, choices for safe and comfortable housing, and opportunities for social contact and community integration (George et al, 2005). The level and nature of the supports change as the person's needs or wants change, and they are provided at an intensity directed by the tenant—not by the tenant's mental health services provider.

To facilitate this delinking of access to housing from decisions about level of support preferred, it is recommended that the mental health agency providing the support services *not* serve as the landlord. As a result, mental health agencies that provide supported housing services often partner or contract with property management companies to handle tenancy issues, while the mental health agency focuses on the provision of the support services.

Custodial housing settings include congregate-living environments that are most often operated for profit by private landlords, including board and care homes and single-room occupancy hotels. The term **board and care home** describes living arrangements that provide shelter, food, and 24-hour supervision or protective oversight and personal care services to residents. Other terms for board and care homes include *homes for the aged, residential care homes, adult foster care, domiciliary care,* and *assisted-living facilities.* Such homes may be licensed or unlicensed and range in size from two residents to more than 200 (Center for Mental Health Services, 2006, p. 35). In 2006, SAMHSA published its *Transforming Housing for People with Psychiatric Disabilities* report, which outlined recommendations for how to reduce the use of board and care homes and increase the number of supported/supportive housing options for persons with psychiatric disabilities. In general, these settings provide little mental health support or rehabilitation interventions, even when required by law to do so, and are understood by occupational therapists to be sites of profound occupational deprivation (Center for Mental Health Services, 2006; Suto & Frank, 1994; Whiteford, 2000).

In the **supportive housing** approach, which began developing in the early years of the 1960s deinstitutionalization movement, staff provide case management, support, and/or rehabilitation in a variety of different housing types, including halfway houses, group homes, and supervised apartments. The idea underlying this approach is to match the needs of the consumer with the appropriate housing type, which is linked to the amount of support necessary. The consumer then moves from one level of care to another as his or her level of support needs change.

Understood as a transitional approach, advocates of the supportive housing approach argue that people who are discharged from psychiatric hospitals need a place to develop the skills for community living before "going it alone." It is believed that skill development is needed because lengthy institutional stays may have either (1) atrophied what skills existed prior to the hospital admission or (2) limited the individual's ability to develop such skills if he or she had not had any tenure in independent living prior to that admission (Glasscote, Gudeman, & Elpers, 1971; Raush & Raush, 1968; Rothwell & Doniger, 1966). In addition, advocates of the supportive housing approach believe that the needs of some people with mental illness are better met in congregate housing settings with onsite services (Rog, 2004).

Woodley House and Fairweather Lodge

Woodley House is one of the earliest halfway houses described in the literature. Located in Washington, D.C., it was developed and staffed by occupational therapists Joan Doniger and Edith Maeda. The initial halfway house established in 1958 housed 10 residents and was expanded in the mid-1970s to include an apartment program as well. Despite its transitional nature, the description of the staff role at Woodley House and the nature of the support provided is strikingly consistent with that of the current approach to supported housing (Doniger, Rothwell, & Cohen, 1963; Kresky, Maeda, & Rothwell, 1976; Rothwell & Doniger, 1966). As Doniger, Rothwell, and Cohen (1963) state:

We give applicants three cautions. The first is that life in the house isn't always beautiful; good times are mixed with bad. Second, we tell them that the house is loosely supervised. During the day, staff members come and go, as do the residents, each of whom has his own key. No staff member sits up at night. If someone needs constant watching, Woodley House is not for him. However, we do tell them that someone is always available to be called at night if a resident is acutely anxious or physically ill. The third caution, and the most difficult to make understood, is that our house is not a treatment facility. By the time all this has been explained, the prospective resident usually wants to know whether there is any point in moving to Woodley House, since it won't treat him, protect him, or keep him happy. Then we say, if you like it, it's a nice place to live, and if you don't like it, it isn't anything (pp. 193–194).

Robert Cohen, in his foreword to the case study of Woodley House published in 1966 (Rothwell & Doniger, 1966), argued that the philosophy and practices of Woodley House were particularly informed by an occupational therapy perspective:

In my opinion, the characteristics of the House derive quite naturally from the training and special experiences of Joan Doniger and Edith Maeda. Both of them were trained professionally as occupational therapists. . . . From her first contact [the occupational therapist] deals with the patient's integrative skills, his ego strengths, and fosters the development of his sense of mastery (p. viii).

Another example of supportive housing is the **Fairweather Lodge model,** developed originally by George Fairweather in the early 1960s. This model is a unique approach to supportive housing because it combines housing and work opportunities. In addition, the Lodge operates from a set of core principles informed by a social psychology perspective that persons with psychiatric disabilities are more likely to succeed in community living if they do so in small, family-like units (Fairweather, Sanders, Cressler, & Maynard, 1969).

The original design of the Lodge involved a small number of people with psychiatric disabilities living together and creating and operating a small business that would provide the necessary work opportunities, such as lawn care. Currently, all members of the Lodge do not necessarily live together; some may live independently and work only for the business component (Onaga, McKinney, & Pfaff, 2000). A key aspect of the Lodge programs is that members assume decision-making authority and responsibility for the Lodge operations, and staff serve as consultants to facilitate the members'/residents' success; as such, its philosophy is more consistent with supported housing in terms of choice and control (Haertl, 2005; 2007).

Supported Housing as Creating a Sense of Home

Models of providing sequential and graded reintroduction into community life (i.e., hospital to halfway house to independent living), which is called the **linear continuum paradigm** (Ridgway & Zipple, 1990), have been replaced with the paradigm of helping persons with psychiatric disabilities to find housing that can become a home for them—a safe home—and that offers a base from which they may be fully engaged in their community as citizens. Tsemberis and Asmussen (1999) noted the weaknesses of the linear continuum model for persons with serious mental illness:

- Moving from one level of care to the next disrupts the formation of interpersonal relationships so necessary for success and satisfaction, and the need to adjust to each new context is stressful. [See also Forchuk, Ward-Griffin, Csiernik, & Turner, 2006.]
- Skills learned for successful functioning in a structured congregate setting are not necessarily transferable to an independent living situation.
- Residents of such settings lack choices and freedoms; residential treatments offer standardized levels of care to which the person must adapt.
- Placement into a level of supervised housing is based on the decision of clinical staff, and clients are afforded little privacy or control (Tsemberis & Asmussen, 1999, p. 116).

George et al (2005) acknowledged that the distinctions between *supported* and *supportive* housing have become less evident as supportive housing providers have worked to adopt practices that are more closely aligned with the promotion of consumer/survivor choice, as advocated by the supported housing approach. They strive for a "values-based" approach to providing housing for persons labeled with psychiatric disabilities that focuses on a set of key values that include:

- Empowerment (consumers have choice and control over housing)
- Resources (financial, professional, housing and social)
- Community integration (Nelson & Peddle, 2005)

These values are consistent with the philosophy and science espoused by occupational therapists. Experiencing a "sense of home" in one's living environment is said to promote a sense of wellbeing and contribute to overall quality of life (Dupuis & Thorns, 1998; Mallett, 2004). A sense of home is particularly important for individuals with psychiatric disabilities, especially given the disruptions to stable housing that they have often experienced (Evans, Wells, & Moch, 2003; Padgett, 2007). Occupational therapy (Hasselkus, 2002; Rowles, 2003) has expanded on its understanding of "homemaking" by drawing on the concept of place from philosophy, geography, and environmental psychology. These perspectives on place distinguish it from the spatial dimensions of a specific environmental context and emphasize the deep meaning and value that particular settings can have for humans (Gieryn, 2000; Tuan, 1977), including the presence of personal objects (Csikszentmihalyi & Rochberg-Halton, 1981).

It is clear from the research on how a sense of place is established that it happens by engaging in occupations in that context (Rowles, 2003). Therefore, it is important to help tenants personalize their space with meaningful items and help them engage in occupations within the units themselves, as well as in the surrounding community, in order to help them establish a sense of home.

It is important to note that "home" is experienced not just within the walls of the unit but also by being a part of one's community. Criticism of community-based efforts are that persons with psychiatric disabilities may be living in the community but are not fully engaged in the life of the local community (Segal & Aviram, 1978 [cited in Wong & Solomon, 2002]). Therefore, attention to facilitating occupational habits, routines, and rituals that engage the person in the local community must be included in any supported housing context. This could include participating in local organizations, attending local social and recreational events, voting, and so on.

Funding for Supported Housing

Funding for supported housing is generally of two broad types: funding for the support services and funding for the housing itself. For the most part, the support services are financed by public mental health funding sources, including Medicaid's Targeted Case Management and/or Rehabilitation Option(s) and state-specific mental health revenue sources such as California's Mental Health Services Act (MHSA, Prop. 63). In some cases, support services are included in HUD-funded new low-income housing construction and rehabilitation initiatives. Most often these support services are provided by nonprofit, community-based agencies specializing in mental health services for persons

Evidence-Based Practice

People with psychiatric disabilities consistently prefer to live in their own apartments rather than in supervised, congregate-living situations. Supported housing can offer this option as well as reduce homelessness and hospitalization and improve the quality of life for persons with psychiatric disabilities.

➤ Occupational therapists can partner with consumer advocates and other mental health professionals to promote the development of supported housing.

➤ Occupational therapists can support individuals with mental illness with whom they are working to obtain and sustain supported housing.

Greenwood, R., Schaefer-McDaniel, N., Winkel, G., & Tsemberis, S. (2005). Decreasing psychiatric symptoms by increasing choice in services for adults with histories of homelessness. *American Journal of Community Psychology, 36*(3), 223–238.

Nelson, G., Hall, G. B., & Forchuk, C. (2003). Current and preferred housing of psychiatric consumers/survivors. *Canadian Journal of Community Mental Health, 22,* 5–19.

Owen, C., Rutherford, V., Jones, M., Wright, C., Tennant, C., & Smallman, A. (1996). Housing accommodation preferences of people with psychiatric disabilities. *Psychiatric Services, 47,* 628–632.

Rosenheck, R., Kasprow, W., Frisman, L., & Liu-Mares, W. (2003). Cost-effectiveness of supported housing for homeless persons with mental illness. *Archives of General Psychiatry, 60*(9), 940–951.

Tanzman, B. (1993). An overview of surveys of mental health consumers' preferences for housing and support services. *Hospital & Community Psychiatry, 44,* 450–455.

Tsemberis, S., Gulcur, L., & Nakae, M. (2004). Housing First, consumer choice, and harm reduction for homeless individuals with a dual diagnosis. *American Journal of Public Health, 94*(4), 651–656.

Warren, R., & Bell, P. (2000). An exploratory investigation into the housing preferences of consumers of mental health services. *Australian and New Zealand Journal of Mental Health Nursing, 9,* 195–202.

with psychiatric disabilities, including comprehensive community mental health centers, psychosocial rehabilitation clubhouses, and agencies that strictly provide supported housing services. State and local mental health authorities contract with these agencies to provide housing support services using whatever funding resources the particular state has authorized for such purposes. The agencies providing these services may also pursue foundation grants as a method to fund new or expanded services that will later be funded through more stable funding sources. Occupational therapy educational programs have often been able to use foundation grants to support student practicum experiences in these settings.

Personal Assistance Services

In addition to Targeted Case Management and rehabilitation services, Medicaid also funds personal care services, also called **personal assistance services (PAS)**. According to the Center for Personal Assistance Services (http://www.pascenter.org), these services assist people with disabilities with tasks essential for daily living. Although initially developed and used primarily by persons with physical and developmental disabilities in response to the independent living movement, persons with psychiatric disabilities are also using such services to sustain themselves in independent living situations (Farkas, Chamberlin, Harding, Kramer, & Kenyon, 2003; Pita, Ellison, & Farkas, 2001).

Since 1975, states have had the option of offering personal care services as a Medicaid benefit. States have considerable discretion in defining these services, but programs typically provide nonmedical assistance with activities of daily living (e.g., bathing and eating) for participants with disabilities and chronic conditions. States vary in the amount and scope of the services provided (e.g., some states provide these services outside the participant's residence). States can provide this service to all eligible persons covered in their state Medicaid plan or can apply for a Home and Community-Based Services waiver and specifically define the population that will be served by the program. To receive the Medicaid-funded personal care services, the person with a psychiatric disability must be a Medicaid recipient and be evaluated by a Medicaid representative to be in need of the service. An important aspect of PAS is that it supports self-determination and personal control of resources, because the person with the disability has sole decision-making authority over who provides the services as well as when and where the services are provided.

Housing

Funding for housing itself includes rent or mortgage payments as well as new construction or rehabilitation of properties. Tenants are responsible for ensuring an income stream that will be sufficient to meet their rent or mortgage obligation. Most tenants of supported housing settings are Social Security Disability Income (SSDI) or Supplemental Security Income (SSI) beneficiaries. They receive this income because they have been found to be disabled as a result of their psychiatric disorder. Persons on SSDI receive an amount based on their past earnings, so the total amount each person receives varies. Persons on SSI receive the federal benefit rate, which was $674 per month in 2010 for an individual, plus any supplement that specific state government contributes. For example, in California in 2010, SSI beneficiaries received $845 per month. In addition to their disability income, some tenants of supported housing settings work part time.

Although some states may provide financial resources for the development of supported housing (e.g., the California Mental Health Services Act supported housing initiative), the primary source of public funds for financing new housing construction or rehabilitation of existing properties that provide rental assistance is the federal-level Department of Housing and Urban Development (HUD) (see Resources at the end of this chapter). Agencies that provide supported housing services to persons with psychiatric disabilities can access both the Section 811 and Section 8 HUD housing programs.

HUD's Section 811 Supportive Housing Program for Persons with Disabilities provides interest-free capital advances to nonprofit agencies to help them finance the development of rental housing, such as independent living projects, condominium units, and small group homes, with the availability of supportive services for persons with disabilities. The capital advance can finance the construction, rehabilitation, or acquisition with or without rehabilitation of supportive housing and does not have to be repaid as long as the housing remains available for very low-income persons with disabilities for at least 40 years.

HUD also provides project rental assistance; this covers the difference between the HUD-approved operating cost of the project and the amount the residents pay—usually 30% of adjusted income. The initial term of the project rental assistance contract is 3 years and can be renewed if funds are available. The available program funds for a fiscal year are allocated to HUD's local offices according to factors established by HUD.

Each project must have a supportive services plan. The appropriate state or local agency reviews a potential sponsor's application to determine and certify that the plan is well designed to meet the needs of persons with disabilities. Services may vary with the target population but can include case management, training in independent living skills, and assistance in obtaining employment. However, residents cannot be required to accept any supportive service as a condition of occupancy (HUD, 2007).

HUD's Section 8 Housing Choice Voucher Program is the federal government's major program for assisting very low–income families, the elderly, and the disabled to afford decent, safe, and sanitary housing in the private market. Since housing assistance is provided on behalf of the family or individual, participants are able to find their own housing, including single-family homes, townhouses, and apartments. The participant is free to choose any housing that meets the requirements of the program and is not limited to units located in subsidized housing projects.

Housing choice vouchers are administered locally by **public housing agencies (PHAs)**. The PHAs receive federal funds from HUD to administer the voucher program. A family that is issued a housing voucher is responsible for finding a suitable housing unit of the family's choice where the owner agrees to rent under the program. This unit may include the family's present residence. Rental units must meet minimum standards of health and safety, as determined by the PHA. A housing subsidy is paid to the landlord directly by the PHA on behalf of the participating family. The family then pays the difference between the actual rent charged by the landlord and the amount subsidized by the program. Under certain circumstances, if authorized by the PHA, a family may use its voucher to purchase a modest home (HUD, n.d.).

Occupational Therapy Assessment

The occupational therapy evaluation process in supported housing settings includes the development of an occupational profile and an analysis of occupational performance (AOTA, 2002; 2008). In the **occupational profile,** the occupational therapist focuses on eliciting the person's occupational history, perception of the need for change, and preferences for the direction of that change as it relates to his or her housing situation.

Following the identification of the person's targeted outcomes related to housing, the occupational therapist conducts an analysis of the person's occupational performance related to those specific targeted outcomes. It is important to identify the person's past successes and difficulties related to domestic and self-care routines and habits as well as his or her preferences for how to perform these activities, including what level of social and environmental support he or she has needed to engage in and sustain their enactment of those habits and routines. The occupational therapist's analysis should include a thorough understanding of the person's illness management strategies as well as the nature of any neurocognitive or sensory disruptions and their impact on the person's functioning.

An assessment of the environmental resources and barriers specific to the targeted outcomes must be completed as well. This should include an assessment of the actual living environment (e.g., both the specific apartment and the apartment building as well as the surrounding neighborhood and community). The occupational therapist must understand to what degree the social and task environments will support the person's enactment of preferred and obligated habits and routines. Specific assessment tools for the occupational profile and the analysis of occupational performance that may be useful in supported housing services are described next.

Tools for Developing an Occupational Profile

The most common assessment approach for developing an occupational profile is an interview. Interviews are particularly valuable in this phase of the occupational therapy evaluation because, when conducted effectively, they allow for the exploratory dialogue necessary for identifying a person's perceived strengths, needs, and preferences for supported housing. In addition, the therapist can elicit the person's subjective experiences related to creating a sense of home, which is necessary for good quality of life.

Self-report checklists that elicit the person's global or specific perspectives related to their independent living strengths, needs, and preferences can also be used to help the occupational therapist develop an individual's occupational profile. Occupational therapists often combine an interview with selected self-report checklists to strengthen their understanding of the person. The tools described in the following sections are well established in occupational therapy practice and informed by clearly articulated frames of reference consistent with the person-environment-occupation perspective.

Occupational Performance History Interview-II

The Occupational Performance History Interview II (OPHI-II) comes from the model of human occupation (MOHO) and uses a semistructured and narrative interview approach to help the occupational therapist understand the individual as an occupational being. The OPHI-II manual provides a set of suggested interview questions organized in five thematic areas: occupational roles, daily routine, occupational behavior settings, activity/occupational choices, and critical life events (Kielhofner et al, 2004).This assessment can be used with adolescents (at least 12 years of age) through older adults, with the main consideration being whether or not the person can meaningfully and effectively participate in a history-taking interview.

An important role for this tool is identification of the person–environment interaction through the use of its assessment of the person's occupational behavior settings, including home and leisure contexts. In addition, given the narrative nature of this assessment and its effort to elicit aspects of meaning in the person's life, the OPHI-II can assist the occupational therapist in helping the person to establish a sense of home.

Use of the OPHI-II requires that the therapist be comfortable and skilled in a narrative interviewing approach and be familiar with MOHO in order to interpret the findings from the interview. Upon completion of the interview, the clinician uses the information collected to complete a set of rating scales and key forms, specifically the occupational identity, occupational competence, and occupational behavior settings. Each scale includes a finite set of items representative of MOHO concepts. Each item is rated using a 4-point adaptive scale, with 4 representing the most adaptive response and 1 representing the least adaptive response. Each rating for each item is operationally defined to facilitate the therapist's interpretation of the information from the interview to assign the rating (Kielhofner et al, 2004). For example, related to occupational competence, should the client reveal that some functional limitations pertaining to the timing of occupations needed to live independently as a tenant (such as not putting out the garbage in time for neighborhood garbage pickup nor writing a rent check when it is due) were consistent challenges, then a score of 2 would be noted. This score would signal the need to develop a case management plan for helping the person to carry out such tasks within the appropriate time parameters, thus supporting the occupational role of tenant.

Reliability and validity of the OPHI-II are demonstrated in several studies, including interrater reliability, concurrent validity, and predictive validity (Kielhofner, Forsyth, Clay, et al, 2007). Further, a study investigating the nature of the interview questions found that the narrative approach to questions effectively generated rich occupational stories and more meaningful information for intervention planning (Apte, Kielhofner, Paul-Ward, & Braveman,

2005). Cross-cultural validity has also been demonstrated (Kielhofner, Forsyth, Clay, et al, 2007)

Occupational Self-Assessment

The Occupational Self-Assessment (OSA) (Baron, Kielhofner, Iyenger, Goldhammer, & Wolenski, 2006; Kielhofner, Forsyth, Suman, et al, 2007) is a self-report checklist that is also derived from MOHO. It facilitates identification of the person's perception of the degree of difficulty he or she is experiencing in targeted areas of occupational performance and the importance of those in daily life. The therapist and consumer can then discuss each area, and then the person prioritizes areas for change.

Studies have demonstrated that the OSA is a valid and reliable measure (Baron et al, 2006; Kielhofner, Forsyth, Suman, et al, 2007). One study found the OSA was useful in eliciting information to facilitate the development of a meaningful occupational therapy intervention for young people in an early intervention psychosis program (Fisher & Savin-Baden, 2001).

Tools for Analyzing Occupational Performance

The analysis of occupational performance in supported housing environments should focus on the person's activities of daily living (ADLs) and instrumental activities of daily living (IADLs), neurocognitive deficits that may impact safe and successful enactment of those ADL/IADLs, and the social/interpersonal skills necessary for maintaining effective neighbor and landlord relationships. Other areas of occupational performance that go beyond tenancy status include the persons' leisure/recreational competencies. The tools described in the following sections are well established in occupational therapy practice and informed by clearly articulated frames of reference consistent with the person-environment-occupation perspective.

Allen Cognitive Level Screen

The Allen Cognitive Level Screen (ACL-5) (Allen et al, 2007) is based on the cognitive disabilities model and is designed to obtain a baseline measure of the person's capacity to learn and the need for environmental compensations. This model describes six hierarchical cognitive levels for understanding how neurocognitive impairments impact a person's occupational performance (Allen, Earhart, & Blue, 1992). This performance-based test is usually administered at the end of the initial interview and establishes an initial level of functioning. The ACL-5 is a visuomotor task that provides an estimate of a person's ability to learn to do other visuomotor tasks. See Chapter 18 for a more in-depth description of the ACL-5 and all cognitive tools.

Reliability and validity studies find the ACL-5 to be a dependable measure of cognitive levels consistent with the model (Allen et al, 1992). Further observation is required to verify the level and is often accomplished using the Routine Task Inventory–Expanded (Katz, 2006), described in the next section, or the Allen Diagnostic Module (ADM). The ADM consists of craft activities that have been organized by the six levels (Allen & Reyner, 2005).

An important contribution of this assessment and its companion tools to the occupational therapist in supported housing settings is that it provides information regarding how to modify the living environment in a way that minimizes the impact of any neurocognitive deficits that are identified. For example, a person functioning at a cognitive level 5 may not anticipate problems that might occur in sharing the common areas of an apartment such as the bathroom, kitchen, and living room. The occupational therapist might assist the individual and his or her roommate to establish agreements as to how they will handle sharing food or chores to prevent later problems from occurring

Routine Task Inventory-Expanded

The Routine Task Inventory–Expanded (RTI-Expanded), which is informed by the cognitive disabilities frame of reference, is an observational guide. It consists of 14 tasks that describe behavioral actions consistent with the cognitive levels. The cognitive levels represent a six-level hierarchical model for understanding how cognitive impairments impact a person's occupational performance (Allen et al, 1992). The RTI-Expanded describes the functional severity of a disability; it is a here-and-now assessment of the impact of a disease.

The 14 routine tasks of the RTI are divided into two scales: physical and instrumental. The six tasks on the physical scale are grooming, dressing, bathing, walking, feeding, and toileting. The eight tasks on the instrumental scale are housekeeping, preparing food, spending money, taking medication, doing laundry, traveling, shopping, and using the telephone. Under each of the 14 tasks, behavioral descriptions are written in connection with each cognitive level.

Administration of the interview requires the identification of an informant who is well acquainted with the individual's performance and willing to provide information. The informant and the occupational therapist review the inventory together. The behavioral description that best matches the individual's routine task performance is noted. The RTI-Expanded takes approximately 1 hour to administer (Allen et al, 1992).

Assessment of Motor and Process Skills

The Assessment of Motor and Process Skills (AMPS) gathers information on skills by observing the person doing selected ADLs, both personal and instrumental. The AMPS is designed so that cross-culturally standardized tasks can be used to measure occupational performance. When administering the AMPS, motor skills (i.e., actions done to move oneself or objects) and process skills (i.e., logical sequencing of actions, selection and appropriate use of tools and materials, and adaptation to problems) are observed simultaneously. The AMPS score takes into consideration the level of difficulty of the task the person is performing and the severity/leniency of the rater.

Scores for the AMPS are computer generated, and occupational therapists using the AMPS must be trained and calibrated for their severity/leniency. Studies support the validity, reliability, internal consistency of the scales, stability of the measure over time, and ability of the measures to remain stable when the AMPS is scored by different raters. Administration and scoring of the AMPS takes 30 to 60 minutes and includes a brief interview and observation of the person performing four or five preferred standardized tasks (Kielhofner, Cahill, et al, 2007), including such IADL tasks as money management, meal preparation, and laundry management. The AMPS is demonstrated to be an effective tool in assessing the occupational performance of persons with psychiatric disabilities in community-based living contexts (Girard, Fisher, Short, & Duran, 1999; McNulty & Fisher, 2001; Pan & Fisher, 1994).

Kohlman Evaluation of Living Skills

The Kohlman Evaluation of Living Skills (KELS) is an evaluation of basic living skills that combines interview and task performance techniques. It is intended to be administered and scored within 30 to 45 minutes. It assesses 18 living skills grouped under five major categories: self-care, safety and health, money management, transportation and telephone, and work and leisure. Scoring criteria are formulated to indicate the minimum standards required for living independently within the community. Items scored as "needs assistance" are given a score of 1 point, with the exception of items in the work/leisure category, which are assessed one-half point. Studies find that the KELS has good interrater reliability and that the scale can correctly differentiate persons living in a sheltered setting from those living independently with an accuracy of 90% (Thomson, 1992)

Test of Grocery Shopping Skills

The Test of Grocery Shopping Skills (TOGGS) is a performance-based assessment conducted in the natural environment to measure the person's grocery shopping skills. The person is asked to find 10 grocery items, and an accuracy score is calculated based on his or her finding items of a particular size and at the lowest cost (Hamera & Brown, 2000). A companion tool, the Knowledge of Grocery Shopping Skills (KOGSS), is a self-report measure that identifies the person's grocery shopping knowledge, with higher scores indicating more grocery shopping knowledge (Brown, Rempfer, Hamera, & Bothwell, 2006). Both tools are demonstrated to reliable and valid measures of their respective aspects of grocery shopping skills (Brown et al, 2006; Hamera & Brown, 2000).

Assessment of Interpersonal Problem Solving Skills

The Assessment of Interpersonal Problem Solving Skills (AIPSS) uses videotaped examples of typical problematic social encounters that a person might experience in daily life. The person being evaluated is shown the videotape and then asked a series of questions to assess receiving skills (problem identification and problem description) and processing skills. One set of problems relates a job interview where a challenging scenario is provided, with the interviewer not available when scheduled.

AIPSS is demonstrated to effectively measure interpersonal problem-solving skills in individuals with schizophrenia (Donahoe et al, 1990) and has also been used in the development of training interventions for interpersonal problem solving skills (Liberman, Eckman, & Marder, 2001).

Interventions to Support Tenancy and Community Integration

Occupational therapists can serve either a generalist or specialist function in supported housing services (Lloyd, King, & McKenna, 2004; Parker, 2001).

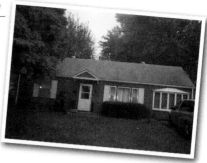

PhotoVoice

My house is a safe haven where I find peace and serenity. Not only is my house a home to me, but a place the squirrels call home as well. I enjoy watching the squirrels. Their interactions and movements relax me. I feel a sense of responsibility to the squirrels. I feed them corn, sunflower seeds, and bread daily. Everyday I know when I get home, they will be waiting for me to feed them. While I am taking care of the squirrels, I am also taking care of myself because I feel peaceful and relaxed. It gives me a sense of recovery.

—Glen

General Services

In a generalist role, the occupational therapist serves as a case manager or services coordinator and provides general mental health support services to the tenants of the housing unit. In this generalist function, the practitioner applies his or her unique perspective on humans as occupational beings, along with occupational therapy values, knowledge, and skill sets related to occupation, participation, and psychiatric disability.

The major responsibility of an occupational therapist in this generalist role is to help people with mental illness meet their tenancy obligations in a manner that ensures their success and satisfaction and minimizes the risk of eviction. These responsibilities include assisting the tenant to:

- Initiate and sustain friendly interpersonal relationships with the apartment manager and other tenants.
- Budget financial resources in order to meet payment deadlines for rent/mortgage and other utilities related to sustained tenancy status.
- Engage in domestic routines and lifestyle practices that maintain the physical interior of the apartment unit in a manner that does not exceed normal wear and tear.
- Engage in leisure and social recreational practices that are satisfying but do not disrupt the quality of life of other tenants or neighbors in the immediate area.
- Manage the symptoms and behavioral manifestations of the psychiatric disorder in a manner that minimizes the risk of psychiatric hospitalization and minimizes its intrusion on the quality of life of other tenants.
- Develop a sense of home.

Building Relationships

Initiating and sustaining friendly relationships with other tenants and the apartment manager facilitates the person's access to support and minimizes tensions that can lead to increased stress. It is equally helpful to maintain friendly relationships with the neighbors in the immediate area, even when the local neighborhood is less than desirable (Boydell, Gladstone, Crawford, & Trainor, 1999). As with any living situation, being able to get along with others is critical to an individual's success and satisfaction (Caslyn & Winter, 2002; Hansson et al, 2002; Perlick et al, 2001), and for many persons with psychiatric disabilities, comfort with and skill in social interaction is often disrupted by the nature of the psychiatric disorder (Dickerson, Boronow, Ringel, & Parente, 1999).

Occupational therapists can facilitate relationship development and may be called upon to help tenants negotiate and resolve conflicts between one another as well as to help tenants in communicating their complaints or needs to the apartment manager or property management company.

Budgeting

In general, most individuals labeled with psychiatric disabilities live on limited incomes, with their main source of income often coming from SSDI and/or SSI. Given the cost of living in most areas of the United States, this means that they are living below the poverty line, which in 2007 was $10,210 for single-person households (USDHHS, 2007). It is critical for tenants to budget their financial resources in order to meet payment deadlines for rent/mortgage and utilities in order to sustain their tenancy status.

When tenants are working, they must monitor the impact of those earnings on their disability benefits. Although both benefit programs (SSDI and SSI) have work incentives, workers must take responsibility to report these earnings or risk benefit repayments. Should this occur, the person's income can be so drastically impacted that he or she may not be able to sustain housing. Assistance with monitoring and reporting can be helpful and prevent future problems. The occupational therapist also may need to assist the person in negotiating reduced pay-back plans.

Because many of the supported housing options are HUD-funded, tenants may also benefit from assistance in understanding how their income and expenses are calculated in order to determine their total rent obligations. Although property management representatives are responsible for providing this information, tenants may still be confused. In addition, SSDI, SSI, and earned wages can change; the tenant is responsible for informing the property management representative of such changes. Managing financial resources is critical to sustaining the person's housing and avoiding eviction. The occupational therapist must understand each of these programs and how they interact in order to provide counsel to consumers.

Housekeeping

As in any living situation, optimizing the upkeep and minimizing damage to the interior spaces of the dwelling are necessary. This includes engaging in domestic routines and lifestyle practices that maintain the physical building in a manner that does not exceed normal wear and tear, alerting the apartment manager or property management company to repair needs, and/or completing minor repair tasks on one's own. Initial and sustained engagement in domestic routines may be difficult for persons with psychiatric disabilities as a result of the volitional and cognitive disruptions associated with various disorders (Allen et al, 1992).

Occupational therapists can help people learn the necessary housekeeping skills, if needed, and/or help them to establish and maintain housekeeping habits that are consistent with their personal preferences and meet at least the minimum requirements (Nolan & Swarbrick, 2002). Since many of the supported housing units available to persons with psychiatric disabilities are HUD-funded, the tenant's apartment likely will be inspected at regular intervals. Tenants often experience these inspections as intrusions into their privacy; in other cases, tenants consider them to be helpful in mediating their volitional difficulties by "keeping them on their toes." Occupational therapists can assist consumers in monitoring their inspection dates and helping them to prepare for each inspection as they occur.

Socializing

It is important for individuals to engage in leisure and social recreational practices that are satisfying but do not disrupt the quality of life of other tenants or neighbors. Occupational therapists can facilitate social and recreational interaction between tenants, such as meeting for coffee or taking a walk in the neighborhood, including the establishment of community rituals and celebrations that promote a "sense of place" and help to mediate the risk of loneliness (Brown, 1996; Chesters, Fletcher, & Jones, 2005).

As in any housing situation, tenants are responsible for establishing a pattern of living that does not disturb their neighbors. The primary issue is noise level, particularly during evening hours. In addition, when using common areas, such as patios and community/recreation rooms, it is also expected that tenants clean up and do not damage property. Many supported housing settings are intentionally designed to include multiuse common areas where tenants can gather as well as host guests, particularly when the individual apartments have limited square footage or are "singles" rather than one- or two-bedroom units.

Managing Symptoms

Consumers need to manage the symptoms and behavioral manifestations of their psychiatric disorders to minimize the risk of psychiatric hospitalization and minimize their intrusion on the quality of life of other tenants. Having the social and mental health support services tied to the housing allows for earlier interventions, such as in-home crisis response interventions, so that admission to a psychiatric hospital or crisis residential setting can be avoided (Bond, Drake, Mueser, & Latimer, 2001; Burns, Catty, & Wright, 2006). This is an important benefit of linking support services to housing, as the disruption and trauma associated with psychiatric hospitalization is profound.

However, should hospitalization or rehospitalization be required, generally the person does not lose his or her housing. In some instances, the individual and the mental health team may decide that returning to the same housing situation is contraindicated. However, as long as arrangements are made for the rent to be paid, which can be facilitated by the occupational therapist, the person will be able to sustain the housing even if he or she is away for an extended period of time.

Specialty Services

In addition to functioning as a generalist mental health provider in a supported housing setting, occupational therapists may also provide specialty services related to the occupational therapy–specific knowledge and skill sets. In this role, the practitioner will primarily serve as a consultant to other mental health providers and the apartment manager in their efforts to facilitate successful community tenure for persons with mental illness. Consultation may occur both before the tenant moves into the housing and during his or her occupancy when functional difficulties are experienced. These consultations will draw on occupational therapy's strengths in functional assessment and activity analysis to identify what skilled actions will spontaneously emerge in response to the environmental demands of the specific housing unit(s) as well as what behavioral responses will require cuing and support.

Occupational therapy's comprehensive perspective on the person-environment-occupation transaction can provide a rich understanding of what the person wants and needs to do to sustain his or her housing as well as the impact of the disability. Occupational therapy practice models informed by cognitive and sensory perspectives are particularly useful here.

Assessing Cognition

The need for assessing cognition is supported by research that has linked neurocognitive deficits, particularly problems with executive functioning, to successful community tenure (Green, 1996). The cognitive disabilities model (Allen, 1985; Allen & Blue, 1998; Allen, Earhart, & Blue, 1997; Allen et al, 1992) with its six levels of cognitive functioning provides specific guidance on the type of social and task supports that the person will require in order to safely sustain housing. Assessment tools informed by this model, described earlier in this chapter, include the ACL-5, the ADM, and the RTI-Expanded. The MOHO cognitive perspective (Kielhofner, 2007) also provides an approach that is embedded in a comprehensive frame of reference for understanding human occupation.

The AMPS (Kielhofner, Cahill, et al, 2007), also described previously, is an assessment developed for use with this frame of reference that has been used with persons with mental illness in supported housing settings (Fossey, Harvey, Plant, & Pantelis, 2006). In addition, the Dynamic Interactional Model (Josman, 2005; Josman & Katz, 2006) provides an approach for understanding the impact of neurocognitive impairments on function that can assist occupational therapists in designing recommendations for needed environmental supports. This model provides guidance to facilitate learning new habits and routines necessary for successful adjustment to the person's supported housing context.

Assessing Sensory Patterns

Assessment of the sensory patterns of individuals with mental illness, particularly the behavioral strategies they employ to manage their sensory difficulties, is also helpful. Sensory difficulties can impact function, and specific sensory patterns have been identified in persons with schizophrenia, particularly a tendency to miss information and to avoid situations with more intense sensory stimuli (Brown, Cromwell, Filion, Dunn, & Tollefson, 2002), including noise level, crowds, and social

Evidence-Based Practice

Neurocognitive functioning, particularly executive functioning, or metacognition, has been linked to successful community functioning, especially independent living skills.

➤ Occupational therapists working in supported housing programs should evaluate independent living skills, habits, and routines, *as well as* the nature of the neurocognitive impairments in order to design optimum supports and minimize safety risks.

➤ Occupational therapists must consider the link between cognition and function when selecting assessment tools. Tools that target both, such as the ACL-5/RTI-E, AMPS, and/or TOGGS, should be considered.

Green, M. (1996). What are the functional consequences of neurocognitive deficits in schizophrenia? *American Journal of Psychiatry, 153*(3), 321–330.
Rempfer, M. V., Hamera, E. K., Brown, C. E., & Cromwell, R. L. (2003). The relations between cognition and the independent living skill of shopping in people with schizophrenia. *Psychiatry Research, 117*(2), 103–112.

interactions that are highly emotional or negative. Tenants with such sensory disruptions may experience very modest noise levels coming from neighboring apartments as highly toxic and uncomfortable. They may initiate complaints to the apartment manager or directly to the tenant who is making the noise. This can result in problematic neighbor relations when the neighbor does not understand how everyday activities are experienced so loudly. In such cases, conflict resolution assistance may be required to help facilitate communications between the two tenants.

With assistance from the occupational therapist, the tenant experiencing the noise levels can better understand the sensory experiences and initiate strategies that will help to mediate their discomforts (Brown, 2001). In addition, the occupational therapist can educate the mental health provider, apartment manager, and possibly other tenants about how sensory disruptions can impact function; this can help promote a community of support within the supported housing setting.

Dunn's sensory processing model describes four patterns of sensory processing—sensory sensitivity, sensation seeking, sensation avoidance, and low registration—and provides a meaningful framework to guide occupational therapy consultations (Dunn, 2001). Chapter 20 provides additional information that may be helpful in addressing sensory issues that might present themselves in a person's living environment. The Adult/Adolescent Sensory Profile (Brown & Dunn, 2002), which is informed by Dunn's model, was developed to identify each of the four sensory patterns. This tool is demonstrated to effectively assess sensory patterns in persons with mental illness.

Whether functioning as a generalist or specialist in a supported housing setting, providing such services involves intimate encounters in the person's home. Such interventions risk being experienced by the tenant as intrusive and disruptive to their privacy. The boundaries of professional relationships become more muted in home-based interventions, and supporting a person's autonomy and self-determination may be difficult, particularly when the person is experiencing serious psychiatric distress. Occupational therapists and other mental health professionals providing services to people in their homes need to be thoughtful and act in ways that takes these issues into consideration (Magnusson & Lutzen, 1999).

Summary

Recovery for persons with mental illness can be facilitated by having a home. However, poverty and stigma are formidable barriers for persons with mental illness in their efforts to access safe, affordable, and permanent housing. Becoming a tenant provides these individuals with a normative social role (Burger, Kimelman, Lurie, & Rabiner, 1978) and, with supported housing, affords them the opportunity for fuller participation in the social life of the community. National, state, and local efforts have been developed to increase the number of supported housing units (O'Hara, 2007), but supported housing still falls far short of meeting the needs of individuals with psychiatric disabilities. Occupational therapists value the importance of having meaningful places to live. They have specific philosophical and theoretical perspectives consistent with the philosophy of supported housing as well as the practical knowledge and skills that facilitate satisfying and successful community integration through housing for persons with psychiatric disabilities.

Active Learning Strategies

1. Self-Reflection on Living Independently

If you have lived independently or are currently living independently, reflect on your experience with meeting the day-to-day obligations of being a tenant.

Reflective Questions

- Have you consistently met all of your rental, mortgage, or utilities payment deadlines?
- Have you ever been evicted or had your utilities turned off as a result of late or failed payments?
- How well are you maintaining the upkeep of your living environment?
- What emotional and physical resources do you need to call upon regularly to maintain the habits and routines related to maintaining your environment in a way that is satisfying to you?
- What supports have you needed or called upon to maintain your living situation?
- What interpersonal and other problem-solving strategies do you use to meet daily challenges?
- Did you feel a sense of home? If so, how did you make that happen?

2. Community Research

Contact your local public housing authority (PHA) and find out how many low-income housing units are available in your community for persons with psychiatric disabilities. Obtain copies of any application forms used by the PHA and review them to determine what information is required. Reflect on the personal and cognitive demands required to complete such forms. Determine if there is a waiting list for Section 8 vouchers in your community. How long is the waiting list? Consider what options people with psychiatric disabilities have if the wait is longer than 30 days.

3. Supported Housing Services

Contact a local community mental health agency that provides supported housing services to persons with mental illness. Learn as much as you can about the services they offer. For example, how many supported housing units do they have available? How many do they need to meet the needs of people with mental illness in your community? If there are not enough housing units to meet those needs, what other types of housing options (e.g., residential care) are available? Talk with the agency representatives about the challenges they have had in locating and establishing housing in your local community. Have they had any experiences with NIMBY-type responses to their efforts? What strategies did they employ, and how effective were they in countering negative reactions?

Resources

Books

Cognitive Disabilities Model Assessments and Resources

- Allen, C. K., Austin, S., David, S. K., Earhart, C. A., McCraith, D. B., & Riska-Williams, L. (2007). *Manual for the Allen Cognitive Level Screen-5 and Large Cognitive Level Screen-5 (2007)*. Camarillo, CA: ACLS and LACLS Committee..
- Allen, C. K., & Blue, T. (1998). Cognitive disabilities model: How to make clinical judgments. In N. Katz (Ed.), *Cognition and Occupation in Rehabilitation: Cognitive Models for Intervention in Occupational Therapy* (pp. 225–279). Bethesda, MD: American Occupational Therapy Association.
- Allen, C. K., Earhart, C. A., & Blue, T. (1992). *Occupational Therapy Treatment Goals for the Physically and Cognitively Disabled*. Bethesda, MD: American Occupational Therapy Association.
- ———. (1997). *Understanding Cognitive Performance Modes*. Colchester, CT: S&S Worldwide.
- Allen, C. K., & Reyner, A. (2005). *How to Start Using the Allen Diagnostic Module* (9th ed.). Colchester, CT: S&S Worldwide.

Model of Human Occupation Assessments

- Baron, K., Kielhofner, G., Iyenger, A., Goldhammer, V., & Wolenski, J. (2006). *A User's Manual for the Occupational Self Assessment (OSA), Version 2.2*. Chicago: Model of Human Occupation Clearinghouse, Department of Occupational

Therapy, College of Applied Health Sciences, University of Illinois.

- Kielhofner, G., Mallinson, T., Crawford, C., Nowak, M., Rigby, M., Henry, A., et al. (2004). *User's Manual for the Occupational Performance History Interview (Version 2.1) OPHI-II*. Chicago: Model of Human Occupation (MOHO) Clearinghouse, Department of Occupational Therapy, College of Applied Health Sciences, University of Illinois.

Adolescent/Adult Sensory Profile

- Brown, C., & Dunn, W. (2002). *Adolescent/Adult Sensory Profile: User's Manual*. San Antonio, TX: Psychological Corporation. Available at: http://www.sensoryprofile.com.

Assessment of Interpersonal Problem Solving Skills

- Psychiatric Rehabilitation Consultants: http://www.psychrehab.com

Websites

- Bazelon Center for Mental Health Law: http://www.bazelon.org
- Center for Personal Assistance Services: http://www.pascenter.org
- Corporation for Supportive Housing offers a toolkit for developing and operating supportive housing: http://www .csh.org/index. fhm:fuseaction=page.viapage&pageID=3663
- Department of Housing and Urban Development (HUD): http:// www.hud.gov
- Homelessness Resource Center: http://homelessness.samhsa.gov/
- Woodley House: http://www.woodleyhouse.org

References

Allen, C. K. (1985). *Occupational Therapy for Psychiatric Diseases: Measurement and Management of Cognitive Disabilities*. Boston: Little Brown.

———. (2004). *Just Like Where You and I Live: Integrated Housing Options for People with Mental Illness*. Washington, DC: Bazelon Center for Mental Health Policy.

Allen, C. K., Austin, S., David, S. K., Earhart, C. A., McCraith, D. B., & Riska-Williams, L. (2007). *Manual for the Allen Cognitive Level Screen-5 and Large Cognitive Level Screen-5 (2007)*. Camarillo, CA: ACLS and LACLS Committee.

Allen, C. K., & Blue, T. (1998). Cognitive disabilities model: How to make clinical judgments. In N. Katz (Ed.), *Cognition and Occupation in Rehabilitation: Cognitive Models for Intervention in Occupational Therapy* (pp. 225–279). Bethesda, MD: American Occupational Therapy Association.

Allen, C. K., Earhart, C., & Blue, T. (1997). *Understanding Cognitive Performance Modes*. Colchester, CT: S&S Worldwide.

———. (1992). *Occupational Therapy Treatment Goals for the Physically and Cognitively Disabled*. Bethesda, MD: American Occupational Therapy Association.

Allen, C. K., & Reyner, A. (2005). *How to Start Using the Allen Diagnostic Module* (9th ed.). Colchester, CT: S&S Worldwide.

American Occupational Therapy Association (AOTA). (2002). Occupational therapy practice framework: Domain and process. *American Journal of Occupational Therapy, 56*, 609–639.

———. (2008). Occupational therapy practice framework: Domain and process (2nd ed.). *American Journal of Occupational Therapy, 62*, 625–683.

Apte, A., Kielhofner, G., Paul-Ward, A., & Braveman, B. (2005). Therapists' and clients' perceptions of the Occupational Performance History Interview. *Occupational Therapy in Health Care, 19*(1–2), 173–192.

Baron, K., Kielhofner, G., Iyenger, A., Goldhammer, V., & Wolenski, J. (2006). *A User's Manual for the Occupational Self Assessment (OSA), Version 2.2*. Chicago: Model of Human Occupation Clearinghouse, Department of Occupational Therapy, College of Applied Health Sciences, University of Illinois.

Bigelow, D. A. (1998). Supportive homes for life versus treatment way-stations: An introduction to TAPS Project 41. *Community Mental Health Journal, 34*(4), 403–405.

Bond, G., Drake, R., Mueser, K., & Latimer, E. (2001). Assertive community treatment for people with severe mental illness: Critical ingredients and impact on patients. *Disease Management and Health Outcomes, 9*(3), 141–159.

Boydell, K., Gladstone, B. M., Crawford, E., & Trainor, J. (1999). Making do on the outside: Everyday life in the neighborhoods of people with psychiatric disabilities. *Psychiatric Rehabilitation Journal, 23*(1), 11–18.

Brown, C. (1996). A comparison of living situation and loneliness for people with mental illness. *Psychiatric Rehabilitation Journal, 20*(2), 59–64.

———. (2001). What is the best environment for me? A sensory processing perspective. *Occupational Therapy in Mental Health, 17*(3/4), 115–125.

Brown, C., Cromwell, R. L., Filion, D., Dunn, W., & Tollefson, N. (2002). Sensory processing in schizophrenia: Missing and avoiding information. *Schizophrenia Research, 55*(1–2), 187–195.

Brown, C., & Dunn, W. (2002). *Adolescent/Adult Sensory Profile: User's Manual*. San Antonio, TX: Psychological Corporation.

Brown, C., Rempfer, M., Hamera, E., & Bothwell, R. (2006). Knowledge of grocery shopping skills as a mediator of cognition and performance. *Psychiatric Services, 57*, 573–575.

Burger, A. S., Kimelman, L., Lurie, A., & Rabiner, C. J. (1978). Congregate living for the mentally ill: Patients as tenants. *Hospital & Community Psychiatry, 29*, 590–593.

Burns, T., Catty, J., & Wright, C. (2006). Deconstructing home-based care for mental illness: Can one identify the effective ingredients? *Acta Psychiatrica Scandinavica, 113*(s429), 33–35.

Carling, P. J. (1993). Housing and supports for persons with mental illness: Emerging approaches to research and practice. *Hospital & Community Psychiatry, 44*, 439–449.

———. (1995). *Return to Community: Building Support Systems for People with Psychiatric Disabilities*. New York: Guilford Press.

Caslyn, R. J., & Winter, J. P. (2002). Social support, psychiatric symptoms, and housing: A causal analysis. *Journal of Community Psychology, 30*, 247–259.

Center for Mental Health Services. (2006). *Transforming Housing for People with Psychiatric Disabilities*. Rockville, MD: U.S. Dept. of Health and Human Services, Substance Abuse and Mental Health Services Administration.

Chesters, J., Fletcher, M., & Jones, R. (2005). Mental illness recovery and place [electronic version]. *Australian e-Journal for the Advancement of Mental Health, 4*, 1–9, Available at: http://www .auseinet.com/journal/vol4iss2/chesters.pdf.

Corrigan, P. W. (2001). Place-then-train: An alternative service paradigm for persons with psychiatric disabilities. *Clinical Psychology: Science and Practice, 8*, 334–349.

Csikszentmihalyi, M., & Rochberg-Halton, E. (1981). *The Meaning of Things: Domestic Symbols and the Self*. Cambridge: Cambridge University Press.

Davidson, L., & Strauss, J. (1992). Sense of self in recovery from severe mental illness. *British Journal of Medical Psychology, 63*, 131–145.

Dickerson, F., Boronow, J. J., Ringel, N., & Parente, F. (1999). Social functioning and neurocognitive deficits in outpatients with schizophrenia: A 2-year follow-up. *Schizophrenia Research, 37*(1), 13–20.

Donahoe, C. P., Carter, M. J., Bloem, W. D., Hirsch, G. L., Laasi, N., & Wallace, C. J. (1990). Assessment of interpersonal problem-solving skills. *Psychiatry 53*(4), 329–339.

Doniger, J., Rothwell, N. D., & Cohen, R. (1963). Case study of a halfway house. *Mental Hospitals*, 194–198.

Dunn, W. (2001). The sensations of everyday life: Empirical, theoretical, and pragmatic considerations. *American Journal of Occupational Therapy, 55*(6), 608–620.

Dupuis, A., & Thorns, D. (1998). Home, home ownership and the search for ontological security. *Sociological Review, 46*, 25.

Evans, G. W., Wells, N. M., & Moch, A. (2003). Housing and mental health: A review of the evidence and a methodological and conceptual critique. *Journal of Social Issues, 59,* 475–500.

Fairweather, G., Sanders, D., Cressler, D., & Maynard, D. (1969). *Community Life for the Mentally Ill.* Chicago: Aldine.

Fakhoury, W. K. H., Murray, A., Shepherd, G., & Priebe, S. (2002). Research in supported housing. *Social Psychiatry and Psychiatric Epidemiology, 37,* 201–315.

Farkas, M., Chamberlin, J., Harding, C., Kramer, P., & Kenyon, A. D. (2003). *Personal Assistance Services for Persons with Serious Psychiatric Disabilities.* Baton Rouge: Louisiana Department of Health and Hospitals, Office of Mental Health.

Fisher, A., & Savin-Baden, M. (2001). The benefits to young people experiencing psychosis, and their families, of an early intervention programme: Evaluating a service from the consumers' and the providers' perspectives. *British Journal of Occupational Therapy, 64,* 58–65.

Forchuk, C., Ward-Griffin, C., Csiernik, R., & Turner, K. (2006). Surviving the tornado of mental illness: Psychiatric survivor's experiences of getting, losing and keeping housing. *Psychiatric Services, 57,* 558–562.

Fossey, E., Harvey, C., Plant, G., & Pantelis, C. (2006). Occupational performance of people diagnosed with schizophrenia in supported housing and outreach programmes in Australia. *British Journal of Occupational Therapy, 69,* 409–419.

George, L., Sylvestre, J., Aubry, T., Durbin, J., Nelson, G., Sabloff, A., et al. (2005). *Ontario Housing Policy Report: Strengthening the Housing System for People Who Have Experienced Serious Mental Illness: A Value-Based and Evidence-Based Approach.* University of Ottawa. Technical report prepared for the Ontario Ministry of Health and Long-Term Care.

Gieryn, T. F. (2000). A space for place in sociology. *Annual Review of Sociology, 26*(1), 463–496.

Girard, C., Fisher, A. G., Short, M. A., & Duran, L. (1999). Occupational performance differences between psychiatric groups. *Scandinavian Journal of Occupational Therapy, 6,* 119–126.

Glasscote, R. M., Gudeman, J. E., & Elpers, J. R. (1971). *Halfway Houses for the Mentally Ill: A Study of Programs and Problems.* Washington, DC: American Psychiatric Association and National Mental Health Association.

Goldstein, J. L., & Godemont, M. M. L. (2003). The legend and lessons of Geel, Belgium: A 1500-year-old legend, a 21st-century model. *Community Mental Health Journal, 39,* 441–458.

Green, M. (1996). What are the functional consequences of neurocognitive deficits in schizophrenia? *American Journal of Psychiatry, 153*(3), 321–330.

Greenwood, R., Schaefer-McDaniel, N., Winkel, G., & Tsemberis, S. (2005). Decreasing psychiatric symptoms by increasing choice in services for adults with histories of homelessness. *American Journal of Community Psychology, 36,* 223–238.

Haertl, K. (2005). Factors influencing success in a Fairweather model mental health program. *Psychiatric Rehabilitation Journal, 28,* 370–377.

———. (2007). The Fairweather mental health housing model: A peer supportive environment: Implications for psychiatric rehabilitation. *American Journal of Psychiatric Rehabilitation, 10,* 149–162.

Hamera, E., & Brown, C. (2000). Developing a context-based performance measure for persons with schizophrenia: The test of grocery shopping skills. *American Journal of Occupational Therapy, 54,* 20–25.

Hansson, L., Middelboe, T., Sargaard, K. W., Gengtsson-Tops, A., Bjarnason, O., Merinder, L., et al. (2002). Living situation, subjective quality of life and social network among individuals with schizophrenia living in community settings. *Acta Psychiatrica Scandinavica, 105,* 343–350.

Hasselkus, B. (2002). *The Meaning of Everyday Occupation.* Thorofare, NJ: Slack.

Housing and Urban Development (HUD). (2007). "Section 811 Supportive Housing for Persons With Disabilities." Available at: http://www.hud.gov/offices/hsg/mfh/progdesc/disab811.cfm (accessed December 26, 2007).

———. (n.d.). "Housing Choice Vouchers Fact Sheet." Available at: http://www.hud.gov/offices/pih/programs/hcv/about/fact_sheet.cfm (accessed December 26, 2007).

Josman, N. (2005). The dynamic interactional model in schizophrenia. In Katz, N. (Ed.), *Cognition & Occupation Across the Life Span: Models for Intervention in Occupational Therapy* (pp. 169–185). Bethesda, MD: American Occupational Therapy Association.

Josman, N., & Katz, N. (2006). Relationships of categorization on tests and daily tasks in patients with schizophrenia, post-stroke patients and healthy controls. *Psychiatry Research, 141,* 15–28.

Katz, N. (2006). *Routine Task Inventory–Expanded Prepared and Elaborated on the Basis of Allen, C. K. (1989 Unpublished).* Unpublished manuscript, available at http://www.allen_cognitive_network.org.

Kielhofner, G. (2007). *Model of Human Occupation: Theory and Application* (4th ed.). Baltimore: Lippincott Williams & Wilkins.

Kielhofner, G., Cahill, S. M., Forsyth, K., de las Heras, C. G., Melton, J., Raber, C., et al. (2007). Observational assessments. In G. Kielhofner (Ed.), *Model of Human Occupation: Theory and Practice* (4th ed.) (pp. 217–236). Baltimore: Lippincott Williams & Wilkins.

Kielhofner, G., Forsyth, K., Clay, C., Ekbladh, E., Haglund, L., Hemmingsson, H., et al. (2007). Talking with clients: Assessments that collect information through interviews. In G. Kielhofner (Ed.), *Model of Human Occupation: Theory and Application* (4th ed.). (pp. 262–287). Baltimore: Lippincott Williams & Wilkins.

Kielhofner, G., Forsyth, K., Suman, M., Kramer, J., Nakamura-Thomas, H., Yamada, T., et al. (2007). Self-reports: Eliciting clients' perspectives. In Kielhofner (Ed.), *Model of Human Occupation: Theory and Application* (4th ed.). (pp. 237–261). Baltimore: Lippincott Williams & Wilkins.

Kielhofner, G., Mallinson, T., Crawford, C., Nowak, M., Rigby, M., Henry, A., et al. (2004). *User's Manual for the Occupational Performance History Interview (Version 2.1) OPHI-II.* Chicago: Model of Human Occupation (MOHO) Clearinghouse, Department of Occupational Therapy, College of Applied Health Sciences, University of Illinois.

Kresky, M., Maeda, E. M., & Rothwell, N. D. (1976). The apartment program: A community-living option for halfway house residents. *Hospital & Community Psychiatry, 27,* 153–154.

Liberman, R. P., Eckman, T. A., & Marder, S. R. (2001). Rehab rounds: Training in social problem solving among persons with schizophrenia. *Psychiatric Services, 52*(1), 31–33.

Link, B. G., Struening, E. L., Neese-Todd, S., Asmussen, S., & Phelan, J. C. (2001). Stigma as a barrier to recovery: The consequences of stigma for the self-esteem of people with mental illnesses. *Psychiatric Services, 52*(12), 1621–1626.

Lloyd, C., King, R., & McKenna, K. (2004). Generic versus specialist clinical work roles of occupational therapists and social workers in mental health. *Australian and New Zealand Journal of Psychiatry, 38,* 119–124.

Magnusson, A., & Lutzen, K. (1999). Intrusion into patient privacy: A moral concern in the home care of persons with chronic mental illness. *Nursing Ethics, 6,* 399–410.

Mallett, S. (2004). Understanding home: A critical review of the literature. *Sociological Review, 52,* 62–89.

McNulty, M., & Fisher, A. (2001). Validity of using the Assessment of Motor and Process Skills to estimate overall home safety in persons with psychiatric conditions. *American Journal of Occupational Therapy, 55,* 649–655.

Meyer, A. (1916/1952). The extra-institutional responsibilities of state hospitals for mental disease. In E. Winters (Ed.), *The Collected Papers of Adolf Meyer: Mental Hygiene* (Vol. IV, pp. 229–236). Baltimore: Johns Hopkins University Press.

Moxham, L. J., & Pegg, S. A. (2000). Permanent and stable housing for individuals living with a mental illness in the community: A paradigm shift in attitude for mental health nurses. *Australian and New Zealand Journal of Mental Health Nursing, 9,* 82–88.

Nelson, G., Hall, G. B., & Forchuk, C. (2003). Current and preferred housing of psychiatric consumers/survivors. *Canadian Journal of Community Mental Health, 22,* 5–19.

Nelson, G., Lord, J., & Ochocka, J. (2001). *Shifting the Paradigm in Community Mental Health: Towards Empowerment and Community.* Toronto: University of Toronto Press.

Nelson, G., & Peddle, S. (2005). *Housing and Support for People Who Have Experienced Serious Mental Illness: Value Base and Research Evidence.* Waterloo, ON: Wilfrid Laurier University.

New Freedom Commission on Mental Health. (2003). *Achieving the Promise: Transforming Mental Health Care in America.* DHHS Pub. No. SMA-03-3832. Rockville, MD: U.S. Department of Health and Human Services.

Nolan, C., & Swarbrick, M. (2002). Supportive housing occupational therapy home management program. *AOTA Mental Health Special Interest Section Quarterly, 25*(2), 1–3.

O'Hara, A. (2007). Housing for people with mental illness: Update of a report to the President's New Freedom Commission. *Psychiatric Services, 58,* 907–913.

Olmstead v L.C. and E.W., 527 U.S. 581, 138 F.3d 893 (1999).

Onaga, E. E., McKinney, K. G., & Pfaff, J. (2000). Lodge programs serving family functions for people with psychiatric disabilities. *Family Relations, 49,* 207–216.

Owen, C., Rutherford, V., Jones, M., Wright, C., Tennant, C., & Smallman, A. (1996). Housing accommodation preferences of people with psychiatric disabilities. *Psychiatric Services, 47,* 628–632.

Padgett, D. (2007). There's no place like (a) home: Ontological security among persons with serious mental illness in the United States. *Social Science & Medicine, 64,* 1925–1936.

Pan, A., & Fisher, A. (1994). The assessment of motor and process skills of persons with psychiatric disorders. *American Journal of Occupational Therapy, 48,* 775–780.

Parker, H. (2001). The role of occupational therapists in community mental health teams: Generic or specialist? *British Journal of Occupational Therapy, 64,* 609–610.

Perlick, D. A., Rosenheck, R. A., Clarkin, J. F., Sirey, J. A., Salahi, J., Struening, E. L., et al. (2001). Stigma as a barrier to recovery: Adverse effects of perceived stigma on social adaptation of persons diagnosed with bipolar affective disorder. *Psychiatric Services, 52,* 1627–1632.

Piat, M. (2000). The NIMBY phenomenon: Community resident's concerns about housing for deinstitutionalized people. *Health & Social Work, 25,* 127–138.

Pita, D. D., Ellison, M. L., & Farkas, M. (2001). Exploring personal assistance services for people with psychiatric disabilities: Need, policy, and practice. *Journal of Disability Policy Studies, 12,* 12.

Raush, H. L., & Raush, C. (1968). *The Halfway House Movement: A Search for Sanity.* New York: Appleton-Century-Crofts.

Rempfer, M. V., Hamera, E. K., Brown, C. E., & Cromwell, R. L. (2003). The relations between cognition and the independent living skill of shopping in people with schizophrenia. *Psychiatry Research, 117,* 103–112.

Ridgway, P., & Zipple, A. (1990). The paradigm shift in residential services: From the linear continuum to supported housing. *Psychosocial Rehabilitation Journal, 13*(4), 11–31.

Rog, D. J. (2004). The evidence on supported housing. *Psychiatric Rehabilitation Journal, 27,* 334–344.

Rosenheck, R., Kasprow, W., Frisman, L., & Liu-Mares, W. (2003). Cost-effectiveness of supported housing for homeless persons with mental illness. *Archives of General Psychiatry, 60,* 940–951.

Rothwell, N. D., & Doniger, J. M. (1966). *The Psychiatric Halfway House.* Springfield, IL: Charles C. Thomas.

Rowles, G. (2003). The meaning of place as a component of the self. In E. Crepeau, E. Cohn, & B. Boyt Schell (Eds.), *Willard & Spackman's Occupational Therapy* (10th ed.) (pp. 111–120). Philadelphia: Lippincott Williams & Wilkins.

Salzer, M.S. (Ed.). (2006). *Psychiatric Rehabilitation Skills in Practice: A CPRP Preparation and Skills Workbook.* Columbia, MD: United States Psychiatric Rehabilitation Association.

Segal, S. P., & Aviram, U. (1978). *The Mentally Ill in Community-Based Sheltered Care: A Study of Community Care and Social Integration.* New York: Wiley.

Sells, D. J., Stayner, D. A., & Davidson, L. (2004). Recovering the self in schizophrenia: An integrative review of qualitative studies. *Psychiatric Quarterly, 75,* 87–97.

Stefancis, A., & Tsemberis, S. (2007). Housing First for long-term shelter dwellers with psychiatric disabilities in a suburban county: A four-year study of housing access and retention. *Journal of Primary Prevention, 28,* 265–279.

Suto, M., & Frank, G. (1994). Future time perspective and daily occupations of persons with chronic schizophrenia in a board and care home. *American Journal of Occupational Therapy, 48,* 7–18.

Tanzman, B. (1993). An overview of surveys of mental health consumers' preferences for housing and support services. *Hospital & Community Psychiatry, 44,* 450–455.

Thomson, L. K. (1992). *The Kohlman Evaluation of Living Skills* (3rd ed.). Bethesda, MD: American Occupational Therapy Association.

Tsemberis, S., & Asmussen, S. (1999). From streets to homes: The pathways to housing consumer preference supported housing model. In K. J. Conrad (Ed.), *Homelessness Prevention in Treatment of Substance Abuse and Mental Illness: Logic Models and Implementation of Eight American Projects* (pp. 113–131). New York: Haworth Press.

Tsemberis, S., Gulcur, L., & Nakae, M. (2004). Housing First, consumer choice, and harm reduction for homeless individuals with a dual diagnosis. *American Journal of Public Health, 94,* 651–656.

Tuan, Y. (1977). *Space and Place: The Perspective of Experience.* Minneapolis: University of Minnesota Press.

Tuntiya, N. (2006). Making a case for the Geel model: The American experience with family care for mental patients. *Community Mental Health Journal, 42,* 319–330.

U.S. Department of Health and Human Services (USDHHS). (2005). *Transforming Mental Health Care in America. The Federal Action Agenda: First Steps.* (DHHS Publication No. SMA-05-4060). Rockville, MD: Author.

————. *Annual Update of the HHS Poverty Guidelines.* (2007). *Federal Register, 72*(15). Available at: http://aspe.hhs.gov/poverty/07fedreg.pdf (accessed December 28, 2009).

Warren, R., & Bell, P. (2000). An exploratory investigation into the housing preferences of consumers of mental health services. *Australian and New Zealand Journal of Mental Health Nursing, 9,* 195–202.

Whiteford, G. (2000). Occupational deprivation: Global challenge in the new millennium. *British Journal of Occupational Therapy, 63,* 200–204.

Wong, Y.-L. I., Filoromo, M., & Tennille, J. (2007). From principles to practices: A study of implementation of supported housing for psychiatric consumers. *Administration Policy in Mental Health and Mental Health Services Research, 34,* 13–28.

Wong, Y.-L. I., & Solomon, P. L. (2002). Community integration of persons with psychiatric disabilities in supportive independent housing: A conceptual model and methodological considerations. *Mental Health Services Research, 4,* 3–28.

Yanos, P. T., Felton, B. J., Tsemberis, S., & Frye, V. A. (2007). Exploring the role of housing type, neighborhood characteristics and lifestyle factors in the community integration of formerly homeless persons diagnosed with mental illness. *Journal of Mental Health, 16*(6), 703–717.

Yanos, P. T., Rosenfield, S., & Horwitz, A. V. (2001). Negative and supportive social interactions and quality of life among persons diagnosed with severe mental illness. *Community Mental Health Journal, 37,* 405–419.

Zippay, A. (2007). Psychiatric residences: Notification, NIMBY, and neighborhood relations. *Psychiatric Services, 58*(1), 109–113.

CHAPTER 34

Early Intervention: A Practice Setting for Infant and Toddler Mental Health

Kris Pizur-Barnekow

> *"Children are the world's most valuable resource and its best hope for the future.*
>
> —John F. Kennedy

Introduction

Many occupational therapists are employed in infant and toddler service settings and typically address the developmental needs of the child. However, the mental health concerns of the infant and toddler may be overlooked. Mental health issues often are considered as problems dealt with by adolescents and adults. Children's mental health is starting to receive more attention, but the mental health needs of infants and toddlers are far less often considered. Problems related to attachment, emotion regulation (e.g., fussiness, sleep problems), and cognitive development (e.g., responsiveness to stimuli) are all issues that can be considered in the realm of mental health or psychosocial functioning. All of these problems are within the domain of concern of occupational therapy and are common issues addressed by occupational therapists working in infant and toddler settings.

This chapter describes early intervention in a service delivery setting or context and incorporates principles of infant and toddler mental health into this setting. The mission, population served, team members, funding sources, role of occupational therapy, assessments, and intervention models used in this setting are reviewed. Building strong working relationships with the child and family members is key to successful early intervention.

Overview of Infant and Toddler Mental Health

For the purposes of this chapter, **early intervention** refers to those services provided under Part C of the Individuals with Disabilities Education Act (IDEA). According to Public Law 108-446 of IDEA, infants and toddlers at risk for or diagnosed with a disability can receive nutritional, educational, therapeutic, and psychological services. Early intervention programs serve families with infants or toddlers from the time they are born through their third birthday.

Before describing a service delivery setting that incorporates infant mental health practice, it is important to define what is meant by **infant mental health**. The concept of infant mental health is often questioned, with many critics asking how infants and toddlers can have mental health deficits or problems. The answer is that infants and toddlers have significant capacities to feel and know about their environment and the people with whom they interact (Sameroff, 2004).

The problems seen in infant and toddler emotional and social development are often related to the characteristics of their early relationships (Kraemer, 1992; Sameroff, 2004). Children thrive with responsive caregiving and a cohesive family. These experiences during development contribute to their sense of self (Gilkerson, 2006). During infancy and the toddler years, the ability to connect with others facilitates regulation of homeostasis, emotions, and cognitive development (Barnekow & Kraemer, 2005). Therefore, it is critical that occupational therapists in pediatric settings attend to those attributes that lead to healthy social and emotional development in addition to healthy physical development.

Infant mental health practice is relationship based. Relationships are an organizing factor in which all other development occurs (Kalmanson & Seligman, 2006). The interactions that occur within the relationship between the infant or toddler and the primary caregiver regulate the child's physiology, behavior, emotion, and cognition (Barnekow & Kraemer, 2005; Kraemer, 1992). For example, when a mother is responsive to her infant, the infant shows greater regulation of heart rate and affect (Haley & Stansbury, 2003). Therefore, the focus of infant or toddler mental health is on therapist–parent/caregiver relationships, parent–child relationships, and family–community relationships.

When working in early intervention, occupational therapists need to foster relationships by embracing complexity, respecting diversity, viewing behavior from the caregiver's perspective or experience, and being attuned to their own emotional responses (Kalmanson, 2006). Providers need to incorporate relationship-based, self-reflective, and theoretically driven practices into their work with infants, toddlers, and their families to promote optimal child mental health. Traditionally, infant and toddler mental health practices have not been embedded in the assessments and interventions provided by pediatric occupational therapists practicing in early intervention, or birth to three, programs. This chapter presents methods of assessment and intervention strategies that focus on infant and toddler mental health in early intervention settings.

Assessments and interventions in infant and toddler mental health practice should focus on early relationships. As Sameroff (2004) states, there is more than one client in infant and toddler mental health practice. The clients are the infants or toddlers and the caregivers within the relational context. A primary assumption underlying this chapter is that therapists use infant and toddler mental health principles when treating children with special health care needs.

Children with special health care needs are those children who have or are at risk for chronic physical, developmental, behavior, or emotional conditions (Fleischfresser, 2004). Often, children with special health care needs present with developmental delays that challenge the relationship between caregiver and child. Therapists who utilize an infant and toddler mental health approach recognize that all children can reach their potential when relationships are optimal. For example, a toddler displaying symptoms of autism may demonstrate stereotypical behavior after being separated from and reunited with his or her caregiver. Instead of giving the caregiver a hug, the toddler hops up and down and loudly vocalizes. The caregiver may not view the behavior as a favorable response and may begin to feel emotionally

detached from the toddler, consequently impairing their relationship. If the parent continues to detach from the child, the opportunities for engagement in activities that promote development decrease.

The following case illustrates how early intervention providers (occupational therapists) can include aspects of infant and toddler mental health into their practice.

Evidence-Based Practice

Research indicates that early relationships that occur within the context of daily routines affect the structure and function of the brain (Kraemer, 1992).

➤ Occupational therapists should assess the transaction between the primary caregiver and the child to understand developmental outcomes.

➤ Occupational therapists should consider co-occupation as an essential part of early intervention practice and evaluate shared physicality, intentionality, and emotionality between the primary caregiver and the child.

➤ Occupational therapists should provide interventions that include the primary caregiver and the child as they engage in daily routines.

Kraemer, G. W. (1992). A psychobiological theory of attachment. *Behavioral and Brain Sciences, 15,* 493–541.

Case

An early intervention provider serving families in an urban setting received a referral for a child who was Hmong. The supervisor contacted the provider and said that the child was discharged from the hospital and his prognosis was poor. Three months earlier, he was admitted to the hospital because of an *E. coli* infection that resulted in severe brain damage. Upon discharge from the hospital, the medical team thought he would not live long, and the referral to early intervention was initiated to help support the family during his final days. Because the family was Hmong and followed the practices of Eastern medicine, they had significant trust issues with professionals who practiced Western medicine. Until the child's admission into the hospital, he was a typically developing young child. The family believed the hospitalization made their healthy son become very ill, and they did not associate the child's outcomes to an infection.

The initial step in treating this child within the context of the family was establishment of the professional–family relationship. The first home visit consisted of talking with the father, who was the boy's primary caregiver, for the entire visit. The early intervention provider did not physically handle the child until she was invited back for a second visit. Over time, the family and the early intervention provider established a relationship, and the parents became great teachers. They taught the early intervention provider about the Hmong culture, Eastern medicine, and the difficulties they encountered with Western health care.

Throughout the assessment and intervention process, the provider came to understand that the child's impairments were significant. He was cortically blind, his ability to localize to sound was inconsistent, and his movement patterns consisted of severe spinal extension with minimal voluntary movement in his arms and legs. His parents told the early intervention provider that they did not know if the child knew who they were. As treatment progressed, the early intervention provider realized that this child *did* know who his parents were, as he would become calm when he heard their voices. The role of the early intervention provider was to help the parents reestablish a relationship with their son.

Upon discharge from the early intervention program into the early childhood program, this young child who was not expected to live thrived because of the loving care he received within the family context. His attachment behaviors were relatively mature in comparison to his motor and sensory development. He displayed separation anxiety from his primary caregiver, and when held by members of his family, he gently nestled into their arms. This experience illustrates the importance of relationships in early intervention practice.

Early Intervention Programs: Mission and Philosophy

Early intervention programs, also known as birth to three programs, provide coordinated services to families with young children. Children referred to early intervention programs are at risk for or diagnosed with a condition that may impair their ability to fully participate in occupations or co-occupations experienced by typically developing peers.

The primary philosophical model used in early intervention practice is family-centered care. **Family-centered care** is a social model that promotes competencies based on the family life style (Dunst, Johanson, Trivette, & Hamby, 1999). This model recognizes that infants and young children depend upon family members for support, nurturance, and survival (Stephens & Tauber, 2005). Early intervention programs that use family-centered care models espouse the concept that families are experts on their child's habits and routines; therefore, family members need to be active team members.

Providers who use a family-centered model must include aspects of the caregiver–child relationship during problem identification and intervention planning. The nature of the early intervention provider's work focuses on relationships and is characterized by the interpersonal realm of therapy (Kalmanson & Seligman, 2006). The provider is then able to address the family's needs and concerns. This model enables providers to recognize the diversity of each family and respect the decision-making of the family.

The degree to which a family is involved in early intervention depends primarily on the structure, roles, beliefs, and family patterns. Providers must reflect on their own value system to ensure that services are responsive to the family's characteristics. This philosophy encompasses provision of intervention services within home and community settings, otherwise known as natural environments.

Population Served

Families become involved in early intervention services if their child has an established risk, a developmental delay, or is at risk for developmental delays. **Established risk** means that a child has a diagnosed condition that places him or her at risk for delays in socioemotional, cognitive, or physical development. For example, a child born with cerebral palsy is a child with an established risk. A child with a **developmental delay** presents with delays in socioemotional, cognitive, communication, motor, or adaptive development. Children with developmental delays, however, do not have a clinical diagnosis that classifies the delay. Children are identified as **at risk** if they are born with significant biological risks or are living in a high-risk environment. For example, a child born

to a teen mother is at greater risk for delay and may qualify for services (Stephens & Tauber, 2005).

Team Members and Models

Occupational therapists who work in early intervention programs collaborate with a variety of team members. Other members of the early intervention team include psychologists, social workers, physicians, special education teachers, physical therapists, nutritionists, and speech-language pathologists.

Two types of teaming, interdisciplinary and transdisciplinary, are common in early intervention practice. **Interdisciplinary teaming** consists of team members who value each other's work and who communicate routinely and effectively. Interdisciplinary teams set goals collaboratively and through consensus. The team members may meet formally and informally to discuss the child's case, and their interactions focus on the needs of the child. The child's family may not be considered team members (McGonigel, Woodruff, & Roszmann-Millican, 1994). As can be seen, interdisciplinary teaming may not be the most optimal in early intervention settings because the family may not be active team members.

Transdisciplinary teams are the second type of teaming model found in early intervention practice. Transdisciplinary teams, like interdisciplinary teams, value team members' expertise and work. All team members working with the child become informed by the theories and strategies of the other disciplines involved (Kalmanson, 2006). The primary difference between an interdisciplinary team and a transdisciplinary team is the process by which the teaming and treatment occur. Transdisciplinary team members are dedicated to learning and working across disciplinary boundaries. Consultation and coaching are commonly used because team members share responsibility for treatment outcomes. The child's family is considered an integral part of the team and is empowered to participate in assessment, goal planning, and treatment. Transdisciplinary teaming is the preferred teaming model in early intervention, because it is responsive to the changing dynamics of families (McGonigel, Woodruff, & Roszmann-Millican, 1994).

Funding Sources

The U.S. government provides funding for early intervention programs under IDEA. Part C of IDEA regulates individual states within the union regarding policies and procedures for early intervention services. Early intervention is an entitlement program, which means that states are not obligated to provide early intervention services. If a state chooses to provide early intervention services, it must follow the regulations established by the federal government. Currently, under Part C, states are required to provide interdisciplinary and transdisciplinary assessments and interventions.

Another requirement is that there must be an **Individualized Family Service Plan** (IFSP) written *with* the family, and services should be family centered, coordinated, and occur within the child's natural environments. The IFSP is a plan of care that identifies the family's resources, desired outcomes for their child, activities to achieve the noted outcomes, developmental strengths and needs of their child, and plans for transition if the child is approaching his or her third birthday.

Role of Occupational Therapy

The role of an occupational therapist in early intervention is to provide family-centered care within the context of the child's natural environment. Occupational therapists address the needs of the family and child in relation to co-occupational and occupational performance. Play, activities of daily living (ADLs), and early educational activities are within the domain of the occupational therapist's practice in early intervention. A key point to remember in early intervention is that performance in these occupational areas occurs within the context of a relationship with a parent or caregiver. Therefore, models of co-occupation, as presented in Chapter 45, may provide a framework when considering aspects of co-occupation important to functional engagement.

The occupational therapist may also serve in the role of service coordinator. Service coordination involves setting up assessment and intervention plans, coordinating services among all disciplines, assuming responsibility for formal documentation on the IFSP, and assisting the family with access to services that help them in their daily lives.

For example, a therapist is working with a family in which English is a second language. The family's child uses a wheelchair for transportation, and the family had a parking permit that allowed them to park in spaces reserved for people with disabilities. The permit was stolen, and the family is having difficulty obtaining another permit due to the language barrier. As service coordinator, the occupational therapist would assist the family with obtaining another permit. If necessary, the occupational therapist may invite an interpreter to assist with communication. Occupational therapists are well prepared to be service coordinators because understanding the family's engagement in meaningful occupations and co-occupations is instrumental in the service coordination role.

Facilitating the Professional–Parent Relationship

The process of evaluation, treatment, and discharge in the field of early intervention has been compared to a dance (Fialka, 2006). The first step of this "dance" is for the provider to develop a working relationship with the family. Occupational therapists working in early intervention should look for patterns of healthy relationships as well as patterns of abuse, neglect, or substance abuse. If parents are in need of assessment and individual treatment, referral to the appropriate professional is recommended. It is essential for occupational therapists to remember that the outcome of their intervention rests strongly on the quality of the parent–provider relationship (Kalmanson & Seligman, 2006). To facilitate the professional–parent relationship, occupational therapy providers should ask the following questions:

- *Would assessment goals be accomplished with multiple providers present or with one or two providers present?* Often, parents are overwhelmed by their child's diagnosis, and interaction with more than one provider may not be effective. Parents and providers need to develop a relationship built on trust, and it may be easier to do that when there are fewer professionals involved.
- *What strategies will the providers use to develop an understanding of infant and family relationships?* Providers should use open-ended questions that can assist with developing an understanding of the relationship between the infant and family. For example, the therapist might ask how the family chose the child's name. In this way, he or she may develop a more thorough understanding of the family's story and their associated cultural perspectives.
- *How does the parent/caregiver feel about receiving services?* Occupational therapists chose their profession. They practice in early intervention because they enjoy working with children and their families. Parents may not want to enter into a relationship with therapists. Parents do not have the same level of choice as the therapists do when involved in early intervention (Fialka, 2006).
- *What type of relationship does the parent want to have with the therapist?* Many times, parents do not even know the therapist's last name, and the therapist may see the parents at their most vulnerable moments. Therapists hear their guilt and see the parents' tears. There is a level of immediate intimacy that may be difficult and awkward for parents. The provider–parent relationship does not develop over time; it develops immediately. The therapist's compassion and nonjudgmental attitudes are essential to build the relationship (Fialka, 2006).
- *Who is leading the therapy process?* The professional and the parent contribute to the "dance," and each partner guides the other partner to the next step. For example, parents may need the professional's assistance with understanding development or with choosing activities and toys that promote play. At the same time, providers need to understand the contributions of the parent (Fialka, 2006).
- *What are the priorities for the parents?* The therapist must know what is most important to the parents. Then, therapy providers can bring relevant ideas and knowledge to the treatment experience. They recommend new approaches and are prepared to assist the family with incorporating agreed-upon approaches. Therapists need to ask if there is anything that they have missed. They also need to develop an understanding of how suggestions may change or complicate daily living (Fialka, 2006).

Screening and Assessment

Child Find activities are methods and procedures adopted by statewide early intervention programs designed to identify and locate children at risk for developmental delay who would benefit from early intervention services (Dunst, Trivette, Appl, & Bagnato, 2004). Child Find activities include standard referral procedures and an organized process to assign a service coordinator for the family. Once children are identified as appropriate for early intervention services, they are eligible for evaluation. There are assessment procedures that are particularly useful in gaining information about the child within the context of the family.

Occupational Profile

When working in early intervention, the occupational profile should include open-ended questions that facilitate responses and allow the parents to elaborate on their responses. The goal of the occupational profile is to understand the family's internal experiences with the child (Kalmanson, 2006). For example, do the parents experience anxiety when they need to feed their infant who uses a nasogastric tube? Do the parents feel sad when they take their child to a playground and notice that their child does not play as the other children play? The therapist encourages parental involvement by forming a team and involving the parents through understanding their experiences and feelings. This team relationship assists in the therapeutic process for the child.

Self-Reflection

Practice in early intervention with a focus on infant and toddler mental health requires providers to be self-reflective (Kalmanson, 2006). Providers need to understand the experiences and feelings of the parents, as their feelings may influence the behavior displayed by a parent. In addition, providers need to pay attention to their own feelings and their feelings in relation to the families they are serving. Self-reflection is at the core of all assessment and intervention strategies in infant mental health practice.

Often, when children have physical challenges, self-reflective practice and the socioemotional development of the child is overlooked. If the parent agrees, videotaping the assessment and how the parent or caregiver interacts with the child may be helpful. The advantage of video-recording is that the tapes can be replayed and used for intervention planning and discussion. The time lapse between the initial assessment and discussion may facilitate self-reflection. In addition, reviewing the tapes with the parent and asking the parent to describe his or her perceptions of the child's response to the interaction may also facilitate self-reflection. Therefore, it is essential to remember that self-reflective practice must be embedded in the pragmatics of assessment and intervention.

Arena-Style Assessment

All team members are present during an **arena-style assessment**. One team member is the evaluation facilitator and is primarily responsible for interacting with the child during the actual assessment. Another team member may serve as coach. This person assists the facilitator during the assessment and facilitates discussion after the evaluation. All other team members observe the child's responses during the evaluation.

The advantages of an arena-style assessment are that team members may share their unique perspectives and little is missed. The child and family only need to attend to the facilitator instead of attending to multiple evaluators. In addition, the entire team is present, reducing the number of evaluations, and a variety of ideas are offered and discussed. Conversely, arena-style assessments require maximal preparation time, forethought, and planning. Coordination among team members is imperative, and the facilitator needs to be highly skilled and committed to the process (McGonigel, Woodruff, & Roszmann-Millican, 1994).

Hawaii Early Learning Profile

The Hawaii Early Learning Profile (HELP) (Furuno, O'Reilly, Hosaka, Zeisloft, & Allman, 1984) is an excellent instrument frequently used during an arena-style assessment. The HELP is a criterion-referenced, curriculum-based assessment used for treatment planning (Stewart, 2005). This assessment is used to develop an understanding of child development in children from birth to age three. The HELP is primarily recommended for use in natural environments because observations of the environment and caregiver interactions are included.

The HELP is divided into seven major sections: regulatory/sensory organization, cognitive, language, gross motor, fine motor, socioemotional, and self-help. Adaptations for disabilities are acceptable, and sample adaptations are included in the administration manual. Developers of the HELP also included a family-centered interview. The interview ensures a family-directed assessment of each family's concerns, priorities, and resources as they relate to the needs of their child. This interview assists providers in determining where to start when using the HELP as an assessment instrument.

Ages and Stages Questionnaires

Developmental screenings are conducted to determine if more comprehensive evaluation is warranted and may be used in Child Find systems (Stewart, 2005). In addition, screening instruments, such as the Ages and Stages Questionnaires (ASQ) are frequently used when a child is receiving early intervention services as a way of empowering the parents.

The ASQ is a parent-completed instrument that screens for developmental delays during the first 5 years of life (Bricker, Squires, & Mounts, 1995). Parents or primary caregivers complete the questionnaires, and professionals assist in the interpretation of the results. The questionnaires are administered at designated intervals.

The advantage of this screening instrument is the ability to assess children in their natural environments. Parents or caregivers may complete each questionnaire in 10 to 15 minutes.

The questionnaires provide screening in five key developmental domains: communication, gross motor, fine motor, problem-solving, and personal-social. Guidelines are provided to the parents so they can identify if their child is at risk in the five domains. The ASQ User Guide provides

---

Evidence-Based Practice

Specialized interventions that focus on the individual needs of children and their families are more effective than generic programs (Brooks-Gunn, Berlin, & Fulgini, 2000; Farran, 2000; Guralnick, 1998).

➤ Occupational therapists should use the information gathered in the occupational profile to plan individualized treatments that meet the needs of the children within the family context.

Brooks-Gunn, J., Berlin, L. J., & Fuligni, A. S. (2000). Early childhood intervention programs: What about the family? In J. P. Shonkoff & S. J. Meisels (Eds.), *Handbook of Early Childhood Intervention* (2nd ed.) (pp. 549–587). New York: Cambridge University Press.

Farran, D. C. (2000). Another decade of intervention for children who are low income or disabled: What do we do now? In J. P. Shonkoff & S. J. Meisels (Eds.), *Handbook of Early Childhood Intervention* (2nd ed.) (pp. 510–548). New York: Cambridge University Press.

Guralnick, M. (1998). The effectiveness of early intervention for vulnerable children: A developmental perspective. *American Journal on Mental Retardation, 102,* 319–345.

parents and caregivers with sample activities to promote development. This screening instrument is recommended for use in public health for early identification and screening (American Academy of Pediatrics, 2006).

The Infant/Toddler Sensory Profile

The Infant/Toddler Sensory Profile (Dunn, 2002) measures the caregiver's perception of children's responses to sensory events that occur during routine activities. The profile consists of 84 questions; 36 of the items evaluate children ages birth to 6 months, and 48 items evaluate children ages 7 to 36 months. This instrument is a parental self-report questionnaire with which parents rate the child's responsiveness on a 5-point Likert scale. The rating identifies how frequently their child responds to sensory stimuli.

Studies have shown that children diagnosed with certain forms of disability have significantly different patterns of sensory processing than children without disabilities (Dunn, 2004). This instrument may assist the occupational therapist in identifying how sensory processing affects the relationship between the primary caregiver and the child. The occupational therapist may identify potential sources of challenging relationships by using the Infant/Toddler Sensory Profile (Dunn, 2002).

Intervention Models

Four intervention models to provide a framework for practice in infant and toddler mental health practice in early intervention settings are discussed. First, the family systems model describes the family as a system composed of subsystems that resides in a larger community and social system. Second, the transactional model outlines three intervention strategies that focus on improving the parent–child relationship. Third, psychobiological attachment theory illustrates how the bond between caregiver and child regulates the child's physiology, behavior, emotion, and cognition. And finally, the sensory processing model describes how the child's degree of processing sensory information during daily routines can influence the parent–child relationship. Using these models in early intervention practice can help the provider focus on mental health aspects of care.

Family Systems Model

The family systems model (Klein & White, 1996) assists providers by creating a framework that examines the complexity and diversity of families. Families experience a wide array of external factors that influence relationships, communication, values, and beliefs. The family systems model is based on four assumptions that provide a useful guide to thinking in early intervention practice.

Families as Systems

The first assumption is that a family is a system composed of interrelated parts. That is, all family members are connected; if one member of the family is having difficulty, it may affect the other family members. For example, a child with special health care needs may affect interactions between the parents, the parents and another sibling, or even a relationship between the parents and extended family. The family is composed of multiple subsystems, including the parent–parent relationship, the parent–child relationship,

and the sibling–sibling relationship. All of these subsystems interact to create the family unit.

Think about working with a family who has two children (ages 2 and 4), and the youngest child is diagnosed with Down syndrome. Both parents are employed, and the mother is primarily responsible for the morning routine of getting ready for the day. The child with Down syndrome requires a longer time to eat and sometimes needs to be fed. The 4-year-old sibling, although fairly independent in dressing and eating, sees how much time the mother is spending with the 2-year-old and refuses to be as independent in dressing. The mother is receiving reprimands from work because she is sometimes late. Her frustration with the 4-year-old escalates, and their relationship is impaired. The mother then becomes angry with the father because he is unable to help in the morning, and their relationship becomes strained.

This example illustrates the "ripple effect" of a child with special health needs. In this case, the occupational therapist needs to be aware of how the morning routine is affecting the family. The therapist may look at the issue of temporality or timing within the routine and work with the mother in establishing a routine that allows her to get to work on time. The therapist may suggest getting the 4-year-old ready first while the 2-year-old is still sleeping. Changes in the temporality of the routine may decrease stress and improve the relationships between the mother and the 4-year-old as well as the mother and the father.

Wholeness

The second assumption within a family systems model states that consideration of the family as an entire unit is more meaningful than considering each individual member. This concept is considered wholeness (von Bertalanffy, 1968). **Wholeness** is the concept that the entire family is greater than the sum of each individual family member. This means that the processes and relationships between family members relate to occupational and co-occupational outcomes more than just evaluation and treatment of individual family members.

For example, an occupational therapist identifies that a child has sensory processing problems and is hypersensitive in the tactile and olfactory sensory systems. This hypersensitivity is creating problems during bathing and feeding. The therapist should observe the processes of bathing and feeding to see how the parent and child interact. Evaluating the child and parent separately would not assist the therapist with understanding the entire situation, or the whole. Observing the bathing and feeding processes allows the therapist to better understand the influence of both the child and the parent. Otherwise, the therapist may assume the outcome is related to a particular characteristic of either the parent or the child, and that assumption may not necessarily be true.

Homeostasis

The third assumption addresses the concept of homeostasis. **Homeostasis** is the family's ability to achieve a sense of balance or equilibrium through the use of rituals and routines. When a child is diagnosed with impairment or disability, families may rearrange their work and leisure interests to accommodate the child's needs. Families use routines and rituals to maintain a sense of balance. Occupational therapists may be instrumental in assisting with engagement in routines and habits that create a sense of balance.

For example, a family with three children, one child who is diagnosed with a serious heart valve defect, enjoys attending the annual holiday parade. The parade signifies the beginning of the holiday season and is fun for everyone. One month before the holiday parade, the child with the heart defect underwent surgery for a valve repair. Because the child was in recovery when the parade was scheduled, the family missed the annual event, and the parents stated that the holiday season did not feel the same. They felt sad; however, they knew that there would be another parade. The following year, everyone was healthy and the family was able to attend the parade. All family members were cheerful, and that year, the family felt joyous with the holiday season approaching. The parade was a ritual that brought cohesion and happiness to all of the family members.

Internal and External Factors

The fourth assumption of the family systems model is that internal and external forces influence the family and how it functions. Some examples of external forces include employment, health insurance, and a change in pediatrician. Internal forces can include personality, values, or beliefs. To be effective, occupational therapists need to develop an awareness and understanding of all of the forces.

For example, the therapist is scheduled to conduct home visits with a family two times per week. The family consists of a mother, live-in boyfriend, and twins born prematurely. One of the twins receives therapy biweekly by an occupational therapist, physical therapist, speech-language pathologist, and special educator. The other twin receives consultation services. During a typical week, five early intervention visits are scheduled in the home. The mother is also pregnant with another child.

During the first month of intervention, the family misses 15 of the 20 visits because they are not at home. At first, the therapist assumes that the family is noncompliant. However, after a discussion with the mother, the occupational therapist discovers that the mother is responsible for all home management tasks, including shopping, banking, cleaning, laundry, and caregiving. In addition, she works outside of the home. The mother talks about her busy schedule and the difficulty she has managing all of the appointments involved in the early intervention schedule. Recognizing the internal and external factors affecting this family, the early intervention team convenes a meeting, and the outcome includes development of a schedule conducive to the mother's schedule. After these changes, attendance in the early intervention program increases dramatically. Success in this example was achieved because the early intervention team understood the internal and external forces affecting therapy attendance.

Clinical Reasoning

The four assumptions in the family systems model relate to using the framework to guide clinical reasoning. This framework provides a way of knowing about the family and helps therapists understand the organization of the family. Through this understanding, therapists are able to provide family-centered intervention that produces the most optimal outcomes.

Evidence-Based Practice

Interventions that are targeted at daily routines and everyday experiences in the infant/toddlers environment improves skill acquisition (Farran, 2000).

➤ The occupational profile should include information that describes everyday routines and experiences.

➤ Occupational therapy treatment should occur within the context of daily routines whenever possible.

Farran, D. C. (2000). Another decade of intervention for children who are low income or disabled: What do we do now? In J. P. Shonkoff & S. J. Meisels (Eds.), *Handbook of Early Childhood Intervention* (2nd ed.) (pp. 510–548). New York: Cambridge University Press.

Transactional Model

Arnold Sameroff introduced the transactional model as way of understanding the process of development. Children develop as a result of the continuous interaction between the characteristics of the child and their experiences in the environment (Sameroff & Chandler, 1975; Sameroff, 1993, 2004). Sameroff identifies risk factors that contribute to poor developmental outcomes. For example, a child born with a genetic anomaly may be at greater risk for poor developmental outcomes. The risk for poor developmental outcomes is due not to the genetic anomaly alone but also to the effect that the genetic anomaly has on the relationship with the parent.

Sameroff also identifies environmental risks that can result in poor developmental outcomes, such as single parenthood, poverty, parental depression, and poor parenting practices. These environmental risks can create a series of interactions that are maladaptive and, over the course of time, may negatively affect the child's development. Social environment and family context contribute to the child's development. The family context includes the parents' characteristics and history. The social environment contributes through supports and barriers, including extended family, poverty, and demographics.

Sameroff (2004) identifies three relationship-focused intervention strategies designed to improve developmental outcomes: remediation, redefinition, and reeducation. **Remediation** is designed to change the child, with eventual changes occurring in the parent. For example, if a child has a known genetic disorder such as Down's syndrome and the child's responsiveness to stimuli is low, remediation would be directed toward changing the child's responsiveness. As the child's responsiveness to stimuli changes, the parents may respond more adaptively to the child.

The premise of the remediation approach is that changes in the child will lead to increased adaptive responses of the parent. Occupational therapists are experts in remediation and have a long history of the use of remediation techniques. The transactional model takes remediation one step further by recommending that therapists look at how remediation affects the child and the parent–child relationship.

Redefinition is directed toward parenting. The goal of redefinition is to alter parental beliefs and expectations so that parents are able and willing to provide nurturing caregiving experiences. For example, parents of a child with extreme sensory defensiveness may believe that the child's behavioral outbursts (tantrums and uncooperativeness; e.g., the child may cry during bathing and dressing) are the result of negative behavior and the child is just being naughty.

An occupational therapist can help the parent understand that the child's behavior is the result a sensory modulation disorder. By redefining the problem, the therapists may then provide some ideas to make bathing and dressing a more pleasant experience. The caregiving experience can be enhanced, and the parent–child relationship may be improved.

Reeducation is directed toward educating the parents in different methods to raise their child. The focus of reeducation is to teach parents what to expect from their child and to teach caregiving practices that are related to positive developmental outcomes. This strategy is preventative in nature and useful in situations in which the parents are at high risk. For example, a teen mother with very little experience in caregiving may benefit from interventions focused on child development and age-appropriate activities. The underlying assumption of reeducation is that parental knowledge about their child will enhance adaptive parent–child relationships. Over time, these adaptive interactions will promote positive child development.

In summary, the transactional model provides a framework for occupational therapists working in early intervention. The transactional model facilitates the combination of more traditional occupational therapy approaches (sensory integration and neurodevelopmental treatment) with infant and toddler mental health practices. The targeted outcome of the transaction model is to focus on strategies that improve the parent–child relationship in order to improve child outcomes.

Psychobiological Attachment Theory

Psychobiological attachment theory (Kraemer, 1992) extends John Bowlby's (1969) attachment theory. Bowlby identified warm, nurturing care as a predictor of childhood health and wellbeing. He introduced two concepts, the secure base and the internal working model. A **secure base** is a caregiver who promotes exploration and learning about the environment by providing a safe, comfortable atmosphere. Through repeated interactions with the caregiver, the child develops a representation of what is and what should be. This internal representation becomes the child's **internal working model**. The child uses the internal working model to regulate behavior during interactions with playmates and other caregivers.

Bowlby's theory informs practice when disruption in attachment is due to inadequate caregiving, as it emphasizes the importance of warm responsive care. Bowlby's theory, however, does not account for disruptions in attachment when the caregiver is nurturing, yet the child responds differently. The variation in a child's response to nurturing care may be a direct result of impairment or disability.

Kraemer (1992) addresses attachment disruptions when the caregiver is nurturing and the child responds differently. Children with disabilities may not express behaviors and emotions in the same fashion as children without disabilities.

They may not respond to nurturing care with the same repertoire of behavior as children without disabilities. The expression of unusual behavior may actually be a part of the attachment behavior repertoire and needs to be recognized as such (Kraemer, 1992). Therefore, psychobiological attachment theory provides a way of thinking about infant and toddler mental health and relationships when a child has a disability or is at risk for developing a delay.

Psychobiological attachment theory includes four tenets that address the child and caregivers' contributions within the context of the infant–caregiver system:

1. Infants are born with adaptive mechanisms that foster attunement.
2. Infants' nervous systems are highly plastic and responsive to caregiving.
3. Caregivers regulate infant neurobiology.
4. Caregiving is characterized by factors within a sociocultural niche.

First, Kraemer (1992) proposes that adaptive mechanisms present at birth foster attunement to a caregiver. Neonates have the unique ability to discriminate their mother's face from a stranger's face, and they tend to orient visually to their mother rather than a stranger (Field, Cohen, Garcia, & Greenberg, 1984). This ability to discriminate facial differences early in life facilitates maternal–infant bonding. Therefore, providers should be aware of the infant's sensory and perceptual abilities that contribute to social attunement, as these may not represent typical signaling strategies.

For example, recall the case presented earlier in this chapter. The occupational therapist provided intervention for a family whose son was typically developing until 9 months of age, when he developed sepsis secondary to an *E. coli* infection. When the boy was discharged from the hospital, the physicians believed he would not survive the year. His motor development skills were that of a newborn. He had severe extensor posturing and was visually and auditorily impaired. His parents believed that he did not know who they were, as he demonstrated no visual gaze toward them, and he did not orient his head to the sound of their voice. Because the child was agitated, he would cry for extended periods of time, and the parents could not console him.

During therapy, the therapist noticed that when she held the boy and when the father spoke, his muscle tone changed. The boy's body would soften slightly in her arms as the father spoke to the boy. The therapist discussed this with the father, and the father was reinforced to engage with his son. Eventually, the father and mother were able to console the child, and their bond grew over time. Upon the transition evaluation into the school setting, the boy's socioemotional development represented that of a child 9 to 12 months old. The growth in this area of development was very rewarding for the parents.

Second, Kraemer (1992) states that the child's nervous system is highly plastic. Nervous system development occurs within the context of the caregiver–child relationship. Social experiences facilitate neuronal connections and pruning (Greenough, Black, & Wallace, 1987). Providers should recognize the significant role the social environment plays in neural maturation. Occupational therapists in early intervention must pay attention to the social processes that occur during play and ADLs. Research has shown that these co-occupational experiences influence the structure and function of the brain. When therapists address the parent–child relationship, they are using evidence-based practice in therapy.

Third, Kraemer (1992) espouses that the caregiver serves as a psychobiological regulator. Caregiving regulates the child's physiology, neurobiology, and behaviors. Postnatal organization occurs in response to the patterned events provided by the caregiver. This point underscores the impact of the caregivers during daily routines. If the parent responds negatively, harshly, or intrusively to the child, that response is shaping the child's neurobiology.

For example, Nicole is a teenage mother who lives with her mother and stepfather in a small rural home. The family has significant financial needs, and they use Nicole's food assistance to feed the entire family. Nicole's baby was born preterm. During a mother–infant play session, the occupational therapist noticed that Nicole's play style was very intrusive. That is, she took toys from the baby and bopped her baby on the face. She roughly patted the baby's cheeks with her hands. Her voice was loud and harsh. She did not wait for the baby to respond. The baby's face was fearful during this interaction, and his movements were sporadic and uncontrolled. Eventually, the baby looked away and shielded his face with his arm. The more the baby looked away, the more Nicole tried to obtain his attention. Finally, the baby began to cry in distress.

This example demonstrates how the mother deregulated the infant's behavior. It is reasonable to assume that the infant's physiology was deregulated as well because the infant was displaying a stress response. If Nicole had responded differently to her son, the infant's behavioral and physiological responses would have also been different.

Occupational therapists in early intervention need to empower parents and caregivers at risk so that they can help their children develop in a more positive manner. Video-recording the play interaction between Nicole and her son would provide an opportunity for the therapist and Nicole to review the videotape. The therapist could ask Nicole about the positive and negative aspects of the interaction. Through probing and problem-solving, Nicole would identify how she could interact with her son to create a different outcome. Also, the occupational therapist should inquire about Nicole's mental health status. If Nicole is demonstrating signs of postpartum depression, the therapist could explain postpartum depression and ask if she has been screened for depression. The therapist should refer Nicole to an appropriate professional for depression screening and treatment if necessary.

Fourth, Kraemer (1992) states that caregiving styles are embedded within a sociocultural niche. Hence, sociocultural factors influence caregiver–child reciprocity. Ethnicity and culture play a significant role in parenting or caregiving characteristics. The most adaptive parenting styles may vary across culture. For example, the Eastern medical traditions of the Hmong culture may be in direct conflict with practices of Western medicine (Fadiman, 1997). Interpretation of caregiving patterns is best understood through the sociocultural influences on caregiving routines. Early intervention

---

Evidence-Based Practice

Interventions focused on specific parenting behaviors are more effective than generic parenting education programs (Brooks-Gunn, Berlin, & Fuligni, 2000).

➤ Occupational therapist should observe parent–infant interactions so that the intervention can target specific parenting behaviors.

➤ Occupational therapists may want to use video-recording of parent–infant interactions to assist the parent with identification of parental behaviors that do not promote exploration and development.

Brooks-Gunn, J., Berlin, L. J., & Fuligni, A. S. (2000). Early childhood intervention programs: What about the family? In J. P. Shonkoff & S. J. Meisels (Eds.), *Handbook of Early Childhood Intervention* (2nd ed.) (pp. 549–587). New York: Cambridge University Press.

---

providers need to be culturally competent in their practice. Learning about caregiving practices in other cultures is essential.

Psychobiological attachment theory contributes to the field of early intervention by identifying the influence of the sociocultural environment on early neurobiological development. Specific therapeutic intervention strategies based on fundamental nurturing and exposure to harmonious interactions may facilitate optimal neurobehavioral regulation, emotional, social, and cognitive development (Kraemer, 1992). When providers integrate their current knowledge of neuromuscular and sensory motor development to promote attachment relationships, they are performing best practice within the context of natural environments. Modeling interactions, offering resources, and developing collaborative relationships with caregivers are important strategies to promote healthy child development.

Sensory Processing

The sensory processing model (Dunn, 1997, 2004) was developed to assist caregivers with understanding their own sensory processing and their infant's sensory processing. The sensory processing model educates caregivers about sensory processing so they can reflect on their own experiences with sensory stimuli and understand their infant's reactions during daily routines. The sensory processing model contains two continuums: the neurological threshold continuum and the self-regulation strategy continuum, which interact and result in behavioral responses.

Neurological Threshold Continuum

Two categories (sensitization and habituation) comprise the neurological threshold continuum. If a child's neurological system primarily responds with sensitization, the child may be readily distracted. Conversely, if a child's nervous system primarily responds to the environment by habituating, then the child may not notice stimuli in the environment (Dunn, 2004).

Self-Regulation Strategy Continuum

Two categories (passive and active) comprise the self-regulation strategy continuum. A child using a passive response strategy is allowing sensory stimuli encountered in daily life to occur without interference. Too much passivity may indicate that the stimuli are overwhelming. A child using an active response strategy is engaging in behaviors to manage the sensory stimuli inherent in his or her daily activities. Active response strategies can include avoidance or approach, and these strategies may interfere with the developing relationship. For example, a toddler who is using avoidance may not interact with his or her caregiver during certain ADLs, such as dressing. This could create stress for the parent and impair their interactions.

Interaction Between High Neurological Threshold and Self-Regulation Strategy Continuums

If an infant has a high neurological threshold, the infant may display passive and active self-regulatory behaviors. Examples of passive self-regulation include being oblivious to events and stimuli in the environment. An infant using this mode of regulation may present with a flat affect or seem self-absorbed. An adult who has low registration may not readily notice the infant's signals. They may be slower to respond to the infant and may need cues to attend to the infant in a timely manner.

Conversely, active self-regulatory behavior of an infant with a high neurological threshold includes sensory-seeking behavior. An infant who is sensory seeking enjoys stimuli. These children tend to be more active and may enjoy play that activates the sensory systems, such as roughhouse play. A caregiver who is sensory seeking may actively engage the infant continuously throughout the day. Infants who are not sensory seeking may become overwhelmed from the continuous stimulation given by the caregiver and withdraw.

Interaction Between Low Neurological Threshold and Self Regulation Strategy Continuums

If an infant has a low neurological threshold, the infant may also demonstrate passive and active self-regulatory behaviors. Passive self-regulatory behaviors include overreaction to stimuli in the everyday environment that other infants may not notice. These infants may be light sleepers or may dislike certain sounds, food textures, and clothing. Caregivers who have sensory sensitivity may be overly concerned with the infant's wellbeing. Their care and concern may result in undue tension and anxiety. These caregivers may be overprotective and overreactive.

Conversely, an infant who is demonstrating active self-regulatory behaviors will avoid certain sensations. These infants may withdraw from stimuli or become more rigid and tense when exposed to uncomfortable stimuli (Dunn, 2004). Caregivers who are sensory avoiding may be more cautious about their interactions with their infants. These caregivers prefer routine and will appreciate an infant who enjoys predictable patterns.

The Parent–Child Relationship

When caregivers and their children have sensory processing styles that are different from each other, it is important for caregivers to understand their own preferences in relation to their child's preferences. For example, if a caregiver has a high neurological threshold and displays low registration behaviors (does not react quickly), and the child has a low neurological threshold and displays sensory sensitivity (overreacts to many stimuli), the child may become overly fussy due to the slow response of the caregiver. Over time, the child may learn that his or her needs are not being met, which can result in difficulty with formation of an attachment bond to the caregiver. Occupational therapists who work in early intervention may use Dunn's (1997, 2004) model of sensory processing to address infant and toddler mental health through parental education and intervention.

Transition to Early Childhood

The early intervention team is responsible for coordinating a smooth transition into early childhood education. Parents may feel abandoned at this time, as their interactions with professionals in relation to their child significantly changes. That is, families may become accustomed to professionals coming into their home and miss the close relationships that have been established with the early intervention team. The school setting differs from early intervention programming because the family loses the service coordination of early intervention settings.

To help alleviate this stress, the early intervention team can begin talking about transition services early. This planning should begin at least 6 months before the child transitions into the school setting. The occupational therapist may be instrumental in setting up visits to the school and addressing the parents' concerns. Parents will need to be strong advocates for their children in school settings. The occupational therapist may assist through empowerment and helping the family find its voice. It is important to remember that when taking a life-cycle approach to the family, transitions may be a time of disturbance. The occupational therapist's role may be to help the family develop a sense of balance and homeostasis by establishing new routines and habits.

Summary

Practice in early intervention requires the therapist to use principles of infant and toddler mental health. In early intervention settings, occupational therapists must pay attention to the relationship between the primary caregiver and the child. The therapist must also develop the professional–parent relationship because a positive professional–parent relationship will enhance occupational therapy outcomes. This chapter provided examples of how an occupational therapist uses assessments and intervention strategies to facilitate the optimum mental health of the infant and toddler.

Active Learning Strategies

1. Reflection

Reflect on your own memories of a time when you were introduced to a new health care provider. What did that health care provider do to facilitate a professional–client relationship? What characteristics did the health care provider have that allowed you as a client to feel comfortable?

 Describe your memories in your **Reflective Journal**.

2. Interview a Parent

Interview a parent regarding relationships with health professionals. Start by asking general questions, such as what qualities they look for in a health care professional that foster trust. Ask them to reflect on good and bad experiences that they have had with health care professionals. What made those experiences good or bad, and how could the health professional have improved the interaction?

3. Family

Reflect on your own family and answer the following questions:

Reflective Questions
- How do you define family? Who is included in your immediate family and your extended family?
- What family routines and rituals bring a sense of balance to your family?
- How does your family cope with difficult events?
- What internal and external factors influence occupational and co-occupational engagement in your family?

 Use your **Reflective Journal** to document your answers.

Resources

- Zero to Three Organization: http://www.zerotothree.org
- The National Mental Health Association: http://www.nmha.org
- Annie E. Casey Foundation: http://www.aecf.org/kidscount

References

American Academy of Pediatrics. Council on Children with Disabilities, Section on Developmental Behavioral Pediatrics, Bright Futures Steering Committee and Medical Home Initiatives for Children with Special Needs Project Advisory Committee. (2006). Identifying infants and young children with developmental disorders in the medical home: An algorithm for developmental surveillance and screening. *Pediatrics, 118*(1), 405–420.

Barnekow, K. A., & Kraemer, G. W. (2005). The psychobiological theory of attachment: A viable frame of reference for early intervention providers. *Physical and Occupational Therapy in Pediatrics, 25,* 3–15.

Bowlby, J. (1969). *Attachment and Loss: Vol. 1. Attachment.* New York: Basic Books.

Bricker, D., Squires, J., & Mounts, L. (1995). *Ages and Stages Questionnaires: A Parent-Completed, Child-Monitoring System* (2nd ed.). Baltimore: Brookes.

Dunn, W. (1997). The impact of sensory processing abilities on the daily lives of young children and their families: A conceptual model. *Infants and Young Children, 9*(4), 23–25.

———. (2002). *The Infant/Toddler Sensory Profile Manual.* San Antonio, TX: Psychological Corp.

Dunn, W. (2004). A sensory processing approach to supporting infant–caregiver relationships. In A. J. Sameroff, S. C. McDonough, & K. L. Rosenblum (Eds.), *Treating Parent–Infant Relationship Problems* (pp. 152–187). New York: Guilford.

Dunst, C. J., Johanson, C., Trivette, C. M., & Hamby, D. (1991). Family-oriented early intervention policies and practices: Family-centered or not? *Exceptional Children, 58*(2), 115–126.

Dunst, C. J., Trivette, C. M., Appl, D. J., & Bagnato, S. J. (2004). Framework for investigating child find, referral, early identification and eligibility determination practices. *Tracelines, 1,* 1–11.

Fadiman, A. (1997). *The Spirit Catches You and You Fall Down.* New York: Noonday Press.

Fialka, J. (2006). The dance of partnership: Why do my feet hurt? Paper presented at the meeting of the Zero to Three 21st National Training Institute, December 1–3, Albuquerque, NM.

Field, T., Cohen, D., Garcia, R., & Greenberg, R. (1984). Mother–stranger face discrimination by the newborn. *Infant Behavior and Development, 7,* 19–25.

Fleischfresser S. (2004). Wisconsin Medical Home Learning Collaborative: A model for implementing practice change. *Wisconsin Medical Journal, 103*(5), 25–7.

Furuno, S., O'Reilly, K. A., Hosaka, C. M., Inatsuka, T. T., Allman, T. A., & Zeisloft, B. (1984). *Hawaii Early Learning Profile.* Palo Alto, CA: Vort.

Gilkerson, L. (2006). Infant and early childhood mental health: Building a family friendly service infrastructure. Paper presented at the meeting of the Zero to Three 21st National Training Institute, December 1–3, Albuquerque, NM.

Greenough, W. T., Black, J. E., & Wallace C. S. (1987). Experience and brain development. *Child Development, 15,* 539–559.

Haley, D. W., & Stansbury, K. (2003). Infant stress and parent responsiveness: Regulation of physiology and behavior during still-face and reunion. *Child Development, 74,* 1534–1546.

Kalmanson, B. (2006). What babies teach us: The transdisciplinary practice of infant mental health and early intervention. Paper presented at the meeting of the Zero to Three 21st National Training Institute, December 1–3, Albuquerque, NM.

Kalmanson, B., & Seligman, S. (2006). Process in an integrated model of infant mental health and early intervention practice. In G. M. Foley & J. D. Hochman, (Eds.), *Mental Health in Early Intervention: Achieving Unity in Principles and Practice* (pp 245–265). Baltimore: Brookes.

Klein, D. M., & White, J. M. (1996). *Family Theories: An Introduction.* Thousand Oaks, CA: Sage.

Kraemer, G. W. (1992). A psychobiological theory of attachment. *Behavioral and Brain Sciences, 15,* 493–541.

McGonigel, M., Woodruff, G., & Roszmann-Millican, M. (1994). The transdisciplinary team: A model for family-centered early intervention. In L. Johnson, R. J. Gallagher, M. LaMontagne, J. Jordan, J. Gallagher, P. Huttinger, & M. Karnes (Eds.), *Meeting Early Intervention Challenges: Issues from Birth to Three.* Baltimore: Brookes.

Sameroff, A. J. (1993). Models of development and developmental risk. In C. H. Zeanah, Jr. (Ed.), *Handbook of Infant Mental Health* (pp. 3–13). New York: Guilford.

———. (2004). Ports of entry and the dynamics of mother–infant interventions. In A. J. Sameroff, S. C. McDonough, & K. L. Rosenblum (Eds.), *Treating Parent–Infant Relationship Problems* (pp. 3–28). New York: Guilford.

Sameroff, A. J., & Chandler, M. J. (1975). Reproductive risk and the continuum of caretaking casualty. In F. D. Horowitz, E. M. Hetherington, S. Scarr-Salapatek, & G. Siegel (Eds.), *Review of Child Development Research* (Vol. 4, pp. 187–244). Chicago: University of Chicago Press.

Stephens, L. C., & Tauber, S. K. (2005). Early intervention. In J. Case-Smith (Ed.), *Occupational Therapy for Children* (5th ed.) (pp. 771–794). St. Louis: Mosby.

Stewart, K. (2005). Purposes, processes, and methods of evaluation. In J. Case-Smith (Ed.), *Occupational Therapy for Children* (5th ed.) (pp. 218–240). St. Louis: Mosby.

von Bertalanffy, L. (1968). The meaning of general system theory. In *General System Theory Foundations, Development, Applications* (pp. 31–53). New York: George Braziller.

CHAPTER 35

Consumer-Operated Services

Margaret Swarbrick

> "*S*elf-help is having a place where we can get rid of our rage and pain, and learn to respect each other—and ourselves—for what we've been through.
> —Judy Banes, Founder of On Our Own, Hackensack, New Jersey

Introduction

The onset of mental illness often occurs during young adulthood, a time when personal developmental goals focus on enhancing productivity, sustaining close relationships at home and in the community, and pursuing education. In addition to the difficult symptoms of the disease, mental illness is associated with many secondary negative effects, such as poverty, substandard housing, inaccessibility of quality health care, isolation, and loneliness (Carling, 1995; Davidson, Hoge, Godleski, Rakfeldt, & Griffith, 1996; del Vecchio, Fricks, & Johnson, 2000). Consumers often encounter stigmatizing attitudes (e.g., the negative stereotype that people with mental illness are violent), which can result in discrimination in social, employment, and housing situations (Chamberlin, 1990, 1995; Ribeiro, 1995). Consumers are often treated as "second-class citizens" (Chamberlin, 1995; del Vecchio et al, 2000) and frequently experience isolation, loneliness, and rejection (Davidson et al, 1996; Solomon, 2004).

Consumer-operated services (COSs) are important community-based resources that can address the secondary effects of mental illness through socialization and participation in meaningful activity (Swarbrick, 2005). COSs, also known as peer-operated, peer-delivered, or consumer-delivered services, are funded through state legislatures and private foundations. These services are considered both a complement and an alternative to traditional mental health services (Clay, 2005; Davidson et al, 1999; Segal, Hardiman, & Hodges, 2002; Van Tosh & del Vecchio, 2000). Although professionals may and do participate, COSs are mostly planned, operated, and evaluated by and for mental health consumers.

The clubhouse model also includes consumers as providers of services, but it is a specific model with unique characteristics and is discussed in Chapter 39. In contrast to traditional modalities that often mandate specific services for consumers and even label them according to their diagnoses, COSs offer a menu of service options to address individual desires, needs, and resources. They promote the empowerment and self-determination of consumers, and continue to develop and grow in the United States and throughout the world.

The final report of the President's New Freedom Commission on Mental Health (2003) suggests that in order to create a mental health system focused on recovery, COSs should be promoted. Occupational therapists working in mental health practice can consider this coming trend and position themselves to work collaboratively with the consumers they support to develop, implement, and evaluate this innovative service model. COSs are designed to address the social and emotional needs of consumer-participants and to empower them.

This chapter highlights the history of the development of COS, including types and categories, research, and core principles. It describes the consumer-operated self-help center model that evolved in one state. Occupational therapy values place mental health practitioners in an ideal situation to work with this promising practice model. Roles and possibilities for practitioners are reviewed. Practitioners are challenged to examine the possibilities in terms of how they can become involved locally with consumer groups to develop, implement, and evaluate COSs.

History of the COS Model

Historically, mental health consumers lived for years in confined institutional environments with little expectation of returning to the community (Goffman, 1961). Mental health system reform in the United States was influenced by a combination of social, political, and economic factors that changed the landscape wherein services are delivered. The COS model grew out of both the patients' rights movement, a civil rights movement against involuntary commitment and forced treatment, and the general self-help movement in the United States (Chamberlin, 1978; Zinman, Harp, & Budd, 1987). Individuals who experienced the inadequacies and indignities that traditional settings engendered helped to form a mental health consumer-survivor movement that was influential in focusing on the reform of the traditional medical model of "care" and helped to spur development of the COS model.

The **consumer-survivor movement** was strengthened by the Community Support Program (CSP) of the National Institute of Mental Health (NIMH), which was established to address the need for organized, community-based systems of care for adults with long-term mental illness

I am vice president of the Board of S.I.D.E. Being a part of the organization has been a successful feeling. S.I.D.E. is a consumer run organization for members diagnosed with a mental illness. S.I.D.E. to me is a place where I feel I totally belong. S.I.D.E. provides leadership skills, educational skills, and fun activities such as Halloween, Christmas, and Super Bowl. A lot of members have no family for celebrations during the year. So, S.I.D.E. compensates for the lack of family gatherings. I feel fortunate to be a member of a wonderful Consumer Run Organization that deeply cares about its members.

—Mary

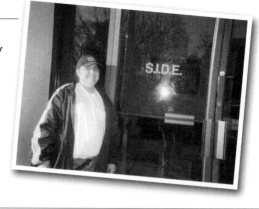

(Stroul, 1986). The CSP aimed to develop a network of community support systems focused on assisting and empowering people with long-term mental illness to meet their needs and help them to develop their personal potentials without being unnecessarily isolated or excluded from their communities (Carling, 1995; Stroul, 1986). The CSP included the active involvement of key stakeholders, including mental health consumers and their family members, in the service delivery design.

The consumer-survivor movement determined that consumers had limited options and involvement in their individual services and in the system as a whole. Consumers were not empowered by the traditional mental health system, which tends to be based on control and acts as the primary decision-maker for persons diagnosed with mental illness (Carling, 1995; Goffman, 1961). The movement viewed the traditional service system as paternalistic and lacking in policy and personal treatment options and opportunities (Campbell, 1997; Chamberlin & Rogers, 1990). Dissatisfaction with the traditional mental health service delivery approach was the impetus for the creation of COSs (Campbell, 1997; Segal et al, 2002; Segal & Silverman, 2002). Reacting to their experiences of the inadequacies of the mental health system and the indignities it engendered, consumers aimed to empower themselves by producing their own consumer-operated self-help alternatives (Chamberlin, 1978; 1984).

Early COS initiatives included the work of Howie the Harp, a prominent consumer who pioneered Project Release, a single-room housing service in New York for consumers, based on principles of service delivery, mutual support, and advocacy (Knight, 1997). Another pioneer, Judi Chamberlin, started the Ruby Rogers Drop-In Center in Boston (Chamberlin, 1978).

The most common type of COS, **drop-in centers**, developed without strict adherence to one specific model and proliferated with different levels of professional involvement (Bond, 1994; Johnson, 1994; Mowbray & Tan, 1992; Silverman, Blank, & Taylor, 1997). Drop-in centers offer a supportive environment where consumers can connect to a peer network, gain practical assistance from peers, relax, and experience freedom, the lack of imposed structure, and a familylike environment (Mowbray & Tan, 1993; Silverman, Blank, & Taylor, 1997).

From 1988 to 1991, the Center for Mental Health Services (CMHS), a branch of the Substance Abuse and Mental Health Services Administration (SAMHSA), funded demonstration

projects to examine the feasibility of COSs (Salzer, 2001; Van Tosh & del Vecchio, 2000). The demonstration projects resulted in expanding the range of COSs from a focus on drop-in centers to a wider array of services, including housing programs (Conrad, 1993), consumer businesses (Page, Lafreniere, & Out, 1999; Van Tosh & del Vecchio, 2000), mutual aid/self-help groups and peer-support programs (Chinman, Weingarten, Stayner, & Davidson, 2001; Mead, Hilton, & Curtis, 2001; Salzer, & Shear, Liptzen, 2002; Weingarten, Chinman, Tworkowski, Stayner, & Davidson, 2000), and case management (Nikkel, Smith, & Edwards, 1992).

COS programs can be organized into three clusters: drop-in centers, peer-support programs, and education programs (Clay, 2005). The first cluster, drop-in centers, provides varied services, such as meals and housing assistance for members, as well as a place to meet friends and relax. Drop-in centers are typically characterized as low-expectation environments where consumers can participate voluntarily in a wide variety of activities, particularly social and recreational pursuits that provide social support (Bond, 1994). Drop-in centers begin by offering socialization, but once they have achieved some longevity, they often begin to provide additional services, as requested by the membership. The centers provide links to a variety of community resources, such as traditional mental health services, food, housing, clothing, and shelter. Drop-in centers may also provide information about mental illness, medication, benefits, and coping skills. Information can be supplied in written form or by sharing "folk wisdom" gathered by consumers over the period of their psychiatric illnesses or experiences in the mental health system (Meek, 1994).

The second cluster, **peer-support programs**, consists of self-help groups and peer-support systems wherein persons in recovery provide services to one another. As the name implies, the emphasis in peer-support programs is the provision of social support by people who share the lived experience of mental illness. This may be in the form of group meetings but frequently is offered as one-on-one services. The location of peer-support programs may also be more individualized. For example, peers may meet in an individual's apartment. An example of a peer-support program offered by the state of New Jersey is highlighted later in this chapter.

The third cluster, **education programs**, includes training programs during which consumers learn recovery and advocacy skills (Clay, 2005). These programs are typically time limited. Using a consumer-led group format, consumers meet to acquire new information or gain new skills. Education programs fall on a continuum of more informal sharing of information to courses that follow an established curriculum. Box 35-1 describes the Fairweather Program.

Core Principles

Core COS principles include the following (Reissman, 1990):

- Consumers develop, control, and provide the services. Peers are involved in the design and delivery of services.
- Participation is completely voluntary. A person does not have to take medications or attend a traditional service program in order to participate.
- Emphasis is on strengths and competencies. The focus is not on symptoms or remediating impairments but on quality of life.

- A goal is mutuality among members instead of a hierarchy of helper and person helped. There is no power differential between the helper and helpee. The person providing the services does not execute any formal or informal control over the person receiving services.
- "Helper-therapy principle" is the notion that the helper and helpee both gain through the support experience.

Some COSs are entirely consumer managed, whereas others incorporate the use of nonconsumer professionals in certain areas of planning, implementation, and evaluation (Kaufmann, Freund, & Wilson, 1989; Solomon, 2004) (Figure 35-1). Nonconsumers are often hired for training and consultation services. This is a great role for occupational therapists. For example, an occupational therapist might provide training to group leaders in an educational program or might make recommendations regarding the physical environment to support participation for all individuals.

BOX 35-1 ■ Fairweather Programs *by Kristine Haertl*

The Fairweather model represents a unique peer-supported environment upholding major principles of rehabilitation and recovery. At the time of deinstitutionalization in the 1960s, under a National Institutes of Health grant, Dr. George Fairweather designed a unique community living environment developed on the premise of the importance of work, mutual support, and personal empowerment whereby individuals with serious and persistent mental illness lived and worked together in a peer-supported environment relatively autonomously from staff (Fairweather, 1964; Fairweather & Fergus, 1988; Fairweather, Sanders, Cressler, & Maynard, 1969). The program sought to empower consumers to take an active role in society and to combat the stigma of mental illness.

Fairweather's model included "lodges," which today are typically community-based homes that house 4 to 8 persons in an interdependent community culture. Residents live together and maintain the household by sharing daily responsibilities. Persons may choose to live in a lodge or may live elsewhere yet receive services through involvement in the work, recreational, and mental health aspects of the program. As the current state of health care focuses on shorter lengths of stay, a unique aspect of the Fairweather program is that persons may remain in the program for as long as they choose provided they meet programmatic expectations, including active participation in the peer culture, productive work, and follow-through with daily responsibilities.

Competitive work is a key aspect of the Fairweather model, as is the emphasis on mutual decision-making and meaningful engagement in daily activity. Typically, each house is supervised by a lodge coordinator who serves to assure the healthy daily functioning of the lodge community. Depending on the program and skill level of the residents, a coordinator may be on site an average of 2 to 10 hours a week. Employees and members of the Fairweather program are given equal decision-making power, and collaboration is emphasized in the running of the household. Basic tenets of the lodge include the following: (a) members have a stake in the system, (b) they are given much autonomy, (c) their role is voluntary, (d) the system offers opportunities for advancement, and (e) individuals are expected to fulfill the roles of society (Onaga, 1994).

The funding for lodge programs varies throughout the country and includes funds from governmental, private, and faith-based organizations. In addition, many of the Fairweather programs have developed their own businesses and hire members at a competitive rate of pay. Currently, various work options available to participants include janitorial services, clerical work, mail room services, construction/home refurbishing, lawn care, printing, and other services. In addition to work and residential programs, various Fairweather sites offer comprehensive services including psychiatric, recreational, vocational, residential, contracted medical (e.g., nursing and occupational therapy), wellness, and chemical dependency support. The wrap-around services enable consumers to receive most of their needs in one organization, a benefit in both efficiency and effectiveness of services.

There are many potential roles for an occupational therapist within the Fairweather model. Therapists have worked in various capacities, including the development of the living skills training curricula, as lodge and basic living skills coordinators, and as special consultants to the program. Additional opportunities exist within the vocational and wellness components of the program, in management, and in program design. As the mental health delivery system has increased emphasis on community-based services, it is vital that occupational therapists market their unique contributions and skill sets to develop and integrate into innovative programs.

Despite its emergence in the 1960s and there being over 100 Fairweather lodges nationwide, other than Fairweather's original research and publication, the model has only recently been highlighted in academic literature (e.g., Haertl 2005, 2007; Haertl & Minato, 2006; Nikelly, 2001; Onaga & Smith, 2000). Research and outcomes monitoring have demonstrated the lodge model's effectiveness in promoting a familylike culture, reducing hospitalization rates, increasing quality of life, decreasing total cost to the community, and increasing number of hours worked and rate of pay (Fairweather, 1964; Fairweather & Fergus, 1988; Haertl, 2005, 2007; Onaga & Smith, 2000). In recent years, as the Fairweather model has regained popularity, the national Fairweather organization Coalition for Community Living (n.d.) has developed fidelity standards outlining criteria to evaluate programs. Key principles within the standards emphasize (1) safe environments, (2) good health and symptom management, (3) long-term services, (4) productive work, (5) meaningful social roles, (6) community culture, (7) autonomy, and (8) the securing of resources. The development of these standards will provide a guide for new programs in development and serve to maintain quality within the existing Fairweather-operated programs.

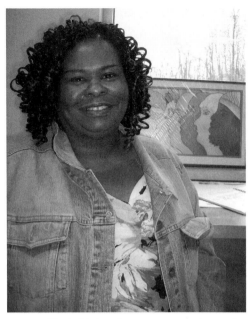

FIGURE 35-1. Cherie Bledsoe is a consumer and executive director of the consumer-operated service known as S.I.D.E. in Kansas City, Kansas. She contributed to the consumer perspective of Chapter 2.

By the nature of their design, COSs offer mental health consumers a setting that fosters empowerment by offering opportunities for all members to participate in an inclusive, democratic process of shared decision-making at their own comfort level. In the COS model, the inclusion of nonconsumer or professional involvement is within the control of the consumer operators (Solomon & Draine, 2001). That is, the consumers make the decision to hire a nonconsumer professional, determine the scope of work, provide feedback, and determine whether to maintain the working relationship. This is quite different from the traditional mental health care system in which staff members act as a surrogate decision-maker for the person who experiences mental illness (Carling, 1995; Goffman, 1961). The COS model has become a vehicle that helps expand consumers' options and opportunities to meaningfully affect policy planning and decision-making (Campbell, 1997; Chamberlin & Rogers, 1990).

Segal et al (2002) found that consumer-operated self-help agencies provide access to longer-term services for social support, although professionals are not fully aware of these social support resources. Occupational therapists can help consumer-leaders with consumer outreach and recruitment of members. For example, occupational therapists working in a mental health setting can provide consumers with information about the local COS.

COS Research

A growing body of COS literature provides information about participant and program characteristics, service usage, and program outcomes (Chamberlin, Rogers, & Ellison, 1996; Clay, 2005; Davidson et al, 1999; Kaufmann, Ward-Colasante, & Farmer, 1993; Salzer, 2001; Segal & Silverman, 2002; Solomon, 2004; Swarbrick, 2005; Yanos, Primavera, & Knight, 2001). In addition, some studies examine program

fidelity (Clay, 2005; Holter, Mowbray, Bellamy, MacFarlane, & Dukarski, 2004; Mowbray, Robinson, & Holter, 2002). Most of the research on COSs is descriptive in nature. Although this research is informative, there is a need for randomized controlled trials to study the efficacy of this service delivery model.

Kaufmann et al (1993) identified the following characteristics of successful drop-in centers:

- Presence of a leader with good organizational skills
- Core group of consumer-volunteers
- Interdependent relationship with the mental health provider system
- Planned social events
- Ongoing recruitment of new members

Consumers reported that they liked centers that had a relaxed atmosphere, offered social activities, and provided the opportunity to interact with people who had similar mental health problems.

Segal et al (1995) examined 310 long-term members of self-help agencies for mental health consumers in San Francisco. These authors found that the predominant demographic characteristics of the self-help agency members were male (72%), African American (64%), homeless or living in a shelter (46%), and never married (49%). Members were primarily interested in obtaining food, shelter, clothing, and other practical necessities rather than counseling or other traditional mental health services.

Chamberlin et al (1996) developed an evaluation method to collect empirical data on the effectiveness of consumer-operated self-help programs, as perceived by members. Six programs in six different states (New Hampshire, New Jersey, Indiana, Arkansas, Washington, and California) were examined. There were 171 respondents, of which 59.8% were male, 56.4% were Caucasian, 36% were African American, and 7.6% identified themselves as "other." The authors found that an array of services were offered, including social/recreational activities, individual and system-level advocacy, assistance with housing and employment, transportation, and assistance with activities of daily living. Respondents rated the overall quality of their programs as good or excellent (48.7% and 35.3% respectively). Respondents reported that participation helped them to feel more in control of their lives (64.2%); most felt that they were treated with respect and courtesy (82.3%); and nearly all would recommend the program to a friend (91.5%) (Chamberlin et al, 1996). Word of mouth is the most common referral method.

COSs seem to offer more tolerant, flexible, and supportive environments than traditional services (Davidson et al, 1999; Mowbray & Tan, 1992, 1993; Nikkel et al, 1992). A study examined COSs and traditional mental health services and found that traditional community mental health centers provide acute treatment-focused service, whereas COSs provided services aimed at fostering socialization, empowerment, and autonomy (Segal et al, 2002). These studies suggest that the COS model is ideally suited to offer services that meet the long-term social needs of consumers living in the community. Individuals who choose to access mental health services on a long-term basis may need an "environmental niche" that can provide ongoing support. The professional system of mental health care is typically not designed to provide long-term support, and such assistance is more effectively provided through a network of natural supporters rather than paid staff.

Other researchers (e.g., Silverman et al, 1997) examined the social environment of consumer-operated drop-in centers and found that members perceived their centers as highly supportive and oriented toward mutual learning, independence, and self-understanding. COSs appear to provide mental health consumers who live in a community with an environment that promotes recovery (Kaufmann et al, 1993; Mowbray et al, 1988; Mowbray & Tan, 1992, 1993; Nikkel et al, 1992).

COSs attract individuals who may or may not access the traditional mental health system. Therefore, consumers may receive both traditional and consumer-oriented services (Bond, 1994; Segal, Silverman, & Temkin, 1994; Segal et al, 2002). Traditional community agencies seem best suited to primarily deliver acute treatment-focused services, whereas COSs can meet longer-term social and emotional needs.

There have been few randomized controlled COS studies. In 1998, the CMHS allocated $19.6 million for a multisite research study designed to examine the extent to which COSs, when used as an adjunct to traditional mental health services, effectively improve outcomes of adults with serious and persistent mental illness (SAMHSA, 1998). The COSP Initiative was a 4-year project using a multisite, random assignment experimental design aimed at generating empirical data to provide a more in-depth understanding of consumer-operated programs and services. This has been the largest such study to date and included more than 1,800 consumer participants. The COSP Initiative investigated the extent to which COSs, when combined with traditional services, are more effective than traditional services alone (Clay, 2005).

The initial analysis indicated that both groups (COS + traditional and traditional only) had improvements over time in wellbeing, but the COS program did not significantly enhance traditional services alone (Campbell, 2005). However, more in-depth analyses revealed differential effects for the different COS models. Those attending a drop-in center type COS (but not educational or mutual support type) did have greater improvements in wellbeing than did the traditional-only group. Furthermore, level of participation regardless of type of program seems to have a positive effect. Those consumers with the greatest use of the COS had the highest levels of wellbeing.

Assessment in COS

Formal assessment of the individual consumer is inconsistent with the philosophy of COSs. Participation is voluntary, and there are no formal assessments used to include and/or exclude individuals. The peer group generally follows a democratic process to develop and reinforce rules of conduct, which serve to monitor behavior that could possibly threaten the safety of the membership. For example, many peer programs will ask a person to leave if they arrive onsite under the influence of alcohol or drugs and/or their behavior becomes threatening after arrival.

Efforts are being made to assess specific consumer-operated programs using standardized **fidelity measures**, which examine the extent to which a program's implementation is true to the program model. Fidelity measures rate programs against

Evidence-Based Practice

One of the primary benefits of COSs is the provision of long-term natural (as opposed to paid staff) social supports (Segal et al, 2002). However, Swarbrick (2005) found that the primary COS referral source is generally word of mouth.

➤ Occupational therapists should have available the necessary information and contacts to refer consumers with whom they are working who need to make such connections. Occupational therapists can also assist the COS leadership in collaborating with traditional mental health programs to establish formalized referral networks.

➤ Occupational therapists can help consumer leaders to plan presentations and outreach activities at traditional mental health facilities to educate mental health professionals and their families about the role of COSs in providing social support environments for mental health consumers who live in the community.

➤ Occupational therapists can use their creative skills and abilities to help consumer leaders develop and adapt marketing materials, such as brochures, to assist mental health consumers in finding their way to a local self-help center.

➤ Occupational therapists can help COSs reach out to more traditional mental health care providers, families, and other new venues in order to connect with additional mental health care consumers.

Segal, S., & Silverman, C. (2002). Determinants of client outcomes in self-help agencies. *Psychiatric Services, 53*, 304–309.

Swarbrick, M. (2005). Consumer-operated self-help centers: The relationship between the social environment and its association with empowerment and satisfaction. Unpublished dissertation, University of Medicine and Dentistry of New Jersey.

an agreed-upon list of components within a program model (Clay, 2005). Researchers in Michigan developed a fidelity instrument to operationally measure the core elements that comprise COS models. They identified an ideal COS program based on a review of literature and expert feedback, creating the Fidelity Rating Instrument for Consumer-Operated Services (FRI) (Holter, Mowbray, Bellamy, MacFarlane, & Dukarski, 2004). The FRI criteria were validated through expert judgments (and consensus) using a modified Delphi method (Holter et al, 2004). Respondents rated structural and process components, emphasizing the value of consumerism: consumer control, consumer choices and opportunities for decision-making, voluntary participation (absence of coercion), and respect for members by staff.

The FRI was examined, and reliability has been very good for almost all items. It was validated by comparing FRI ratings to what consumers themselves said about the same aspects of their drop-ins. Holter et al (2004) found that the fidelity criteria showed excellent interrater agreement, with generalizability coefficients of 0.85 or above. Generalizability coefficients fell below 0.60 for only three criteria, suggesting that improvement may be needed on conceptualization or specification of criteria for facilitating referrals; housing, transportation, education, and job assistance; and social-recreational activities. Further testing needs to be done to refine the FRI and examine it in relation to member outcomes.

In addition, as part of the COSP Initiative, the Fidelity Assessment Common Ingredients Tool (FACIT) was developed (Clay, 2005). FACIT describes and quantifies COSs rather than suggesting what a program should be. The FACIT is a valuable tool in helping to identify the current characteristics of a program. Both the FRI and FACIT provide descriptions of the common program ingredients of consumer-service models, and both are at initial phases in terms of evaluating and establishing their psychometric properties. These instruments have the potential for use in future research and program development. Occupational therapists interested in collaborating with consumers to develop, monitor, and/or evaluate the COS model should refer to these fidelity instruments.

Links to Traditional Mental Health Services

COS is considered both a complement and an alternative to the traditional mental health services system. A COS acts as a complement when the individual receives services from both a traditional mental health center and a COS. For example, a person in recovery may receive outpatient services for medication monitoring and counseling and then participate in a COS for social and emotional support or educational purposes. Many services that are rarely provided by traditional mental health programs are a primary offering of a COS. A COS can offer a place where people can occupy their time productively with peers. It offers a sense of belonging among people with shared experiences. A COS can also serve as a resource for people transitioning from time-limited mental health services such as day treatment programs.

Some people choose not to seek traditional mental health services and receive services only from the COS. Although typically individuals first receive traditional services and then access the COS, sometimes the opposite is true. For example, the COS may serve individuals experiencing homelessness or near crisis, and then the COS becomes the avenue by which the person can safely access traditional services through the support of a peer. Table 35-1 outlines differences between traditional and consumer-operated services.

Limitations of COS

COSs seem to be a great resource, but they have limitations. A common concern among COS programs is funding. COSs are not well funded, so hours of operations may be limited. In addition, fiduciary requirements of the main funding source can influence the extent to which a center has full control over budgetary and operational decisions. Fiscal and legal parameters are imposed by the funding source (generally state, federal entities, or private foundations) and a sponsoring agency. In some instances COSs have foundered and faded because of fiscal mismanagement.

COSs are not for everyone, and there is great variability in the amount and quality of services offered by each COS program. Like any organization that is heavily based on social interaction, it is likely that cliques will form, and some people will find it easier than others to feel a part of the organization. Again, like other organizations, the COS may be less open or sensitive to the needs of cultural groups that are not a part of the predominant COS community.

Another limitation of the COS is the lack of rigorous empirical data that demonstrates specific outcomes and efficacy of this service model. More research is needed to help COS programs identify the needs best addressed by the COS and core features that contribute to a successful program.

Example of a COS Self-Help Center in New Jersey

This section describes a successful consumer-operated program offered in the state of New Jersey. Most New Jersey COSs are run as self-help groups, which fall within the peer-support model of COS. Self-help groups provide social and emotional benefits for people who are experiencing a wide range of mental, physical, and social health challenges. Self-help programs help consumers deal with the everyday problems they face. Included in this section is information about the program's mission, population served, members of the team, funding, goals, and outcomes

Table 35-1 ● Differences Between Traditional and Consumer-Operated Services

	Traditional Services	Consumer-Operated Services
Services Provided	Medications Psychotherapy Skills training Housing and employment services Case management	Peer support Education Advocacy Socialization Recreation
Service Providers	Mental health professionals	Individuals with mental illness
Length of Service Provision	Shorter term; services typically end when outcomes are achieved, program deadlines are met, or reimbursement guidelines so specify	Long term and voluntary; individual receives services for as long as desired
Assessment	Formalized assessment of the individual	No use of formal assessments of individuals; assessment focuses on fidelity of the program
Outcomes Targeted	Symptom relief, increased community tenure, employment, skill acquisition	Empowerment, improved quality of life, enhanced social support, wellness and recovery

Mission and Guidelines

Self-help centers are designed to empower mental health consumers to realize a lifestyle centered on wellness. The self-help center offers an environment for learning and growth in a comfortable, relaxed, and supportive setting that is easily accessible to mental health care consumers. The atmosphere and daily operations are provided through the efforts of the membership, leadership, and sponsoring agency. Self-help centers provide environments where a consumer can feel respected and accepted and can develop a support network. Self-help centers offer a place where consumers can relax and access resources and support that promote recovery and wellness. Consumers grow in the spirit of giving and gaining through mutual aid and support.

Collaborative Support Programs of New Jersey (CSP-NJ), a COS agency, sponsors 21 of the 27 centers in the state. The New Jersey Division of Mental Health Services (DMHS) worked with consumer leaders to expand the scope of COSs by developing a *Self-Help Center Policy and Procedure Guideline* (NJDMHS, 1998; 2002; 2005). The self-help center model evolved from the drop-in center model. From 1985 to 1997, drop-in centers developed and were funded in New Jersey. By 1997, a group of consumers organized and, through consultation with occupational therapists, developed a manual for operating a safe, accessible, empowering social environment. An occupational therapist was very involved in the development of the *Self-Help Center Policy and Procedure Guideline* and was involved in researching this service model (Swarbrick, 2005). The New Jersey consumer-operated self-help center model includes the socialization and recreation components of the drop-in center model with an expanded focus on self-help, advocacy, training and education, and wellness and recovery (Swarbrick & Duffy, 2000).

Population Served

Self-help centers are open to adults 18 years of age and older who live in the nearby community and are current or past recipients of public mental health services (Swarbrick & Duffy, 2000). Participation is voluntary, and people can choose to attend and choose to participate in activities at the level at which they feel comfortable. Centers are open on weekends, evenings, and holidays, which are often the loneliest times for mental health consumers. In New Jersey, all counties have at least one publicly funded self-help center (New Jersey Department of Health & Human Services, 2001), providing mental health consumers with a social setting in which to form friendships and become involved and empowered in an environment of peers (Swarbrick, 2005). Centers serve individuals who may or may not access traditional mental health services, and the self-help center is often a means for an individual to learn about available services. Centers can be considered a complement or alternative for peers. Some peers attend a center in addition to receiving outpatient services. Others may only participate in a center and not seek services from the traditional mental health service delivery system.

Self-help centers are designed to reach a wide range of individuals, and leaders are making a conscious effort to reach out to individuals from different backgrounds to expand the ethnic and cultural diversity of the centers. The self-help center leaders have consulted with the Self-Help Technical Assistance Resource (STAR) Center, funded through SAMHSA, to assist in organizing a cultural competency and diversity workgroup. The workgroup is an outreach and marketing initiative to assure that the self-help centers are reaching the diversity reflected in their local community. As part of this project, self-help center leaders have developed a Web-based tracking system called Self-Help Outcomes and Utilization Tracking (SHOUT), which is helping the consumer leadership groups to examine the extent to which centers are serving the local communities. SHOUT was developed through a participatory action research approach involving consumer leaders in all phases of the design, implementation, and evaluation.

Members of the Team and Funding

The COS model is based on peer support, mutuality, shared governance, and a focus on ability rather than disability. Organizational decisions, including hours of operation and program planning within budgetary constraints, are shared among all members. Members can assume a peer leader (facilitator) role, either on a volunteer or a paid-stipend basis. Facilitators open and close the center; meet, greet, and support members; plan and run groups and activities; and transport members in the center's van. Members are responsible for following the rules and regulations established by the membership and participate at a level they determine to be comfortable for them (CSP-NJ, 2005).

Self-help center members and leaders work as equals in planning and implementing center operations. The core decision-making is accomplished through a democratic decision-making process. For example, in New Jersey, the Department of Mental Health Services funds a not-for-profit sponsoring agency. The majority of COSs in New Jersey are allocated through state block grant funding, and the sponsoring agency is responsible for the fiscal and legal matters. Many states have a consumer liaison position within the state bureaucracy; these individuals can be helpful contacts regarding the availability of COSs in a local community or state.

The self-help center model in New Jersey has not only survived but also thrived because of a strong focus on fiscal responsibility. This has not been the situation throughout the country.

PhotoVoice

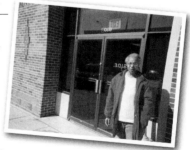

I come to S.I.D.E., our drop-in center, on Tuesdays. I study and take notes at this center. I also eat lunch. I paint, sew, and visit with my friends. I've been thinking better. After eating lunch, painting, and visiting, I can go home and live independently in the community.

—Barbara

Goals and Outcomes

Self-help centers play an important role in addressing the need for support and connection by providing a supportive community that is available to address the long-term social needs of mental health consumers living in the community (Swarbrick, 2005).

Typical activities offered at self-help centers include self-help activities, social and recreational activities, advocacy, community outreach and public relations, and training (Figure 35-2).

Self-Help Activities

Each center schedules a minimum of one self-help activity per week, including, but not limited to, Dual Recovery Anonymous; Alcoholics Anonymous (AA); GROW; support groups for individuals diagnosed with schizophrenia, depression, and bipolar disorder; member-run support groups; and a range of other mutual-aid support groups that the membership decides best address members' needs.

Social and Recreational Activities

Social and recreational activities are important features of centers because many consumers lack the ability to engage in these types of activities due to economic and transportation barriers. At a center, members can socialize and engage in recreational activities. Types of activities conducted at or sponsored by the center may include, but are not limited to, meals, drop-in center hours, dances, picnics, movies, bowling, trips (e.g., day and overnight trips to the beach or camping trips), and educational conferences. In terms of socialization, sharing meals is an important activity. For many consumers, peers at a center serve as surrogate families. As with any family, meals can be a focal point for sharing time together. In addition, centers work with local food banks, which enable them to obtain low-cost food for meals and holiday events.

Advocacy

Self-help centers collaborate with other state advocacy efforts in support of enhanced consumer participation in mental health planning and policymaking. Centers provide a hub of information and processes for activities; members work together to develop strategies to address issues such as health care reform, entitlements, and other ongoing mental health issues. Members have opportunities to work within the state's advocacy efforts that support enhanced consumer participation in mental health planning. Members are encouraged and provided opportunities to take part in local and national advocacy initiatives and participate in local, state, and national advocacy groups.

Community Outreach and Public Relations

Outreach to boarding and rooming houses is a priority, because individuals in these settings feel isolated and lonely. Other outreach activities can include, but are not limited to, visits to members at their homes or while in the hospital; presentations to staff and consumers at hospital and day program settings; visits or phone calls to members or individuals in the community in need of additional support; and operation of a warm line, a peer-run service that people can call in for support in nonemergency situations. In terms of public relations, the membership organizes presentations at local mental health boards, community agencies, family groups, and other settings for membership recruitment.

Training

Consumer leaders are given training and technical support by CSP-NJ staff during facilitator meetings, regular visits, conferences, and regional training sessions. Center staff meets on a regular basis with the facilitators to define the leadership training needs and receive technical support for the day-to-day operations. Many centers allocate funding to provide the membership with opportunities to attend national and local workshops and conferences.

Training offered at centers may include, but is not limited to, financial literacy, computer training, employment assistance, and wellness and recovery workshops. Consumers are encouraged to pursue continuing education, and many take advantage of the range of psychiatric rehabilitation academic and certification opportunities. The center leadership has been encouraged to pursue the Certification for Psychiatric Rehabilitation Practitioner (CPRP) offered by the United States Psychiatric Rehabilitation Practitioners (USPRA).

Member Satisfaction

Self-help centers are a type of COS designed to promote empowerment and satisfaction by providing members with an active role in their programmatic planning and day-to-day operations. A study was conducted to examine the associations between the social environment and empowerment and satisfaction within the CSP-NJ-sponsored self-help centers (Swarbrick, 2005). All 144 study participants identified themselves as having a diagnosed psychiatric-related condition and had current or past involvement with the traditional mental health system. In this study, findings indicated that participants are more satisfied with an environment that is orderly and predictable and not chaotic. Participants reported higher levels of satisfaction when the peer leaders direct the center activities, enforce rules, involve the members in decision-making, and promote diversity and change in the center functioning. It appeared from this

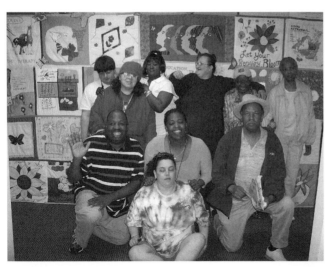

FIGURE 35-2. Members of the consumer-operated program S.I.D.E. in Kansas City, Kansas, standing in front of a quilt they created that depicts recovery.

study that participants' sense of satisfaction can be enhanced when the center provides explicit expectation, order and organization, and leadership control and when it promotes innovation.

In the study, participants reported higher levels of satisfaction associated with the self-help centers that offered opportunities to form social relationships and become part of a group of peers (Swarbrick, 2005). This finding is consistent with other reported studies that demonstrate associations between social environment variables (in both self-help groups and peer-operated drop-in centers) and satisfaction. This finding is similar to Moos (1994), who found that when a group is reported to be moderate to high on the relationship dimension (Moos Group Environment Scale), participants tend to be more satisfied with participation. 1992).

Consumer-Providers

Consumers do not only provide services to other consumers via COSs, but they frequently work as consumer-providers within the traditional mental health system as well. A consumer-provider is an employee or staff member who has a history of living with a mental illness. The notion of a consumer-provider is similar to that recognized in the field of substance abuse counseling, which long ago recognized the benefits of having individuals in recovery serve as service providers.

The mental health field has been slower to accept the consumer-provider role. Mowbray, Moxley, Jasper, and Howell (1997) identified some reasons for using consumer-providers:

1. Inclusion of consumers as mental health workers can increase the sensitivity of programs and services about [consumers].
2. [Consumers] can serve as effective role models for other [consumers].
3. The inclusion of consumers is an expression of affirmative action and consistent with contemporary civil and disability rights policies.

Evidence-Based Practice

A number of studies of COSs have found that the social environment offers a more tolerant and flexible environment for individuals at various phases of their recovery. Mowbray and Tan's (1992) study of drop-in centers found that participants are more satisfied when they perceive that the drop-in centers are highly supportive and oriented toward independence. Participants reported higher levels of satisfaction associated with the self-help centers that offered opportunities to form social relationships and become part of a group of peers (Swarbrick, 2005). This finding is consistent with other reported studies that demonstrate associations between social environment variables (in both self-help groups and peer-operated drop-in centers) and satisfaction. Members of supportive, cohesive, and well-organized self-help groups tend to report more satisfaction (Moos, 1994).

➤ Occupational therapists can use their skills to provide training and mentoring for peer leaders in terms of creating environments that are welcoming and foster recovery and wellness.

➤ If there are no consumer-operated programs available in their area, practitioners can consider advocating for funding for these highly efficient and effective services.

➤ Occupational therapists should be familiar with existing consumer-operated organizations and services in their communities.

➤ Occupational therapists can contact the local or state department of mental health to identify programs that receive public funding and visit these programs to meet with the clients.

Moos, R. (1994). *The Social Climate Scales: A User's Guide* (2nd ed.). Palo Alto, CA: Consulting Psychologists Press.

Mowbray, C., & Tan, C. (1992). Evaluation of an innovative consumer run service model: The drop in center. *Innovation and Research, 1,* 33–42.

Swarbrick, M. (2005). Consumer-operated self-help centers: The relationship between the social environment and its association with empowerment and satisfaction. Unpublished dissertation, University of Medicine and Dentistry of New Jersey.

The Lived Experience

Steve

The Moving Forward Self-Help Center provided an opportunity for me to learn and exercise new skills and increased my chances to become gainfully employed in the near future. These skills could not have been fostered in any of my previous work environments. Practices I learned in college are exercised at the Center.

My business skills help with the administration of the Center. Psychiatric Rehabilitation classes help with peer advocacy. I help people with their problems by leading them to find their own solutions within themselves. In addition, my experience with showmanship is demonstrated when I strum a guitar or read poetry at a coffeehouse. I use my public-speaking experience when I speak in front of high school and college students about the Reducing Stigma Project. When driving for the Center, I have responsibilities for getting gas, washing the van, turning in receipts of tolls to the Fiscal Department, getting the van serviced, making phone calls to schedule members coming into the Center. I learn to navigate through unknown streets and follow directions on a map or MapQuest. I must also demonstrate my patience during rush hours or when sitting in traffic jams. I am able to do all these things thanks to my self-help center.

My future looks bright. I am confident that the outcomes from applying myself and living up to the wellness and recovery principles will bear much fruit. There is no telling how one's life may wind up—and that is just it . . . up!

Effectiveness studies of consumer-providers have demonstrated that consumers can provide effective mental health service. Solomon and Draine (1995; 1996) compared outcomes of consumers who had been assigned to teams with either consumer case managers or nonconsumer case managers. The studies demonstrated that consumers who received services from the consumer case management team did as well as those who received services from the nonconsumer team. Other studies have shown that consumer-providers can be more effective than nonconsumers in providing mental health services. A randomized study by Robert Paulson et al (1999) compared assertive community treatment teams containing consumer-providers with teams made up of nonconsumers. The study found equivalent results between the two teams and a stronger working alliance between the recipient of service consumers and the team in the consumer-provider team versus the nonconsumer team.

Although consumer-providers do possess direct experience living with a psychiatric disability, they may lack the training and important skills, attitudes, and knowledge necessary to be an effective supporter. Some consumers pursue traditional academic routes for gaining credentials, such as in the fields of social work, psychiatric rehabilitation, occupational therapy, and other rehabilitation sciences. In recent years, a variety of training approaches have developed to specifically prepare and support consumer-providers. Specific training programs for consumer-providers are identified in the resources section at the end of the chapter.

Occupational therapists who work with consumers who desire to become consumer-providers can help them explore career and training options that may best suit their abilities, potentials, and interests.

Roles and Opportunities for Occupational Therapy Practice

There are many opportunities for occupational therapy practitioners to collaborate with consumer organizations, grassroots groups, and COSs. Practitioners who work in all aspects of mental health practice (in-patient state and county hospital settings, Veterans Administration services, and community-based settings) have the requisite knowledge and skills to work directly within the COS model described in this chapter. Practitioners are challenged to create opportunities where they can collaborate with consumers to develop, implement, and/or evaluate COSs regardless of the service setting.

The first step in getting involved is to determine what is available in your community. Contact the state consumer liaison at your local or state mental health authority. Become familiar with existing COSs and self-help groups in your local community. Contact the local, state, or county department of mental health to identify programs that receive public funding, and call or visit these programs. You can also contact one of the technical assistance centers to learn about any local groups that are listed in the database. If no COSs are available in a given area, then practitioners could consider advocating for funding for this service model, as it is an effective resource for helping people connect with supportive peers and role models. Occupational therapists can invite COS participants to visit settings where occupational therapists are employed to inform clients and staff

about the availability of COSs in the community. For example, in New Jersey, the local self-help centers work with occupational therapists and other rehabilitation staff to make regular visits to individuals who are currently at state facilities to help them learn about the free resources that are available in the community where the person will relocate when discharged.

At one facility, the occupational therapists have arranged for patients to visit their local consumer-operated self-help center as part of the occupational therapy community integration program. For example, the local Depression and Bipolar Support Alliance and other consumer advocacy groups have been making regular visits to the state-run hospitals to educate patients and staff about these resources.

Occupational therapists can join with like-minded providers from other disciplines, such as psychiatric rehabilitation, rehabilitation counseling, psychology, and social work to promote the development of and access to COS for mental health consumers living in the community (Swarbrick & Pratt, 2006).

Occupational therapists can assist COS leadership in collaborating with traditional mental health programs to establish formalized referral networks. Along witch student interns, they can help develop and adapt marketing materials, such as brochures, to assist mental health consumers in finding their way to a local self-help center. Occupational therapists can help COSs reach out to more traditional mental health care providers, families, and other venues in order to connect with mental health consumers. COSs can be an excellent nontraditional student field worksite (Swarbrick & Pratt, 2006).

Occupational therapists working at research centers or universities can contribute to COS research endeavors (Swarbrick & Pratt, 2006). Participatory action research (PAR) is an empowering form of applied research whereby the people being studied are fully engaged in the process of investigation. PAR is a method of inquiry consistent with the consumer-self-help ethos that explores practical problems and issues of concern to constituents (Rogers & Palmer-Erbs, 1994). The PAR approach involves maximum participation of stakeholders—those whose lives are affected under study—in the systematic collection and analysis of information for the purpose of taking action and making change (Nelson, Ochocka, Griffith, & Lord, 1998; Rogers & Palmer-Erbs, 1994). Using this approach, researchers can play an important role in assisting consumer groups in research to examine aspects of COS fidelity and efficacy.

Summary

Consumer operated services provide an exemplar of the recovery model and demonstrate the benefits that can be gained when the expertise of consumers is recognized. COS often address social and emotional needs that are left unmet by more traditional service delivery models. Occupational therapy values of client-driven services make occupational therapists suited for work within this practice model. Although the consumer must always remain the primary administrators and service providers, occupational therapists can assist in the development, implementation and evaluation of COSs.

Active Learning Strategies

1. Experience a COS

Spend time at a local COS, such as a drop-in center or self-help center, or interview leaders at such a center over the telephone. Listen and observe to determine whether the following principles of COS are evident:

- Consumers develop, control, and provide the services.
- Participation is completely voluntary.
- Emphasis is on strengths and competencies of participants and leaders.
- A goal is mutuality among members instead of a hierarchy of helper and person helped.
- "Helper-therapy principle" (Reissman, 1990) is the idea that past and present recipients of mental health services provide unique perspective and expertise to design and implement services to improve the quality of life of peers through peer support, advocacy, and education.

Reflective Questions

After interviewing members or spending time at a particular COS, how would you answer these questions?

- Which principles of COS were present, and which were not? What examples support your conclusions?
- What did you see as primary benefits for consumers?
- What role might occupational therapy play at the COS?

 Write about the experience in your **Reflective Journal**.

2. Creating a Wellness Recovery Action Plan

Get a copy of Mary Ellen Copeland's (2002) Wellness Recovery Action Plan (typically called a WRAP). This booklet is very reasonably priced and an excellent resource. Although developed for consumers with psychiatric disabilities, it can be used by anyone who is interested in creating a more healthy lifestyle. Step by step, follow the instructions and create a WRAP for yourself.

Reflective Questions

- What did you learn about yourself by creating a WRAP?
- Do you think formalizing the process for creating a healthy lifestyle will help you change behaviors? Why or why not?
- What aspects of your plan will be easiest to follow, and what will be difficult? How might you become motivated to address the more difficult parts of the plan?
- Consider populations that might benefit from WRAP. As an occupational therapist, how might you incorporate WRAP into your practice?

Resources

Books

- Clay, S. (2005). *On Our Own Together*. Nashville, TN: Vanderbilt University Press. This book provides an in-depth description of eight programs, including examples of drop-in centers, educational programs, and peer supports.

Conferences

- The Alternatives Conference offers in-depth technical assistance on consumer/survivor-delivered services and self-help/recovery methods. The Alternatives Conference also offers a forum for mental health consumers and survivors from across the nation to meet and exchange information and ideas. SAMHSA's Center for Mental Health Services sponsors the conference. http://www.mentalhealth.samhsa.gov/calendar/advisorycouncil.asp

Consumer as Provider Training

Although consumer-providers have experience living with psychiatric disabilities, they may lack the training and important skills, attitudes, and knowledge necessary to be an effective COS supporter. In recent years, a variety of training approaches have developed to specifically prepare and support consumer-providers. The following are examples of such training programs.

- The Kansas Consumers as Providers Training Program teaches consumers of mental health services the skills and knowledge necessary to work in the mental health or human service field. The training program consists of 15 weeks of classroom instruction and Educational Support Group followed by 104 hours (7 weeks) of internship activities. http://www.socwel.ku.edu/projects/SEG/cap.html
- The Georgia Certified Peer Specialist Project's mission is to identify, train, certify, and provide ongoing support and education to consumers of mental health services to provide peer support as part of the Georgia mental health service system.

Consumer-providers are trained to assist consumers in skill-building, goal-setting, problem-solving, conducting recovery dialogues, setting up and sustaining mutual self-help groups, and helping consumers build their own self-directed recovery tools (including the Wellness Recovery Action Plan [WRAP]). http://www.gacps.org/Home.html

- The META Peer Support Training Recovery Innovations is a 60-hour intensive training program for individuals with psychiatric disabilities who wish to work as peer providers. The program utilizes a learning community in which individuals are encouraged to engage in a process of self-exploration, growth, and acquisition of knowledge about recovery from mental illness (Hutchinson et al, 2006). Students who complete the class and pass the competency tests are eligible for employment as peer-support specialists. http://www.recoveryinnovations.org
- Vet-to-Vet programs have been established from Albuquerque, New Mexico, to Madison, Wisconsin. The Vet-to-Vet program is run by veterans who have a psychiatric diagnosis (Resnick, Armstrong, Sperrazza, Harkness, & Rosenheck, 2004). The Vet-to-Vet hour-long group meetings are egalitarian, with conversations loosely organized around books written by consumer-provider mental health experts, including Moe Armstrong (Moe Armstrong, personal communication, June 22, 2006). www.veteranrecovery.med.va.gov and www.vettovetusa.com

National Organizations

- The National Mental Health Consumers' Self Help Clearinghouse is a technical assistance center that provides online training materials and resources and a directory of COSs to connect consumers with their local programs. The directory can be searched by location, program name, or program type. http://www.mhselfhelp.org
- The Depression and Bipolar Support Alliance is consumer run and provides online educational resources and a call-in center.

It has a network of nearly 1,000 support groups and holds an annual conference. http://www.dbsalliance.org

Wellness Recovery Action Plan (WRAP)

• Consumer-providers can be trained to assist peers to develop a WRAP, which is a self-designed plan that can help consumers assume personal responsibility and improve their quality of life (Copeland, 1997). The WRAP approach is frequently used in consumer-operated programs and empowers people to take control of their own health and wellness. Since its development, WRAP has been shared with thousands of people through the *Wellness Recovery Action Plan* (1997); *Winning Against Relapse* (1999); the *Winning Against Relapse* audiotape; the *Creating Wellness* video series; numerous support groups, workshops, and seminars; and through the following website: http://www .mentalhealthrecovery.com

References

Bond, G. (1994). The role of drop-in centers in mental health services. *Innovations and Research, 3,* 46–47.

Campbell, J. (1997). How consumer/survivors are evaluating the quality of psychiatric care. *Evaluation Review, 21,* 357–363.

———. (2005). Effectiveness findings of the COST Multisite Research Initiative. In *Grading the Evidence for Consumer-Driven Services* [webcast]. University of Illinois–Chicago, December 20, NRTC Webcast.

Carling, P. (1995). *Return to Community: Building Support Systems for People With Psychiatric Disabilities.* New York: Guilford.

Chamberlin, J. (1978). *On Our Own: Patient Controlled Alternatives to the Mental Health System.* New York: McGraw-Hill.

———. (1984). Speaking for ourselves: An overview of the ex-psychiatric inmates' movement. *Psychiatric Rehabilitation Journal, 2,* 56–63.

———. (1990). The ex-patient movement: Where we've been and where we're going. *Journal of Mind and Behavior, 11,* 323–336.

———. (1995). Rehabilitating ourselves: The psychiatric-survivor movement. *International Journal of Mental Health, 24,* 39–46.

Chamberlin, J., & Rogers, J. A. (1990). Planning a community-based mental health system: Perspectives of service recipients. *American Psychologist, 45,* 1241–1244.

Chamberlin, J., Rogers, E. S., & Ellison, M. L. (1996). Self-help programs: A description of their characteristics and their members. *Psychiatric Rehabilitation Journal, 19,* 33–42.

Chinman, M., Weingarten, R., Stayner, D., & Davidson, L. (2001). Chronicity reconsidered: Improving person-environment fit through consumer run services. *Community Mental Health Journal, 37,* 215–229.

Clay, S. (2005). *On Our Own Together: Peer Programs for People with Mental Illness.* Nashville, TN: Vanderbilt Press.

Coalition for Community Livint (n.d.) *Fairweather Lodge Fidelity Standards.* http://theccl.org/FairweatherStandards.htm (accessed March 2, 2010).

Collaborative Support Programs of New Jersey (CSP-NJ). (2005). *Self-Help Center Policy and Procedure Guideline–Revised.* Freehold, NJ: Author.

Conrad, E. (1993). Consumer-run housing in the Bronx. *Innovations and Research, 2,* 53–55.

Copeland, M. E. (1997). *Wellness Recovery Action Plan.* West Dummerston, VT: Peach Press.

———. (1999). *Winning Against Relapse: A Workbook of Action Plans for Recurring Health and Emotional Problems.* Oakland, CA: New Harbinger.

———. (2002). *Wellness Recovery Action Plan: A System for Monitoring, Reducing, and Eliminating Uncomfortable or Dangerous Physical or Emotional Difficulties.* West Dummerston, VT: Peach Press.

Davidson, L., Chinman, M., Kloos, B., Weingarten, R., Stayner, D., & Tebes, J. (1999). Peer support among individuals with severe mental illness: A review of evidence. *Clinical Psychology: Science and Practice, 6,* 165–187.

Davidson, L., Hoge, M., Godleski, L., Rakfeldt, J., & Griffith, E. (1996). Hospital or community living? Examining consumer perspectives on deinstitutionalization. *Psychiatric Rehabilitation Journal, 19,* 49–58.

del Vecchio, P., Fricks, L., & Johnson, J. R. (2000). Issues of daily living for persons with mental illness. *Psychiatric Rehabilitation Skills, 4,* 410–423.

Fairweather, G. W. (Ed.). (1964). *Social Psychology in Treating Mental Illness: An Experimental Approach.* New York: Wiley.

Fairweather, G. W., & Fergus, E. O. (1988). *The Lodge Society: A Look at Community Tenure as a Measure of Cost Savings.* East Lansing: Michigan State University.

Fairweather, G. W., Sanders, D. H., Cressler, D., & Maynard, D. (1969). *Community Life for the Mentally Ill.* Chicago: Aldine.

Goffman, E. (1961). *Asylums: Essays on the Social Situation of Mental Patients and Other Inmates.* New York: Anchor Books.

Haertl, K. L. (2005). Factors influencing success in a Fairweather model mental health program. *Psychiatric Rehabilitation Journal, 28,* 370–377.

———. (2007). The Fairweather mental health housing model—A peer supported environment: Implications for psychiatric rehabilitation. *American Psychiatric Rehabilitation Journal, 3,* 149–162.

Haertl, K., Minato, M. (2006). Daily occupations of persons with mental illness: Themes from Japan and America. *Occupational Therapy in Mental Health, 22,* 19–32.

Holter, M., Mowbray, C., Bellamy, C., MacFarlane, P., & Dukarski, J. (2004). Critical ingredients of a consumer run services: Results of a national survey. *Community Mental Health Journal, 40,* 47–63.

Hutchinson, D., Anthony, W., Ashcraft, L., Johnson, E., Dunn, E., Lyass, A., & Rogers, E. S. (2006). The personal and vocational impact of training and employing people with psychiatric disabilities. *Psychiatric Rehabilitation Journal, 29,* 205–213.

Johnson, D. (1994). Drop-in centers are a great idea, but do they work? *Innovations and Research, 3,* 43–44.

Kaufmann, C., Freund, P., & Wilson, J. (1989). Self-help in the mental health system: A model for consumer-provider collaboration. *Psychosocial Rehabilitation Journal, 13,* 6–21.

Kaufmann, C., Ward-Colasante, C., & Farmer, J. (1993). Development and evaluation of drop-in centers operated by mental health consumers. *Hospital and Community Psychiatry, 44,* 675–678.

Knight, E. (1997). A model of the dissemination of self-help in public mental health systems. *New Directions for Mental Health Services, 74,* 43–51.

Mead, S., Hilton, D., & Curtis, L. (2001). Peer support: A theoretical perspective. *Psychiatric Rehabilitation Journal, 25,* 134–141.

Meek, C. (1994). Consumer-run drop-in centers as alternatives to mental health services. *Innovations and Research, 3,* 49–51.

Moos, R. (1994). *The Social Climate Scales: A User's Guide* (2nd ed.). Palo Alto, CA: Consulting Psychologists Press.

Mowbray, C. (1997). Benefits and issues created by consumer role innovation in psychiatric rehabilitation. In C. T. Mowbray, D. P. Moxley, C. A. Jasper, & L. L. Howell (Eds.), *Consumers as Providers.* Columbia, MD: International Association of Psychosocial Rehabilitation.

Mowbray, C., Chamberlain, P., Jennings, M., & Reed, C. (1988). Consumer-run services: Results from five demonstration projects. *Community Mental Health Journal, 24,* 151–156.

Mowbray, C., Robinson, E., & Holter, M. (2002). Consumer drop-in centers: Operations, services and consumer involvement. *Health Social Work, 27,* 248–261.

Mowbray, C., & Tan, C. (1992). Evaluation of an innovative consumer-run service model: The drop-in center. *Innovation and Research, 1,* 33–42.

———. (1993). Consumer-operated drop-in centers: Evaluation of operations and impact. *Journal of Mental Health Administration, 20,* 8–19.

Mowbray, C. T., Moxley, D. P., Jasper, C.A., & Howell, L.L. (Eds.). (1997). *Consumers as Providers.* Columbia, MD: International Association of Psychosocial Rehabilitation.

National Institute of Mental Health. (1982). *A Network of Caring: The Community Support Program of the National Institute of Mental Health.* Rockville, MD: Author.

Nelson, G., Ochocka, J., Griffith, K., & Lord, J. (1998). "Nothing without me without me": Participatory action research with self-help/mutual aid organizations for psychiatric survivors. *American Journal of Community Psychology, 26,* 881–912.

New Freedom Commission on Mental Health. (2003). *Achieving the Promise: Transforming Mental Health Care in America. Final Report.* DHHS Pub. No. SMA-03-3832. Rockville, MD: U.S. Department of Health and Human Services.

New Jersey Department of Health and Human Services. (2001). *Healthy People 2010: A Public Health Agenda for the New Millennium.* Trenton, NJ: Author.

New Jersey Department of Mental Health Services (NJDMHS). (1998, 2002, 2005). *Self Help Center Policy and Procedure Guideline.* Trenton, NJ: Author.

Nikelly, A. G. (2001). The role of environment in mental health: Individual Empowerment through social restructuring. *Journal of Applied Behavioral Science, 37,* 305–323.

Nikkel, R., Smith, G., & Edwards, D. (1992). A consumer-operated case management project. *Hospital and Community Psychiatry, 43,* 577–579.

Onaga, E. (1994). The fairweather lodge as a psychosocial program in the 1990s. In IAPSRS (Ed.), *An Introduction to Psychiatric Rehabilitation* (pp. 206–214). Columbia, MD: The International Association of Psychosocial Rehabilitation Services

Onaga, E., & Smith, B. A. (2000). Reinvention of the lodge program: A case study of program changes to promote full-time employment. *Psychiatric Rehabilitation Skills, 4*(1), 41–60.

Page, S., Lafreniere, K., & Out, J. (1999). An evaluation of the ten friends diner: A collaborative community project. *Psychiatric Rehabilitation Journal, 23,* 171–173.

Paulson, R., Herinckx, H., Demmler, J., Clark, G., Cutler, D., & Birecree, E. (1999). Comparing practice patterns of consumer and non-consumer mental health service providers. *Community Mental Health Journal, 35,* 251–269.

Reissman, F. (1965). The helper-therapy principle. *Social Work, 10,* 26–32.

Reissman, R. (1990). Restructuring help: A human service paradigm for the 1990s. *American Journal of Community Psychology, 18,* 221–230.

Resnick, S., Armstrong, M., Sperrazza, M., Harkness, L., & Rosenheck, R. (2004). A model of consumer-provider partnership: Vet-to-Vet. *Psychosocial Rehabilitation Journal, 28,* 185–187.

Ribeiro, K. (1999). The labyrinth of community mental health: In search of meaningful occupation. *Psychiatric Rehabilitation Journal, 23,* 143–152.

Rogers, S., & Palmer-Erbs, V. (1994). Participatory action research: Implications and evaluation in psychiatric rehabilitation. *Psychosocial Rehabilitation Journal, 18,* 3–12.

Salzer, M. (2001). *Best Practice Guidelines for Consumer-Delivered Services.* Unpublished manuscript, Behavioral Health Recovery Management Project.

Salzer, M., & Liptzen Shear, S. (2002). Identifying consumer provider benefits in evaluation of consumer-delivered services. *Psychiatric Rehabilitation Journal, 25,* 281–288.

Segal, S., Hardiman, E., & Hodges, J. (2002). Characteristics of new clients at self-help and community mental health agencies in geographic proximity. *Psychiatric Services, 53,* 1145–1152.

Segal, S., & Silverman, C. (2002). Determinants of client outcomes in self-help agencies. *Psychiatric Services, 53,* 304–309.

Segal, S., Silverman, C., & Temkin, T. (1994). Consumer-run drop-in centers as alternatives to mental health services. *Innovations and Research, 3,* 47–49.

Silverman, S., Blank, M., & Taylor, L. (1997). On our own: Preliminary findings from a consumer run service model. *Psychiatric Rehabilitation Journal, 21,* 151–159.

Solomon, P. (2004). Peer support/peer provided services: Underlying processes, benefits, and critical ingredients. *Psychiatric Rehabilitation Journal, 27*(4), 392–402.

Solomon, P., & Draine, J. (1995). The efficacy of a consumer case management team: Two-year outcomes of a randomized trial. *Journal of Mental Health Administration, 22*(2), 135–146.

———. (1996). Perspectives concerning consumers as case managers. *Community Mental Health Journal, 32*(1), 41–46.

———. (2001). The state of knowledge of the effectiveness of consumer provided services. *Psychiatric Rehabilitation Journal, 25,* 20–27.

Stroul, B. (1986). *Approaches to Helping Persons with Long-Term Mental Illness.* Rockville, MD: National Institute of Mental Health.

Substance Abuse and Mental Health Services Administration (SAMHSA). (1998). GFA No. SM 98-004. Cooperative agreements to evaluate consumer-operated human service programs for persons with serious mental illness. Rockville, MD: Author.

Swarbrick, M. (2005). Consumer-operated self-help centers: The relationship between the social environment and its association with empowerment and satisfaction. Unpublished dissertation, University of Medicine and Dentistry of New Jersey.

Swarbrick, M., & Duffy, M. (2000). Consumer-operated organizations and programs: A role for occupational therapists. *Mental Health Special Interest Quarterly, 23*(March), 1–4.

Swarbrick, P., & Pratt, C. (2006). Consumer-operated self-help services: Roles and opportunities for occupational therapy practitioners. *OT Practice, 11*(5), CE1–CE8.

Van Tosh, L., & del Vecchio, P. (2000). *Consumer-Operated Self-Help Programs: A Technical Report.* Rockville, MD: U.S. Center for Mental Health Services.

Weingarten, R., Chinman, M., Tworkowski, S., Stayner, D., & Davidson, L. (2000). The welcome basket project: Consumers reaching out to consumers. *Psychiatric Rehabilitation Journal, 24,* 65–68.

Yanos, P., Primavera, L., & Knight, E. (2001). Consumer-run service participation, recovery of social functioning, and the mediating role of psychological factors. *Psychiatric Services, 52,* 493–500.

Zinman, S., Harp, H., & Budd, S. (1987). *Reaching Across: Mental Health Clients Helping Each Other.* Riverside, CA: California Network of Mental Health Clients.

After-School Programs

Ann E. McDonald

> "Most of the time, people think that regular girls you know go to the movies [after school] with their friends or over to their friend's house. But it seems like, all of us here [in the shelter] really don't do nothing. We just like go up and sit inside our rooms.
>
> —Geri, 11-year-old girl

Introduction

Research has shown that a youth's use of time after school impacts his or her **occupational competence** (or the personal sense of achievement in performance of daily activities) in everyday leisure, personal-social, and academic tasks. This has been documented largely for youths without disabilities and to a lesser degree for youths with mental health concerns (Durlak & Weissberg, 2007; Jackson & Arbesman, 2005).

After-school program (ASPs) can promote academic, personal, social, and recreational development by providing children and teens the opportunity to participate in structured and/or targeted activities. Although there is limited research into the benefits of ASPs for youths with social or behavioral problems, occupational therapy can play an integral role in helping youths with mental health concerns to benefit from participation in ASPs.

Whether the youth is homeless or in a home where parental or adult supervision and assistance in after-school hours is limited, it is important to address the youth's safe and meaningful engagement in choosing occupations that promote health and adaptation (Zemke & Clark, 1996). For the purposes of this chapter, *after-school time* refers to time spent after the school day and before going to bed. This chapter explores:

- Time use and occupational engagement for children and teens in the after-school hours.
- Evidence-based benefits of participation in ASPs.
- Occupational therapy assessments and intervention for youths with mental health concerns in ASPs.
- Future directions in after-school, occupation-based intervention and research.

Time Use in After-School Hours

Increasing evidence suggests that where and how youths spend their time outside of normal school hours has important implications for their development. An estimated 8 million children in the United States were reported to be without adult supervision for some period of time after school in 1999 (National Institute on Out-of-School Time, 2003). Unsupervised time has been associated with greater risk for negative outcomes such as academic and behavioral problems, drug use, and other health-compromising behaviors (Elliott, 1993; Weissman & Gottfredson, 2001). Conversely, additional research suggests that after-school time use plays an important part in promoting personal and social development as well as positive health outcomes (Bodilly & Beckett, 2005; Durlak & Weissberg, 2007; Elliott, 1993).

Although it is important to know the benefits of participation in structured adult-directed ASPs (presented later in this chapter), it is first helpful to understand the varied contexts within which after-school occupations occur and the occupational patterns in which youths engage,

Over the past 15 years, studies of children's time use have identified five consistent domains that typify out-of-school life for school-aged children (Copperman & Bhat, 2007; Medrich, Roizen, Ruben, & Buckley, 1982; Meeks & Maudlin, 1991). The five categories are not mutually exclusive but are generic types of childhood occupations that cross class and ethnicity:

1. Activities alone or with friends
2. Activities with parents
3. In-home and out-of-home chores, jobs, and responsibilities
4. Organized activities, including participation in lessons, formal team sports, and recreational and cultural programs supervised by adults (other than their parents)
5. Television viewing and use of other media

The last category has received the most attention by researchers because it is associated with an increased risk of obesity (Copperman & Bhat, 2007; Office of the Surgeon General, 2007).

The data from the 2002 Child Development Supplement (CDS) to the Panel Study of Income Dynamics (PSID) reveal the types of activities in which youths engage. This study provided data on a nationally representative sample of individuals and households, including demographic, employment, and health information. The CDS included a survey of 2,500 children (ages 5–18 years) through health and achievement test surveys, primary caregiver and child interviews, and a 2-day time-use diary (one weekday and one weekend day). The time-use diary collected information on the type, number, duration, and location of activities for each 24-hour survey day beginning at midnight. Survey results were obtained on a total of 1,970 children. Eleven activity types were derived from these data:

1. Work (for pay)
2. Household chores (including nonpaid child care)
3. Meals (including snacks)
4. Organized activities (e.g., lessons, meetings, clubs)
5. Studying
6. Recreation (e.g., hobbies and sports, outings, reading, playing, television viewing, and music)
7. Social activities (including conversations, being intimate, parties, visiting, and religious services)
8. Personal business (e.g., shopping, obtaining services, writing e-mails or letters)
9. Personal care
10. Receiving child care (e.g., daycare, with baby-sitter)
11. School

These data are useful in tracking some of the trends of children's time use during nonschool hours. As expected, almost every child in this survey eats, recreates, and pursues personal care activities each day. Children on average invest time in recreation, totaling about 3.5 hours on weekdays and 6.5 hours on weekend days. Television or movie viewing and playing video or computer games were the most dominant forms of recreation found among children in this study.

The participation rates and mean durations of social activities and personal business increase substantially over the weekend days. Also, as children get older and decrease time spent in day care, the participation rates and mean durations increase in organized activities, social activities, and personal business (e.g., shopping). In addition, adolescents (15–18 years old) spend approximately 4.5 hours in paid work on weekdays and 6 hours on a weekend day.

Another finding from the CDS survey was the data specific to "where" and "with whom" these out-of-home occupations took place. A substantial amount of time is spent either at school or at someone else's home on both the weekdays and weekends. Children reported they participate with other children (rather than alone) in out-of-home activities, and a significant proportion of these occupational pursuits are with nonfamily members. However, home is by far the most common location for activity participation, especially on the weekdays (Copperman & Bhat, 2007).

What is unknown from many children's time use studies is the meaning of these daily occupational pursuits during nonschool hours to the child or adolescent. The occupational therapist plays a valuable role in identifying the meaning of these activities, as described in the Assessment section of this chapter.

ASPs as Intervention

An **after-school program** is an intervention offered to children between the ages of 5 and 18 during the school year and after normal school hours. ASPs typically focus on providing youths with various growth-enhancing opportunities and often include adult-directed, structured activities and experiences to promote academic, personal, social, and recreational development (Durlak & Weissberg, 2007).

ASP staff may include professionals (e.g., psychologists, early childhood educators, recreation therapists, occupational therapists) as well as individuals who have some work-related experience with children but lack a professional degree. ASPs are funded both publicly and privately, with the federal government investing $3.6 billion in ASPs in 2002 (The Finance Project, 2003). More recently, studies are focused on a clearer picture of the cost of programs, which range from $1.17 per child per hour at the lowest cost to specialized intensive programs at $8.36 (Beckett, 2008), with emphasis on quality outcomes (Grossman, Lind, Hayes, McMaken, & Gersick, 2009).

Where and how youths spend their time outside of regular school hours is increasingly found to have important implications for their development, leading to strong public support for ASPs from working parents who cannot be with their children immediately after school. Consequently, the number of ASPs has steadily risen over the past decade.

According to research conducted by the Rand Corporation, as of the late 1990s, one of every six children ages 6 to 12 with employed mothers was participating in a before- or after-school program. However, the literature on after-school time use largely does not identify if youths with disabilities are being served within these programs but instead focuses primarily on the benefits of participation (Bodilly & Beckett, 2005; Durlak & Weissberg, 2007; Harvard Family Research Project, 2003). The psychological and occupational therapy literature mention after-school interventions that focus on the development of specific social and recreational skills (Jackson & Arbesman, 2005). However, these are not typically **inclusive programs**; that is, children without disabilities do not normally attend these focused interventions.

Evidence-Based Benefits

Although many ASPs aim to provide a safe and supportive adult-supervised environment with opportunities to enhance growth, few have provided formal evaluations of the program's effectiveness and the factors associated with positive outcomes (Harvard Family Research Project, 2003; Vandell, Pierce, & Dadisman, 2005) because of the multiple variables in conducting these studies. Apsler (2009) further verified that few studies meet the criteria for being methodologically sound. However, quasi-experimental and experimental research designs from multiple disciplines document the value of ASPs for the school-age child (Bodilly & Beckett, 2005; Durlak & Weissberg, 2007; Jackson & Arbesman, 2005).

Durlak and Weissberg (2007) conducted a meta-analysis of ASPs focused on the personal and social development of children and adolescents. Their study involved a systematic review of 73 ASPs that were described in 49 reports from both published and unpublished sources. Although most of the 73 studies reviewed did not specify the ethnicity of the participants, 27 programs included the following participants, listed in order of predominance: African American, Latino, Asian or Pacific Islander, and American Indian.

Programs reviewed were predominantly in community settings (56%) rather than on school grounds (41%), and many had an academic component such as tutoring or homework assistance. Youths had participated for less than 1 year at the time of the program evaluation in the majority of the reports. Participating youths were not known to be experiencing problems (Durlak & Weissberg, 2007).

This meta-analysis revealed three major findings:

- ASPs have an overall positive and statistically significant impact on participating youths.
- Youths who participate in ASPs improve significantly in three major areas: feelings and attitudes, indicators of behavioral adjustment, and school performance. (The only outcome that failed to reach statistical significance was the mean effect for school attendance [0.10]. However, participants showed a statistically significant increase in positive feelings and attitudes about themselves and their school and an increase in positive social behaviors.)
- Programs that used evidence-based skill-training procedures were the only types of programs that were associated with positive outcomes.

In the study, Durlak and Weissberg (2007) identified four characteristics of evidenced-based ASPs based on theory and research in social skills training:

1. The program involved teaching a sequenced set of activities to achieve the program objectives related to skill development. That is, skills to be taught were broken down into observable units of action, from least to most complex.
2. The program involved active learning, or *doing*, by the participant.
3. The program's content contained at least one component devoted to developing personal or social skills.
4. The program's content was explicit in targeting specific personal or social skills with clear and specific objectives.

Thus, effective programs were identified as those including skill-development activities aimed at promoting personal and social skills and characterized by a sequential, active, focused, and explicit training process and agenda. Figure 36-1 shows the staff, students, and family members at Carver Elementary School in St. Louis, Missouri, viewing the products of a 10-week after-school art program.

The findings from Durlak and Weissberg's analysis provide support for the basic tenets of occupational science and occupational therapy. That is, active engagement in purposeful and meaningful occupations or activities promotes healthy development (Clark, 1997; Mandel, Jackson, Zemke, Nelson, & Clark, 1999). The evidence-based ASPs were purported to provide structured opportunities for positive interactions with adults and peers and to encourage initiative and decision-making by the participants. Although it is unknown if participants in the ASPs were allowed to decide which activities to engage in, this is inferred from the description of evidence-based programs.

Finally, activities involving challenging tasks that developed new skills and personal talents were identified as most effective. This finding is a critical part of the occupational therapy intervention process—that is, to meet "the just right challenge" to develop personal skills and talents within the context of personally meaningful after-school activities.

Barriers to Participation

Durlak and Weissberg (2007) describe some of the benefits of participation in ASPs, but there are also barriers to participation for youths both with and without mental health concerns. Some of the variables influencing time use in the after-school hours for all youths include the family's socioeconomic background, the sponsorship of the activity format (e.g., YMCA, Boy's or Girl's Club, Scouts), availability and access to programs, and parental attitudes and actions (Durlak & Weissberg, 2007). After dealing with many challenges as a child with special needs, Lily was able to successfully participate in an after-school softball league (Figure 36-2).

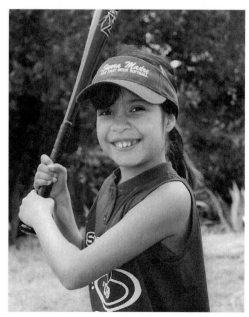

FIGURE 36-2. After dealing with many challenges as a child with special needs, Lily was able to successfully participate in an after-school softball league.

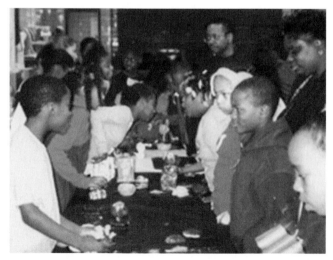

FIGURE 36-1. The staff, students, and family members at Carver Elementary School in St. Louis, Missouri, view the products of a 10-week after-school art program.

The Lived Experience

Barriers to Participation in After-School Programs: A Parent's Story

My daughter Sara is eight years old. She has a diagnosis of attention deficit, hyperactivity disorder (ADHD) and borderline developmental delay. She has been through so many after school programs, I have lost track. The reason she has not been able to stay with one program has often been related to the inflexibility and lack of awareness by staff to understand her disability and know how to best meet her needs.

Sara is really a very loving, affectionate child, but she can sometimes get upset and have difficulty calming herself. For example, she may become defiant when asked to do a simple task like cleaning up or moving along to the next activity. If she gets very frustrated on a task she may destroy her work or lash out at another child by pulling hair or slapping. She also can get upset by loud or unexpected noises in her environment. She enjoys all the same activities as other children her age. But, she just needs more time to understand what is being expected of her and a better way of expressing herself. I just want her to fit in but the usual reply I get from program directors is that Sara may not remain in the program unless she has an aide to accompany her. How can I afford to pay for that on top of the cost for the after-school program? I just want her to have the same socialization experiences and opportunities as other children in after-school programs.

Youths with mental health concerns are often faced with an additional disadvantage due to limited or lack of social acceptance of individuals with significant learning, emotional, or behavioral challenges. According to the Surgeon General's report (Office on Disability, 2005; Office of the Surgeon General, 2002), 80% of American children who have mental health disorders do not receive the services they need due to a range of factors, with limited access and availability of programs often identified as key deterrents. Although publicly funded programs may not discriminate on the basis of disability, programs may limit participation for youths with disabilities by requiring the presence of an adult assistant or excluding them if there is substantial risk to the health and safety of others (U.S. Department of Justice, 2007). One parent's account of the barriers to inclusion her daughter encountered in an ASP is provided above and illuminates some of the obstacles faced by families. These variables need to be considered when evaluating the after-school needs of youths with mental health concerns.

The Role of Occupational Therapy

Occupational competence, or the personal sense of achievement in one's performance of daily activities, is an integral component of the occupational therapy evaluation and intervention process for youths with behavioral and psychosocial needs (Jackson & Arbesman, 2005; Kannenberg & Greene, 2003). Occupational therapy practitioners who use ASP as intervention provide a wide variety of options that allow for choice and meet the physical, social, emotional, and academic needs of the youth. Children and youth considered to be at greatest risk for problems such as isolation, low academic achievement, and behavioral issues such as conduct, aggression, and drug use require more comprehensive and intensive programs.

The quote that opened this chapter and the following statements describe the range of feelings regarding after-school time use by young teens residing in a homeless shelter with their families (McDonald, 2001; 2006). When asked to describe a typical day after school, Marta, a 12-year-old

Latina who resides in a homeless shelter with her family, named each activity as if reading a monotonous list: "I do my homework, watch TV, then play a game, go and eat, and then come back in here [the homeless shelter]." Marta often appeared either upset or bored while discussing her use of after-school time at the shelter (McDonald, 2001).

Conversely, John, a 13-year-old African American male also living in a homeless shelter, described his after-school activities in a different way: "I catch the bus home, do my homework, eat dinner, take a shower, iron my clothes, and get ready for school the next day. I play with my sisters—we play tag, have swinging contests, everything." John appeared to be excited and eager to share his involvement in after-school activities.

These statements provide a glimpse into the after-school time use for young teens residing in a homeless shelter. Whether youths are homeless or at risk, occupational therapists should be skilled at providing assessment and interventions to youths with mental health concerns in ASPs.

Case: Occupational Therapy in After-School Programming for Youths Residing in a Homeless Shelter

Mary, a 10-year-old Latina, often spent long hours in the shelter's after-school child care program because of her single mother's seven-day-a-week work schedule. Mary often appeared despondent, and her affect was often flat or constrained. She frequently complained of headaches to child care staff. During the occupational therapy evaluation, Mary was asked semistructured, open-ended questions to determine her feelings and needs regarding her time use in the after-school hours.

Since Mary spent a large part of her after-school hours in child care, she was asked what she thought of her daily routine. Mary described how she accepted the routines imposed by the staff, although she often felt "bored." She stated, "You need to have time for yourself

. . . and someone to talk to because if you just keep your things inside they'll just stay there . . . like it affects your health and you're really sad and angry. It makes you feel . . . like you're not breathing. Like on the weekends I'm more free to do things and [during the week] it's like I'm trapped . . . you know I have to stay in my room. We can't go out. Then my weekends I have all free and I feel more emotionally happy and I could do more things." When asked who or what helped her to do what she wanted to do after school, Mary described how her mother helped her cope with boredom at the shelter. She stated, "When it was a boring time, my mom always tried to make the best out of it. She tried to give us games or tell us how to play a new game."

Mary was also asked to describe some of her favorite play activities. She became animated when describing her favorite play activities as "playing pirates or school" or "having a pumpkin carving contest." When asked if she engaged in any of the shelter's activities, she stated she enjoyed going to art therapy and counseling. When asked how she would like to spend her time after school, Mary said she would like to have time to spend with a friend, then do her homework and, if possible, "play baseball."

As part of the assessment process, Mary was given a 1-week time-use journal to obtain further information about her typical time use on weekdays after school and on the weekends. The journal provided a written log of how she spent her time in hourly increments, identifying where the activity occurred, who was present, how she felt while performing the activity, and her motivation for the activity (i.e., obligatory, voluntary, or both). For example, in the time column for 4:00–5:00 p.m., she wrote: "doing homework" (occupation); "in child care" (location); "with kids from shelter and child care staff" (people present); "bored" (feeling); "have to and want to" (motivation).

The results of Mary's individual interview, her time-use journal, and observation of Mary in child-care activities were reviewed with input from her mother, child care staff, and counselors. In designing an effective ASP, Mary reported needing more time to develop friendships and to spend time engaged in novel play activities. Due to her mother's absence after school, Mary needed more attention from a caring, consistent adult who would be able to "check-in" with her about her day. The child-care staff structured her after-school time differently so she would be able to choose games or play activities before doing her homework. Her affect improved considerably, and she became more animated in child care, engaging in conversations with other peers. Mary continued her participation in art therapy and counseling. Occupational therapy in conjunction with child-care staff provided a Girl's Club group with weekly meetings as well as opportunities for outdoor games, craft activities, and dramatic play.

Occupational Therapy Assessments

Occupational therapists, with their expertise in activity analysis, disability, occupational adaptation, and human development, are vital in identifying not only the psychosocial

needs of youths with mental health concerns but also the importance of everyday occupations to these youths. Knowledge of the personal meaning of an activity or occupational pursuit not only provides the motivation for participation but also assists in individualizing the intervention to best meet the client's needs and personal goals.

Depending on the goals of the ASP or intervention, the occupational therapy assessment process requires gathering relevant data specific to the present and future desired after-school occupations. It is important to learn the present after-school routine of the child or teen and the subjective meanings the youth ascribes to these occupations or activities This knowledge provides insight into the youth's motivation for pursuing or avoiding certain occupations as well as the perceived importance of these daily occupations.

Occupational therapists often utilize skill-based assessments to gather data on clients' cognitive, perceptual, sensory, and socioemotional development. Several tools may be helpful in identifying youths' needs in ASPs and interventions. The assessments listed in Table 36-1 include both standardized and semistructured tools to gather information regarding daily routine, time use, and the youth's perception of daily tasks.

The assessments in Table 36-2 are standardized and semistructured specific skill-based and sensory-processing assessments.

Occupational Therapy Intervention

The extent to which youths with mental health concerns attend structured ASPs is unknown, but the role of occupational therapy in facilitating inclusion for youths with mental health concerns is significant. Because the literature in occupational therapy does not specifically note the placement of their interventions in ASPs for children and youths with behavioral and psychosocial needs, a broader review of 69 studies by Jackson and Arbesman (2005) resulting in the *AOTA Practice Guidelines for Children with Behavioral and Psychosocial Needs* is reported here. Their findings provide

---

Evidence-Based Practice

Research evidence shows that addressing the sensory needs for youths with both sensory and mental health concerns benefits the child's self-regulation and modulation of stressful stimuli during everyday activities (Schaaf & Roley, 2005).

➤ Occupational therapists need to assess the youth's sensory processing needs, when appropriate, using the Sensory Processing Measure (SPM) (Kuhaneck, Henry, Glennon, Parham, & Ecker, 2007) or the Sensory Profile (Dunn, 1999; Brown & Dunn, 2002).

➤ Occupational therapists can help educators, parents, and other after-school providers to better understand the youth's sensory difficulties at home and school and can recommend appropriate sensory strategies and environmental modifications to improve occupational performance.

Schaaef, R., & Roley, S. S. (2005). *Sensory Integration: Applying Clinical Reasonings to Diverse Populations*. Bethesda, MD: AOTA Press.

Table 36-1 ● Tools for Gathering Information on Youth's Daily Routine, Time Use, and Perception of Daily Tasks

Assessment	Description	Appropriate Ages
Time-Use Journal (McDonald, 2001)	A written description of the youth's time use. Each weekday, the youth records his or her experiences in half-hour increments from 3:00 p.m. until bedtime, responding to five questions for each activity: 1. What are you doing? 2. Where are you? 3. Who is with you? 4. Why are you doing this activity (i.e., you have to, you want to, or both)? 5. How do you feel while you are doing this activity?	8–18 years
Children's Assessment of Participation and Enjoyment (CAPE) and Preferences for Activities of Children (PAC) (King et al, 2004)	Both measures provide information regarding an individual's participation in activities with the assistance of a parent or caregiver.	6–21 years
Perceived Efficacy and Goal Setting System (PEGS) (Missiuna, Pollock, & Law, 2004)	Utilizes a child's self-reported performance on everyday tasks to establish and prioritize goals for intervention. Provides the child's perception of ability to perform daily activities at home, school, and in the community. Parent and teacher versions are also available.	5–21 years

Table 36-2 ● Tools for Assessing Skills and Sensory Processing

Assessment	Description	Appropriate Ages
Dynamic Occupational Therapy Cognitive Assessment for Children (DOTCA-Ch) (Katz & Parush, 2004)	Measures the cognitive abilities and learning potential for children with special needs. Twenty-two subtests assess five cognitive areas: orientation, spatial perception, praxis, visual motor organization, and thinking operations.	6–12 years
Social Skills Rating System (SSRS) (Gresham & Elliott, 2007)	Assesses the social behavior of children and adolescents based on standardized, norm-referenced data. Parent, teacher, and student questionnaires provide information about perceived social skills, problem behaviors, and academic competence.	3–18 years
Sensory Processing Measure (SPM) (Kuhaneck, Henry, Glennon, Parham, & Ecker, 2007)	Generates norm-referenced scores of a child's social participation, sensory systems, and motor planning in home, classroom, and school environments. Parent and teacher versions are available.	5–12 years
Sensory Profile (Dunn, 1999)	Examines sensory processing patterns in children who are at risk for or have specific disabilities relating to sensory processing abilities. Parent and teacher versions are available.	3–10 years
Adolescent/Adult Sensory Profile (Brown & Dunn, 2002)	A self-report questionnaire providing information about six sensory processing categories: taste/smell, movement, touch, vision, activity level, and auditory processing.	11 years and older

information that will help occupational therapists to shape interventions toward the best outcomes.

In general, Jackson and Arbesman's review demonstrated that activity-based interventions aided in improving peer and social interactions in children and youths across a range of *Diagnostic and Statistical Manual of Mental Disorders,* Fourth Edition, Text Revision, diagnoses. The review was considered extremely broad and included a wide range of activity-based interventions, treatment sizes, ages of participants, and diagnoses and conditions. Often, the studies were conducted by a wide variety of professional disciplines; four studies incorporated occupational therapy into the intervention. However, successful interventions had several common features:

- Direct instruction geared toward targeted skills.
- Activities to teach and encourage practice of new skills.
- Peers to model and promote practice of new skills.
- A supportive adult to provide coaching and reinforcement for appropriate behavior.
- A sufficient duration of time, allowing children ample opportunity to experience the intervention and practice-emergent skills.

Interestingly, these are some of the same characteristics that Durlak and Weissberg (2007) identified for successful evidenced-based ASPs aimed at improving personal and social skills.

The activity-based studies in the *AOTA Practice Guidelines* identified a variety of activities "commonly and rarely used . . . in the course of occupational therapy intervention with children and adolescents." These included "play, arts and crafts, role-playing, puppets, board games, computer games, sports skill training, art/movement programs, music activities, team-/cooperation building exercises, camping, life skills training, drama and fairy tale enactment groups, conversational skills training, bibliotherapy (short stories, poems, films), supported employment, physical challenges programs, and other types of recreational and leisure activities" (Jackson & Arbesman, 2005, p. 31). Although the authors indicated the focus of the treatment was often on improving social cooperation, children's achievement in these activities or occupations was identified as a legitimate goal in itself, building on the child's sense of competency as an occupational being.

For the occupational therapist, intervention may include involvement at either the macroscopic or microscopic level. A macroscopic view may entail influencing program directors and public policymakers with facilitating access and availability of ASPs for youths with or at risk for mental health concerns. At the microscopic level, the occupational therapist may help youths participate in desired after-school occupations such as individual or small-group therapy aimed at improving the youth's specific skill development. The latter focus predominates the evidenced-based literature reviews in occupational therapy and related disciplines (Jackson & Arbesman, 2005).

Occupational Therapist as Advocate

Because youths with behavioral and social problems often face barriers to inclusion in many community programs (Office on Disability, 2005), occupational therapists play an integral role in advocating for the needs of youths with mental health concerns. Advocacy may involve assisting clients with how to access services and supports within their community. Occupational therapists and other professionals need to educate consumers about their legal entitlements under the Americans with Disabilities Act (ADA, 1990). For example, community-based programs that receive state and/or federal funding must abide by the federal mandate under the ADA to provide access to publicly funded community programs for individuals with disabilities. Knowledge regarding the legal rights for inclusion in these community programs can be obtained from specific state agencies serving the consumer and from the ADA website (see Resources section).

In California, for example, the Department of Developmental Services contracts with Regional Centers for the Developmentally Disabled to provide service coordination and legal advocacy to ensure that persons with developmental disabilities have the opportunity to lead more independent, productive, and satisfying lives. Regional Centers for the Developmentally Disabled provides consumers who have developmental disabilities with the opportunity to participate in inclusive social and recreational programs within the community. Unfortunately, youths who have not been diagnosed as developmentally disabled often do not receive comparable opportunities for inclusion.

Access to free legal advice and inclusion support for ASPs can be found through nonprofit agencies that work in partnership with people with mental health disabilities. These agencies vary by state but may include Protection and Advocacy, Inc. (PAI), the Association for Retarded Citizens (ARC), and the National Alliance on Mental Illness (NAMI).

Finally, occupational therapists as advocates can assist in educating insurance companies on the cost effectiveness of occupational therapy services through prevention and promotion of healthy lifestyles.

Occupational Therapist as Innovative Practitioner and Program Director

Occupational therapy as a discipline has historically identified the importance of addressing the play and leisure concerns for individuals with mental health disorders (Reilly, 1974). Provision of occupational therapy services has traditionally been in the context of the psychiatric hospital but is now increasingly found in private practice clinics during after-school hours. An advantage to occupational therapy intervention over traditional psychotherapy approaches is the utilization of active engagement in carefully designed occupations or activities to maximize the individual's play and social skills. In addition, the occupational therapist has the expertise to address the child's sensory processing needs within the context of play and social interaction.

Unfortunately, there are some disadvantages to clinic-based occupational therapy. Although occupational therapists serving in private practice clinics may receive funding from state agencies, there is usually little or no reimbursement from insurance companies. Consequently, caregivers often must pay out-of-pocket expenses for participation in psychosocial interventions. Additionally, most clinic-based services provided by mental health professionals do not include youths without disabilities to serve as role models and allow only a limited amount of time for these interventions, usually meeting only once a week for an hour. To counter these disadvantages, it is essential that the occupational therapist consult with other after-school providers, such as sports and recreation leaders in the child's community, to ensure that the skills learned in the clinic are carried over into other activities (Reynolds, 2006).

A model social skills program developed and directed by occupational therapists for youths with mental health concerns would ideally (1) include components of an evidence-based, social skills group (Frankel, Myatt, Cantwell, & Feinberg, 1997; Jackson & Arbesman, 2005) and (2) address the individual's occupational interests and sensory motor needs through carefully tailored occupation-based activities. Many pediatric occupational therapists focus on meeting the sensory processing needs of youths through active engagement in movement-based activities. Incorporating sensory motor activities within the session would provide the youth with the level of sensory input likely to facilitate attentiveness and self-calming while acquiring new play and social skills. Yoga is one occupation that addresses the sensory motor needs of youths (Mollo & Schaaf, 2007). This activity may be taught within the social skills program and can be shared with parents for use at home.

Innovative roles for occupational therapy practitioners include providing consultation to and development of community-based ASPs. An example of an inclusive ASP model that could be developed by an occupational therapist is the S.M.I.L.E.-A-While Day Camp in Pasadena, California. This program is contracted with the Eastern Los Angeles Regional Center for the Developmentally Disabled and serves children with and without disabilities from 3.5 to 12 years of age. The ASP runs weekdays between 12:00 p.m. and 6:00 p.m. The program's mission is to foster the development of the skills necessary to function successfully in society through real-life experiences. The goals of the day camp are to encourage and facilitate character building, healthy peer relationships, spontaneous communication and interaction, and individual talents and creativity.

The after-school day camp is run by two directors with extensive clinical training in both regular and special education. Camp counselors are trained by the camp directors, and the counselor/staff-to-child ratio is dependent on the age of the group (i.e., one adult for every 6 to 8 youths ages 3–7 years; one adult for every 10 youths ages 7–14 years). In addition, a one-on-one aide may be provided if necessary. Examples of onsite activities include friendship circle/ greetings, songs and stories, share time, arts/crafts, swimming, horseback riding, and games to encourage cooperation and team spirit. A wide variety of developmentally appropriate activities are offered, and while activities are structured, they allow for individual creativity, needs, and attention span. Occupational therapists do not work directly within the camp but, along with other contractors such as speech pathologists and school psychologists, provide assistance as needed for comprehensive and individualized developmental plans for each child.

Future Directions

According to the Office on Disability (2005), the need for more inclusive after-school opportunities is identified as a high priority at the state and national levels. Occupational therapists can develop a unique, comprehensive, occupation-based ASP for youths with and without mental health concerns either in collaboration with an existing program or in response to focused needs within the community. Providing opportunities for youths to be in inclusive settings after school requires therapists to step out of familiar and comfortable professional roles so they may advocate for and address the needs of youths with mental health concerns across wider service delivery settings. Working side by side with school social workers and other community workers, occupational therapists can promote an image of youths as building on their strengths (as opposed to being viewed as inadequate or incapable), having peers work with peers to support their growth, sharing interests, and making friends— all developmental activities of importance to this population (Ngai, Cheung, & Ngai, 2009).

Examples of occupation-based service delivery settings include aquatic therapy and hippotherapy (Engel & MacKinnon, 2007). Novel service delivery can also include development of community-based violence-prevention programs and acting as a consultant to a homeless shelter program (McDonald, 2001; Miller, Herzberg, & Ray, 2006). Reynolds (2006) describes the strategies and benefits for consulting in after-school team sports for youths on the autism spectrum. Bazyk (2006) also describes an innovative, occupation-based social skills group for low-income urban youths in after-school care.

Occupational therapists can engage in a wider scope of practice by considering the many different occupations in which youths participate after school. Specifically, daily occupations including self-care, prevocational work, and community involvement are valued and important arenas for intervention that were not addressed in this chapter.

Health promotion and prevention for at-risk youths is also a growing concern in the United States given the increased incidence of obesity and, for some youths, sedentary lifestyles (Office of the Surgeon General, 2007; Schmelzer, 2006). Evidence-based research is growing within the field of occupational therapy and related disciplines, but more research is needed to continue supporting the efficacy of occupation-based interventions driven by the needs of the consumer.

Summary

Occupational therapists who work with school-aged children and youths can provide integrated services through various after-school agencies. Engagement in meaningful and purposeful occupations after the structure of the school day can help youths with mental health concerns gain competence, health, and adaptation. Programs can directly include occupational therapy assessment and intervention, or the occupational therapist can serve as an advocate or as a program director of community-based programs. Research and future program development to enhance the physical, social, emotional, and academic performance of youths experiencing or at risk for mental health conditions through the expertise of an occupational therapist in ASPs will more fully promote participation in all the occupational roles associated with adolescence.

Active Learning Strategies

1. Advocating Against Barriers to Inclusion

Review The Lived Experience narrative by Sara's mother. Consider the following questions:

Reflective Questions
- What barriers to inclusion can you identify?
- How could you help consult with the ASP to provide Sara with more successful inclusion opportunities?
- How could you help her mother advocate for her daughter's inclusion in an ASP?
- What resources are available for her mother to obtain legal advice on her rights to have her child attend a publicly funded program?

 Capture your responses to these questions in your **Reflective Journal**.

2. Time-Use Study

Interview a child or adolescent about his or her after-school time. Start by asking general, open-ended questions, such as "What activities to do you usually do after school?" Ask more detailed questions to gain more information about a particular activity, such as, "Where and with whom do you do this activity?" and "How do you feel when you are doing this activity?"

3. Examining Your After-School Time Use

Insight into your own use of after-school time can provide you with a better understanding of the barriers to inclusion for youths with mental health concerns and an awareness of the resources that may be utilized to adapt to their unique situation. Reflect on your own memories of time spent after school at different ages. What resources (intrapersonal or extrapersonal) helped you to do what you wanted or needed to do? Examples of intrapersonal resources may include your personality traits, problem-solving abilities, and emotional state when engaged in making occupational choices. Extrapersonal resources may include the significant people in your family or community as well as your socioeconomic status and gender.

 Record your memories and the resources that you utilized in your **Reflective Journal**.

4. Case Example: "Max"

Max is a 14-year-old boy with Asperger syndrome. He is attending a full-inclusion ASP on site at his school. The program is fairly structured, including time for snack, homework, and sports activities. However, Max often persists in doing his homework and shows less interest in participating with other children, especially during the sports program. Consider the following questions:

Reflective Questions

- As an occupational therapist hired to consult with the ASP, what recommendations can you give them to help Max develop his socialization with peers?
- Is it best to allow Max to persist in his homework if this is his desired activity?
- What input will you gather from his teachers, parents, and program staff to guide your consultation?
- Describe a successful inclusion activity you may implement to promote Max's socialization with peers in his ASP.

 Capture your responses to these questions in your **Reflective Journal**.

Resources

- The Finance Project is focused on "helping leaders finance and sustain initiatives that lead to better futures for children, families and communities." It is an independent, nonprofit research, consulting, technical assistance, and training firm for public- and private-sector leaders nationwide. http://www.financeproject.org
- The Wallace Foundation "seeks to support and share effective ideas and practices that expand learning and enrichment opportunities for all people." Its three current objectives are to strengthen education leadership to improve student achievement, improve after-school learning opportunities, and build appreciation and demand for the arts. http://www.wallacefoundation.org
- National Institute on Out-of-School Time (NIOST), Wellesley College: "Our mission is to ensure that all children, youths, and families have access to high-quality programs, activities, and opportunities during nonschool hours. We believe that these experiences are essential to the healthy development of children and youths, who then can become effective and capable members of society. Our work bridges the worlds of research and practice." This site provides links to NIOST Clearinghouse, yearly fact sheet on out-of-school time, and other resources. http://www.niost.org

References

Apsler, R. (2009). After-school programs for adolescents: A review of evaluation research. *Adolescence, 44*(173), 1–19.

Americans with Disabilities Act (1990). Available at: http://www.ada/gov/pubs/ada.htm (accessed January 3, 2010).

Bazyk, S. (2006). Creating occupation-based social skills groups in after-school care. *OT Practice, 11*(17), 13–18.

Beckett, M. K. (2008). *Current-Generation Youth Programs: What Works, What Doesn't, and at What Cost?* Santa Monica, CA: Rand.

Bodily, S. J., & Beckett, M. K. (2005). *Making Out-Of-School Time Matter: Evidence for an Action Agenda.* Santa Monica, CA: Rand.

Brown, C., & Dunn, W. (2002). *The Adolescent/Adult Sensory Profile.* San Antonio: Harcourt Assessment.

Clark, F. (1997). Appendix III: Occupational science. In P. Crist & C. B. Royeen (Eds.), *Infusing Occupation into Practice: Comparison of Three Clinical Approaches in Occupational Therapy* (pp. 101–111). Bethesda, MD: American Occupational Therapy Association.

Copperman, R. B., & Bhat, C. R. (2007). An exploratory analysis of children's daily time use and activity patterns using the child development supplement (CDS) to the US Panel Study of Income Dynamics (PSID). Available at: http://www.caee.utexas.edu/prof/bhat/full_papers.htm (accessed January 3, 2010).

Dunn, W. (1999). *The Sensory Profile.* San Antonio, TX: Harcourt Assessment.

Durlak, J. A., & Weissberg, R. P. (2007). *The Impact of After-School Programs That Promote Personal and Social Skills.* Chicago: Collaborative for Academic, Social, and Emotional Learning.

Elliott, D. S. (1993). Health enhancing and health compromising lifestyles. In S. G. Millstein, A. C. Petersen, E. O. Nightingale (Eds.), *Promoting the Health of Adolescents* (pp. 119–145). New York: Oxford University Press.

Engel, B. T., & MacKinnon, J. R. (2007). *Enhancing Human Occupation Through Hippotherapy: A Guide for Occupational Therapy.* Bethesda, MD: AOTA Press.

The Finance Project, (2003). *Funding Guide.* Available at: http://www.financeprojectinfo.org/Publications/FundingGuide2003.pdf (accessed September 27, 2009).

Frankel, F., Myatt, R., Cantwell, D., & Feinberg, D. (1997). Parent assisted transfer of children's social skills training: Effects on children with and without attention deficit disorder. *Journal of the American Academy of Child and Adolescent Psychology, 36,* 1056–1064.

Gresham, F. M., & Elliott, S. N. (2007). *Social Skills Rating System (SSRS).* Los Angeles: Western Psychological Services.

Grossman, J. B., Lind, C., Hayes, C., McMaken, J., & Gersick, A. (2009). The cost of quality out-of-school-time programs: Executive summary. Commissioned by the Wallace Foundation. Available at: http://www.financeproject.org/publications/

CostofQuality OSI-ExecSummary.pdf (accessed September 27, 2009).

Harvard Family Research Project. (2003). *A Review of Out-of-School-Time Program Quasi-Experimental and Experimental Evaluation Results*. Cambridge, MA: Author.

Jackson, L. L., & Arbesman, M. (2005). *Occupational Therapy Practice Guidelines for Children with Behavioral and Psychosocial Needs*. Bethesda, MD: AOTA Press.

Kannenburg, K., & Greene, S. (2003). Infusing occupation into practice: Valuing and supporting the psychosocial foundation of occupation. *OT Practice, 8,* CE1–CE8.

Katz, N., & Parush, S. (2004). *Dynamic Occupational Therapy Cognitive Assessment for Children*. San Antonio, TX.: Harcourt Assessment.

King, G., Law, M., King, S., Hurley, P., Hanna, S., Kertoy, M., Rosenbaum, P., & Young, K. (2004). *Children's Assessment of Participation and Enjoyment (CAPE) and Preferences for Activities of Children (PAC)*. San Antonio, TX: Harcourt Assessment.

Kuhaneck, H. M., Henry, D. A., Glennon, T. J., Parham, L. D., & Ecker, C. (2007). *The Sensory Processing Measure*. Los Angeles: Western Psychological Services.

Mandel, D. R., Jackson, J. M., Zemke, R., Nelson, L., & Clark, F. (1999). *Lifestyle Redesign: Implementing the Well-Elderly Program*. Bethesda, MD: AOTA Press.

McDonald, A. E. (2001). *The After-School Occupations of Homeless Youth: Implications for Occupational Science, Occupational Therapy and Public Policy*. Unpublished doctoral dissertation, University of Southern California, Los Angeles.

McDonald, A. E. (2006). The after-school occupations of homeless youth: Three narrative accounts. *Occupational Therapy in Health Care, 20*(3,4), 115–133.

Medrich, E. A., Roizen, J. A., Rubin, V., & Buckley, S. (1982). *The Serious Business of Growing Up: A Study of Children's Lives Outside of School*. Los Angeles: University of California Press.

Meeks, C. B., & Maudlin, T. (1990). Children's time in structured and unstructured leisure activities. *Lifestyles, Family and Economic Issues, 11*(3), 257–259.

Miller, K. S., Herzberg, G. L., & Ray, S. A. (2006). *Homelessness in America: Perspectives, Characterizations, and Considerations for Occupational Therapy*. New York: Haworth.

Missiuna, C., Pollock, N., & Law, M. (2004). *The Perceived Efficacy and Goal Setting System*. San Antonio, TX: Harcourt Assessment.

Mollo, K., & Schaaf, R. (2007). *Use of Kripalu Yoga to Decrease Sensory Reactivity to Individuals with Sensory Defensiveness*. Poster session presented at American Occupational Therapy Association Annual Conference, St. Louis, Missouri.

National Institute on Out-of-School Time. (2003). *Fact Sheet on School-Age Children's Out-Of-School Time*. Wellesley, MA: Wellesley College, Center for Research on Women.

Ngai, S. S.-Y., Cheung, C.-K., & Ngai, N.-P. (2009). Building mutual aid among young people with emotional and behavioral problems: The experiences of Hong Kong social workers. *Adolescence, 44,* 447–464.

Office of the Surgeon General. (2007). *The Surgeon General's Call to Action to Prevent and Decrease Overweight and Obesity in Children and Adolescents*. Available at: http://www.surgeongeneral.gov/topics/obesity (accessed January 3, 2010).

Office of the Surgeon General. (2002). *Youth Violence: A Report of the Surgeon General*. Available at: http://www.surgeongeneral.gov/library/youthviolence (accessed January 3, 2010).

Office on Disability. (2005). *A Report of the Summit. State-Community Response to Barriers for Children with Co-occurring Developmental Disabilities and Emotional/Substance Abuse Disorders*. U.S. Department of Health & Human Services. Available at: http://www.hhs.gov/od/whitepaper_appendix_a.pdf (accessed January 3, 2010).

Reilly, M. (1974). *Play as Exploratory Learning*. Beverly Hills: Sage.

Reynolds, S. (2006). Get in the game: Participation in sports for children on the autism spectrum. *OT Practice 11*(20), 13–17.

Schmelzer, L. (2006). Occupation-based camp for healthier children. *OT Practice, 11*(16), 19–23.

United States Department of Justice. (2007). *Commonly Asked Questions about Child Care and the ADA*. Available at: http://www.ada.gov/childq&a.htm (retrieved March 10, 2010).

Vandell, D. L., Pierce, K. M., & Dadisman, K. (2005). Out-of-school settings as a developmental context for children and youth. *Advances in Child Development Behavior, 33,* 43–77.

Weissman, S. A., & Gottfredson, D. C. (2001). Attrition from after school programs: Characteristics of students who drop out. *Prevention Science, 2,* 201–205.

Wong, G. (2003). *Eastern Los Angeles Regional Center Consumer Handbook*. Alhambra, CA: Eastern Los Angeles Regional Center.

Zemke, R., & Clarke, F. (1996). *Occupational Science: The Evolving Discipline*. Philadelphia: F.A. Davis.

Mental Health Practice in Forensic Settings

Jaime Phillip Muñoz

> "The ordinary person, no matter how sympathetic or liberal, cannot be expected to visualize the circumstances of a mentally ill offender. People find it hard to think of inmates as people, or their disorders as very often caused, or at least aggravated, by contemporary public and social attitudes towards the mentally ill.
>
> —Peter Thompson, 1972

Introduction

Roger was 42 and had been in and out of jail, mostly on drug possession charges, since the age of 18. Roger had completed an occupational therapy supported employment program for ex-offenders at the local county jail and was back visiting his occupational therapist. At the time, Roger was drug free and had been out of jail for almost 2 years. Roger began talking about his life growing up and told a story about learning a lesson in trust from his father.

Roger's father and other relatives were in and out of jails and prisons throughout Roger's childhood, and his father drifted in and out of his life. When Roger was in fifth grade, his father rejoined the family after being released from prison. One day, Roger came home from school to find his father repairing a window with an 8-foot stepladder set up next to the house. When he saw Roger, his father called him over and told him to put down his bookbag and climb to the top of the ladder. Roger did as he was told, and when he got to the top, his father instructed him to jump, assuring Roger that he would catch him. Roger jumped, but his father did not catch him. Roger recalled how his father then beat him, and when the beating stopped, his father hugged him and told him, "Son, I just taught you a very important lesson—trust no one. When you do a job, do it alone, because you can keep your own secret, but you can never, ever trust a partner." The "job" Roger's father was referring to was criminal activity.

Everyone has a story. Occupational therapists are challenged to elicit and understand each person's story, to situate the story in sociocultural and environmental context, and to recognize the meanings inherent in the experiences and events the storyteller shares. However, as Peter Thompson's quote suggests, it is difficult for most people to connect with "bad guys" or criminal characters in a story. Working in a **forensic setting** (a setting pertaining to or connected with the correctional system) requires a unique skill set, attitude, and perspective. As in all settings of occupational therapy practice, we are most effective when we get to know the people we work with emotionally and spiritually. We can also make better treatment decisions when we seek to understand the socioenvironmental context that influences the person's day-to-day occupations.

Forensic occupational therapy is the application of mental health specialty practice in legal contexts. Forensic mental health occupational therapists work with individuals with mental disorders who have committed a crime and are consigned by law into custody at a correctional setting. In some ways, the practice of forensic mental health in occupational therapy is not that different from other forms of mental health specialty practice. On the other hand, correctional settings are unique practice settings with unique contextual features. This chapter examines occupational therapy mental health practice in forensic settings. It begins by presenting a broad picture of incarceration in the United States and a description of the various correctional settings. The lived experience of incarceration is then considered through a lens of occupation and environment. The chapter closes with a review of occupational therapy programming in correctional settings.

Incarceration in the United States

In the early 1970s, the incarceration rate in the United States began to grow by 6% each year; it has continued to grow at this pace for nearly 35 years (Travis, 2005). As of January 2008, the number of men and women incarcerated in the United States is nearly 2.3 million, or 1 in every 100 Americans (Pew Charitable Trust, 2008). If you add the number of people who are serving probation sentences or are on parole, then that number jumps to nearly 7.5 million (Bureau of Justice Statistics, 2009). The rate of incarceration in the United States easily exceeds every other nation in the world (King's College, 2007). As shown in Figure 37-1, the U.S. incarceration rate is four times higher than the imprisonment rate in the United Kingdom; six and seven times higher than the rates in China and France, respectively; more than 10 times the rate in Japan; and 20 times the rate in India.

More prisoners require more correctional facilities. To accommodate this incredible growth, the number of state prisons in the United States has nearly doubled in the past 30 years, expanding from 592 in 1973 to over 1,023 in 2000 (Lawrence & Travis, 2004). A number of factors might

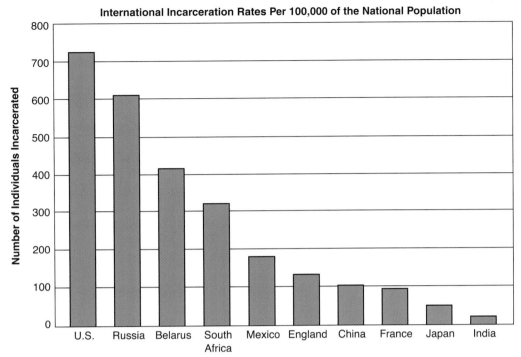

FIGURE 37-1. International incarceration rates per 100,000 of the national population. *Data from King's College, London, International Centre for Prison Studies Prison Brief—lowest to highest rates. Available at: http://www.kcl.ac.uk/depsta/rel/icps/worldbrief (accessed May 5, 2007).*

explain this sustained growth in the prison population; however, a considerably higher rate of crime is not one of them. A primary contributing factor is the shift toward tougher sentencing and corrections policies, which include mandatory sentencing guidelines and "three strikes" laws that require life sentences for those who commit violent crimes. Other factors include the abolition of parole boards in many states, stricter approaches to drug enforcement, and tougher supervision of persons who had been incarcerated after their release from prison (Travis, 2005). Imprisonment rates have leveled off in some states recently, but the overall number of incarcerated persons in the United States continues to grow despite evidence that increased imprisonment does not reduce crime (Magnani & Wray, 2006).

Table 37-1 provides a list of common terms used in the correctional system.

Table 37-1 ● A Corrections Vocabulary

Term	Definition
Acquitted	A judgment that the defendant is not guilty of the offense(s).
Adjudication	The formal pronouncement of a judgment.
Appeal	A defendant's (person charged with a crime) petition for a rehearing in an appellate court (a court that has the jurisdiction to review decisions of a lower court).
Bail bond	A financial obligation signed by the accused to ensure he or she appears at trial. The accused will lose this money if he or she does not appear for the trial.
Bench warrant	A judge's order for the arrest of a person.
Community reintegration planning	Planning a prisoner's return to the community in a law-abiding role. Effective planning requires interagency coordination. Ideally, community reintegration planning should begin when the person is incarcerated, follow the offender through release, and provide aftercare.
Correctional officer (CO)	A person who maintains custody and security of offenders, usually within the confines of a correctional institution.
Deposition	Testimony of a witness or a party taken under oath outside the courtroom.
Disposition, Court	The action taken as a result of the defendant's court appearance (e.g., dismissed, acquitted, convicted or sentenced, placed on probation).
Diversion	A disposition before or after adjudication but before sentencing; the court diverts the defendant from incarceration to participation in a work, educational, or rehabilitation program.
Felony	A crime punishable by imprisonment or death in a state prison.
Forensic psychiatry	The branch of psychiatry focusing on the study of crime and criminality.

Continued

Table 37-1 ● A Corrections Vocabulary—cont'd

Term	Definition
Halfway or transitional house	A transitional facility where the offender lives and is involved in school, work, training, and so on, while stabilizing for reentry to the community.
Misdemeanor	An offense that is less serious than a felony but punishable by a fine and/or incarceration, usually in a local confinement facility, typically for a year or less.
Parole	A period of control and monitoring that follows an offender's release from incarceration.
Probation	A judicial sentence of community-based supervision or a requirement that a person fulfill certain conditions of behavior in lieu of incarceration; probation may sometimes include a fine, a jail sentence, or both.
Recidivism	Repetition of criminal behavior resulting in a return to incarceration.
Recidivism rate	The percentage of offenders who were released from incarceration and rearrested for a new crime.
Relapse prevention	Strategies aimed at training substance abusers in coping and other skills that help them to diminish stress and ignore environmental triggers that can lead them back into drug use or other criminal activity.
Work release	An alternative to continuous incarceration whereby offenders work for pay in the community but return to the correctional institution during nonworking hours.

Note: Definitions were adapted and based on information from multiple sources, including Cybrary files provided by Frank Schmalleger retrieved from http://talkjustice.com/files/ glossary.htm; About.com Criminal Justice Glossary retrieved from http://crime.about.com/od/g_criminal/Criminal_Justice_Glossary.htm; Criminal Justice Profile retrieved from http://www.plsinfo.org/ healthysmc/12/glossary.html; and Criminal Justice Glossary retrieved from http://www.nicic.org/Downloads/PDF/WWGlossary.pdf.

Correctional Settings

Broadly speaking, a correctional setting could be a prison or penitentiary, jail, boot camp, prison farm, forestry or conservation camp, youth offender facility, forensic hospital, drug and alcohol treatment facility, state-operated local detention center, halfway house, or community corrections facility. Jails, prisons, forensic hospitals, and community corrections settings are each briefly described here.

Jails

Jails often serve as a person's entry point into the correctional system. In most states, jails are local correctional facilities operated by a city, a county, or a consortium of counties rather than by the federal or state government. Jails confine persons before or after adjudication (that is, before or after they have been convicted). Adjudication is often a complex process of criminal court proceedings that results in sentencing. Therefore, people in jail may be awaiting arraignment or a trial, or they may be in the process of being tried. Others may be jailed while waiting for a hearing on parole, probation, or bail revocation. Some people are confined in jails temporarily while they await transfer to a juvenile facility, a state or federal prison, or an immigration facility. Some people in jails have been convicted, while others may be awaiting sentencing. Jails typically confine individuals who have been convicted and given a short sentence (i.e., less than 2 years).

In some ways, jails are like a correctional distribution hub, filtering people to and from courts, community programs, and other correctional institutions while simultaneously holding a segment of the population who have already been convicted and sentenced. In addition to those arrested or convicted, there is a steady stream of family members; visitors; and legal, social, and faith-based human service personnel moving in and out of jails, all of whom must adhere to visitation protocols and are subjected to scrutiny and searches. This constant movement of people in and out can make jail settings very busy.

The physical environment varies among jails, but most are structured so that minimum-, medium-, and maximum-security-level inmates are housed on different floors. Depending on the facility, there will be more or less designated areas for medical, mental health, educational, or drug and alcohol programs. Each floor includes space for staff offices and some have an open multi-purpose or gym area.

Eggers, Muñoz, Sciulli, and Crist (2006) described the physical structure of a county jail where occupational therapy is a key component of a community reintegration program. In this setting, each floor of the jail was subdivided into cellblocks or "pods." A common area allowed for some interaction among offenders. In general, activities were limited to watching television, playing cards or table games, reading, writing letters, talking on the payphone, and playing basketball or walking in the small gym area on the pod. Jails are mandated to provide basic mental health screening, and some jails have beds designated for inmates with mental illness, but the availability of comprehensive mental health services in jails (e.g., crisis intervention, referral services, ability to segregate consumers) varies considerably (American Psychiatric Association, 2000).

Prisons

State and federal prisons are secure institutions that confine offenders who, in general, have been convicted of a felony and have been sentenced for at least 1 year of incarceration. Whether the person is sentenced to a state or federal prison is primarily a function of whether he or she is convicted of committing a state or federal offense. Compared to jails, prisons are generally more stable environments with much less movement in and out of the facility. A primary objective of any prison facility is to confine the offender and protect the safety of the public, the prisoners, and the correctional staff.

People in prison experience a longer separation from the community than those who are incarcerated in jails or in community programs. Thus, the social and psychological adjustment of incarceration, as well as issues relating to

The Lived Experience

Joel

The following comments come from an ex-offender who successfully completed the Community Reintegration Project. He was asked to write a story for this chapter but chose instead to deliver a tape with his musings and commentary on topics he had reviewed in the occupational therapy program. His comments therefore do not appear in a sequential story but instead are organized topically. He hopes they provide some insights to the lived experience of community reintegration for an ex-offender.

Joel (a pseudonym) is a 43-year-old white male who has been convicted and sentenced for various crimes since he was a teenager. He has been diagnosed with bipolar disorder and has battled substance abuse for 27 years. He is the single father of a 14-year-old son. His wife died of an overdose when the child was 7 years old. Joel has been clean and sober for nearly 4 years. A multitude of factors are necessary to support successful reentry into the community. The following comments are provided by Joel and are a collection of his thoughts on community, family, work, and the social environment.

Joel's Strategies for Reintegration

"I avoid my relatives. Anybody, any of my friends in the past that used drugs."

"In the program, the counselors would tell you, 'There's 20 of you in here, maybe one or two of you might make it.' They were right. I used to see the same faces coming back in. I told myself right then and there, I'm going to be the one [who remains out of jail]."

"I know people's gonna sit up there and say, 'Oh, I can't find a job, no one will hire me, you can't find this, you can't find that. . . .' You got to make your own way."

"You have to work hard. Everybody is proud of a paycheck. I know mine's not gonna equal theirs [from selling on the street], but who has to walk around and worry? Not me, 'cause all mine is legal. All his is illegal."

"When you want to plant a flower, you can't just stick a seed in dirt and expect it to grow. You gotta put it in the right dirt, gotta have a good seed, you have to water . . . combination of things have to happen. The first thing that has to happen is that you have to want to inside. That'll get you clean, but it won't keep you clean. Now, to stay clean, you gotta discipline yourself."

Joel's Comments on his Family and Social Environments

"My dad was in prison for armed robbery, drugs' and alcohol, but he's been 28 years of sobriety and, uh, he didn't want nothing to do with me . . . and my mother once told me, 'Why don't you fill out a donor's card?' and so I say, 'What for?' and she says, 'Sell your arms—you got thousands of dollars invested in them. Maybe when you die someone will want to get high off of them.' You know, all things considered, I think I am doing pretty good. If you plant a turnip you get a turnip, if you plant a carrot you get a carrot. I come from two nuts, what did you expect to get?"

"My dad was into numbers and used to collect money for people. . . . He used to hurt people and he always had card games at the house. My uncles were cocaine dealers and drug dealers, and when I was 14 years old, I bought a brand new truck, car, motorcycle. I quit school. I come from basically a family of criminals."

"I can't keep running in and out my son's life. 'Cause how you think a kid feels when their dad is not around? 'Oh, there goes dad, he's gone again.' It's not good for the kid, I can speak from experience on that one."

"People, places, and things. You can't go back into the same environment. You can't go into a bar and drink a pop. I cannot go to, like, my relatives still sell drugs, use drugs. I haven't visited them since I got outta jail. No. People, places, and things will get you in trouble."

---

transitions to and from prison, are often different for those in prison. Prisons are mandated to provide a basic level of psychiatric service, but the frequency, quality, and availability of these services can vary among institutions (Beck & Maruschak, 2001). Basic services in prisons typically include screening at intake and psychotropic medications (Thigpen, Hunter, & Ortiz, 2001). Only about 10% of all inmates identified as mentally ill receive 24-hour care in specialized psychiatric units (Beck & Maruschak, 2001). In fact, the majority of prisons do not have dedicated beds for prisoners with mental illness. Mentally ill prisoners are managed within the prison milieu, or the prison arranges for services at state-operated or other forensic hospitals, which provide treatment then return the offenders to prison when they are stabilized.

Prisons are classified by their level of security. The U.S. Federal Bureau of Prisons (2006) designates levels of security as high, medium, low, and minimum security according to the presence of various security features in the institution. Security features include armed external patrols, security towers, fences and other security barriers, electronic detection devices, and staff-to-prisoner ratios. Health care service delivery, including mental health care, is determined by both physical and procedural limitations these security levels designate.

High-Security Prisons

Some of the most dangerous offenders are housed in high-security prison facilities. The physical environment at such facilities is usually set up with the prisoners' cells and facilities in the center of the institution with a series of physical and structural barriers between these facilities and the outer perimeter of the institution. Beginning in the 1990s, several states constructed administrative-maximum, or "super-maximum," prisons with the sole function of incapacitating offenders, particularly those with violent histories and records of escape. These super-max prisons are designed with very limited space for treatment programs. It is not unusual for prisoners to be detained in their 8-foot by 10-foot cell for all but 1 hour each day (Banks, 2005).

In high-security and super-maximum prisons, offenders can be confined for long periods of the day, and when they are allowed out of their cells, they remain in the cellblock or in an exterior cage. Each cell has a toilet bolted to the floor, and prisoners are typically allowed up to three 10-minute showers a week. Movement is tightly restricted, and movement out of the cellblock does not occur without further restrictions such as handcuffs, leg irons, and correctional officer escorts. These facilities have both multiple- and single-prisoner cells and the highest staff-to-inmate ratio of all prisons.

Medium-Security Prisons

Medium-security prisons provide more opportunity for movement, activity, and interaction among prisoners. Inmates typically have access to a prison yard and exercise areas, libraries, showers, health care services, and other facilities. The perimeter of a medium security prison is usually double fenced, patrolled by armed guards, and set with electronic detection systems (U.S. Federal Bureau of Prisons, 2006). Medium-security prisons often have a wide variety of work-oriented and treatment programs. In some medium-security prisons, offenders sleep in dormitories and have access to communal showers, toilets, and sinks. Given these opportunities for movement within the facility, correctional officers primarily monitor the population through a head count, which occurs several times throughout the day.

Low-Security and Minimum-Security Prisons

Low- and minimum-security prisons also have consistent security routines, but prisoners generally have many opportunities for movement and interaction. Work and treatment programs are common. There is often more open space, and some institutions even have windows. While the perimeter in a low-security prison may be double fenced, it is not usually patrolled by armed guards; minimum-security prisons may not have perimeter fencing at all. Offenders in these settings may work on agricultural, transportation, or conservation projects. Low- and minimum-security prisons are often situated close to higher-security institutions or on military bases. This placement in a complex of correctional institutions allows opportunities for inmates to serve the labor needs of the other institutions while also allowing for efficient training and use of prison staff (U.S. Federal Bureau of Prisons, 2006).

Beck and Maruschak (2001) reported that nearly one-third of the correctional settings that reported offering no mental health services were minimum-security confinement facilities. This finding may reflect the expectation that offenders will receive mental health services in the community upon release. However, the lack of transitional mental health services between correction facilities and the community is cited as a notable weakness in mental health service for prisoners (Beck & Maruschak, 2001, Massaro, 2005; Thigpen et al, 2001).

Forensic Hospitals

In a 2000 census of mental health treatment in state prisons, less than 10% of the 1,558 adult correctional facilities in the United States reported that they specialized in mental health psychiatric confinement. Less than 1% ($n = 12$) of all adult correctional facilities identified mental health psychiatric confinement as their primary function. (Beck & Maruschak, 2001). Approaches for managing the prisoner who is severely mentally ill vary considerably among facilities. Some correctional settings house such prisoners separately only when the inmate is in crisis or acutely symptomatic; when the prisoner exhibits severe decompensation in the general population; or when the person is considered dangerous, suicidal, or at significant risk of self-harm (Thigpen et al, 2001).

Many prisons and jails transfer the most severely mentally ill offenders to secure units in state mental hospitals or private or public secure psychiatric hospitals. Secure forensic hospitals also treat offenders who are judged incompetent to stand trial, who are not guilty because of insanity, or who are found guilty but mentally ill (Snively & Dressler, 2005). Within secure forensic hospitals there is great diversity in the mental health treatment programming; some facilities have considerable resources and space directed toward mental health services and programming, while others have much less (Thigpen et al, 2001). Some forensic units are housed in state hospitals, and here occupational therapists will encounter many of the same resources found in large mental health institutions. Security concerns will always add a layer of watchfulness, protection, and safety, but occupational therapists may offer comprehensive programming such as life skill, prevocational, or social skills training (Snively & Dressler, 2005).

Community Corrections

Community-based correctional settings may be considered in two ways:

1. As a residential or nonresidential setting where offenders are sent as an alternative to incarceration; this approach is called **diversion**.
2. As a residential reentry setting where offenders may be placed just prior to or upon release; **reentry centers** provide a structured, supervised environment and support in job placement, counseling, and other services.

Diversion

People who commit less serious crimes, first-time offenders, and offenders with mental illnesses can be diverted from prosecution and incarceration provided they meet guidelines for completing work, drug, or mental health treatment programs. Upon successful completion of the treatment, their records may be expunged or the original charges against them may be dropped. Decisions on diversion occur locally by a judge or, in some cases, jail wardens and trained correctional staff. Diversion programs can take many forms. An offender can be sentenced to community service or a weekend reporting program; can be monitored electronically; or can be referred to a mental health treatment program or work release program. These types of programs monitor offenders to ensure they complete victim restitution or community service, follow through with educational or vocational training, or participate in the drug or mental health treatment as sentenced. Failure to complete the program results in incarceration.

A more recent development in the U.S. correctional system that directly addresses the needs of the mentally ill offender is the emergence of mental health courts. In mental health courts, the criminal justice system and the mental health system collaborate to address the needs of nonviolent offenders diagnosed with mental illnesses (Bureau of Justice Assistance, 2007). There are over 150 mental health courts operating in the United States (Bureau of Justice Assistance, 2007), and their primary goal is to use mental health treatment options instead of criminal sanctions to address the needs of the mentally ill offender (Brazelton Center for Mental Health Law, 2007). The basic idea of the mental health court is to connect people with mental illness to the resources they need for medication, employment, social functioning, housing, or other support services in lieu of incarceration.

To understand how mental health courts work, consider the story of Rondell, a thin man in his 40s who was found pacing in front of the local convention center. The convention center was closed and locked, but Rondell repeatedly shook and banged on the doors. He carried with him a set of crumpled folders containing various papers; periodically, he took one out and read from it in a loud, angry voice. To passers-by, he appeared to be a one-man demonstration. After a while, he began kicking at one of the doors. Police were called, and when Rondell failed to identify himself and accused the officers of collaborating with the "landlord," they moved in and informed him he was under arrest. Hearing this, Rondell cowered down with his hands over his head, and as they approached, he flailed wildly, striking one of the officers in the side.

Rondell was taken to jail to await a court appearance on charges of vagrancy and unlawful trespass, resisting arrest, and assaulting a police officer. If he goes to mental health court instead of criminal court, it is likely that this contact with the police will not result in extended incarceration and that Rondell will be connected to mental health services. Rondell can expect to agree to voluntary inpatient or outpatient treatment, case management services, and continued supervision for at least as long as he would have been sentenced to incarceration. If Rondell complies with these conditions, his charges will be dismissed or his sentence will be reduced. Rondell's other choice is to be incarcerated and await trial. While he waits, he will likely be offered a more basic level of mental health services.

Community Reentry Centers

Reentry centers provide a structured and supervised residential setting for offenders just prior to or after their release from prison. These settings assist residents with reintegration planning, job placement, and financial management; help them to locate permanent housing; and connect residents with an array of community services that can support their return to the community.

Such facilities may be particularly helpful for offenders with extensive criminal histories who are returning to the community after a prolonged period of incarceration. For these individuals, the social and psychological adjustment to community reintegration can be particularly difficult. For example, one ex-offender related a story of how out of touch he felt when he boarded a bus to attend a job interview after spending 20 years in prison. He had not taken public transportation for decades and felt disoriented when he realized the bus was "talking to him." He was not having an auditory hallucination. He was just unaccustomed to the electronic monitoring and voice systems on the bus, which told him to move away from the door and announced the next stop. He got so unnerved that he got off the bus and returned to the reentry center.

While the level of security at community reentry centers varies, it is like a minimum-security setting, and multiple strategies are used to monitor the movements of the residents. Like jail and prison settings, community reentry centers expect rigid adherence to a strict schedule, and periodic head counts are common. Residents must sign in and out of the facility, and random calls or visits to employment sites are used to monitor their whereabouts. Random drug and alcohol tests can also be administered to people sentenced to a community reentry center.

Community reentry centers provide assistance and training that support employment by providing job-seeking classes, organizing job fairs, and developing connections with local employers and industries willing to hire people with criminal histories. These settings also support residents as they look for housing. Once suitable housing is found, a resident can be released from the reentry center but will continue to be monitored.

A critical component of community reentry center programming is substance abuse and mental health treatment and counseling. Such services can be offered on site, or the reentry center may contract with local providers to deliver these services. Community-based corrections settings may provide one of the best contexts for authentic occupational therapy intervention. The focus on reintegrating into the daily routines of community life and the development of the skill sets necessary to support reintegration resonate with the basic mission and philosophy on which the profession was founded.

Mental Illness and Incarceration

In 2000, the American Psychiatric Association, summarizing research reports available at the time, estimated that as many as 20% of all prisoners were seriously mentally ill and that 5% were actively psychotic at any given moment (American Psychiatric Association, 2000). More recent data from the U.S. Department of Justice, Bureau of Statistics (James & Glaze, 2006), reveals two disturbing facts: (1) more than half of the offenders in U.S. jails and prisons have a recent history or symptoms of mental illness, and (2) the majority do not receive adequate treatment during their incarceration (Box 37-1). The data in the Bureau of Statistics report were compiled from the Department of Justice 2004 *Survey of Inmates in State and Federal Correction Facilities,* the 2002 *Survey of Inmates in Local Jails,* and over 25,000 face-to-face interviews where symptoms were measured using selected questions from the *Diagnostic and Statistical Manual of Mental Disorders,* Fourth Edition, Text Revision structured clinical interviews. These interviews primarily focused on identifying symptoms associated with major depression, mania, and psychotic disorders. Inmates who refused or were unable to complete the survey were excluded from the studies, which suggests that these data may not be reflective of those with the most severe and persistent mental illnesses.

BOX 37-1 ■ Prevalence of Mental Health Problems in Prison/Jail Inmates

The data reported here are based on a December 2006 Bureau of Justice Statistics Report that summarized findings from the *2004 Survey of Inmates in State and Federal Correction Facilities* and the *2002 Survey of Inmates in Local Jails.*

■ Inmates with mental health problems most frequently reported symptoms of mania (44.3%), major depression (23.1%), and psychosis (18.5%) in the 12 months prior to being interviewed.

■ Women inmates in both prisons (73%) and jails (75%) had higher rates of mental health problems than did men in prisons (55%) or jails (63%).

■ Approximately three fourths of all inmates in prisons and jails with mental health problems met DSM criteria for substance abuse or substance dependence.

■ Inmates in jails (60%) had a higher rate of mental health problems than did inmates in state (49%) or federal (40%) correctional facilities.

Data summarized from U.S. Department of Justice (2006). "Mental Health Problems of Prison and Jail Inmates." Bureau of Justice Statistics Special Report, December 14. Available at: http://www.ojp.usdoj.gov/bjs/pub/pdf/mhtppji.pdf (accessed March 2, 2007).

BOX 37-2 ■ Mental Health Treatment in U.S. Correctional Facilities

The data reported here are based on the *2000 Census of State and Federal Adult Correctional Facilities,* which includes data from nearly 1,700 federal, state, and private correctional facilities.

■ State correctional facilities (95%) reported available mental health screening and treatment services more often than community-based facilities (82%).

■ On average, 10% of all offenders in all facilities were receiving psychotropic medications. This rate was 20% in five states and was reduced by half (5%) in community-based facilities.

■ Most of the inmates (66%) receiving therapy, counseling, or medications were housed in facilities that did not specialize in providing mental health services in the correctional setting.

■ Approximately two-thirds (63%) of all correctional facilities were equipped to provide 24-hour mental health care. Community settings were least likely to provide 24-hour care; referral to community mental health services was the most common mental health care provided by community settings.

Data summarized from U.S. Department of Justice. (2001). "Mental Health Treatment in State Prisons." Bureau of Justice Statistics Special Report, July. Available at: http://www.ojp.usdoj.gov/bjs/pub/pdf/mhtsp00.pdf (accessed March 2, 2007).

Jails and prisons operate as de facto front-line mental health providers but are often ill-equipped to provide quality mental health care (Box 37-2). The most likely type of psychiatric treatment inmates with mental illness receive during their incarceration is medication (James & Glaze, 2006). Recent studies have reported a higher number of offenders with documented mental illness in jails than in prisons (James & Glaze, 2006; Magnani & Wray, 2006). Jail environments in particular, being more transient in nature than prisons, typically lack adequate mental health screening and mental health services (Human Rights Watch, 2003). As a result, offenders in jails are less likely than offenders in prisons to receive mental health treatment.

There is clear evidence that the number of people with mental illness in U.S. jails and prisons is substantial. The information reported in Box 37-2 reflects criminal justice institutions' inability to provide sufficient mental health services to offenders. It also provides evidence of an inadequate community mental health system that lacks the resources to serve some of the neediest segments of the population, including people who are poor, mentally ill, and/or homeless. For many people, prison may present them with their first opportunity to access substance abuse treatment or mental health counseling as well as other aspects of health care. However, health services and service delivery is generally inadequate (Human Rights Watch, 2003), and any meager efforts at mental health care service can be abruptly terminated once a person leaves the correctional institution.

Sociocultural Context of Incarceration

The term *criminal justice* usually refers to the network of police, who enforce laws; the courts, which interpret and apply the laws; and correctional institutions, which hold those accused or convicted of breaking the law. **Social justice** refers to the ideal of a just society, one in which social relations and social conditions are fair and equal, particularly in regard to the poorest and most marginalized members of society. "**Occupational justice** has been described as the recognition of, and provision for, the occupational needs of individuals and communities, as part of a fair and empowering society" (Watson, 2005, p. 56). Occupational therapists working in correctional systems must have a clear grounding in these three dimensions of justice.

Magnani and Wray (2006) advocate that criminal behavior be examined from a broad social and ecological perspective.

Incarceration is big business with increasing resources spent to warehouse poor behind bars rather then addressing issues of violence, affordable housing, equal quality education and universal healthcare as a human right or other healthcare resources that would improve daily life in marginalized communities. Instead incarceration has a ripple effect that further strains and debilitates individuals, families, and communities with the fewest resources. (p. 36)

When occupational therapists examine criminal behavior, and more important, how to diminish such behavior, from a broad sociocultural perspective, it requires practitioners to consider the complex social, political, psychological, and economic realities that impact criminal behavior law enforcement and penal responses to such behaviors. We can start this examination by asking ourselves, "What type of person is incarcerated in our jails and prisons?"

The burgeoning prison population in the United States can be easily described by attending to key sociocultural demographics such as gender, race, and economics. For the most part, people in U.S. correctional systems are poor, male, racial and ethnic minorities. The typical offender has a history of poverty, substance abuse, mental illness, and learning disability (Box 37-3). It is likely that the offender grew up in a poorer community with few environmental resources, limited access to quality health care and education, and diminished political power (Magnani & Wray, 2006). People in prison are more likely to have dropped out of and been unsuccessful in school and are less likely to have pursued vocational education or college (Bernstein & Houston, 2000). People who are incarcerated often come from marginalized communities with high rates of crime. When they are released, they often return to these same communities, adding to the already heavy concentrations of previously incarcerated persons (Travis, 2005).

In every state in the United States, the proportion of blacks in prison exceeds the proportion of blacks in the general population (Human Rights Watch, 2002). Estimates suggest that racial and ethnic minorities make up two-thirds of the prison population, and three-fourths of all persons in prison for nonviolent drug offenses are people of color (The Sentencing Project, 2003). In 2008, the national rate of incarceration for white males was estimated to be 1 per 106. Hispanic males were incarcerated at a rate of 1 per 36, and black males at a rate of 1 per 15 (Pew Charitable Trust, 2008). Incarceration rates for white, Hispanic, and black women followed the same trend and were 1 per 355, 1 per 297, and 1 per 100, respectively (Pew Charitable Trust, 2008).

The typical female offender is a poor woman of color with substance dependence and mental health issues who is unemployed, undereducated, and a single mother of young children. She likely comes from a poor community that is disproportionately affected by acts of violence. Her family lacks financial and often emotional resources, and she has other family members who have also been incarcerated

(Bloom, Owen, & Covington, 2003). Some studies have reported that the rate of serious mental illness for women in jails is nearly double the rate for men (National GAINS Center, 2002). The constellation of problems that women in jails and prisons present is complex and can include issues relating to child rearing, parenting, physical and mental health, violence, physical and sexual abuse, and trauma. Teplin, Abram, and McClelland (1996) estimated that up to one-third of the women entering jails have been diagnosed with posttraumatic stress disorder at some point in their lives. Since 1990, the population of female prisoners in U.S. jails and prisons has doubled, and the growth rate of female prisoners is expected to outpace the growth rate of male prisoners by 2011 (Beck & Harrison, 2001).

A growing proportion of the offender population in the United States is incarcerated youths. While the age of 18 is still the threshold for a person to automatically come under the jurisdiction of the adult criminal justice system, a person who is at least 14 years old can be tried and convicted as an adult in almost every state in the union (Griffin, Torbet, & Szymanski, 1998; Sickmund, 2003). In 10 states, youths may be tried and convicted as adults at the age of 17, and in three other states, the age is set at 16 (Hartney & Silva, 2007). Youths in adult correction systems can expect a difficult road. They often do not receive the same level of rehabilitation services that are mandated in juvenile systems, and they are more likely to become victims when housed with adults in correctional facilities (Hartney & Silva, 2007). When they leave the correctional setting, these young people can have a very difficult time expunging their criminal record, which can limit educational and employment opportunities (Western, Kling, & Weiman, 2001). The ethnic and racial disparities seen in the adult offender population are also reflected in youths who are incarcerated.

The U.S. correctional system is also full of offenders who reoffend. Reoffense behavior is called **recidivism**. Travis (2005) uses the term *churners* to refer to people who slip into a cycle of release and reentry into the correctional system. Churners repeatedly agitate in, around, and through the correctional system. Current estimates suggest that two-thirds of offenders released from U.S. prisons are rearrested within 3 years of their release (Travis, 2005). The first year postrelease is a particularly critical time period. Nearly one-third of those who return to a correctional institution do so within 6 months of their release, and nearly half return within the first year (Langan & Levin, 2002). These statistics are alarming and should prompt occupational therapists to consider whether occupational therapy can help ex-offenders develop prosocial occupational patterns that can reduce these high recidivism rates. The bottom line is that nearly every prisoner is eventually released. Unless an offender is sentenced to life imprisonment without parole, dies while incarcerated, or is given a death sentence, he or she will be released; occupational therapy can be an effective intervention to support reintegration.

BOX 37-3 ▓ Contextual Factors of Incarceration

The data reported here is based on a December 2006 Bureau of Justice Statistics Report that summarized findings from the *2004 Survey of Inmates in State and Federal Correction Facilities* and the *2002 Survey of Inmates in Local Jails*.

- Inmates with mental health problems were twice as likely to have been homeless before incarceration (13% compared to 6%), twice as likely to have lived in a foster home or institution while growing up (18% compared to 9%), and three times as likely to report a past history of physical or sexual abuse (24% compared to 8%) than inmates without mental health problems.

- Over one third (37%) of inmates with mental health problems reported that they grew up with a parent who abused alcohol, drugs, or both. This rate was nearly twice that of inmates without mental health problems (19%).

- Incarceration of other family members was a common experience for all inmates; however, inmates with mental health problems (52%) reported past family history of incarceration more often than state prisoners (41%) or jail inmates (36%) without mental health problems.

Data summarized from U.S. Department of Justice (2006). "Mental Health Problems of Prison and Jail Inmates." Bureau of Justice Statistics Special Report, December 14. Available at: http://www.ojp.usdoj.gov/bjs/pub/pdf/mhtppji.pdf (accessed March 2, 2007).

An Occupational Perspective on Incarceration

Under the best of environmental conditions, a person with mental illness experiencing prolonged confinement may feel isolated, bored, and frustrated at the lack of basic comforts.

Evidence-Based Practice

Pope, Lovell, and Hsia (2002) completed a meta-analysis (intensive, critical review of more than 30 studies) that examined studies on race and the juvenile system published in professional academic journals and scholarly books from 1989 through 2001. The authors focused on empirical research studies that addressed the processing of minority youths within the juvenile justice system to examine the impact of race on decisions made in the juvenile justice system.

Key findings included the following:

➤ Nearly three-quarters of the studies (74%) showed negative "race effects," direct or indirect, at one stage or another in the juvenile justice system process.

➤ A youth's racial status made a difference at selected stages of juvenile processing.

➤ Substantial differences were identified in how minority youths were processed within many juvenile justice systems.

➤ These findings were consistent across many of the studies and were independent of the type of research design that was employed.

➤ The results of this meta-analysis supported the existence of disparities in the juvenile justice processing but could not specify the causes and mechanisms of these disparities.

Hartney and Silva (2007) updated a report originally published in 2000 that examined the extent to which minority youths are overrepresented in the criminal justice system. The authors drew on previously published analyses and generated their own original analyses. They also examined national databases including statistics from the National Center for Health Statistics, the FBI's Uniform Crime reporting Program, and U.S. Department of Justice reports.

Key findings included the following:

➤ After controlling for the type of offense, the authors found that black youths are dealt with more severely at every stage of the juvenile justice process than are white youths.

➤ Minority youths are more likely than white youths to be detained by police, to be formally charged by prosecutors, and to be sent to prison by a judge.

➤ The negative impact of race is a cumulative effect that gets compounded at every successive step in the criminal justice system (from arrest to detainment to disposition to sentencing, etc).

➤ Black youths charged with a violent crime but who had not previously been to juvenile prison were nine times more likely than white youths to be sentenced to prison.

➤ Black youths convicted of a drug offense and without a prison record were 48 times more likely than white youths to be sentenced to prison.

Hartney, C., & Silva, F. (2007). And justice for some: Differential treatment of youth of color in the justice system. Washington DC: National Council on Crime and Delinquency. Available at: http://www.nccd-crc.org/nccd/ pubs/2007jan_justice_for_some.pdf (accessed March 1, 2007).

Pope, C. E., Lovell, R., & Hsia, H. M. (2002). Disproportionate minority confinement: A review of the research literature from 1989 through 2001. Washington, DC: Office of Juvenile Justice and Delinquency Prevention. Available at: http://ojjdp.ncjrs.org/dmc/pdf/dmc89_01.pdf (accessed March 1, 2007).

At its worst, the environment is one where a person may be routinely victimized by others or constantly bombarded with sensory stimulation.

> *They [prisons] are tense and overcrowded places in which all prisoners struggle to maintain their self-respect and emotional equilibrium despite omnipresent violence, exploitation, and extortion; despite an utter lack of privacy; stark limitations on family and community contacts; and the paucity of opportunities for education, meaningful work, or other productive, purposeful activities. Prisoners with mental illness must survive as best they can in frequently brutal and brutalizing environments that they may be particularly ill-equipped to navigate. (Human Rights Watch, 2003)*

A small, cramped cell is an ineffective refuge from an overcrowded prison environment that lacks opportunities for engagement in meaningful activity. The images in Figure 37-2 provide two visual examples of confinement spaces. Compare and contrast the physical structure and the objects pictured in these environments to those that you have in your own bedroom.

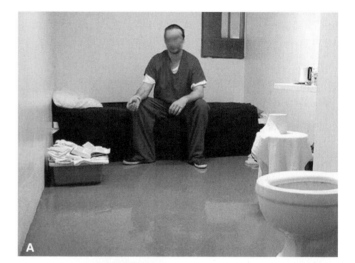

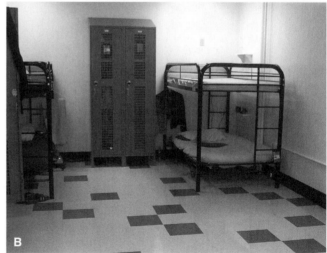

FIGURE 37-2. Two examples of confinement spaces. (A) Individual cell at a county jail. (B) Dormitory room in community corrections site.

Mentally ill offenders may also have to endure corrections personnel and other offenders who stigmatize them, view their mental illness as suspect, and label them as malingerers. In a book documenting his experiences in prison, Victor Hassine (1996) describes the difficulties people with mental illness have coping with day-to-day prison life. Correctional officers often intimidate these prisoners into snitching on other offenders, which is a violation of the prisoners' code, while other offenders threaten or manipulate persons with mental illness into activities that result in serious prison rule infractions. Some offenders try to avoid trouble by isolating themselves in their cells, which often only serves to magnify their disability and the stigmatization that accompanies it (Hassine, 1996).

The occupational science literature contains useful concepts for deepening your understanding of how correctional environments limit engagement in occupation and for designing individual and environmental interventions to address these limitations. These concepts include occupational imbalance, occupational alienation, and occupational deprivation (Wilcock, 1998); occupational restriction and reconciliation (Galvaan, 2005); occupational apartheid (Kronenberg & Pollard, 2005); and occupational enrichment (Molineux & Whiteford, 1999). You are encouraged to examine the references cited here for a deeper understanding of each of these concepts. Brief definitions of each concept and examples of how they may be applied to incarcerated populations are listed in Table 37-2.

Although each of these concepts has relevance for understanding and intervening with offenders in correctional settings, occupational deprivation and occupational engagement provide useful conceptual frameworks for designing skill-building and role-development interventions that support successful community reintegration postrelease and, as such, necessitate further discussion here.

Occupational Deprivation

Occupational deprivation has been defined as "the influence of an external circumstance that keeps a person from acquiring, using, or enjoying something" (Wilcock, 1998, p. 145). It is a tacit dimension of the environment in correctional institutions. Whiteford (1997) completed an occupational needs assessment in a high-security Australian prison and concluded that occupational deprivation not only limited opportunities for participation in occupation while the person was incarcerated but could also pose significant barriers to successful community reintegration postrelease. She asserted that prisoners can become so estranged from the occupational roles of community life that they lose the capacity to structure their time to meet the challenges of community participation, which in turn significantly diminishes the likelihood of adaptive community reintegration. Two primary functions of correctional environments are to confine and to control. As a result, offenders are often deprived of opportunities to engage in occupations that are

Table 37-2 ● **Occupational Science Concepts Applied to Incarceration**

Concept	Definition	Example of Concept Applied to Incarcerated Populations
Occupational alienation (Wilcock, 1998)	"Sense of isolation, powerlessness, frustration, loss of control, estrangement from society or self as a result of engagement in occupation which does not satisfy inner needs" (p. 257).	The primary need for correctional settings to control inmate behavior inevitably limits occupational choices and creates conditions in which the everyday activities of life lack meaning or purpose. It is difficult to feel connected, to create, to feel productive, or to have a sense of purpose in environments where the daily rhythm of life is monotonous and repetitive. Even occupations that may be allowed and that once provided pleasure and meaning, such as reading or physical activity, lose meaning when they become the only choice in a mundane routine.
Occupational apartheid (Kronenberg & Pollard, 2005)	"Refers to the segregation of groups of people through the restriction or denial of access to dignified and meaningful participation in occupations of daily life on the basis of race, color, disability, national origin, age, gender, sexual preference, religion, political beliefs, status in society, or other characteristics" (p. 67).	Applied to incarcerated populations, this concept challenges occupational therapists to examine the social, economic, and political conditions that deny or restrict opportunities for occupational and social participation for some populations, such as the undereducated, the poor, immigrants, and the mentally ill. In addition, there is growing recognition that the high recidivism rates for offenders in the U.S. correctional systems demands a reexamination of correctional policies. Nonetheless, many U.S. citizens continue to believe that prison environments should restrict access to activity and that prisoners should be denied such occupations.
Occupational deprivation (Wilcock, 1998)	"Deprivation of occupational choice and diversity because of circumstances beyond the control of individuals or communities" (p. 257). "Deprivation is distinguished from a disruption in occupational choice because it is a process that occurs over a long period of time" (Whiteford, 1997).	Occupational deprivation is an implicit characteristic of correctional settings, particularly those with higher security levels. That is, restriction in occupational choice is the standard operating procedure of institutions that confine prisoners, systematically denying an offender's need for meaningful and health-promoting occupations.
Occupational enrichment (Molineux & Whiteford, 1999)	"The deliberate manipulation of environments to facilitate and support engagement in a range of occupations congruent with those that the individual might normally perform" (p. 127).	Relative to prisoner populations, occupational enrichment refers to direct interventions in the social, physical, and cultural environment that address occupational deprivation.
Occupational imbalance (Wilcock, 1998)	"A lack of balance or disproportion of occupation resulting in decreased well-being" (p. 257).	In correctional institutions, the environment creates conditions that can significantly limit the opportunity for a person to be involved in a balance of physical, mental, social, and restful occupations. The constriction of both choice of occupations and opportunities to engage in occupations can negatively influence an offender's health and wellbeing

Continued

Table 37-3 ● **Occupational Science Concepts Applied to Incarceration—cont'd**

Concept	Definition	Example of Concept Applied to Incarcerated Populations
Occupational reconciliation (Galvaan, 2005)	This concept describes a person's submissive response to stifling environmental conditions.	Prisoners' lack of opportunity to develop their potential as a result of loneliness, lack of stimulation, and limited resources can lead them to "give way to their circumstances and engage in limited occupations because of their restricted opportunities" (p. 436).
Occupational restriction (Galvaan, 2005)	This concept describes a sense of devaluation experienced by domestic workers whose occupational choices are severely controlled by their employers' needs. Occupational restriction leaves a person feeling as if they have no control, no choices, and no options for engaging the environment except as organized and controlled by the correctional institution's needs.	In prison environments, systematic denial of occupation and the external control over basic choices can lead many offenders to devalue themselves and the occupations in which they engage.

necessary or meaningful. The end result of occupational deprivation can include diminished capacities, reduced self-efficacy, and significant loss of identity as a citizen of the community (Whiteford, 1997; 2000). Whiteford's needs assessment of a maximum-security prison concluded that for mentally ill offenders, occupational deprivation may actually increase psychiatric symptoms.

It was our assessment that the environment that had been created to ensure the safety of inmates and wardens and to better manage acute disorientation and brief psychotic episodes had in itself contributed to a situation where vulnerable inmates were more likely to experience these phenomenon. (1997, p. 129)

Occupational Enrichment

Close your eyes for a moment and envision the ideal therapeutic environment for offenders with severe and persistent mental illness. Make special note of the social environment. Who is there, what do they look like, and what are they doing? How do they interact with one another? Pay attention to the details of the physical environment. What materials are used in the built environment? How are they arranged? What opportunity for activity does the physical space invite? What colors are used? How are plants or natural light part of the context? What are the prominent symbols and artifacts in the environment? Now compare what you visualized with your understanding of what the physical and social environment of a correctional institution might be like. It is critical for occupational therapists to consider how to influence the environmental context of correctional institutions to provide opportunities for meaningful engagement in occupation.

Molineux and Whiteford (1999) offer the concept of occupational enrichment as a guiding principle to enhance correctional settings where occupational deprivation is a consistent characteristic of the environment. **Occupational enrichment** is "the deliberate manipulation of environments to facilitate and support engagement in a range of occupations congruent with those that the individual might normally perform" (p. 127). Criminal justice settings place significant restrictions on inmates' opportunities for engagement in meaningful activities. The typical daily routine in all correctional settings, but particularly in the most secure settings, is structured by a strict schedule for meals,

showering, security checks, staff shift changes, and lights out. In some settings, in-house jobs such as cooking or washing dishes in the staff cafeteria, janitorial tasks, laundry, and assisting in a library may be available to well-disciplined offenders on the recommendation of correctional officers. Classes (such as adult literacy, GED, or computer instruction), religious services, recovery support groups, and reintegration education may also offer some diversion from the consistent routine.

As occupational therapists, however, we know that activities that lack personal and cultural meaning for an individual cannot be considered occupation. Simply adding objects or opportunities in the physical or social environment will not necessarily result in a sense of meaning or purpose. Meaningful occupation is in the mind and being of the individual. Films about prison life often provide excellent examples of this point. For example, the Stephen King story *The Green Mile* describes a year in the lives and deaths of guards and inmates on a death row in a Louisiana prison in the 1930s. One inmate awaiting death, named Del, captures and trains a small mouse to do tricks. For Del, the training of this mouse is his meaningful occupation. The training occupies his time, provides him immense pleasure, and even offers opportunities for socialization with the other prisoners and guards as Del encourages others to watch his mouse, Mr. Jingles, perform tricks.

This example illustrates that the underlying principle of individualizing occupational interventions to the person and his or her unique environmental context applies to men and women in correctional settings as well. Expanding opportunities for engagement in self-care, leisure, and productive activities is one strategy for occupational enrichment. However, there are several unique challenges to incorporating occupational enrichment in correctional settings. To begin with, it is difficult to find ways to individualize interventions in a context where conformity is valued as a method for confinement and control. Another challenge lies in finding ways to influence the physical and social environment when a consistent characteristic of the environment is to severely restrict the offender's capacity to gain any measure of control over the environment. Finally, it is difficult to define ways for offenders to have choice over how they orchestrate their daily routine in an environmental context where nearly every activity is completed in a manner dictated by the correctional institution. The following quote from Whiteford's analysis of a medium-security prison environment should help you see both the necessity of enabling occupations in correctional environments and the impact that even simple changes in the environment can produce.

> There was, however, one very bright spot on the daily occupation horizon. That was the fish tank, which some enlightened prison administrator had had installed a year before we arrived. Such was the power of being involved in any of the occupations associated with the fish (e.g., feeding and cleaning) that the inmates would swap privileges, food, and even the main currency of the prison—cigarettes—in order to have more time on fish care. Staff reported inmates being up before 4:30 a.m., dressed and waiting for their turn to feed the fish. (p. 128)

In the United Kingdom, where occupational therapists have a long history of contributing to the rehabilitation of offenders, practitioners were part of an interdisciplinary team that defined standards of quality care in four medium-security units (Allured, 2005). The standards were developed and fine-tuned on the basis of 2-day onsite visits to each medium-security unit in the region. Many of these standards, listed in Box 37-4, specifically addressed the environmental context and opportunities for meaningful engagement in daily occupations. The standards were used to evaluate 17 medium-security units across England. If the environmental standards were met, these interventions could alleviate some of the effects of occupational deprivation.

Future Directions

Although occupational deprivation and engagement may be very relevant conceptual frameworks for occupational therapists to contribute to intervention and policy within

---

BOX 37-4 ■ Quality Standards for Medium-Security Units in the United Kingdom

1. Clear process for admission
2. Clear process for discharge, transfer, and follow-up
3. Clear process for workforce planning
4. Clear process, including advocacy, to encourage inmates to contribute to their own care
5. Clear arrangements for comprehensive clinical governance
6. Opportunity for inmate input to quality improvement
7. Local liaisons with referring agencies
8. Suitable physical environment
9. Availability of therapeutic interventions
10. Availability of interventions to assess and meet health needs
11. Opportunity to engage in vocational, leisure, educational, and living skill activities
12. Opportunity to maintain contact with family and social relations
13. Respect for cultural differences
14. Staff guidance on managing positive relationships on the unit

Source: Allured, I. (2005). Quality in medium secure units. *Mental Health Review, 10*(3), 21–24.

---

correctional settings, these concepts need to be further defined (O'Connell & Farnworth, 2007). Occupational therapists will need to generate the research evidence that bolsters arguments that humans have occupational natures and that deprivation negatively influences health and well-being. Research evidence is also needed that demonstrates that occupational enrichment can result in observable and measurable outcomes that mitigate the negative effects of incarceration and support successful reentry for prisoners postrelease.

Occupational Therapy Programming in Correctional Settings

Forensic mental health is an area of practice that is beginning to be discussed more frequently in occupational therapy professional journals, textbooks, and educational programs within the United States. It is easy to find entire journals specifically addressing forensic practice in the disciplines of nursing, psychology, or psychiatry (e.g., *Journal of Forensic Psychology Practice, American Journal of Forensic Psychiatry,* and *Journal of Forensic Nursing*). In occupational therapy, however, the evidence-based literature in corrections is relatively small, but descriptions of individual practitioner's experiences as well as group interventions with various subsets of prisoner populations can be found (O'Connell & Farnworth, 2007). In addition, occupational therapists in the United Kingdom, Canada, Australia, and Africa have been developing and describing some of their intervention methods with incarcerated populations for some time (Eggers et al, 2006; Mountain, 1998). Despite the cultural and correctional system differences in these countries, these descriptions serve as important resources for the development of occupational therapy practice in U.S. forensic settings.

The Role of the Occupational Therapist

In many ways, forensic mental health in occupational therapy is not that different from other forms of mental health specialty practice in occupational therapy (Chackersfield & Forshaw, 1997). An obvious difference between mental health specialty practice and forensic mental health is that intervention occurs in a secure environmental context. The forensic occupational therapist can practice in a broad multidisciplinary environment that can include health care professionals (e.g., nurses, social workers, psychologists) and professionals from legal and nonmedical arenas (e.g., lawyers, judges, correctional officers, parole officers). The occupational therapist's unique contribution to the forensic team comes from his or her training to apply participation in occupations as a healing modality and his or her ability to consider characteristics of the person and of the environment in any rehabilitation intervention.

Martin (2001) has suggested that forensic nurses seek additional training in criminal justice and counseling skills, and this is a recommendation that may also be relevant for occupational therapists. In a similar vein, nurses in the United States and in other countries have developed a set of forensic competencies, including risk assessment for forensic populations; understanding professional, legal, and ethical issues related to incarceration; psychoeducational and cognitive behavioral approaches; gender-specific interventions; and enhanced interpersonal competencies required for working with prisoner populations (Watson 2002; Watson & Kirby, 2000; Woods, 2004). O'Connell and Farnworth (2007) reported that some of the roles of occupational therapists in a forensic setting include activities of daily living and instrumental activities of daily living skills training for community reintegration and the capacity to participate in court proceedings as necessary. Table 37-3 lists some of the knowledge and skill sets needed for practice in correctional settings based on descriptions of competencies within and outside the occupational therapy profession, descriptions of forensic occupational therapy practice culled from the literature, and consultations with U.S. practitioners working in forensic settings.

Models of Practice

There are several models of practice for occupational therapy that could effectively be used to address the needs of offenders. The model of human occupation (MOHO) is frequently defined as a practice framework for assessment and/or program design (Couldrick & Aldred, 2003; Eggers et al, 2006, Forsyth, Duncan, & Mann, 2005; Farnworth, Nikitin, & Fossey, 2004; Tayar, 2004). Other models that have been described as providing the structure for program design and intervention include the Canadian model of occupational performance (Clarke, 2003; Duncan, 2004), the Role Acquisition Model (Schindler, 2004) and the Occupational Adaptation Model (Stelter & Whisner, 2007). It is important to note that each of these models can be described as comprehensive models of occupational functioning that provide multiple constructs for conceptualizing occupational function and dysfunction. Similarly, each, to a greater or lesser degree, offers specific concepts for considering the physical and social environment. Finally, each provides assessment tools for evaluation.

Assessment of Forensic Populations

Duncan, Munro, and Nicol (2003) asked more than 70 practitioners with an average of 3 or more years working in forensic settings in the United Kingdom to identify assessment tools they routinely employed. The vast majority of the tools identified by these therapists were grounded in MOHO:

- Observation tools included the Assessment of Motor and Process Skills, the Assessment of Communication and Interaction Skills, the Model of Human Occupation Screening Tool, the Occupational Therapy Task Observation Scale (Margolis, Harrison, Robinson, & Jayaram, 1996), the Comprehensive Occupational Therapy Evaluation (Kunz & Brayman, 1999), and the Volitional Questionnaire.
- Self-report instruments included the Interest Checklist (Matsutsuyu, 1969), the Role Checklist, and the Occupational Self-Assessment.
- Interviews included the Assessment of Occupational Functioning, the Canadian Occupational Performance Measure (Law, et al, 2005), the Occupational Circumstances Assessment Interview and Rating Scale, and the Occupational Performance History Interview II (Kielhofner, 2008).

Each of these MOHO tools is briefly described in Kielhofner's latest text (2008), and some are discussed elsewhere in this book.

The only tool specifically designed to assess the explicit needs of incarcerated populations is the Occupational Circumstances Assessment Interview and Rating Scale (OCAIRS). The OCAIRS is a semistructured interview based on MOHO. Interview questions have been modified for use with forensic populations. Questions are designed to elicit data on roles, habits, personal causation, values, readiness for change, interests, skills, goals, interpretation of past experiences, and the physical and social environment

Table 37-3 ● **Knowledge and Skill Set for Forensic Mental Health Practice**

Type of Skill	Specific Skills
Interpersonal	• Ability to initiate therapeutic relationships with inmates • Capacity to collaborate with correctional staff • Effective listening skills • Effective de-escalation strategies • Strong communications skills
Knowledge	• Appreciate correctional systems structure and functioning • Be familiar with corrections subculture • Know and use effective outcome measures to evaluate interventions • Understand process and methods for risk assessment and risk management • Recognize postrelease options for continuity of care • Understand social, occupational, and restorative justice perspective
Practical	• Ability to document clearly and concisely • Capacity to maintain confidentiality • Coping skills for managing institutional and environmental stressors • Self-defense for maintaining personal safety • Familiarity with how to access community services, particularly those with expertise serving ex-offenders
Professional development	• Consistent professionalism • Clear professional identity • Cultural competency • Strong commitment to ongoing professional development

(Parkinson, Forsyth, & Kielhofner, 2006). To date, no published studies have examined the usefulness of this tool in practice (O'Connell & Farnworth, 2007).

The ability to effectively interview an occupational therapy client is an essential skill for every practitioner. Regardless of what tool is used to elicit a person's occupational profile, a practitioner working in correctional settings must approach the interview process with the mind of a scientist. Look for data, withhold assumptions, and verify conclusions when the data supports your reasoning. The following quote from Candice DeLong, a psychiatric nurse and 20-year veteran of the FBI, exemplifies this point:

Chances are, when you are dealing with a patient under stress, what you hear them saying is not necessarily what happened. In stressful situations, some people deliberately lie, or they minimize their involvement in anything that makes them look bad or suspicious. As a forensic nurse, you must be circumspect about the first interview. It has been my experience that people under duress, whether they are in a law enforcement setting or a clinical setting, are worked up because they have been victimized in some way. You should not believe everything you hear and you should not necessarily believe your own eyes. Just be very scientific and look at the data you are getting. What is the patient really saying? Ask the patient the same question from different angles and be prepared to accept that the first story you get from the patient may not be accurate. (as cited in Pyrek, 2006, p. 412)

Risk Assessment

One area of assessment specific to the forensic mental health setting is risk assessment. Risk assessment is a crucial function in correctional institutions because it is viewed as a means to gauge an offender's potential to commit another offense. For offenders with mental illness, it is also used to evaluate the risk of violence.

Assessment of risk is determined by considering the presence and relevance of certain conditions assumed to be risk factors (Elbogen, 2002). Two broad categories of risk factors are typically considered. **Static risk factors** are unchanging characteristics of the individual, such as his or her age at first offense, gender, or history of prior convictions or violence. **Dynamic risk factors** are variables of risk that can change over time and can include socioeconomic, marital, or employment status; family support; criminal network; and substance abuse (Lindsay & Beail, 2004). Hanson and Harris (2000) suggested that dynamic factors can be further subdivided into stable and acute factors. In their model, **stable dynamic factors** are characteristics that remain unchanged for longer periods of time but are treatable, such as alcoholism, drug abuse, or attitudes toward violence. **Acute dynamic factors** are those characteristics that can change extremely quickly, such as the deterioration in mood or thought processing often seen in the exacerbation of mental illness or negative behavioral outcomes as a result of alcohol intoxication.

Risk assessment is typically performed by psychologists and psychiatrists. Widely used risk assessment measures include the following tools:

■ The Psychopathy Checklist-Revised (PCL-R) is a structured professional judgment assessment used to measure criminal recidivism, violence, and sexual violence (Hare, 1991). The clinician measures psychopathology by rating 20 items on a 3-point scale: 0 (absent), 1 (some indication of the variable), and 2 (clear evidence of the variable).

■ The Level of Service Inventory-Revised (LSI-R) is a structured professional judgment assessment that assesses eight broad risk factors: antisocial attitudes; antisocial thoughts; cognitions and ways of thinking; antisocial personality; antisocial history; employment, family, leisure, and recreational activities; substance abuse problems; and antisocial peers or criminal associates (Andrews & Bonta, 1995).

■ The Violence Risk Appraisal Guide (VRAG) has 12 variables, including the Psychopathy Checklist–Revised (PCL-R) score, which is weighted most heavily in the analysis (Quinsey, Harris, Rice, & Cromier, 1998). Historical (e.g., age at first offense, history of violence) and diagnostic variables (e.g., personality disorder, alcohol abuse, schizophrenia) also influence the VRAG score. It is noteworthy to consider that a diagnosis of schizophrenia has an inverse relation to risk of violence.

Occupational therapists should have a working understanding of the purpose and intent of risk assessment and some of the primary tools used to measure risk. When appropriate, practitioners can contribute their observations to improve the interdisciplinary team's clinical judgment. From a person–environment interaction perspective, it is essential to note the significance of sociodemographic factors environmental influences, especially the presence of substance abuse, in predicting recidivism and violence (Lindsay & Beail, 2004). On the other hand, relatively little is known about how clinical variables and contextual or environmental factors interact to influence recidivism or violence in offender populations (Norko & Baranoski, 2005). Occupational therapists might use a person–environment perspective to examine whether interventions directed at influencing occupation and the social and interpersonal environments where ex-offenders engage in occupation offer a productive risk-management strategy to reduce recidivism.

Occupational Therapy Interventions

Nearly 30 years ago, Penner (1978) provided an overview of the U.S. criminal justice system and concluded the profession had a unique contribution to make to the rehabilitation of incarcerated populations. In her textbook on community-based practice, Scaffa (2001) suggests that services that focus on skill development, relapse prevention, community reintegration, and employment are appropriate interventions for occupational therapy programming in correctional settings. In another textbook, Snively and Dressler (2005) share a few examples of occupational therapy programming in jails, prisons, and community correctional settings. Descriptions of forensic occupational therapy first emerged in the United Kingdom in the 1980s (Chackersfield & Forshaw, 1997; Mountain, 1998), and a National Forensic Occupational Therapy Conference has been taking place annually in the United Kingdom since 1999 (Duncan, Munro, & Nicol, 2003). Despite this, the international occupational therapy literature has relatively few examples of contemporary, evidence-based programs in correctional settings (O'Connell & Farnworth, 2007).

Interventions addressing employment and education issues with offenders have appeared in the occupational therapy literature for over two decades (Chackersfield & Forshaw, 1997; Farnworth, 1987; Garner, 1995; Lloyd, 1985, 1987a, 1987b). These programs tend to use group interventions to address problem-solving and social skills (Garner, 1995), to evaluate the employability of the offender, and to develop work-related skills to reenter the competitive job market (Lloyd, 1988). Many of the older references to occupational therapy programming in correctional settings suggest the challenges of and intervention strategies for providing services to specific subgroups of the prisoner population. Examples include programs designed to help sex offenders develop parenting skills (Lloyd, 1989) and programs that address addiction issues (Chackersfield & Forshaw, 1997). In a more recent edited textbook on forensic occupational therapy, Couldrick and Aldred (2003) include several chapters describing interventions with various subgroups of the offender population.

Duncan, Munro, and Nicol (2003) surveyed more than 70 practitioners with an average of 3 or more years of experience working in forensic settings to identify the titles they assigned to groups included as part of their intervention services. These titles were then thematically categorized by the researchers. Groups that addressed effective communication and social skills training were, by far, the most frequently occurring group, followed by life skills groups. Other types of groups relatively frequently focused on drug and alcohol addiction, anxiety management, mental health awareness/education, and anger management. Baker and McKay (2001) surveyed occupational therapists working in Regional Secure Units in the United Kingdom about their perceptions of the needs of incarcerated women and found over 70% of the programs included interventions addressing functional life skills, social skills, assertiveness training, stress management, problem-solving, and recreational skills.

The more recent literature provides encouraging evidence that practitioners are beginning to apply occupational therapy practice models to guide their interventions and are using valid and reliable assessments to evaluate occupational performance patterns of offenders (Crist et al, 2005; Duncan, 2004; Forsyth et al, 2005; Farnworth et al, 2004). Eggers et al (2006) provide one of the most complete descriptions of occupational therapy programming in a county jail available in the occupational therapy literature. These authors describe the Community Reintegration Project, a program at the Allegheny County Jail in Pittsburgh, Pennsylvania, that grew out of a community university partnership in which faculty from Duquesne University collaborated with the correctional staff at the local county jail and Goodwill Industries of Pittsburgh to bring occupational therapy programming into the county jail. This program is designed to decrease recidivism and support successful community reintegration. A multidisciplinary staff, directed by the occupational therapist, addresses these overall goals by focusing on four key domains of reintegration: wellness, family and support structure, skills for living, and education and employment. This structured program begins with group and individual interventions while the offender is incarcerated and follows the offender for up to 1 year postrelease using an intensive case management model to support successful reintegration. Case managers are referred to as reintegration specialists and collaborate with each offender to develop an Individualized Reintegration Plan, which identifies specific and realistic goals in each domain area.

Other programs exist but as yet are not described in the published literature. For example, for the last few years, Dr. Barbara Hooper and Johanna Cubra, a community-based occupational therapy practitioner in New Mexico, have been developing gender-specific programming at Dismas House, a community-based transitional program for female offenders. The group intervention protocols developed for Dismas House focus on work acquisition, work maintenance, leisure, citizenship, community reintegration, and empowerment. These protocols served as the basis for a program Dr. Toby Hamilton at the University of Oklahoma has been developing and delivering for the past 3 years with her students at the Oklahoma Halfway House, a nonprofit correctional residential facility (personal communication, Dr. Toby Hamilton, June 26, 2007). These programs recognize that incarcerated women have different needs than men (Bloom, Owen, & Covington, 2003). The interventions address these gender differences by focusing on the maintenance of a safe environment (physical and emotional) and addressing the skills needed to build and sustain healthy relationships with children and family. These programs also seek to provide opportunities for women to improve their socioeconomic status and develop connections to their community and to services that support reintegration. Brief descriptions of other programs described in the occupational therapy literature are listed in Table 37-4.

Table 37-4 ● **Occupational Therapy Programming in Correctional Settings**

Authors	Setting	OT Role	Type of Interventions
Clarke (2003)	Forensic hostel, UNITED KINGDOM	Uses Canadian model of occupational performance for assessment and intervention	Daily living skills; psychological issues; work, education, and leisure engagement; community reintegration. Environmental focus to consider offender's physical and social environment.
Baker & McKay (2001)	Medium-secure unit, UNITED KINGDOM	Varied by setting but generally integrated into correctional system with skills building, one-to-one and group interventions	Most common service delivery was one to one, then group interventions addressing skills development in instrumental activities of daily living, interpersonal relations, assertiveness, stress management, problem-solving, work, leisure, community reintegration, and gender-specific issues.
Duncan (2004)	Prison prerelease program for women, SOUTH AFRICA	Occupational coaching for women offenders' postprison adjustment	Occupational storytelling to facilitate collaborative goal setting and to reveal patterns of occupational engagement. Develop interpersonal and self-maintenance strategies, including self-defense; prepare vitae; practice job interview skills and journal writing.

Table 37-4 ● Occupational Therapy Programming in Correctional Settings—cont'd

Authors	Setting	OT Role	Type of Interventions
Duncan (2004)	Youth diversion program, SOUTH AFRICA	Addresses self-efficacy and personal control through doing and identifies community service tasks for the youth	Variety of services focused on academic and/or practical skills training, community service, life skills training, prosocial leisure and physical recreation.
Eggers et al (2006)	County jail, UNITED STATES	Supports community reintegration, vocational exploration, and work	Individual and group interventions focused on four domains: wellness, family support/structure, living skills, and education and employment.
Jones & McColl (1991)	Forensic inpatient service unit, CANADA	Addresses interpersonal skill and intrapersonal growth	Biweekly life skills program; group interventions featuring facilitated self-disclosure and feedback, self-evaluation in context of individual, and group task participation and interpersonal skills and effect on others.
Schindler (2004)	Maximum-security psychiatric facility, UNITED STATES	Supports role development	Group interventions focused on supporting persons with schizophrenia to internalize social roles and develop prosocial task and interpersonal skills.
Snively & Dressler (2005)	Community program, UNITED STATES	Prevents relapse and/or reoffense while stabilizing the client in the community	Address work skills, independent living skills, and development of social supports. Group and one-on-one interventions addressing skills building, symptom recognition, acceptance of mental illness, substance abuse prevention, social skills training, stress management, life skills, and problem solving.
Tayar (2004)	Rural women's prison, UNITED STATES	Educates about relapse prevention, develops skills set for coping	Substance abuse relapse prevention program delivered by occupational therapists and psychology students. Activities to identify values and interests, develop resources for leisure and employment, time management, social and assertiveness skills using psychoeducation, individual writing exercises, group discussions, narratives, and role-playing techniques.

Summary

In an ideal world, every correctional setting would have established policies for screening the mental health of offenders and a wide array of mental health services provided by well-trained, professional staff. The current state of services for offenders who are mentally ill have not reached this ideal. Nonetheless, mental health services in forensic settings should strive to equal best practices in community-based service delivery—that is, to support and facilitate the highest level of recovery and to help the individual develop a skill set that supports full community integration and participation and meaningful quality of life.

From the earliest days of its inception, the profession of occupational therapy has been grounded in concepts that support every person's full integration into society (Kielhofner, 2008). Occupational therapists work with a number of populations that experience challenges to full community integration (e.g., children with autism, individuals diagnosed with AIDS, people who experience a traumatic brain injury). Individuals who have been incarcerated represent another large and growing population, and occupational therapists have the potential to significantly impact the quality of the reintegration experience.

Active Learning Strategies

1. "Boxed In": A Simulation in Confinement

This exercise is designed to help you experience confinement emotionally and physiologically and better understand the occupational deprivation that goes along with confinement.

Choose a time when you can be reasonably assured of being alone in your living space for at least a few hours. Find a space in your apartment or home where you cannot see or hear a clock, phone, television, or audio equipment. Use masking tape or tape and string to mark an 8-foot by 10-foot rectangle so that the boundaries are clearly visible. If possible, arrange your rectangle in a corner of your room so that there are blank walls on two sides. Do not put your rectangle next to a window, but if you have no choice, draw the shades so you cannot look out. This is your box.

Now choose any two, but only two, of the following items: one book, one pad of paper and something to write with, a deck of cards, a photo album, a bottle of water, or one small snack. Put these in your box. Do not bring anything else into your box. This means no electronics, cell phone, computer, camera, clock, TV remote, or other items.

Before you step into your box, remove any jewelry you may be wearing and take off your watch. Check the time on a clock in another room and record the time on a piece of paper. Enter your box and remain in the box for as long as you can, but for at least 2 hours. Do not ever let your body or any of the items you brought in with you stretch beyond the boundaries of your box. When you feel you can no longer remain in the box, record the time you left and consider the following guided reflections.

Reflective Questions
- What did it feel like getting into your box?
- What criteria did you use when deciding what two things to bring in with you?
- What was your mood like at the start, middle, and end of your "confinement"?
- What did you miss the most, and what did it feel like to be denied access to your favorite things?
- How did you mark time?
- How do you feel you might react if you had to live in this amount of space for the next 365 days?
- Did this simulation provide insights into the experience of confinement? Explain.

 Record your responses to these questions in your **Reflective Journal**.

2. Reflection on Personal and Professional Boundaries

Occupational therapists working in correctional settings may find themselves in a very isolated and sometimes stressful environment. Practitioners are providing a service to offenders in a correctional setting—cultural context that may be very different from clinical or community settings where they have trained or practiced before. This exercise is designed to help you to reflect on your ability to develop and maintain professional boundaries that ensure safe interactions between you and consumers with mental illness in correctional settings. Provide an answer for each of the five directives listed below, then share your responses with one other peer or in a small group.

1. Define "personal boundaries" and give an example of another's behavior when that person crossed one of your personal boundaries.
2. Define "professional boundaries" and explain similarities and/or differences between personal and professional boundaries.
3. Generate a list of reasons that we need boundaries.
4. The definition of boundary suggests there is a clearly defined line of demarcation. Identify a situation or interaction that could occur in a correctional setting between a practitioner and an offender in which boundaries are crystal clear. Identify a situation or interaction that could occur in a correctional setting between a practitioner and an offender in which boundaries are less clear.
5. Review your responses to question 3 and determine if you have considered all of the following possibilities: personal comfort; knowing what to do in certain situations to maintain clarity in relationships, to maintain a professional stance, to ensure safety, to ensure confidentiality, to protect from legal issues, and to abide by professional codes of ethics so others know what to expect from us.

3. Reflection on Safety and Security

Occupational therapists working with prisoners and with persons recently released from a correctional setting should be aware that there are some risks, and this is particularly true of postrelease work. However, the chances of a significant problem arising and the risk of being put in a seriously dangerous situation are small. You can reduce risk by knowing and following all security and safety procedures. This reflective exercise is designed to help you to consider knowledge, attitudes, and skill sets that can support success in correctional settings. Review the two lists of strategies with another peer or in a small group. Discuss how each strategy represents a specific method for maintaining personal safety and security.

General Strategies for Working With Offenders
- Wear appropriate, modest clothing.
- Do not make promises that you may not or will not keep.
- Know the consumer; seek out information about any risk that any consumer may represent.
- Do not give or accept gifts.
- Guard personal information (e.g., personal circumstances, family details, home address, telephone number).
- If an offender is distressed or escalating at the end of your therapy session, make sure to communicate this to corrections staff.
- Always share information when an offender discloses any intention of self-harm, suicide, physical violence, uprising, or escape.
- Always disclose to staff if an offender at your setting is a personal friend or relative.
- Do not do favors (e.g., run errands, mail letters, make phone calls) for offenders or ask them to do a favor for you.
- In community corrections settings, do not agree to transport a resident anywhere if you have not read a detailed risk assessment; even then, make sure you carry a mobile phone and that other staff know your travel plan, including expected departure and arrival times.
- Avoid meetings in your own community, and do not give details that disclose where you live.

Strategies for Reducing Risk and Maintaining Security
- Any keys should be concealed and secured. Never put keys down anywhere.
- Educate yourself to know how offenders can use keys, tools, food, chemicals, cleaning or medical supplies to escape or cause injury to self or others.
- Know how to call for emergency assistance if needed, and be clear on how you should respond should an alarm sound.
- Understand procedures for maintaining and controlling materials and tools within the occupational therapy environment.
- Organize workspace to always maintain clear access to an exit and to emergency alarm systems.
- Always double check gates, doors, cabinets, windows, and so on, to confirm that the lock is functioning.
- It is your responsibility to fully understand security procedures and requirements, to find out when you are not sure, to ask when you visit a new facility, and to make sure you always follow procedures (e.g., policies for escape prevention, emergency response, custody escorts, lockup units, tool control, syringe counts, key control).
- Strictly observe rules for what can and cannot be taken into a correctional setting, and limit the personal possessions you carry as much as possible.
- If you are at all instinctively uncomfortable about working with an offender, especially in the community, it is prudent to follow that instinct.

Resources

- The Federal Bureau of Prisons website provides an excellent overview of various types of prison facilities, updated statistics on the U.S. prison population, and research reports on a variety of topics such as prison populations, mental health and drug treatment, and postrelease employment. http://www.bop.gov/about/index.jsp
- The Legal Action Center website has a variety of resources that reflect this organization's mission to (1) improve the criminal justice system by helping offenders fight stigma and discrimination related to employment, housing, education, and political activity; (2) advocate for just sentencing laws, particularly for nonviolent offenders, and for reasonable alternatives to incarceration; and (3) research the barriers to community reentry and programs to address these barriers. http://lac.org/index.php/lac/category/criminal_justice_programs
- The PEW Center on the States: Corrections and Public Safety collects and analyzes data on sentencing and correction policies and practices to advance prison reform and reduce recidivism in the U.S. corrections system. Multiple resources are available for free download, and two recent useful guides include *One in 100: Behind Bars in America* (February 2008) and *One in 31: The Long Reach of American Corrections* (March 2009). http://www.pewcenteronthestates.org/topic_category.aspx?category=528
- The Sentencing Project is a national organization that has advocated for a fair and effective criminal justice system for over 20 years. This website provides a wealth of research, publications, and policy reviews on a variety of topics, including inequities in the U.S. criminal justice system, sentencing laws and practices, and alternatives to incarceration. http://www.sentencingproject.org/template/index.cfm

References

Allured, I. (2005). Quality in medium secure units. *Mental Health Review, 10*(3), 21–24.

American Psychiatric Association. (2000). *Psychiatric Services in Jails and Prisons: A Task Force Report of the American Psychiatric Association* (2nd ed.). Washington, DC: Author.

Andrews, D. A., & Bonta, J. (1995). *LSI-R: The Level of Service Inventory–Revised.* Toronto: Multi-Health Systems.

Baker, S., & McKay, E. A. (2001). Occupational therapists' perspectives of the needs of women in medium secure units. *British Journal of Occupational Therapy, 64*(9), 441–448.

Banks, C. (2005). *Punishment in America: A Reference Handbook.* Santa Barbara, CA: ABC CLIO.

Beck, A. J., & Harrison, P. M. (2001). *Prisoners in 2000.* Washington, DC: U.S. Department of Justice, Bureau of Justice Statistics.

Beck, A. J., & Maruschak, L. M. (2001). *Mental Health Treatment in State Prisons.* U.S. Department of Justice, Bureau of Justice Statistics Special Report, July. Available at: http://www.ojp.usdoj.gov/bjs/pub/pdf/mhtsp00.pdf (accessed March 2, 2007).

Bernstein, J., & Houston, E. (2000). *Crime and Work: What Can We Learn From the Low Wage Labor Market?* Washington, DC: Economic Policy Institute.

Bloom, B., Owen, B., & Covington, S. (2003). *Gender-Responsive Strategies: Research, Practice, and Guiding Principles for Women Offenders.* Washington, DC: National Institute of Corrections.

Brazelton Center for Mental Health Law. (2007). "The Role of Mental Health Courts in System Reform." Available at: http://www.bazelon.org/issues/criminalization/publications/mentalhealthcourts (accessed May 2, 2007).

Bureau of Justice Assistance. (2007). "Mental Health Courts Program." Washington, DC: U.S. Department of Justice. Available at: http://www.ojp.usdoj.gov/BJA/grant/mentalhealth.html (accessed April 22, 2007).

Bureau of Justice Statistics (2009). Correctional populations. Key facts at a glance. http://bjs.ojp.usdoj.gov/content/glance/tables/corr2tab.cfm (accessed March 10, 2010).

Chackersfield, J., & Forshaw, D. (1997). Occupational therapy and forensic addictive behaviors. *British Journal of Therapy and Rehabilitation, 4*(7), 381–386.

Clarke, C. (2003). Clinical application of the Canadian model of occupational performance in a forensic rehabilitation hostel. *British Journal of Occupational Therapy, 66*(4), 171–174.

Couldrick, L., & Aldred, D. (2003). *Forensic Occupational Therapy.* London: Whurr.

Crist, P., Fairman, A., Muñoz, J. P., Hansen, A. M., Sciulli, J., & Eggers, M. (2005). Education and practice collaborations: A pilot case study between a university faculty and county jail practitioners. *Occupational Therapy in Health Care, 19*(1/2), 193–210.

Duncan, E. A., Munro, K., & Nicol, M. M. (2003). Research priorities in forensic occupational therapy. *British Journal of Occupational Therapy, 66*(2), 55–64.

Duncan, M. (2004). Occupation in the criminal justice system. In R. Watson & L. Swartz, (Eds), *Transformation Through Occupation* (pp. 129–142). London: Whurr.

Eggers, M., Muñoz, J. P., Sciulli, J., & Crist, P. A. H. (2006). The community reintegration project: Occupational therapy at work in a county jail. *Occupational Therapy in Health Care, 20*(1), 17–37.

Elbogen, E. B. (2002) The process of violence risk assessment: A review of descriptive research. *Aggression & Violent Behaviour, 7,* 591–604.

Farnworth, L. (1987). Prison-based occupational therapy. *Australian Occupational Therapy Journal, 34*(2), 40–46.

Farnworth, L., Nikitin, L., & Fossey, E. (2004). Being in a secure forensic psychiatric unit: Every day is the same, killing time or making the most of it. *British Journal of Occupational Therapy, 67*(10), 430–438.

Forsyth, K., Duncan, E. A. S., & Mann, L. S. (2005). Scholarship of practice in the United Kingdom: An occupational therapy service case study. *Occupational Therapy in Health Care, 19*(12), 17–29.

Galvaan, R. (2005). Domestic workers' narratives: Transforming occupational therapy practice. In F. Kronenberg, S. S. Algado, & N. Pollard (Eds.), *Occupational Therapy Without Borders: Learning From the Spirit of Survivors* (pp. 429–439). London: Elsevier Churchill Livingstone.

Garner, R. (1995). Prevocational training within a secure environment; A programme designed to enable the forensic patient to prepare for mainstream opportunities. *British Journal of Occupational Therapy, 58*(1), 2–6.

Griffin, P., Torbet, P., & Szymanski, L. (1998). *Trying Juveniles as Adults in Criminal Court: An Analysis of State Transfer Provisions.* Washington, DC: U.S. Office of Juvenile Justice and Delinquency Prevention.

Hanson, R. K., & Harris, A. J. R. (2000) Where should we intervene? Dynamic predictors of sexual offence recidivism. *Criminal Justice & Behaviour, 27,* 6–35.

Hare, R. (1991). *The Hare Psychopathy Checklist–Revised.* Toronto: Multi-Health Systems.

Hartney, C. & Silva, S. (2007). *And Justice for Some: Differential Treatment of Youth of Color in the Justice System.* Washington, DC: National Council on Crime and Delinquency.

Hassine, V. (1996). *Life Without Parole: Living in Prison Today.* Los Angeles: Roxbury.

Human Rights Watch. (2002). "Race and Incarceration in the United States." Available at: http://hrw.org/backgrounder/usa/race (accessed May 17, 2007).

———. (2003) *Ill-equipped: U. S. Prisons and Offenders with Mental Illness.* New York: NY Human Rights Watch. Available at: http://www.hrw.org/reports/2003/usa1003 (accessed March 14, 2007).

James, D. J., & Glaze, L. E. (2006). *Mental Health Problems of Prison and Jail Inmates.* U.S. Department of Justice, Bureau of Justice Statistics Special Report, December 12. Available at: http://www.ojp.usdoj.gov/bjs/pub/pdf/mhtppji.pdf (accessed March 2, 2007).

Jones, E. J., & McColl, M. A. (1991). Development and evaluation of an interreactional life skills group for offenders. *Occupational Therapy Journal of Research, 11,* 80–92.

Kielhofner, G. (2008). *The Model of Human Occupation: Theory and Application* (4th ed.). Philadelphia: F.A. Davis.

King's College. "International Centre for Prison Studies Prison Brief—Lowest to Highest rates." Available at: http://www.kcl.ac.uk/depsta/rel/icps/worldbrief (accessed May 5, 2007).

Kronenberg, F., & Pollard, N. (2005). Overcoming occupational apartheid: A preliminary exploration of the political nature of occupational therapy. In F. Kronenberg, S. S. Algado, & N. Pollard (Eds.), *Occupational Therapy Without Borders: Learning from the Spirit of Survivors* (pp. 58–86). London: Elsevier Churchill Livingstone.

Kunz, K. R., & Brayman, S. J. (1999). The comprehensive occupational therapy evaluation. In B. J. Hemphill (Ed.), *Assessments in Occupational Therapy Mental Health: An Integrated Approach* (pp. 259–278). Thorofare, NJ: Slack.

Langan, P. A., & Levin, D. J. (2002). *Recidivism of Prisoners Released in 1994.* Washington, DC: U.S. Department of Justice, Bureau of Justice Statistics.

Law, M., Baptiste, S., Carswell, A., McColl, M. A., Polatajko, H., & Pollock, N. (2005). *Canadian Occupational Performance Measure* (4th ed.). Ottawa: Canadian Association of Occupational Therapist.

Lawrence, S., & Travis, J. (2004). *The New Landscape of Imprisonment: Mapping America's Prison Expansion.* Washington, DC: The Urban Institute.

Lindsay, W. R., & Beail, N. (2004). Risk assessment: Actuarial prediction and clinical judgment of offending incidents and behaviour for intellectual disability services. *Journal of Applied Research in Intellectual Disabilities, 17*, 229–234.

Lloyd, C. (1985). Evaluation and forensic psychiatric occupational therapy. *British Journal of Occupational Therapy, 48*(5), 137–140.

———. (1987a). The role of occupational therapy in the treatment of the forensic psychiatric patient. *Australian Occupational Therapy Journal, 34*(1), 20–25.

———. (1987b). Working with a female offender: A case study. *Australian Occupational Therapy Journal, 50*(2), 42–48.

———. (1988). A vocational rehabilitation programme in forensic psychiatry. *British Journal of Occupational Therapy, 51*(4), 123–126.

———. (1989). Parenting: A group programme for abusive parents. *Australian Occupational Therapy Journal, 36*(1), 24–33.

Magnani, L., & Wray, H. L. (2006). *Beyond Prisons: A New Interfaith Paradigm for Our Failed Prison System.* Minneapolis: Fortress Press.

Margolis, R. L., Harrison, S. A., Robinson, H. J., & Jayaram, G. (1996). Occupational therapy task observation scale (OTTOS): A rapid method for rating task group function of psychiatric patients. *American Journal of Occupational Therapy, 50*(5), 380–385.

Martin, T. (2001). Something special: Forensic psychiatric nursing. *Journal of Psychiatric Mental Health Nursing, 8*, 25–32.

Massaro, J. (2005). *Overview of the Mental Health Service System for Criminal Justice Professionals.* Delmar, NY: GAINS Technical Assistance and Policy Analysis Center for Jail Diversion.

Matsutsuyu, J. (1969). The interest checklist. *American Journal of Occupational Therapy, 23*, 323–328.

Molineux, M. L., & Whiteford, G. (1999). Prisons: From occupational deprivation to occupational enrichment. *Journal of Occupational Science, 6*(3), 124–130.

Mountain, G. (1998). *Occupational Therapy in Forensic Settings. A Preliminary Review of the Knowledge and Research Base.* London: College of Occupational Therapists Research and Development Group.

National GAINS Center. (2002). *The Prevalence of Co-occurring Mental Illness and Substance Use Disorders in Jails.* Delmar, NY: Author.

Norko, M. A., & Baranoski, M. V. (2005). The state of contemporary risk assessment research. *Canadian Journal of Psychiatry, 50*, 1, 18–26.

O'Connell, M., & Farnworth, L. (2007). Occupational therapy in forensic psychiatry: A review of the literature and a call for a united and international response. *British Journal of Occupational Therapy, 70*(5), 184–191.

Parkinson, S., Forsyth, K., & Kielhofner, G. (2006). *A User's Manual for the MOHOST; The Model of Human Occupation Screening Tool (Version 2.0).* Chicago: Model of Human Occupation Clearinghouse.

Penner, D. A. (1978). Correctional institutions: An overview. *American Journal of Occupational Therapy, 32*(8), 517–524.

Pew Charitable Trust (2008). More than one in 100 adults are behind bars. Pew study finds http://www.pewtrusts.org/news_room_detail.aspx?id=35890. (Retrieved March 10, 2010)/

Pope, C. E., Lovell, R., & Hsia, H. M. (2002). *Disproportionate Minority Confinement: A Review of the Research Literature From 1989 Through 2001.* Washington, DC: Office of Juvenile Justice and Delinquency Prevention. Available at: http://ojjdp.ncjrs.org/dmc/pdf/dmc89_01.pdf (accessed March 1, 2007).

Pyrek, K. M. (2006). *Forensic Nursing.* Boca Raton: Taylor & Francis.

Quinsey, V. L., Harris, G. T., Rice, M. E., & Cromier C. A. (1998). *Violent Offenders: Appraising and Managing Risk.* Washington, DC: American Psychological Association.

Scaffa, M. (2001). *Occupational Therapy in Community-Based Practice Settings.* Philadelphia: F.A. Davis.

Schindler, V. P. (2004). *Occupational Therapy in Forensic Psychiatry: Role Development and Schizophrenia.* New York: Haworth Press.

The Sentencing Project. (2003). "U.S. Prison Populations: Trends and Implications." Available at: http://www.sentencingproject.org/pubs_02.cfm (accessed January 25, 2004).

Sickmund, M. (2003). *Juveniles in Court, 6–10.* Washington, DC: U.S. Department of Justice.

Snively, F., & Dressler, J. (2005). Occupational therapy in the criminal justice system. In E. Cara, & A. MacRae (Eds.), *Psychosocial Occupational Therapy: A Clinical Practice* (pp. 568–590). Clifton Park, NY: Thompson Delmar Learning.

Stelter, L., & Whisner, S. M. (2007). Building responsibility for self through meaningful roles: Occupational adaptation theory applied in forensic psychiatry. *Occupational Therapy in Mental Health, 23*(1), 69–84.

Tayar, S. G. (2004). Description of a substance abuse relapse prevention programme conducted by occupational therapy and psychology graduate students in a United States women's prison. *British Journal of Occupational Therapy, 67*(4), 159–166.

Teplin, L. A., Abram, K. M., & McClelland, G. M. (1996). The prevalence of psychiatric disorder among incarcerated women: Pretrial jail detainees. *Archives of General Psychiatry, 53*, 505–512.

Thigpen, M. L., Hunter, S. M., & Ortiz, M. (2001). *Provision of Mental Health Care in Prisons.* Longmont, CO: U.S. Department of Justice, National Institute of Corrections Information Center.

Travis, J. (2005). *But They All Come Back: Facing the Challenges of Prisoner Reentry.* Washington, DC: Urban Institute Press.

U.S. Department of Justice. (2001). "Mental Health Treatment in State Prisons." Bureau of Justice Statistics Special Report, July. Available at: http://www.ojp.usdoj.gov/bjs/pub/pdf/mhtsp00.pdf (accessed March 2, 2007).

———. (2006). "Mental Health Problems of Prison and Jail Inmates." Bureau of Justice Statistics Special Report, December 14. Available at: http://www.ojp.usdoj.gov/bjs/pub/pdf/mhtppji.pdf (accessed March 2, 2007).

U.S. Federal Bureau of Prisons. (2006). "Prison Types and General Information." Available at: http://www.bop.gov/locations/institutions/index.jsp (accessed April 4, 2007).

Watson, C. (2002). Exploring the interface of competence and clinical effectiveness. In A. Kettles, P. Woods, & C. Collins (Eds.), *Therapeutic Intervention for Forensic Mental Health Nurses* (pp. 51–73). London: Jessica Kinglsey Publishers.

Watson, C., & Kirby, S. (2000). A two nation perspective on issues of practice for professionals caring for mentally disordered offenders. In D. Robinson & A. Kettles (Eds.), *Forensic Nursing and Multi-Disciplinary Care of the Mentally Disordered Offender* (pp. 37–55). London: Jessica Kingsley Publishers.

Watson, R. (2005). A population approach to transformation. In R. Watson & L. Swartz (Eds.), *Transformation Through Occupation* (pp. 51–65). London: Whurr.

Watson, R., & Swartz, L. (2004). *Transformation Through Occupation*. London: Whurr.

Western, B., Kling, J. R., & Weiman, D. F. (2001). The labor market consequences of incarceration. *Crime & Delinquency, 47,* 410–427.

Whiteford, G. (1997). Occupational deprivation and incarceration. *Journal of Occupational Science, 4*(3), 126–130.

———. (2000). Occupational deprivation: Global challenge in the new millennium. *British Journal of Occupational Therapy, 63*(5), 200–204.

Wilcock, A. (1998). *An Occupational Perspective of Health.* Thorofare, NJ: Slack.

Woods, P. (2004). The person who uses forensic mental health services. In I. Norman & I. Ryrie (Eds.), *The Art and Science of Mental Health Nursing: A Textbook of Principles and Practices* (pp. 594–623). Maidenhead, UK: Open University Press.

State Hospitals

Stephanie Megan Exley, Catherine Annette Thompson, and Carole Ann Hays

> *In the midst of winter, I finally learned that there was an invincible summer in me.*
>
> —Albert Camus, "Return to Tipasa," 1954

Introduction

State mental health facilities are generally thought of as places of last resort, where individuals with serious mental illness are kept sequestered from the rest of society because they are often viewed by the general public as peculiar, dangerous, and even unwelcome in the community (Link, Phelan, Bresnahan, Stueve, & Pescosolido, 1999). These stigmatizing views deny the humanity of the individual and do not recognize the current practices of many state hospitals, which are no longer warehouses but places where those with the most severe mental illnesses can stabilize and receive services that promote successful transitions to community life. To be successful in the state hospital, occupational therapists must be empathetic and provide the consumer with hope and a continuous therapeutic relationship. Staff members must recognize the frequent, episodic nature of mental illness and the importance of a consistent, therapeutic approach to meet the consumer's needs.

This chapter provides an overview of state mental health facilities in the United States and explores the functions of other members of the treatment team. The recovery-oriented approach to assessment and treatment interventions for occupational therapy in state hospitals is described, and the expanded opportunities available to occupational therapists in this area of mental health are explored.

Overview of State Hospitals in the United States

State hospitals are public institutions that provide inpatient services to those with serious mental illness. Those admitted to state hospitals are often on public assistance and may be admitted involuntarily because they are considered a danger to themselves or others or are committed by criminal courts because their competency to stand trial is questioned (Fisher, Geller, & Pandianini, 2009). Significant changes have occurred in state mental health facilities in the United States since their inception. It is helpful to understand the evolution

of state mental health hospitals to better appreciate their current state.

A Brief History

Before state-run mental health facilities were established, individuals with mental illness were either cared for by their families or treated at private hospitals. In the late 1700s and early 1800s, facilities were established to treat individuals with mental illness who could not afford to pay for care at private hospitals. The first state hospital, named the Public Hospital for Persons of Insane and Disordered Minds, opened in Williamsburg, Virginia, in 1773 (Benjamin & Baker, 2004).

In their early days, state mental health facilities featured the words *asylum* and *insane* in their titles, a naming convention that continued until the 1900s, when these terms were recognized as negative and demeaning. As a result, facilities were renamed to *state hospitals,* reflecting a shift from confinement to care and treatment. The treatment at this time was called moral therapy. Moral treatment aimed to remove the inhumane conditions of the state hospital where individuals were often kept in prisonlike conditions, chained to walls, and beaten (Peloquin, 1989). Principles of moral treatment included creating a pleasant living situation and providing therapeutic activities that combined rest and manual work.

During the late 1700s, Phillip Pinel, who wrote on the harsh treatment of individuals with mental illness in French asylums, advocated for structured, individualized, and humane treatment with the goal of returning individuals to the community (Benjamin & Baker, 2004). Pinel's influences in mental health treatment during the late 1700s and early 1800s is still evident in the 21st century, as state hospitals strive to remain structured, individualized, and humane with a goal of returning individuals to the community. The moral treatment movement contributed to the development of new asylums and an increase in the number of individuals residing in these institutions. In 1955, the greatest number of state hospital residents was reached, approximately 559,000 (Mandersched, Atay, & Crider, 2009).

The Lived Experience

Shane

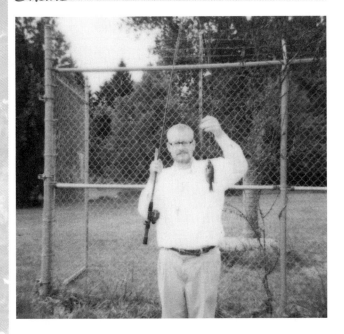

Shane is a 46-year-old single male Caucasian who currently resides in a state psychiatric hospital in the behavioral management program. Shane attends the treatment mall program Monday through Friday and is involved in a variety of multidisciplinary groups at the treatment mall. His occupational therapy groups have included team-building, fishing, explore your world, mural painting, needlecraft, and money management. The interview with Shane took place in a quiet dining room area at the treatment mall. Shane works with the occupational therapist who interviews him on a regular basis and has established rapport. The purpose of the interview was explained to Shane before the meeting took place, and he agreed to participate. Some dialogue has been left out for brevity.

OT: Shane, I thought first we could talk about your hospitalizations. I was wondering if you could tell me how many times you have been hospitalized?

Shane: *I can't really remember—it has been a lot.*

OT: How old were you when you were first hospitalized?

Shane: *Twenty-three.*

OT: Do you remember how many times you have been in a state hospital?

Shane: *Yeah, I think so. I was at Crownsville for three years and now I have been here for two.*

OT: Do you think you have benefited from your time in the hospital?

Shane: *Yes, in some ways. I have time to read the Bible, and from 8:00 a.m. till 2:30 it [the treatment mall] keeps me from smoking cigarettes. I quit now. I went four months.*

OT: Shane, could you tell me a little about your hobbies and interests?

Shane: *I like preaching, singing hymns, and reading the Bible.*

OT: Is there anything else you enjoy?

Shane: *Yeah, I like painting but it can be expensive. You know, buying all of the paint and things. I like fishing . . . it's good to be in the sunlight and good to look at the water . . . you know you get baptized in the water. I also like swimming.*

OT: Shane, can you tell me about your experiences with the rehabilitation department and occupational therapy?

Shane: *Yes, I like those things. They give me something to do during the day.*

OT: What do you think of mural painting group? I thought that was a group you really enjoyed.

Shane: *It makes people think about what is really important in this world and that Jesus can save. If it wasn't for God, there wouldn't be clothes, food, or water. . . .*

OT: Do you think your groups and experiences with rehabilitation improve your quality of life while you are at the hospital?

Shane: *Yes, I like team building, playing games, bowling, and throwing darts. I'm ready to work. but the lady wants me to sit at a table and I don't want to do that. I don't have to sit at a chair or a table.*

OT: What kind of work have you done in the past?

Shane: *I worked for a surveyor, and at an electrical shop, and cut grass. Things like that.*

OT: So you like to be up and about at hands-on activities?

Shane: *Yes. You get tired of being in the same place, so when I was 18, I joined the Army. I changed tires on trucks and fixed brakes.*

OT: Shane, what are some of your goals for the future?

Shane: *I would like to be a disciple and travel around and preach and heal the sick and blind.*

OT: Other than that, Shane, is there anything else you might like to do?

Shane: *I could be a janitor at a church and be a groundskeeper.*

OT: What about housing, Shane? Where would you like to live?

Shane: *All over the place—people get tired of being in the same place. Are we done now? I need to get up now.*

OT: Yes, we can be done now. Thank you for meeting with me today.

Shane: *You're welcome. Thank you.*

At that time, state hospitals were virtually self-sufficient, often located in rural areas where hospital residents contributed to maintaining buildings, growing food, and the general operations of the facility such as laundry, food preparation, and janitorial service. Overcrowding was a major issue.

In 1961, the Joint Commission on Mental Illness and Mental Health (1961) emphasized deinstitutionalization and promoted community-based treatment. Two years later, the federal government passed the Community Mental Health Centers Act (Benjamin & Baker, 2004). The impact of these events led to a shift in funding from state hospitals to community-based programs, resulting in a dramatic decrease in residents in state facilities (Mandersched, Atay, & Crider, 2009). From the peak of 559,000 in 1955, the numbers dramatically decreased to less than 200,000 by 1980 and less than 50,000 in 2005—despite overall population growth in the United States.

The history of Springfield Hospital Center in Maryland illustrates the changes in state hospital systems. Originally named The Second Hospital for the Insane of Maryland, it was founded in 1896 by an act of the Maryland State Legislature. The first residents were temporarily housed in renovated farm buildings. The first buildings constructed were three wards and a service building. In rapid succession, additional buildings were completed, and a building for the treatment of the mentally ill with tuberculosis was completed in the 1930s. By the late 1940s and early 1950s, the population of Springfield had grown to approximately 3,400 patients. Buildings were overcrowded and poorly maintained. Public pressure caused the State Legislature to appropriate more funds to relieve the overcrowding, resulting in the construction of eight new buildings.

Beginning in the late 1960s, however, the hospital redirected its efforts toward returning individuals to the community, a practice that accelerated through the 1970s and early 1980s. During this time, Springfield Hospital Center saw its inpatient census fall to the present level of 335. Despite the reduction in census, the hospital continues to build additional modern facilities (Springfield, 2004).

Current Profile of State Hospitals

The population at Springfield Hospital Center mirrors that for state facilities across the United States. Currently, according to the National Association of State Mental Health Program Directors (NASMHPD) Research Institute (2004), 29% of individuals in state hospitals are voluntarily admitted, 27% are involuntarily civilly committed, and 39% are involuntarily criminally committed. State facilities serve children, adolescents, adults, and older adults. Some hospitals serve all age groups, while others have separate facilities for children and adolescents. More than 80% of all adults served in psychiatric facilities have at least one of the following disorders (NASMHPD Research Institute, 2002):

- Schizophrenia (53%)
- Affective disorders (22%)
- Personality disorders (17%)
- Anxiety disorders (3%)
- Other psychoses (7%)

One study of children and adolescents found that depression was the most common diagnosis (20%), followed by posttraumatic stress disorder (15%), attention deficit-hyperactivity disorder (12%), and bipolar disorder (10%) (Romansky, Lyons, Lehner, & West, 2003). Many of the children were undiagnosed.

The number of nonwhite residents, particularly African Americans and Latinos, has increased (Fisher et al, 2009).

The funding sources for state mental health hospitals usually include state general funds, state special appropriations, federal mental health block grants, Medicaid and Medicare revenues, plus other federal funds such as research and demonstration grants (NASMHPD Research Institute, 2003).

The Recovery Model and the State Hospital

Although the recovery model is most often associated with noninstitutional settings, recovery-oriented practices are still relevant and essential in the state hospital environment. Currently, state hospitals across the country are moving toward the recovery model paradigm (Fisher & Chamberlin, 2004). This is a strengths-based, holistic, person-centered model, which fits naturally with the profession of occupational therapy. It is important for occupational therapists to adopt practices and language that are strengths-based, holistic in nature, person centered, and self-directed. Principals such as instilling hope; promoting empowerment through choice, individual responsibility, and decision-making; and peer-run services can all be implemented, thereby enhancing the services in the state hospital (National Technical Assistance Center, 2002). Many state hospitals are implementing recovery-oriented services. For example, an academic and state hospital collaboration in New Jersey targets the most discharge-resistant individuals (Mayerhoff & Schliefer, 2008). In this program, staff are trained to address individual needs of consumers and move from a medical to a wellness and recovery model. In addition, evidence-based practices such as illness management and recovery and independent living skills modules are implemented. At Napa State hospital in California, individuals work with their Wellness and Recovery Planning team to develop individualized recovery plans upon admission (California Department of Mental Health, 2009).

Interventions centered on the recovery model provide individuals with choice, support them in achieving self-identified goals, address all aspects of life, and empower them to make decisions and do for themselves. With all the restrictions and precautions that may be placed on consumers in state hospitals, occupational therapists are often in a unique position to help clients maximize their individuality and choice during intervention. Examples include allowing clients to choose the menu during cooking group, inviting a client to serve as a representative on a hospital committee, or helping an individual identify which de-escalation technique works best for him or her.

The Treatment Team

The treatment team is the most vital component of integrated and quality care for persons with mental illness in the state hospital setting. Occupational therapy practitioners are an essential part of the team. Although the size and complexity varies among facilities, the treatment team should include, at a minimum, the consumer, a psychiatrist, a registered nurse, and a social worker. Roles often overlap

Evidence-Based Practice

The recovery model is becoming recognized as the national model for all mental health service delivery systems (U.S. Department of Health and Human Services, 2004). Increasing research demonstrates that people with severe and persistent mental illness, such as schizophrenia, can live productive and satisfying lives (Bellack, 2006). Longitudinal studies, varying in criteria, measures, samples, and time frame, have shown that between 20% and 70% of people diagnosed with schizophrenia have positive outcomes, such as decreased symptoms and improved role function (Bellack, 2006). Evidence supports recovery-based intervention such as family intervention (Bellack, 2006; Glynn, Cohen, Dixon, & Niv, 2006), supported employment, and skills training (Bellack, 2006). The values and suggested interventions outlined by the recovery model resonate closely with those of occupational therapy.

➤ Occupational therapists should use their expertise in client/family education, role development, and skill training to offer recovery-based intervention and to support clients' overall recovery.

➤ Occupational therapists should consider ways to provide increased choice for clients within the restricted context of locked psychiatric units and empower clients by helping them do as much for themselves as possible within the hospital context.

➤ Occupational therapists should use their expertise as holistic, client-centered therapists to serve as role models in organizations adopting the recovery model.

Bellack, A. (2006). Scientific and consumer models of recovery in schizophrenia: Concordance, contrasts, and implications. *Schizophrenia Bulletin, 32,* 432–442.

Glynn, S., Cohen, A., Dixon, L., & Niv, N. (2006). The potential impact of recovery movement on family interventions for schizophrenia: Opportunities and obstacles. *Schizophrenia Bulletin, 32,* 451–464.

U.S. Department of Health and Human Services, Substance Abuse and Mental Health Services Administration. (2004). "National Consensus Statement on Mental Health Recovery." Available at: http://mentalhealth.samhsa.gov/publications/allpubs/sma05-4129 (accessed September 23, 2009).

in mental health facilities, yet primary roles are fairly consistent across the country:

■ The consumer's role is to help establish the goals for his or her treatment program, recommend interventions, question the direction of his or her treatment program, and accept responsibility for the recovery process.
■ The psychiatrist is the diagnostician, team leader, medication manager, and primary therapist for the consumer.
■ The registered nurse is responsible for the day-to-day operation of the client's inpatient unit, providing a safe and therapeutic environment 24 hours a day, 7 days a week. The nursing staff administers medication, assures that activities of daily living (ADLs) are completed, monitors changes in the client's response to medication, and provides interventions such as group sessions on topics such as medication information, understanding your mental illness, and wellness.
■ The social worker focuses on the supports available to the consumer, including family, financial, spiritual, and cultural, and provides housing assistance. The social worker may also provide case management and mental health therapy.

In all cases, the clinical staff is responsible for assessment, intervention, and reassessment.

The effectiveness of the overall treatment program is dependent on the additional clinicians working as a team to provide services for the consumer. Table 38-1 describes the roles and interventions used by other clinicians working in this context.

In addition, most state mental health facilities have an addiction service to meet consumers' needs. An addiction service is often an interdisciplinary addictions team, which includes social workers, addiction counselors, psychologists, occupational therapists, and recreational therapists. The team is responsible for evaluating the consumer for substance abuse problems, reviewing family history, and conducting a review of prior recovery efforts. The addiction service then recommends services to the individual and the treatment team, such as individual recovery-oriented counseling, Alcoholics Anonymous, Narcotics Anonymous, or group counseling.

Table 38-1 ● Additional Clinicians on the State Hospital Client Treatment Team

Team Member	Role	Type(s) of Intervention
Psychologist	Performs psychological evaluations and assessments; helps consumers identify their worries, concerns or needs; and helps the team recognize risk factors, including suicidal ideation, self-injurious behavior, anger or low frustration tolerance, violence or homicidal ideation, and history of impulsivity	Individual therapy, group therapy, and family/couples therapy; consultation with the team on a behavioral plan or trauma recovery services
Certified recreational therapy specialist	Provides information on the consumers' leisure interests, ability to structure free time, attention span, and interpersonal social skills	Leisure education, exercise programs, and recreation skills development
Board-certified music therapist	Assesses clients and uses music as the treatment method; focuses on developing interpersonal skills and improving concentration and self-esteem.	Improvisation, drumming, lyric analysis, music listening, and singing
Art therapist	Uses art as the modality for treatment; art therapists are an excellent addition to the treatment team because they provide consumers the opportunity to explore conflicts and use nonverbal methods for expression	Example modalities are pottery, watercolors, collages, freehand drawing
Dance/movement therapist	Uses movement as a therapeutic process to help with the emotional and physical integration of the individual	Focuses on movement, posture, breathing, and interaction with the environment

Forensic services have become an integral component of the mental health treatment team, because up to 30% of hospitalized individuals with mental illness have some sort of involvement with the legal system (NASMHPD Research Institute, 2004). The forensic staff evaluates individuals to determine if they are competent to stand trial or are criminally responsible. They may also advocate for clients to receive a conditional release from the hospital to a less restrictive environment. In some cases, the forensic staff determines that the individual is competent and returns him or her to the legal system to stand trial. The forensic service relies on the input from the multidisciplinary treatment team to assist in the determination.

Vocational adjustment services in state facilities teach and reinforce work habits and behaviors such as time management, workmanship, attention span, work tolerance, and dependability. Providers teach basic job-related and workmanship skills and provide feedback to the client regarding work attitudes, working relationships, and habits. They provide clients with the opportunity to practice interpersonal behaviors that comprise essential worker relationship skills, and then work with the team to assist and support community reintegration for clients in the worker role.

Occupational Therapy in State Hospitals

Occupational therapists in a state psychiatric facility have the opportunity to provide to individuals with severe and persistent mental illness services that improve their function and the quality of their lives. Occupational therapists in mental health provide direct service in this context, which includes:

- Performing evaluations and screenings.
- Establishing an intervention.
- Selecting relevant occupations.
- Implementing the intervention.
- Modifying the plan as necessary.
- Terminating the intervention when objectives are accomplished.

Each component of the occupational therapy process requires communication with the consumer, his or her family/significant other, and the treatment team. Documentation of services is a necessary and vital part of the occupational therapist's responsibilities.

The opportunities for occupational therapists in a state mental health facility are broad and exciting. The therapist may be an evaluator of consumers, providing direct services and serving as a client advocate with the treatment team. The opportunity to shape the facility toward a recovery model and to alter the client's role expectations from that of a passive recipient to one who is able to influence events and have some control over his or her daily living experience should be the occupational therapist's primary role. This may happen as a direct service provider.

Yet other opportunities exist for occupational therapists to create an atmosphere that is conducive to client and staff growth. For example, an occupational therapist can serve on the construction oversight committee to help ensure that all new construction or remodeling meets the requirements for access for persons with disabilities. The therapist would need to be familiar with the federal and state laws regarding accessibility.

An Americans with Disabilities Act (ADA) officer for the facility is appointed to ensure that employees are provided reasonable accommodations when they have permanent or temporary disabilities that affect their work performance. This position is often held by an occupational therapist.

Occupational therapists may serve on medical records committees. This committee is responsible for the content, format, and review of medical records. The committee determines if the facility's records are complete and accurate and that they meet legal requirements and accreditation requirements.

All hospitals have a strategic planning committee, and occupational therapists can be a great asset to this committee by assuring that the needs of the consumers are given first priority in all stages of the planning process.

Occupational therapists can also serve as the liaison between the facility and community mental health programs. In this role, occupational therapists have the opportunity to advocate for clients in the discharge planning process. As a liaison, the occupational therapist gains firsthand knowledge of the skills needed by the individual to be successful in a community placement. They then work with the client to modify the treatment intervention plans to bridge the gap between the hospital and the community.

Occupational Therapy Assessments

Just as the profession of occupational therapy has progressed, developed, and changed over the years, so has the assessment process in the state psychiatric hospital. As evidence-based practice has grown increasingly important, informal assessment has decreased, and the use of standardized assessments supplemented with informal assessment has become common practice. Frequently in the state hospital environment, a structured, formal assessment process is implemented and includes initial assessment, continual informal reassessment, and an annual formal reassessment. Additionally, as the profession has evolved from the use of uniform terminology to the Occupational Therapy Practice Framework, the assessment process has become more holistic focusing on global functioning of the individual, performance patterns, environment in the hospital and the discharge environment, as well as the occupations that are of value and interest to the consumer (American Occupational Therapy Association [AOTA], 2002). The assessment guides interventions to improve quality of life while in the hospital, promote health and wellness, prepare for discharge into the community, and prevent further hospitalizations.

This section examines the admission assessment and reassessment process, and then describes the standardized assessment tools available.

The Admission Assessment

When an individual is admitted to a state psychiatric hospital, the assessment process begins informally through observation and interaction with the client. Additional data for the occupational therapy assessment should be gathered through input from other members of the treatment team and a holistic screening with observation of functional performance and interview components.

There are many areas of particular interest in the initial assessment in a psychiatric hospital: prior living conditions, activities of daily living (ADLs), instrumental activities of daily living (IADLs), mental functions, social participation (including roles, routines and habits, cultural influences, substance abuse history, vocational history, educational history, legal history, and current legal issues), particular interests of the clients, and volition to participate in occupational therapy. A screening to determine functional reading level may also be completed and shared with the treatment team to assist in better understanding what forms, written treatment materials, educational materials, and other possible papers the client will be able to read and understand and how much assistance he or she might need. This screening will decrease confusion and frustration for the individual during his or her stay in the hospital.

Interpretations of the assessment should be immediately documented and filed in the medical record to ensure the most accurate information and quick communication with the treatment team. The formal process is typically completed within the first 72 hours so the treatment team can collaborate and design the individual's plan of care, including treatment recommendations and discharge plans. The occupational therapy assessment should be used to guide the treatment team's decisions for discharge planning from the initial assessment and throughout the hospitalization.

Informal Reassessment

As with all populations with whom the occupational therapist works, reassessment with the psychiatric population is a continual process. The therapist continually observes the individual's behaviors in the milieu, in one-to-one interactions, and in therapy groups. These observations and treatment interactions are noted in weekly and monthly progress notes. The reassessment process guides changes in treatment focus and interventions.

Formal Reassessment

Because of the severity of illness seen in state psychiatric hospitals, it is common to work with people who have had multiple long-term hospitalizations throughout their life span. These hospitalizations can affect the person's self-care skills and ability to perform IADLS; they also may hinder the client's ability to perform time management tasks and to make choices and decisions. Therefore, a formal reassessment similar to the initial assessment is completed for long-term-stay clients on an annual basis. The therapist can than gauge progression and regression in each of these areas and guide treatment to assist the individual in relearning or adapting for these skills. Comparisons from initial and annual assessments should be made, changes and progress should be noted, and interventions modified as appropriate.

Standardized Assessments

Because of the nature of mental illness and possible comorbid diagnoses, a multitude of standardized assessments are available that may be relevant for the state psychiatric setting. Standardized assessments provide an in-depth look at performance in areas of occupation, performance skills, and performance patterns of particular concern or interest (AOTA, 2002). For example, performing the Kohlman Evaluation of Living Skills (KELS) (Thomson, 1992) assessment with a client upon admission gives the therapist insight into the individual's ability to perform particular IADLs and assists in making recommendations for discharge. Standardized assessments are also important in guiding treatment and measuring outcomes. The KELS can determine, for example, particular areas that a person needs to improve in order to live in a more independent setting; these areas, if important to the individual, would then be used as a focus of treatment. The KELS can be readministered to determine outcomes of treatment, such as preparedness to be discharged to a more independent setting. The assessments most commonly used in the state psychiatric hospital are discussed in this section; however, this list is not comprehensive, and the frequency and variety used differs among hospitals.

One example of a recovery-oriented assessment is the Canadian Occupational Performance Measure (Pollock, 1993). This assessment is useful in the initial stages of the assessment process because it is self-directed and person centered and assists the individual in determining what life areas are important to focus on. It also allows the client to indicate his or her level of satisfaction with current performance in the previously identified life areas. This client-centered assessment approach allows intervention to be guided by what the client finds meaningful. It is then used after an intervention has been implemented to detect change in the client's perception over time (Asher, 1996).

The Occupational Performance History Interview II (OPHI-II) (Kielhofner et al, 2004) is an interview designed to gain a history of the client's work, play, and self-care performance. It provides insight into the individual's perception of his or her life and his or her ability to adapt (Asher, 1996). The Role Checklist (Oakley, Kielhofner, Barris, & Reichler, 1986) assesses productive roles by indicating the individual's perception of his or her past, present, or future roles.

Cognitive assessments are also used in the state psychiatric setting. Two examples of cognitive assessments are the Allen Cognitive Level (ACL) test (Allen, 1982) and the Kitchen Task Assessment (KTA) (Baum & Edwards, 1993). The ACL uses a variety of leather-lacing activities to look at cognitive function, assess cognitive disabilities, and suggest treatment approaches (Asher, 1996). The KTA uses a common kitchen task to evaluate cognitive skills such as organization, planning, and judgment (Asher, 1996).

Other assessments directly assess ADLs. The KELS (Thomson, 1992) evaluates the consumer's ability to perform certain basic living skills such as self-care, money management, transportation, safety, work, and leisure. It can assist in determining his or her level of independence and discharge recommendations. The Street Survival Skills Questionnaire (SSSQ) assesses adaptive skills for prevocational evaluation (McCaron, Cobb, Smith, & Barron, 1982). It consists of nine sections: Basic Concepts, Functional Signs, Tools, Domestic Management, Health and Safety, Public Services, Money, Time, and Measurement.

The Motor-Free Visual Perceptual Test Revised (MVPT-R) (Colarusso & Hammill, 1996) is a motor-free evaluation of visual perception, looking at the following components of visual perception: spatial relations, figure ground, visual discrimination, visual closure, and visual memory.

Along with the change to the recovery model, naturally, comes a change in the use of seclusion and restraints in the psychiatric setting. The long-term goal is to have seclusion- and restraint-free hospitals. Occupational therapists' knowledge of sensory integration and sensory processing can aid hospitals in achieving the recovery-oriented goal of ultimately being seclusion and restraint free. "The ability to offer alternative forms of stimulation and environmental modifications, identified as helpful by the consumer, may help to decrease or more skillfully help the individual manage difficult thoughts, arousal states, emotions, and cravings when they occur and may contribute to the decreased need for the use of restraint and seclusion" (Champagne, 2005, p. 2). The knowledge gained through the assessment of sensory processing can be used to educate staff on how best to work with each client, to educate the client on his or her sensory needs, and to adapt the environment to meet those sensory needs. One particular assessment useful in this area is the Adolescent and Adult Sensory Profile (Brown, Tollefson, Dunn, Cromwell, & Filion, 2001).

The Adolescent/Adult Sensory Profile is a self-administered questionnaire of sensory experiences organized around four quadrants derived from the intersection of a neurological threshold continuum and a behavioral response continuum: (1) low registration, (2) sensation seeking, (3) sensory sensitivity, and (4) sensation avoiding (Brown et al, 2001). There is support for the reliability and validity of the Adolescent/Adult Sensory Profile in determining sensory preferences, making recommendations for environmental adaptations and environmental fit, and teaching individuals ways to cope with their sensory environment.

Assessing Special Populations

Many special populations exist within the psychiatric population in the state hospital, including individuals who are deaf, older adults, children and adolescents, individuals with a criminal history, and individuals with dual diagnoses such as mental illness and substance abuse or mental illness and developmental disabilities. There are also individuals with developmental disabilities, physical injuries, physical health problems, and those who do not speak or understand the English language. Due to the holistic nature of occupational therapy and our ability to look at the person, the environment, and the occupations of life, we must adapt our assessments and assessment processes to assist the team in working with all of these populations. We must also keep competencies in all of these areas in order to best assess and treat the individual.

Occupational therapists provide unique contributions in working with the treatment team for these special populations in the state psychiatric hospital. These unique contributions include our ability to recommend and make environmental adaptations and to use techniques such as sensory integration. Occupational therapists focus on performance patterns, occupation in the context of the life span, motivation, volition, and quality of life, which add a unique perspective in working with these individuals.

The occupational therapist also provides a role in assessing the need for speech and physical therapy, and referring consumers to these services when necessary.

Following are some key points to remember when assessing special populations:

■ When working with a person who is deaf or who does not speak English, an interpreter must always be present to assure accurate communication.

■ When assessing an older adult, the Parachek Geriatric Rating Scale (Parachek, 1986) can be used in addition to the normal assessment process to examine the affects of aging on function. The rating scale assists clinicians in planning treatment programs for older adults. The clinician rates the individual in three categories: physical capabilities, self-care skills, and social interaction skills. Rated over time, the assessment reveals strengths and problem areas so the clinician can plan goal-oriented treatment.

■ Many consumers with mental illness are admitted with upper extremity injuries due to self-injurious behaviors and accidents. The occupational therapist should assess the need for a referral for hand therapy and splinting. A hospital should have on staff at least one occupational therapist who has the competencies to perform splinting and hand therapy as needed.

Occupational Therapy Intervention

The assessment and reassessment process guides discharge planning and intervention. Accurate, person-centered, holistic evaluation provides the information needed to build meaningful and successful interventions for the individual receiving state psychiatric services. Intervention is an exciting process by which the therapist utilizes his or her creativity, capitalizes on the therapeutic use of self, and builds rapport with clients.

Although there are broad trends in occupational therapy intervention in state psychiatric hospitals, it is important to remember that any occupational therapy intervention should be as unique as the individual to which it is provided. In order to provide occupation-based, client-centered services, interventions must be centered on the client's identified needs, goals, and context (AOTA, 2002): there are as many different types of interventions as there are consumers. However, in order to provide an accurate description of the state psychiatric practice setting, it is necessary to identify common trends in occupational therapy intervention. This section addresses the general goals of intervention, considerations for intervention planning, use of group intervention, types of rehabilitation programming, interventions for special populations, and emerging areas of focus in state hospitals.

General Goals of Intervention

The goals of occupational therapy intervention should be tailored to the client's identified strengths, needs, and context, but general goals remain the same in all inpatient psychiatric settings. Although the criteria for medical necessity is unique to each state system, the acute inpatient psychiatric setting is designed for clients who make direct threats or infer serious harm to self or others and/or demonstrate violent or uncontrolled behavior that presents potential harm to self or others Because of the acute stage of illness experienced by inpatients, they often present with paranoid or delusional thinking and aggressive behaviors (Fisher et al, 2009). Occupational therapists in acute care units must therefore work on multidisciplinary teams with the common goal of providing a safe, stable daily routine for individuals whose internal worlds are filled with turmoil. Acute care intervention strategies center on improving orientation functions, impulse control, and emotional functions and seek to establish medication routine and diagnosis education, all while preparing the client for discharge (AOTA, 2002).

In addition to acute mental illness, many individuals admitted to state hospitals have forensic, or legal, involvement. Many people with mental illness are first diagnosed following an arrest due to bizarre or violent behavior stemming from symptoms of their illness (Fisher et al, 2009). In this context, intervention may also focus on helping clients cope and manage themselves within the legal system.

With the increased availability of community rehabilitation settings, consumers who become stable on medication are able to reenter the community with more frequency and efficiency than ever before. Therefore, many individuals are discharged within days or weeks after being admitted to state hospitals. The remaining clients in the state hospital system are those whose mental illness is so chronic and severe that they often require inpatient care for many years. These individuals are transferred to long-term stay programs, such as psychiatric rehabilitation or behavioral management programs, which are often unique to state psychiatric hospitals. Long-term institutionalization creates additional challenges for reentry into the community. As required, the hospital provides for many of the consumers' needs, such as meal preparation and medication management, and may even assist with basic ADLs. While staff encourages individuals to be as independent as possible in the setting, the opportunities for independence are limited, which can result in loss of skills and learned helplessness. However, to successfully reenter the community, clients are expected to be able to care for themselves to varying degrees, depending on the placement context. Therefore, intervention in long-term programs is focused on building the functional living skills people will need upon discharge to community settings, such as home with family, residential rehabilitation programs, or nursing homes. Goal areas in long-term programs at state hospitals are similar to those in any psychiatric setting, such as improving ADLs (e.g., grooming and hygiene) and IADLs (e.g., financial management, home establishment and management, meal preparation/clean-up, safety procedures and emergency responses). Other goal areas include developing employment interests/acquisition, improving job performance, participating in volunteer activities, pursuing play and leisure activities, and improving social participation (AOTA, 2002). Even though the general goal areas in state hospitals are very similar to those in other psychiatric settings, the course of intervention to achieve them is often much slower and more basic.

Considerations for Intervention Planning

The unique setting of a state hospital requires special considerations for intervention planning. The diverse population includes clients in acute and clients in chronic phases of illness, and the level of impairment of hospitalized individuals is typically severe. In addition, state hospitals typically have limited resources because of the financial structure of the setting and the safety considerations. These issues must be considered when developing interventions.

Qualities of Successful Intervention

Because of the severity of illness experienced by individuals in the state hospital setting, most continue to have active symptoms, such as delusions, hallucinations, and disorganized thoughts even while on medications. Others continue to experience severe negative symptoms, such as catatonic behavior, impoverished speech, and slowed cognitive and motor responses. Such symptoms often result in difficulty attending to activities, organizing tasks and speech, and thinking abstractly, and they may manifest as cognitive impairments such as decreased memory and problem-solving skills.

As in other occupational therapy settings, it is important to match interventions with the performance level of the consumer. However, taking into account the effects of severe mental illness, many of the most successful interventions in state hospitals share similar qualities regardless of the performance skill or client factor being addressed by an intervention.

One common quality of successful interventions in state hospitals is that information is presented in a concrete manner. Consumers with severe mental illness often have difficulty processing auditory information alone because it is abstract. For example, a verbal discussion about stress management techniques may result in the client speaking off-topic, misunderstanding information, or falling asleep. However, when information is delivered in a more concrete way (e.g., through visual examples on a video, pictures and words on a worksheet, or hands-on activities), individuals are more engaged and integrate the information more thoroughly. Generally, people with disorganized thought are more likely to process information successfully if several of their senses are stimulated. Therefore, it is important for therapists to provide information in ways that allow clients to hear, see, do, and say as much as possible. Methods for providing extremely concrete information often seem elementary. Therefore, therapists need to be sure that the interventions they provide are age appropriate even though individuals may require overexaggerated, obvious examples of information in order to process it successfully.

Next, successful interventions are usually very basic and involve breaking down tasks into one- or two-step subtasks and chaining tasks for client success. When chaining, the next step of a task is not attempted until the first step is successfully accomplished, and when the next step is presented, supports are in place to promote success. For example, during an intervention related to meal preparation, the therapist often needs to provide visual demonstration of a subtask (such as breaking an egg into a bowl) before expecting the client to do so correctly. Only after this step is accomplished is the client encouraged to move on to the next step (using a fork to scramble the egg). Also, the therapist may need to do large segments of the activity (e.g., actually cook the egg) in order for the client to engage in the subtasks appropriate for his or her current level of ability.

Many consumers with extreme negative symptoms, such as catatonic behavior, have severely decreased verbalization. For these individuals, it is important to incorporate motor activities in addition to verbal activities whenever possible so they may successfully engage in intervention. For example, during group introductions, the therapist might throw a ball to members of the group when it is their turn to introduce themselves. This provides motor engagement for those who are nonverbal. The added motor stimulation also provides an alerting response that may trigger clients to verbalize when they otherwise might not.

It is also important to remember that most clients who have lived in state hospitals for many years have not kept up with technology. This affects intervention because they are often unfamiliar with resources we take for granted. For example, clients often need several lessons on using a microwave oven before they can complete a simple task such as making popcorn. Others might want to communicate with family via e-mail but have never seen a computer or used the Internet before. Long-term, graded intervention on the use of such technology is generally required before the occupation can be independently performed.

Limitations of Context

Because consumers in state hospital settings continue to remain potentially dangerous to themselves or others, therapists must address certain contextual considerations when planning intervention. For example, some individuals are unable to leave their locked units without close supervision, if at all. Also, in areas such as the occupational therapy clinic, potentially dangerous materials such as scissors and knives must be counted carefully before and after an activity and stored in locked cabinets. Finally, many items we take for granted, such as pipe cleaners and aluminum foil, are identified as contraband in the hospital setting. Therefore, therapists must carefully consider the materials and modalities used for intervention during the planning process. For example, a therapist running a task group must ensure that all project ideas are free of contraband materials so that clients will be allowed to keep their project once finished. The therapist must check individuals' privilege levels before taking them off the unit for a group held in the clinic. If a project requires sharp objects, they must be carefully counted before, during, and after group sessions to ensure safety.

Because context is an important aspect of meaningful occupation, therapists try to provide intervention in the most natural context possible. However, therapists are often limited in where interventions can take place because of safety restrictions. For example, the most effective context in which to teach money-handling skills would be in a setting such as a grocery store. For a client who is unable leave the building, however, a therapist might start by helping him or her figure out the correct change needed to purchase a snack from the lobby vending machine instead.

Types of Intervention

The most common types of interventions in the state hospital setting are group intervention, rehabilitation programming, treatment mall approach, and sensory approaches.

Group Intervention

While group intervention has both benefits and drawbacks, it continues to be the most common intervention technique used in state hospital systems. Logistically, group intervention offers efficient services in a setting where staffing is quite often limited. Groups are less expensive to provide, allow therapists to see more clients at one time, and deliver services to a larger population than individual interventions.

Group sessions also provide benefits to the consumer. Those in state hospital settings typically have very limited social networks. Those with disorganized thought often have decreased awareness of the people around them and have difficulty forming social relationships. Group intervention encourages individuals to talk with each other, cooperate, and help one another, thus offering opportunities for social participation and feedback. In addition, offering a variety of intervention groups throughout the day provides a structured routine for clients. And as occupational therapists, we know that balanced routines are a healthy and organizing part of daily life.

Although group intervention is commonly used, it has some drawbacks. While many individuals benefit from the social nature of groups, those who experience severe paranoia or anxiety often find it difficult to engage in group activity. Also, even as therapists attempt to help clients meet their individual goals in the group setting, group intervention can never be as tailored to individual needs as a one-to-one session. Despite these disadvantages, as long as group intervention provides the most effective and efficient services, it will continue to be a hallmark of intervention in the state hospital setting.

Rehabilitation Programming

In addition to typical group intervention, many state settings provide hospitalwide rehabilitation programming designed to assist clients in acquiring and/or maintaining as many occupational roles as possible before discharge. Those with long-term hospitalizations often lose touch with new technologies. They have not performed home management tasks, driven a vehicle, or used community resources for long periods of time. Many of their ADLs, such as laundry, cooking, grocery shopping, and budgeting, have been done for them.

Rehabilitation programming is usually reserved for individuals who are likely to be discharged in 6 months to a year. These programs are often delivered in various locations throughout hospital grounds so clients have the opportunity to function in a broader context than the confined hospital unit. Rehabilitation programs may include vocational services in which clients can build job skills through supported employment on or off hospital grounds, day programs that help clients become familiar with activities and routines similar to those found in community mental health settings, intensive home management training in which clients can engage in meal preparation and cleaning, and community reentry in which clients take trips to begin interacting with people and resources outside the hospital setting.

Treatment Mall Approach

Another area gaining popularity and efficacy is the **treatment mall approach**. The treatment mall is a decentralized program, meaning that clients come from different areas of the hospital to attend the program. It is structured around an educational or classroom model, with a large selection of courses available to clients. The treatment mall supports many recovery practices, such as individualized care, self-determination, and choice.

As of 2001, there were 28 public psychiatric hospital treatment malls across the country, according to the *Directory of Public Psychiatric Hospital Treatment Malls* (Bopp, 2001), and this number continues to grow. The treatment mall approach was designed as an alternative to ward-based programming. A highly structured locked unit tends to increase clients' dependence on staff, isolation from the community, and general boredom (Chovil, 2005). On a locked unit, individuals must rely on staff to schedule and oversee everyday activities, which confines clients to a limited context. This results in a cyclical process in which lowered expectations from both the staff and the client become reinforcing (Bopp, Ribble, Cassidy, & Markoff, 1996) Also, individuals with the most severe illness often receive the fewest rehabilitation services, usually because they are not easily accessible from the ward (Bopp et al, 1996). Treatment malls offer an alternative environment for clients in much the same way that work, school, or volunteering does for members of the general community. The mall is typically held in an easily accessible, locked building or location separate from the unit on which clients live. While programs offered by treatment malls varies among hospitals, they are all based on an academic or psychoeducational model in which clients participate in groups or courses designed to assist them in improving life skills (Ballard, 2008). A wide variety of multidisciplinary groups are offered, and clients can help create their own schedule to address their personal goals and intervention needs. In addition to activity rooms and classrooms, many treatment malls offer resources such as a fitness center, boutique, hair salon, and kitchen. Such resources allow not only for a change of context but also for broader social opportunities, as several units may attend the same treatment mall program.

Individuals attending a treatment mall program often demonstrate a higher level of engagement and participation than those receiving treatment only in a confined hospital unit. A measure of efficacy implemented at Middletown Psychiatric Center in New York showed that clients had improved in all areas of an effectiveness-of-functioning scale after 1 year of treatment mall attendance (Markoff, 1999). Individuals in this program demonstrated the greatest improvement in basic survival skills and stability of mental status (Markoff, 1999). Western State Hospital in Virginia

has had a 90% drop in seclusion and restraint since opening its treatment mall program (Ferrie, 2002). Occupational therapists providing intervention in a treatment mall program frequently find themselves cofacilitating groups with other disciplines, such as nursing, social work, psychology, music therapy, art therapy, and therapeutic recreation. This cooperation strengthens the occupational therapy intervention by providing a wider scope of expertise and resources to more fully support individuals' engagement in occupation. Occupational therapists working within this model may also be called upon to help manage and assess treatment mall programming and develop new groups or courses to more fully meet consumer needs.

Sensory Approaches

Another emerging area is the use of sensory approaches in state hospitals as a component of crisis prevention planning. The Massachusetts Department of Mental Health, the National Association of State Mental Health Program Directors, and the Joint Commission for Accreditation of Healthcare Organizations have all recognized the need for responsible and skilled use of sensory approaches,

---

Evidence-Based Practice

Several published articles support the use of treatment mall programs within state hospitals. These articles suggest that treatment mall programs (1) provide consumers with a structured "working day" away from the unit (Markoff, 1999); (2) bring the hospital context closer to that of the outside community (Bopp et al, 1996); (3) encourage the matching of expert staff to clients in need of that expertise (Markoff, 1999); (4) improve overall functioning in participants (Markoff, 1999); and (5) may contribute to decreased use of seclusion and restraint (Ferrie, 2002).

➤ Occupational therapists can use their expertise to develop the structured, daily routine of treatment mall programs.

➤ Occupational therapists can use their knowledge of the effect of context on occupations to help develop the space used for treatment malls to more effectively create a "community feel."

➤ Occupational therapists can use their expertise of group facilitation to create and develop group protocols, lead groups within the treatment mall, and serve as role models and trainers for other staff in the program.

➤ Occupational therapists can use their expertise of functional assessment to accurately refer clients to relevant groups and provide outcomes data regarding effectiveness of treatment mall program.

Bopp, J., Ribble, D., Cassidy, J., Markoff, R. (1996). Re-engineering the state hospital to promote rehabilitation and recovery. *Psychiatric Services*, 47(7), 3–5.

Ferrie, B. (2002). Changing the environment. *Advance for Nurses*, 4(12), 15–16, 28.

Markoff, R. (1999). Innovations: "Treatment mall" at Middletown Psychiatric Center. *Treatment Mall Best Practices Directory*, 6–7. (Reprinted from *Quality of Care Newsletter, 75,* Spring 1999.)

Evidence-Based Practice

Research evidence shows that use of sensory approaches in inpatient psychiatric facilities provides an important component of person-centered crisis prevention tools (Champagne, 2005), helps clients self-organize, reduces levels of distress, and reduces episodes of seclusion and restraint (Champagne & Stromberg, 2004).

➤ Occupational therapists should assess clients' individual sensory preferences and needs using the Adolescent and Adult Sensory Profile (Brown & Dunn, 2002).

➤ Occupational therapists should work with clients to plan and implement individualized sensory diets to help them improve coping skills and crisis prevention.

➤ Occupational therapists should use their expertise in environmental modifications to develop and implement the safe use of multisensory treatment rooms that can be readily available to clients.

Brown, C., & Dunn, W. (2002) *Adolescent/Adult Sensory Profile*. Psychological Corporation, San Antonio, TX.

Champagne, T. (2005). Expanding the role of sensory approaches in acute psychiatric settings. *Mental Health Special Interest Section Quarterly, 28*, 1–4.

Champagne, T., & Stromberg, N. (2004). Sensory approaches in inpatient psychiatric settings: Innovative alternatives to seclusion and restraint. *Journal of Psychosocial Nursing, 42*, 35–44.

identifying occupational therapists as the professionals most qualified to provide consultation in order to create and carry out these services (Champagne, 2005). As mentioned previously, the use of sensory approaches for crisis prevention may greatly reduce the need for seclusion and restraint (Champagne, 2005; Champagne & Stromberg, 2004). Sensory approaches can also be used to help prevent clients from engaging in self-injury (Champagne, 2005). Intervention centered on sensory processing might include assisting clients in developing and practicing individualized sensory diets; making recommendations for environmental modification, such as the development and implementation of multisensory rooms; and educating other treatment team members on the responsible use of sensory experiences before, during, or after a crisis (Champagne, 2005).

Summary

State hospitals have changed dramatically over the last 50 years; however, they continue to provide an important service in the continuum of care for people with serious mental illness. Occupational therapy can play a significant role in enhancing quality of life in the state hospital environment and providing interventions that allow for the successful transition to community life.

Active Learning Strategies

1. Limited Freedoms and Choices

Imagine you have been admitted to a state psychiatric hospital. You want to go outside but realize the doors are locked and you cannot go out until other people think is safe for you; even then, your time outside will be limited to a few hours a day. You would like to eat but are told that meals are served only at certain times, and there is no food available right now. You decide you would like some time to lie down alone, so you go into your bedroom. However, you now share a room with two other people, and they are talking, so you cannot lie down and rest as you would like to. You really need a cigarette because you are a smoker, but then you realize that smoking time is not for another 3 hours. A shower might feel good, but you realize the showers are being cleaned, and you will not be able to take one any time soon. You want to watch television, but the group decides together what to watch, and you are not very interested in the show they have chosen. How frustrated do you feel right now?

 In your **Reflective Journal**, describe how living with these limited freedoms and choices would make you feel.

Reflective Questions

● If you were working on such a unit, what could you do to give the clients greater freedom and more choices?
● As an occupational therapist, how could you assist a client in a situation like this? How could you assist the other staff working on the unit?

● Do you think the treatment team can ensure safety and set appropriate limits yet still allow individuals as many choices and freedoms as possible? If so, how?
● What do you think may happen to a person's ability to problem-solve and make choices if he or she lives with limited opportunities to do so for a long period of time? How do you think this would affect a person's self-esteem?
● What activities might a therapist do with individuals to give them opportunities to problem-solve and make choices so they may improve upon these skills?

2. Time Warp Interview

Imagine the situation of someone who has been hospitalized for the last 30 years with limited personal access to new technologies. Identify the technologies that have become commonplace in the last 30 years. You may need to interview someone who is older than yourself to help you with this.

 Make a list of the most important technologies and how they are used in everyday practice. Then reflect on the following questions.

Reflective Questions

● Without knowledge of or familiarity with these technologies, what barriers would be present for an individual transitioning from the state hospital to the community? How would life be affected in terms of work, home management, and communication?

- What skills and training would the individual need to understand and use the technology?
- What additional challenges would someone with severe mental illness face in learning these new skills? How could these skills be adapted to assist the individual with severe mental illness in learning how to use new technology in community life?

3. Shopping on a Budget

Your assignment is to go shopping for a pair of men's jeans, size 50 waist, 36 length. You have $12.00 to spend.

 Describe your experience in your Reflective Journal.

Reflective Questions

- What skills were required to plan the shopping trip? To use transportation? To find the pants? To pay for the pants? Did you feel competent in these skills?
- Did you ask others for any kind of assistance? If so, were the individuals helpful?
- What challenges did you experience during this shopping trip?
- What feelings did you experience during the shopping trip?
- What other challenges would an individual with severe mental illness who has not lived in the community for 10 years have faced?

References

Allen, C. K. (1982). Independence through activity: The practice of occupational therapy (psychiatry). *American Journal of Occupational Therapy, 36*(11), 731–739.

American Occupational Therapy Association (AOTA). (2002). Occupational therapy practice framework: Domain and process. *American Journal of Occupational Therapy, 56,* 609–639.

Asher, I. E. (1996). *Occupational Therapy Assessment Tools: An Annotated Index* (2nd ed.). Bethesda, MD: American Occupational Therapy Association.

Ballard, F. A. (2008). Benefits of a psychosocial rehabilitation program in a treatment mall. *Journal of Psychosocial Mental Health Services, 46,* 26–32.

Baum, C., & Edwards, D. (1993). Cognitive performance in senile dementia of the Alzheimer's type: The Kitchen Task Assessment. *American Journal of Occupational Therapy, 47,* 431–436.

Bellack, A. (2006). Scientific and consumer models of recovery in schizophrenia: Concordance, contrasts, and implications. *Schizophrenia Bulletin, 32,* 432–442.

Benjamin, L. T., Jr., & Baker, D. B. (2004). *From Seance to Science: A History of the Profession of Psychology in America.* Belmont, CA: Wadsworth/Thomson.

Bopp, J. (2001). *Directory of Public Psychiatric Hospital Treatment Malls, 2001.* 122 Dorothea Dix Dr. Middletown, NY: author.

Bopp, J., Ribble, D., Cassidy, J., & Markoff, R. (1996). Re-engineering the state hospital to promote rehabilitation and recovery. *Psychiatric Services, 47*(7), 3–5.

Brown, C., & Dunn, W. (2002). *Adolescent/Adult Sensory Profile.* Psychological Corporation, San Antonio, TX.

Brown, C., Tollefson, N., Dunn, W., Cromwell, R., & Filion, D. (2001). The adult sensory profile: Measuring patterns of sensory processing. *American Journal of Occupational Therapy, 55,* 75–82.

California Department of Mental Health. (2009). "Treatment Programs and Recovery Services." Available at: http://www.dmh.ca.gov/Services_and_Programs/state_hospitals/Napa/Treatment.asp (accessed September 25, 2009).

Camus, A. (1954). "Return to Tipasa." In *Selected Essays and Notebooks* (pp. 147–154). Trans. and ed. Philip M. W. Thody. Middlesex, England: Harmondsworth, Penguin, 1970.

Champagne, T. (2005). Expanding the role of sensory approaches in acute psychiatric settings. *Mental Health Special Interest Section Quarterly, 28,* 1–4.

Champagne, T., & Stromberg, N. (2004). Sensory approaches in inpatient psychiatric settings: Innovative alternatives to seclusion and restraint. *Journal of Psychosocial Nursing, 42,* 35–44.

Chovil, I. (2005). Reflection on schizophrenia, learned helplessness/dependence, and recovery. *Psychiatric Rehabilitation Journal, 29,* 69–71.

Colarusso, R. P., & Hammill, D. D. (1996). *Motor-Free Visual Perception Test-Revised.* Nonato, CA: Academic Therapy Publications.

Ferrie, B. (2002). Changing the environment. *Advance for Nurses, 4*(12), 15–16, 28.

Fisher, D. B., & Chamberlin, J. (2004). *Consumer-Directed Transformation to a Recovery-Based Mental Health System.* Lawrence, MA: National Empowerment Center.

Fisher, W. H., Geller, J., & Pandianini, J. A. (2009). The changing role of the state psychiatric hospital. *Health Affairs, 28,* 676–685.

Glynn, S., Cohen, A., Dixon, L., & Niv, N. (2006). The potential impact of recovery movement on family interventions for schizophrenia: Opportunities and obstacles. *Schizophrenia Bulletin, 32,* 451–464.

Joint Commission on Mental Illness and Mental Health. (1961). *Action for Mental Health: Final Report, 1961.* New York: Basic Books.

Kielhofner, G., Mallinson, T., Crawford, C., Nowak, M., Rigby, M., Henry, A., & Walens, D. (2004). *Occupational Performance History Interview II (OPHI-II).* Chicago: Model of Human Occupation Clearinghouse.

Link, B. G., Phelan, J. C., Bresnahan, M., Stueve, A., & Pescosolido, B. A. (1999). Public conceptualizations of mental illness: Labels, causes, dangerousness and social distance. *American Journal of Public Health, 89,* 1328–1333.

Manderscheid, R. W., Atay, J. E., & Crider, R. A. (2009). Changing trends in state psychiatric hospital use from 2002 to 2005. *Psychiatric Services, 60,* 29–34.

Markoff, R. (1999). Innovations: "Treatment mall" at Middletown Psychiatric Center. *Treatment Mall Best Practices Directory,* 6–7. (Reprinted from *Quality of Care Newsletter, 75,* Spring 1999.)

Mayerhoff, D. I., & Schliefer, S. J. (2008). Academic-state hospital collaboration for a rehabilitation model of care. *Psychiatric Services, 59,* 1474–1475.

McCarron, L., Cobb, G., Smith, C., & Barron, P. (1982). *Curriculum Guides for the Street Smart Survival Skills Questionnaire.* Dallas: Texas Tech University, Research and Training Center in Mental Retardation.

National Association of State Mental Health Program Directors (NASMHPD) Research Institute. (2002). *Public Report: Diagnostic Profile of Clients Served.* Alexandria, VA: Author.

———. (2003). *Funding Sources and Expenditures of State Mental Health Agencies: Fiscal Year 2003.* Alexandria, VA: Author

———. (2004). *State Mental Health Agency Profiling System: 2004.* Alexandria, VA: Author.

National Technical Assistance Center (NTAC). (2002). Mental health recovery: What helps and what hinders? Available at: http://www.nasmhpd.org/general_files/publications/ntac_pubs/reports/MHSIPReport.pdf (accessed September 25, 2009).

Oakley, F., Kielhofner, G., Barris, R., & Reichler, R. K. (1986). The role checklist: Development and empirical assessment of reliability. *Occupational Therapy Journal of Research, 6*(3), 157–169.

Paracheck, J. F. (1986). *Parachek Geriatric Rating Scale* (3rd ed). Phoenix: Center for Neurodevelopmental Studies.

Peloquin, S. M. (1989). Moral treatment: Contexts considered. *American Journal of Occupational Therapy, 43,* 537–544.

Pollock, N. (1993). Client-centered assessment. *American Journal of Occupational Therapy, 47*(4), 298–301.

Romansky, J. B., Lyons, J. S., Lehner, R. K., & West, C. M. (2003). Factors related to psychiatric hospital readmission among children and adolescents in state custody. *Psychiatric Services, 54,* 356–362.

Springfield Hospital Brochure. (2004). More than 100 years of quality service to the community with a commitment to the future. Sykesville, MD: Springfield Hospital Center.

Thomson, L. K. (1992). *The Kohlman Evaluation of Living Skills* (3rd ed.). Bethesda, MD: American Occupational Therapy Association.

U.S. Department of Health and Human Services, Substance Abuse and Mental Health Services Administration. (2004). "National Consensus Statement on Mental Health Recovery." Available at: http://mentalhealth.samhsa.gov/publications/allpubs/sma05-4129 (accessed September 23, 2009).

Psychosocial Clubhouses

Virginia Carroll Stoffel

> "The inspiration comes in when you see "I can work" at the club. For many of us, all we could do is either have the succession of failed jobs or succession of failed school, then hang around the apartment for some time, years . . . then you come to the club and you say "I am somebody because I can contribute" and that's a big part of it. The clubhouse responsibility is to provide a way to inspire people to say, not only can we engage you here, but you can go to school, you can work elsewhere.
>
> —Clubhouse member cited in Stoffel (2008), p. 108

Introduction

Psychosocial clubhouses comprise an international community of people who share the lived experience of mental illness and recovery. Clubhouses offer a physical place where people are afforded respect and varied opportunities to pursue valued and chosen occupations that hold meaning and purpose. The clubhouse model of psychosocial rehabilitation has evolved over time, from 1944, when several people joined together in New York City to form a self-help group called We Are Not Alone (WANA) (Anderson, 1998), to today, when there are more than 310 clubhouses worldwide associated with the International Center for Clubhouse Development (ICCD) (ICCD, 2004, 2008b; Propst, 1997).

In contrast to consumer-operated services (see Chapter 35), clubhouses operate with a blend of staff and members who assume leadership for all clubhouse operations in an egalitarian and strength-based context in which members pursue personal goals related to their recovery. A variety of mental health professionals are employed by psychosocial clubhouses worldwide, including occupational therapists and occupational therapy assistants.

This chapter provides a picture of the international clubhouse movement, from its inception in New York City to its current worldwide status. It identifies meaningful occupational roles offered by the clubhouse model where occupational therapy practitioners can and do contribute.

Description of Psychosocial Clubhouses: The Fountain House Model

Fountain House, the early prototype for psychosocial clubhouses, was first established in New York City in 1948. Meeting the needs of people with mental illness so that vocational and educational goals would prepare members for the "normal processes of training and work" (Anderson, 1998, p. 29), Fountain House was supported by funding from philanthropists and from the New York State Department of Vocational Rehabilitation. In the early years, Fountain House offered its members a mix of sheltered workshop experiences fabricating small items facilitated by an occupational therapist, clerical job training, and social and recreational activities.

John Beard, a social worker from Michigan, was hired as the executive director of Fountain House in 1955. Program development evolved with an emphasis on daytime work-related activities. During the evenings and weekends, activities such as arts, crafts, and drama and choral groups were offered, along with holiday and seasonal events. By 1957, daily lunch was added as a clubhouse offering, and the development of social relationships was emphasized with the hope that as members interacted, they would provide healthy and constructive influences on one another (Anderson, 1998).

Although some Fountain House members were able to successfully obtain and keep a job, many were not successful. In an effort to provide support for those members who had difficulties with employment stability and success, Beard (1987) developed agreements with local businesses (e.g., a supermarket, brokerage firm, printing company, and clothing store) that Fountain House would ensure that a member would fill a position, and should the regularly assigned member be unable to work, the position would be filled by a Fountain House staff or other member who could fulfill the job duties. This practice continues today and is known as transitional employment (further described later in this chapter) (Anderson, 1998; Henry, Barreira, Banks, Brown, & McKay, 2001).

Program development at Fountain House was based on helping members meet the challenges of living successfully in the community. When members found that they needed assistance with securing leases for housing during 1958 and 1959, Fountain House intervened by working with landlords and real estate agents. Providing assistance with initial deposits and assisting members to share living space in order to keep living expenses affordable expanded the types of services offered by Fountain House to its members (Anderson, 1998). A thrift shop was developed at the Fountain House to offer members donated household goods and clothing in an affordable manner.

As Beard interacted with others from across the country and shared his experiences with Fountain House, interest in how the various programs operated and could be replicated was expressed. A training program was developed in which staff from other programs observed and interacted at Fountain House for 3 to 4 weeks, carrying out programming side by side with members and staff (Anderson, 1998). A combination of observation, engagement, and instruction across all of the clubhouse work units (clerical, food service, housekeeping, building maintenance, outreach) and those involved in transitional employment provided the training participants with a working knowledge of successful practices employed at Fountain House. This model of training continues through the ICCD, with training locations throughout the world (ICCD, 2008a).

As interest in developing psychosocial clubhouses across the globe widened during the 1980s, clubhouse members and staff joined together for international seminars held every 2 years. These gatherings offered sessions in which clubhouse members and staff shared their experiences and successes with one another. Ultimately, in 1989, Standards for Clubhouse Programs were developed on the basis of the consensus of participants involved in clubhouse programs around the globe. In 1994, the ICCD was formed with representatives from clubhouses worldwide.

The International Standards for Clubhouse Programs continue to be carefully reviewed and updated biannually so that these principles are globally understood and universally applied to programs that adopt the psychosocial clubhouse model. The term *work-ordered day*, coined when the first Standards for Clubhouse Programs were developed in 1989, reflects how staff and members are mutually involved in operating and enhancing the clubhouse community (Anderson, 1998; Propst, 1992).

Clubhouse Mission and Goals

The vision of the ICCD is that men and women with mental illness throughout the world will have access to the respect and dignity offered by clubhouses, and to the full range of clubhouse opportunities, as they rebuild their lives. The mission of the ICCD is to promote and protect the rights, opportunities and future of psychiatrically disabled men and women who are members of clubhouses all over the world. Today, as mental health services delivery systems around the world are facing new crises, the ICCD is here to insist on a future with respect and opportunity for those who have been denied them for too long. (ICCD, 2008b)

The mission and vision of the ICCD and clubhouses throughout the world are linked and further reflected in the International Standards for Clubhouse Programs. The ICCD emphasizes that clubhouses should be developed in a manner that is culturally sensitive and holistic, offering "respect, hope, mutuality and unlimited opportunity to access the same worlds of friendship, housing, education and employment as

the rest of society" (2008b). The ability to live and work in the community as full participants who contribute to society is part of the ICCD vision, providing an environment of hope, support, acceptance, and commitment to building capacity.

Beard, Propst, and Malamud (1982) reflected on their Fountain House experience and stated that the broad goals of clubhouses include keeping people with mental illness out of the hospital and in the community in order to achieve social, financial, educational, and vocational goals important to the individual. The ways in which clubhouses facilitate these goals are best understood by reading the 36 standards, available at http://www.iccd.org and summarized here, as well as the first-person accounts in Flannery and Glickman's 1996 book, *Fountain House: Portraits of Lives Reclaimed from Mental Illness*.

International Standards

The principles embedded in the Clubhouse Standards have been tested across time. Some can clearly be traced back to the early Fountain House experience, whereas others have been shaped by the international clubhouse community through the biannual review of Standards conducted through the ICCD, with the most recent update in October 2008. The Standards (ICCD, 2008a) provide members and staff with clarity about membership, staff and member relationships, space, the work-ordered day, employment (transitional, supported, and independent), education, clubhouse functions, funding, governance, and administration. They are also the criteria to which clubhouses seeking ICCD accreditation are held accountable.

Membership

The Standards emphasize the voluntary nature of membership and the absence of time limits. Clubhouses are open to anyone with a history of mental illness who does not pose a safety threat, with freedom of choice and full access to all clubhouse opportunities and records. In addition, members who are hospitalized, isolate, or drop their attendance are assured that the clubhouse has a system of reaching out to reengage members so they realize the clubhouse is still fully available.

Relationships

With regard to staff–member relationships, the Standards emphasize that all clubhouse meetings are open (e.g., there are no exclusive meetings for staff) and that the number of staff employed should be only enough to engage members in the real work of running the clubhouse. Clubhouse responsibilities are jointly filled and dependent on member involvement. All clubhouse staff are expected to have generalist roles that are not defined by any professional credentials they might possess, such as social work, occupational therapy, or vocational rehabilitation. Staff members share all responsibilities across the clubhouse, including evening, weekend, and holiday programming, as well as unit, employment, and housing responsibilities.

Space

The Standards require that each clubhouse have its own name, address, and telephone number and be separate from

PhotoVoice

The bus slowed, wheezed and coughed the rider onto the street. She took timid steps toward the tall building. The sun rose from her slumber. Birds flocked toward sidewalks scattered with bread. Indecisive, she nearly turned back several times, back to the warmth of her hearth, back to the safety of her bed, back to the known. Even when the familiar reeks with pain, even when the routine suffocates with fear, even when the day is filled with dread, some prefer it to—change.

It took all her courage to place one foot in front of the other. Then she did it again and again and again. Moments passed. Emotions ranged from dread to anxiety to calm to wonder. She grasped the handrail and ascended the stairs. Slowly opening the heavy wooden door, she peeked inside. The sound "Welcome to the Grand Avenue Club" bounced off her tiny frame. She gathered her courage, moved inside and joined the others.

When the grandfather clock boomed twelve, she was busily carving meat. Sharing the work of the day, she created culinary cuisine for the colleagues. Members came and went. Meetings were announced, commenced and ended. She endured. She met everyone and remembered no one.

It was unlike any other day. For just this once, she was not managing her madness. Just for today she was not consumed with fear. The focus was not on symptoms, side effects and sickness. She hoped she found the remedy. Removing her hair net and discarding her gloves, she strode downstairs. Smiling broadly, she said good-bye to the greeter. "Perhaps," she thought, "work is it's own reward."

—Neil

a mental health institution. The design of the clubhouse is expected be attractive, convey respect and dignity, be fully accessible to all members and staff (e.g., no exclusive areas), and facilitate the work-ordered day.

Work-Ordered Day

When the Standards were first written in 1989, the concept of the **work-ordered day** was named (Anderson, 1998; Beard et al, 1982). It conveys the expectation that members and staff run the clubhouse, side by side, at least 5 days per week during typical working hours (Vorspan, 1992). The clubhouse is expected to be organized in member- and staff-engaged work units that perform the real work of enhancing the clubhouse community. Members are neither paid nor receive artificial rewards but gain self-worth, purpose, and confidence through their contributions. The work of the clubhouse is expected to include:

- Intake and orientation of new members, staff, and volunteers
- Hiring, training, and evaluation of staff
- Outreach
- Advocacy
- Public relations
- Research
- Evaluation of clubhouse effectiveness
- Administration of the clubhouse

All of these tasks are opportunities that are open to all members. Each unit is expected to conduct meetings that organize and plan the day as well as foster unit relationships. Many clubhouses have culinary, education and employment, communication, and clubhouse services units, although each clubhouse may organize these uniquely according to the volume of work and number of members/staff available.

Employment

The Standards address facilitating member engagement in paid work through three employment programs: transitional employment, supported employment, and independent employment, all of which must take place outside of the clubhouse.

Transitional employment (TE) is defined as a right of clubhouse membership for those who desire to work and offers opportunities to be placed in clubhouse-contracted positions in business and industry. The clubhouse guarantees the position is covered should a member be absent, and the member is paid the prevailing wage by the employer in a part-time and time-limited position (typically 15–20 hours/week for 6–9 months). TE placement and job training are provided by the clubhouse generalist staff and members.

Supported employment (SE) positions may be full time or part time and are "owned" by the person holding the position, typically after an interview at which the employer (not the clubhouse) selects the employee (McKay, Johnsen, Banks, & Stein, 2006). The member and staff jointly determine the specific needs of the employed member, with the clubhouse maintaining a relationship with both the employer and the employee. **Independent employment (IE)** occurs when a member obtains and maintains a job without the direct support of the clubhouse. Members who are independently employed have full access to all other clubhouse services and programs.

Education

As indicated in the Standards, members who want to participate in adult education opportunities in the community are supported by the clubhouse, which might also include pursuit of a GED, vocational technical education, or higher education. When tutoring service is available, clubhouse members are taught by other members to be successful in reaching their educational goals.

Clubhouse Functions

The Standards guide such functions as ensuring the clubhouse and TE locations are accessible via local transportation or effective alternatives and that the clubhouse provides (through its work units) community support services such as entitlements, housing and advocacy, health promotion, and assistance in connecting with needed medical, psychological, and pharmacological and substance abuse services. Although not all clubhouses are expected to offer their own housing programs, they are expected to help members secure safe, suitable, and affordable housing.

Other functions outlined in this section of the Standards include regularly conducting an objective evaluation of clubhouse effectiveness; participation of the director, members, and staff in the 3-week clubhouse model training at an ICCD-certified center; and provision of evening and weekend social and recreational programs, including celebration of holidays on the actual day observed.

Funding, Governance, and Administration

The final section of the Standards addresses the functions of the clubhouse's independent board of directors (or separate advisory board), annual budget development and monitoring, appropriate mental health licenses, accreditation, and community support. Staff members are expected to be paid competitively comparative with other mental health positions. The clubhouse is expected to hold open forums with full engagement of members and staff in arriving at consensus decisions guiding clubhouse direction and development.

Given that the clubhouse standards are continually evolving, clubhouses worldwide continually explore other ways in which they can impact the health and wellbeing of their members. Exploring better ways to meet the nutritional needs of members by changing their culinary practices in offering healthier meals is one current focus of clubhouses, along with smoking cessation programs, stress management, dental care, improving sleep habits, health screenings and risk assessments, and HIV/AIDS education (McKay & Pelletier, 2007). In addition, finding that members are challenged by issues associated with inactivity and obesity, programs that engage members in fitness and exercise are being explored, with early studies finding that members increased their aerobic capacity and mental wellness (Pelletier, Ngyuen, Bradley, Johnsen, & McKay, 2005). How and where to position exercise, stress reduction, and fitness programs with the clubhouse emphasis on the work-ordered day is noted as a challenge (Stoffel, 2008).

Population Served

Clubhouses are open to anyone with a history of mental illness who wishes to be voluntarily involved in the clubhouse. Typically, clubhouses are directed to adults, yet some clubhouses have outreach programs connecting with young adults nearing their 18th birthday so as to offer support and involvement in aiding the person's transition to adulthood while coping with a mental illness. Although members simply need to provide documentation of a mental illness from a physician, membership is not restricted "based on diagnosis or level of functioning" and "unless that person poses a significant and current threat to the general safety of the Clubhouse community" (ICCD, 2008a, p. 1). The latter quote might include members who are actively abusing alcohol or other drugs, whose behavior might be deemed as endangering others. Consistent with clubhouse culture, members with active substance misuse would be aided in connecting with substance abuse services and self-help groups.

Several studies have identified characteristics of clubhouse members (Macias et al, 2006; Mowbray, Woodward, Holter, MacFarlane, & Bybee, 2008; Pernice-Duca, 2008; Stoffel, 2008) as a part of reported study results. For example, in the Macias et al study, which included 89 clubhouse members from two Massachusetts ICCD certified sites, 49% of clubhouse members were male, 82% were Caucasian, baseline age was 39 years, and 44% had a diagnosis of schizophrenia, 32% with a substance use disorder. Sixty-seven percent had a high school diploma.

Stoffel (2008) completed a phenomenological study conducted at one clubhouse in Milwaukee, Wisconsin, with 463 members ages 18 to 70 years, where 43% were female, 35% were African American, and 60% were Caucasian.

In Mowbray et al (2008), a sample of 31 clubhouses in Michigan representing 892 members, revealed a mean age of 44.43 years; 17% were African American, 55% were male, and average education level was high school plus some postsecondary education. Twenty-four percent reported a substance abuse history, and 82% self-reported a mental illness, with 90% receiving Social Security or Social Security Disability income. Thirty-seven percent reported living with schizophrenia, 15% with bipolar disorder, and 9.6% with depression. Seventy-two percent considered themselves to be in recovery from a mental health problem, had a moderate sense of hopefulness, and experienced a moderate level of global quality of life.

Pernice-Duca (2008) profiled 221 clubhouse members across 15 clubhouse programs in Michigan, with 53% reported as female, 82% Caucasian, 52.5% with schizophrenia, and 32.6% with a major affective disorder.

These studies show that adult men and women with a variety of mental illness and substance use disorders, from a number of ethnic and cultural groups, become members of psychosocial clubhouses, reflecting the population in each country where it exists.

Composition of Clubhouse Staff

Clubhouse staffing includes the position of executive director and staff who operate as generalists throughout the clubhouse work units. The Clubhouse Standards do not set any specific criteria for staff credentials, simply governing the nature of member–staff relationships noted earlier. Although it is not required to have an academic degree in one of the following, the professions of social work, vocational rehabilitation, occupational therapy, counseling, and nursing are commonly indentified in the clubhouse literature. In addition, because the number of staff members employed by psychosocial clubhouses is intended to be only enough to engage members in the running of the clubhouse, it is carefully monitored, consistent with the International Standards (ICCD, 2008a).

The Lived Experience

Rather than share one person's perspective on clubhouse engagement, these narratives are drawn from the four clubhouse members who participated in a series of in-depth phenomenological interviews (Stoffel, 2008). Together they create a feeling for clubhouse programs and the ups and downs associated with the experience of living with a mental illness and clubhouse engagement, and they provide an insider perspective of how clubhouse engagement impacts mental health recovery. Pseudonyms are used to share the voices of these four participants: Shana, Jake, Mary and Matthew.

Shana, a single 52-year-old female of mixed heritage (African American, Hispanic, and Native American) shared how she first came to the clubhouse:

I had fallen on hard times—lost my home, lost family, had financial supports removed. I was battle-scarred and my mind was dead, so my case manager asked me to get involved. After a tour of the clubhouse, I thought "Maybe I can do this." (Stoffel, 2008, p. 92)

Later, she shared her ambivalence about the warm and welcoming environment of the clubhouse:

I felt like they were patronizing, like they were equating my mental illness with me needed to be coddled or something. I'm not sure right now if that was because I was in a survival mode, or whether some of them were actually patronizing . . . maybe I did need a little pampering. (Stoffel, 2008, p. 93)

Jake, a single 36-year-old African American male shared his start at the clubhouse:

I didn't have any place to go, to relax or to get away from drugs. My probation officer told me about the clubhouse. I had no money, no place to go, was down and out, so I started coming here. (p. 92)

I thought, wow, a kitchen, tutoring, jobs where I could earn money, food. I need to be here. It can be my second home . . . but, will I be the laughing stock in the streets? (p. 94)

Mary, a single 53-year-old Caucasian female, had been involved in the clubhouse and was returning after many years away:

I think I came back because I didn't know what else to do. I didn't know where to put myself. . . . I tend to think I can't do anything and because I've done some jobs that were kind of menial and didn't have a lot of dignity to it, I thought that was all I could do and would hate myself. I'd have problems with medications and side effects and different things like that. So I just wanted to give the clubhouse another chance and see what I could do. (Stoffel, pp. 92–93)

She also reflected on the Standards regarding membership:

You have to have a handle on your illness. You have to have a handle on your emotions to be successful (in the clubhouse), because if you have anger issues like I

do, you have to learn how to express your anger in a way that won't damage anyone or something like that. (p. 93)

Matthew, a divorced 43-year-old Caucasian male, shared that he came to the clubhouse after his father discovered the clubhouse program:

I can remember coming and treating it like a job. Coming in right around 8:30 or 9 and then be there for the 9:30 meetings and staying for the whole day. (p. 97)

I was still involved but then I started feeling discouraged. . . . I was sort of going home earlier and then coming in later. (p. 98)

He recounted how the staff re-engaged him by inviting him to join a group of members who were preparing to attend an out-of-town clubhouse coalition meeting. This seemed to spark a new level of involvement and commitment, ultimately leading to assuming a position on the clubhouse board of directors (one of two members who served on the board) and trying out several TE positions, one leading to independent employment.

For **Shana,** finding a place where one can contribute and feel comfortable in the clubhouse was important:

I found I felt safer in culinary. It was more fun to be there at that time. Even though we had a lot of hard work to do, we had a rhythm about how we worked together. (p. 95)

Jake, who received a letter inviting him to return to the clubhouse after completing his 2-week orientation when he didn't return for several weeks, shared:

I was very eager to meet people on the third floor . . . just went to the library and see all the books and computers. . . . I thought that was great. I could pick up a book and sit back, read something with help because I'm slow a little bit, you know. My schizophrenia triggers me every now and then . . . but everyone appreciated me for being there, doing a good job. I could name a whole bunch of things I got credit for. I was working really hard just to be me, the new me, actually. (p. 96)

He tried a group TE placement cleaning a local church and earning some money:

It gave me a sense of responsibility when I started with the church. People look at me different now . . . there was a lot of people who cheered me on. I was like "yeah, this is a good opportunity for me." So I stuck with it. And now it's a year later. Actually, I'm the supervisor! (p. 101)

Mary talked about some of the challenges and hopefulness that she found in her clubhouse experiences:

I like to work at the reception desk. I briefly worked in the kitchen in the beginning. I'm not really much of a cook and I don't always like to be around food. Instead of preparing it, I'm afraid I'm going to eat it right on the job. So now the other two units are where I spend time. . . . They give you the

Continued

The Lived Experience—cont'd

impression that you can do something . . . as a contrast to other places where I was told I could never work. . . . They give you the structure you need if you have an unstructured life. It's a place where the unit gives you some work to do during the day, it's not for pay, but it's meant to get you back in the swing of things if you've been out of practice with a job or school. I think it's a very positive place to be. (pp. 96–97)

She later reflected on her experience on a TE:

I was nervous about it, then I was confident for the most part. I was nervous about it because I thought, "well, gee, it's going to fail" and then, "what'll I do and what'll happen and how will it affect the club" and all that, so actually last week was tough. I was nervous about it. . . . Life was different when I had my transitional employment position in the sense that I had to get there every day, even when I didn't have a good night's sleep. I had to get up and go. It was the discipline that I need. It's been very hard to function, but it was a different feeling in a sense that I had to get out there and go someplace. I had to be responsible. (pp. 105–106)

Matthew reflected on his TE:

There's one real nice guy and he's real friendly with me. And there's two other guys, both supervisors—they don't treat me very well. They don't mistreat me but they're not very friendly, being either aloof or quiet. I always try to greet them. I'm starting to give up now because there is never a real good response from them . . . there's never any warmth to their greeting . . . the only thing that makes sense is that they treat me this way because I'm mentally ill and they know that. So it could be that they are rude people, but I see them interacting with other people in friendly ways, so they're not rude people. . . . It's seeing people for who they are, knowing that they have a weakness and accepting them anyway. Much like I want to be accepted because I have a weakness. (p. 107)

Jake spoke about his clubhouse engagement and his recovery:

There's many a thing I could be doing right now but trying to motivate myself more by being in a recovery program (for alcohol and drug abuse) really helps me to learn what things I need to be around. So I chose the clubhouse and it works for me . . . with my schizophrenia and anxiety, there's lots of things that can trigger me back . . . so I need to be in a safe place like this. (p. 115)

For me, recovery is based on making good decisions by keeping the consequences in mind. . . . I'm telling you, being on drugs is a very easy thing to get with, but it's hard to get off . . . drugs was my first love and now I have to divorce it. Becoming part of the clubhouse, I felt like it was a chance, a chance for me to stop getting high. I felt motivated because I felt part of something. I felt the clubhouse was the gateway for me to clean myself up. By being wanted by the clubhouse, I can stand proudly. (p. 119)

Matthew spoke of his views on the clubhouse and his recovery:

Recovery is not a destination, not a fixed place. . . . I think it is part of a journey, our life long journey . . . a process of recovering. I'll always be taking my medications. I'll always visit a psychiatrist a few times a year for check-ins. I'll have a therapist for a period of time while I work on closure for some of the major wounds in my life. But recovery is about becoming and for me, especially, it's about becoming more whole as a person. (p. 114)

You know how they talk about the revolving door of mental illness, well I think about the revolving door of the clubhouse and how we bring in recovery through the revolving door. Some people come to stay for a while and leave. Sometimes when we're out of the club, we find isolation and a lack of community. When I return, I get sustenance. I take a deep breath to take in all the sustenance, and then go out into the world. (p. 118)

Shana, like other clubhouse members who serve as informal leaders shaping the dynamic clubhouse environment and the surrounding community, speaks to the future and her hopes for change:

We need to be advocating for the community to do the very best for us, not the very least. We are not second-class or third-class citizens. I think we have too many times been recipients of the very least that people can do. If I can't do anything else but to embark that message, I'll be satisfied. (p. 137)

When dissatisfied with what she sees as an overemphasis on the work-ordered day and the business environment of the clubhouse, she said:

Wouldn't you really want to have options after two o'clock, rather than working all day? You've done your work since 8:30 and you've picked up papers, you've hung countless clothes, you've sorted and made sure everything is in good repair, and you've thrown away stuff. You bagged it yourself, helped somebody else do it, dealt with membership and the staff, heard complaints about your inventory even though you do not have a say since we are operating on donations. We've done all that back breaking work and now it's time to get ready to leave. But the phone is still ringing off the hook. . . . I feel like it doesn't help the recovery of people who need a nurturing place, not a business atmosphere. They keep stressing the work-ordered day in such a way that it's almost like a mantra, which is kind of how Hitler did his work. (p. 138)

Shana's hope was to be able to access recreational and leisure pursuits in the clubhouse prior to the end of the work-ordered day (4:30 p.m.), not having to return in the evenings or on weekends.

These four clubhouse members shared their perspectives in the hopes that others will understand their experience of clubhouse, mental illness, mental health recovery, and the challenges they look to in the future.

Funding and Costs

Several articles have analyzed sources of funding and costs associated with psychosocial clubhouses (McKay, Yates, & Johnsen, 2007; Plotnick & Salzer, 2008). Representing an international perspective, McKay et al (2007) analyzed data from clubhouses in 12 countries to determine the costs associated with the delivery of various services, including the overall cost of programs, annual cost per member, and the cost per visit. Data in their study were derived from the 2000 International Survey of Clubhouses, which is a biennial survey regularly collected by the ICCD. Given an overall worldwide response rate to this survey of 68%, a total of 89 clubhouses (55 from the United States, 34 from other parts of the world) met the study criteria of having been in operation for at least 3 years, operating with professional staff, and having more than 15 and less than 500 active members (active membership means attending the clubhouse once every 90 days).

Core services offered by the majority of clubhouses included

- Work-ordered day
- Low-priced meals
- Social activities
- Transitional, independent, and supported employment
- Outreach
- Help with entitlements
- Housing
- Supported education
- Links to health services
- Political advocacy
- Medication links
- Volunteer work to benefit the clubhouse
- Arbitration to settle disputes involving landlords, family members, employers, and benefits)
- Transportation to and from the clubhouse
- Money management
- Case management
- Mobile outreach
- Transportation to work

To ensure that cost comparisons were not influenced by the significant costs associated with housing or formal residential programs, those numbers were removed from the cost information prior to analysis. Primary sources of funding included monies from the state or province in which the clubhouse was located (41%); Medicaid (13%); county/borough funding (9%); and a number of grants, social services, and private sources. Based on the 2000 data, total annual costs ranged from $40,145 to $1,461,100, with a mean of $408,082 and a median of $350,000. Mean cost per member ($3,203) and per visit ($27.12) were computed, both of which were found to significantly influence one another as well as the overall budget.

The study concluded that clubhouse costs reflect the country in which the clubhouse is located as well as the length of time the clubhouse has been in operation and certification status. In comparing clubhouse costs with those incurred by assertive community treatment (ACT) settings (Macias, DeCarlo, Wang, Frey, & Barreira, 2001), the annual costs per person are substantially higher in ACT programs than in clubhouse programs, a finding that is consistent with comparing individual place and support (IPS) programs with clubhouse programs (Clark, Xie, Becker, & Drake, 1998), in which IPS costs were three times higher. Community mental health centers (CMHC) programs (Baker & Woods, 2001) were reported to be almost twice that of clubhouse programs (McKay et al, 2007).

Clubhouse costs in the state of Pennsylvania were the focus of Plotnick and Salzer (2008) as they looked at mental health system transformation, with services moving from day treatment and partial hospitalization toward clubhouses and reflecting mental health recovery and community integration. Three consecutive years (2003–2006) of cost data were analyzed from the 29 clubhouses in the Pennsylvania Clubhouse Coalition to compute cost per member and per contact. These results were then compared with rates incurred in the partial hospitalization programs. The average annual cost of each clubhouse was found to be $318,000 (range $100,000 to $770,000). The average annual cost per member was $3,454, and average cost per daily contact was less than $48. These costs were in contrast with an average daily cost of $84 for partial hospital programs in the state, a difference of 43%.

The Occupational Therapy and Clubhouse Fit

This chapter reviewed the history of the development of psychosocial clubhouses and the resultant ICCD Standards and programs that have been implemented across the worldwide community of clubhouses. Like contemporary programs in occupational therapy mental health settings, clubhouses are centered around meeting the needs of their members, who join the clubhouse and gain a sense of belonging, community, purpose, and meaning, which is important to mental health recovery.

The goals of helping to engage members in the meaningful work of running the varied clubhouse work units; getting involved in advocacy, education, employment; and, during evenings and weekends, engaging in culturally relevant social and recreational interests are consistent with the occupational therapy domain of engagement in occupation to support participation and health (AOTA, 2008). Clubhouses offer an environment that facilitates occupational role performance in instrumental activities of daily living, school, work, leisure, and social participation, and through such engagement, clubhouse members find opportunities to experience mental health recovery (Stoffel, 2008).

In summarizing what the clubhouse members described as their engagement in the clubhouse community, Stoffel (2008) noted that clubhouses were seen as a desirable environment, a warm and welcoming place where members could choose what they wanted to do, where they could contribute, and with whom they could spend time engaged in clubhouse activities. Building self-efficacy toward recovery goals such as employment, education, and advocacy attracted people to the clubhouse setting, which also met social needs and established a foundation of hopefulness, success, and a shared sense of mental health recovery.

PhotoVoice

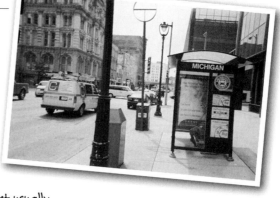

Here we see a common feature of life for a person who has experienced a mental illness.

Public transportation is deliberately considered when clubhouse sites are selected. Without proper transportation, access to the clubhouse, transitional employment, and independent employment, as well as medication clinics and low-income housing, would be impossible.

There are difficulties in recovery here as well. Stigma is attached to all who make use of public transit. Transportation of personal property is limited. One is more likely to be exposed to communicable disease, and there is always the reality that some people on a bus may be, though not usually dangerous, untreated for mental illness or alcohol and other drug abuse.

These and other problems have roots in poverty, racism, and the absence of an educated society which could emphasize what the clubhouse community calls "strengths, talents, and abilities."

We must educate our leaders and the general public about these realities. If we do not, we can expect more apathy and not much more. Consequently, clubhouses perform advocacy and participate in social change.

—Brian

Assessment and Intervention

Specific assessments that measure function and performance are considered to be incompatible with clubhouse practices. Building on the interests, goals and desires of members, and matching people with available opportunities is the primary work of the clubhouse staff. Given that the Standards (ICCD, 2008a) provide that the clubhouse members choose the manner in which they participate, with no agreements, contracts, schedules or rules, members can choose to set their own goals. Members have access to all opportunities available at the clubhouse, without limits placed on them based on diagnosis or functional level.

At the facility level, assessment of clubhouse operations is focused on adherence to the clubhouse model (Macias, Harding, Aiden, Geertsen, & Barreira, 1999). Two fidelity instruments (Lucca, 2000; Macias, Propst, Rodican, & Boyd,

2001) have been used to determine such adherence. Macias, Barreira, Alden, and Boyd (2001) identified ICCD certification as a valid indicator of program quality after examining 71 certified and 48 noncertified programs.

Intervention is simply clubhouse engagement: providing a warm and welcoming place for members to gather, carry out the work-ordered day, engage in the clubhouse activities side by side with other members and staff, seek employment opportunities, and provide advocacy in the community to promote community inclusion for all individuals with mental illness as well as to meet member needs.

Evidence-Based Practice

The evidence-based literature is just beginning to build on outcomes associated with clubhouses. Primary attention has been directed toward employment outcomes associated with clubhouses, such as comparing clubhouse members engaged in one type of work (transitional employment placements) with models of supported employment and measuring differences in longer-term employment and earnings over time (Cook et al, 2005; Johnsen, McKay, Henry, and Manning, 2004; Macias, 2001; Macias et al, 2006; McKay, Johnsen, & Stein, 2005; Schonebaum, Boyd, & Dudek, 2006). Macias, Kinney, and Rodican (1995) described 295 Fountain House members who participated in TE over a 6-year period and reported no relationship between diagnosis or prior hospitalizations with tenure on the first TE. A positive correlation was found with attendance at Fountain House prior to their TE placement. Mean reported tenure across all TE positions was 4.5 months, with more than one-half of the members achieving 6 months of tenure on at least one TE. Independent employment beyond the TE was not reported.

In a subsequent study, Macias, Jackson, Schroeder, and Wang (1999) surveyed 173 U.S. clubhouses and found that just under 20% of active clubhouse members were in TE placements, and 17.5% were in independent competitive

---

Evidence-Based Practice

Given the significant association between leisure motivation and recovery, more emphasis should be given to supporting clubhouse members to fully participate in community leisure and recreational activities. Intellectual and social components were the strongest associations with motivation for leisure engagement.

➤ Occupational therapists should structure and facilitate leisure activities that build on the interests of clubhouse members and provide social and intellectual stimulation.

➤ A rich variety of opportunities within the clubhouse and links to community leisure environments should be jointly developed by members and clubhouse staff.

Lloyd, C., King, R., McCarthy, M., & Scanlan, M. (2007). The association between leisure motivation and recovery: A pilot study. *Australian Occupational Therapy Journal, 54,* 33–41.

Evidence-Based Practice

The following factors are important to mental health recovery and consistent with clubhouse culture: members directing their recovery process, finding meaning in life, skill development, assumption of and success in social roles, available crisis assistance, involvement in meaningful activities, belonging to a larger community, and recognition of and building on personal strengths. Specific clubhouse practices found to be supportive of mental health recovery include warm and hopeful greeting to members, an orientation process that stimulates interest and self-efficacy via meaningful clubhouse activities, clear and realistic feedback that conveys hope, employment and educational opportunities, housing assistance, and access to entitlements and mental health treatment. Member outreach, recognition of member contributions, providing choices and a balance between self-determination and support, along with opportunities to serve, leadership, and the just right level of challenge are all understood as supportive of mental health recovery.

Factors impeding mental health recovery include being belittled or patronized by staff, offering little information for self-determining decision-making, and the lack of feedback from others. Lack of outreach and expectations that are too high or too low are also seen as impediments to recovery.

➤ Occupational therapists and clubhouse staff should continually monitor the clubhouse environment to ensure that members experience warm welcomes toward one another and provide regular outreach to other members.

➤ Staff should ensure that a sufficient variety of opportunities for clubhouse engagement are available and be ready to supply just the right challenge that fully engages members in activities that have meaning for them.

➤ Realistic feedback and encouragement of self-reflection should be incorporated into unit meetings so that members can benefit from their unit experiences.

➤ Belittling or patronizing statements, especially by staff, should be mindfully avoided.

Stoffel, V. C. (2008). Perception of the clubhouse experience and its impact on mental health recovery. *Dissertation Abstracts International Section A: Humanities and Social Sciences, 68*(8-A), 3300.

employment. Bond, Drake, Becker, and Mueser (1999) found that rates of employment for adults with serious mental illness were higher in clubhouse programs than in the general population of people with serious mental illness but also called into question whether TE promotes dependence and limits movement to competitive employment.

Henry, Barreira, Banks, Brown, and McKay (2001) studied 138 clubhouse members who participated in TE over a 6-year period using retrospective data and found that members' average TE tenure was 131.26 days, with older members, those with a longer membership at the clubhouse before their last TE job, and those working more days per week averaging longer tenure on TE. In addition, they found that average tenure was unrelated to disability severity, and 30% of members found competitive independent employment in the 12 months following their last TE job. Henry et al also found a relationship between those members who worked more total hours on TE and their likelihood of obtaining competitive employment. McKay, Johnsen, Banks, and Stein

(2006) found that movement among transitional, supported, and independent employment positions, when tracked over a 4-year period, tended to occur in the direction of moving from a position associated with more support to one that offered less support.

Several studies have contrasted clubhouse TEs with other forms of supported employment in ACT settings. For example, Macias (2001) studied 175 clients over a 24-month period who were randomly assigned to programs of assertive community treatment (PACT) or clubhouse TE programs, finding that both programs supported clients entering the workforce and raised client interest in competitive work, with competitive jobs being accessed by 50% within 6 months. In addition, Macias found that although PACT programs retained their clients in the work-oriented programs more than did clubhouses, clubhouse participants were employed more calendar days, with higher wages, and with jobs of higher quality when compared with PACT participants. Clubhouse jobs were nearly twice as long as PACT jobs, as the PACT positions had much higher turnover.

In a related study with contrasting results, Cook et al (2005) found that when 1,273 participants were randomly assigned to supported employment positions or control conditions, the superiority of supported employment over control conditions, which included clubhouse programs, was demonstrated. The authors suggested that tailoring clinical services with vocational services may prove to be more effective than usual services.

Macias et al (2006) studied 121 adults with serious mental illness who were interested in work and found that both ACT and clubhouse supported employment programs had outcomes that met or exceeded the benchmark for exemplary supported employment programs over the 24-month period of the study. Although there were no significant differences in employment rates, participants in the ACT sites ($n = 63$) were more likely to be engaged in other services offered by the ACT and retained in their programs; participants in the clubhouse sites ($n = 58$) worked significantly longer, for more total hours, and earned more money. These findings were confirmed by Schonebaum, Boyd, and Dudek, (2006), who reviewed the same data set using different methods and a different choice of variables but arrived at the same conclusion as the Macias et al (2006) study.

Several researchers studied the benefits of clubhouse involvement, including rates of and time between rehospitalizations, empowerment, quality of life, changes in psychosocial characteristics, and quality of social network support, constructs believed to have some relationship to mental health recovery. Beard, Malamud, and Rossman (1978) conducted two longitudinal studies comparing rehospitalizations for individuals who were clubhouse members with controls who did not access clubhouse programs. Over a 9-year period, 252 clubhouse participants were compared with 81 control participants who had a rate of rehospitalization of 75% within 5 years. Much lower rates were reported for the clubhouse members who received systematic outreach services (home visits, telephone or letter contact). The need for rehospitalization was not eliminated but was delayed: the clubhouse participants spent twice as long in the community and needed 40% fewer hospital days then their control counterparts.

In Beard et al's (1978) second study, which took place over a 5-year period and included 40 clubhouse participants and 34 control participants who did not have access to a clubhouse, similar results were found, with one half the rate of rehospitalizations for those participants who had 100 or more clubhouse visits (37%).

Rosenfield and Neese-Todd (1993) interviewed 157 members of a clubhouse in New Jersey and measured empowerment and quality of life (satisfaction with living arrangements, family relations, social relations, leisure activities, work status, financial status, safety, health, and prevocational activities) related to various clubhouse services in which members engaged. They found that perception of empowerment was associated with most of the aspects of quality of life, with the exception of work status and financial status, which might be considered to be outside of the control of the individual.

Warner, Huxley, and Berg (1999) found that clubhouse users were more likely to have a reasonable employment status, good social relations, and subjective wellbeing with less treatment and lower costs when compared with nonclubhouse users who had similar mental illness conditions.

Yau, Chan, Chan, and Chui (2005) studied 17 new clubhouse members and contrasted them with 22 existing clubhouse members who served as the control group to explore the changes in psychosocial abilities and work-related abilities during 12 weeks of clubhouse programs by conducting repeat measures at baseline and 12 weeks later. Emotional-coping abilities (impulsive-frustration and depression-withdrawal) and work personality (task orientation, social skills, and team work) showed significant improvement in all skills after 12 weeks for those new to the clubhouse. These changes were further studied and found to relate to their performance in simulated typing and cleaning tasks.

Pernice-Duca (2008) studied 221 members across 15 clubhouses and examined sources of social support. Family members were the most common source of such support, whereas fellow clubhouse members were least likely to be nominated. However, when clubhouse staff was combined with clubhouse peers, they formed the second-most common source of support. Overall, clubhouse participation was associated with the level of satisfaction with their social network. Community inclusion was evidenced by the extent of friendships outside of the clubhouse. Those members with schizophrenia were less likely to cite family and were more likely to rate their support as more important to their lives, finding such support outside of family and more likely within the clubhouse.

In addition to the quantitative studies reported, other researchers have conducted qualitative studies of employment perspectives in an effort to understand the relationship between clubhouse work and mental health recovery. Occupational therapists Kennedy-Jones, Cooper, and Fossey (2005) conducted in-depth interviews of four clubhouse members who found that "support from significant others, the personal meaning of work, experiences within the Clubhouse programme, and the ongoing struggle with illness" (p. 116) provided their sense of self as worker. Support from peers, supervisors, case managers, health professionals, and family were noted as important. Being able to work, receive remuneration for work, have regular activity and structure each day, and have a social context with a sense of belonging were all aspects of personal meaning. Different aspects of the clubhouse, such as a sense of acceptance, social supports and networks, as well as the assistance the clubhouse provided in obtaining and maintaining competitive employment were all noted as significant contributions. Motivation, managing persistent symptoms, coping with stress, and managing fatigue were all factors related to the struggle while maintaining employment. Norman (2006) also found that clubhouse members were engaged when meaningful relationships, meaningful work tasks, and supportive environments were a part of the clubhouse culture.

Studies like these contribute to a deeper understanding of what may impact clubhouse members as they enter the world of work, TEs, and competitive or supported employment, as well as noting what kinds of supports mental health programs might offer their clients who work.

Summary

This chapter explained the unique environment of the psychosocial clubhouse as a place for people with mental illness who seek to connect with a community rich with opportunities and engage in meaningful and productive occupations that are important in a journey toward mental health recovery. Occupational therapists and occupational therapy assistants contribute to clubhouse communities worldwide and join with other professional staff and members with the lived experience of mental illness. The vibrant environment of psychosocial clubhouses offers an option for people to find a context that supports their participation in everyday life while positively impacting their health and wellbeing, consistent with the domain of occupational therapy (AOTA, 2008).

Active Learning Strategies

1. Visit a Clubhouse

Go to the ICCD website (http://www.iccd.org) and explore the resources available. Note the location of clubhouse nearest to where you study, live, or vacation. Visit that location using the Internet (most clubhouses have websites), and find a way to set up either a face-to-face or virtual visit by contacting the clubhouse, asking for a tour, and meeting with members. Plan for what you will intentionally observe (perhaps the International Standards in action or the factors that support or impede mental health recovery in the Evidence-Based Practice boxes will help focus your observations).

Reflective Questions
● What was your sense of the clubhouse environment (warm, welcoming, aloof)?

- What did you notice about the relationships between and among members and staff?
- What opportunities for occupational engagement on the varied units within the clubhouse did you see, and how meaningful did these seem to the members?
- If you were employed at the clubhouse, what would you be able to contribute, given your background in occupational therapy?
- Do you see any barriers or reasons this setting might not be a good fit for you?
- Are there consumers you think would be a good fit for the clubhouse environment? Any you think would not be a good fit?

 Describe your visit and document your reflection in your **Reflective Journal**.

2. The Lived Experience

Reread the first-person narratives in The Lived Experience in this chapter.

Reflective Questions

- What conclusions do you draw from their insights about the nature of clubhouses, clubhouse engagement, the challenges they experience living with mental illness, their pursuit of recovery?
- If you were a staff member working with Shana, Jake, Mary, and Matthew, what do you think you would encourage them to do through the clubhouse in their pursuit of recovery? Might there be opportunities outside of the clubhouse environment that you would refer them to?

 Use your **Reflective Journal** to capture your thoughts and feelings.

Resources

- The website for the ICCD (http://www.iccd.org) has a wealth of information about the vision, mission, and history of the organization and provides up-to-date standards, publications, research, and training available to those who are interested in supporting and implementing the clubhouse model. The international clubhouse directory provides links to the clubhouse locations worldwide.
- The website for Fountain House (http://www.fountainhouse .org) provides descriptions, pictures, and testimonies of how this founding clubhouse impacts recovery in the lives of its current members.

References

American Occupational Therapy Association (AOTA). (2008). Occupational therapy practice framework: Domain & process (2nd ed.). *American Journal of Occupational Therapy, 62,* 625–683.

Anderson, S. B. (1998). *We Are Not Alone: Fountain House and the Development of Clubhouse Culture.* New York: Fountain House, Inc.

Baker, B. C., & Woods, S. W. (2001). Cost of treatment failure for major depression: Direct costs of continued treatment. *Administration and Policy in Mental Health, 28,* 263–277.

Beard, J. H. (1987). The rehabilitation services of Fountain House. In L. Stein & M. A. Test (Eds.), *Alternatives to Mental Hospital Treatment.* New York: Plenum Press.

Beard, J. H., Malamud, T. J., & Rossman, E. (1978). Psychiatric rehabilitation and long-term rehospitalization rates: The findings of two research studies. *Schizophrenia Bulletin, 4,* 622–635.

Beard, J. H., Propst, R. N., & Malamud, T. J. (1982). The Fountain House model of psychiatric rehabilitation. *Psychosocial Rehabilitation Journal, V,* 47–53.

Bond, G. R., Drake, R. E., Becker, D. R., & Mueser, K. T. (1999). Effectiveness of psychiatric rehabilitation approaches for employment of people with severe mental illness. *Journal of Disability Policy Studies, 10,* 18–52.

Clark, R. E., Xie, H., Becker, D. R., & Drake, R. E. (1998). Benefits and costs of supported employment from three perspectives. *Journal of Behavioral Health Services & Research, 25,* 22–34.

Cook, J. A., Leff, S. E., Blyler, C. R., Gold, P. B., Goldberg, R. W., Mueser, K. T., Toprac, M. G., McFarlane, W. R., Shafer, M. S., Blankertz, L. E., Dudek, K., Razzano, L. A., Grey, D. D., & Burke-Miller, J. (2005). Results of a multisite randomized trial of supported employment interventions for individuals with severe mental illness. *Archives of General Psychiatry, 62,* 505–512.

Flannery, M., & Glickman, M. (1996). *Fountain House: Portraits of Lives Reclaimed From Mental Illness.* Center City, MN: Hazelden.

Henry, A. D., Barreira, P., Banks, S., Brown, J., & McKay, C. (2001). A retrospective study of clubhouse-based transitional employment. *Psychiatric Rehabilitation Journal, 24,* 344–354.

International Center for Clubhouse Development. (2004). "What Is a Clubhouse?" Available at: http://www.iccd.org/whatis.html (accessed March 10, 2010)

———. (2008a). *International Standards for Clubhouse Programs.* New York: Author.

———. (2008b). Home page. Available at: http://www.iccd.org. (accessed March 10, 2010)

Johnsen, M., McKay, C., Henry, A. D., & Manning, T. D. (2004). What does competitive employment mean? A secondary analysis of employment approaches in the Massachusetts Employment Intervention Demonstration Project. In W. Fisher (Ed.), *Employment for Persons with Serious Mental Illness, Vol. 13, Research in Community and Mental Health* (pp. 43–62). Oxford, UK: Elsevier.

Kennedy-Jones, M., Cooper, J., & Fossey, E. (2005). Developing a worker role: Stories of four people with mental illness. *Australian Occupational Therapy Journal, 52,* 116–126.

Lloyd, C., King, R., McCarthy, M., & Scanlan, M. (2007). The association between leisure motivation and recovery: A pilot study. *Australian Occupational Therapy Journal, 54,* 33–41.

Lucca, A. M. (2000). A clubhouse fidelity index: Preliminary reliability and validity results. *Mental Health Services Research, 2,* 89–94.

Macias, C. (2001). "An Experimental Comparison of PACT and Clubhouse Fountain House." Available at: http://files .fountainhouse.org/samhsa_final.pdf (accessed March 21, 2006).

Macias, C., Barreira, P., Alden, M., & Boyd, J. (2001). The ICCD benchmarks for clubhouses: A practical approach to quality improvement in psychiatric rehabilitation. *Psychiatric Services, 52,* 207–213.

Macias, C., DeCarlo, L. T., Wang, Q., Frey, J., & Barreira, P. (2001). Work interest as a predictor of competitive employment: Policy implications for psychiatric rehabilitation. *Administration and Policy in Mental Health, 28,* 279–297.

Macias, C., Harding, C. Alden, M., Geertsen, D., & Barreira, P. (1999). The value of program certification for performance contracting: The example of ICCD clubhouse certification. *Administration & Policy in Mental Health, 26,* 345–360.

Macias, C., Jackson, R., Schroeder, C., & Wang, Q. (1999). What is a clubhouse? Report on the ICCD 1996 survey of USA clubhouses. *Community Mental Health Journal, 35,* 181–190.

Macias, C., Kinney, R., & Rodican, C. (1995). Transitional employment: An evaluative description of Fountain House practices. *Journal of Vocational Rehabilitation, 5,* 151–157.

Macias, C., Propst, R. N., Rodican, C., & Boyd, J. (2001). Strategic planning for ICCD clubhouse implementation: Development of the Clubhouse Research and Evaluation Screening Survey (CRESS). *Mental Health Services Research, 3,* 155–167.

Macias, C., Rodican, C. F., Hargreaves, W. A., Jones, D. R., Barreira, P. J., & Wang, Q. (2006). Supported employment outcomes of a randomized controlled trial of ACT and clubhouse models. *Psychiatric Services, 57,* 1406–1415.

McKay, C. E., Johnsen, M., Banks, S., & Stein, R. (2006). Employment transitions for clubhouse members. *Work, 26,* 67–74.

McKay, C. E., Johnsen, M., & Stein, R. (2005). Employment outcomes in Massachusetts clubhouses. *Psychiatric Rehabilitation Journal, 29,* 25–33.

McKay, C. E., & Pelletier, J. R. (2007). Health promotion in clubhouse programs: Needs, barriers, and current and planned activities. *Psychiatric Rehabilitation Journal, 31,* 155–159

McKay, C. E., Yates, B. T., & Johnsen, M. (2007). Costs of clubhouses: An international perspective. *Administration and Policy in Mental Health and Mental Health Services Research, 34,* 62–72.

Mowbray, C. T., Woodward, A. T., Holter, M. C., MacFarlane, P., & Bybee, D. (2008). Characteristics of users of consumer-run drop-in centers versus clubhouses. *Journal of Behavioral Health Services & Research, 36,* 361–371.

Norman, C. (2006). The Fountain House movement, an alternative rehabilitation model for people with mental health problems, members' descriptions of what works. *Scandinavian Journal of Caring Sciences, 20,* 184–192.

Pelletier, J. R., Nguyen, M., Bradley, K., Johnsen, M., & McKay, C. (2005). A study of a structured exercise program with members of an ICCD certified clubhouse: Program design, benefits, and implications for feasibility. *Psychiatric Rehabilitation Journal, 29,* 89–96.

Pernice-Duca, F. M. (2008). The structure and quality of social network support among mental health consumers of clubhouse programs. *Journal of Community Psychology, 36,* 929–946.

Plotnick, D. F., & Salzer, M. S. (2008). Clubhouse costs and implications for policy analysis in the context of system transformation initiatives. *Psychiatric Rehabilitation Journal, 32,* 128–131.

Propst, R. N. (1992). The Standards for Clubhouse Programs: Why and how they were developed. *Psychosocial Rehabilitation Journal, 16*(2), 25–30.

———. (1997). Stages in realizing the international diffusion of a single way of working: The clubhouse model. *New Directions for Mental Health Services, 74,* 53–66.

Rosenfield, S., & Neese-Todd, S. (1993). Elements of a psychosocial clubhouse program associated with a satisfying quality of life. *Hospital & Community Psychiatry, 44,* 76–78, 497–498.

Schonebaum, A. D., Boyd, J. K., & Dudek, K. J. (2006). A comparison of competitive employment outcomes for the clubhouse and PACT Models. *Psychiatric Services, 57,* 1416–1420.

Stoffel, V. C. (2008). Perception of the clubhouse experience and its impact on mental health recovery. *Dissertation Abstracts International Section A: Humanities and Social Sciences, 68*(8-A), 3300.

Vorspan, R. (1992). Why work works. *Psychosocial Rehabilitation Journal, 16,* 49–54.

Warner, R., Huxley, P., & Berg, T. (1999). An evaluation of the impact of clubhouse membership on quality of life and treatment utilization. *International Journal of Social Psychiatry, 45,* 310–320.

Yau, E. F. Y., Chan, C. C. H., Chan, A. S. F., & Chui, B. K. T. (2005). Changes in psychosocial and work-related characteristics among clubhouse members: A preliminary report. *Work, 25,* 287–296.

Community-Based Case Management

Jeanenne Dallas

> *One of the greatest weapons in the battle against discrimination is the powerful example of hope we see in the lives of those PACT serves.*
>
> —Laurie Flynn, NAMI Executive Director

Introduction

Occupational therapists work with people who have mental illness in a variety of environments—homeless shelters, psychosocial clubhouse programs, group homes, and case management organizations, to name a few. Working with clients in their "real-life" environment brings about a number of rewards and challenges for these practitioners. Client-centered occupational therapy practice assists clients in a number of ways to achieve their potential. The rewards of working with people in the community includes the unique opportunity to develop close relationships and contribute in a meaningful way to the client's quality of life through skills training, providing environmental adaptations, and providing emotional support and coaching. Helping clients identify and work with their strengths is an integral part of working in the community with this population.

All professionals face challenges associated with working in the community. For example, occupational therapists generally do not receive a great deal of training regarding social service agencies, entitlement programs, and other issues that clients living in the community deal with on a daily basis. This chapter describes models of community-based case management, the primary features of programs for assertive case management, and the role of occupational therapy in case management. It also features the lived experience of a consumer who has worked with an occupational therapist as his case manager. The personal narrative highlights the working relationship of the client and therapist and the rewards and challenges of working in the community setting.

Psychiatric Rehabilitation

Psychiatric rehabilitation (or **psychosocial rehabilitation**; the terms are used interchangeably) is the model most commonly used by practitioners who work in the community with people who have psychiatric disabilities. **Psychiatric rehabilitation (PsyR)** is a comprehensive strategy for meeting the needs of people diagnosed with psychiatric disabilities. The U.S. Psychiatric Rehabilitation Association (USPRA) states that psychiatric rehabilitation

promotes recovery, full community integration and improved quality of life for persons who have been diagnosed with any mental health condition that seriously impairs functioning. Psychiatric rehabilitation services are collaborative, person directed, and individualized, and an essential element of the human services spectrum and should be evidence-based. They focus on helping individuals develop skills and access resources needed to increase their capacity to be successful and satisfied in the living, working, learning and social environments of their choice. (USPRA, n.d.)

Studies show that through the use of psychiatric rehabilitation, there is a 65% reduction in hospital stays, a 70% decline in homelessness, 70% fewer incarcerations, and an 80% increase in employment (USPRA, 2006). PsyR practitioners include (but are not limited to) psychiatrists, psychologists, social workers, psychiatric nurses, occupational therapists, vocational counselors, consumers, and peer counselors. Each practitioner is valued for the experience, expertise, and knowledge he or she brings to the individual client and the team.

Case management is a process or method for ensuring that a consumer is provided with needed services in a coordinated, effective, and efficient manner (Baker & Intagliata, 1992; Pratt, Gill, Barrett, & Roberts, 2002). Case managers serve many functions: they assess client's needs, link clients to appropriate community resources, coordinate services, advocate for the client, monitor progress toward recommendations, and provide supportive services when needed. Baker and Intagliata describe the roles of a case manager in psychiatric rehabilitation as "integrator, expeditor, broker, ombudsman, advocate, primary therapist, patient representative, personal program coordinator, systems agent and continuity agent" (1992, p. 217).

Case management is an individualized process. The case manager must first understand the needs of the person and develop a level of trust. The two should develop a plan together to meet the client's needs. The plan should take into account the client's strengths and weaknesses and any environmental concerns that may impact the person's ability to meet goals. The case manager then helps the client connect with agencies or services needed to achieve the goals. The case manager should form and maintain a professional relationship with the agencies and services utilized by the client. Next, the case manager monitors, advocates, and evaluates as needed for the client to achieve his or her goals.

Case Management Models

Various case management models are used when working with people in the community who have a psychiatric disability. These models are sometimes called by different names when described by various authors. This chapter describes the brokerage model, strengths model, and programs for assertive community treatment (PACT) model. Each of these case management models has been used to coordinate services for persons with severe and persistent mental illness. Brief descriptions of some of the models that have generated the most discussion and research are provided. The PACT model is described in more detail because it is the most well-defined, evidenced-based model of community-based case management and because occupational therapists are designated mental health practitioners on PACT teams (Rosen, Mueser, & Teeson, 2007).

The Brokerage Model

The brokerage model is also known as the traditional or generalist model. Practitioners working in this model depend on referrals to other agencies and services in the community for most of the basic services provided to their clients (Pratt et al, 2002). The case manager serves the functions of assessment, planning, linking, and advocating. He or she acts as an agent for the client and connects the client with resources in the community, such as the Social Security Administration to apply for Social Security Insurance (SSI) or Social Security Disability Insurance (SSDI) benefits; the Division of Family Services to apply for food stamps or Medicaid; shelters or churches for housing, clothing, or food; and health care providers.

In this model, the case manager does not serve in a direct clinical role and typically has a large caseload, sometimes up to 60 or more clients. The clients are typically expected to meet the case manager in an office setting or agency. Due to the level of responsibility this model places on the individual client, it may not be the best fit for clients who have difficulty staying organized, keeping schedules, or getting to locations in the community on their own, or for clients who distrust health care systems.

The Strengths Model

The strengths model was developed in response to criticism that practitioners were too focused on the impairments of people with mental illness and that the consumer's personal assets and natural community supports were often overlooked when planning interventions (Barry, Zeber, Blow, & Valenstein, 2003). This model specifically focuses on building on the strengths and abilities of individuals with mental illness and intentionally seeks out environmental supports that facilitate the person's self-determination and community

integration. There are two primary assumptions of the strengths model (Pratt et al, 2002; Rapp, 1998):

1. To be a successful person, you must be able to use, develop, and access your own potential and have the resources to do this.
2. A person's behavior is dependent on the resources the person has available.

Intervention in the strengths model is guided by six basic principles (Rapp, 1993).

1. Focus on strengths, not deficits.
2. Look for natural supports in the community; it is an oasis of resources.
3. The case manager–consumer relationship is primary.
4. Helping processes are guided by the consumer's self-determination.
5. Care occurs in the community.
6. People with severe and persistent mental illness continue to learn, grow, and change.

These principles of focusing on strengths, collaborating to emphasize consumer empowerment, and providing intervention in context are consistent with occupational therapy models of person-centered care. A few studies have demonstrated positive effects of this approach, usually in terms of self-perceived improvements in quality of life and reductions in rates of hospitalization (Barry et al, 2003; Björkma, Hansson, & Sandlund, 2002; Rapp & Chamberlain, 1985). This approach shows promise and is consistent with occupational therapy practices, but more controlled research would help practitioners reach conclusions about the efficacy of this approach.

Assertive Community Treatment

Many of the principles underlying the strengths model are also utilized by case managers who work on a PACT team. A primary difference between the strengths model and PACT teams is the team approach to case management in PACT teams. The acronyms PACT and ACT (assertive community treatment) are used interchangeably to identify this model. PACT was developed in the early 1960s by a group of mental health researchers and clinicians, including Arnold Marx, Leonard Stein, and Mary Ann Test, at Mendota State Hospital in Madison, Wisconsin. They designed interventions that would help people with major mental illness improve to the point at which they could be discharged from the hospital (Stein & Test, 1980). This research team noted improvements made by the individuals in the hospital did not transfer into community living and that these individuals were not connected with the services that could support successful community integration (Morse & McKasson, 2005). In fact, the discharged individuals soon began to require hospital readmission. As a result, the researchers designed the **PACT** approach, a comprehensive, intensive approach to providing services to this population.

This approach provides community-based treatment, rehabilitation, and support services, 24 hours a day, 365 days a year, by a multidisciplinary team (Allness & Knoedler, 1998). The PACT approach has been identified as one of the few evidenced-based practices for this population (Phillips et al, 2001; Salyers & Tsemberis, 2007). It has been found to be moderately effective in reducing rehospitalization rates and increasing housing stability while showing more modest effect on reducing symptomatology or improving consumers' quality of life (Mueser, Bond, Drake, & Resnick, 1998; Salyers & Tsemberis, 2007). The National Alliance on Mental Illness (NAMI) has supported the establishment of PACT teams in every state, and today PACT teams operate in nearly every state. An increasing number of occupational therapists are working in PACT teams as case managers, team leaders, or consultants.

Principles of Assertive Community Treatment

Occupational therapy is one of several disciplines that comprise the multidisciplinary PACT team. To understand the nature of PACT, practitioners must understand the underlying philosophy and principles that guide interactions between the consumer and the PACT team members. The principles

identified in this chapter are gleaned from a start-up manual written by Allness and Knoedler (1998) and published by NAMI. The role of occupational therapy is included in each principle.

Primary Provider of Services and Fixed Point of Responsibility

The team acts as the primary service provider and has responsibility for helping clients meet their needs in all aspects of community living. This approach minimizes the need for coordination of numerous service providers within the mental health or social services organizations in the community. The same team members provide both treatment and rehabilitation services. PACT teams typically include staff members representing a variety of mental health and rehabilitation disciplines (psychiatry, nursing, social work, occupational therapy, vocational rehabilitation) that offer the competence and skills to meet the clients' multiple needs. PACT members carry individual caseloads, but the team

---

Evidence-Based Practice

PACT has been based in research since its development over 30 years ago. NAMI's *PACT Advocacy Guide* (n.d.) reports the following findings:

> PACT clients spend much less time in hospitals and more time in independent living, spend less time unemployed, earn more from competitive employment, have more positive social relationships, enjoy greater satisfaction with life, and have fewer symptoms of severe mental illness. (p. 12)

The Schizophrenia Patient Outcomes Research Team (PORT), funded by the National Institute of Mental Health (NIMH), completed a review of research documenting the most effective treatments for schizophrenia (Lehman & Steinwachs, 1998). Assertive community treatment/intensive case management was identified as one of seven recommendations for effective treatment of schizophrenia.

Numerous research studies have been conducted on the effectiveness of the PACT model (Bond, Drake, Mueser, & Latimer, 2001; Burns & Santos, 1995; Mueser, Bond, Drake, & Resnick, 1998). Generally, the findings have been that the model demonstrates superior results for decreasing hospitalizations, improving stable housing, producing positive consumer satisfaction, facilitating positive family satisfaction and cost effectiveness, decreasing psychiatric symptoms, improving social functioning, improving vocational functioning, improving quality of life, and taking medications as prescribed (Morse & McKasson, 2005).

Specific subgroups of this population, such as populations that are homeless or have records of incarceration, may have specific challenges to their recovery and community integration that may be effectively addressed using PACT approaches.

Results of Coldwell and Bender's (2007) study concluded that PACT models, when compared with other case management models, significantly reduced rates of homelessness and levels of psychiatric symptoms but showed no difference in the rate of rehospitalization for persons who are homeless. Cosden, Ellens, Schnell, and Yamini-Diouf (2003) completed a randomized controlled clinical trial and found that persons with serious mental illnesses in a county jail who were processed through a mental health court and received assertive community treatment model of case management showed reduced levels of substance abuse, developed more

independent living skills, and experienced reductions in criminal activity when compared with inmates who received standard criminal processing and mental health care.

➤ Occupational therapist working in homeless shelters may want to explore the structure and processes of assertive case management to consider whether such approaches can support positive outcomes in their programs.

➤ Occupational therapist working in correctional settings may want to use and study whether assertive case management approaches impact a person's ability to develop independent living skills and to maintain stability in the community.

➤ Occupational therapists should explore whether the evidence supports using ACT approaches with other subpopulations of community-dwelling persons with severe and persistent mental health such as persons with co-occurring (substance abuse/mental illness) disorders, homeless teens, veterans with disabilities, and so on.

Bond, G. R., Drake, R. E., Mueser, K. T., & Latimer, E. (2001). ACT for people with severe mental illness. *Disease Management and Health Outcomes, 9,* 141–159.

Burns, B. J., & Santos, A. B. (1995). ACT: An update of randomized trials. *Psychiatric Services, 46,* 669–675.

Coldwell, C. M., & Bender, W. S. (2007). The effectiveness of assertive community treatment for homeless populations. *Cochrane Database of Systematic Reviews,* AN: 00075320-100000000-01089.

Cosden, M., Ellens, J. K., Schnell, J. L., Yamini-Diouf, Y., & Wolfe, M. M. (2003). Evaluation of a mental health treatment court with assertive community treatment. *Behavioral Sciences and the Law, 21,* 4, 415–427.

Lehman, A. F., Steinwachs, D. M. (1998). Patterns of usual care for schizophrenia: Initial results form the schizophrenia patient outcomes research team (PORT) client survey. *Schizophrenia Bulletin, 24,* 11–32.

Morse, G., & McKasson, M. (2005). Assertive community treatment. In R. E. Drake, M. R. Merrens, & D. W. Lynde (Eds.), *Evidence-Based Mental Health Practice* (pp. 317–347). New York: W.W. Norton.

Mueser, K. T., Bond, G. R., Drake, R. E., & Resnick, S. G. (1998). Models of community care for severe mental illness: A review of research on case management. *Schizophrenia Bulletin, 24,* 37–74.

National Alliance for the Mentally Ill (NAMI). (n.d.). *The PACT Advocacy Guide.* Arlington, VA: Author.

members share the responsibility for treating and supporting all clients. The case manager serves as the "record keeper" for a specific number of clients, specifically to monitor and ensure that documentation requirements such as individualized treatment plans and quarterly reports are met and to keep the clients' medical records up to date. Individual team members and case managers are all responsible for documenting care. A typical caseload is 10 clients. A small caseload is necessary because of the intense demand on a case manager's time in serving the clients' various needs.

Occupational therapists as a case managers coordinate services, such as assisting a client with accessing medical care or social service assistance, while also providing occupational therapy rehabilitation services such as activities of daily living (ADL) training and support. Occupational therapists may not be familiar with social service agencies in the community, which presents a learning opportunity for the practitioner to tap into the expertise of other team members. The team approach relies on close coordination and communication with other team members.

Services Provided Out of the Office

The majority of PACT services (typically 70–80%) are provided in vivo—in the community where clients work, play, and live. Interventions are focused on assisting the client with living a "normal" life in the community. Stein and Test (1980) found in their early research that clients are more likely to successfully learn and apply new skills when taught in the actual environment where they are needed instead of in an institutionalized setting, which requires having to generalize learned skills to a new setting. Interventions take place in a client's home environment and in their neighborhood grocery store, bank, restaurant, employment sites, and so on.

An occupational therapist often works with a client on basic ADL and instrumental ADL (IADL) skills in the person's own apartment or other living situation. Here the focus may be on teaching home management tasks, assisting the client with task adaptations, or role-modeling negotiations with the landlord. Teaching budgeting and grocery shopping skills would also occur in context at a grocery store in the client's neighborhood. These real-life interventions provide opportunities to assess the client's abilities and difficulties performing everyday activities in their natural context.

Highly Individualized Client Services

Team members place a great deal of importance on getting to know the client, learning about the person's values, wishes, goals, strengths, and problems. Each member of the team works with the person. It is important that each team member spends time getting to know the person so that the client is comfortable with a number of team members. Treatment interventions are tailored to address the current needs and preferences of the client rather than assigning the client to existing programs or groups, which typically occurs in the hospital setting.

The content, amount, timing, and types of interventions, rehabilitation, and supports provided vary widely among clients. Some clients receive services on a daily basis for brief contacts; others are seen once or twice a week for a longer period of time. For example, if a client is experiencing

difficulty remembering to take medication on a daily basis, the team would set a schedule of daily contacts to ensure the client takes his or her medication and understands more about the medications. After a period of time, when the client feels comfortable with remembering and taking medication, the team members may reduce the number of times they go to the client's home to bring medication (perhaps 3 times a week versus daily). This service provision model is a fluid approach that allows the team to tailor services to a person's need at particular points in time.

The nature of intervention in PACT teams is assertive and comprehensive. The case management team works from an office base, but the clients are not expected to come to the office. The team member drives to the client's home and often drives the client or rides public transportation with the client to places in the community for skills training and support. This "assertive" approach lessens the dropout rate of clients. Clients receive service intervention from the team throughout the week according to their specific needs. A typical client receives an average of four face-to-face contacts with the team and approximately 2 hours of individual contact each week (Morse & McKasson, 2005). These numbers are determined by the specific needs of clients. Those clients in crisis may need more than one contact per day, whereas a client who is stable may need only 1 to 2 brief visits per week for support. When a case manager is off duty for a period of time, the client continues to receive services from other team members.

An occupational therapist may not need to work directly with a client on skills training several times a week but may rely on the other team members to monitor the ADL needs of the client. If the person is experiencing difficulties with symptoms or with following everyday routines, the team will increase the time spent with the client. A client's service plan is monitored on a daily basis, and adjustments are made on the basis of the client's needs and changing circumstances.

The PACT team needs to coordinate many clients and interventions, so communication among team members is integral to the model. As part of the model, a daily morning meeting is held with all team members present. Each client's status is reviewed, a brief report is given regarding team contact with the client during the past 24 hours, and the client's needs and schedule for the day are reviewed. This information is documented in a log system to provide communication with team members who are off or working a different shift. The team members then assign themselves to visit or carry out services for clients during the day.

There may be a team member responsible for coordinating efforts during the day. It is each team member's responsibility to communicate throughout the day with the coordinator or other team members to provide assistance when needed. The nature of this work is dynamic; crises occur and changes in client needs occur. All team members must be flexible in their approach and willing to help other team members when needed.

An Assertive, "Can Do" Approach

The team accepts responsibility to do whatever needs to be done to assist the client to meet his or her goals and desires. This client-centered approach is essential to the model. The team works to adapt the environment and their approaches to meet the needs of the client rather than expecting the

The Lived Experience

Derek

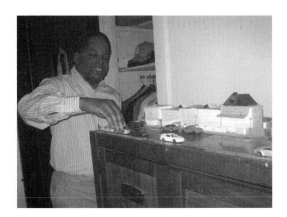

I was staying in empty houses, in cars and on the streets for about 3 years. My father had put me out because I wasn't doing right. . . . I was using drugs and I wasn't working so I couldn't pay rent. Some friends of mine told me about a church where I could go to stay. I met the ROADS team (a PACT team in St Louis, MO) when I was staying there. Some of the caseworkers came to see me at the shelter.

They helped me come to their office. I told them I wanted help with getting housing and getting off of drugs—cocaine and alcohol. I didn't have any income so they helped me apply for SSI. They got me to see a psychiatrist and I starting taking medications. I went into drug treatment after awhile. I went to drug treatment a few times over a couple of years. It was really hard to stay off of the drugs and alcohol. After I left one of the treatment centers I went to live at a Christian housing program. The team helped me find people to help me pay my rent. I had to wait until my SSI got approved—that took a long time, I think about 2 years.

I did OK at the house but I didn't like it. The case managers from the team came to see me a lot. I would get my medications from them and go to the office sometimes to see the doctor and go to groups. My main case worker told me she was an occupational therapist, I didn't know what that meant but I liked working with her. She would come over to my room and help me get it organized and made sure that I kept it clean. I had a roommate who would come in drunk and give me trouble. She helped me get away from him and stay away from the house during the day. I stopped using drugs and drinking when I was there.

When my SSI came through she helped me find a payee to help me with my money. We found an apartment and I moved in. I was so happy to have my own place again. My payee would pay my bills and give me a check every week. The team helped me spend my money every week. I got some money and bought furniture and stuff. My main case manager (the occupational therapist) helped me go shopping; she showed me how to take care of my apartment. I already knew how to do some of those things, but I hadn't had my own apartment in a long time and forgot how to do some things. She helped me learn those things again. I finally had a place to put my Hot Wheels collection, I like to set them up around the apartment. I have about 200 cars. I like to move them around like I am going out somewhere and people are coming to see me. That is my main hobby.

I am in another apartment now. I don't have the payee anymore. I did real good at spending my money so my case manager said I didn't need a payee anymore. Now the team helps me go cash my check when it comes and we pay my bills with money orders. I sometimes have them help me with shopping, but my sister likes to take me. I see my family a lot more now that I am better. We are real close. I go out of town with my sister to see my baby sister a few times a year. My father is sick now and in a home, I go and see him and help take care of him.

I go to church meetings every week; that helps me. I work with a guy sometimes, but he doesn't like to pay me right. The people on the ROADS team helped me tell him that he needs to pay me better. I go to GED classes now and I am going to take the test pretty soon. I want to go to college after I get my GED. The team helps me with my medications every week; I fill up a weekly pill box and they come to see me once a week to help me with that. I have only been in the hospital one time in the past 3 years. I still hear voices a little bit, I am very paranoid, and I think people are behind me talking about me. The doctor says I have schizophrenia. When I start having trouble I play with my cars, listen to music, call my sister or the ROADS team. The medicines help me. I don't like going away from the apartment without people, I think people are watching me. It helps me when the team goes places with me.

I think I do real good with my apartment, I keep it clean and my case managers say that I keep my place real nice. I have worked with the ROADS team for about 6 years. I think I am doing a lot better than when I started with them. I don't know where I would be without them; I would probably be in my grave. I am doing great.

client to adapt to the team or follow rules of a treatment program. A primary responsibility for all team members is to reach out and engage the clients and to develop trusting relationships. Team members are persistent in attempts to serve the client and do not give up on clients because of missed appointments or other difficulties that may interfere with treatment or needed services. Role flexibility is an essential characteristic for all team members. An occupational therapist will perform activities deemed "occupational therapy" but may also accompany a client to medical appointments, advocate for the client to receive entitlement benefits, or provide medication education. The same is true for other members of the team; for example, a social worker may help a client plan a monthly budget or learn grocery-shopping skills.

Team members each assess the strengths, needs, and goals of the individual from their own disciplinary perspective and share their analyses with the team. Together with the client, the team establishes a treatment plan to address the client's goals and needs. This "transdisciplinary" approach depends on the members of the team being comfortable providing services outside of their professional background (within legal limits) or comfort zone. Team members are cross-trained to meet the individual needs of the clients. For example, the occupational therapist will assess a client's living skills and make suggestions for environmental adaptations or teaching strategies. Coaching or training other team members in the strategies to best teach or role-model for the client may be how the expertise of the occupational therapy practitioner is implemented. When other team members meet with the client, they will carry out the strategies suggested by the occupational therapist or attempt other techniques. The team will discuss issues and brainstorm suggestions together.

All team members are responsible for all aspects of the interventions, with just a few exceptions. Nursing and psychiatry are specifically responsible for diagnosis, hospital admissions, medication prescription, and administration of injection medications. The team collaborates with the psychiatrist regarding diagnosis and medication, but the psychiatrist is ultimately responsible for medication management.

Continuous, Long-Term Services

Another feature of PACT services is that they are not time-limited service. Services are offered continuously for as long as the client wants and needs the service and are adjusted as the needs and goals of the client change. Further, the client is empowered to terminate services if desired. The goal of providing continuous, long-term service is to have a positive impact on the course of the client's mental illness so episodes are less frequent and prolonged and functioning between episodes is improved.

PACT is an intensive case management model. Services are provided 24 hours a day, 7 days a week. Team members are on duty throughout the day. Typically, there is a case manager on duty 10 to 12 hours during the day and part time during the weekends. After hours is covered by an on-call type of system, and all case managers share in this responsibility. The case manager may respond to crisis situations either by phone or in person when necessary. Occupational therapists serving as case manager are also responsible for handling crisis and after-hours calls. Training on crisis intervention is provided to all team members who cover the on-call pager, and a line of communication is established to ensure that one case manager is not solely responsible for crisis intervention. For example, teams have a backup system in case the person on call is not able to completely handle the situation, and other team members will be available for consultation or physical assistance.

Targeted Population

PACT services target specific populations; the team enrolls clients who fit a specific set of criteria depending on the focus of the team. These individuals are diagnosed with a severe and persistent mental illness (e.g., schizophrenia or bipolar disorder) and have a high level of need for services in the community. These programs target clients with one or more of the following characteristics: high-risk for hospitalization, frequently in crisis and requiring emergency intervention, severe and disabling symptoms and unresponsive to traditional outpatient programs, homeless,

co-occurring substance abuse disorders, and at-risk of involvement with the criminal justice system (Allness & Knoedler, 1998; Morse & McKasson, 2005). Clients targeted by PACT are often consumers who have not been successful in case management using a brokerage model.

PACT works with client families to provide support to the family and advocate with the client. Family members are viewed as partners in the treatment process. With the client's consent, the team consults with family members and collaborates with the family to improve or maintain family relationships. The overarching goal of PACT is the recovery of the individual with mental illness. PACT service strives to support the client in his or her efforts to recover from mental illness and live a productive, fulfilling life.

Funding Sources

When compared with standard community services, PACT consistently leads to better outcomes for clients (Bond, Drake, Mueser, & Latimer, 2001). In 1999, *Mental Health: A Report of the Surgeon General* (U.S. Department of Health and Human Services, 1999) highlighted PACT as an effective service for people with severe and persistent mental illness (Morse & McKasson, 2005). The federal Health Care Financing Administration issued an advisory letter in 1999 to state governments that clarified and encouraged the use of Medicaid to fund PACT services. Medicaid provisions vary widely among states; practitioners should contact their state's Medicaid statutes to ascertain the funding for PACT services in the state.

According to the *Assertive Community Treatment: Implementation Resources Kit*, the Substance Abuse and Mental Health Services Administration (SAMHSA) determined that the presence of PACT services is one of three indicators of the quality of a state's mental health system (SAMHSA, 2002). SAMHSA identified PACT as one of its six evidenced-based services. Funding for PACT teams has also come from grants awarded from private foundations. NAMI has also been involved in developing funding sources for PACT teams.

Role of Occupational Therapy

Occupational therapy is specifically listed by Allness and Knoedler (1998) as one of the mental health professions represented on PACT teams. As a case manager on the team, the occupational therapist is responsible for coordinating care with the other team members, carrying a caseload, and carrying out all the duties of a team member. The occupational therapist offers the profession's strength in assessment of functioning in natural environments and task analysis, especially for those clients with cognitive limitations associated with their mental illness. The occupational therapist is often responsible for evaluating the client's ADL functional skills and deficits as related to living independently in the community. The results of the ADL evaluation become part of the comprehensive assessment compiled by the team typically within the first 30 days of enrolling a client on the team.

The occupational therapist may also evaluate a client to determine an appropriate level of care when the client is having difficulty living in independent housing. A client's housing preference is paramount to the client-centered approach. For example, if a client living in a residential care facility states that he or she would like to live in an apartment, the team does whatever is needed to help make this a reality. Each discipline is involved in various aspects of assisting the client to fulfill this goal. The social work team members investigate and assist the client with finding housing assistance, and the occupational therapist further assesses the client's ADL and IADL skills to determine what assistance and environmental adaptations may be needed to help the client successfully reach this goal. Through the efforts of the team and client, this change in living situation may be accomplished in time.

Occupational therapists believe that engagement in meaningful occupations contributes to successful community living. The occupational therapist assists clients with identifying meaningful occupations and helps them pursue these occupations while finding ways to remain productive during the day. This may include finding resources for leisure pursuits within a limited budget, volunteer opportunities, or opportunities for paid employment. Many PACT teams include a position for a vocational specialist. An occupational therapist may be able to fill this position in order to specifically target vocational goals and pursuits of the clients.

An occupational therapist may also work as a consultant to a PACT team, which may be more economical for a team with limited finances. The team and the organization determine with the occupational therapist what specific needs may be served through the consultant relationship. The occupational therapy consultant may be called upon to conduct ADL functional assessments, identify intervention strategies targeting specific issues, or train other professionals or paraprofessionals (e.g., consumer-workers or assistants) to carry out task adaptations to enable clients' successful performance of ADL tasks. The occupational therapist may also provide information or training to other team members working with clients who have physical limitations by training them in, for example, joint protection and energy conservation techniques.

Occupational therapy assistants may be working on a PACT team as a cost-effective way of including occupational therapy on a team. An occupational therapist consultant may provide supervision for the occupational therapy assistant employed on the team. The occupational therapy practitioner may serve as a clinical instructor for occupational therapy students working on a PACT team as part of a fieldwork level I or II experience. Many occupational therapy educational programs include contemporary mental health field experiences for students. An occupational therapist seeking a position as a consultant to a PACT team would benefit both the organization and the educational programs by designing a fieldwork program for the team. Many occupational therapy programs have clinical faculty members working part time in community organizations in order to develop fieldwork sites or potential occupational therapy positions in community settings. A PACT team is an excellent place for this in vivo training to take place. The educational program may enter into a mutually beneficial relationship with the organization to provide occupational therapy service to the organization and fieldwork sites for the occupational therapy program.

Assessments

Newly enrolled clients in PACT receive a comprehensive assessment that is conducted by members of the team. The PACT Comprehensive Assessment, as recommended in the PACT start-up manual (Allness & Knoedler, 1998), includes seven parts:

1. Psychiatric History, Mental Status, and Diagnosis conducted by a psychiatrist
2. Physical Health completed by the team nurse
3. Use of Alcohol and Drugs conducted by the team member designated as the substance abuse specialist
4. Education and Employment conducted by the team member designated as the vocational specialist (this could be the occupational therapist)
5. Social Development and Functioning conducted by a mental health professional (typically a social worker) member of the team
6. Activities of Daily Living conducted by a mental health professional (typically the occupational therapist) member of the team
7. Family Structure and Relationships conducted by a mental health professional (typically a social worker) member of the team

Each discipline brings its profession's expertise to this process.

The Activities of Daily Living (ADL) assessment is typically an interview, and the occupational therapist further contributes to this process by conducting a performance-based assessment. The clients seen by a PACT team typically have issues developing trust with health care professionals and may be difficult to engage in the beginning of the relationship with the team. Thus, formal assessment may be difficult to accomplish within the first 30 days.

The occupational therapist may begin with an interview to help establish rapport. The Canadian Occupational Performance Measure (COPM) (Law et al, 1998) is a semistructured interview instrument that measures a client's self-perception of occupational performance. This instrument allows clients the opportunity to set goals for themselves and describe the performance areas that they identify as priorities. Another assessment that may be useful for a client to establish goals is the Occupational Self Assessment (OSA) (Baron, Kielhofner, Lyenger, Goldhammer, & Wolenski, 2002), a tool developed from the model of human occupation (MOHO). This assessment allows the client to rate how competently he or she performs a number of tasks related to occupational life (Kielhofner, 2002).

In order to conduct an assessment of everyday function in the natural environment, the occupational therapist observes the client performing typical daily activities in his or her home, such as how the client prepares meals or safely heats and cools his or her apartment. In the grocery store, observation of task performance, managing money, selection of items to be purchased, and overall reaction to the environment allow the occupational therapist to identify occupational performance issues needing further assessment. Brown, Moore, Hemman, and Yunek (1996) found that mental health consumers may perform instrumental ADL tasks inconsistently between simulated and natural environments; therefore, whenever possible, assessments should be conducted in the environment in which the client will be performing the skill (e.g., home kitchen for cooking assessment, local grocery store for grocery shopping and money management, a local laundromat to assess laundry skills). Chapter 47 reviews numerous IADL assessment tools that are appropriate to use in this practice setting.

Interventions

PACT is an evidenced-based case management model developed from the psychosocial rehabilitation movement; the focus is client centered and reflects the goals and desires of the client. Much of the work of the case manager is to assist clients through the maze of entitlement programs and help them obtain the psychiatric and medical care they need in order to fully participate in community life.

ACT interventions have been categorized by various authors (Allness & Knoedler, 1998, Morse & McKasson, 2005) into three areas: treatment, rehabilitation, and support and direct assistance.

Treatment

Treatment may include engaging the client with the services of the team. As explained previous, ACT targets those clients who have not been engaged in services or who have been unsuccessful in other case management programs. Treatment interventions might include medical evaluation and management, counseling, and crisis intervention.

Medical evaluation and management occurs when the team psychiatrist evaluates the client and, together with the client and team members, determines a course of medical management agreeable to the client. Due to the frequent contact with case managers, the team can assess problems with medications and make recommendations to the psychiatrist; therefore, the client may be more willing to take medications. Medical management strategies are developed with the client's input. The occupational therapist may use strategies to help the client be compliant with medications, such as developing environmental strategies to help clients remember to take medications, setting up a weekly medication box, or using signs or other visual reminders. Chapter 18 describes cognitive skills strategies that the occupational therapists may use to develop the habit of taking medications.

Counseling is another treatment intervention used by team members. This involves the use of active listening skills and helping clients manage psychiatric symptoms. Occupational therapists are trained in therapeutic communication techniques and should be able to counsel clients along with other members of the treatment team.

Many of the clients engaged in ACT services also have an addiction to either drugs and/or alcohol. The case manager must deal with co-occurring disorders along with the client's mental illness symptoms. By integrating treatment, the team can provide substance abuse counseling and motivational strategies to focus on the client's willingness and goals to stop using substances or can develop relapse prevention strategies. An occupational therapist working in this setting may seek further education on substance abuse counseling and motivational interviewing.

Crisis intervention as a treatment intervention is available to the clients 24 hours a day, 7 days a week. Responding swiftly to client crises and concerns is an effective strategy to decrease emergency department visits and hospitalizations. All members of the PACT treatment team typically receive crisis intervention training and continuing education in this area.

Rehabilitation

Rehabilitation is focused on helping the client learn skills necessary for everyday community living. This area should be the primary focus of the occupational therapist on the treatment team. ADL assessment and training are areas in which occupational therapy can add value to the treatment team. Many clients may be living in apartments for the first time and have not learned the skills necessary to cook for themselves or to manage a household. The occupational therapist intervenes with skills training and role and habit development. Since each member of the PACT team is cross-trained, the occupational therapist may not be the only team member working with a client on ADL training. Task analysis and adaptation are strengths of occupational therapy. Educating other team members about the best strategies for the client to learn or practice the skill (e.g., various cueing systems or repetition of task) is an important contribution of occupational therapy to the PACT team.

Social skills training is another intervention that all team members will use while in the community with the client. Many mental health clients served by a PACT team may not have the communication skills or the confidence to be assertive with others in the community. The team may serve as an advocate and coach to the client to assert his or her rights and desires. Work and leisure activities should also be included in the rehabilitation services provided to the client. Many PACT teams assign one team member to focus primarily on work reintegration, and the occupational therapist may serve in this role. The client may need to learn other skills before applying for a job; the occupational therapist may help the client identify work interests and aptitudes, conduct a job search, fill out applications, and talk to prospective employers. The team also helps the client deal with the issues involved in working for pay while receiving entitlements.

Support and Direct Assistance

Support and direct assistance is another service of a PACT team. The ultimate focus of this approach is for the client to learn skills to enable successful, independent community living. Many clients have difficulty learning all the necessary skills and need ongoing direct assistance to accomplish tasks. The client may need ongoing support to take medications, to cook meals on a routine basis, to budget finances, and so on. The team provides the supports necessary for the client and encourages the client's independence whenever possible. The team may provide direct assistance to the client with finding housing, resources in the community such as food baskets, and utility assistance. If a client requires hospitalization, the team provides support and attempts to coordinate discharge plans with the hospital staff.

Basically, the members of a PACT team do whatever is needed to assist the client with successful community living. This places a great deal of pressure on the team members to have good communication and team work skills. This work is demanding of the staff's time during the day. The pace of the day is typically busy, with most of the day spent in and out of automobiles, homes, and businesses. The team members have to be flexible and ever ready to "switch gears" when needed. The schedule a team member sets for himself or herself often changes frequently during the day: clients may not be home, may have other things they want to accomplish, or may refuse to do anything with the team member as planned. When this happens, the team member must accommodate the client and either negotiate other plans with the client or contact other clients.

Some clients demand more time than staff seem able to give. The team members need to check in with each other on a daily basis to guard against burn-out. This is one of the benefits of having a daily meeting to review the clients' status. The team can adjust service strategies and priorities. For example, if an occupational therapist has worked daily with a client on home management training and is feeling tired and less than therapeutic with the client, he or she may ask the team for a "break" from working with the client. In that case, another team member will see the client and carry out the training activities.

Safety in the community may be another concern for the team members. Many of the clients live in substandard housing, and the team may need to be mindful of the neighborhoods in which the clients live. The team should communicate with each other if they have witnessed any suspicious or seemingly dangerous situations in the client's neighborhood. Sometimes, it may be safer for two team members to go into an area of town together rather than one member going alone. Close communication with other team members or the daily coordinator throughout the day is also an important safety precaution.

"Role blurring" is part of the PACT model's philosophy. The occupational therapist may not "feel" as if he or she does occupational therapy every day. Practitioners often must carry out duties that are traditionally identified with social work. When working in a PACT model, the occupational therapist must be secure in knowing that whatever he or she is doing to assist a client to live productively in the community is indeed "occupational therapy." Clients may not know what the professional background is of any of the team members; all they know is that the team members are there to work with them, teach them skills, and support them each day.

Summary

Case management has been used for decades to coordinate services for persons with mental illness. Various models of case management have been practiced by a variety of disciplines. Regardless of the variability in case management models and practitioners, the goal of case management is the same: to coordinate the complex, often fragmented mental health services to meet the needs and desires of consumers

with mental illness in ways that encourage integration and participation in the community.

This chapter described models of community case management with particular emphasis on PACT. Occupational therapists can serve as case managers and as members of assertive case management teams. The role of occupational therapy in assessment, care planning, implementation, and ongoing review of a consumer's community integration were discussed. Occupational therapy practitioners have a commitment to person-centered collaboration with consumers and expertise in addressing both personal and environmental factors impinging on participation and occupational functioning that prepare them to function effectively as case managers for persons with severe and persistent mental illness.

Evidence-Based Practice

Since its inception in the 1980s, the effectiveness of assertive community treatment (ACT) has been systematically evaluated. Practitioners searching the evidence will find more than two dozen random clinical trials and some systematic reviews that, collectively, help to identify ACT as an evidenced-based approach. Studies of ACT are aided by the fact that the developers and supporters of ACT have rigorously articulated the structural and functional features of this model and have created widely used fidelity scales to ensure services and staffing adhere to ACT standards.

➤ Occupational therapists who seek to join PACT teams can feel confident about the processes used in ACT but should also keep abreast of new research that helps refine specific approaches that may address housing, independent living, community participation, and so on, to ensure their practices are effective.

➤ Occupational therapists can develop strong, person-centered, helping relationships as a PACT case manager or team member because consumers frequently identify the quality of the helping relationship as a critical ingredient in their success in the community.

Source: Marshall, M., & Lockwood, A. (2009). Assertive community treatment of people with severe mental disorders. *Cochrane Database of Systematic Reviews,* AN: 00075320-100000000-01089.

Active Learning Strategies

1. Research Local Resources

Contact your local NAMI office and determine if your state or community has a PACT team. Contact the team and ask to visit or set up an interview to determine what services they offer. Ask if an occupational therapist is employed by the team. If not, ask for a job description of the case manager and vocational specialist positions and determine if an occupational therapist or occupational therapy assistant would qualify for a position. Provide educational materials about occupational therapy to the agency or team.

2. Research State Resources

Research your state's mental health service program (Department of Mental Health) to determine if PACT is offered. Find out if your state's Medicaid program funds community support and/or ACT services. Read the regulations regarding your state's definition of a qualified mental health provider (or similar language) to determine if occupational therapy is included as one of the professions.

3. Psychiatric Rehabilitation Model

Visit the U.S. Psychiatric Rehabilitation Association website (http://www.uspra.org) to familiarize yourself with the psychiatric rehabilitation model.

4. Fieldwork

Ask your school's academic fieldwork coordinator to pursue fieldwork experiences with a PACT team in your community.

Resources

- Allness, D. A., & Knoedler, W. H. (1998). *The PACT Manual of Community-Based Treatment for Persons with Severe and Persistent Mental Illness: A Manual for PACT Start-up.* Waldorf, MD: National Alliance on Mental Illness. This manual is designed to assist agencies or organizations with starting and operating a PACT program. Occupational therapy is listed as a mental health profession that may be included on a PACT. The manual can be purchased from the online NAMI store at http://www.nami.org.
- The National Alliance on Mental Illness (NAMI) offers information about mental illness and resources for education, family support, advocacy, and research. NAMI is a national organization with state affiliates. The site contains links to each state's NAMI office and other helpful website. NAMI has been instrumental in advocating for PACT teams in all states. Also on this website you will find information on the PACT model and publications available through NAMI to learn how to start a PACT team: http://www.nami.org
- The U.S. Psychiatric Rehabilitation Association (USPRA) is committed to improving psychiatric rehabilitation practice. This website has up-to-date information about psychiatric rehabilitation and evidence-based practices in mental health practice. Consumers and their families will also find useful resources, such as links to state chapters and information on how to become a member of USPRA (many occupational therapists belong to this organization): http://www.uspra.org
- SAMHSA's National Mental Health Information Center is a component of the SAMHSA Health Information Network. On this site is a wealth of educational resources on various mental health topics, such as children's mental health, suicide prevention, youth violence prevention, consumer/survivor resources, and homelessness. It also offers links to local mental health services in the states and hotline information: http://mentalhealth.samhsa.gov
- Mental Health America (MHA), a nonprofit organization, has lived its mission to "inform, advocate and enable access to quality behavioral health services for all Americans" for over 100 years. The site provides many resources for advocacy, public education, and support services for people who have mental health conditions. It is a great site for mental health advocacy and for following U.S. legislation that impacts mental health care: http://www.mentalhealthamerica.net
- The Assertive Community Treatment Association (ACTA) website provides information on the ACT model, the national ACT conference, model fidelity, ACT trainings, and other resources. ACTA organizes and supports a yearly conference on assertive community treatment services, which encourages consumers and their families to join with practitioners and researchers to promote and improve ACT services. The resource links on this page is particularly helpful for finding ACT toolkits and summaries of evidence-based research on ACT. http://www.actassociation.org

References

Allness, D. A., & Knoedler, W. H. (1998). *The PACT Manual of Community-Based Treatment for Persons with Severe and Persistent Mental Illness: A Manual for PACT Start-up.* Waldorf, MD: National Alliance on Mental Illness.

Baker, F., & Intagliata, J. (1992). Case management. In R. P. Liberman (Ed.), *Handbook of Psychiatric Rehabilitation* (pp. 213–243). Boston: Allyn & Bacon.

Baron, K., Kielhofner, G., Lyenger, A., Goldhammer, V., & Wolenski, J. (2002). *The Occupational Self Assessment (OSA), Version 2.0.* Chicago: Model of Human Occupation Clearinghouse, Department of Occupational Therapy, College of Applied Health Sciences, University of Illinois at Chicago.

Barry, K. L., Zeber, J. E., Blow, F. C., & Valenstein, M. (2003). Effect of the strengths model versus assertive community treatment model on participant outcomes and utilization: Two-year follow-up. *Psychiatric Rehabilitation Journal, 26*(3), 268–277.

Björkma, T., Hansson, L., & Sandlund, M. (2002). Outcome of case management based on the strengths model compared to standard care: A randomized controlled trial. *Social Psychiatry Psychiatric Epidemiology, 37,* 147–152.

Bond, G. R., Drake, R. E., Mueser, K. T., & Latimer, E. (2001). ACT for people with severe mental illness. *Disease Management and Health Outcomes, 9,* 141–159.

Brown, C., Moore, W. P., Hemman, D., & Yunek, A. (1996). Influence of instrumental activities of daily living assessment method on judgments of independence. *American Journal of Occupational Therapy, 50,* 202–206.

Burns, B. J., & Santos, A. B. (1995). ACT: An update of randomized trials. *Psychiatric Services, 46,* 669–675.

Coldwell, C. M., & Bender, W. S. (2007). The effectiveness of assertive community treatment for homeless populations. *Cochrane Database of Systematic Reviews,* AN: 00075320-100000000-01089.

Cosden, M., Ellens, J. K., Schnell, J. L., Yamini-Diouf, Y., & Wolfe, M. M. (2003). Evaluation of a mental health treatment court with assertive community treatment. *Behavioral Sciences and the Law, 21,* 4, 415–427.

Kielhofner, G. (2002). *A Model of Human Occupation: Theory and Application* (3rd ed.). Baltimore: Lippincott Williams & Wilkins.

Law, M., Baptiste, S., Carswell, A., McColl, M., Polatajko, H., & Pollock, N. (1998). *Canadian Occupational Performance Measure (COPM)* (3rd ed.). Thorofare, NJ: Slack.

Lehman, A. F., Steinwachs, D. M. (1998). Patterns of usual care for schizophrenia: Initial results form the schizophrenia patient outcomes research team (PORT) client survey. *Schizophrenia Bulletin, 24,* 11–32.

Marshall, M., & Lockwood, A. (2009). Assertive community treatment of people with severe mental disorders. *Cochrane Database of Systematic Reviews,* AN: 00075320-100000000-01089.

Morse, G., & McKasson, M. (2005). Assertive community treatment. In R. E. Drake, M. R. Merrens, & D. W. Lynde (Eds.), *Evidence-Based Mental Health Practice* (pp. 317–347). New York: W.W. Norton.

Mueser, K. T., Bond, G. R., Drake, R. E., & Resnick, S. G. (1998). Models of community care for severe mental illness: A review of research on case management. *Schizophrenia Bulletin, 24,* 37–74.

National Alliance for the Mentally Ill (NAMI). (n.d.). *The PACT Advocacy Guide.* Arlington, VA: Author.

Phillips, S. D., Burns, B. J., Edgar, E. R., Mueser, K. T., Linkins, K. W., Rosenheck, R. A., Drake, R. E., & McDonel Herr, E. C. (2001). Moving assertive community treatment into standard practice. *Psychiatric Services, 52*(6), 771–779.

Pratt, C. W., Gill, K. J., Barrett, N. M., & Roberts, M. M. (2002). *Psychiatric Rehabilitation.* San Diego: Academic Press.

Rapp, C. A. (1993). Theory, principles, and methods of the strengths model of case management. In M. Harris & H. C. Bergman (Eds.), *Case Management for Mentally Ill Patients: Theory and Practice* (pp. 143–164). Langhorne, PA: Harwood Academic Publishers.

———. (1998). *The Strengths Model: Case Management with People Suffering from Severe and Persistent Mental Illness.* New York: Oxford University Press.

Rapp, C. A., & Chamberlain, R. (1985). Case management services for the chronically mentally ill. *Social Work, 30,* 417–422.

Rosen, A., Mueser, K. T., Teeson, M. (2007). Assertive community treatment: Issues from scientific and clinical literature with implications for practice. *Journal of Rehabilitation Research & Development, 44*(6), 1–13.

Salyers, M. P., & Tsemberis, S. (2007). ACT and recovery: Integrating evidence-based practice and recovery orientation on assertive community treatment teams. *Community Mental Health Journal, 43*(6), 619–641.

Stein, L. I., & Test, M. A. (1980). Alternative to mental hospital treatment, I: Conceptual model, treatment program and clinical evaluation. *Archives of General Psychiatry, 37,* 392–397.

Substance Abuse and Mental Health Services Administration (SAMHSA). (2002). *Assertive Community Treatment: Implementation Resources Kit, Draft Version 1.* Rockville, MD: Author.

U.S. Department of Health and Human Services. (1999). *Mental Health: A Report of the Surgeon General.* Rockville, MD: U.S. Department of Health and Human Services, Substance Abuse and Mental Health Services Administration, Center for Mental Health Services, National Institutes of Health, National Institute of Mental Health.

U.S. Psychiatric Rehabilitation Association (USPRA). (n.d.). Core principles and values. http://www.uspra.org/files/public/USPRA_CORE_PRINCIPLES2009.pdf (accessed March 10, 2010).

Hospital-Based Mental Health Care

Lisa Mahaffey and Brian Holmquist

> "A well-functioning occupational milieu requires the development of routines that create optimal occupational demands for patients. These demands should be systematically planned and formally recognized as a responsibility of the entire team. Occupational therapists have a major role to play in identifying opportunities within usual care routines that allow patients to take a more active role.
>
> —Fortune & Fitzgerald, 2009, p. 87

Introduction

In contemporary mental health care, admission to a hospital is typically reserved for people in crisis who require rapid restabilization of their mental status (American Psychiatric Association, 2006). A person is admitted to a psychiatric hospital after consideration of multiple factors, but a primary factor is the level of risk the person presents to himself or herself or others. Additional factors include the person's level of insight, willingness to seek care, and the legal criteria in the state where the person lives (McCormick & Currier, 1999).

For the past several decades, there has been a notable shift away from long inpatient hospitalization and toward community-based psychiatric rehabilitation (Wang et al, 2005). Nonetheless, on the continuum of mental health care, hospitalization remains an important treatment option for persons with severe and persistent mental illnesses. This chapter explores some of the contextual factors that influence mental health care in hospital-based settings. After a brief discussion of voluntary and involuntary admission to hospitals, historical and contemporary discussions of the therapeutic environment of hospitals are presented, a variety of specialized hospital-based inpatient settings are identified, and the role of occupational therapy in these contexts is discussed.

Inpatient Hospital Admission

On the continuum of hospital-based mental health care, involuntary inpatient hospitalization on a locked unit represents the most restrictive treatment environment. In most states, a decision for **involuntary commitment** is made because there is clear and convincing evidence the person is a danger to self or others and/or because the individual is judged to be incapable of taking care of his or her basic needs to maintain health and safety (Weiner & Wettstein, 1993). It is often a family member or mental health professional who recognizes the person is in need of

hospitalization and begins the process of involuntary hospitalization.

All states also have the right to involuntarily hospitalize a person in an emergency situation. In an **emergency hospitalization** situation, the state can order a person detained against his or her will for, on average, 3 to 5 days while a hearing is convened to evaluate whether there is probable cause to hold the individual (Weiner & Wettstein, 1993). In these cases, the criteria to hold a person against his or her will are the same as those for involuntary commitment.

Involuntarily outpatient commitment is a less restrictive, court-ordered mechanism that requires a consumer to submit to outpatient services. These decisions are usually made because the person has a history of decompensation that has required involuntary commitment to inpatient facilities, has a history of severe and persistent mental illness and lacks insight into the need for treatment, and/or has a demonstrated risk of homelessness or incarceration (Appelbaum, 2001).

About two-thirds of all mental health hospital admissions are **voluntary admissions** (Healthcare Cost and Utilization Project, 2008). When an individual voluntarily presents for treatment, he or she agrees to stay as long as treatment is deemed necessary and may sign out at any time unless the mental health providers determine that the admission status be changed from voluntary to involuntary status. In these cases, the health professionals must again demonstrate due cause for their decision (Weiner & Wettstein, 1993). When an individual directly applies for voluntary admission, an initial assessment is completed and a suggestion is made for level of care based on factors such as safety, need for medication titration, and symptomology.

At times, payers will agree with the assessment, but at other times, they will suggest another, less costly course of treatment. Individuals who qualify for state- and federal-funded programs may be referred to community settings that provide support for continued recovery or may follow up in a less restrictive program. Most are referred to outpatient therapy for counseling and a psychiatrist for medication management (National Association of Psychiatric Health Systems, 2008; Sturm & Bao, 2000).

The Hospital as a Therapeutic Environment: A Brief History

The following brief history provides some historical perspective to the treatment context within hospitals. Historical milestones in mental health practice are discussed in Chapter 2, major legislation impacting mental health service delivery is detailed in Chapter 27, and historical perspectives specific to state hospitals are detailed in Chapter 38. The goal of this chapter is to specifically examine historical conceptualizations of the therapeutic environment in hospitals in order to consider how they may be applied in contemporary practice.

Most occupational therapists are aware of the dismal environmental conditions that existed in European asylums during the 18th century because they are aware of the work of people such as Philippe Pinel and others who fought for more humane treatment that linked activity to recovery (Stein & Cutler, 2002). In the 19th century, Dorothea Dix fought to improve the treatment of persons with mental illness, and the creation of a system of state mental hospitals in the United States can be directly attributed to her tireless calls for reform (Greenstone, 1979). The physical environment of many of these state hospitals followed an architectural style based on the Kirkbride Plan, which emphasized structures with features such as sunlight, fresh air, landscaped and well-kept grounds, and physical spaces that provided opportunities for socialization as well as privacy.

Reforms also led to the redesign of social and treatment environments of these institutions, and many of these efforts were guided by moral treatment perspectives (Stein & Cutler, 2002). **Milieu therapy** is the process of establishing a planned treatment environment where everyday interactions and therapeutic events are designed and integrated into the institution's daily routine with the goal of providing consumers with opportunities for socialization and productivity. The idea that the treatment environment or milieu could support and enhance the functioning of persons with mental illness in their recovery has been a central organizing tenet of most inpatient settings since the middle of the 20th century (Weiner, 2003). A primary assumption of milieu therapy was that all relationships were part of the milieu (Rice & Rutan, 1987). Various models of milieu therapy have been developed, but five critical variables common to all models are structure, support, validation, involvement, and containment (Gunderson, 1978).

Around the same time that many practitioners in the mental health field began considering how best to structure the hospital as a therapeutic institution (Whiteley, 2004), new classes of psychotropic drugs were being created that significantly decreased some of the most disabling symptoms of severe mental illness. These new medications offered many individuals the opportunity to effectively interact within the therapeutic environment of the hospital. The deinstitutionalization movement in the mid-1960s, the steady discovery of more effective psychiatric medicine in the 1980s and 1990s, and the advent of managed mental health care in the 1990s all influenced current trends of decreased use

of hospitalization for people with mental illness and the imposition of limits on hospital length of stay (Torrey, Entsminger, Geller, Stanley, & Jaffe, 2004).

In the early 1980s, inpatient stays averaged 4 weeks, with treatment focused on medication stabilization and exploration of thought and lifestyle patterns (Sturm & Bao, 2000). In 2006, one of every five hospital admissions included a mental health condition as either a primary or secondary diagnosis, and the average inpatient stays was 8.2 days (Healthcare Cost and Utilization Project, 2008). The median length of stay in inpatient mental health facilities in community hospitals for children and adolescents also fell from 12.2 days in 1990 to 4.5 days in 2000 (Case, Olfson, Marcus, & Siegal, 2007).

The current trend in mental health care is for frequent, short hospital admissions for people with serious mental illness (Marshall, Gray, Lockwood, & Green, 1999). This pattern challenges practitioners to consider how best to apply the concepts of therapeutic environment in the context of brief hospitalizations. Fortune and Fitzgerald (2009) suggest that the hospital setting continues to provide opportunities for occupational engagement and that interdisciplinary collaboration is a key to maximizing the therapeutic potential of hospital-based treatment settings.

Evidence-Based Practice

Several studies support using client-centered evaluation. As the length of stay in acute care settings has decreased, priorities for use of time and goals for acute care have had to change. Long, involved evaluation procedures no longer make sense. Client-centered evaluations that guide people toward goals specific to the treatment focus make sense, and several studies support the efficacy of this sort of evaluation.

➤ The Canadian Occupational Performance Measure (Law et al, 1994; Law et al, 1998) has validity and also provides information that cannot be determined with current standard assessments.

➤ Research on client-centered evaluation can focus treatment to the client's priorities and improves the person's motivation and drive toward their treatment (Kielhofner, 2002; Law, Baum, & Dunn, 2001; Law et al, 1990).

➤ Client-centered evaluations allow for the collection of outcomes data that determine if the person perceives an improvement or change in his or her mental health status (Kielhofner, 2002; Law et al, 1990).

Kielhofner, G. (2002). *A Model of Human Occupation: Theory and Application* (3rd ed.). Baltimore: Williams & Wilkins.

Law, M., Baum, C., & Dunn, W. (Eds.). (2001). *Measuring Occupational Performance: Supporting Best Practice in Occupational Therapy.* Thorofare, NJ: Slack.

Law, M. C., Baptiste, S., Carswell, A., McColl, M. A., Polatajko, H., & Pollock, N. (1998). *The Canadian Occupational Performance Measure* (3rd ed.). Toronto: CAOT Publications.

Law, M., Baptiste, S., McColl, M., Opzoomer, A., Polatajko, H., & Pollock, N. (1990). The Canadian Occupational Performance Measure: An outcome measure for occupational therapy. *Canadian Journal of Occupational Therapy, 57,* 82–87.

Law, M., Polatajko, H., Plock, N., McColl, M. A., Carswell, A., & Baptiste, S. (1994). Pilot testing of the Canadian Occupational Performance Measure: Clinical and measurement Issues. *Canadian Journal of Occupational Therapy, 61,* 191–197.

Inpatient Mental Health Settings

An individual's stay in an acute care setting is typically very brief, but it is often the beginning of a person's recovery. From the moment a person comes into the hospital, the focus must be on discharge and the follow-up care that will help the individual continue his or her recovery. Little has been formally written about inpatient mental health in the past 10 years. According to a study published by the Substance Abuse and Mental Health Services Administration (SAMHSA) in 2001, only about 7% of all adults who seek treatment for mental health problems utilize inpatient services (Barker et al, 2002; Centers for Disease Control and Prevention [CDC], 2008). Although this is a small percentage, it is a service that cannot be eliminated because of the serious consequences of acute mental crisis on personal and psychological safety.

The primary mission of the inpatient mental health setting is to save lives (CDC, 2007). Data from the 2006 National Vital Statistics Report identifies intentional self-harm as the 11th highest cause of death overall and the third highest for ages 10 to 44 (CDC, 2009). Even more alarming is the disproportionate number of elderly people who successfully take their lives. People over the age of 65 commit 18% of all suicides, yet this group makes up only 13% of the population (CDC, 2007). The inpatient setting allows people to work through their crises in a safe environment, identify with others who share similar problems, understand and come to terms with their illness, and begin treatment. For individuals and families who seek effective inpatient treatment, fears and resistance are challenged, problems are presented as surmountable, and a vision of mental health recovery is made possible.

The focus for inpatient hospitalization is to structure a brief intervention focused on transitioning into less restrictive care environments (Wang et al, 2005). Inpatient intervention is a combined effort of a team of care providers including a psychiatrist, medical doctors, and nurses to manage psychotropic medications and other medical therapies (Antai-Otong, 2008). Social workers, counselors, occupational therapists, and other therapists work to facilitate recovery, educate clients about how to navigate a complicated mental health system, help identify needed supports, and introduce clients and families to available resources that can support the recovery process.

Additionally, inpatient treatment works to empower people to advocate for the help they need and ultimately for a stronger mental health system without stigma. Introducing empowerment and self-determination strategies can help consumers normalize their condition, be more accepting of the recovery process, and participate in self-advocacy occupations that specifically address limitations to their options for mental health care (Bradshaw, Roseborough, & Armour, 2006; McLean, 2003; Onken, Dumont, Ridgway, Dornan, & Ralph, 2002).

Case: Derek

Derek, a 23-year-old male, presented to the hospital after he was found wandering the streets in shorts and combat boots in 20-degree temperatures. He was seen talking to himself, and he scared people with bizarre threats. He complained that there were strange messages on his cell phone and that he was afraid someone was trying to kill him. This was Derek's second admission. His first hospitalization followed a situation in which he became agitated, threatening his mother with a knife when she suggested he get help for many of the same symptoms. Although the symptoms abated with medication, he reportedly stopped taking it several weeks after discharge.

Derek was fired from several jobs because of sporadic attendance. On the job, he had trouble getting along with peers, preferring to stay to himself. He was unable to organize his behavior and, when given feedback, overreacted with agitation. Derek's family was supportive but had difficulty understanding his illness and was fearful that he might become threatening again. Although they agreed to allow him to return home, they stipulated that he must stay on his medication and have something to do during the day. He was referred to occupational therapy for help with organizing his day and improving his independence.

Derek completed a daily living assessment and was interviewed to determine his interests, values, work history, and daily routine. He described the responsibilities of his various roles and what kept him from meeting them. He also identified specific goals for himself, both for his hospital stay and long term. He was assessed to determine any cognitive and/or sensory challenges.

Derek's evaluation indicated he lacked understanding of the responsibilities of the work role and his relationship roles. He had few friends. He did not go out much, and when he did, it was to a club where he drank too much. As a worker, he struggled with organization, motivation, and self-control. He misinterpreted the social interactions of his coworkers and personalized the feedback from his boss. When asked about his long-term goals, he said he wanted to go to college, get a job, and marry. He was unable to identify the process for any of these goals. He blamed others for not understanding that he is different and suggested that the expectations should be easier for him. He identified very few interests and spent his days watching TV, smoking, drinking coffee, and occasionally going out for walks.

After completing the sensory processing evaluation, Derek showed difficulty with auditory sensitivity and a tendency to underreact to all other sensory input. When his psychotic symptoms increased, Derek tended to go from nervous system underarousal to overarousal, and it took a long time for him to calm down.

Derek's OT program consisted of life skills groups focusing on social interaction, recovery and symptom management, community resources for supported education, and employment. Derek began to understand his illness and the concept of symptom management. One to one, Derek was taught about sensory regulation and recognizing his level of alertness. He was assessed in the sensory room and was able to identify several sensory strategies that helped him be more alert and less agitated. With regular use of the sensory room and groups, he became increasingly active and more motivated for recovery.

Upon discharge, the occupational therapist worked with the social work staff to identify a program in the community that would provide him with daily structure and help him move toward his goals of supported education and competitive employment. He also worked with the occupational therapist to identify some sensory strategies he could use at home to help him get to his day program and eventually to his jobs on time. He and his family agreed to attend some of the programs sponsored by the National Alliance for the Mentally Ill (NAMI) to improve their understanding as well (Kannenberg & Dufresne, 2001; American Occupational Therapy Association [AOTA], 2002).

Many inpatient mental health programs have separate, specialized acute care units. Private hospital systems, such as Sheppard Pratt (see http://www.sheppardpratt.org), often have specialized inpatient hospital programs subdivided by life stage (child, adolescent, young adult, adult, geriatric) or by disability (crisis stabilization, eating disorder, psychotic disorder, co-occurring disorders, etc). Public and general hospitals may also have specialized programs for children and adolescents, substance abuse, eating disorders, and dementia. Although all programs share the goals of safety, education, motivation, and transition, there are additional goals specific to the program specialty. For example, programs for children and adolescents must include working with parents/guardians for education, parenting and exploration of family systems, as well as communication with the education systems to which the youth will return (Jackson & Arbesman, 2005; Case et al, 2007).

People addicted to chemicals may be placed on special inpatient units with specific protocols to monitor the physical problems associated with detoxification (Denton & Skinner, 2001). People diagnosed with eating disorders require carefully monitored refeeding protocols, dietary support, and programs focusing on distorted body image (Spearing, 2001). Programs addressing self-injury must establish an environment and treatment philosophy that address interpersonal behavior and emotion as well as thought management (Linehan, 1993; National Institutes of Health, 2003).

Case: Shayla

Shayla, a 47-year-old woman, presented to the hospital with a blood alcohol level of 0.18 and a plan to overdose. Shayla has struggled with depression and alcoholism for several years, and although she completed two chemical dependency treatment programs, this is the first time she has been treated for depression. Her husband decided he cannot handle her drinking and has asked for a divorce and custody of their two children, ages 10 and 13. Shayla lives in a suburb of a large city with a number of community resources that she could use to help her recover. Although her husband is filing for divorce, he wants to support her sobriety and involvement in the children's lives. She also has the support of extended family. Shayla was referred to occupational therapy to assess her ability to manage her daily responsibilities and incorporate self-care strategies to help her maintain sobriety.

Shayla was assessed using a client-centered interview to determine what her daily routine was and what activities were associated with her drinking behaviors. The therapist also elicited information from Shayla about her interests, what she values in her day, and her understanding of the responsibilities of her chosen roles. In addition, the therapist strived to determine what Shayla believes is keeping her from recovery and her goals for hospitalization and long term.

Shayla described a very disorganized daily routine. She worked as a waitress in a bar several nights a week. On working nights, she drank, got home late, and struggled to get up in the morning to get the kids off to school. She rarely prepared a meal, and when not at work, she watched TV. More recently, she spent a lot of her time sleeping. She stated that when the kids were younger, she volunteered at their school and enjoyed talking with the other mothers. During those years, she rarely drank, and her marriage was much better. She identified past interests but engages in few. She lost track of most of her friends. She has one neighbor she likes but interacts with her only outside in the summer. She enjoys the people she works with but also drinks the most when with them.

The therapist worked with Shayla to create a schedule to help her meet her role responsibilities and increase participation in activities not associated with drinking and encouraged regular attendance at the support groups suggested by her treatment team. Shayla was encouraged to consider other waitressing jobs where drinking is not prevalent. She identified several interests that she would like to engage in to build her support network and develop healthy friendships. She was also encouraged to include activities she can do with her children. She expressed a wish to return to school as a long-term goal and was provided with resources to explore her options. Lastly, she was encouraged to attend life skills groups that teach symptom management as part of her ADLs, the connection between self-esteem and occupation, and developing meaning in her life.

Shayla was discharged with a plan to return home and attend an outpatient dual diagnosis program to address her depression and substance abuse. She formulated a schedule with healthy, nondrinking activities throughout the day. She plans to participate in a quilting group that she contacted during her hospitalization and set up a lunch date with a few friends she lost contact with during the past 3 years. She remains uncertain about her job, as the earnings from tips are important. She is willing to explore other options while she completes the treatment program (Denton & Skinner, 2001; AOTA, 2002).

Geriatric staff must be well versed in the safety aspects and communication skills required for working with people with dementia, including educating and supporting family members who serve as care providers. Practitioners in geriatric specialty units are expected to communicate with long-term care facilities to share techniques and approaches that worked best with the person they are accepting into their care (Corcoran, 2001b). Many elderly people with mental health issues other than dementia need help dealing with mourning and managing an increasing number of losses, a decreased sense of control, and other difficult end-of-life issues (Corcoran, 2001a; French & Hanson, 1999; Hay et al, 2002).

The Lived Experience

Grant Bell

I was first treated for depression in 1980. I was 16 and working in a restaurant at a local resort. I began to have angry outbursts, crying spells, and generally felt really depressed. I went to my Dad's psychiatrist to get checked out and was put on Lithium and an antidepressant. This was my first experience taking medication and I didn't see any benefit. I was still depressed and had a lot of medication side effects, like dizziness and dry mouth. I eventually stopped the medicine.

For five years I lived with my condition. Then in 1985, things got worse. I was attending a college in Prescott, Arizona. This was my first time living away from home and at first things went okay. Then I began to have psychotic symptoms. I was confused, disoriented, and became disorganized. I would call home every day and cry. I had more angry outbursts. I threw a stereo out the window of my apartment and I broke my mountain bike that was worth three hundred dollars. It felt like my mind was splitting in half. Near the end of the semester I had a particularly bad night . . . I hit myself with an iron rod in the head. My academic advisor called my home and I left to go back home to Illinois the next day. When I got home I felt broken inside. I wanted to escape and join a commune somewhere in another state. My parents intervened and drove me to a psychiatric hospital where once again I was put on medication. This would be my first hospitalization.

During the six years that followed I would be hospitalized four times. My worst experience in a hospital was a state hospital. I was overmedicated and slept in the hall the first night. I was then put into a room with 6 other people. At one point, my shoes and clothes were stolen. I was there three days before my mom found a research hospital where I got some quality help. I was there for 4 months. When I was first admitted I was hearing voices, seeing visions, and I thought I was president. I was psychotic. As a result of the new medicine, the therapy and other services of the hospital, the visions, voices, and delusions subsided. Although I eventually improved, it took what seemed to me a very long time. My experiences at the hospital were mostly helpful but there were some things I won't forget. Being in seclusion twice, ECT (electroconvulsive therapy) and being in a locked ward made me feel frightened, vulnerable, and out of control. Sometimes the medications made me tired and dizzy. There were many things that I thought were helpful. The staff members were very helpful and attentive. Some of the things that helped me the most were the therapy groups, dance therapy, occupational therapy, and back in those days we could have passes to go outside and even to go home on weekends.

Also helpful were the opportunities to visit with family and friends. There was a church service we could go to on Sunday and a library. There was a quiet hour every day where you could rest in your room and relax. They also had dances on the weekend where all the units would meet in the gym, although at first I was afraid to leave the unit because of my delusions. There were some vending machines in the lobby downstairs and when I had a grounds pass I would go there. It's been 15 years since I was last in the hospital.

Mental illness recovery is a complicated process and sometimes a hard road. I have learned with proper care, recovery is possible. It means asking and accepting help and making a commitment. The emotional, physical, and spiritual help requires a team effort between the patient, doctors, nurses, therapists, family and friends, the church and other community organizations. Working has really helped me in my recovery. By accepting the help of a job coach, I have been able to work, allowing me to feel like a contributing member of society as well as a sense of accomplishment.

I am still on the road to recovery. It can still be difficult at times but I know I am on a path of healing. Between my faith in God, my friends and family, and the professional help I have received and continue to receive, I am able to stay out of the hospital. Mental health is a journey but we do not have to be on it alone.

Admissions
Grant Bell

I answered a lot of questions
Defensively
Who is President?
What day is it?
I am not sure
I know
But I can't remember
I am afraid
In this white room
With no pictures
Just faded paint
Now the next step
Take your clothes off
Someone gives me a physical
I leave my family behind
To go up the stairs
To the ward
I wonder how long I will stay
I sit alone and pray

Members of Treatment Team

The composition of the treatment team depends on patient demographics and the philosophy of the setting. Funding sources require that all settings provide medical and psychiatric intervention requiring physicians, psychiatrists, and nurses. Social workers or licensed counselors provide family intervention, process group therapy, and provide placement and referral support. Other team members can include occupational therapy, recreational therapy, and expressive therapies such as art, music, and dance or movement. In addition, facilities employ staff members to provide structure on the unit, help with meals and daily scheduled activities, and lead psychoeducational groups.

Team members may hold bachelor's degrees and receive additional training at the facility (Sederer, 1986). Programs that serve people with dementia employ team members who are specially trained in personal care techniques and provide ADL care, feeding, and other such needs (Corcoran, 2001b). Dieticians are integral team members on units treating people with eating disorders. Many programs also include staff who care for spiritual needs, volunteers from programs such as Alcoholics Anonymous, and psychologists who provide psychiatric or neuropsychiatric testing who may or may not be a part of the core team.

Funding Sources

Each state provides public inpatient beds for their residents funded through Medicaid, Medicare, and state subsidies. (NAMI, 2006; Onken et al, 2002). Consumers with private insurance, the bulk of which is provided by managed care organizations, make up less than one-quarter of all individuals receiving mental health services (National Association of Psychiatric Health Systems, 2008; Substance Abuse and Mental Health Services Administration [SAMHSA], 2006). In 2006, Medicare and Medicaid were billed for over 60% of all mental health-related hospital stays (Healthcare Cost and Utilization Project, 2008). Both government and managed care payments lag behind the true costs of inpatient hospitalization, and many argue that one factor behind the closure or downsizing of mental health beds is that hospitals are no longer willing to make up the differences in costs in their own budgets (Case et al, 2007; Martin & Leslie, 2003; Wang et al, 2005). In some situations, facilities fund mental health programs with grant monies, although recent years have seen a decrease in available grants (National Institute of Mental Health, 2007).

Partial Hospitalization Programs

Partial hospitalization programs (PHPs) and **intensive outpatient programs (IOPs)** are considered in this discussion of hospital-based settings even though not all of these types of programs are physically located in a hospital setting. However, like inpatient hospital settings, PHPs and IOPs are structured mental health treatment, albeit with a reduction in the level of structure and care found in inpatient hospitals. PHPs and IOPs are appropriate treatment settings for consumers who can be treated in a less restrictive environment.

Typically, PHPs function Monday through Friday for an average of 6 hours a day, whereas IOPs operate Monday through Friday for an average of 3 hours a day (Association for Ambulatory Behavioral Health, 2007). In most cases, the only difference between a PHP and an IOP is the length of time a person spends at the facility. Although there may be separate IOP programs, for example, for chemical dependency, most people in IOPs are simply encouraged to choose the days and hours of the program that most effectively address their needs. Whether someone participates in a PHP or IOP may be determined by insurance (Whitelaw & Perez, 2004).

The primary mission of PHPs and IOPs is consistent with inpatient care: medication titration, education, and support for recovery. It is assumed that participants are safe outside of the hospital. This allows for people to practice new skills while participating in many of their life roles at home. Participants are treated by a team including physicians who see them weekly for medication management. Psychiatric nursing staff members do not distribute medication but are available to monitor vital response to medication changes, provide education both individually and in groups, and assist with overall health needs. Social workers, counselors, and occupational, recreational, and expressive therapists lead group therapies.

Many people are referred to PHPs and IOPs from inpatient programs; others are admitted directly to the PHP or IOP because their assessment indicates a need for the intense daily treatment but not for the level of safety characteristic of the inpatient unit. Populations served in PHPs and IOPs are much the same as those in inpatient programs and typically reflect the inpatient demographics. Depending on the facility, there can be PHP/IOP programs geared for any age and/or diagnosis. Some programs combine their outpatient PHP/IOP clients with their inpatient population for treatment groups. Funding for PHP/IOP programming is primarily managed care and Medicare, although Medicaid does pay for some child and adolescent programs (SAMHSA, 2006; Whitelaw & Perez, 2004).

Evidence-Based Practice

Research in the mental health community supports function for people struggling with mental illness. Much of the recent work on the recovery model of mental health is about active participation in a person's community. This concept fits with occupational therapy theory and belief of participation in roles and development of sense of meaning.

➤ The President's New Freedom act states that people with mental illness have a right to live and participate in the community, and supports must be put in place to help people be able to do that. In acute care, occupational therapy can assess individuals to determine what supports are needed for them to be most involved and independent. Being aware of the programs available and empowering people to ask for what they need is very much a part of inpatient care (New Freedom Commission on Mental Health, 2003).

➤ Knowledge of community treatment programs for people with persistent mental illness allows therapists in the acute care situation to help clients understand the challenges they face in navigating the system and asking for help (SAMHSA, 2005; 2006).

➤ Understanding the focus of programs such as assertive community treatment can allow the therapist in the acute setting to begin the process by introducing the idea of self-reliance and responsibility for making use of available programs. There is also precedent for the benefits of social interaction and communication programs, support network building, and other beginning skills, making acute care the beginning of a continuum of care (National Association of Psychiatric Health Systems, 2008; SAMHSA, 2005).

National Association of Psychiatric Health Systems. (2008). "Behavioral Healthcare Delivery Today: 2005 Annual Survey Report. Psychotherapies for Children and Adolescents." No. 86. Available at: http://www.aacap .org/page.ww?section=Facts+for+Families&name=Psychotherapies+For+ Children+And+Adolescents (accessed March 17, 2010).

New Freedom Commission on Mental Health. (2003). *Achieving the Promise: Transforming Mental Health Care in America. Final Report.* DHHS Pub. No. SMA-03-3832. Rockville, MD: Author.

Substance Abuse and Mental Health Services Administration (SAMHSA). (2005). *Evidence-Based Practices: Shaping Mental Health Services Toward Recovery: Assertive Community Treatment Toolkit.* Available at: http://mentalhealth.samhsa.gov/cmhs/communitysupport/toolkits/ community (accessed May 2007).

———. (2006). *Mental Health Transformation Trends: A Periodic Briefing.* Department of Health and Human Services. Available at: http://www .samhsa.gov/Matrix/MHST/TransformationTrendsMay05.pdf (accessed May 2007).

Role of Occupational Therapy

As in all mental health settings, the primary role of occupational therapy hospital-based settings is to help people identify what interferes with their ability to participate in valued occupations, intervene with education, assist with generating solutions, and recommend environmental supports for after discharge. The therapist can help people identify the relationship between actions and choices, the impact of those actions on their primary roles, and the demands and opportunities presented in different social and physical environments. Problems with cognition and sensory regulation can contribute to poor management of daily role responsibilities and negatively impact recovery.

Occupational therapy intervention focuses on exploring solutions for the identified problems and helping the person establish a plan that will eventually lead to a satisfying level of role participation. In treatment settings where a consumer's length of stay is limited, assessment and treatment are ongoing processes. Once people are introduced to the relationship between the effect of their illness symptoms and their valued occupations and sense of meaning, they can better understand the steps of recovery. Woven throughout this process is education on the resources available to them in the discharge environment. Much of the groundwork in treatment can be accomplished in group settings where concepts can be taught, and structured discussions among participants help them apply the information and learn from one another.

Occupational therapy provides a unique contribution to the team when the focus is on the impact of illness on a person's ability to carry out meaningful occupations. In addition, the occupational therapist's knowledge of cognitive and sensory needs can help the team determine the best approach in treatment as well as the best discharge environment.

The case studies presented in this chapter draw from a theoretical practice model grounded in occupation in order to guide assessment and treatment. When therapists combine occupation with concepts from developmental theory to determine a person's life stage, and apply concepts from cognition, learning theories, sensory integration, and the factors within their environments, they provide a unique and practical contribution to the person's treatment team and ultimately to their recovery (AOTA, 2002; Kielhofner, 2002; Law et al, 1996;).

Assessments

Evaluation in hospital-based settings is challenging because of the shortened length of stay, the acuity of illness, and the high turnover in patient population. For many years, surveys of therapists practicing in inpatient settings yielded reports that many practitioners created and administered their own site-specific assessment tools. In addition, observation was used in groups and with activities to address task and interpersonal skills. Information that was collected included a history of occupation, interests, support network, skill sets, cognitive dysfunction, and goals, to name a few (Hemphill-Pearson, 1999). A number of reliable and useful instruments have been developed over the years, and some of these can be effectively used in settings with high turnover rates and short treatment stays.

Creating an evaluation protocol and choosing specific assessments requires sound clinical reasoning. A critical step in this process is to select a theoretical practice model and become well versed in its components. This selection guides the process of choosing appropriate assessments, allows the therapist to explain the rationales for his or her choices to treatment members, and supports the production of outcomes evidence. There are a number of theoretical models to consider; choosing the most appropriate one becomes a product of experience, preference, and perceived ease of use. Although therapists will benefit from choosing an occupation-based model to guide decisions about evaluations, treatment, and program development, using concepts and techniques from other models, both from within the profession and from other mental health disciplines, is not only reasonable, it is necessary

Another way that clinical reasoning impacts the development of an evaluation protocol is as a guide to support reflection on the ultimate goals for the evaluation process. The process is meant to gather information of interest to occupational therapists and to produce a report for the client's record, but if the therapist wants to use the assessment results to drive treatment, the evaluation process must reveal the issues that can be reasonably addressed within the context of the setting. Further, it should support the therapist's ability to make appropriate recommendations for environmental adaptations and follow-up interventions.

The development of a sound evaluation protocol can also be informed by a thorough needs assessment, taking into consideration the population being treated as well as the length of stay. Other considerations include age range and occupational expectations for that life stage, primary diagnostic features, and common cognitive and sensory processing difficulties associated with age and diagnosis. The actual choice of assessment tools is likely to be most appropriate when the practitioner researches available assessments tools and tries them to determine if they can be easily integrated into daily practices and provide the type and depth of data that supports treatment planning (Hemphill-Pearson, 1999; Kielhofner, 2002). Tables 41-1 through 41-4 list a variety of tools that may be considered for use in hospital-based settings. Many of these are discussed in more detail in other chapters.

Client-centered assessment gives the therapist the opportunity to combine assessment and treatment by improving the client's awareness of the effect of his or her illness on occupation and sense of meaning. It also allows for use of instruments that are reliable, valid, and useful for measuring programmatic outcomes (Dedding, Cardol, Eyssen, Dekker, & Beelen, 2004; Kielhofner, 2002; Law & Mills, 1998).

Table 41-1 ● **Assessments That Build an Occupational Profile**

Test	Population	Description
Occupational Circumstances Assessment–Interview and Rating Scale Version 4.0 (OCAIRS) (Forsyth et al, 2005)	Adult/geriatric	A semistructured interview designed to measure occupational adaptation. When scored, it can discriminate between clients who do not require intervention and those who do.
Occupational Performance History and Interview, second edition (OPHI-II) (Keilhofner et al, 1997)	Adult/geriatric/adolescent	A semistructured interview designed to collect historical information on occupation and then create a life history narrative.
Canadian Occupational Performance Measure (COPM) (Law et al, 1990)	Adult/geriatric	A semistructured interview designed to gather information on an individual's perception of his or her occupational performance over time.
Interest Checklists and Pediatric Interest Profile (PIP) (Beard & Ragheb, 1980; Driver, Tinsley, & Manfredo, 1991; Henry, 2000)	Adult/geriatric/adolescent/child	There are a number of interest profiles. PIPs cover all ages from 6 to 21. Ratings cover interest, sense of enjoyment, and competence.
Occupational Self-Assessment (OSA); Child Occupational Self-Assessment (COSA) (Baron, Kielhofner, Iyenger, Goldhammer, & Wolenski, 2002)	Adult/geriatric/adolescent	A client-centered self-report that identifies problem areas in occupations. The client is helped to set goals based on the results. The OSA may be used to measure intervention outcomes. The COSA is adapted to allow children to complete the assessment.
Model of Human Occupation Screening Tool (MOHOST) (Parkinson, Forsyth, & Kielhofner, 2006)	Adult/geriatric/adolescent	A screening tool on which ratings can be made after chart review, observation, and participation in a brief interview process.
Short Child Occupational Profile (SCOPE) (Bowyer, Ross, Schwartz, Kielhofner, & Kramer, 2005)	Children	Assesses the child through observation in typical child roles and determines problem areas. This is the child version of the MOHOST.
School Setting Interview (Hoffman, Hemmingsson, & Kielhofner, 2000)	Adolescent/child	Allows children who struggle with emotional/behavioral issues to identify problems in their schools and determine needed accommodations.
Role Checklist (Oakley, Kielhofner, Barris, & Reichler, 1986)	Adult/geriatric/adolescent	Identifies 11 major life roles and asks that the person check whether he or she participates in the role now, has in the past, or plans to in the future. Allows for a comprehensive role interview.
School Function Assessment (Coster, Deeny, Haltiwanger, & Haley, 1998)	Children	Allows for ratings on all activities associated with school function, including class work, mobility, ADLs, and socialization. Each team member completes the appropriate section.
Worker Role Inventory (Velozo et al, 1999)	Late adolescent/adult	A semistructured interview that measures aspects of disability that interfere with participation in work—specifically for someone who was working in the recent past.

Table 41-2 ● **Assessments That Measure Performance Skills**

Test	Population	Description
Allen Battery (Allen, 1990; Penny, Musser, & North, 1995)	Adult/geriatric	Assesses problem-solving and direction-following to determine cognitive disability and needed accommodation.
Assessment of Motor and Process Skills (AMPS); School AMPS (Atchinson, Fisher, & Bryze, 1998; Doble, Fisk, Lewis, & Rockwood 1999; Fisher et al, 1995; Fisher, 1999)	Adult/geriatric/children	Rates a set of motor skills and process skills based on observation of familiar IADL tasks. Considers the relationship between the skill and occupational performance. The School AMPS is specific to school tasks.
Kitchen Task Assessment (Baum & Edwards, 1993)	Adult/geriatric	Eleven items rated on a 5-point scale based on observation of a cooking task. Ratings cover safety, initiation, organization, and follow-through.
Assessment of Communication and Interaction Skills (ACIS) (Forsyth, Salamy, Simon, & Kielhofner, 1998)	Adult/adolescent	An observation tool with 20 items that measure social interaction skills in people with mental illness.
Sensory Integration and Praxis Test (SIPT) (Ayers, 1989)	Children	A standardized assessment that includes visual subtests and somatosensory subtests on vestibular and proprioceptive sensation.
Bruinicks–Oseretsky Test of Motor Proficiency, 2nd edition (BOT-2) (Bruinicks & Bruinicks, 2006)	Children	Uses a number of tasks that require gross and fine motor skills and motor planning to establish proficiency on task. Takes into account client factors.
Motor Free Visual Perceptual Test (MVPT-2) (Colarusso & Hammill, 2003)	Children	A series of subtests that determine problems with such factors as visual acuity, visual interpretation, and visual perception.
Bay Area Functional Performance Evaluation (BaFPE) (Bloomer & Lang Williams, 2002)	Adult/late adolescence	An assessment battery with two scales. The first measures cognitive, affective, and performance skills, and the second measures social interaction skills. This scale is also designed to help determine the effectiveness of occupational therapy intervention.

Table 41-3 ● **Assessments That Measure Activities of Daily Living and Instrumental Activities of Daily Living**

Test	Population	Description
Functional Independence Measure (FIM) (Linacre, Heinemann, Wright, Granger, & Hamilton, 1994)	Geriatric	Observation of 18 activities to determine the level of assistance needed for self-care tasks.
WeeFIM (Ottenbacher et al, 1996)	Children	The version of the FIM for children 6 months to 7 years of age. Items are the same as on the adult version.
Kohlman Evaluation of Living Skills (KELS) (McGourty, 1999)	Adult	Ratings are made after observing performance on 17 items grouped into self-care, safety, money management, transportation, and telephone use. Results help determine if a person is able to live independently.
Routine Task Inventory (Heimann, Allen, & Yerxa, 1989)	Adult	Based on Allen's Cognitive Levels, this assessment establishes a level of function using 32 items that cover ADL and IADL tasks and major roles.

Table 41-4 ● **Assessments That Measure Sensory Processing**

Test	Population	Description
Adolescent/Adult Sensory Profile (Brown & Dunn, 2002)	Adult/geriatric/ adolescent	Client self-report with a 4-point rating scale. Assesses sensory sensitivity, sensory avoidance, and sensory seeking behaviors.
Child Sensory Profiles (Dunn, 1999; 2006)	Children	Inventory completed by parent and/or care providers that measures the same areas as the Adult Sensory Profile.
Sensory Inventories (Champagne, 2006)	Different groups	Several inventories ask clients, parents, and other caregivers to identify reactions to a variety of sensory inputs to create a picture of sensory sensitivities.
Sensory Processing Measure (Miller-Kuhaneck et al, 2005; Parham & Ecker, 2005)	Children	Three integrating rating scales for home, school, and community to create a picture of a child's sensory processing. Covers two higher levels of function (praxis and social participation) and five sensory systems (visual, auditory, tactile, proprioceptive, and vestibular).

Summary

The chapter explored some of the contextual factors that influence mental health care in hospital-based settings. Inpatient hospitalization of persons with mental illness has declined dramatically, and the number of hospital beds in both government and private hospitals has also dropped precipitously. Nonetheless, millions of people are admitted for inpatient hospitalization, and millions more are treated in less structured outpatient settings. Occupational therapists have a vital contribution to make not only in the variety of specialized hospital-based inpatient settings that continue to exist but also in helping lead the transformation of the mental health system and a reconsideration of the therapeutic environment despite the short stays that are common in contemporary practice.

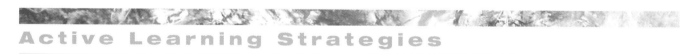

Active Learning Strategies

1. Know Your State

Every state is different in terms of how much money it allocates for care of the mentally ill and how those funds are distributed. Services for people vary widely from county to county. For those with mental illness, this means trying to figure out where to go to get the support consumers need to continue their recovery. They are forced to rely on mental health professionals; however, the knowledge of the professionals in the acute setting about additional support is limited to what they themselves take the time to learn. Occupational therapists have the ability to consider what kinds of environmental supports will best assist the person to function and engage in meaningful life roles.

Take time to explore the services available to people with mental illness in your area. Identify the following information and put together a handout with a description of the available service and contact numbers. Frame your resource by considering the needs of those in the cases described earlier in this chapter. What supports will they need to live, work, eat, go to school, attend church, and maintain their everyday life in the community?

Important Information to Gather

- Obtain a copy of *Achieving the Promise: Transforming Mental Health Care in America* (New Freedom Commission on Mental Health, 2003), available at http://www.nicic.org/Library/020228. Locate and learn how your state mental health organization is responding to this initiative.
- Identify the difference between Social Security Insurance (SSI) and Social Security Disability Insurance (SSDI) as

well as the difference between Medicaid and Medicare funding for services.

- Develop an understanding of the state's system for calculating and distributing monies for food and other needs.
- Identify special programs that qualify people for additional monies such as circuit breaker funds, support programs for medications, and stipulations for working on disability.
- Understand the procedure that drug companies use in their indigent programs that distribute free medications.
- Learn about the community mental health programs in your local county and statewide. Include group homes, supported employment, supported work, supported living, and office of rehabilitation services. Get information on whom to contact, what they offer, how they are funded or what kind of funding they offer, and what criteria the person must meet to benefit from these services.
- Develop a list of support groups in the area. Look for groups for chemical dependence, mental illness, ADHD, autism, self-injury, caregiver support groups, Alzheimer's education programs, and so on.
- Develop a list of supports for those in the process of career changes or needing additional role support, such as volunteer opportunities, leisure opportunities, church-related activities, sports or other hobby groups, and so on.

Choose one or more of the above areas to gather information. Get together with others and split up the items so that you can share the information with each other. Begin with the premise that these programs exist. How would you go about this process?

 Describe the experience in your Reflective Journal.

Reflective Questions

- What process did you use to gather the information?
- How many different sources did you need to access before you felt you had all the information you needed?
- What skills did you need to be able to gather this information?
- What resources did you use to be able to complete this task?
- Did you have to ask for help from others in the community? Were they helpful?
- What was most challenging? How did you feel during this process?
- What would it be like to go through the process of gathering this information while struggling with the symptoms of mental illness and the side effects of medication and stigma?
- What process can the occupational therapist engage in to help the person connect with community services that will be most supportive?
- How much more successful will a person be in recovery if he or she has someone in the inpatient setting who has explored the community and mental health system thoroughly and can provide contacts for those organizations that are most likely to support successful recovery?
- How might an understanding of the mental health system affect your treatment goals while the person is in the hospital?

Resources

- The Association of Therapeutic Communities (ATC) website is a professional organization in the United Kingdom. Its mission is to support the work and continued development of therapeutic communities within the United Kingdom and internationally. You can learn more about different types of therapeutic communities and find resources for education and training: http://www.therapeuticcommunities.org
- The McLean Hospital Behavioral Health Partial Hospital Program website describes the goals of and services provided at McLean Hospital in Belmont, Massachusetts, a private psychiatric institution. Specialized programs for persons with mood and anxiety disorders or borderline personality disorder, as well as a life skills–oriented program, are featured: http://www.mclean.harvard.edu/patient/adult/bhphp.php
- The SAMHSA Therapeutic Communities Training Program offers a free online training package including a trainer's manual and PowerPoint slides intended to orient new workers into the concepts and practices of a therapeutic community. It is a comprehensive, 11-module learning process that supports understanding and application of the therapeutic community concepts: http://www.kap.samhsa.gov/products/manuals/tcc/index.htm
- The Sheppard Pratt Inpatient Services website describes some of the many specialized inpatient mental health services provided at Sheppard Pratt. It is not intended as an endorsement of this particular health care system but can provide the opportunity to broaden your awareness of the range of specialized inpatient services that can be offered in hospital settings: http://www.sheppardpratt.org/sp_htmlcode/sp_services/sp_serv.aspx#hsp

References

Allen C. (1990). *Allen Cognitive Level Test Manual.* Colchester, CT: Worldwide.

American Occupational Therapy Association (AOTA). (2002). Occupational therapy practice framework: Domain and process. *American Journal of Occupational Therapy, 56,* 609–639.

American Psychiatric Association. (2006). *Practice Guidelines for the Treatment of Psychiatric Disorders: Compendium 2006.* Arlington, VA: Author.

Antai-Otong, D. (2008). *Psychiatric Nursing: Biological and Behavioral Concepts.* Clifton Park, NY: Thompson Delmar Learning.

Applebaum, P. S. (2001). Thinking carefully about outpatient commitment. *Psychiatric Services, 52,* 347–350.

Association for Ambulatory Behavioral Health. (2007). "Fast Facts About Partial Hospitalization." Available at: http://aabh.org/about-aabh/fast-facts/ (accessed March 10, 2010).

Atchinson, B. T., Fisher, A. G., & Bryze, K. (1998). Rater reliability and internal scale and person response validity of the School Assessment of Motor and Process Skills. *American Journal of Occupational Therapy, 52,* 843–850.

Ayers, J. (1989). *Sensory Integration and Praxis Test Manual.* Los Angeles: Western Psychological Services.

Barker, P. R., Epstein, J. F., Hourani, L. L., Gfroerer, J., Clinton-Serrod, A. M., West, N., & Shi, W. (2002). Patterns of mental health service utilization and substance use among adults, 2000 and 2001 (DHHS Publication No. SMA 04-3901, Analytic Series A-22). Rockville, MD: Department of Health and Human Services, Substance Abuse and Mental Health Services Administration.

Baron, K., Kielhofner, G., Iyenger, A., Goldhammer, V., & Wolenski, J. (2002). *The Occupational Self Assessment (OSA), Version 2.0.* Chicago: Model of Human Occupation Clearinghouse, Department of Occupational Therapy, College of Applied Health Sciences, University of Illinois.

Baum, C., & Edwards, D. (1993). Cognitive performance in senile dementia of the Alzheimer's type: The Kitchen Task Assessment. *American Journal of Occupational Therapy, 47,* 431–436.

Beard, J. G., & Ragheb, M. G. (1980). Measuring leisure satisfaction. *Journal of Leisure Research, 12,* 20–30.

Bloomer, J. S., & Lang Williams, S. (1987). *BaFPE—Bay Area Functional Performance Evaluation.* Wayne, NJ: Maddak.

Bowyer, P., Ross, M., Schwartz, O., Kielhofner, G., & Kramer, J. (2005). *The Short Child Occupational Profile (SCOPE)* (version 2.1). Chicago: Model of Human Occupation Clearinghouse, Department of Occupational Therapy, University of Illinois.

Bradshaw W., Roseborough D., & Armour, M. P. (2006). Recovery from severe mental illness: The lived experience of the initial phase of treatment. *International Journal of Psychosocial Rehabilitation, 10,* 123–131.

Brown, C., & Dunn, W. (2002) *Adolescent/Adult Sensory Profile.* San Antonio, TX: Psychological Corporation.

Bruinicks, R. H., & Bruinicks, B. D. (2006). *BOT-2: Bruinicks-Oseretsky Test of Motor Proficiency* (2nd ed.). San Antonio, TX: Pearson Assessments.

Case, B. G., Olfson, M., Marcus, S. C., & Siegal, C. (2007). Trends in the inpatient mental health treatment of children and adolescents in the US community hospitals between 1990 and 2000. *Archives of General Psychiatry, 64,* 89–96.

Centers for Disease Control and Prevention (CDC). (2008). "Depression in the United States Household Population 2005–2006." Available at http://www.cdc.gov/nchs/data/databriefs/db07.htm (accessed March 10, 2010).

———. (2007). *Suicide: Fact Sheet.* Available at: http://www.cdc.gov/nchs/datawh/statab/unpubd/mortabs/lcwk9_10.htm (accessed February 2007).

———. (2009). "Deaths: Final data for 2006." National Vital Statistics Report. Available at: http://www.cdc.gov/nchs/fastats/lcod.htm (accessed October 12, 2009).

Champagne, T. (2006). *Sensory Modulation and Environment: Essential Elements of Occupational. General Handbook and Reference* (2nd ed.). Southampton, MA: Champagne Conferences and Consultation.

Colarusso, R. P., & Hammill, D. D. (2003). *Motor-Free Visual Perception Test–3 (MVPT-3).* Novato, CA: Academic Therapy Publications.

Corcoron, M. (2001a). *Fundamentals of Occupational Therapy for Individuals with Dementia.* Online course materials. American Occupational Therapy Association.

———; American Occupational Therapy Association, Commission on Practice. (2001b). *Occupational Therapy Practice Guidelines for Adults with Alzheimer's Disease.* AOTA Practice Guidelines Series. Bethesda, MD: American Occupational Therapy Association.

Coster, W., Deeny, T., Haltiwanger, J., & Haley, S. (1998). *School Function Assessment.* San Antonio, TX. Psychological Corp.

Dedding, C., Cardol, M., Eyssen, I. C., Dekker, J., & Beelen, A. (2004). Validity of the Canadian Occupational Performance Measure: A client-centered outcome measurement. *Clinical Rehabilitation, 18,* 660–667.

Denton, P., & Skinner, S. (2001). *Occupational Therapy Practice Guidelines for Adults with Mood Disorders.* Bethesda, MD: American Occupational Therapy Association.

Doble, S. E., Fisk, J. D., Lewis, N., & Rockwood, K. (1999). Test–retest reliability of the Assessment of Motor and Process Skills in elderly adults. *Occupational Therapy Journal of Research, 19,* 203–215.

Driver, B. L., Tinsley, H. E., & Manfredo, M. J. (1991). The paragraphs about Leisure and Recreation Experience Preference Scales: Results from two inventories designed to assess the breadth of the perceived psychological benefits of leisure. In B. L. Driver, P. J. Brown, & G. L. Peterson (Eds.), *Benefits of Leisure* (pp. 263–286). State College, PA: Venture.

Dunn, W. (1999). *Sensory Profile.* The Psychological Corporation, San Antonio, TX: Psychological Corporation.

———. (2006). *Sensory Profile School Companion.* San Antonio, TX: Harcourt Assessment.

Fisher, A. G. (1993). Functional measures: Part 1: What is function, what should we measure and how should we measure it? *American Journal of Occupational Therapy, 46,* 183–185.

———. (1999). *Assessment of Motor and Process Skills* (3rd ed.). Fort Collins, CO: Three Star Press.

Fisher, A. G., Kielhofner, G., Bernspang, B., Bryze, K., Doble, S., Englund, B., Salamy, M., & Simon, S. (1995). Skill in occupational performance. In G. Kielhofner (Ed.), *A Model of Human Occupation* (2nd ed.) (pp. 113–137). Baltimore: Williams & Wilkins.

Forsyth, K., Deshpande, S., Kielhofner, G., Henriksson, C., Haglund, L., Olson, L., Skinner, S., & Supriya, K. (2005). Occupational Circumstances Assessment Interview and Rating Scale Version 4.0 (OCAIRS. Available at MOHO Clearing House: http://www.moho.uic.edu/assess/ocairs.html (accessed March 17, 2010).

Forsyth, K., Salamy, M., Simon, S., & Kielhofner, G. (1998). *Assessment of Communication and Interaction Skills (Version 4.0).* Chicago: Model of Human Occupation Clearinghouse, Department of Occupational Therapy, University of Illinois.

Fortune, T., & Fitzgerald, M. H. (2009). The challenge of interdisciplinary collaboration in acute psychiatry: Impacts on the occupational milieu. *Australian Occupational Therapy Journal, 56,* 81–87.

French, D., & Hanson, C. (1999). Survey of driver rehabilitation programs. *American Journal of Occupational Therapy, 53,* 394–397.

Grant, B. (1992). *Silver Linings.* Available from NAMI of DuPage, 1430 N. Main St., Suite 301, Wheaton, IL 60187, 630-752-1064.

Greenstone, D. J. (1979). *Dorothea Dix and Jane Addams: From Transcendentalism to Pragmatism in American Social Reform.* Chicago: University of Chicago Press.

Gunderson, J. (1978). Defining the therapeutic processes in psychiatric milieus. *Psychiatry, 41,* 327–335.

Hay, J., LaBree, L., Luo, R., Clark, F., Carlson, M., Mandel, D., Zemke, R., Jackson, J., & Azen, S. P. (2002) Cost-effectiveness of preventive occupational therapy for independent-living older adults. *Journal of the American Geriatric Society, 50,* 1381–1388.

Healthcare Cost and Utilization Project. (2008). "Hospital Stays Related to Mental Health, 2006." Statistical Brief #62. Available at: http://www.hcup-us.ahrq.gov/reports/statbriefs/sb62.pdf (accessed October 12, 2009).

Heimann, N. E., Allen, C. K., & Yerxa, E. J. (1989). The Routine Task Inventory: A tool for describing the functional behavior of the cognitively disabled. *Occupational Therapy Practice, 1,* 67–74.

Hemphill-Pearson, B. J. (Ed.). (1999). *Assessments in Occupational Therapy Mental Health: An Integrative Approach.* Thorofare, NJ: Slack.

Henry, A. D. (2000). *The Pediatric Interest Profiles: Surveys of Play for Children and Adolescents.* San Antonio, TX: Therapy Skill Builders.

Hoffman, O. R., Hemmingsson, H., & Kielhofner, G. (2000). *A User's Manual for the School Setting Interview (SSI) (Version 1.0).* Chicago: Model of Human Occupation Clearinghouse, Department of Occupational Therapy, College of Applied Health Sciences, University of Illinois.

Jackson, L. L., Arbesman, M.; American Occupational Therapy Association. (2005). *Occupational Therapy Practice Guidelines for Children with Behavioral and Psychosocial Needs.* AOTA Practice Guidelines Series. Bethesda, MD: American Occupational Therapy Association.

Kannenberg, K., Dufresne, G.; American Occupational Therapy Association. (2001). *Occupational Therapy Practice Guidelines for*

Adults with Schizophrenia. Bethesda, MD: American Occupational Therapy Association.

Kielhofner, G. (2002). *A Model of Human Occupation: Theory and Application* (3rd ed.). Baltimore: Williams & Wilkins.

Keilhofner, T., Mallinson, T., Crawford, C., Novak, M., Rigby, M., Henry, A., & Walens, D. (1997). *A User's Guide to the Occupational Performance History Interview II (OPHI-II) (Version 2.0)*. Chicago: Model of Human Occupation Clearinghouse, Department of Occupational Therapy, College of Applied Health Sciences, University of Illinois.

Law, M. C., Baptiste, S., Carswell, A., McColl, M. A., Polatajko, H., & Pollock, N. (1998). *The Canadian Occupational Performance Measure* (3rd ed.). Toronto: CAOT Publications.

Law, M., Baptiste, S., McColl, M., Opzoomer, A., Polatajko, H., & Pollock, N. (1990). The Canadian Occupational Performance Measure: An outcome measure for occupational therapy. *Canadian Journal of Occupational Therapy, 57,* 82–87.

Law, M., Baum, C., & Dunn, W. (Eds.). (2001). *Measuring Occupational Performance: Supporting Best Practice in Occupational Therapy*. Thorofare, NJ: Slack.

Law, M., Cooper, B., Strong, S., Stewart, D., Tigby, P., & Letts, L. (1996). The person-environment-occupation model: A transactive approach to occupational performance. *Canadian Journal of Occupational Therapy, 63,* 9–23.

Law, M., & Mills, J. (1998). Client-centered occupational therapy. In M. Law (Ed.), *Client-Centered Occupational Therapy* (pp. 1–18). Thorofare, NJ: Slack.

Law, M., Polatajko, H., Plock, N., McColl, M. A., Carswell, A., & Baptiste, S. (1994). Pilot testing of the Canadian Occupational Performance Measure: Clinical and measurement Issues. *Canadian Journal of Occupational Therapy, 61,* 191–197.

Linacre, J. M., Heinemann, A. W., Wright, B. D., Granger, C. V., & Hamilton, B. B. (1994). The structure and stability of the Functional Independence Measure. *Archives of Physical Medicine and Rehabilitation, 75,* 127–132.

Linehan, M. (1993). *Skills Training Manual for the Borderline Personality Disorder*. New York: Guilford Press.

Marshall, M., Gray, A., Lockwood, A., & Green, R. (1999). Case management for people with severe mental disorders. *Cochrane Database of Systematic Reviews, 3,* No. CD000050. DOI: 10.1002/14651858.CD000050.

Martin, A., & Leslie, D. (2003). Psychiatric inpatient, outpatient and medication utilization and costs among privately insured youths, 1997–2000. *American Journal of Psychiatry, 16,* 757–764.

McCormick, J. J., & Currier, G. W. (1999). Emergency medicine and mental health law. *Topics in Emergency Medicine, 21,* 28–37.

McGourty, L. K. (1999). Kohlman Evaluation of Living Skills. In B. J. Hemphill-Pearson (Ed.), *Assessments in Occupational Therapy Mental Health: An Integrative Approach* (pp. 231–242). Thorofare, NJ: Slack.

McLean, A. (2003) Recovering consumers and a broken mental health system in the United States: Ongoing challenges for consumers/survivors and the New Freedom Commission on Mental Health. *International Journal of Psychosocial Rehabilitation, 8,* 58–70.

Miller-Kuhaneck, H., Henry, D. A., & Glennon, T. J. (2005). *Sensory Processing Measure—School*. Los Angeles: Western Psychological Services.

National Alliance on Mental Illness. (2006) "Grading the States: A Report on America's Health Care System for Serious Mental Illness." Available at: www.nami.org/gtstemplate,cfm? section= grading_the_states&lstid=701 (accessed April 2007).

National Association of Psychiatric Health Systems. (2008). "Behavioral Healthcare Delivery Today: 2005 Annual Survey Report. Psychotherapies for Children and Adolescents." No. 86. Available at: http://www.aacap.org/page.ww?section=Facts+for+Families& name=Psychotherapies+For+Children+And+Adolescents (accessed March 17, 2010).

National Institutes of Health. (2003). *Older Adults: Depression and Suicide Facts*. (NIH Publication No. 03-4593). Washington DC: U.S. Government Printing Office.

National Institute of Mental Health. (2007). "FY 2007 Funding Strategies for Research Grants." Available at: http://www.nimh.nih .gov/grants/fypolicy.cfm (accessed May 2007).

New Freedom Commission on Mental Health. (2003). *Achieving the Promise: Transforming Mental Health Care in America. Final Report*. DHHS Pub. No. SMA-03-3832. Rockville, MD: Author.

Oakley, F., Kielhofner, G., Barris, R., & Reichler, R. K. (1986). The Role Checklist: Development and empirical assessment of reliability. *Occupational Therapy Journal of Research, 6,* 157–170.

Onken, S. J., Dumont, J. M., Ridgway, P., Dornan, D. H., & Ralph, R. O. (2002). *Mental Health Recovery: What Helps and What Hinders? A National Research Project for the Development of Recovery Facilitating System Performance Indicators*. Paper, Fifth Annual International Inter-Centre Network for Evaluation of Social Work Practice Workshop, Columbia University, New York, October.

Ottenbacher, K. J., Taylor, E. T., Msall, M. M., Braun, S., Lane, S. J., Granger, C. V., Lyons, N., & Duffy, L. C. (1996). The stability and equivalence reliability of the Function Independence Measure for Children (WeeFIM). *Developmental Medicine and Child Neurology, 38,* 907–916.

Parham, L. D., & Ecker, C. (2005). *Sensory Processing Measure—Home*. Los Angeles: Western Psychological Services.

Parkinson, S., Forsyth, K., & Kielhofner, G. (2006). *A User's Manual for the Model of Human Occupation Screening Tool (MOHOST) (Version 2.0)*. Available at MOHO clearinghouse: http://www .moho.uic.edu/assessments.html (accessed March 17, 2010).

Penny, N. H., Musser, K. T., & North, C. T. (1995). The Allen Cognitive Level Test and social competence in adult psychiatric patients. *American Journal of Occupational Therapy, 49,* 420–427.

Rice, D., & Rutan, J. S. (1987). *In-patient Group Psychotherapy: A Psychodynamic Perspective*. New York: McGraw Hill Professional.

Sederer, L. I. (1986). *Inpatient Psychiatry: Diagnosis and Treatment* (2nd ed.). Baltimore: Williams & Wilkins.

Spearing, M.; National Institute of Mental Health. (2001). *Eating Disorders and the Search for Solutions: Facts About Eating Disorders and the Search for Solutions*. Public Information and Communications Branch, National Institute of Mental Health, NIH Publication No. 01-4901. Bethesda, MD: Department of Health and Human Services, Public Health Service, National Institutes of Health, National Institute of Mental Health.

Stein, F., & Cutler, S. K. (2002). *Psychosocial Occupational Therapy: A Holistic Approach*. Albany, NY: Delmar Thompson Learning.

Sturm, R., & Bao, Y. (2000). Datapoints: Psychiatric care expenditures and length of stay: Trends in industrialized countries. *Psychiatric Services, 51,* 295.

Substance Abuse and Mental Health Services Administration. (2005a). *Evidence-Based Practices: Shaping Mental Health Services Toward Recovery: Assertive Community Treatment Toolkit*. Available at: http://mentalhealth.samhsa.gov/cmhs/communitysupport/ toolkits/community (accessed May 2007).

———. (2005b). *Evidence-Based Practices: Shaping Mental Health Services Toward Recovery: Illness Management and Recovery Toolkit*. Available at: http://mentalhealth.samhsa.gov/cmhs/ communitysupport/toolkits/illness (accessed May 2007).

———. (2006). *Mental Health Transformation Trends: A Periodic Briefing*. Department of Health and Human Services. Available at: http://www.samhsa.gov/Matrix/MHST/TransformationTrends May05.pdf (accessed May 2007).

Torrey, E. F., Entsminger, K., Geller, J., Stanley, J., & Jaffe, D. J. (2004). "The Shortage of Public Hospital Beds for Mentally Ill Persons: A Report of the Treatment Advocacy Center." Available at: http://www.treatmentadvocacycenter.org (accessed October 10, 2009).

Velozo, C., Kielhofner, G., Gern, A., Lin, F., Azhar, F., Lai, J., & Fisher, G. (1999). Worker role interview: Toward validation of a psychosocial work-related measure. *Journal of Occupational Rehabilitation, 9*(3), 153–168.

Wang, P. S., Lane, M., Olfson, M., Pincus, H. A., Wells, K. B., & Kessler, R. C. (2005). Twelve-month use of mental health services in the United States: Results from the National Comorbidity Survey Replication. *Archives of General Psychiatry, 62,* 629–640.

Weiner, B. A., & Wettstein, R. M. (1993). *Legal Issues in Mental Health Care.* New York: Plenum Press.

Weiner, C. (2003). Holding American hospitals accountable: Rhetoric and reality. *Nursing Inquiry, 11,* 82–90.

Whiteley, S. (2004). The evolution of the therapeutic community. *Psychiatric Quarterly, 75,* 233–248.

Whitelaw, C. A., & Perez, E. L. (2004). Partial hospitalization programs: A current perspective. *Administration and Policy in Mental Health and Mental Health Services Research, 15*(2), 62–72.

Mental Illness in the Workplace: Policies and Practices That Impact Disability

Nancy Spangler

> "[Lincoln] had learned from severe experience that suffering had to be acknowledged and tolerated and that it might, with patience, lead to something "purer, and holier" than could be known without it. The same progression can be seen in his presidency. The qualities associated with his melancholy—his ability to see clearly and persist sanely in conditions that could have rattled even the strongest minds; his adaptations to suffering that helped him to be effective and creative; and his persistent and searching eye for the pure meaning of the nation's struggle—contributed mightily to his good work.
>
> —Joshua Wolf Shenk, 2005.

Introduction

To work is a human drive and a primary life role for most adults. The world of work provides a setting for people to use interpersonal, cognitive, and self-management skills and to develop a sense of effectiveness. Bandura (1997, 1977) suggests that people's beliefs in self-efficacy are influenced particularly by personal mastery experiences, observations of other people managing tasks successfully, encouragement from others, and the physiological perception of challenge. All of these components can be highly abundant in work settings.

Opportunities to develop a sense of self-efficacy through work are extremely important for people with mental illness, and most people with mental illness report that they would like to work (Henry, 2005). The importance of work is underscored by the following observation:

> Work participation provides most adults with daily structure, economic stability, and social opportunities. To be unemployed is to be cut off from a valued social role. In the words of one consumer participant, "If you have a mental illness and you can work, it decreases the stigma a lot, because this society puts a great value on working . . . you see somebody on the street, the first question they ask you is, 'Are you working? . . . What are you doing?'" (Henry & Lucca, 2003, p. 177)

The role of work is perceived as so valuable that an individual's right to pursue work has been protected by two important acts of legislation, the Rehabilitation Act (1973) and the Americans with Disabilities Act (ADA) (1990). "In the ADA, Congress declared that the nation's policy regarding people with disabilities is to offer them equal protection of the laws, and, thereby, the opportunity to fully participate in the community, to live independent lives there, and to become economically self-sufficient contributors" (Stowe, Turnbull, & Sublet, 2006, p. 86). These and other core concepts underlying the development and enforcement of disability policies (Turnbull, Beegle, & Stowe, 2001) are meant to open the doors to the workplace for individuals with mental illness.

Society, however, has only inconsistently included individuals with disabilities in the workplace. In fact, historically, people with mental illness have been highly marginalized by societal fears and stigma and, at times, relegated to institutional living and menial labor at best (Braddock, 2002). Although treatments for mental illness have improved radically, and access to the workplace has increased, challenges remain in ensuring that people with mental illness are able to exercise their rights to participate successfully in the important role of work. Workplaces, however, typically do not exist for lofty humanitarian purposes nor solely to provide opportunities for self-fulfillment for employees. On the contrary, employers focus on the work itself (i.e., making products, providing services, and returning profits to shareholders). Therefore, accommodating people with mental illness represents a particular challenge in the workplace.

Many occupational therapists work with individual employees who have mental impairments in both work and clinical settings. This chapter, however, examines mental health from the broader frameworks of population-based health and health policy and addresses issues for occupational therapists to consider as they work with employers in nontraditional and innovative ways to address mental health in the workplace. Topics include:

- Historical barriers to employment due to the competing interests of society with those of individuals with mental illness.
- Legislation intended to protect employment rights of those with mental illness and judicial interpretation of those laws.
- Current practice in treatment of workers with mental illness.
- Emerging roles for occupational therapists in the workplace mental health arena.

Historical Barriers to Employment

There is a longstanding history of challenges to employment for individuals with mental illness in the United States. In the past, society was likely to discriminate against and isolate people who had symptoms of mental illness that were obvious and potentially frightening to others, such as the hallucinations, delusions, and disordered social behaviors of some people with schizophrenia.

Early attribution of sin or witchcraft to aberrant behaviors eventually gave way to the understanding that these behaviors were the result of illness and out of the control of the individual. The resulting medical model justified keeping people with mental illness separate from the rest of society for their protection and the protection of society (Braddock, 2002; Szasz, 1970). Outrage, however, at the deplorable conditions in institutions for people with mental and intellectual impairments and a growing recognition that the basic human rights and principles of liberty and equality guaranteed in the United States Constitution were being violated have led to a progressive movement toward deinstitutionalization and enhanced community treatment. (For more information, see Chapter 2.)

Even so, conflicts between the interests of individuals and those of American institutions remain, and many people with mental illness are unemployed or underemployed. People with mental illness have higher rates of unemployment than any other disability group. Fifty percent of individuals with some form of mental illness are unemployed, and only 12% of individuals with schizophrenia are working full time (Mechanic, Bilder, & McAlpine, 2002). Two-thirds of individuals on Social Security Insurance (SSI) or Social Security Disability Insurance (SSDI) are persons with mental illness. Similarly, unemployment rates in the United Kingdom range from 80% to 90% for individuals with schizophrenia (Marwaha & Johnson, 2004).

In an update to a report for the New Freedom Commission on Mental Health (NFCMH), barriers to employment for people with serious mental illness were reviewed (Cook, 2006). Barriers include issues such as low educational attainment (attributed at least partially to illness onset during high school or college years), lack of effective vocational services, discrimination in the workplace, and employment disincentives (e.g., losing health insurance if an individual goes off SSDI to work). Another barrier noted was the failure of legislation, particularly the American's with Disabilities Act, to protect individuals with mental illness. Claims filed by people with mental illness are more likely to be identified as low priority, and individuals filing these claims are less likely to receive benefits from the claim than are individuals with physical disabilities.

Mental Illness in the Workplace Today

The disorderly behaviors associated with some mental conditions may continue to limit employment due to fears and stigma, even though people with mental illness and substance abuse are no more likely than others in the community to commit violent acts (Levin, 2001). The most common mental conditions in the workplace, however, are those that are not highly obvious to others or even readily recognizable to the individual. Depressive and anxiety disorders are highly prevalent, can be as debilitating as any major chronic illness, and often occur comorbidly with other disabling medical conditions, such as back pain, cancer, and heart disease (Langlieb & Kahn, 2005).

Reports from the U.S. Surgeon General (U.S. Department of Health and Human Services, 1999) and the World Health Organization (2002) describe depression as a major public health problem affecting major facets of life, including work attendance and performance. Productivity losses of up to 20% have been attributed to the behavioral changes commonly associated with depression, including poor concentration, difficulty with memory and decision-making, fatigue, and lowered self-confidence (Greenberg et al, 2003). Other symptoms, such as withdrawal, flat affect, and problems with cognitive processing, can reduce social interaction and increase marginalization of people with these traits.

The diagnosis of mental illness alone, without any knowledge of the individual or the person's abilities, can create stigma that impacts employment. A study of small business owners found that although employers believed individuals with mental illness should work, these employers had a high degree of concern regarding the work potential of individuals with mental illness (Hand & Tryssenaar, 2006). Few of the employers had ever hired anyone with a mental illness. There was more concern for social issues such as controlling emotions and handling criticism than there was for work competence. In a study of employees with anxiety and depression, most individuals reported that they were reluctant to disclose their disability because of concerns related to stigma (Haslam, Atkinson, Brown, & Haslam, 2005). Ironically, when individuals with mental illness are employed, attitudes toward mental illness become more positive (Perkins, Raines, Tschopp, & Warner, 2009).

Although the majority of people with serious mental illness express a desire to work, it is estimated that only about 10% to 20% of this group is engaged in competitive employment (McGurk, Mueser, & Pascaris, 2005) despite implementation of legislative and policy changes to protect rights of those with mental illness.

Legislation and Definition of Disability

The U.S. government initially established the Social Security system in order to protect people who were struggling economically during the Great Depression. Certainly, people with disabilities were highly represented in this group, but in 1956, services provided by Social Security were expanded to specifically support people disabled by mental or physical impairments that prevented work (Social Security Advisory Board, 2006). This prompted questions regarding the definition of disability and determination of who qualifies as disabled. This process of **classification**, which generally identifies those diagnoses and conditions that qualify an individual as disabled, form a core concept of disability policy. "Classification is frequently seen as a means by which difficult-to-serve subpopulations can be ensured of access to individualized and appropriate services" (Turnbull, Beegle, & Stowe, 2001, p. 137).

The Lived Experience

Tom Johnson
Former Chairman and CEO, CNN; Former Publisher and CEO, Los Angeles Times

Depression invaded my life in my mid 40s. It sapped me of my strength and robbed me of my energy. It brought me inexplicably to the brink of suicide. Every day was incredibly difficult. Just the act of getting out of bed and into the shower each morning was tough.

At work, I did all I could to keep my depression a secret from my staff. At home, I shared my intense pain only with my wife, Edwina, our two children, and fewer than six friends.

I was ashamed to admit I had a mental illness. I was reluctant to see a psychiatrist, and I hated the idea of taking a mood-altering antidepressant medication.

But, fighting depression without professional help did not work. My condition worsened. At times I would try to recharge by lying on the floor of my office. I was baffled by the sadness I felt, by the loss of self-confidence, by a feeling of being trapped at the bottom of a deep, dark well.

Only after my wife forced me to begin seeing physicians at UCLA did I receive a clear diagnosis of chronic depression. And only after a roller-coaster ride of several different medications did I begin to move from the darkness back into the light. Based on my own experiences, I am convinced that most serious cases of depression can be treated successfully. All depression sufferers need to receive a diagnosis by a trained professional.

Many depression sufferers will benefit from a combination of talk therapy and medication to deal with the chemical imbalances and emotional issues.

I care most about the millions of people of all ages who have depression and cannot afford treatment and medication—the uninsured and the underinsured. We need insurance plans that cover mental health as thoroughly as general health. In my opinion, healing a broken mind is more critical than healing a broken arm or leg. We need to remove the stigma associated with depression. More of us need to speak out. We need to demonstrate that workers will become more productive and that absenteeism will be reduced if corporate America and government provide mental health benefits.

We also must not slash state and federal funds for mental health. I believe we are on the verge of finding new medications and treatments. Now is not the time to retreat.

Two acts of legislation further expanded on the classification concept established by the Social Security process and added concepts of antidiscrimination and integration, essentially protecting the civil rights of people with disabilities. Section 504 of the Rehabilitation Act of 1973 (with amendments in 1991 and 1992) protected qualified individuals from discrimination based on disability in any institution receiving federal funds. The legislation specifies that disability is "a natural part of the human experience and in no way diminishes the right of individuals to (A) live independently; (B) enjoy self-determination; (C) make choices; (D) contribute to society; (E) pursue meaningful careers; and (F) enjoy full inclusion and integration in the economic, political, social, cultural, and educational mainstream of American society" (Rehabilitation Act, 1973).

In 1990, the Americans with Disabilities Act (ADA) further expanded on the Rehabilitation Act's national mandate against discriminating against people with disabilities and defined as *disabled* a person who (1) has a physical or mental impairment that substantially limits one or more of major life activities, (2) has a record of such impairment, or (3) is regarded as having such an impairment (Americans with Disabilities Act, 1990).

Although considered important legislation for protecting people with disabilities, Section 504 of the Rehabilitation Act and the ADA present yet another conflict of interest between individuals and institutions, particularly for those with mental impairments. That is, classification as being disabled is required in order for individuals to receive the benefits and accommodations that may help them be successful in the workplace. However, the very act of defining oneself as "disabled" can begin a disabling process. This progression from impairment to disability is impacted by interaction among complex biological,

behavioral, and environmental factors, and quality of life is reduced as disability increases (Pope & Tarlov, 1991) as dependence on institutions increases and personal autonomy decreases.

The classification and definition of disability built on a medical model of differential diagnosis and specific protocols of care helps many people get needed care, but it necessitates control by medical institutions rather than the individual and may result in dependence on systems of care rather than autonomy and self-reliance. Furthermore, interpretation of the level of impairment that must be evident in order to receive benefits has not been clear cut, as court cases challenging the legislation illustrate (see later in this chapter).

Legislation in addition to the ADA protects core concepts of classification, equality, antidiscrimination, privacy/confidentiality, empowerment, autonomy, protection from harm, family integrity and unity, and prevention for people with mental illness. The Family and Medical Leave Act (FMLA) of 1993 requires employers to allow unpaid leave of absences for employees to care for their own medical problems, for birth or adoption, or to care for the health of a family member with a serious health condition. The Health Insurance Portability and Accountability Act of 1996 (HIPAA) prohibits employers and insurers from disrupting health care when workers change jobs, and it protects private employee health information retained by employers and health care providers. Hailed as a patients' rights bill protecting employee privacy, HIPAA can also inhibit managers from discussing behaviors reflecting mental illness at early stages when simple accommodations could help employees better manage their work (i.e., prior to the progressive disabling process). Instead, the mental illness may progress to the point at which the employee's work performance declines, social support from supervisors and coworkers wanes, and his or her continued employment is placed at risk.

The Ticket to Work and Work Incentives Improvement Act of 1999 was drafted to expand work opportunities for people with disabilities without risking loss of Social Security disability payments. The Act unfortunately has not yet increased the number and quality of employment service providers because of the complexity of eligibility and reimbursement regulations (Social Security Administration, 2004).

Numerous acts of legislation, summarized in Table 42-1, have attempted to preserve the rights of individuals with disabling mental conditions to allow them to remain employed or, when that is not possible, to provide financial assistance for independent living.

Judicial Interpretations

In drafting protective legislation, the reality of reconciling what is best for the individual with the collective good, the individual's responsibility, and the collective responsibility of employers is rarely straightforward. A number of court cases related to the ADA have ruled in favor of employers' rights over employees' rights despite legislative protections for individuals with mental illness. Although some of these cases did not directly involve mental health issues, they set a precedent for interpreting future cases, and many continue the debate over the definition of disability. Consider the examples in Table 42-2.

These cases illustrate that while framers of legislation have set out to protect individuals with disabilities, employers still hold a great deal of power and expect high levels of personal responsibility from their employees. Consequently, employers denying employment or accommodations have been able to justify their cases by arguing either that the individual was not truly disabled or that the disability interferes with the core requirements of the job. As Stowe, Turnbull, and Sublet (2006) pointed out:

The Court has diminished the core concepts of antidiscrimination, integration, accountability, and productivity by using the core concept of classification to define narrowly the scope of ADA's protection. If individuals with impairments seek ADA protections from discrimination by a prospective employer, they now face considerable additional hurdles. Do their impairments substantially affect activities central to daily life even when considering mitigating measures? If not, they *may not be classified as persons with a disability who qualify for ADA protection. . . . If so, the request for accommodation is unreasonable, and the ADA will offer no protection. (p. 93)*

This imbalance of power and interests presents a dilemma for disability policymakers as they consider mental illness and the future of mental health services. Psychosocial impairments are frequently "hidden" disabilities, particularly those that are context specific (e.g., panic attacks that occur in response to stressful situations, cognitive changes following depressive episodes that make problem-solving difficult, or reduced attention levels with excessive environmental noises). Symptoms can wax and wane or become increasingly chronic and more disabling over time. Mental illness can cause periodic changes in behavior or cognitive processing.

At least one court has ruled that the unique features of mental illness must be considered, and the employer must bear the burden of responsibility for initiating accommodations for the employee if the mental illness makes requesting accommodation difficult for the employee (*Bultemeyer v. Fort Wayne Community Schools,* as cited in Emens, 2006). However, in other cases, rulings have favored the employers.

Korn (2003) points out that the language of the ADA tends to reflect physical conditions more strongly than mental conditions, and judicial authorities view disability as "an observable, physical limitation." Although mental illness does have neurophysiological and organic correlates, diagnosis and classification still tend to be based on highly specific behavioral symptoms rather than biological markers. The ADA's example of major life activities (caring for oneself, performing manual tasks, walking, seeing, hearing, speaking, breathing, learning, and working) "neatly captures the notion that basic physical tasks are really what distinguish people with disabilities from the rest of the population. . . . Orderly cognitive thinking, the ability to get along with people, and the ability to react in an emotionally appropriate manner should be added," according to Korn (Section VI, para 5).

Perhaps underlying the conflict inherent in these court decisions is the belief of some employers that many people with mental disabilities are being manipulative, lying about the extent of their impairments, and trying to be paid for work they would rather not do (Cook, 2006). When employees do take disability leaves, it is usually the claims adjuster for their disability insurance who has the most frequent contact with the employee. Training for claims adjusters includes

Table 42-1 ● **Summary of Legislation Related to Mental Illness in the Workplace**

Year	Legislation	Summary
1956	Revision of Social Security Act	Provides support for people with mental or physical impairments.
1973	Rehabilitation Act	Section 504 of this Act is considered the first civil rights legislation for people with disabilities. Provides protections in the workplace and authorizes programs associated with vocational rehabilitation.
1990	Americans with Disabilities Act	Defines disabilities, prevents discrimination, and requires employers to accommodate individuals with disabilities.
1993	Family & Medical Leave Act	Allows leaves of absence to care for health.
1999	Health Insurance Portability & Accountability Act	Protects patients' rights to privacy and health coverage.
1999	Ticket to Work Act	Attempts to expand work opportunities for people with disabilities.

Table 42-2 ◉ **Court Decisions Related to the ADA**

Case	Description
School Board of Nassau County v. Arline (1973)	Established there must be a relative assignment of risk when considering accommodations in the workplace, and employers may not put others at risk (direct threat) just to accommodate a disabled worker.
Sutton v. United Airlines (1999)	Challenged the definition of disability and brought a paradox to the surface in the concepts of classification and due process. Twin sisters sued United Airlines when not hired as pilots because of vision impairments, contending United violated ADA by discriminating against them. Supreme Court ruled in favor of United, saying lack of visual acuity disqualified the job applicants. Paradoxically, visual correction, while not allowable as an accommodation to qualify them for the job, actually worked against these individuals, as the court ruled corrective lenses served to mitigate their visual deficits; thus, they could not be defined as handicapped and protected under the ADA (i.e., persons who are able to mitigate their impairment are not considered to be disabled). Furthermore, employers were allowed to deny employment to individuals with impairments when public safety could be jeopardized. Interests of the greater public fell in line with employers' interests.
Toyota v. Williams (2002)	Challenged Supreme Court to decide just how disabled a person must be in order to be classified as disabled. Ms. Williams was fired for poor attendance after a dispute about her physical condition and abilities to carry out newly assigned duties (increased physical labor). Ms. Williams was limited in her ability to work, garden, lift objects, and play with her grandchildren, yet she was able to complete household chores, bathe, and brush her teeth, and thus did not meet criteria for being disabled. Court determined an employee must be severely limited in a broad range of basic functions needed to meet demands of everyday life to be defined as disabled. Furthermore, the condition must be permanent or long term to be considered a disability.
Chevron v. Echazabel (2002)	A man's liver disease disqualified him from a job that exposed him to solvents and chemicals that could directly threaten his health. Thus, employers may refuse to hire someone with a disability to a job that might exacerbate the impairment.
Baxter v. Wisconsin Department of Natural Resources (1991) (Wisconsin Court of Appeals, 1991, as cited in Miller, 1997).	Although employers have been required to provide readers for people with visual disabilities and environmental accommodations for physical disabilities, in this case the Court denied an employee with severe depression a job coach to help with illness-related productivity (e.g., difficulties following through with directions), even at no cost to the employer. (The ADA's requirement of reasonable accommodations by employers for people with disabilities is interpreted differently for psychiatric disabilities.)
Bultemeyer v. Fort Wayne Community Schools (as cited in Emens, 2006)	A janitor's mental illness interfered with his ability to complete work at a fast pace in a new and intimidating work environment, and difficulties with communication due to the mental illness prevented him from requesting accommodations for the speed of his work. Seventh Circuit court ruled the employer is responsible for facilitating communication in cases where difficulty with communication is a feature of the disability and must help determine the necessary accommodations.

recognizing, preventing, and investigating fraud (Bureau of Labor Statistics, 2006), yet training to understand human behavior and facilitating the return to work is lacking from many training programs.

It is important for employers who are fearful of accommodating people with psychiatric disabilities to know that initial fears about accommodating physical disabilities were largely unfounded. Many employers see accommodations for people with psychiatric disabilities as unnecessary. As Miller (1997) notes,

> Accommodations that are not of a physical nature may also be perceived less as a necessary tool to allow the individual to work than as special or easier treatment of the individual with a psychiatric disability. Non-physical accommodations such as flexible scheduling, time off for therapy, or increased supervision and positive feedback are more likely than physical accommodations to be seen as favorable treatment or as something everyone will want if they can get it. . . . As difficult as physical barriers are to get past, the social barriers to full integration of people with disabilities are the most pervasive and pernicious. (Section II, C, I, para 2)

In most of the legal cases described here, employers and employees are challenged to determine if the person is qualified for the job (i.e., justifying hiring or firing decisions by the employer) or whether the person is disabled and therefore protected by the ADA. The power of this role in determining disability is typically given to physicians and psychiatrists. An entrenchment in the medical model for identification and treatment of disability with a focus on disease categories may contribute to the lack of protection provided by the ADA. A disability model with a focus on functional abilities could potentially better identify factors that are most associated with employment.

Vocational Rehabilitation

As legislation such as the Rehabilitation Act and ADA established expectations that people with mental disabilities would receive supports for working outside of mental institutions and become more integrated in the community, the scope of practitioners who provide services to people with mental illness has expanded beyond medical professionals to vocational rehabilitation professionals. However, the vocational rehabilitation system has tended to create jobs that are unskilled and low paying, and the process to qualify has been slow and arduous for people with disabilities.

In its report, "A Legacy of Failure: The Inability of the Federal-State Vocational Rehabilitation System to Serve People with Mental Illness," the National Alliance for the Mentally Ill strongly criticized the state system, saying that "the federal-state vocational rehabilitation system has achieved dismal outcomes in serving people with severe mental illness. It achieves a lower rate of closure into meaningful jobs as compared to others with physical disabilities and mental retardation" (Noble, Honberg, Hall, & Flynn, 1997, p. 11). The report concluded that "most state vocational rehabilitation agencies show little initiative to revise existing procedures or to adopt systems that would create real incentives for counselors to serve consumers with complex needs, including those with severe mental illness (p. 11)." As an example, the Ticket to Work and Work Incentives Act of 1999, in which new employment service providers, or employment networks (ENs), would be recruited and a new system developed for returning those on Social Security disability rolls to work, has been far from successful (Social Security Administration, 2004). Clearly, the original intention of building systems capacity has not been met. The vocational rehabilitation and Social Security disability systems operate outside of the mainstream of typical work, resulting in closed systems that can perpetuate a disability culture and keep people segregated and isolated from society.

Some programs have been designed to help individuals with serious mental illness work in typical settings (i.e., competitive jobs, not segregated workshops) with the help of job coaches, arranged transportation, and assistive technology (U.S. Department of Labor, 1993). Known as **supported employment**, ongoing natural supports (i.e., from supervisors and coworkers rather than mental health service providers) facilitate longer-term job retention (McGurk, Mueser, & Pascaris, 2005). Other successful strategies for enhancing work opportunities for those with mental illness include the clubhouse and assertive community treatment (ACT) models, which are described in Chapter 39 and Chapter 40.

Supportive Workplaces for People With Mental Illness

Finding solutions to the problems of mental illness in the workplace has become a high priority in the United States and other countries. Numerous reports over the past several years from authorities, including the U.S. Surgeon General (U.S. Department of Health and Human Services, 1999), the NFCMH (2003), the National Business Group on Health (Finch & Phillips, 2005), the Social Security Advisory Board (2006), the Partnership for Workplace Mental Health (2005), and the World Health Organization (Saxena, Jane-Llopis, & Hosman, 2006), have identified suggestions for changing our approach to mental health care. These changes affect employer policies and practices, health care providers, and even employees themselves. Figure 42-1 depicts benefits that are provided by some employers to address mental health concerns. The following section summarizes some of these changes, explains how they correspond with core disability concepts, and suggests changing roles for care delivery in workplace mental health.

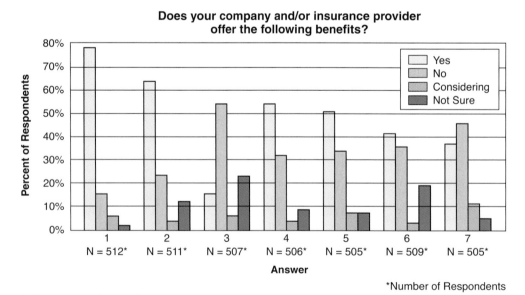

Does your company and/or insurance provider offer the following benefits?

*Number of Respondents

1. Employee Assistance Program
2. Return-to-work assistance for employees on disability
3. Screening for mental illness as part of treatment for chronic physical illness
4. Equivalent medical and behavioral health benefits
5. Behavioral health education programs and/or materials for employees
6. Reimbursement for primary-care doctors screening for mental illness and substance abuse
7. Regular monitoring of employee morale, satisfaction, stress levels, etc.

FIGURE 42-1. A survey of 500 employers depicts the benefits most often provided to address mental health issues in the workplace. *Adapted with permission from The Partnership for Workplace Mental Health.*

Early Detection and Treatment

Earlier detection and treatment of mental illness is important, particularly for individuals with co-occurring chronic medical and mental conditions. It is also important for individuals who are injured in the workplace, because the length of time away from work after injury is associated with the risk of developing depression (Green, 1996; Stice & Moore, 2005). Unfortunately, the act of labeling may create stigma, as the label sets people apart based on their differences (Minow, 1990), and our expectations of individuals, once identified, may affect the person's self-confidence and consequently his or her behavior (Goffman, 1962).

However, earlier identification and access to effective treatment may ultimately reduce the negative impact of mental illness. Employers can use brief, evidence-based tools that are readily available to screen worker populations for conditions such as depression, anxiety, and bipolar disorder (Finch & Phillips, 2005). Therapeutic approaches using empowerment strategies and supporting individuals with or at risk for depression may help them retain active work roles and reduce the likelihood of impairments becoming disabling. In addition, more proactive and better integrated disability management programs offered by employers could enhance earlier identification, increase collaborative care, and support employees in resuming work roles as quickly as possible (Spangler, 2006).

Financial Assistance

Financial issues are also important to address. Authorities recommend equalizing benefits (mental health parity) by providing medical and mental health coverage at the same levels to reduce financial barriers to treatment. Employers who equalized medical and mental benefits found that overall health care costs did not increase (Finch & Phillips, 2005). Equalized benefits may also help to diminish stigma for mental illness, putting core disability concepts of antidiscrimination and integration into practice.

Effective Treatment

Effective treatment depends on qualified and knowledgeable providers using evidence-based practices, common metrics for measurement, collaborative care, and referral systems. Both individual providers of mental health services and systems of care can benefit from consultation, education, and training that promotes best practices. Dissemination of information and increased training for mental health professionals are critical (NFCMH, 2003). In addition, treatment providers are encouraged to consider contextual factors, risk and protective factors, family needs and cultural practices, and individual consumer preferences in their approaches to treatment (Saxena, Jane-Llopis, & Hosman, 2006), incorporating core concepts of *autonomy*, empowerment, participatory decision-making, family centeredness, and antidiscrimination.

Employee Assistance Programs

Employee assistance programs (EAPs) are additional supports built within mainstream workplaces that can help employers address mental health issues more proactively.

Initially created to address substance abuse in the workplace, many EAPs now offer assistance in a wide variety of work-life areas, including psychological counseling, financial management, child care, elder care, and wellness programs (Thomas & Hersen, 2004). The mental health providers in EAPs are typically master's-level social workers and doctoral-level psychologists.

Most EAP services are provided at no cost to employees for assessment or short-term counseling. If the issue is not resolved in a few sessions, the employee is then typically referred to another mental health provider in the health plan for additional counseling. A number of employers encourage use of the EAP as a first point of intervention and for coordination of care for behavioral health treatment. Work can be important to the recovery process. Thus, EAPs that proactively assist workplace managers with strategies for successful support and motivation of individuals with mental health conditions may be able to keep employees working (Thomas & Hersen, 2004).

EAP professionals can help managers recognize declining job performance that can result from changes in cognitive skills, social interaction, and mood regulation due to mental illness or to identify more systemic issues, such as conflicts between workers or between worker and supervisor. EAPs can also help address issues of productivity (such as effective supervisory practices) and absenteeism (such as health promotion, health care education, and stress-related intervention) (Finch & Phillips, 2005).

The Society for Human Resources Management (2006) reports that approximately 70% of all employers provide EAP services to their employees. Many employees, however, remain unaware of the employer resources available to them. For example, in a 2001 survey of employees of 11 Kansas City–based employers, the Mid-America Coalition on Health Care (2004) found that while all of the employers offered a number of resources for depression treatment, 49% of the 6,399 respondents reported their employer offered "few" resources (Charbonneau et al, 2005). An additional 20% reported they did not know if their employer offered any resources, suggesting there were opportunities to improve awareness. A large number of respondents reported either they themselves (52%) or family members (74%) had suffered from depression in the past, yet only 38% of those who had experienced depression had sought professional assistance. An additional study with one of these employers found that workplace communication and awareness programs could improve care-seeking through EAP programs (Spangler, 2005).

Mental Health–Friendly Workplaces

A recent program from the Substance Abuse and Mental Health Services Administration (SAMHSA), Center for Mental Health Services, provides support to human resource personnel and managers to help create "mental health–friendly workplaces." Information on assessing the workplace and descriptions of policies and promising practices is provided, along with in-depth portraits of actual mental health–friendly workplaces and training modules for supervisors (Center for Mental Health Services, 2004). This resource describes ways to stay in touch with employees during or as they return from an extended absence and strategies for using peer mentors or peer advocates to help people with

People who have experienced mental illness retain a vulnerability to future problems, since mental illness is highly episodic. Some may never be entirely symptom free. The recovery model, however, embodies the "democratic principle of self-determination" (Mulligan, 2003) in that it is based on the voice of consumers of mental health services. Recognizing and building on strengths, retaining hope, and identifying sources of support are key features of this model. The recovery model is described as "the process in which people are able to live, work, learn, and participate fully in their communities. For some individuals, recovery is the ability to live a fulfilling and productive life despite a disability. For others, recovery implies the reduction or complete remission of symptoms" (NFCMH, 2003).

A number of states have participated in a process to move away from more traditional day rehabilitative treatment programs toward recovery-oriented programs that encourage illness self-management (instead of excessive dependence on clinical personnel) and supported employment in typical jobs with competitive wages (Becker, Torrey, Toscano, Wyzik, & Fox, 1998; Fisher & Chamberlin, 2004). Recovery-oriented programs focus on actively coping with stressors, reclaiming a positive sense of self by honoring strengths and talents, finding a sense of purpose and meaning, and acknowledging the importance of positive social support (Ridgway, 2001).

➤ Workplace education to build resilience uses concepts similar to recovery-oriented programs to help individuals, including those without diagnosed mental illness, proactively take responsibility for their health by learning more adaptive patterns of thinking and responding.

➤ Exercises and structured interactions help empower participants to reinterpret the world around them, understand their natural reactions to life events, and effectively connect and communicate with others for valuable social support.

Becker, D. R., Torrey, W. C., Toscano, R., Wyzik, P. F., & Fox, T. S. (1998). Building recovery-oriented services: Lessons from implementing individual placement and support (IPS) in community mental health centers. *Psychiatric Rehabilitation Journal, 22*(1), 51–54.

Fisher, D. B., & Chamberlin, J. (2004). "Consumer-Directed Transformation to a Recovery-Based Mental Health System." SAMHSA'S National Mental Health Information Center. Available at: http://mentalhealth.samhsa.gov/publications/allpubs/NMH05-0193/default.asp (accessed February 22, 2006).

Mulligan, K. (2003). Recovery movement gains influence in mental health programs. *Psychiatric News, 38*(1), 10.

New Freedom Commission on Mental Health (NFCMH). (2003). *Achieving the Promise: Transforming Mental Health Care in America. Final Report.* DHHS Pub. No. SMA-03-3832. Rockville, MD: U.S. Department of Health and Human Services.

Ridgway, P. (2001). ReStorying psychiatric disability: Learning from first person recovery narratives. *Psychiatric Rehabilitation Journal, 24*(4), 335–343.

- Difficulty in problem-solving or making decisions.
- Withdrawing from group interaction or excessive irritability.
- Requiring time off for medical appointments or counseling.
- Drowsiness due to medications (especially in the morning) or other medication side effects, such as blurred vision or trembling hands.

Bruyere (1994) at the Cornell University Program on Employment and Disability makes the following recommendations for supervisors:

Good management practices will produce many of the workplace accommodations needed by people with psychiatric disabilities. Like all employees, workers with psychiatric disabilities may benefit from supervisors who:

- *approach each employee with an open mind about his/her strengths and abilities,*
- *clearly delineate expectations for performance,*
- *deliver positive feedback along with criticisms of performance in a timely and constructive fashion, are available regularly during the workday for consultation with employees,*
- *demonstrate flexibility and fairness in administering policies and work assignments. (p. 3)*

In addition, the Partnership for Workplace Mental Health's Taskforce on Disability and Return to Work has developed materials for assessing functional abilities for workplace tasks and tools for clinicians treating employees with psychiatric disabilities to assist in successful return to work. Figure 42-2 shows an excerpt of the Work Function Assessment Form, and Figure 42-3 shows an excerpt of the Treatment Recommendation & Management Form.

The U.S. Equal Employment Opportunity Commission (EEOC), which is responsible for clarifying the rights and responsibilities of employers and individuals with disabilities, has also addressed reasonable accommodations for people with psychiatric disabilities. These include changes in workplace policy to help employees who have difficulty concentrating, modifying methods for communicating work assignments or providing training, and assistance from temporary job coaches.

The ability to interact effectively with role models and meet challenges successfully can encourage an individual's sense of self-efficacy and simultaneously enhance work performance and meet employer goals. Interestingly, employers have reported that accommodation for people with mental health disabilities is an area where the least training has been conducted, and 65% of private-sector employers surveyed identified this as an area on which they would like more information (Bruyere, 1994).

Improving Social Security Disability Programs

The Social Security Advisory Board suggests that Social Security disability programs are not appropriately aligned with national disability policy, and definitions of disability should better align with the concepts and values of the ADA,

mental illness remain fully integrated in the culture of the workplace.

Because of HIPAA privacy legislation, most employers will know of an impairment related to mental illness only if the employee chooses to disclose it (e.g., to request a job accommodation) or if the illness begins to interfere with the employee's job performance in obvious ways. The following are examples of what employers may observe:

- Difficulty concentrating or processing verbal instructions, particularly in noisy or visually distracting environments.

| Work Function Assessment Form | (EXCERPT) | PWMH-5 |

This form is designed to correlate the job tasks that the patient/employee has not been able to do (disability) with the mental functions (impairment) the assessor physician has determined are the medical basis for each functional disability.

The form shown below identifies categories of work functions generally used in the workplace.

Key objectives of this form are to ask the assessor to identify:
• categories of work function generally used in the workplace that the employee cannot perform (disability), and
• the mental and functional impairment(s) that form the medical bases for the disability.

Assessment of Work Functions: Please provide your opinion on the employee's level of impairment, taking into consideration impairment in daily functioning and job-like functions.

Patient Name: _____   As of ___ /___ /___

Please base this assessment on your visit with the patient as it relates to work functioning according to the following scale:

Functional Impairment Scale	None 1	Mild 2	Moderate 3	Severe 4
Can the employee	Yes	Usually	Occasionally	Rarely
Cognition				
Comprehend and follow instructions?				
Maintain work focus/concentration in spite of usual disruptions?				
Organize complex information?				
Mood				
Organize and sustain energy to attend work regularly and timely?				
Sustain realistic energy through a regular workday?				
Affect				
Capable of working on his/her own much of the time				
Maintain stable relationships in the face of usual stresses?				
Insight				
Communicate appropriately socially in appearance, speech, and actions?				
Take responsibility for solving routine work problems?				
Judgment				
Make effective independent decisions?				
Set appropriate boundaries on authority and relationships				

Signature _____   Date _____

FIGURE 42-2. Work Function Assessment Form (excerpt). *Reprinted with permission. Partnership for Workplace Mental Health, Taskforce on Disability and Return to Work. (2007). Assessing and Treating Psychiatric Occupational Disability: New Behavioral Health Functional Assessment Tools Facilitate Return to Work.*

such as integration, empowerment, autonomy, productivity, and contribution. The process of being supported through payment systems instead of working "tends to make an individual who might have been able to work at an earlier point in time less and less capable of doing so. Attachment to an employer, the maintenance and improvement of skills, the sense of belonging to the workforce, the mindset that work is possible—the loss of all of these factors, combined with the passage of time and with the program requirements that reward inability to work, conspire to transform a person

| Treatment Recommendation and Management Form | (EXCERPT) | PWMH-6a |

This form utilizes the information already gathered to develop the treatment plan that focuses on the key medical impairments that limit the patient's capacity to perform their usual essential job functions. Although the complete form is not shown here, the excerpt below illustrates the listing of key medical impairments that interfere with the patient's ability to perform as they previously did.

Key elements in this form are:
- The form is organized to identify the specific job duties that the patient is unable to perform and relates them to the mental impairment that is a basis for that deficit.
- The form asks how long the recommended treatment should take to have its intended clinical and functional effects.
- The form requires that the treatment plan specify treatment approach(es), intensity of treatment, kind of provider who should deliver a treatment, and an estimate of when the patient should return to baseline function and transition to work given adherence to the recommended plan.

Name: _____   **Date:** _____

Please list as you see: (Take into consideration both their current daily function in life tasks and job-like tasks)

List job duties **you** believe the patient cannot currently do	What specific mental impairment is the basis for this?	If no specific mental impairment, please indicate if the limitation is due primarily to distress, need for time for other problems, or job conflict?	Expected duration with recommended treatment

Please list as you see: (Take into consideration both their current daily function in life tasks and job-like tasks)

Duties the **patient** says they cannot do	Describe if there is a specific mental impairment associated	Note if this represents distress, time needed for other problems, or job conflict	Expected duration with recommended treatment

RECOMMENDATIONS FOR TREATMENT OF ISSUES CAUSING WORK DYSFUNCTION

TREATMENT FOCUS	Describe treatment needed. BE SPECIFIC: For example,		Frequency—duration	When should significant improvement be expected?
Symptoms underlying impairments	❑ Med management ❑ Stressor management ❑ Coping skills training for work problems ❑ IPT ❑ Interpersonal skills coaching	❑ Cognitive restructuring ❑ Safety planning ❑ Coping skills training for nonwork problems ❑ Vocational placement ❑ Other		
Symptoms affecting cognitive function				
Symptoms affecting affective stability				
Life stressors that require new coping skills				
Work issues that require new coping skills				

Signature _____   **Date** _____

FIGURE 42-3. Treatment Recommendation & Management Form (excerpt). *Reprinted with permission. Partnership for Workplace Mental Health, Taskforce on Disability and Return to Work. (2007). Assessing and Treating Psychiatric Occupational Disability: New Behavioral Health Functional Assessment Tools Facilitate Return to Work.*

Evidence-Based Practice

Research suggests resilient employees have higher levels of coworker cohesion and supervisor support, use more problem-focused and fewer emotion-focused coping strategies, and have higher levels of immune system functioning (Aitken, 1999; Dolbier et al, 2001).

➤ Education programs can be used in workplaces to proactively develop higher-level adaptive skills within individuals and groups, perhaps reducing the stress responses that can trigger symptoms and relapse in people vulnerable to mental and emotional problems and enhancing their abilities to cope.

Aitken, S. (1999) How Motorola promotes good health. *Journal for Quality and Participation, 22*(1), 54–57.

Dolbier, C. L., Cocke, R. R., Leiferman, J. A., Steinhardt, M. A., Nehete, P. N., Schapiro, S. J., et al. (2001). Differences in functional immune responses of high vs. low hardy healthy individuals. *Journal of Behavioral Medicine, 16,* 219–229.

from an 'impaired individual' with potential into an individual who, in fact, has come to meet the definition 'unable to work'" (2006, p. 8). Encouraging and enabling people to remain employed by better use of rehabilitation science and technology, the Board suggests, can help increase our country's economic productivity and add to, rather than detract from, our tax coffers.

Role of Occupational Therapy

Current systems for addressing mental illness in the workplace are far from optimal. Occupational therapists, with experience and training in enabling people with mental impairments to participate effectively in numerous occupational roles, including work, are in a strong position to help employers address this problem more effectively. The Occupational Therapy Practice Framework (American Occupational Therapy Association, 2002) can guide occupational therapists working with employers to develop strategies, programs, and policies for mentally healthy workplaces and to support employees in the areas of work and social participation. The process for working with employers as clients is similar to working with individual clients and includes

evaluation, intervention, and outcomes measurement, as described in the Framework.

Evaluation

A client-centered approach allows the consulting therapist to gather information that is meaningful to the client and encourages client engagement in the assessment and intervention planning process. In the case of workplace consultation, the client is typically representatives from management and/or teams that represent the employees. The consultant begins by learning about the work setting, current policies and practices, and stated priorities and values as they relate to employee health and safety in general and mental health and work performance in particular.

Information can be gathered through individual or group interviews, including a broad sample of organizational representatives from as many departments as possible, such as human resources/benefits, EAP, wellness, safety, occupational health, corporate communications, and first-line supervisors. Observation of work groups in natural settings helps the consultant assess contextual issues, such as healthy environmental supports and opportunities for employee interpersonal interaction.

Outcomes Measurement

Measurement of long-term outcomes should be established with the client's management team using existing data, such as work attendance, health care utilization and costs, and disability indicators. Shorter-term indicators can be obtained through health risk appraisal aggregate reports (Centers for Disease Control, 2006) and other screening tools. Challenges to consultants include multiple data sets and limited access to data from outside carriers (e.g., third-party administrators of health plans, external employee assistance programs, and disability contractors).

Partnering with academic institutions for outcomes measurement should also be considered. For example, the Work Limitations Questionnaire is a tool available to researchers interested in assessing the effects of physical and mental conditions on the ability to perform typical work functions as well as the impact of interventions to prevent impairment and disability (Lerner et al, 2001). Table 42-3 outlines tools for evaluation and outcomes measurement.

Table 42-3 ● **Tools for Evaluation and Outcomes Measurement**

Data	Source of Data
Cost information	
• Projected costs	• Depression calculator
• Actual health care costs	• Insurance audits
• Disability costs and return to work indicators	• Pharmacy costs
• Workers compensation costs	• Human resources, worker's compensation, and disability carrier data
Management information	
• Absenteeism	• Human resources data
• Benefit design (parity)	

Continued

Table 42-3 ● **Tools for Evaluation and Outcomes Measurement—cont'd**

Data	Source of Data
Health and mental health status indicators	
• Symptoms of mental illness • Functional status and work abilities	• Health risk appraisals, including questions about stress and mental health • Behavioral Risk Factor Surveillance System (BRFSS): Centers for Disease Control and Prevention's surveillance system for physical and mental health • PHQ-9: Screening tool for depression; for research purposes only (Spitzer, Kroenke, & Williams, 1999) • Work Limitations Questionnaire (Lerner et al, 2001) • Treatment Recommendation and Management Forms (Partnership for Workplace Mental Health, 2005) • WHO Health and Work Performance Questionnaire (HPQ; Kessler et al, 2004)
Indicators of employee engagement	
• Work satisfaction • Work skills • Goal attainment • Work participation • Peer interaction	• Employee opinion and satisfaction surveys • Employee involvement in planning and interacting with supervisors and peers • Periodic and annual reviews of work performance • Work skills assessment and training

Occupational therapists may work with employers as independent consultants, through benefits consulting groups that provide a wide variety of services to employers, or through health provider and managed care groups, such as health insurance plans or hospitals. Those interested in working with employers may find it useful to participate in local business groups, such as business coalitions, chambers of commerce, human resource and training professional organizations, organizational development, management consulting organizations, and the Workplace Special Interest Section of the American Occupational Therapy Association. In addition, area public health and wellness organizations may be useful for establishing collaborative relationships with workplaces.

Intervention Strategies

Encourage integration among the various functions within a workplace, such as human resources, employee benefits, EAP, disease management, health promotion, safety, occupational health, workers compensation, disability management, communications, and training. Integrated planning, problem-solving, collaboration, and data sharing can promote and enhance employee recognition of services and allow for earlier identification and intervention for people with mental health problems.

Advocate for policy changes to enhance employee involvement in planning and completing work tasks, and provide adequate training and peer mentoring to enhance skills and develop mastery as well as enhance psychosocial skills and coping abilities. Such skills can reduce stressful triggers for onset or relapse of mental conditions.

Encourage changes in workers compensation and disability management to include transitional duties and accommodations of work process, schedules, or environmental factors to allow earlier return to work. Disability leaves that extend past the time of biological need (e.g., to adjust initially to new psychotropic medications or to recover from co-occurring physical injury or illness) can contribute to deconditioning and other maladaptive processes (McGrail, Lohman, & Gorman, 2001). One employer found that early identification, a focus on goals for returning to work by medical providers, and a collaborative approach may reduce the disabling process and help with the return of workers to previous jobs (Spangler, 2006).

Advocate for inclusion of psychosocial interventions for individuals with chronic pain conditions to avoid disablement.

Assess environments for features that may be distracting or distressing for some individuals, and encourage universal design features that modulate noise and vibration, provide adequate lighting and temperature regulation, and enhance safe and efficient work process abilities. Encourage employers to provide access to environmental spaces for self-replenishing activities, such as exercise and relaxation areas.

Provide information to employers on the evidence base for group education and self-help approaches for reducing symptom levels (e.g., MoodGym) and advocate providing onsite programs and access to online programs (Christensen, Griffiths, & Jorm, 2004).

Advocate for equalizing, or parity, of benefits (i.e., mental health coverage that is equal to medical coverage).

Summary

Solutions to the problems of mental illness in the workplace need to balance the needs of the institutions (employers) with the individual values our society holds dear, such as freedom, autonomy, and equal opportunity. Proactive and innovative approaches to mental health are necessary to help individuals participate in the workplace.

Policymakers, employers, and health care providers need to consider how core disability concepts interact as they develop solutions for addressing mental health in the workplace. Specifically, *systems capacity, prevention, classification, individualized and appropriate services, least restrictive environment, integration, empowerment, and participatory decision-making* are concepts that may play a role in improving employee mental health while helping employers manage cost and productivity issues. Occupational therapists with insights into the role of work in enhancing self-efficacy and health processes have opportunities to bring an innovative focus to mental health in the workplace.

Active Learning Strategies

1. Employer Innovations

Visit the Employer Innovations online database at the Partnership for Workplace Mental Health's website, http://www.workplacementalhealth.org/search.aspx. Review the case studies for several of the employers.

- In what ways have these employers supported prevention or enhanced treatment of mental illness?
- What role might strong organizational leadership and interdisciplinary communication play in improving employee mental wellbeing in these workplaces?
- How might occupational therapists who work in occupational settings help employers to understand the importance of integrating interventions for both mental and physical health together?

 Record your observations and ideas in your **Reflective Journal**.

2. Return to Work

Imagine that you are an occupational therapist working with a client who has been on disability for several months because of a mental illness.

- Review the symptoms of the particular illness in the corresponding chapter of this book and make a list of the work abilities that might be affected.
- How might you advise your client or his or her supervisor in ways to accommodate work tasks to ensure a successful return-to-work experience? See the ideas at the Job Accommodation Network website, http://www.jan.wvu.edu/media/Psychiatric.html.

3. Resilience Building

Some workplaces offer resilience-building programs to help employees avoid or minimize the negative effects of stress. Reflect on how you build your own resilience.

Reflective Questions

- Do you recognize how you respond to stress?
- Do you regularly engage in activities that replenish and relax you?
- Do you have strong social connections through friends, family, faith-based organizations, and other groups that help support you through challenging times?
- Do you try to cultivate a positive, hopeful outlook on life and its circumstances?
- Do you have challenging but realistic goals for your life? Do you take actions toward those goals each day?
- Do you recognize strong emotions? Are you able to experience emotions without being consumed by them? Can you express yourself to others even when you are experiencing strong emotions?
- See suggestions from the American Psychological Association at http://www.apahelpcenter.org/featuredtopics/feature.php?id=6 or the Center for Positive Organizational Scholarship at http://www.bus.umich.edu/Positive/POS-Research/Pods/Resilience.

 Use your **Reflective Journal** to examine your own resilience.

Resources

- Assertive Community Treatment Association: http://www.actassociation.org
- Bazelon Center for Mental Health Law: http://www.bazelon.org
- Center for Psychiatric Rehabilitation, Boston University: http://www.bu.edu/cpr
- Depression Calculator: see link at http://www.phrma.org/news_room/press_releases/web-based_depression_calculator_benefits_employers_and_employees
- Disability Management Employer Coalition: http://www.dmec.org
- Equal Employment Opportunity Commission: http://eeoc.gov
- Families and Work Institute: http://www.familiesandwork.org/index.html
- Institute for Health & Productivity Management: http://www.ihpm.org
- Integrated Benefits Institute: http://www.ibiweb.org
- International Center for Clubhouse Development: http://www.iccd.org/default.aspx
- Job Accommodation Network: http://www.jan.wvu.edu
- Mental Health America (formerly the National Mental Health Association): http://www.nmha.org
- Mid-America Coalition on Health Care: see "Depression Resources" at http://www.machc.org
- MoodGym: http://moodgym.anu.edu.au
- National Alliance on Mental Illness: http://www.nami.org
- National Institute on Disability and Rehabilitation Research: http://www.ed.gov/about/offices/list/osers/nidrr/index.html
- Partnership for Workplace Mental Health: http://www.workplacementalhealth.org
- Substance Abuse and Mental Health Services Administration: http://www.samhsa.gov
- U.S. Department of Justice, Americans with Disabilities Act homepage: http://www.ada.gov
- Work Fitness & Disability Roundtable: http://educ.webility.md/wf/wfdr-join.tcl

References

Aitken, S. (1999). How Motorola promotes good health. *Journal for Quality and Participation, 22*(1), 54–57.

American Occupational Therapy Association. (2002). Occupational therapy practice framework: Domain and process. *American Journal of Occupational Therapy, 56,* 609–639.

Americans with Disabilities Act of 1990, 42 U.S.C. § 12101 *et seq.*

Bandura, A. (1977). Self-efficacy: Toward a unifying theory of behavioral change. *Psychological Review, 84,* 191–215.

———. (1997). *Self-Efficacy: The Exercise of Control.* New York: W.H. Freeman.

Becker, D. R., Torrey, W. C., Toscano, R., Wyzik, P. F., & Fox, T. S. (1998). Building recovery-oriented services: Lessons from implementing individual placement and support (IPS) in community mental health centers. *Psychiatric Rehabilitation Journal, 22*(1), 51–54.

Braddock, D. (2002). *Disability at the Dawn of the 21st Century and the State of the States.* Washington, DC: American Association on Mental Retardation.

Bruyere, S. M. (1994). *Employing and Accommodating Workers with Psychiatric Disabilities.* Goleta, CA: Cornell University Program on Employment and Disability.

———. (2000). *Disability Employment Policies and Practices in Private and Federal Sector Organizations.* Ithaca, NY: Cornell University, School of Industrial and Labor Relations Extension Division, Program on Employment and Disability.

Bureau of Labor Statistics. (2006). *Occupational Outlook Handbook, 2006–07 Edition.* "Claims Adjusters, Appraisers." U.S. Department of Labor. Available at: http://www.bls.gov/oco/ocos125.htm (accessed November 19, 2006).

Center for Mental Health Services. (2004). *Workplaces That Thrive: A Resource for Creating Mental Health-Friendly Work Environments.* Rockville, MD: Department of Health & Human Services, Substance Abuse and Mental Health Services Administration.

Centers for Disease Control and Prevention. (2006). "Healthier Worksite Initiative: Health Risk Appraisals." Available at: http://www.cdc.gov/nccdphp/dnpa/hwi/program_design/health_risk_appraisals.htm#top (accessed December 30, 2006).

Charbonneau, A., Bruning, W., Titus-Howard, T., Ellerbeck, E., Whittle, J., Hall, S., et al. (2005). The community initiative on depression: Report from a multiphase work site depression intervention. *Journal of Occupational and Environmental Medicine, 47*(1), 60–67.

Christensen, H., Griffiths, M., & Jorm, A. F. (2004). Delivering interventions for depression by using the Internet: Randomized controlled trial. *British Medical Journal,* doi:10.1136/bmj.37945.566632.EE, 1–5. http://www.bmj.com/cgi/content/abridged/328/7434/265 (accessed March 15, 2004).

Cook, J. A. (2006). Employment barriers for persons with psychiatric disabilities: Update of a report for the President's Commission. *Psychiatric Services, 57*(10), 1391–1405.

Dolbier, C. L., Cocke, R. R., Leiferman, J. A., Steinhardt, M. A., Nehete, P. N., Schapiro, S. J., et al. (2001). Differences in functional immune responses of high vs. low hardy healthy individuals. *Journal of Behavioral Medicine, 16,* 219–229.

Emens, E. F. (2006). The sympathetic discriminator: Mental illness, hedonic costs, and the ADA. *Georgetown Law Journal, 94,* 399.

Finch, R., & Phillips, K. (2005). *An Employer's Guide to Behavioral Health Services: A Roadmap and Recommendations for Evaluating, Designing, and Implementing Behavioral Health Services.* Washington, DC: National Business Group on Health, Center for Prevention and Health Services.

Fisher, D. B., & Chamberlin, J. (2004). "Consumer-Directed Transformation to a Recovery-Based Mental Health System." SAMHSA'S National Mental Health Information Center. Available at: http://mentalhealth.samhsa.gov/publications/allpubs/NMH05-0193/default.asp (accessed February 22, 2006).

Goffman, E. (1962). *Stigma: Notes on the Management of Spoiled Identity.* Englewood Cliffs, NJ: Prentice-Hall.

Green, J. F. (1996). Management of debilitating injuries in a large industrial setting. *Journal of Back and Musculoskeletal Rehabilitation, 7,* 167–174.

Greenberg, P. E., Kessler, R. C., Birnbaum, H. G., Long, S. A., Lowe, S. W., Berglund, P. A., & Corey-Lisle, P. K. (2003). The economic burden of depression in the United States: How did it change between 1990 and 2000? *Journal of Clinical Psychiatry, 64,* 1465–1475.

Hand, C., & Tryssenaar, J. (2006). Small business employers views on hiring individuals with mental illness. *Psychiatric Rehabilitation Journal, 29,* 166–173.

Haslam, C., Atkinson, S., Brown, S. S., & Haslam, R. A. (2005). Anxiety and depression in the workplace: Effects on the individual and organization (a focus group investigation). *Journal of Affective Disorders, 88,* 209–215.

Henry, A. D. (2005). Employment for people with serious mental illness: Barriers and contemporary approaches to service. *OT Practice, 10*(5), CE1–CE8.

Henry, A. D., & Lucca, A. M. (2003). Facilitators and barriers to employment: The perspectives of people with psychiatric disabilities and employment service providers. *Work, 22,* 169–182.

Kessler, R. C., Ames, M., Hymel, P. A., Loeppke, R., McKenas, D. K., Richling, D., Stang, P. E., & Ustun, T. B. (2004). Using the WHO Health and Work Performance Questionnaire (HPQ) to evaluate the indirect workplace costs of illness. *Journal of Occupational and Environmental Medicine, 46*(Suppl 6), S23–S37.

Korn, J. B. (2003). Crazy (mental illness under the ADA). *University of Michigan Journal of Law Reform, 36,* 585.

Langlieb, A. M., & Kahn, J. P. (2005). How much does quality mental health care profit employers? *Journal of Occupational and Environmental Medicine 47*(11), 1099–1109.

Lerner, D., Amick, B. C., Rogers, W. H., Malspeis, S., Bungay, K., & Cynn, D. (2001). The Work Limitations Questionnaire. *Medical Care, 39*(1), 72–85.

Levin, A. (2001). Violence and mental illness: Media keep myths alive. *Psychiatric News, 36*(9), 10. Available at: http://pn.psychiatryonline.org/cgi/content/full/36/9/10 (accessed November 4, 2006).

Marwaha, S., & Johnson, S. (2004). Schizophrenia and employment: A review. *Social Psychiatry and Psychiatric Epidemiology, 39,* 337–349.

McGrail, M. P., Lohman, W., & Gorman, R. (2001). Disability prevention principles in the primary care office. *American Family Physician, 63*(4), 679–684.

McGurk, S. R., Mueser, K. T., & Pascaris, A. (2005). Cognitive training and supported employment for persons with severe mental illness: One-year results from a randomized controlled trial. *Schizophrenia Bulletin, 31*(4), 898–909.

Mechanic, D., Bilder, S., & McAlpine, D. D. (2002). Employing persons with serious mental illness. *Health Affairs, 21*(5), 242–253.

Mid-America Coalition on Health Care. (2004). "Human Resource Executive Worksite Strategies for Depression Management." Available at: http://www.machc.org/documents/3_Strategies%20for%20worksite1.pdf (accessed January 21, 2007).

Miller, S. P. (1997). Keeping the promise: The ADA and employment discrimination on the basis of psychiatric disability. *California Law Review, 85,* 701.

Minow, M. (1990). *Making All the Difference: Inclusion, Exclusion, and American Law.* Ithaca, NY: Cornell University Press.

Mulligan, K. (2003). Recovery movement gains influence in mental health programs. *Psychiatric News, 38*(1), 10.

New Freedom Commission on Mental Health (NFCMH). (2003). *Achieving the Promise: Transforming Mental Health Care in America. Final Report.* DHHS Pub. No. SMA-03-3832. Rockville, MD: U.S. Department of Health and Human Services.

Noble, J. H., Honberg, R. S., Hall, L. L., & Flynn, L. M. (1997). "A Legacy of Failure: The Inability of the Federal-State Vocational Rehabilitation System to Serve People with Severe Mental Illness." National Alliance on Mental Illness. Available at: http:// www.nami.org/PrinterTemplate.cfm?Template=/Content Management/HTMLDisplay.cfm&ContentID=6050 (accessed November 4, 2006).

Partnership for Workplace Mental Health, Taskforce on Disability and Return to Work. (2005). "Assessing and Treating Psychiatric Occupational Disability: New Behavioral Health Functional Assessment Tools Facilitate Return to Work." Available at: http://www.workplacementalhealth.org/disabilityreportpart1.pdf (accessed March 17, 2010).

Perkins, D. B., Raines, J. A., Tschopp, M. K., & Warner, T. C. (2009). Gainful employment reduces stigma toward people recovering from schizophrenia. *Community Mental Health Journal, 45,* 158–263.

Pope, A. M., & Tarlov, A. R. (Eds.). (1991). "Disability in America: Toward a National Agenda for Prevention." National Academies Press. Available at: http://books.nap.edu/catalog/1579.html (accessed December 11, 2006).

Rehabilitation Act of 1973, 29 U.S.C. § 504 *et seq.*

Ridgway, P. (2001). ReStorying psychiatric disability: Learning from first person recovery narratives. *Psychiatric Rehabilitation Journal, 24*(4), 335–343.

Saxena, S., Jane-Llopis, E., & Hosman, C. (2006). Prevention of mental and behavioural disorders: Implications for policy and practice. *World Psychiatry, 5*(1), 5–14.

Shenk, J. S. (2005). *Lincoln's Melancholy: How Depression Challenged a President and Fueled His Greatness.* Boston: Houghton Mifflin.

Social Security Administration, Ticket to Work and Work Incentive Advisory Panel. (2004). "Advice Report to Congress and the Commissioner of the Social Security Administration: The Crisis in EN Participation—A Blueprint for Action." Available at: http://www.socialsecurity.gov/work/panel/panel_documents/pdf_versions/CrisisEnParticipation.pdf (accessed October 19, 2006).

Social Security Advisory Board. (2006). "A Disability System for the 21st Century." Available at: http://www.ssab.gov/documents/disability-system-21st.pdf (accessed November 19, 2006).

Society for Human Resource Management. (2006). *Benefits Survey Report.* Alexandria, VA: Author.

Spangler, N. (2005). Workplace depression information and care-seeking. Dissertation, University of Kansas. Pub. # 1430292, vol. 44-03M, Proquest.

———. (2006). American Airlines soars with integrated disability program. *Mental HealthWorks,* 4th Quarter, 2006, 3–5. Available at: http://www.workplacementalhealth.org/pdf/MHW4qtr2006.pdf (accessed March 20, 2007).

Spitzer, R. L., Kroenke, K., & Williams, J.B.W. (1999). Validation and utility of a self-report version of PRIME-MD: the PHQ primary care study. *JAMA, 282,* 1737–1744.

Stice, D. C., & Moore, C. L. (2005). A study of the relationship of the characteristics of injured workers receiving vocational rehabilitation services and their depression levels. *Journal of Rehabilitation, 71*(4), 12–22.

Stowe, M. J., Turnbull, R., III, & Sublet, C. (2006). The Supreme Court, "Our Town," and disability policy: Boardrooms and bedrooms, courtrooms and cloakrooms. *Mental Retardation, 44*(2), 83–99.

Szasz, T. (1970). *The Manufacture of Madness: A Comparative Study of the Inquisition and the Mental Health Movement.* New York: Harper Row.

Thomas, J. C., & Hersen, M. (2004). *Psychopathology in the Workplace: Recognition and Adaptation.* New York: Brunner-Routledge.

Turnbull, H., Beegle, G., & Stowe, M. (2001). The core concepts of disability policy affecting families who have children with disabilities. *Journal of Disability Policy Studies, 12,* 133–143.

U.S. Department of Health and Human Services. (1999). *Mental Health: A Report of the Surgeon General.* Rockville, MD: U.S. Department of Health and Human Services, Substance Abuse and Mental Health Services Administration, Center for Mental Health Services, National Institutes of Health, National Institute of Mental Health.

U.S. Department of Labor, Office of Disability Employment Policy. (1993). "Supported Employment." Available at: http://www.dol.gov/odep/archives/fact/supportd.htm (accessed October 29, 2006).

World Health Organization (2002). Mental Health Global Action Programme. http://www.who.int/mental_health/actionprogramme/en/(accessed March 17, 2010).

Homeless and Women's Shelters

Christine A. Helfrich

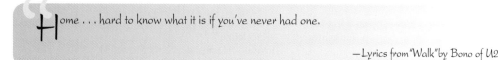

Home . . . hard to know what it is if you've never had one.

—Lyrics from "Walk" by Bono of U2

Introduction

Individuals with mental illness are seen in a wide range of settings, including homeless shelters and transitional living programs. The individuals seen in these settings may have experienced acute or persistent psychological symptoms. They have often been through a series of housing arrangements and, by the time they reach a shelter, experienced severe disruptions to their habits and daily routines. This chapter explores the lives of individuals who enter homeless shelters or transitional living programs, the types of services they often receive while they are there, and the role of occupational therapy in this environment.

Homelessness

Homelessness is often complicated by a variety of physical (Substance Abuse and Mental Health Services Administration, 2003) and psychological (First, Rife, & Kraus, 1990; Folsom & Jeste, 2002; Robertson & Winkleby, 1996) problems and may be a risk factor for emotional disorders (Goodman, Saxe, & Harvey, 1991). Although psychiatric symptoms are often linked to homelessness, the link to functional impairment is often overlooked. Mental illness and homelessness create a cycle of functional impairment that results in an inability to achieve and retain the basic skills necessary for living independently and can result in the need for institutional care. Functional impairments impact an individual's personal health, productivity in personal and vocational areas, and ability to maintain social relationships (Goodman et al, 1991; Gorde, Helfrich, & Finlayson, 2004; Sullivan, Burnam, Koegel, & Hollenberg, 2000). Homeless individuals identify occupational performance problems related to finances, housing, personal care, difficulties satisfying basic needs, and health concerns (Tryssenaar, Jones, & Lee, 1999).

Persons with mental illness are at risk for homelessness because they encounter many barriers when accessing housing services such as strict eligibility criteria, lack of transportation, inadequate resources, and cost (Gallop & Everett, 2001). Barriers also include lack of culturally appropriate or problem-specific services, distrust or fear of the "system,"

geographic isolation, and poverty (Fisk & Frey, 2002; Krishnan, Hilbert, & Pase, 2001; Rowe, Benedict, & Falzer, 2003; Woods, 2000). Mental health service referrals may only be made if there is a mental health crisis severe enough to require hospitalization (Drury, 2003).

While providing housing improves cognitive functioning (Seidman et al, 2003) and decreases rehospitalization (Rosenfield, 1991), the acquisition of life skills may allow more individuals with psychiatric disabilities to live in the least restrictive environment of their choice. Providing supportive services to people with mental illness in housing programs can help them achieve and maintain residential stability, improve mental health, and engage in substance abuse recovery as well as decrease the cost of homelessness to communities (Culhane, 2002; Hurlburt, Hough, & Wood, 1996; Kuno, Rothbard, Averyt, & Culhane, 2000; Schutt & Goldfinger, 1996). The occupational therapy literature has demonstrated the need for, and effectiveness of, life skills interventions with homeless individuals in shelters (Aviles & Helfrich, 2006; Davis, Hagen, & Early, 1994; Gutmann, 1975; Helfrich, 2001; Herzberg, Ray, & Swenson Miller, 2006; Johnson, 2006; Kannenberg & Boyer, 1997; Livingston & Swenson Miller, 2006; Munoz, Dix, & Reichenbach, 2006; Munoz, Garcia, Lisak, & Reichenbach, 2006; Petrenchik, 2006; Schultz-Krohn, Drnek, & Powell 2006; Shordike & Howell, 2001; Tryssenaar et al, 1999).

Several examples of practical and direct supports for community living with the provision of temporary housing exist in the literature. These programs provide traditional case management in combination with life skills training, such as financial management and assistance; grocery shopping, meal preparation, living on a budget and food safety; home management and cleaning; practical job skills training; and self-care skills (Calsyn, Morse, Klinkenberg, Yonker, & Trusty, 2002; Harp, 1990; Morse, Calsyn, Allen, Tempelhoff, & Smith, 1992; Shern et al, 1997; Wasylenki, Goering, Lemire, Lindsey, & Lancee, 1993). Research suggests including life skills training within service agencies that address homelessness helps individuals with mental illness to locate and maintain housing.

Mission and Goals of Homeless Shelters and Transitional Housing

A range of housing programs may all be grouped into the categories of **homeless shelters** and **transitional housing**. The primary mission of shelters is to provide temporary safe housing, while transitional housing programs are designed to promote housing stability. A detailed explanation of these types of settings is beyond the scope of this chapter, but Swenson Miller, Herzberg, and Ray's *Homelessness in America: Perspectives, Characterizations, and Considerations for Occupational Therapy* (2007) is an informative reference. In general, shelters are temporary, safe housing that typically provide a place to stay for one night to 30 days. The specific arrangements at each shelter vary. Some places require a person to arrive by a specified time (e.g., 5:00 p.m.) in order to get a bed for that night and to exit the shelter by a specified time in the morning (e.g., 7:00 a.m.). The person then must return to wait in line the next night for another bed. Other shelters admit a person for up to 30 days and provide a small locker for personal belongings. These settings vary in whether they serve meals, offer showers, or offer other services.

In contrast, transitional housing programs are defined as temporary housing for up to 2 years (U.S. Department of Housing and Urban Development [HUD], 2003). They often offer services, and each program may have a specific focus, such as persons with mental illness or women and children survivors of domestic violence. Participants in transitional housing programs most often have other requirements they must meet while they are living there, such as participation in a job training or educational program, paid employment or participation in treatment services for substance use, mental illness, recovery, and so on. Transitional housing programs often include their own services, which may focus on skills building and rehabilitation, behavioral changes, education, and/or addressing barriers to occupational performance (Petrenchik, 2006).

Populations Served

The McKinney-Vento Homeless Assistance Act is the most commonly used definition of homelessness used by federally funded programs (Livingston & Swenson Miller, 2006). The McKinney-Vento Act defines a homeless person as "an individual who lacks a fixed, regular, and adequate nighttime residence; and a person who has a nighttime residence that is (a) supervised publicly or privately in an operated shelter designed to provide temporary living accommodations (including welfare hotels, congregate shelters, and transitional housing for the mentally ill); (b) an institution that provides a temporary residence for individuals intended to be institutionalized; or (c) a public or private place not designed for, nor ordinarily used as, a regular sleeping accommodation for human beings" (McKinney-Vento Homeless Assistance Act [P.L. 100-77], 1987).

Despite this federal definition, it is difficult to describe a specific population that is served in homeless shelters. The "homeless" are not a homogeneous group. They differ in demographics, subgroups, and their patterns of homelessness. It is generally believed that about 50% of the homeless population are episodically homeless, meaning for one night or a few nights, and the other 50% are chronically homeless (National Coalition for the Homeless, 2009). The Department of Housing and Urban Development (HUD, n.d.) provides a working definition of the "chronically homeless," stating that this group consists of single disabled individuals who have been continuously homeless for over 1 year. Demographically, single men account for the largest number of homeless individuals, although an adult with children is more likely to be female. Children under the age of 18 accounted for 39% of the homeless population in a 2003 report (National Coalition for the Homeless, 2009). All of these statistics are simply estimates and probably reflect numbers that are lower than what actually occurs. It is extremely difficult to count people who are homeless, and the research is especially difficult to understand because different researchers use different definitions and different methods for counting. For the purposes of this chapter, four subgroups of the homeless population are described because they represent the range of people who may be seen by occupational therapists.

Adults With Mental Illness

Adults with mental illness are at risk for becoming homeless, and those who are homeless are more likely to remain so without intervention. Of the 3.5 million people in the United States who experience homelessness each year (The Urban Institute, 2000), 61% to 91% present with psychiatric disabilities. These individuals spend more days homeless, rate their quality of life lower than those without mental illness, and have marked problems meeting basic needs for daily living (Sullivan, Burnam, Koegel, & Hollenberg, 2000). Mental health consumers and their families report a need for improved independent housing skills (Hatfield, Fiersten, & Johnson, 1982; Solomon & Marcenko, 1992). The primary reasons mental health consumers lose housing are (1) not paying rent either because of inadequate finances or cognitive or behavioral limitations, (2) inability to successfully

---

Evidence-Based Practice

The "homeless" are not a homogeneous group. They differ in demographics, subgroups, and their patterns of homelessness. It is generally believed that about 50% of the homeless population are episodically homeless, meaning for one night or a few nights, and the other 50% are chronically homeless (National Coalition for the Homeless, 2009).

➤ People who are homeless have followed a variety of paths to becoming homeless.

➤ Occupational therapists need to understand each person's individual history and experience of homelessness.

➤ It is important to identify the needs of people related to their homeless history.

National Coalition for the Homeless. (2009). "Fact Sheet: Who Is Homeless?" Available at: http://www.nationalhomeless.org (accessed September 22, 2009).

complete instrumental activities of daily living (IADLs), and (3) inadequate preparation, isolation, and lack of meaningful occupations such as role participation (Jones, Quilgars, & Wallace, 2001). Although psychiatric symptoms are identified as being associated with homelessness, the relationship to functional impairment is often overlooked. The effects of mental illness are varied and often impair the individual's ability to engage in social interactions (Goodman et al, 1991; Gorde et al, 2004; Wasylenki et al, 1993), perform activities of daily living (Calsyn et al, 2002; Constantino, Sekula, Rabin, & Stone, 2000; Gilson, DePoy, & Cramer, 2001; Nedd, 2001; Schutt & Goldfinger, 1996; Silverstein, Schenkel, Valone, & Nuernberger, 1998), and manage individual and community responsibilities (Brush, 2000; Harp, 1990; Sosin & Grossman, 1991; Sullivan et al, 2000; Woods, 2000).

Earlier estimates of substance abuse appear to greatly overrepresent the rates of addiction among people who are homeless (National Coalition on Homelessness, 2009). A recent survey found that 38% of adults who are homeless have a problem with alcoholism and 26% have a problem with other drugs.

Survivors of Domestic Violence

Nearly 5 million women experience **domestic violence** in the United States (Tjaden & Thoennes, 2000), impacting them medically and functionally. While the psychological consequences of abuse are broad, the most common disorders are depression and/or posttraumatic stress disorder (PTSD) (Kocot, 2001; Marais, de Villiers, Moller, & Stein, 1999; Skupien, 1998). Depression is noted in 35% to 70% of domestic violence victims (Adelstein & Nelson, 1985; Gerlock, 1999; Marais et al, 1999; McCauley et al, 1995; Nelson, Peterson, Smith, Boughton, & Whalen, 1988; Roberts, Lawrence, Williams, & Raphael, 1998) compared to 12% (National Institute of Mental Health, 2000) of women in the general population. Fifty-five to ninety-two percent of domestic violence survivors experience mild to severe PTSD (Astin, Lawrence, & Foy, 1993; Eisenstat & Bancroft, 1999; Gallop & Everett, 2001; Gorde et al, 2004; Humphreys, Lee, Neylan, & Marmar, 2001; Saunders & Kindy, 1993; Vitanza, Vogel, & Marshall, 1995) compared to 10.4% of women in the general population (Carlson & Ruzek, 2003).

Women report substantial difficulty with daily activities because they have not acquired life skills; because their abusers controlled the household, allowing them little opportunity for responsibility and decision-making; or because of medical conditions (Gorde et al, 2004). Over 44% of domestic violence survivors living in a shelter (compared to only 2.6% of U.S. women) reported their mental conditions resulted in difficulties functioning in work, school, and social environments.

Work limitations due to psychological symptoms can interfere with the ability to satisfy agency requirements and to become and remain independent of one's abuser (Wettersten et al, 2004). Women's abilities to interact effectively with their coworkers and supervisors may also be limited by psychological symptoms. Their behavior may be misunderstood by employers, coworkers, and service providers as attitudinal rather than resulting from treatable symptoms. This misunderstanding contributes to stigma and feelings of powerlessness (Helfrich, Fujiura, & Rutkowski, 2008).

The symptoms of PTSD that interfere with function are compounded with each act of abuse (Jones, Hughes, & Unterstaller, 2001; Mayer & Coulter, 2002). These symptoms limit a woman's ability to develop and maintain life skills that will enable her to be self-sufficient and live independently. Without housing or employment, women with mental illness are more dependent on their partners for the satisfaction of their basic life needs and are thus reluctant or unable to report the abuse or leave their abusers (O'Brien, 2002; Wettersten et al, 2004; Zink & Sill, 2004).

Families With Children

Families with children are the fastest growing subgroup of the homeless population in the United States (Morris & Strong, 2004). Transient or homeless children often experience significant developmental delays in language, gross motor, fine motor, and psychosocial milestones (Bassuk & Rosenberg, 1988; Bassuk & Rubin, 1987; Bassuk, Rubin, & Lauriate, 1986). There is a 30% higher infant mortality rate and 50% higher incidence of elevated blood levels for lead, upper respiratory infections, lice and skin lesions, and trauma for homeless children compared to children with stable housing (Di Marco, 2000; Rafferty & Shinn, 1991; Wright, 1990). Children who are homeless also manifest higher rates of sleepiness, shyness, withdrawal, anxiety, and aggression as well as low-self esteem, emotional stress, depression, and dependent and demanding behaviors (Bassuk & Rosenberg, 1988; Morris & Strong, 2004). This population often experiences behavior problems and depression that may be related to the lack of routines or supervision associated with being homeless (Morris & Butt, 2003). There is little research describing the impact of homelessness experienced as a child on the development of lifelong skills. It is recognized that adverse childhood experiences (including being homeless as a child) are strong predictors of homelessness in adulthood (Burt, 2001). The nature of transitional housing and homelessness causes families to renegotiate routines, living environments, and family roles, impacting life skills development in children (Ray, 2006). The physical setting and materials are instrumental in shaping the interactions that support children's participation in play activities that foster life skills development (Ray, 2006). Children who are homeless frequently have difficulty routinely attending school, causing delays in basic skills learned in elementary education that ultimately impact the development of skills necessary for adult roles.

Youth

Youth homelessness in the United States has reached epidemic proportions with estimates reaching 2 million (Ensign & Santelli, 1997). Youths become homeless for a variety of reasons, including abuse and neglect in their biological or foster care families (American Academy of Pediatrics, 1996; Bassuk & Rubin, 1987; Kurtz, Hick-Coolick, Jarvis, & Kurtz, 1996; Robertson, 1998). Older youths may become homeless when they are separated from their mothers at a shelter if children of their age are not permitted. While minors may become state wards, making them eligible for services, many remain nonwards, fending for themselves on the streets. Youths living on the streets are at risk for unsafe situations, including physical or sexual assault. They may acquire survival skills, such as prostitution, theft, drug use, and gang membership, while living on the street. These marginalized skills are at the expense of life skills needed to become independent, self-supporting adults, integrated into the larger society. These situations limit opportunities to develop life skills that promote mainstream roles such as student, family member, or worker (Aviles & Helfrich, 2006).

Stereotypes of People Who Are Homeless

In general, it is important to note that there are many stereotypes regarding people who are homeless, including that they are all mentally ill, lazy, or dangerous; that they choose to be homeless; and that they use drugs. There is not room for a thorough discussion of those stereotypes here. While some people may exhibit some of these characteristics, they do not define the homeless population. Many people who are homeless are well-educated, clean and sober, have solid work histories, and so on, but for a variety of reasons have become homeless. At The Road Home homeless shelter in Salt Lake City, Utah, the mission includes the statement: "We envision a community that recognizes the inherent dignity of those who live in poverty and homelessness" (Figure 43-1).

When working with individuals who are homeless, it is essential that biases are addressed and that a nonjudgmental attitude prevail. First impressions can be distorted before the person is fully appreciated and understood. For example, some individuals may describe their homelessness as a choice. It may be difficult to comprehend this choice without recognizing some of the issues associated with living in a shelter, such as a loss of freedom and requirements to follow strict rules. Furthermore, many individuals who are homeless have a history of unstable housing that dates back to childhood. For the therapist who has never experienced homelessness, these personal experiences and their impact may be difficult to grasp. Neglected self-care may be another

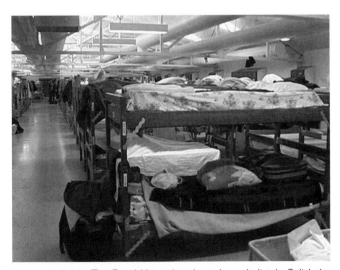

FIGURE 43-1. The Road Home is a homeless shelter in Salt Lake City, Utah. Its mission: "We envision people moving seamlessly from the cold streets into warm housing from despair and alienation toward hope and inclusion. We envision a community that recognizes the inherent dignity of those who live in poverty and homelessness. The Road Home will work with all of our important partners to realize this vision." *Courtesy The Road Home, Salt Lake City, Utah.*

issue that can be challenging initially. Acquiring information regarding a lack of available resources, such as a place to shower, the cost of personal hygiene items, limited privacy, and a loss of daily routines, can improve understanding regarding the individual's difficult circumstances.

Individuals who are homeless come from a variety of backgrounds. The ethnic backgrounds of individuals in homeless shelters typically reflect the geographic location, with larger minority populations in urban areas and Native Americans and migrant workers being more common in rural locations (National Coalition for Homelessness, 2009). As in all practice settings, it is important that occupational therapists are sensitive to cultural differences and practice in a culturally competent fashion. See Chapter 30.

External Factors Affecting Homelessness

Policies and societal events play a significant role in homelessness rates. Changing distributions of employment wages, affordable housing, and federal **entitlement programs** are often cited as factors that influence the prevalence of homelessness in the United States (Petrenchik, 2006). In 2007, the U.S. Senate voted to increase the federal minimum wage for the first time in a decade, while the estimated "living wage"—the hourly wage needed in order to spend no more than 30% of your income on housing costs—has increased steadily (National Low Income Housing Coalition [NLIHC], 2006). In 1999, nearly 28 million American households (25%) failed to earn a living wage and spent more on their housing costs than is considered "affordable" (Bipartisan Millennial Housing Commission, 2002). In 2006, the national average wage needed to afford fair-market rent for a two-bedroom unit was over three times as much as the federal minimum wage (NLIHC, 2006).

During the 1990s, housing costs rose while employment wages were stagnant, with opportunities for federal housing and income assistance more scarce and difficult to access. Between 1997 and 2001, there was a 13% decrease in the number of units affordable to very-low-income renters (HUD, 2003). Additionally, since federal rental assistance is not considered an entitlement, less than a third of eligible households have historically received aid of this kind (U.S. Congressional Budget Office, 1995). While public entitlement programs, such as SSI, can help assuage the costs of housing, homeless persons with mental illness often do not claim these types of subsidies even though they are more likely than other homeless people to receive them (Burt et al, 1999).

During the more recent economic crisis, housing rates have declined, but unemployment and foreclosures have increased, contributing to homelessness. Although the people most vulnerable to homelessness are not homeowners, more than 20% of the properties facing foreclosures in 2008 were rentals (NLIHC, 2009). These rental properties often house multiple families, resulting in a larger number of individuals being affected. A report from the National Alliance to End Homelessness (2009) found that loss of a job was the most common reason for homelessness in several large metropolitan areas. Rising

The Lived Experience

I am 53 years old and I have a diagnosis of personality disorder. I've been homeless about 23 times, sometimes only for just a few days, weeks or months, sometimes it's years at a time. The first episode was when I was 18. My stepfather was abusing me, and my mother didn't believe me. I stayed at a girlfriend's house until she kicked me out. I was on the streets, slept under bridges, piers, parks, backyards, dumpsters, laundromats, sold myself. Anything to just get a place to sleep. You do what you have to. After about five months I went home to mama. Got a job, lost the job—homeless again. I stayed with my sister for awhile and worked. My family was not in a position to help me. Then I met somebody and got pregnant. I went to an old boss and asked him to help me. He put me up in his wife's hotel. I worked for my rent, six months pregnant. I had a place to stay, a roof over my head, a place to wash and shower and stuff like that. But I didn't have anything else, no food. I went and applied for welfare.

My boss introduced me to my ex-husband. I married him, to keep from going on the streets again. We moved to Virginia. But I got tired of all the abuse and fights. That marriage didn't work out so I was homeless again.

I got tired of Virginia. I was lonely for my family. My daughter was there but it's different than having brothers and sisters. So I went back to California and stayed with my sister until I got my own apartment and I was doing okay. I was working at a bank, but lost the job for reporting the staff. The word was out, nobody would hire me. I couldn't get a job so I lost my apartment. I bounced from place to place to place for about a year. I went to friends, in fact a friend from the bank actually took me in. I left their house to work for a lady taking care of her personal care for a year and a half, started therapy, and I left.

I went to see this person, and she helped me realize that I was abused when I was younger. I didn't handle it very well. I had all these emotions. I can't describe all the chaos—you have to feel that for yourself. I couldn't work. I couldn't take care of myself. I didn't know what was going on, and there was no help whatsoever. No counseling. I'm sure there were counselors but I mean, no sliding scale, nothing like that.

I was acting out really violently and physically. I just left my job, went to Alabama, stayed with my brother and his wife. Went back to California, didn't have a job, couldn't find nothing, didn't have a place to stay, stayed with friends or stayed in shelters. And basically you stayed up all night, and slept during the day. That's when I started really cutting. I was dissociating—walking down the street and then waking up and don't know where I am. That type of stuff. So the police caught me and sent me to the Mental Health Facility. They kept me for 24 hours and released me to a shelter. I called my daughter. My daughter sent me money to go back to Virginia. I couldn't get a job and I was having all these emotions again. And I was cutting and I was stabbing myself, I was breaking my bones, I was burning myself.

They put me into the state mental hospital for three months. Then I went to a transitional home for ten months. I paid rent—30% of whatever I made. I didn't pay for food or electricity or anything. While I was there, I started to get my life together because

they put me into a mental health day program when I finished. I had the best therapist ever. The transitional housing asked me to leave, because I wasn't doing the program, I was so busy I was not paying my bills on time, or doing what I was supposed to do. I was so tired from running all that time, I got lazy, and I quit school.

When I left there I went to live in the YWCA. It was $200 a month for a huge room with a couch, chair, T.V. and a bed. We weren't supposed to have microwaves in there but I hid it. Staff cleaned my room. You weren't allowed to have anybody outside the Y in your room. They had a reception hall for visitors. The place was kept clean. I was working 5 jobs to keep a roof over my head. Some of them didn't pay money, they paid food or bus passes, stuff like that.

I did not have the support. I did not have therapists. I worked from 5am–10pm. I was never home. I had a breakdown. I started working, more hours just to keep my house and everything. It was very stressful for me. Then I was doing nothing but working all the time. I started doing a lot of behavior (cutting). I lost a lot of my jobs, but, I was never more than two weeks without work. That's when they would carry me, at the Y because they knew I would pay 'em. I left the Y because I couldn't pay rent and I went to a shelter. I wasn't really asked I went, I left on my own so I was allowed to come back. I got a job as a cake decorator.

I had my disability check coming in so I got my own apartment. It was a bad situation. People broke in and raped me. I could just swear somebody was stealing money and putting it back when I complained. I was thinking it was me. You know, dissociating. That's when they put me on Geodon. I would complain to the police but they didn't even listen after awhile. Nobody wanted to talk to me on the crisis line. The apartment manager said that I never paid my rent, yet I have receipts. They said I set fires to the apartment, but I wasn't. That's when I left Virginia to go to California in 2002. I found out the guys that was living there also did it to other people that lived in that building.

I went to California without a place. I found me a transitional shelter that you pay for 30 days, then you gotta move out for two days, then you can come back and pay for another month. I got tired of transferring from caseworker to caseworker and I was determined to figure out what was going on. I wasn't getting what I needed there so I came out here to do this program I found near Chicago for cutters.

I found out the program was in the suburbs and I couldn't get in. Chicago is very expensive. When I got here I had no money and no place to live. I went to the state hospital here—I started to injure myself. They helped me find this YMCA. I went to the hospital here for six months to get them to help me with my cutting. They never did. I didn't have Medicare at the time 'cause I was a newly disabled person.

My goal is to move into a studio by the end of the year. I'm hoping the doctor will let me. I'm hoping he can let me go back to work, so I can get outta here. He don't want me lifting anything real heavy, he don't want me overdoing. Because of my heart surgery.

unemployment rates therefore can lead to more homelessness. Petrenchik (2006) provides a thorough discussion and analyses of the social, cultural, and intrapersonal factors that contribute to homelessness and the theories that help explain these factors.

Team Members

Shelter and transitional living program staff may include individuals with varying amounts of education and experience. Generally, if a shelter or program aims to serve a specific population type (e.g., survivors of domestic violence), the staff receives additional training about that population. The number, credentials, titles, and roles of staff vary greatly according to funding and availability. There is often a greater need than supply. Staff turnover tends to be high in these settings because of the high stress level placed on frequently overworked and underpaid staff.

Staff involved in the ongoing treatment of an individual may include case managers, social workers, advocates, treatment coordinators, medical personnel, mental health professionals, and occupational therapists; however, medical personnel, such as doctors and nurses, and mental health professionals, such as psychologists and psychiatrists, are often accessed through referral or consultation as opposed to direct care being provided on site. Occupational therapists may provide direct services through group or individual interventions or indirect services in the form of program development and consultation.

Some shelters and programs offer other services through the inclusion of additional staff. **Certified alcohol and drug counselors** (CADC) assist clients affected by the use of alcohol or other drugs by focusing on gaining and maintaining skills for a substance-free lifestyle. Employment counselors discuss employment and disability laws and help individuals explore options for part-time or full-time employment. Housing specialists offer expertise in housing laws, options, and funding. Legal advocates help women obtain orders of protection and address custody issues and other legal matters. Recreational, art, and music therapists provide shelter and program residents with activities that aid in the increased emotional wellbeing of participants.

Most shelters and transitional programs depend on volunteers and administrative/office staff for completion of the daily tasks that maintain shelter functioning. Transitional programs often employ housing supervisors or managers to ensure residents are able to pay rent and follow other housing rules and obligations. Additionally, shelters and programs use intake coordinators or crisis managers to determine if an individual is appropriate for the services and to help the individual transition to the new housing situation. Table 43-1 identifies the types of staff and associated responsibilities often found within these settings.

Funding Sources

The majority of shelters receive funding from several sources, including government, foundation, and private fundraising. HUD is the primary federal agency that provides funding to

---

Table 43-1 ● Shelter and Program Staff Roles and Responsibilities

Case Managers, Social Workers, Advocates and Treatment Coordinators

- Collect functional, environmental, psychosocial, financial, employment, housing, educational, and health information as appropriate to develop and create a care plan
- Develop support systems to meet client needs by identifying and coordinating a variety of available services
- Evaluate client risk and assess need for immediate intervention
- Prepare written reports for funding agency, city, and cooperating agencies
- Assist in the recruitment, training, supervision, and support of volunteers
- Interpret and explain laws, regulations, and service programs
- Determine need for and conduct interagency and/or family conferences
- Provide supportive counseling and advocacy for clients
- Determine quality and effectiveness of services provided and, if necessary, develop and implement new processes and procedures

Medical Personnel (Doctors, Nurses, etc.)

- Prescribe/dispense medications
- Triage
- Health education: individual and, as appropriate, group
- Immunizations, lead tests, tuberculosis and other screening
- Family planning counseling, testing, and treatment
- HIV counseling/testing
- Coordinate health services
- Serve as liaison with onsite case managers and other social service providers

Mental Health Professionals (Psychologists, Psychiatrists, etc.)

- Complete comprehensive biopsychosocial evaluations and intake
- Prescribe medications
- Provide psychotherapeutic interventions
- Provide program consultation as needed
- Assess consumer needs and provide appropriate treatment and recommendation.

Continued

Table 43-1 ● **Shelter and Program Staff Roles and Responsibilities—cont'd**

Occupational Therapists

- Collect functional, environmental, psychosocial, financial, employment, housing, educational, and health information as appropriate to develop and create a care plan
- Assess activities of daily living and instrumental activities of daily living (employment skills, budgeting skills, parenting skills, home management skills, stress management skills, and anger management skills)
- Perform safety assessments and identify barriers in the physical environment
- Initiate referrals
- Provide both direct and indirect services
- Program consultation

Additional Services

- Certified alcohol and drug counselor: assist clients affected by the use of alcohol or other drugs with a focus on gaining and maintaining skills for a substance-free lifestyle through the use of assessment and treatment planning; individual, group, and family counseling
- Employment counselor: discuss employment laws, options for part-time or full-time employment, disability accommodations, job coaching
- Housing specialist: discuss housing laws, housing options, funding sources, maintaining housing stability, disability accommodations in housing
- Legal advocates: discuss orders of protection, custody issues; accompany people to court; assist with appealing SSI/SSDI claim denials
- Recreational, art and music therapists: provide activities that aid in the increased emotional wellbeing of participants

Additional Staff

- Administrative staff
- Volunteers
- Housing supervisors/managers
- Intake volunteers/crisis managers

---

shelters. The U.S. Department of Health and Human Services, which includes a number of specific branches such as the Health Resources and Services Administration, Bureau of Primary Health Care; Substance Abuse and Mental Health Services Administration, Center for Mental Health Services; Centers for Disease Control and Prevention; Administration for Children and Families; the U.S. Department of Labor, and the U.S. Department of Education all provide funding for various programs. In addition, state, regional, county, and city governments may also provide government funding.

Because most shelters and transitional living programs are operated by not-for-profit agencies, they also exert a great deal of effort in seeking funding from foundations and private contributors, including businesses and individuals. Some shelters are funded by a particular religious organization or by other social welfare groups.

Occupational therapists who work in shelter settings may be funded by the agency itself as a paid staff member or consultant, or they may be funded on "soft money" through grant allocations that provide for occupational therapy services. Another innovative method that has been used to "fund" positions in shelters has been through a partnership between an academic occupational therapy department and a local shelter. These arrangements usually involve a faculty member being paid from a grant or as a consultant from the agency to supervise occupational therapy staff or students (e.g., Helfrich et al, 2006).

Role of Occupational Therapy

Occupational therapists can play a central role in homeless shelters by providing training in important independent living skills. Homeless shelters generally focus on meeting basic needs such as food and housing and may have few

resources for individuals with special needs, including those related to disability or independent living skills. People with mental illness may welcome support for daily activities such as budgeting, shopping, and cleaning, which improve their ability to manage their lives independently (Calsyn et al, 2002; Schutt & Goldfinger, 1996). This type of practical assistance and skills training can enhance their ability to retain housing when the training emphasizes relevant skills such as being a responsible tenant and managing routine finances (Harp, 1990; Sosin & Grossman, 1991). Likewise, many women who have experienced domestic violence can benefit from independent skills training and employment interventions (Helfrich, Badiani & Simpson, 2006; Helfrich & Rivera, 2006). See Chapter 47 for more information on skills training and Chapter 50 for more information on employment interventions.

When educational and practical components are integrated into service programs for adults with mental illness who are homeless, the transition from institutional living to community living becomes an attainable goal (Kuno et al, 2000). Successful programs that merge practical and direct supports for community living with the provision of temporary housing include programs that provide traditional **case management** in combination with life skills training (Calsyn et al, 2002; Harp, 1990; Morse et al, 1992; Wasylenki et al, 1993). Programs that include life skills training within service agencies that address homelessness and mental illness result in greater success at assisting individuals to locate and maintain housing. The impact of adding services appears to be greatest for those individuals who are more severely impaired (Clark & Alexander, 2003).

Proactive personalized interventions are also effective in helping homeless individuals with mental illness acquire and retain housing. It is beneficial to provide targeted and specific skills training depending on the particular needs and wants of the client. For example, some individuals may need information regarding money management, whereas for others, home management is a larger issue. Intensive case management and transitional housing often use this approach with significant results (Calsyn, 2002; Harp, 1990; Morse et al, 1992; Washington, 2002). Programming factors are often based on psychiatric rehabilitation principles (Cnaan, Blankertz, & Saunders, 1992), including flexibility, advocacy, increased contact with staff, and an emphasis on teaching independent living skills. Providing practical skills interventions in small groups with consistent staff correlates with higher client satisfaction and greater success in maintaining housing (Calsyn et al, 2002; Campanelli & Sacks, 1992; Morse et al, 1992; Schutt & Goldfinger, 1996; Shern et al, 2000; Wasylenki et al, 1993). Sometimes these approaches are designed and run by mental health consumers.

The increase in families with children in homeless shelters (Morris & Strong, 2004) and the prevalence of children in domestic violence shelters suggests a need for child care skills for the parents. Occupational therapists can play a role in providing either individual or group-based skills training related to child development, play, and parenting. For example, Project SUPPORT, a program that provides emotional and instrumental support along with training in child management skills within a domestic violence shelter environment was effective in reducing conduct problems in children (McDonald, Jouriles, & Skopp, 2006). Another area of need for families relates to routines and habits. Family rituals are typically disrupted in shelter situations, and the occupational therapists can work with both shelter residents and shelter staff to promote family rituals such as eating meals together, supervised homework time, bedtime routines, and celebrations of holidays and special events.

The role of occupational therapy in shelters is diverse and may be determined by the setting, funding issues, and the specific population for each shelter. The previous section described the types of staff who work in shelters and their roles. The role of occupational therapy follows a similar pattern. The most involved role is that of **direct service provider.** In that role, the occupational therapist first evaluates the client holistically, assessing all areas of functioning including ADLs and IADLs; designs a treatment plan; provides intervention, which might include referrals to other services; and eventually discharges the client. Examples of specific treatment areas might include basic self-care skills such as bathing, grooming, and personal medical management; food and nutrition management; IADLs needed to live independently in the community, including money management and community integrations skills; job skills; and housing management skills, to name a few (Figure 43-2).

The role of **consultant** is very common for occupational therapists in shelters. This role usually includes working with clients and staff. The occupational therapist may provide consultation to the shelter in general, offering recommendations for environmental management or programming, or the services may be more focused on individuals, where the therapist evaluates and treats a portion of the shelter residents. In these cases, the treatment is often focused on a particular skill area, and the clients involved are those who need to develop that particular skill. For example, an occupational therapist may offer a group on employment skills or money management to women living in a domestic violence shelter; a group on job-seeking skills to adolescents; or a

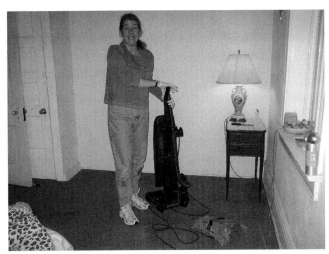

FIGURE 43-2. Occupational therapists can provide skills training in home management. In this photograph, Cynthia has just finished housecleaning. "It's a good feeling."

food and nutrition group to adults in an emergency housing program (Helfrich, Aviles, Walens, Badiani, & Sabol, 2006; Helfrich & Rivera, 2006). Occupational therapists working in a consulting role conducting groups such as these may not have a complete picture of the clients he or she is working with. The occupational therapist may be on site only once a week and see clients only during that group. It is therefore important that the occupational therapist communicate as needed with other staff to acquire additional information. Other areas of consulting may include completing functional evaluations on shelter clients and making recommendations for service plans or referrals. Finally, another consultative function that occupational therapist may provide is broader programmatic recommendations or evaluation. The occupational therapist might work with staff to help structure the routines or environment to enhance functioning by promoting normative routines and habits.

Assessments

The assessments that are used in a shelter setting are numerous and cannot all be discussed in this chapter. The general areas of assessment are discussed, and other chapters in this text that discuss assessments in more detail are referenced.

The hallmark of the occupational therapy assessment in shelters is holism. The goal of the occupational therapy assessment in this setting is to identify the client's strengths and limitations as they relate to independent functioning and determine what the client needs to do or get to manage within different environments of choice. The occupational therapist may be the only professional who has the background to look at the medical, functional, and social aspects of the client as well as how the environment impacts the client. It is important to conduct a broad screen for the range of physical, mental, cognitive, social, and functional challenges that a person might encounter in the environments in which he or she will need to function. Likewise, it is vital to assess each individual's strengths in these areas so that both the client and the staff can be aware of them. Several tools are useful to begin

Evidence-Based Practice

Homeless individuals identify occupational performance problems related to finances, housing, personal care, difficulties satisfying basic needs, and health concerns (Tryssenaar, Jones, & Lee, 1999). Programs that include life skills training within service agencies that address homelessness and mental illness result in greater success at assisting individuals to locate and maintain housing (Clark, 2003).

➤ Occupational therapists have the skills to screen and assess occupational performance.

➤ Group and individual treatment are effective methods for increasing life skills.

➤ Adults, children, and youth are all impacted by the experience of being homeless and can benefit from intervention.

➤ Occupational therapists may assume a variety of roles when working with people who are homeless.

Clark, C. R., & Alexander, R. R. (2003). Outcomes of homeless adults with mental illness in a housing program and in case management only. *Psychiatric Services, 54*(1), 78–83.

Tryssenaar, J., Jones, E. J., & Lee, D. (1999). Occupational performance needs of a shelter population. *Canadian Journal of Occupational Therapy, 66*(4), 188–196.

this broad screen. The Model of Human Occupation Screening Tool (MOHOST) uses interview and observation to determine an individual's baseline functioning and need for further assessment in a wide range of areas (Parkinson & Forsyth, 2002). The Allen Cognitive Level Screen (ACLS) is a leather-lacing task that identifies an individual's cognitive functioning and their need for assistance in the environment (Ansell & Casey Family Programs, 2000, 2002; Nollan, Horn, Downs, & Pecora, 2000, 2002). The Independent Living Skills Survey (ILSS) uses self-report and/or caregiver report to determine an individual's level of independence in ADLs and IADLs (Cyr, Toupin, Lesage, & Valiquette, 1994). The Canadian Occupational Performance Measure (COPM) is a more detailed interview that assesses a person's involvement in occupations (Law et al, 1994). Finally, the Occupational Self Assessment (OSA) is a self-report tool that allows an individual to identify areas of strength and limitations related to self and the environment (Kielhofner et al, 1999). Each of these tools can identify areas that the client needs to work on as well as his or her strengths. The MOHOST, COPM, and OSA all directly invite the client to identify areas that are important to address. Once a thorough screening has been completed, the therapist may identify additional areas that need further evaluation. Some of these areas may require a referral to another health care or social service professional for psychiatric or medical evaluations, for example.

Intervention Models and Techniques

A variety of intervention models can be used effectively in homeless shelters. The overarching principle in selecting a model of practice for this population is to choose one that

will assist the person to return to self-sustaining, independent living. Therefore, most of the models you will see include a holistic perspective that focuses on strengths and self-empowerment. These approaches are consistent with the broader view of recovery in mental illness and with the self-empowerment approaches used in the domestic violence service delivery system. Within this broader framework, occupational therapists use specific approaches to guide their treatment approaches, such as the model of human occupation (Kielhofner, 2002; Bruce & Borg, 2002b) or the cognitive disabilities model (Bruce & Borg, 2002a). Because other chapters in this book cover models that come from occupational therapy, this chapter focuses on the two models borrowed from other disciplines: empowerment theory and situated learning.

Empowerment Theory

Homeless consumers with psychiatric disabilities often feel alienated and disconnected from decision-making about their health, living arrangements, and wellbeing because of a mismatch between service provider recommendations and individual client goals (Fisk & Frey, 2002; Tsemberis & Elfenbein, 1999). Their lack of personal choice is linked to a decreased ability to maintain housing and meet their basic needs, indicating that consumer involvement may be essential to provide successful and relevant services (Rowe et al, 2003; Tsemberis & Elfenbein, 1999). There is a positive association between the ability of consumers to choose and control their services and their ability to function independently (Nelson, Walsh-Brown, & Hall, 1998).

An empowerment approach to service delivery is appropriate for oppressed groups such as homeless consumers and domestic violence survivors because of its emphasis on social action, individual justice, and active participation that give people voice by actively involving them in service design and giving them control over their involvement in treatment (Carling, 1989; Tsemberis & Elfenbein, 1999). Empowerment theory has been used successfully to develop programs for homeless consumers with psychiatric disabilities. Examples include a collaborative community development project among homeless tenants of a shelter and staff, an outreach program that employed homeless peers, a service project that trained homeless consumers for internships on service boards, and a **Housing First** program that offered increased consumer choice in service delivery (Fisk & Frey, 2002; Greenwood, Schaefer-McDaniel, Winkel, & Tsemberis, 2005; Hoch, 2000; Rowe et al, 2003). Despite the evidence to support collaboration between consumers and service providers, this population is often excluded from full involvement in service design, implementation, and research (Gordon, 2005; Minogue, Boness, Brown, & Girdlestone, 2005; Rutter, Manley, Weaver, Crawford, & Fulop, 2004). Reasons cited for this exclusion include consumers' dissatisfaction with the level of collaboration offered, difficulty working within existing organizational structures, logistical difficulties such as inadequate support, and service provider reluctance to share the decision-making process (Gordon, 2005; Rutter et al, 2004).

Occupational therapists can use an empowerment approach with clients by providing opportunities for the client to direct his or her own care. For example, asking clients to

Table 43-2 ● Application of Situated Learning Principles

Principle	Example
Client choice and involvement to address those skills the individual wants and needs to learn	• Clients identify their own goals and priority areas on assessments • Clients choose from a list of activities to work on during a therapy session
Didactic learning with modeling and practice in a context preferred by the individual	• Group session on money management techniques followed by a visit to the bank • Principles of handwashing discussed and then practiced at a sink chosen by the client with the soap of his or her choice
Evaluation of the skill in a specific context to identify barriers and supports needed to be successful in the skill	• Grocery shopping reviewed in the context of what types of food sources are available in the neighborhood, such as food pantries, soup kitchens • Laundry assessed using the washers provided in the shelter
An individualized process that considers the individual's level of functioning	• Group handouts provided to allow for varying levels of literacy • Prompts provided for facilitator to grade activities

identify goal areas, then working on the client's identified list, gives them control over how they spend their therapy session. Helping clients learn how to be assertive and get the information or resources they need from other health or social service providers is also empowering. One client in our life skills program was very distrustful of authority figures and institutions. When she entered therapy, she was having her social security check mailed to her sister's house, which was a 90-minute bus ride away. She worked with the occupational therapist to learn about banking and direct deposit. After making significant changes in therapy she reported, "It was a positive experience. . . . I used to have my social security check mailed to my sister's house, but since then I've gotten direct deposit. I write a check for the rent and then get enough to do a little extra shopping, and then I don't have a lot of money in my room." Through her therapy sessions, she became empowered to learn about community resources, which allow her to be more independent.

While it is more difficult to use empowerment approaches in a group setting, it is very feasible to do so during individual sessions. Clients notice this, and as one person said, "The individual sessions were helpful. . . . [I] appreciated being asked what do you want to work on and being able to list the topic that I wanted to work on."

Situated Learning Theory

Social learning theory using a situated learning approach provides an intervention model wherein adult learners gain knowledge and skills by immersing themselves in a social learning community (Lam, 1995; Lave, 1988; Wilson, 1993). Situated learning places the client learner in contexts that reflect the real world with application to everyday situations (Adelstein & Nelson, 1985). The process follows a logical sequence of providing information, seeing the skill performed, and practicing the skill in a desired context (Nemec & McNamara, 1992). Situated learning allows for (1) client choice and involvement to address those skills the individual wants and needs to learn, (2) didactic learning with modeling and practice in a context preferred by the individual, (3) evaluation of the skill in a specific context to identify barriers and supports needed to be successful in the skill, and (4) an individualized process that considers the client's level of functioning. Research supports the use of this approach to teach social skills, but situated learning has not yet been studied in relation to life skills interventions for homeless persons

with mental illness (Liberman & Kopelowicz, 2002; Liberman et al, 1986; Wallace, 1998; Wong et al, 1988).

Table 43-2 outlines the application of situated learning principles.

These approaches each allow the occupational therapist to look at the individual holistically and collaboratively to determine his or her treatment needs and priorities. They are consumer driven where the client is the central force in determining the direction that treatment should go. Therefore, none of these models specifically dictate treatment priorities. Rather, they identify the things a person wants to change about himself or herself, the environmental adaptations or changes that are needed, and the occupations in which the person desires to engage.

It is important to recognize that many of these treatment foci are the same as those occupational therapists engage in with persons with a wide variety of disabilities; however, the approach is significantly different. People who are homeless, for whatever reason, most likely have very few, if any, material or social resources. They have often exhausted the majority of their support system and have been forced to sell or discard their personal possessions. People living in a shelter may have a small bag that includes all of their belongings, while those living in transitional housing may have a small apartment, though the objects in the apartment may not belong to them. Therefore, it is important for the occupational therapist not only to assist the person with meeting current goals but also to help him or her project into the future and prepare for a more permanent living arrangement. For many consumers, this is a very difficult task. Using concrete tasks rather than talking about future possibilities is most effective. As noted in the assessment section, it is also very important to understand, and to keep in mind throughout treatment, the reasons that a person does not currently have effective skills for living independently.

Summary

Homeless and women's shelters are emerging practice areas for occupational therapists. Individuals living in these temporary settings frequently have significant needs related to independent living, child care skills, and work skills. Occupational therapists can provide interventions that lead to the successful transition of supporting oneself and one's family in a place called home.

Active Learning Strategies

1. Life Skills Acquisition Exercise

Listed in the following table are five common instrumental activities of daily living that most people are expected to complete. Please consider each one and complete the worksheet on the basis of your own experience. *After* you have filled in each box, answer the questions that follow the table.

• Life Skill	• Where did you learn this?	• Who taught you?	• When did you learn this?	• Do you currently receive any assistance with this activity?
1. How to write a check				
2. How to grocery shop on a budget				
3. How to repair your clothing				
4. How to manage your health care needs				
5. How to avoid identity theft				

Reflective Questions

- How would having a serious mental illness impact learning these skills?
- How would living in an institution impact learning these skills?
- How would living with an abusive partner who controlled all of your actions impact learning these skills?
- How would growing up living on the street or in a shelter impact your ability to learn these skills?

 Record your thoughts about this exercise in your **Reflective Journal**.

2. Count Your Losses

The experience of women who are in a domestic violence situation can be very challenging. This exercise will help you get a glimpse of what it might feel like to become homeless because of domestic violence.

- Take out a piece of paper and number it 1 to 5.
- Write down the name of your best friend after number 1.
- Write down your most supportive coworker after number 2.
- Write down your closest family member after number 3.
- Write down your favorite possession after number 4.
- Write down your dream for the future after number 5.

You are in an abusive relationship that you have tried to keep hidden from your friends, family, and coworkers. Last night, your partner came home in a rage and punched your face until you were bleeding because you did not have the house clean. Your 2-year-old daughter's toys were not all put away. After beating you, he threatened to beat your daughter for being so messy with her toys. You keep your daughter safe from him (at the expense of a few more bruises) and vow to yourself that you will leave the relationship as soon as it is safe to go.

1. You call your best friend that night and ask her if you and your daughter can come and stay with her because your partner has beaten you and threatened to hurt your daughter. She asks you why he beat you, and after you explain, she tells you that your partner is a really good person and that you must have deserved to be hit. She advises you to stay in the relationship and keep your house cleaner. You end the phone call feeling ashamed and hurt, and wonder why your friend cannot understand what you are going through.
   You have just lost your best friend. Tear your best friend's name off of your paper and crumple it up.
2. You decide to stay at home that night even though you feel very afraid for the safety of both you and your daughter. In the morning, you try to cover your bruises and cuts with makeup. You take your daughter to day care and go to work. When you get there, your coworkers ask you what happened. You decide to tell them, and they respond similarly to your friend the night before. During lunch with coworkers, they give you the cold shoulder and tell you that you should not be making such accusations about your partner. When you try to explain, they tell you that it is probably your fault for not being a better spouse.
   You have just lost your support system at work. Tear off your most supportive coworker's name and crumple up the paper.
3. You go home very upset; fortunately, your partner is not there, so you call your closest family member (say, your sister) and explain why you are upset. When she has finished listening to you, she tells you that you're crazy and asks what you expected by trying to work full time, go to school, and maintain a household for your partner. She tells you she is sorry and wishes she could help, but she just can't. You need to learn to be a better partner and mother yourself. You're going to have to figure out what to do with this one: maybe reparative therapy is an option.
   You've just lost your closest family member and what you thought would be an option for shelter. Tear off your family member's name and crumple up the paper.
4. You see your partner walking up to the front door with flowers, and you realize you have to leave now or never. As you start to gather your things frantically in a bag, you wonder where you will spend the night. As your partner walks in the front door, you walk out the back. You realize that you have left behind your favorite possession, but you are too afraid to turn back.
   You've just lost your favorite possession. Tear off your favorite possession and crumple up the paper.
5. You now realize that your dreams are being destroyed: your most basic needs are not even being met, you have no money, no financial support, only the clothes on your back and a few personal belongings in a grocery bag. You wonder if you should just go back and try to make it work.
   You have just lost all of your hopes and dreams for the future. Tear off your dreams and crumple up the last piece of paper.

Reflective Questions
- How did it feel to do this exercise?
- How did it feel to lose the things you lost?
- Were some things more difficult to lose than others?
- How will you help a client dealing with these issues?

 Using your **Reflective Journal**, document your feelings and thoughts about this exercise.

Learning strategies adapted by Christine Helfrich, 2007, from http://members.tripod.com.

Resources

Books
- Helfrich, C. A. (2001). *Domestic Abuse across the Lifespan.* Binghamton, NY: Haworth Press.
- Swenson Miller, K., Herzberg, G. L., & Ray, S. A. (2007). *Homelessness in America: Perspectives, Characterizations and Considerations for Occupational Therapy.* Philadelphia: Taylor & Francis.

Organizations
- The National Alliance to End Homelessness works to prevent and end homelessness by advocating for improved federal homelessness policy, building capacity to assist communities to develop best practices, and educating policymakers, practitioners, and the public about homelessness and its solutions: http://www.endhomelessness.org
- The National Coalition on Homelessness (NCH) is a national network of people who are currently experiencing or who have experienced homelessness, activists and advocates, community-based and faith-based service providers, and others committed to a single mission. The NCH engages in public education, policy advocacy, and grassroots organizing with work in the following four areas: housing justice, economic justice, health care justice, and civil rights: http://www.nationalhomeless.org

Government Publications
- "Applicability of Housing First Models to Homeless Persons with Serious Mental Illness" is a publication from the U.S. Department of Housing and Urban Development that describes several programs that use the housing first model: http://www.huduser.org/Publications/pdf/hsgfirst.pdf

References

Adelstein, L. A., & Nelson, D. L. (1985). Effects of sharing versus non-sharing on affective meaning in collage activities. *Occupational Therapy in Mental Health, 5,* 29–45.

American Academy of Pediatrics. (1996). Health needs of homeless children and families. *Pediatrics, 98*(4), 789–791.

Ansell, D. I., & Casey Family Programs. (2000, 2002). *The Ansell Casey Life Skills Assessment III (ACLSA III–Youth Form).* Seattle, WA: Dorothy I. Ansell and Casey Family Programs.

Astin, M. C., Lawrence, K. J., & Foy, D. W. (1993). Posttraumatic stress disorder among battered women: Risk and resiliency factors. *Violence and Victims, 8*(1), 17–28.

Aviles, A. M., & Helfrich, C. A. (2006). Homeless youth: Causes, consequences and the role of occupational therapy. *Occupational Therapy in Health Care, 20*(3/4), 99–114.

Bassuk, E. L., & Rosenberg, L. (1988). Why does family homelessness occur? A case-control study. *American Journal of Public Health, 78,* 783–788.

Bassuk, E. L., & Rubin, L. (1987). Homeless children: A neglected population. *American Journal of Orthopsychiatry, 57,* 278–287.

Bassuk, E. L., Rubin, L., & Lauriate, A. S. (1986). Characteristics of sheltered homeless families. *American Journal of Public Health, 76,* 1097–1101.

Bipartisan Millennial Housing Commission. (2002). *Meeting Our Nation's Housing Challenges.* Washington, DC: Author.

Bruce, M. A. G., & Borg, B. (2002a). Cognitive disability frame of reference: Acknowledging limitations. In *Psychosocial Frames of Reference: Core for Occupation-Based Practice* (3rd ed.) (pp. 244–264). Thorofare, NJ: Slack.

———. (2002b). Model of human occupation: Systems perspective of occupational performance. In *Psychosocial Frames of Reference: Core for Occupation-Based Practice* (3rd ed.) (pp. 210–240). Thorofare, NJ: Slack.

Brush, L. D. (2000). Battering, traumatic stress, and welfare-to-work transition. *Violence Against Women, 6*(10), 1039–1065.

Burt, M. R. (2001). Homeless families, singles, and others: Findings from the 1996 National Survey of Homeless Assistance Providers and Clients. *Housing Policy Debate 12*(4):737–780.

Burt, M. R., Aron, L. Y., Douglas, T., Valente, J., Lee, E., & Iwen, B. (1999). Homelessness: Programs and the people they serve. Findings of the National Survey of Homeless Assistance Providers and Clients. Available at: http://www.urban.org/publications/310291.html (accessed October 14, 2006).

Calsyn, R. J., Morse, G. A., Klinkenberg, W. D., Yonker, R. D., & Trusty, M. L. (2002). Moderators and mediators of client satisfaction in case management programs for clients with severe mental illness. *Mental Health Services Research, 4*(4), 267–275.

Campanelli, P. C., & Sacks, J. Y. (1992). Integrating psychiatric rehabilitation within a community residence framework. *Psychosocial Rehabilitation Journal, 16*(1), 135–147.

Carling, P. J. (1989). Access to housing: Cornerstone of the American dream. *Journal of Rehabilitation* (July–Sept.), 6–8.

Carlson, E. B., & Ruzek, J. (2003). "Effects of Traumatic Experiences: A National Center for PTSD Fact Sheet." National Center for Post-Traumatic Stress Disorder: Department of Veteran Affairs.

Clark, C. R., & Alexander, R. R. (2003). Outcomes of homeless adults with mental illness in a housing program and in case management only. *Psychiatric Services, 54*(1), 78–83.

Cnaan, R. A., Blankertz, L., & Saunders, M. (1992). Perceptions of consumers, practitioners, and experts regarding psychosocial rehabilitation principles. *Psychosocial Rehabilitation Journal, 16*(1), 95–114.

Constantino, R. E., Sekula, L. E., Rabin, B., & Stone, C. (2000). Negative life experiences, depression, and immune function in abused and non-abused women. *Biological Research for Nursing, 1,* 190–198.

Culhane, P. (2002). New strategies and collaborations target homelessness. *Housing Facts and Findings, 4*(5), 4–7.

Cyr, M., Toupin, J., Lesage, A. D., & Valiquette, C. A. (1994). Assessment of independent living skills for psychotic patients: further validity and reliability. *Journal of Nervous and Mental Disease, 182,* 91–97.

Davis, L. V., Hagen, J. L., & Early, T. J. (1994). Social services for battered women: Are they adequate, accessible, and appropriate? *Social Work, 39*(6), 695–704.

Di Marco, M. A. (2000). Faculty practice at a homeless shelter for women and children. *Holistic Nursing Practice, 14*(2), 29–37.

Drury, L. J. (2003). Community care for people who are homeless and mentally ill. *Journal of Health Care for the Poor and Underserved, 14*(2), 194–207.

Eisenstat, S. A., & Bancroft, L. (1999). Primary care: Domestic violence. *New England Journal of Medicine, 341*(12), 886–892.

Ensign, J., & Santelli, J. (1997). Shelter-based homeless youth: Health and access to care. *Archives of Pediatrics & Adolescent Medicine, 151*(8), 817–823.

First, R. J., Rife, J. C., & Kraus, S. (1990). Case management with people who are homeless and mentally ill: Preliminary findings from an NIMH demonstration project. *Psychosocial Rehabilitation Journal, 14*(2), 87–91.

Fisk, D., & Frey, J. (2002). Employing people with psychiatric disabilities to engage homeless individuals through supported socialization: The Buddies project. *Psychiatric Rehabilitation Journal, 26*(2), 191–196.

Folsom, D., & Jeste, D. V. (2002). Schizophrenia in homeless persons: A systematic review of the literature. *Acta Psychiatrica Scandinavica, 105*(6), 404–413.

Gallop, R., & Everett, B. (2001). Recognizing the signs and symptoms. In B. Everett & R. Gallop (Eds.), *The Link between Childhood Trauma & Mental Illness: Effective Interventions for Mental Health Professionals* (pp. 57–79). Thousand Oaks, CA: Sage.

Gerlock, A. (1999). Health impact of domestic violence. *Issues in Mental Health Nursing, 20*, 373–385.

Gilson, S. F., DePoy, E., & Cramer, E. P. (2001). Linking the assessment of self-reported functional capacity with abuse experiences of women with disabilities. *Violence Against Women, 7*(4), 418–431.

Goodman, L., Saxe, L., & Harvey, M. (1991). Homelessness as psychological trauma: Broadening perspectives. *American Psychologist, 46*(11), 1219–1225.

Gorde, M., Helfrich, C. A., & Finlayson, M. L. (2004). Trauma symptoms and life skill needs of domestic violence victims. *Journal of Interpersonal Violence, 19*(6), 691–708.

Gordon, S. (2005). The role of the consumer in the leadership and management of mental health services *Australasian Psychiatry, 13*(4), 362–365.

Greenwood, R. M., Schaefer-McDaniel, N. J., Winkel, G., & Tsemberis, S. J. (2005). Decreasing psychiatric symptoms by increasing choice in services for adults with histories of homelessness. *American Journal of Community Psychology, 36*(3/4), 223–238.

Gutmann, D. (1975). Parenthood: A key to comparative study of life cycle. In N. Datan & L. E. Ginsberg (Eds.), *Lifespan Development Psychology*. New York: Academic Press.

Harp, H. (1990). Independent living with support services: The goal and future for mental health consumers. *Psychosocial Rehabilitation Journal, 13*(4), 85–89.

Hatfield, A. B., Fiersten, R., & Johnson, D. M. (1982). Meeting the needs of families of the psychiatrically disabled. *Psychosocial Rehabilitation Journal, 6*(1), 27–40.

Helfrich, C. A. (2001). *Domestic Abuse across the Lifespan: The Role of Occupational Therapy*. West Hazelton, PA: Haworth Press.

Helfrich, C. A., Aviles, A., Walens, D., Badiani, C., & Sabol, P. (2006). Life skills interventions with homeless people: Youth, domestic violence and mental illness. *Occupational Therapy in Health Care, 20*(3/4), 189–207.

Helfrich, C. A., Badiani, C., & Simpson, E. K. (2006). Worker role identity development of women with disabilities who experience domestic violence. *Work, 27*, 319–328.

Helfrich, C. A., Fujuira, G., & Rutkowski, V. (2008). Mental health characteristics of women in domestic violence shelters. *Journal of Interpersonal Violence, 23*, 437–453.

Helfrich, C. A., & Rivera, Y. (2006). Employment skills and domestic violence survivors: A shelter-based intervention. *Occupational Therapy in Mental Health, 22*(1), 33–48.

Herzberg, G. L., Ray, S. A., & Swenson Miller, K. (2006). The status of occupational therapy: Addressing the needs of people experiencing homeless. *Occupational Therapy & Health Care, 20*(3/4), 1–8.

Hoch, C. (2000). Sheltering the homeless in the US: Social improvement and the continuum of care. *Housing Studies, 15*(6), 865–876.

Humphreys, J., Lee, K., Neylan, T., & Marmar, C. (2001). Psychological and physical distress of sheltered battered women. *Health Care for Women International, 22*, 401–414.

Hurlburt, M. S., Hough, R. L., & Wood, P. A. (1996). Effects of substance abuse on housing stability of homeless mentally ill persons in supportive housing. *Psychiatric Services, 47*(7), 731–736.

Johnson, J. (2006). Describing the phenomenon of homelessness through the theory of occupational adaptation. *Occupational Therapy & Health Care, 20*(3/4), 63–80.

Jones, L., Hughes, M., & Unterstaller, U. (2001). Post-traumatic stress disorder (PTSD) in victims of domestic violence: A review of the research. *Trauma, Violence, & Abuse, 2*(2), 99–119.

Jones, A., Quilgars, D., & Wallace, A. (2001). *Lifeskills Training for Homeless People: A Review of the Evidence*. Edinburgh: Scottish Homes.

Kannenberg, K., & Boyer, D. (1997). Occupational therapy evaluation and intervention in an employment program for homeless youth. *Psychiatric Services, 48*(5), 631–633.

Kielhofner, G. (2002). *A Model of Human Occupation: Theory and Application* (3rd ed.). Baltimore: Lippincott Williams and Wilkins.

Kielhofner, G., Braveman, B., Baron, K., Fisher, G., Hammel, J., & Littleton, M. (1999). The model of human occupation: Understanding the worker who is injured or disabled. *Work, 12*, 3–12.

Kocot, T. G. (2001). Mental health outcomes and coping in battered women: The role of social support. *Dissertation Abstracts International, 61*(8-B), 4410.

Krishnan, S. P., Hilbert, J. C., & Pase, M. (2001). An examination of intimate partner violence in rural communities: Results from a hospital emergency department study from Southwest United States. *Family and Community Health, 24*(1), 1–24.

Kuno, E., Rothbard, A. B., Averyt, J., & Culhane, D. (2000). Homelessness among persons with serious mental illness in an enhanced community-based mental health system. *Psychiatric Services, 51*(8), 1012–1016.

Kurtz, P., Hick-Coolick, A., Jarvis, S., & Kurtz, G. L. (1996). Assessment of abuse in runaway and homeless youth. *Child and Youth Care Forum, 25*(3), 183–194.

Lam, T. C. M. (1995). *Fairness in Performance Assessment*. Greensboro, NC: ERIC Clearinghouse on Counseling and Student Services.

Lave, J. (1988). *Cognition in Practice*. New York: Cambridge University Press.

Law, M. B., Baptiste, S., Carswell, A., McColl, M., Polatajko, H., & Pollock, N. (1994). *Canadian Occupational Performance Measure* (2nd ed.). Toronto: CAOT Publications ACE.

Liberman, R. P., & Kopelowicz, A. (2002). Teaching persons with severe mental disabilities to be their own case managers. *Psychiatric Services, 53*(11), 1377–1379.

Liberman, R. P., Mueser, K. T., Wallace, C. J., Jacobs, H. E., Eckman, T., & Massel, H. K. (1986). Training skills in the psychiatrically disabled: Learning coping and competence. *Schizophrenia Bulletin, 12*(4), 631–647.

Livingston, B. S., & Swenson Miller, K. (2006). Systems of care for persons who are homeless in the United States. *Occupational Therapy & Health Care, 20*(3/4), 31–46.

Marais, A., de Villiers, P. J., Moller, A. T., & Stein, D. J. (1999). Domestic violence in patients visiting general practitioners: Prevalence, phenomenology, and association with psychopathology. *South African Medical Journal, 89*, 635–640.

Mayer, B. W., & Coulter, M. (2002). Psychological aspects of partner abuse. *American Journal of Nursing, 102*, 24AA-24CC, 24EE-24GG.

McCauley, J., Kern, D., Kolodner, K., Dill, L., Schroeder, A., De Chant, H., et al. (1995). The "battering syndrome": Prevalence and clinical characteristics of domestic violence in primary care internal medicine practices. *Annals of Internal Medicine, 123*(10), 737–746.

McDonald, R., Jouriles, E. N. & Skopp, N. A. (2006). Reducing conduct problems among children brought to women's shelters: Intervention effects 24 months after termination of services. *Journal of Family Psychology, 20,* 127–136.

Minogue, V., Boness, J., Brown, A., & Girdlestone, J. (2005). The impact of service user involvement in research. *International Journal of Health Care Quality Assurance, 18*(2), 103–112.

Morris, R. I., & Butt, R. A. (2003). Parents' perspective on homelessness and its effects on the educational development of their children. *Journal of School Nursing, 19*(1), 43–50.

Morris, R. I., & Strong, L. (2004). The impact of homelessness on the health of families. *Journal of School Nursing 20*(4), 221–227.

Morse, G. A., Calsyn, R. J., Allen, G., Tempelhoff, B., & Smith, R. (1992). Experimental comparison of the effects of three treatment programs for homeless mentally ill people. *Hospital and Community Psychiatry, 43*(10), 1005–1010.

Munoz, J. P., Dix, S., & Reichenbach, D. (2006). Building productive roles: Occupational therapy in a homeless shelter. *Occupational Therapy & Health Care, 20*(3/4), 167–188.

Munoz, J. P., Garcia, T., Lisak, J., & Reichenbach, D. . (2006). Assessing the occupational performance priorities of people who are homeless. *Occupational Therapy & Health Care, 20*(3/4), 135–148.

National Alliance to End Homelessness. (2009). "Foreclosure and Homelessness." Available at: http://endhomelessness.org/section/data/interactivemaps/foreclosure (accessed September 22, 2009).

National Coalition for the Homeless. (2009). "Fact Sheet: Who Is Homeless?" Available at: http://www.nationalhomeless.org (accessed September 22, 2009).

National Institute of Mental Health. (2000). *Depression: What Every Woman Should Know.* Bethesda, MD: U.S. Department of Health and Human Services.

National Low Income Housing Coalition. (2006). "Out of reach: 2006." Available at: http://www.nlihc.org/oor/oor2006/?CFID=8353486&CFTOKEN=20965733 (accessed February 19, 2007).

——— (2009). "Housing Assistance for Low Income Families: States Don't Fill the Gap." Available at: http://www.nlihc.org/doc/PATCHWORD.pdf (accessed September 22, 2009).

Nedd, D. M. (2001). Self-reported health status and depression of battered black women. *Association of Black Nursing Faculty Journal, 12,* 32–35.

Nelson, D. L., Peterson, C., Smith, D. A., Boughton, J. A., & Whalen, G. M. (1988). Effects of project versus parallel groups on social interaction and affective responses in senior citizens. *American Journal of Occupational Therapy, 42,* 23–29.

Nelson, G., Walsh-Brown, R., & Hall, G. B. (1998). Housing for psychiatric survivors: Values, policy, and research. *Administration and Policy in Mental Health, 25*(4), 455–462.

Nemec, P. B., & McNamara, S. (1992). Direct skills teaching. *Psychosocial Rehabilitation Journal, 16*(1), 13–22.

Nollan, K. A., Horn, M., Downs, A. C., & Pecora, P. J. (2000, 2002). *Ansell-Casey Life Skills Assessment (ACLSA) and Life Skills Guidebook Manual.* Seattle, WA: Casey Family Programs.

O'Brien, S. M. (2002). Staying alive: A client with chronic mental illness in an environment of domestic violence. *Holistic Nursing Practice, 16,* 16–23.

Parkinson, S., & Forsyth, K. (2002). *Model of Human Occupation Screening Tool (Version 1.0).* Chicago: Model of Human Occupation Clearinghouse.

Petrenchik, T. (2006). Homelessness: Perspectives, misconceptions, and considerations for occupational therapy. *Occupational Therapy & Health Care, 20*(3/4), 9–30.

Rafferty, Y., & Shinn, M. (1991). The impact of homelessness on children. *American Psychologist, 46,* 1170–1179.

Ray, S. A. (2006). Mother–toddler interactions during child-focused activity in transitional housing. *Occupational Therapy in Health Care, 20*(3/4), 81–98.

Roberts, G. L., Lawrence, J. M., Williams, G. M., & Raphael, B. (1998). The impact of domestic violence on women's mental health. *Australian and New Zealand Journal of Public Health, 22*(7), 796–801.

Robertson, M. J., & Winkleby, M. A. (1996). Mental health problems of homeless women and differences across subgroups. *Annual Review of Public Health, 17*(1), 311–336.

Robertson, P. (1998). "Homeless Youth: Research, Intervention, and Policy." Available at: http://www.aspe.hhs.gov (accessed October 3, 1998).

Rosenfield, S. (1991). Homelessness and rehospitalization: The importance of housing for the chronic mentally ill. *Journal of Community Psychology, 19*(1), 60–69.

Rowe, M., Benedict, P., & Falzer, P. (2003). Representation of the governed: Leadership building for people with behavioral health disorders who are homeless or were formally homeless. *Psychiatric Rehabilitation Journal, 26*(3), 240–248.

Rutter, D., Manley, C., Weaver, T., Crawford, M. J., & Fulop, N. (2004). Patients or partners? Case studies of user involvement in the planning and delivery of adult mental health services in London. *Social Science & Medicine, 58*(10), 1973–1984.

Saunders, D. G., & Kindy, P. (1993). Predictors of physicians' responses to woman abuse: The role of gender, background, and brief training. *Journal of General Internal Medicine, 8,* 606–609.

Schultz-Krohn, W., Drnek, S., & Powell, K. (2006). Occupational therapy interventions to foster goal setting skills for homeless mothers. *Occupational Therapy in Health Care, 20*(3/4), 135–148.

Schutt, R. K., & Goldfinger, S. M. (1996). Housing preferences and perceptions of health and functioning among homeless mentally ill persons. *Psychiatric Services, 47*(4), 381–386.

Seidman, L. J., Schutt, R. K., Caplan, B., Tolomiczenko, G. S., Turner, W. M., & Goldfinger, S. M. (2003). The effect of housing interventions on neuropsychological functioning among homeless persons with mental illness. *Psychiatric Services, 54*(6), 905–908.

Shern, D. L., Felton, C. J., Hough, R. L., Lehman, A. F., Goldfinger, S. M., Valencia, E., et al. (1997). Housing outcomes for homeless adults with mental illness: Results from the Second-Round McKinney Program. *Psychiatric Services, 48*(2), 239–241.

Shern, D. L., Tsemberis, S., Anthony, W., Lovell, A. M., Richmond, L., Felton, C. J., et al. (2000). Serving street-dwelling individuals with psychiatric disabilities: Outcomes of a psychiatric rehabilitation clinical trial. *American Journal of Public Health, 90*(12), 1873–1878.

Shordike, A., & Howell, D. (2001). The reindeer of hope: An occupational therapy program in a homeless shelter. *Occupational Therapy & Health Care, 15,* 57–68.

Silverstein, S. M., Schenkel, L. S., Valone, C., & Nuernberger, S. W. (1998). Cognitive deficits and psychiatric rehabilitation outcomes in schizophrenia. *Psychiatric Quarterly, 69*(3), 169–191.

Skupien, M. B. (1998). Domestic violence on the San Carlos Apache Indian Reservation: Incidence and prevalence, associated depression and post-traumatic stress symptomology, and cultural considerations. *Dissertation Abstracts International, 59-05*(B), 2159.

Solomon, P., & Marcenko, M. (1992). Families of adults with severe mental illness: Their satisfaction with inpatient and outpatient treatment. *Psychosocial Rehabilitation Journal, 16*(1), 121–132.

Sosin, M. R., & Grossman, S. (1991). The mental health system and the etiology of homelessness: A comparison study. *Journal of Community Psychology, 19,* 337–350.

Substance Abuse and Mental Health Services Administration. (2003). Blueprint for change: Ending chronic homelessness for persons with serious mental illness and/or co-occurring substance abuse disorders. Rockville, MD: U.S. Department of Health & Human Services.

Sullivan, G., Burnam, A., Koegel, P., & Hollenberg, J. (2000). Quality of life of homeless persons with mental illness: Results from the course-of-homelessness study. *Psychiatric Services, 51*(9), 1135–1141.

Swenson Miller, K., Herzberg, G. L., & Ray, S. A. (2007). *Homelessness in America: Perspectives, Characterizations and Considerations for Occupational Therapy*. Philadelphia: Taylor and Francis, Inc.

The Urban Institute. (2000). "A New Look at Homelessness in America." Available at: http://www.urban.org/url.cfm?ID= 900302&renderforprint=1 (accessed January 17, 2010).

Tjaden, P. G., & Thoennes, N. (2000). *Extent, Nature and Consequences of Intimate Partner Violence: Findings from the National Violence against Women Survey*. Washington, DC: U.S. Department of Justice, Office of Justice Programs, National Institute of Justice.

Tryssenaar, J., Jones, E. J., & Lee, D. (1999). Occupational performance needs of a shelter population. *Canadian Journal of Occupational Therapy, 66*(4), 188–196.

Tsemberis, S., & Elfenbein, C. (1999). A perspective on voluntary and involuntary outreach services for the homeless mentally ill. *New Directions in Mental Health Service, 82*, 9–19.

U.S. Congressional Budget Office. (1995). "Statement of Nancy M. Gordon, Assistant Director for Health and Human Resources, Congressional Budget Office." Available at: http://www.cbo.gov/ftpdocs/47xx/doc4771/1995doc20.pdf (accessed February 19, 2007).

U.S. Department of Housing and Urban Development (HUD). (n.d.). "Chronic Homelessness." Available at: http://www.hud.gov/offices/cpd/homeless/chronic.cfm (accessed July 24, 2007).

———. (2003). "A Report to Congress on Worst Case Housing Needs." Available at: http://www.huduser.org/publications/PDF/trends.pdf (accessed February 19, 2007).

Vitanza, S., Vogel, L. C. M., & Marshall, L. L. (1995). Distress and symptoms of posttraumatic stress disorder in abused women. *Violence and Victims, 10*, 23–34.

Wallace, C. J. (1998). Social skills training in psychiatric rehabilitation: Recent findings. *International Review of Psychiatry, 10*(1), 9–19.

Washington, T. A. (2002). The homeless need more than just a pillow, they need a pillar: An evaluation of a transitional housing program. *Families in Society: Journal of Contemporary Human Services, 83*(2), 183–188.

Wasylenki, D. A., Goering, P. N., Lemire, D., Lindsey, S., & Lancee, W. (1993). The Hostel Outreach Program: Assertive case management for homeless mentally ill persons. *Hospital and Community Psychiatry, 44*(9), 848–853.

Wettersten, K. B., Rudolph, S. E., Faul, K., Gallagher, K., Trangsrud, H. B., & Adams, K., et al. (2004). Freedom through self-sufficiency: A qualitative examination of the impact of domestic violence on the working lives of women in shelter. *Journal of Counseling Psychology, 51*(4), 447–462.

Wilson, A. (1993). The promise of situated cognition. In S. B. Merriam (Ed.), *An Update on Adult Learning* (pp. 71–79). San Francisco: Jossey-Bass.

Wong, S. E., Flanagan, S. G., Kuehnel, T. G., Liberman, R. P., Hunnicutt, R., & Adams-Badgett, J. (1988). Training chronic mental patients to independently practice personal grooming skills. *Hospital and Community Psychiatry, 39*(8), 874–879.

Woods, S. J. (2000). Prevalence and patterns of posttraumatic stress disorder in abused and post-abused women. *Issues in Mental Health Nursing, 21*, 309–324.

Wright, J. D. (1990). Homelessness is not healthy for children and other living things. In N. A. Boxill (Ed.), *Homeless Children: The Watchers and the Waiters* (pp. 65–86). New York: Haworth Press.

Zink, T., & Sill, M. (2004). Intimate partner violence and job instability. *Journal of American Medical Women's Association, 59*(1), 32–35.

Wraparound Services: Children and Families

Pamela Erdman

> *Never doubt that a small group of thoughtful, committed citizens can change the world; indeed, it's the only thing that ever does.*
>
> —Margaret Mead

Introduction

This chapter describes a philosophy of care called wraparound services, which is an approach to working with children and families who are affected by mental illness and other disabilities. The wraparound approach has been integrated into programs staffed by occupational therapists and other health and human service practitioners.

Description of the Approach

The word *wraparound* provokes an image of someone or something being wrapped or enveloped. **Wraparound** is not a service, program, or funding source but a philosophy of care with guiding principles rooted in providing strengths-based community care that is needs driven, culturally sensitive, individualized, and unconditional. Individuals and families are surrounded or "wrapped" in a caring, supportive environment that promotes psychological healing, growth, esteem building, empowerment, and hope.

In the wraparound approach, all aspects or domains of a person's life are addressed with the belief and understanding that each "piece" can impact the functioning of the "whole." Wraparound is a "planning process that brings people together from different parts of the whole family's life. With help from one or more facilitators, people from the family's life work together, coordinate their activities, and blend their perspectives of the family's situation" (Miles, Bruns, Osher, Walker, & the National Wraparound Initiative Advisory Group, 2006, p. 4).

In this approach, formal (i.e., traditional, clinical) and informal (i.e., friends, family, faith-based community) supports are included in the care, and the client and family are actively involved in every stage of care and decision-making. To ensure success, communities must be willing and able to support (both theoretically and financially) this client and family–centered model of care. Collaboration between system partners, such as mental health providers, juvenile justice, social welfare, and education, contribute significantly to the success of this model.

Wraparound is a systems model for organizational and operational change (Miles & Franz, 2001). Although the emphasis of this approach has traditionally been focused on caring for youths with complex mental health needs who have a diagnosis of **severe emotional disturbance (SED)** and their families, it has been adapted for use in early intervention programs with adults who are developmentally delayed and/or experiencing psychiatric disorders and with older adults coping with chronic conditions such as Alzheimer's or Parkinson's disease (Literacy Network of Durham Region, n.d.). Juvenile offenders (Pullman et al, 2006) and children in foster care (McGuiness, 2009) are also targeted populations for use of wraparound programs.

History

The implementation of the wraparound process and philosophy has its roots in Europe and Canada. Some of the formative works in this field were carried out by John Brown and his colleagues, who operated the Brownsdale programs in Canada prior to 1975. These programs promoted the concepts of needs-driven services that were individualized and unconditional. Roots of the Brownsdale efforts are said to be influenced by the Larch movement, a European approach that encourages normalization and societal support to keep individuals with complex needs in their community (VanDenBerg, Bruns, & Burchard, 2003).

In 1975, under the guidance of Karl Dennis, these concepts drove the design of Kaleidoscope, a program in Chicago that implemented private, agency-based, individualized services. In 1985, the mental health, education, and social services departments of Alaska sought consultation from Kaleidoscope, and the Alaska Youth Initiative was formed. Managed by John VanDenBerg, this program successfully returned to the community almost all of the Alaskan youths with complex needs who had been placed in out-of-state institutions.

In the late 1980s, the Robert Wood Johnson Foundation funded major efforts based on the wraparound approach and its system-of-care principles. These efforts enriched further development of the wraparound movement. State-level grantees and programs involved in the National Institute of Mental Health's Child and Adolescent Services System Program (CASSP) utilized the wraparound process during the late 1980s and early 1990s.

In 1993 and 1994, the Substance Abuse and Mental Health Services Administration (SAMHSA) Comprehensive Community Mental Health Services for Children and Families awarded 22 grants to communities that proposed to use the wraparound process to serve youths and their families. As of 2006, 121 communities have been funded (Macro International, n.d.).

Foundations and Core Principles

How do you know if you are implementing the wraparound approach? Since its introduction as a human services practice strategy, the concept and its application have evolved and grown. Miles and Franz (2001) identified four basic assumptions on which wraparound practice and structural components are based:

1. Destructive behaviors are usually driven by unmet needs.
2. The biggest unmet need for many people with destructive behavior is loneliness.
3. Receiving a service does not necessarily mean your needs are being met.
4. It is harder to institutionalize new ideas than to institutionalize people.

Interventions based on wraparound principles and the degree to which they are applied can differ from one community to another. When an individual's social, physical, emotional, or developmental needs are not being met, communities can reject, eject, or provide a mechanism to re-involve those individuals in a social atmosphere that generates access, support, relationship building, and hope. The wraparound approach embraces the latter.

The structural/philosophical base of the wraparound approach is fully explained in the *Ten Principles of the Wraparound Process* (Bruns, Walker, & The National Advisory for Wraparound Initiative Group, 2008), which provides the groundwork for understanding the model. The principles are defined at the client, family, and team levels in an effort to ground the organizational and system supports in the fundamental components. Table 44-1 defines those principles.

Description of Service Delivery

How and to whom wraparound services are delivered are described next. Given that wraparound services reflect primarily a philosophy of care, the essence of how services are delivered are presented.

Population Served

Although the use of wraparound principles are now being employed in a variety of service arenas and with a variety of clients, the primary recipients of wraparound services have traditionally been youths with multidimensional, complex mental health/SED needs and their families. Programs generally serve children/youths from birth to age 18. Communities served by wraparound programs engage youths and families from a multitude of diverse cultures, races, religions, preferences, and socioeconomic groups. The provision of wraparound as a philosophy of care has no cultural boundaries or limitations.

Guidelines for recipient enrollment criteria are usually identified, in part, by the program's funding source. For those wraparound programs primarily serving youth with complex needs, examples of recipient enrollment are:

- A disability that has persisted for 6 months and can be expected to persist for 1 year or longer.
- A condition of severe emotional disturbance, as defined in the *American Psychiatric Association Diagnostic and Statistical Manual of Mental Disorders* (DSM-IV).

Table 44-1 ● **Ten Principles of the Wraparound Process**

Core Principles	Definition
1. Family Voice and Choice	Client and family perspectives are intentionally sought and prioritized. Planning is grounded in family members' perspectives. The team works toward providing options and choices. The plan reflects family values and preferences.
2. Team based	The team is composed of individuals chosen by and committed to the family's wellbeing.
3. Natural supports	Active participation from the family's network of interpersonal and community resources (e.g., neighbors, extended family, faith-based relations) are sought and encouraged. These supports are sustainable after formal services have ended.
4. Collaboration	The team works cooperatively and shares responsibility for developing, implementing, monitoring, and evaluating the family's plan.
5. Community-based	Services and supports are provided in the most inclusive, most responsive, most accessible, and least restrictive setting possible.
6. Culturally competent	The process must demonstrate respect for and build upon the values, preferences, beliefs, culture, and identity of the client/family and their community.
7. Individualized	Each family's plan is tailored to fit them. The team creates and implements a customized plan of strategies, supports, and services.
8. Strengths based	The process and plan identify, build on, and enhance the capabilities, knowledge, skills, and assets of the youth/family, their community, and other team members.
9. Persistence	Despite challenges, the team works toward achieving the goals in the plan until they reach an agreement that a formal wraparound process is no longer required.
10. Outcome based	The team ties the goals and strategies of the plan to observable or measurable indicators of success, monitors indicator progress, and revises the plan as needed.

Data from Bruns, E. J., Walker, J. S., & The National Wraparound Initiative Advisory Group. (2008). Ten principles of the wraparound process. In E. J. Bruns & J. S. Walker (Eds.), The Resource Guide to Wraparound (pp. 2.1.1–2.1.9). Portland, OR: National Wraparound Initiative, Research and Training Center for Family Support and Children's Mental Health.

The Lived Experience

Mary and John

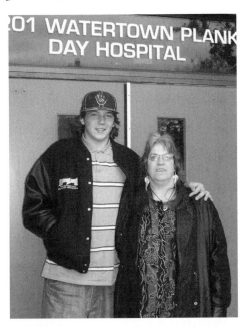

Mary is an educated, single parent of Native American descent who is the mother of three boys. The youngest, John, age 14 at the time, was enrolled into the Wraparound Milwaukee (WM) program in October 2004. Wraparound Milwaukee is a public, county-run wraparound program serving severely emotionally disturbed youth and their families in Milwaukee, Wisconsin. Youths enter the program on a court order either through the juvenile justice system (delinquency order) or through the Bureau of Milwaukee Child Welfare (BMCW) on a Child in Need of Protective Services (CHIPS) order.

A "stressed-out" Mary sought enrollment into WM after receiving services from another community program that was less intensive and could offer services for only a brief period of time. John was enrolled into WM on a delinquency order facing theft, criminal damage to property, and disorderly conduct charges. He was diagnosed at the time with oppositional defiant disorder and attention deficit disorder with hyperactivity. He was a special education student at a Milwaukee public school, had a history of marijuana usage, and was physically aggressive, impulsive, and disrespectful of authority. John had a history of psychiatric inpatient hospitalizations. The family vision at the time of enrollment was for "John to change his behavior, go to school, set goals for himself, and avoid any new charges."

Mary described her view of WM: "Wraparound is a program designed to 'wrap' services around the family and bring these service providers and others together to work toward meeting the needs of the family." Mary spoke briefly of her family's initial referral/screening process, meeting her care coordinator for the first time, identification of her family's strengths and needs, composing the Child and Family Team that would help her family get their needs met, her introduction to the family advocacy program that works with WM, and her own and her family's growth over time. Mary spoke of feeling more empowered as a parent and program participant as her family's enrollment in WM continued. She took on a more "hands on" role within the Child and Family Team, feeling she now had the knowledge and strength to do so.

Mary described how her outlook of her family, self, and the future changed positively as she grew more knowledgeable about the program philosophy and how to implement that philosophy of care. She mentioned that her increased involvement in family advocacy tasks, being a facilitator at WM program trainings and family orientations, and being an active member on several WM committees has allowed her to develop into a more confident, optimistic, and strong individual. "If things don't work, that's OK. Just try something else."

Mary indicated that her parenting skills have strengthened over time. "Our roles are more defined now. I am stronger at following through and being more consistent. The children know what to expect now." Mary identified respite services and involvement in the family advocacy program as being the most beneficial to her. Mary stated that she feels John's self-esteem has improved and that he originally viewed himself as a "problem child" but now realizes that everyone has weaknesses and that's all right. She feels John is now able to identify "triggers" that result in his acting out and has learned more healthy ways to cope and deal with his anger. Mary commented that the mentoring and crisis services her son has received have been instrumental in his development over the past 3 years.

When asked what was the most helpful part of the wraparound process to her and her family, Mary remarked, "Knowing that there are people out there that care, and they are not going to judge you. The care coordinators take this to heart. It is not just a job to them. It becomes who they are, not just what they do. It has changed my family and my life."

Mary has dreams of her children finishing high school and going to college. She has her own aspirations of returning to school and possibly becoming a professional speaker or lecturer.

- Functional symptoms (e.g., psychotic symptoms, dangerous to self/others/property)
- Functional impairments in areas such as self-care, behavioral controls, decision-making skills, judgment, social relationships and norms, family relationships, school, and/or work.
- Receiving services from two or more service systems, such as mental health, social services, child protective services, juvenile justice, and special education.

Funding Sources

The primary funding source for the youth/family-focused wraparound initiatives is grants through the Center for Mental Health Services (CMHS). CMHS is the federal agency within SAMHSA of the U.S. Department of Health and Human Services. SAMHSA also provides mental health block grant monies for other philosophically based wraparound systems, such as community-based systems of care

Evidence-Based Practice

There is research evidence indicating that youth who received wraparound services in a child welfare system exhibited superior outcomes related to movement to less restrictive environments and with family members and more positive outcomes regarding school attendance, school disciplinary actions, and academic performance when compared with youth who received usual mental health services (Bruns, Rast, Walker, Bosworth, & Peterson, 2006).

➤ Occupational therapists can work to influence adoption of a wraparound philosophy of care to impact student occupational outcomes, such as school attendance, behavior, and academic performance through strategies that are strengths based, persistent, and that build on goals grounded in client and family perspectives.

Bruns, E. J., Rast, J., Walker, J. S., Peterson, C. R., & Bosworth, J. (2006). Spreadsheets, service providers, and the statehouse: Using data and the wraparound process to reform systems for children and families. *American Journal of Community Psychology, 38,* 201–212.

for adults with co-occurring substance abuse and mental health disorders. In addition to federal grants, many programs receive monies from state and local funds; Medicaid waivers; child welfare, juvenile justice, education dollars; and other public and private funds.

Two other organizations engaging in the mission to improve health care for youths, families, and adults in the United States are the Annie E. Casey Foundation and the Robert Wood Johnson Foundation. Both of these organizations fund initiatives that address access to health care and promote healthy communities and lifestyles.

Administrative Bodies

Wraparound programs are administered by a variety of entities, including state- or county-based behavioral health systems, public health departments, private health providers, child protective services/child welfare departments, mental health centers/departments, juvenile justice entities, tribal organizations, and departments of education, among others. Although there is always a designated body to administer a program and monitor its funds, the wraparound process/philosophy cannot be carried out by a single community entity. It takes a "system of care" to rally together and meet the needs of an individual or family. Miles and Franz (2001) identified six service technologies that need to be enhanced in order for wraparound to be a successful community and administrative endeavor:

1. A planning process that provides a common vocabulary to help participants from widely varying backgrounds unite in coherent and creative circles of support and provides these teams with reliable steps for moving quickly from discussion to action.
2. A commitment to creative, strengths-based, needs-driven action plans that is supported and reinforced by a management information system that reflects the core values of wraparound and ensures accountability for both process and outcomes.

3. A cross-system funding and service access infrastructure that enables support teams to develop and implement unified, comprehensive plans that incorporate and align the actions and resources of all of the service systems with which an individual or family is involved.
4. Consistent and sustained training, support, and guidance for team facilitators, family members, and service systems staff who may be asked to be members of teams to ensure that the planning and implementation process is undertaken in a culturally competent way and that action plans incorporate community-based, normalized living opportunities for individuals and families.
5. An operational orientation and quality assurance system that ensures that the individuals and families who are at the focus of wraparound circles of support are able to have access, voice, and ownership in the preparation and implementation of each action plan.
6. An explicit commitment expressed in policy and contracts that wraparound teams will remain in place to support individuals and families despite whatever setbacks may occur until the team is not needed or the person or family is able to transition to a more natural or informal supportive context.

Wraparound Care Coordination

Care coordination is a collaborative, culturally sensitive, needs-driven, strength-based process of assessing, planning, implementing, coordinating, monitoring, and evaluating options and services to meet an individual's or family's needs. The process promotes quality care and cost-effective outcomes. The care coordinator (a role that might be filled by an occupational therapist) is the conduit between the client/family, the administrative body, and all system-of-care entities, providers, and natural/informal supports. Their role

Evidence-Based Practice

Youths involved in juvenile justice settings who received conventional mental health services were three times more likely to commit a felony offense and 28% more likely to serve detention time compared with youth who received wraparound services. Wraparound participants showed "significant improvement on standardized measures of behavioral and emotional problems, increases in behavioral and emotional strengths, and improved functioning at home, at school, and in the community" (Pullman et al, 2006, p. 388).

➤ Occupational therapists working with wraparound delinquent youths can provide community-based individual or group therapy focusing on anger management and development of positive coping skills, impulse control, peer relations, and recreational/social skills training. The youth's wraparound plan of care would be the guiding force for the specific services the occupational therapist would render.

Pullmann, M. D., Kerbs, J., Koroloff , N., Veach-White, E., Gaylor, R., & Sieler, D. (2006). Juvenile offenders with mental health needs: Reducing recidivism using wraparound. *Crime and Delinquency, 52,* 375–397.

is to assist the client/family in achieving an optimal level of wellness and functioning, thus enhancing both psychological and physical health, self-worth, productivity, life satisfaction, and quality of life.

Care coordinators promote client self-advocacy, empowerment, and independent decision-making. They must be effective collaborators, communicators, mediators, and delegators. Occupational therapists who assume the role of care coordinator are well trained to meet the complex needs of the client and his or her family, as these are consistent with connecting people with their needed environmental supports in order to carry out their daily occupations and achieve optimal wellness and functioning, consistent with the person-environment-occupation orientation of this text.

The Wraparound Care Coordinator Tool Kit (Miles, 2004) identifies the skills necessary for effective care coordination. The list of skills is divided into four phases that typically occur in the wraparound process: engagement, planning, implementation, and transition. Figure 44-1 shows the phases and associated outcomes that ideally occur during the wraparound process. These phases and their major tasks and activities are described in further detail in the "Phases and Activities of the Wraparound Process" (Walker et al, 2004).

Engagement

The **engagement phase** is the initial stage of involvement, which focuses on team development through face-to-face contact with the family and either personal or telephone contact with potential team members. Care coordinators must be able to effectively introduce themselves and speak to their role; explain the wraparound process; solicit the client/family to tell "their story"; analyze that story in an effort to identify strengths, unmet needs, other potential team members; summarize the story verbally and in writing; solicit the participation of the identified team members; and provide stabilization resources for any immediate crisis situation that the client/family may be experiencing.

Planning

The **planning phase** occurs when the team is brought together to review family strengths, develop a collaborative mission statement, identify needs across all life domains, prioritize those needs, and identify strategies and actions to meet those needs. In this phase, the care coordinator must be able to effectively analyze information gathered during the engagement phase; strategically organize people and information to move ahead with planning (coordinate the first team meeting); communicate the information gathered during the engagement phase; solicit feedback from team members; synthesize all perspectives; facilitate agreement in decision-making; define the ongoing process (e.g., team meetings, strengths orientation, needs, actions, and team rules); and define the future wraparound process and solicit long-term team commitment. Care coordinators must be able to thoroughly and accurately document the meeting results in the form of a plan of care, distribute this plan to all

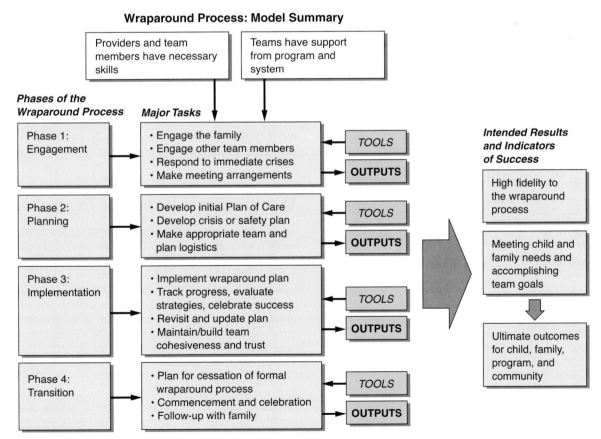

FIGURE 44-1. Phases and associated outcomes that ideally occur during the wraparound process.

team members in a timely fashion, schedule ongoing team meetings, and anticipate any crisis/safety needs.

Implementation

During the **implementation phase**, the team meets regularly to discuss the effectiveness of the interventions and adjust the plan accordingly. This phase continues until the team identifies adequate progress and begins to move ahead with the final phase of transition. During implementation, the care coordinator must work at maintaining and facilitating participation from the team over time and/or introducing new team members as needed; lead the team in searching for an understanding about unmet needs; track, assess, and communicate the family's progress; begin to substitute natural supports and resources for those that have been paid for; maintain the focus on the family's strengths and creative solutions; and empower team members to implement tasks and to take ownership of and make modifications to the plan while maintaining a focus on the original direction established in the plan.

Transition

The **transition phase** occurs when the initial plan of care has been implemented and modified over time and the appropriate interventions have been successfully delivered to produce the desired outcomes. This phase occurs in a thoughtful manner that engages the entire team in decision-making, supports rather than abandons, and helps people move to a life free of system interference—rather than simply moving people from services. In this phase, the care coordinator must analyze progress toward meeting the goals; assess the usefulness of interventions; increase participation by family and natural supports; empower paid providers to create nonsubsidized alternatives for their activities or interventions; implement individual transition plans; set up and practice crisis response drills; build linkages to follow-up resources; and recognize and thank the team for its participation and accomplishments.

Efficacy of Wraparound Programs

The efficacy of an intervention is typically judged according to the research available. Evidence-based practices can be defined as programs or practices that are proven to be successful through research methodology and have consistently produced positive patterns of results and have established generalizability (Waters, n.d.). There are many clinical approaches that appear to work well but have not been studied enough or in the manner necessary to prove that they are evidenced based. Evidence-based practices may not be the only ones that work; however, they are the only ones that are supported by scientific evidence that proves they work to produce specific outcomes when used with the intended populations (Hyde, Falls, Morris, & Schoenwald, 2003).

Compared with many of the more traditional methods of treatment (i.e., cognitive and behavioral therapies), the wraparound model is a newer method of intervention. Thus, in comparison, the number of wraparound evidence-based

research studies is limited. Because wraparound is a highly individualized process rather than a specific modality of treatment, it is harder to standardize and study. Evidence for wraparound's effectiveness at this time lies more in its "face validity": service providers believe in it and families like it versus clinically driven, controlled research studies (Sheehan, Walrath, Bruns, & Meyers, 2005). Though limited, the research published in peer-reviewed journals relevant to the wraparound process is promising and worthy of consideration.

Occupational Therapy Roles and Opportunities

The philosophical values of the wraparound process and its holistic, adaptive, restorative approach of care are complementary to the foundation and beliefs of occupational therapy. As the occupational therapist strives to empower clients to achieve their maximum level of independent functioning in all life areas by employing strategies and techniques applicable to the clients' needs, so does the wraparound care coordinator address all identified needs and employ strategies and services to meet those needs. All "domains" of a wraparound client's life are assessed during the beginning stages of program involvement. These domains include family, mental health/psychological, educational/vocational, cultural/spiritual, social/recreational, living situation, legal, medical, safety/crisis, systems barriers, and transitional planning.

The occupational therapist has all of the necessary educational, philosophical, and experiential "tools" to perform all care coordinator duties with a level of confidence and expertise that would lend itself to successful client outcomes. In addition, more traditional occupational therapy services are often available to the client and family through the program's network of mental health community providers. Occupational therapists have also assumed administrative roles within wraparound programs, such as deputy directors, quality improvement directors, provider network coordinators, HIPPA compliance officers, supervisors, administrative coordinators, and consultants.

Wraparound Program Evaluation

As the expectation intensifies to report clinical/behavioral, social/environmental, client satisfaction and fiscal outcomes to program members, funding sources, governmental bodies, and the community at large, the importance of being able to evaluate a program in a comprehensive and meaningful way becomes paramount. Communities should base the development, implementation, and refinement of their system of care on assessment of the outcomes for the clients served within their communities (Vroon VanDenBerg LLP, n.d.).

In an effort to accomplish this task, every program must identify the program components that need to be evaluated and measured, for what reason and for whom; what processes, tools, and staff need to be acquired and implemented for accurate measures; validity and reliability of the measures; a description of how the data will be analyzed and interpreted; a plan for how the data will be presented in a manner that is respectful, effective, and client and stake-holder driven; a description of how the data will be used to make programmatic changes and improve the quality of care and service delivery; and a plan for program sustainability, including ongoing evaluation and outcome-based research efforts. Evaluating a wraparound program encompasses all of these components.

An example of an extensive longitudinal wraparound evaluation effort involving a multimethod and multilayer design is being undertaken by Macro International, a research company headquartered in the Washington, D.C., area. This evaluation effort is being funded through the SAMHSA Comprehensive Community Mental Health Services for Children Program's Children's Mental Health Initiative (CMHI). Core components of this national evaluation consist of the following (Macro International, 2004):

- *System of Care Assessment Study* examines whether programs have been implemented according to the system-of-care program theory and documents how systems develop over time to meet the needs of the children and families they serve.
- *Cross-Sectional Descriptive Study* describes the children enrolled in the funded systems of care in terms of their demographics, functional status, living arrangement, diagnosis, risk factors, and mental health service history.
- *Child and Family Outcomes Study* examines how the system affects child clinical and functional status and family life. Outcome data are used to assess change over time in symptomatology, diagnosis, social functioning, substance use, school attendance and performance, delinquency, and stability of living arrangements.
- *Services and Costs Study* describes the types of services used by children and families, their utilization patterns,

and associated costs. The study assesses also the extent to which information about various services is captured through local management information systems.

- *Service Experience Study* examines data about the characteristics of services received and child and family ratings of service experiences, including the cultural competence of service providers and satisfaction with services provided.
- *Sustainability Study* explores the extent to which systems of care are maintained after funding from the CMHS grant program has ended. The study identifies features of systems of care that are more likely to be sustained and factors that contribute to or impede the ability to sustain the systems of care developed with grant support.

Several evaluation and data collection instruments have been utilized over time in the national evaluation endeavor. A sampling of the instruments used as a part of the CMHS National Evaluation process is shown in Table 44-2 (Macro International, 2004). Copp, Bordnick, Traylor, and Thyer (2007) report on their pilot evaluation conducted in Georgia and offer a clear description of how the outcome process was implemented with the participating families.

Intervention Models and Techniques

Wraparound intervention techniques at the care coordinator level were briefly identified in the section "Wraparound Care Coordination." Strengths discoveries, goal/needs identification graphs, bubble planning, story boarding, and timelines or clock planning are used to guide the child and family through all four phases of the wraparound process. These

Table 44-2 ● Wraparound Program Evaluation Instruments

Type of Data Collected	Caregiver Interview	Youth Interview
Longitudinal Youth and Family Outcome Instruments		
Descriptive information	Caregiver Information Questionnaire (CIQ)	Youth Information Questionnaire (YIQ)
Youth behavioral and emotional strengths	Behavioral and Emotional Rating Scale-2: Parent Rating Scale (BERS-2C)	Behavioral and Emotional Rating Scale-2: Youth Rating Scale (BERS-2Y)
Youth clinical symptomatology	Child Behavior Checklist (CBCL 1.5–5, CBCL 6–18)	Revised Children's Manifest Anxiety Scale (RCMAS), Reynolds Adolescent Depression Scale (RADS-2)
Youth's social functioning	Columbia Impairment Scale (CIS)	Substance Use Survey–Revised (SUS-R), GAIN Quick Substance Dependence Scale (GAIN Quick-R), Delinquency Survey–Revised (DS-R)
Youth development	Vineland Screener (VS1, VS2, VS3)	NA
Youth's living arrangement	Living Situations Questionnaire (LSQ)	NA
Youth's education information	Education Questionnaire–Revised (EQ-R)	NA
Caregiver's strain related to the care of a youth with special needs	Caregiver Strain Questionnaire (CGSQ)	NA
Service Experience Instruments		
Service contacts in multiple settings	Multi-Sector Service Contacts–Revised (MSSC-R)	NA
Cultural competence of service	Cultural Competence and Service Provision Questionnaire (CCSP)	NA
Client satisfaction with services	Youth Services Survey for Families (YSS-F)	Youth Services Survey (YSS)

Evidence-Based Practice

Urban youths with serious mental health issues who were returned from or diverted from residential care and were receiving wraparound services were compared with youths receiving traditional mental health services. At the 24-month follow-up, the wraparound youths were found to be more likely to be living in regular community placements, attending school and/or work more often, and exhibiting fewer than 3 days of serious behavior problems during the course of the previous month (Hyde, Burchard, & Woodworth, 1996).

➤ With wraparound youths either returning from residential care and/or being diverted from residential care, the occupational therapist might be sought out through a provider referral process or through services rendered under an Individualized Education Plan (IEP). The wraparound process would encourage the establishment of an individualized, strength-based treatment plan that would guide the occupational therapist as to what the specific needs of the youth/family might be and how those needs are to be met.

Hyde, K. L., Burchard, J. D., & Woodworth, K. (1996). Wrapping services in an urban setting. *Journal of Child & Family Studies, 5,* 67–82.

Evidence-Based Practice

A study by Reay, Garbin, and Scalora (2003) evaluated the impact of rendering wraparound services to a rural group of youths at different points in time. Based on an analysis of five behaviors (compliance, peer interactions, physical aggression, alcohol and drug use, and extreme verbal abuse), the multiple baseline case study design found that immediately following the introduction of wraparound, dramatic improvements occurred in all five behaviors despite when the introduction occurred (12, 15, 19, and 22 weeks).

➤ Occupational therapists providing wraparound services in a rural setting are often faced with challenges related to access, transportation, and adequate insurance coverage. Flexibility and adaptability in the provision of individualized, strength-based therapy is of utmost importance in this setting. The occupational therapist would provide services based on the needs identified on the youth's plan of care.

Reay, W. E., Garbin, C. P., & Scalora, M. (2003). The Nebraska evaluation model: Practice and policy decisions informed by case and program specific data. In C. Newman, C. J. Liberton, K. Kutash, & R. M. Friedman (Eds.), *A System of Care for Children's Mental Health: Expanding the Research Base: 15th Annual Research Conference Proceedings, March 2–6, 2002* (pp. 49–52). Tampa, FL: Research & Training Center for Children's Mental Health, Louis de la Parte Florida Mental Health Institute, University of South Florida.

are all consistent with the philosophy and principles of the strengths-based and culturally competent focus of building innovative and practical solutions with and for each family.

The Wraparound Milwaukee (WM) program based in Milwaukee, Wisconsin, is one example of a nationally recognized children's wraparound model. In 1994, Milwaukee County received its initial grant through SAMHSA's Comprehensive Community Mental Health Services for Children and Families. WM has since become a self-sustaining wraparound program, successfully serving emotionally and behaviorally challenged Milwaukee County youths and their families. In 2009, WM received recognition from Harvard University's Kennedy School of Government as one of six top government innovations (*Milwaukee Journal Sentinel*, 2009).

In 2003, the President's New Freedom Commission on Mental Health Report identified WM as an "exemplary program that expressly targets children with serious emotional disturbances and their families." In 2005, WM was named as one of the five "Most Promising Approaches in Public Sector Managed Care Systems" through the Health Care Reform Tracking Project cofunded by SAMHSA and the National Institute on Disability and Rehabilitation Research of the Department of Education. Since 2005, WM has been identified as one of three national training and learning centers for the Center for Mental Health Services grant sites that are

either currently or in the beginning stages of implementing a wraparound-based program in their community.

The DAWN Project in Indianapolis, Indiana, and Westchester, New York's System of Care are the other designated learning communities. Other children's wraparound-based system-of-care models can be identified through the National Wraparound Initiative website at www.rtc.pdx.edu/ nwi.

Summary

This chapter provided a look at the development of wraparound programs based on a philosophy and principles that, when applied to children and families coping with complex issues associated with their child's serious emotional disturbance, provide creative ways to wrap the child and family with the supports and services that allow them to fully participate in their desired roles. Occupational therapy practitioners share their expertise in key staff roles such as care coordinators and supervisors in wraparound programs given the compatibility of their background oriented to this strengths-based family approach matching them to the services and supports in their environment.

Active Learning Strategies

1. Plan of Care

The care coordinator is a key individual with whom the client/family engages during their enrollment in a wraparound program. Although care coordinator training within wraparound programs is tailored to meet the needs of the specific population and community being served, one

important and constant activity engaged in during training is the creation of strong, strengths-based, needs-driven, individualized client plan of care. Care coordinators often state that if they can speak to some similar life experience when initially engaging with the client/family, the opportunity to more quickly bond and develop a trusting relationship increases. In an effort to identify, acknowledge, and process an identified need in an individual's life, it is helpful to complete a mini plan of care for yourself. Remember, because the plan of care is the driving force behind the provision of wraparound service and achievement of the client/family vision, it is imperative that it be thorough, individualized and responsive to the changing needs of the client and family.

Answer the following questions, and then reflect on your answers.

1. What is the "vision" (similar to a long-term goal) you have for yourself or your family during the next 6 to 12 months? Example: For John to finish high school and graduate as planned.
2. What is a current identified need that will help you achieve your vision? Example: John needs to improve his study habits to get passing grades.
3. What life domain does this fall under? Example: Family, social/recreational, education/vocation.
4. What is your start date and your target or accomplish by date?
5. What strengths do you have that can be utilized to help you meet your need and achieve your vision? Example: John is able to pay attention in class. John is willing to accept help from others. John is motivated to graduate.
6. What strategies are you going to put into place to meet that need? Example: John will attend homework club after school 3 days per week. John will work with a tutor for 3 hours per week. John's mother and brother will review his homework nightly for completeness and accuracy.
7. Which team members will help with this? Example: Homework club staff, Nicole (tutor), Lisa (mother), and Rick (brother).

Reflective Questions

● What was difficult for you in completing this process?
● What was easy?
● Take away half of the strategies and/or identified team members that you have helping you with your strategies. How much more difficult would it be to achieve your goal?

● Who could you turn to, and/or what other strategies could you put in place if these helping individuals were no longer available and/or if the current strategies did not result in desirable outcomes?

 Describe your feelings about this exercise in your **Reflective Journal**.

2. Cultural Diversity

Wraparound providers must be cognizant of the cultural beliefs and values of the clients/families they serve. In an effort to respect those values and beliefs, individuals must have some insight into their own values and belief system. Initial impressions and predisposed beliefs of a race, religion, gender, and so on, can impede the provision of culturally sensitive and competent care. Mental health providers often engage in cultural diversity, competency, and sensitivity training and workshops in an effort to learn more about themselves and the people they serve. Try the following:

1. Break into groups of two and introduce yourself by name only.
2. Look at each other for 2 to 3 minutes without saying a word.
3. Ask yourself these questions:
   a. What race/nationality is this person?
   b. Is this person religious? If so, what religion does he or she practice?
   c. What kind of job might this person have?
   d. What kind of music does this person like?
   e. Where is this person likely to vacation?
   f. What kind of car does this person drive?
   g. What kind of hobbies might this person have?

Find out how accurate your assumptions were and have a group discussion about the implications of making assumptions and how such assumptions may impede quality of care. Talk about how, if services were to be wrapped around your partner, his or her cultural background might impact that plan of care.

Resources

- Annie E. Casey Foundation: http://www.aecf.org
- National Center for Mental Health and Juvenile Justice: http://www .ncmhjj.com
- National Federation of Families for Children's Mental Health: (240) 403-1901; http://www.ffcmh.org
- National Wraparound Initiative: http://www.rtc.pdx.edu/nwi
- E. J. Bruns & J. S. Walker (Eds.). (2008). *The Resource Guide to Wraparound*. Portland, OR: National Wraparound Initiative, Research and Training Center for Family Support and Children's Mental Health: complete copy is available at http://www.rtc.pdx .edu/NWI-book/Chapters/COMPLETE-RG-BOOK.pdf
- Robert Wood Johnson Foundation: http://www.rwjf.org
- Systems of Care, Substance Abuse and Mental Health Services Administration: http://www.systemofcare.samhsa.gov
- Website/forum for those interested in dialoguing and learning about more wraparound philosophy and systems of care: http:// www.Paperboat.com
- Wraparound Milwaukee Program: http://www.county.milwaukee .gov (search for Wraparound)

References

Bruns, E. J., Rast, J., Walker, J. S., Peterson, C. R., & Bosworth, J. (2006). Spreadsheets, service providers, and the statehouse: Using data and the wraparound process to reform systems for children and families. *American Journal of Community Psychology, 38*, 201–212.

Bruns, E. J., Walker, J. S., & The National Wraparound Initiative Advisory Group. (2008). Ten principles of the wraparound process. In E. J. Bruns & J. S. Walker (Eds.), *The Resource Guide to Wraparound*. Portland, OR: National Wraparound Initiative, Research and Training Center for Family Support and Children's Mental Health.

Copp, H. L., Bordnick, P. S., Traylor, A. C., & Thyer, B. A. (2007). Evaluating wraparound services for seriously emotionally disturbed youth: Pilot study outcomes in Georgia. *Adolescence, 42*, 723–732.

Hyde, K. L., Burchard, J. D., & Woodworth, K. (1996). Wrapping services in an urban setting. *Journal of Child & Family Studies, 5*, 67–82.

Hyde, P. S., Falls, K., Morris, J. A., & Schoenwald, S. K. (2003). *Turning Knowledge Into Practice: A Manual for Behavioral Health*

Administrators and Practitioners About Understanding and Implementing Evidence-based Practices (p. 14). Boston: Technical Assistance Collaborative.

Literacy Network of Durham Region. (n.d.). "Wraparound in Durham Region." Available at: http://www.lindr.on.ca/wrap/gen-info.pdf (accessed April 3, 2007).

Macro International. (n.d.). Comprehensive Community Mental Health Services for Children and Their Families Program: Funded Communities Grant Sites Map. Available at: http://www.orcmacro.com/projects/cmhi (accessed April 27, 2007).

———. (2004). "Core Components of the National Evaluation." Available at: http://www.orcmacro.com/projects/cmhi/study-components (accessed February 27, 2007).

McGuiness, T. M. (2009). Youth in the mental health void: Wraparound is one solution. *Journal of Psychosocial Nursing, 47*(6), 23–26.

Miles, P. (2004) Wraparound Care Coordinator Toolkit. Available at: http://www.rtc.pdx.edu/nwi/tools/pgTools.php?page=jobs (accessed April 15, 2007).

Miles, P., Bruns, E. J., Osher, T. W., Walker, J. S., & the National Wraparound Initiative Advisory Group. (2006). *The Wraparound Process User's Guide: A Handbook for Families.* Portland, OR: National Wraparound Initiative, Research and Training Center on Family Support and Children's Mental Health, Portland State University.

Miles, P., & Franz, J. (2001). "Foundations of Wraparound: Values, Practice Patterns and Essential Ingredients." Training article. Available at: http://www.paperboat.com (accessed April 11, 2007).

Milwaukee County: County mental health program wins award. Milwaukee Journal Sentinel (2009, September 23). Available at http://www.jsonline.com/news/wisconsin/60467712.html. (Retrieved March 8, 2010).

Pullmann, M. D., Kerbs, J., Koroloff, N., Veach-White, E., Gaylor, R., & Sieler, D. (2006). Juvenile offenders with mental health needs: Reducing recidivism using wraparound. *Crime and Delinquency, 52,* 375–397.

Reay, W. E., Garbin, C. P., & Scalora, M. (2003). The Nebraska evaluation model: Practice and policy decisions informed by case and program specific data. In C. Newman, C. J. Liberton, K. Kutash, & R. M. Friedman (Eds.), *A System of Care for Children's Mental Health: Expanding the Research Base: 15th Annual Research Conference Proceedings, March 2–6, 2002* (pp. 49–52). Tampa, FL: Research & Training Center for Children's Mental Health, Louis de la Parte Florida Mental Health Institute, University of South Florida.

Sheehan, A., Walrath, C. M., Bruns E. J., & Meyers, M. J. (2005). Knowledge, training and supports for evidence-based treatments: Differences between wraparound and non-wraparound providers. Power Point presentation. Personal communication, May 1, 2007 Mary Jo Meyers, Deputy Director, Wraparound Milwaukee Program, Wisconsin.

VanDenBerg, J., Bruns, E., & Burchard, J. (2003). History of the Wraparound Process. *Focal Point: Research, Policy and Practice in Children's Mental Health, 17,* 4–7.

Vroon VanDenBerg LLP. (n.d.) "Research, Evaluation, and Quality Improvement." Available at: http://www.vroonvdb.com (accessed March 19, 2007).

Walker, J., & Bruns, E., for the National Wraparound Initiative. (2007) "Wraparound: Key Information, Evidence, and Endorsements." Available at: http://www.rtc.pdx.edu/nwi (accessed April 26, 2007).

Walker, J. S., Bruns, E. J., Rast, J., VanDenBerg, J. D., Osher, T. W., Koroloff, N., et al. (2004). *Phases and Activities of the Wraparound Process.* Portland, OR: National Wraparound Initiative, Research and Training Center on Family Support and Children's Mental Health, Portland State University.

Waters, P. (n.d.) "Evidence-based Practices (A Three-Part Series), Part 1." Available at: http://www.scattc.org (accessed April 4, 2007).

Occupation

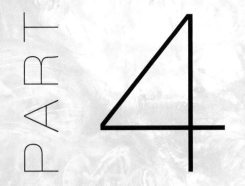

Few occupational therapy texts attempt to comprehensively address areas of occupational performance. This part of the text covers the more familiar occupations of work, self-care, and leisure along with some areas of occupation that have been neglected, such as sleep and spirituality. Attention is paid to the character or purpose of different occupations across the lifespan. Many of these chapters include descriptions of specific assessments and intervention models and techniques.

Introduction to Occupation and Co-occupation

Kris Barnekow and Noralyn Davel Pickens

> "How we spend our days is, of course, how we spend our lives.
>
> —Annie Dillard

Introduction

So much of who we are is associated with what we do. The philosophical founder of occupational therapy, Adolf Meyer (1922), wrote

> *Our conception of man is that of an organism that maintains and balances itself in the world of reality and actuality by being in active life and active use. . . . It is the use that we make of ourselves that gives the ultimate stamp to our every organ. (p. 5)*

As a psychiatrist, Meyer recognized that a lack of participation in the rhythms of daily life contributed to mental illness and that the return to participation had many positive outcomes, including pride in achievement, hopefulness, a balanced use of time, and a sense of a worthwhile existence.

In some ways, Meyer's writings foreshadowed the recovery movement, which de-emphasizes the relevance of symptoms and speaks to the importance of living a full life, engaged in activities that provide meaning and purpose, with an interconnectedness to the community and others (Warner, 2009). For clients with mental health issues, engaging in occupation can provide moments of sanity, calm, and normality. How to help our clients engage in occupation is a major emphasis of this text.

Occupation is the core construct of the profession, yet its meaning has evolved over time and continues to be elusive. To help frame the discussion of occupational engagement, it is important to define and discuss the construct of occupation. This chapter presents several perspectives on occupation and describes dimensions and components of occupation, including an in-depth discussion of the related construct of co-occupation.

Defining Occupation

The use of the term *occupation* originated in the early papers of our profession. In discussing the early work of occupational therapy with clients with mental illness, Meyer writes, "A pleasure in achievement, real pleasure in the use and activity of one's hands and muscles and a happy *appreciation of* time began to be used as incentives in the management of our patients" (1922, p. 3).

While some might argue we lost our focus on occupation during the Progressive Era of scientific medicine, it could be argued that the occupational therapy carried out in mental health facilities never lost the "occupation" in therapy. With the reduction in mental health resources in the United States, occupational therapists and scholars recognized a need to reclaim occupation across all areas of occupational therapy practice. In the late 1980s, the call to re-emphasize occupation began with a group of scholars introducing a discipline: occupational science.

The founders of occupational science first described occupation as "specific 'chunks' of activity within the ongoing stream of human behavior which are named in the lexicon of the culture . . ." (Yerxa et al, 1990, p. 5). This definition and others are widely debated within the occupational therapy community. In capturing the general essence of the word, we might suggest occupation is "everyday life activity" (American Occupational Therapy Association [AOTA], 2002). While this is succinct, it is rather broad and creates challenges to define the scope of practice for occupational therapists. Scholars in the field have noted that occupation is perhaps too complex to define in one sentence (Golledge, 1998; Wood, 1996) and that occupation may be better understood by elaborating on its dimensions.

In 1995, the American Occupational Therapy Association (AOTA) defined occupation as "the ordinary and familiar things that people do every day" (AOTA, 1995, p. 1015). Additionally, AOTA listed dimensions of occupation as performance and context as well as psychological, spiritual, social, temporal, and symbolic. Other related concepts frequently associated with occupation in the literature are health and wellbeing, productivity and adaptation (Canadian Association of Occupational Therapists [CAOT], 1994; Christiansen & Baum, 1997; Hammell, 2004; Hasselkus, 1998, 2000; Nelson, 1996; Pierce, 2003; Whiteford, Townsend, & Hocking, 2000).

In the 2002 Occupational Therapy Practice Framework: Domain and Process, the authors (AOTA) use the Canadian Association of Occupational Therapists (CAOT) definition: "activities . . . of everyday life, named, organized, and given value and meaning by individuals and a culture. Occupation is everything people do to occupy themselves, including looking after themselves . . . enjoying life . . . and contributing to the social and economic fabric of their communities . . ." (1997, p. 32). The framework and integrated terms and definitions are aimed at establishing the domain of occupational therapy practice for clinicians, payers, and clients alike.

One of the problems in defining and communicating the understanding of occupation is its use in the literature and practice as both an end and a means (Gray, 1998; Hasselkus, 2000; Laliberte-Rudman, Yu, Scott, & Pajouhandeh, 2000). Occupation as a means refers to occupation as an agent of change in clinical practice, as in the use of therapeutic occupation in rehabilitation to address regaining homemaking abilities through a culturally significant and meaningful occupation, perhaps cooking. Occupation as an end focuses on occupation as an end-product, meaning the ability to perform meaningful occupations, restoration of "occupational lives" (Gray, 1998, p. 357). In 2000, the American Occupational Therapy Foundation invited leaders in the field of occupational therapy to discuss practice and research issues of occupation. This group of educational and clinical leaders was unable to reach consensus on a definition of occupation. Broad dimensions of the term, such as being, doing, and becoming; everyday tasks; and engagement, were debated (Hasselkus, 2000). These dimensions and the different definitions of occupation reflect the means and end uses of the term.

As noted in the OT Practice Framework (AOTA, 2002), the Canadian model of occupational performance (CMOP) emphasizes the interrelated and interdependent dimensions of occupation. The CMOP is a model of a "dynamic relationship between persons, environment and occupation. The CMOP provides a framework for enabling occupation for all persons." The central focus of the CMOP is the client, placing emphasis on client-centered practice. The 2002 revised CAOT definition of occupation is the following:

> *Everything people do to occupy themselves, including looking after themselves (self-care), enjoying life (leisure) and contributing to the social and economic fabric of their communities (productivity). (CAOT, 2002)*

The CAOT definition reflects the traditional three-pronged self-care–leisure–productivity approach that has been maintained in occupational therapy since Meyer's early writings (1922).

Hasselkus (2002) and Pierce (2001) move away from this traditional approach to suggest that occupation is about experience, that it is complex and embedded in meaning. In her 2001 paper, Pierce suggests a definition for occupation:

> *An occupation is a specific individual's personally constructed, non-repeatable experience. That is, an occupation is a subjective event in perceived temporal, spatial, and socio-cultural conditions that are unique to that one-time occurrence. An occupation has a shape, a pace, and beginning and an ending, a shared or solitary aspect, a cultural meaning to the person. . . ." (p. 139)*

This language encompasses the dynamic nature of occupation and depicts the contextual elements of occupation. Pierce does well in providing a basic description and analysis for educators and students in her text *Occupation by Design* (2003). Hasselkus's 2002 text, *The Meaning of Everyday Occupation*, richly explores the nuances and complexities of occupation and how it is embedded in our being.

Exploring Dimensions of Occupation

In this chapter, we explore dimensions of occupation to further our understanding of this complex construct and its grounding in our practice. The dimensions presented in this chapter include space and place; temporality; sociocultural habits and routines; and doing, being, and becoming.

Space and Place

According to Tuan (1977), space is freedom, movement, and openness. Alternatively, place is endowed with value and meaning, security, attachment, and intimacy. "Space is transformed into place as it acquires definition and meaning" (p. 136). Hasselkus (1998) extends Tuan's theory in her study on wellbeing and dementia care. In her study, Hasselkus found that the day-care staff worked to create for their clients occupational space within the day-care center. In her model of occupational space, Hasselkus suggests occupational place is created during engagement in occupation.

How we experience space and place allows for occupational engagement. Seamon (2002) and Rowles (1991) offer insights into how our individual and cultural use of space can both create and limit interaction. Our training as occupational therapists incorporates understanding of the physical environment. How we experience the small spaces we live in or the larger geographic community either supports or hinders our wellbeing. Occupationally enriched environments foster occupational place for our clients.

Temporality

Tuan (1977) suggests that place and time are connected. Place is a pause in the "temporal current," a marker of time. Cottle and Klineberg (1974) suggest that humans have a "temporal connectedness" in which they experience the past, present, and future at one time. This connectedness means that choices made in the present are reflections of experiences in the past and anticipations for the future. Flaherty

(1993, 1994, 1999) developed a theory of the experience of lived time. Flaherty describes three experiences of time: **protracted duration, synchronicity**, and **temporal compression**. Protracted duration is "experienced during situations of either high or low levels of embedded activity." The passage of time is perceived as too slow. In this temporal experience, the person has high emotional concern and great cognitive engrossment. Temporal compression occurs when the passage of time seems to have quickened. According to Flaherty's theory, this occurs during habitual activity, with a low degree of emotion or cognitive involvement. Synchronicity is a normal relationship between experience and time passage. The situation is unproblematic; there is moderate cognitive and emotional involvement. The result is routine.

Another theory developed to explain the experience of time is Csikszentmihalyi's psychological theory of flow (1990). **Flow** is defined as a timeless experience where a person's skill just meets the challenge of the situation. Two other temporal variations identified by Larson (2004) include temporal rupture—an overwhelming life-changing event that distorts time and deconstructs daily life—and interstitial time. Interstitial time is explained by uncertainty and expectation, engrossment with time, intense experience, and a feeling of expanded time resulting in discomfort or dissatisfaction, such as when expecting an important phone call regarding the results of a diagnostic test.

Sociocultural Habits and Routines

Pierce's third element following the spatial and temporal aspects is the sociocultural dimension of context (2001, 2003). This is a broad heading that can encompass cultural beliefs, institutional power, relationships, co-occupation, and much more. (An in-depth discussion of co-occupation follows this discussion.) Townsend (1993, 1997, 2003) and others (Townsend & Wilcock, 2004; Whiteford, 2001; Wood, 1997) have long championed our role in fostering occupational justice through addressing the societal role enabling occupation.

Doing, Being, Belonging, and Becoming

Health and wellbeing is proposed to be a dynamic balance of doing, being, and becoming (Wilcock, 1998b). In her keynote address at the 1998 World Federation of Occupational Therapists Conference, Wilcock reflected on occupation as doing, being, and becoming. **Doing**, perhaps best understood as "purposeful action," is acting on the environment and interacting with other beings. Doing creates the world in which humans live (Fidler & Fidler, 1983; Wilcock, 1998b). By doing, humans develop and integrate sensory, motor, cognitive, and psychological systems (Wilcock, 1998b). Doing also affirms competence and self-worth (Hammell, 2004).

According to Wilcock, it is in **being** that occupation has meaning. Being allows for reflection, contemplation, and discovery (Wilcock, 1998b). In her paper on aging and "sageing," DoRozario (1998) suggests that being is "enjoying and celebrating our achievements" and "finding a sense of 'enoughness' from within . . ." (p. 119). Rowles (1991) states

that there is too much emphasis on doing and not enough understanding of being in the human perspective. He suggests fully self-actualizing involves being, an awareness of experiencing life and one's surroundings.

Rebeiro, Day, Semeniuk, O'Brien, and Wilson (2001) add the concept of **belonging** to the Wilcock triad. In their paper on mental health programming, they suggest that the need for mutual support, interaction, and sense of belonging are aspects of occupation that demonstrate the interconnectedness that occupation can support. Also important is the idea of reciprocity, unconditional acceptance, and being valued beyond the intrinsic value of self.

Wilcock's concept of **becoming** relates to a person's sense of future or potential, transformation and self-actualization. Fidler and Fidler (1983) state that through doing (investigating) and being (experiencing), a person *becomes*. In other words, through creating, exploring, and reflecting on the experiences of life, a person becomes or is transformed. Some suggest occupation is a source of personal transformation (Townsend, 1997; Wilcock, 1998b). For Hammell (2004), becoming is about envisioning future selves and exploring new opportunities.

Occupational Performance Areas

Occupational therapists have a long history of addressing the occupational performance areas related to productive activities such as work and school, activities of daily living, socialization, and play/leisure. Refinement of occupational therapy's domain of concern through the Occupational Therapy Practice Framework (AOTA, 2002) and the second edition of the Occupational Therapy Practice Framework (AOTA, 2008), as well as influences from the recovery movement (Russinova & Cash, 2007), have further expanded the profession's consideration of performance areas into health and wellbeing, spirituality, and restorative occupations, such as rest and sleep.

Evidence-Based Practice

Clients with mental health issues often lack opportunities for occupational engagement.

➤ Supportive work environments such as Northern Initiative for Social Action (NISA) can provide social outlets, opportunities for health risk taking and address the being and belonging needs of clients with mental illness (Rebeiro, Day, Sememiuk, O'Brien, & Wilson, 2001).

➤ Accomplishment of daily life tasks and care for others creates a sense of competence and meaning. Clients have an improved subjective quality of life (Aubin, Hackey, & Mercier, 1999).

Rebeiro, K. L., Day, D., Semeniuk, B., O'Brien, M., & Wilson, B. (2001). Northern initiative for social action: An occupation-based mental health program. *American Journal of Occupational Therapy, 55,* 493–500.

Aubin, G., Hackey, R., & Mercier, C. (1999). Meaning of daily activities and subjective quality of life in people with severe mental illness. *Scandinavian Journal of Occupational Therapy, 6,* 53–62.

Health and Wellbeing

A basic tenet in the study of occupation is that occupation has a positive effect on personal health and wellbeing (CAOT, 2002; Clark et al, 1997; Hasselkus, 1998, 2002; Law, Steinwender, & Leclair, 1998; Rebeiro et al, 2001; Wilcock, 1993, 1999; Yerxa, 1998). Health and wellbeing are often linked. Yerxa suggests health is "an encompassing, positive, dynamic state of 'well-beingness,' reflecting adaptability, a good quality of life, and satisfaction in one's own activities" (1998, p. 412). "Health is defined in the World Health Organization's constitution as a state of complete physical, mental and social well-being and not merely the absence of disease or infirmity" (WHO, 2006). Emphasized in WHO documents are living in harmony with others and the environment, focusing self-determination for everyday life activities. Scholars of occupational science have resonated with this definition. It reflects broad dimensions of occupation: self-directedness, everyday routines and environment, and accomplishment.

Wilcock (1993) has argued that occupation is a basic human need. Without occupation, humans as individuals and as a society would not survive. Townsend (1997) and Townsend and Wilcock (2004) suggests occupation is transformative in enabling humans to order their lives through routine, thereby allowing for contemplation and decision-making to exert control in everyday and new experiences. The outcome of all this is wellbeing.

Wellbeing is defined as positive psychological functioning, including the dimensions of acceptance of self, positive relations with others, autonomy, environmental mastery, purpose in life, and personal growth (Ryff & Singer, 1996). Additionally, wellbeing is defined as "a perception of one's condition . . . an internal construct . . . independent of external conditions" (Law et al, 1998, p. 83). In their critical review of research on the relationship between occupation and health and wellbeing, Law et al found a positive relationship among daily activity, social activity, and life satisfaction. In their study of an occupation-based mental health program, Rebeiro et al (2001) found that clients attained a sense of wellbeing. However, they warned that the experience was a substitute for "real" community and acceptance.

Not engaging in occupation has received some attention. Yerxa (1998) reviewed research findings that suggested the loss of occupation is more devastating to those with physical disabilities than are their physical losses. Wilcock (1993, 1999) further argues that decreased engagement in occupation could be directly related to inability to survive, both as an individual and more globally as a society. She suggests that the loss of self-sustaining occupations and increased reliance on technology could create a vacuum of self-preservation abilities. From their review, Law et al (1998) found that the removal of occupation from a person's daily life led to increased stress, physiological changes, and decreased health status and wellbeing. Occupational deprivation (Whiteford, 2001, 2005) stresses the complexity and interaction between institutional (cultural, political, and otherwise) and individual power in enabling occupationally enriched environments and opportunities.

The discourse on socially viewed negative occupations, such as self-injurious behaviors or committing violent acts toward others (Mocellin, 1995), or even nonproductive/passive occupations (Farnworth, 2000; Passmore, 2003) and their relationship to health and wellbeing is minimal but an important topic for occupational therapy. Chapter 46 contains more detailed information on this topic.

Activities of Daily Living

Those simple and not so simple things that we do every day to care for ourselves, our homes, and our loved ones make up activities of daily living. Brushing your teeth, preparing a meal, making a bank transaction, tying your child's sneakers, taking the bus to work, sweeping the floor—these are the occupations that are most often taken for granted until there comes a problem.

Activities of daily living are sometimes divided into two categories: basic activities of daily living (BADLs) and instrumental activities of daily living (IADLs) (Stedman, 2005). **BADLs** are those activities that focus on care of the self, such as bathing, dressing, and toileting. **IADLs** are more complex activities that require interaction with the environment and/or others, such as grocery shopping, using public transportation, and money management.

For people with mental illness, there can be many barriers to participation in either BADLs or IADLs. The despair and inertia associated with depression can make it difficult to engage in even the most simple BADLs (Dunlop, Manheim, Song, Lyons, & Chang, 2005). Caring for one's own mental illness often involves complex medication routines; however, cognitive impairments such as those associated with schizophrenia can interfere with successful medication management (Heinrichs, Goldberg, Miles, & McDermid, 2008). Narrow food preferences for children with autism create problems with adequate nutritional intake as well as disrupt family mealtimes. The routines of daily living give life order a predictability, and there is evidence that disruption of those routines are predictive of symptoms of depression in people with bipolar disorder (Sylvia et al, 2009). For more information on activities of daily living, see Chapter 47.

Work, Rest, and Play

Returning to the writings of Adolf Meyer (1922), there is an emphasis on the balance of daily life. This balance includes productive activities, relaxation, and play and leisure. Work (both paid and volunteer) often contributes significantly to a person's identity and allows individuals to see themselves as contributing to the larger society. In addition, productive activity incorporates the role of student for children and adults. Relaxation has received less attention but is essential for health and restoration. Play and leisure activities rejuvenate the individual, provide outlets for pleasure, and often allow for connectedness to others.

Unemployment rates in people with mental illness are higher than in any other disability group (Mechanic, Bilder, & McAlpine, 2002), yet work can play an important role in the recovery process. In a qualitative study, participants identified work as a means to recovery and wellness (van Niekerk, 2009), while a quantitative study found that paid work was associated with higher scores on recovery and empowerment scales (Lloyd, King, & Moore, in press). Likewise, adults with serious mental illness are often left out of higher education, and lack of education can contribute to difficulties with work (Nuechterlein et al, 2009). Psychiatric disabilities in children are often diagnosed and evidenced in the school environment (Preston, Heaton, McCann, Watson, & Selke, 2009).

Disturbance in play/leisure and sleep are also concerns for individuals with mental illness. Mood disorders like depression and bipolar disorder include sleep disturbances as part of the symptomatology (American Psychiatric Association, 2000). Time-use patterns among people with serious mental illness can be very different than patterns of the general population. For example, people with schizophrenia are more likely to spend greater amounts of time sleeping and to engage in solitary and passive activities such as watching television (Minato & Zemke, 2004). Restricted play is common in childhood psychiatric disabilities such as autism. Children with autism lack reciprocal play which in turn limits social interaction (Taylor, Hoch, Potter, Rodriguez, & Kalaigian, 2005).

See Chapters 48 and 49 for information on student roles (child and adult respectively); Chapter 50 for information related to work; Chapter 52 for information on play, leisure, and recreation; and Chapter 53 on rest, sleep, and restorative occupations.

Spirituality and Meaning

Occupational scientists acknowledge that humans are meaning makers: they act on their worlds, seeking and creating meaning. Some have suggested that spirituality is the experience of making meaning in everyday life (CAOT, 2002; Christiansen & Baum, 1997; McColl, 2003; Unruh, Versnel, & Kerr, 2002). Christiansen and Baum (1997) define "activities of spirit" as the occupations engaged in when nourishing the soul and creating meaning. This means reveling in simple everyday occupations, being aware of their place in the rhythm and routine of one's life. Occupation gives meaning to life and is connected to spirituality in that, through occupation, individuals can make a difference in their lives, the lives of others, and the community. Humans live out meaning, and thus their spirit, through occupation. Occupations are engaged in for both material needs and spiritual needs, and through engagement in occupation, a person connects with his or her inner spirit (Christiansen & Baum, 1997; Egan & DeLaat, 1997). "Meaning is constructed through our relationships with ourselves, other humans, other inhabitants of the earth, the earth itself, and for many individuals, a higher power or Creator" (Egan & DeLaat, 1997, p. 116). Humans thus have opportunities to create meaning for themselves and enrich others through activities of spirit, occupations of meaning.

In coming to understand spirituality, many researchers in and outside of occupational therapy have identified categories or expressions of spirituality. These are generally broken into two groups: sacred/theistic or secular. Sacred or theistic are expressions of values and beliefs in a higher power, often in relationship to God. The sacred expressions have a more existential nature and are about connectedness to others and nature. (Unruh, Versnel, & Kerr, 2002 provide an in-depth review.)

Specifically addressing spirituality in occupational therapy practice has been a challenging issue. McColl (2000) discussed the ambivalence therapists felt about spirituality in their practice. This is partly due to the interrelationship with religion, a particular concern in parts of the world where religion and "state" issues are held to be separate. As such, the CAOT defined spirituality as "a pervasive life force, manifestation of a higher self, source of will and self-determination, and a sense of meaning, purpose and connectedness that people experience in the context of their environment" (1997, p. 182). This is acknowledged as a very secular view and purposely so (Townsend, DeLaat, Egan, Thibeault, & Wright, 1999). In their workbook on spirituality, Townsend et al emphasize the human need for meaning and connectedness that is often bereft in the lives of those who are marginalized, abused, or otherwise disadvantaged.

Understanding one's own spirituality is essential to addressing the issue with clients, or at a minimum, recognizing the spiritual needs of clients. When there are questions from clients of a sacred/theistic nature, occupational therapists must make referrals to the appropriate counselor or religious leader. However, coming to understand the client's spiritual self underlies client-centered practice. How a client is motivated and views the world and his or her place in it will drive therapeutic relationships and occupational interventions. The concepts of occupational alienation and deprivation (Whiteford, 2005; Wilcock, 1998a) are inherently related to a spiritual vacuum in the occupational lives of clients. Coming to understand the occupational expressions and needs of our clients is about understanding their spirit. Spirituality as an occupation is further addressed in Chapter 54.

Co-occupation

Social participation is another area of occupational performance. In this chapter, social participation is explored through the concept of co-occupation, and a significant portion of this chapter is dedicated to this concept due to both its importance and limited attention. By its very name, **co-occupation** means mutually engaging in occupation. Meaning and shared experience are essential when defining co-occupation. Occupational scientists have constructed definitions of co-occupation in conceptually different ways. Zemke and Clark (1996) identified a continuum of social occupations ranging from parallel occupations to the most interrelated social occupation as being co-occupation. Parallel occupations are those occupations in which individuals may share the same physical context, such as standing in a grocery line. The individuals are involved in their own occupation and do not share an interaction. Shared occupations may be completed individually, but there is an interchange among people who may share a common goal. According to Zemke and Clark, examples of shared occupations include quilting bees, harvesting, and barn-raising. Zemke and Clark espouse that co-occupations necessitate involvement of two or more individuals who are deeply interrelated. Both individuals must be active in the process, and to best understand the nature of the co-occupational experience, research should explore the active engagement of both co-occupational partners.

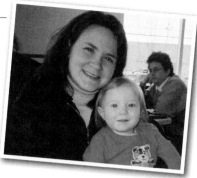
Pierce (2003) builds upon the work of Zemke and Clark by using research findings to construct a theoretical framework of occupation. As discussed previously, Pierce identifies the contextual dimensions of occupation, which include spatial, temporal, and sociocultural. Co-occupations are highly interactive occupations that are categorized under the sociocultural dimension of occupation. Pierce depicts the flow of social occupations in a continuum. The continuum includes solitary occupations, shared occupations, and co-occupations. Co-occupation occurs when two or more individuals share engagement in an occupation. The emergence of a co-occupation from an occupational experience is explained in the following example of kite flying. In this story, kite flying is the activity that has the potential to become a co-occupation. Depending on the context, kite flying can be a co-occupation or a solitary or shared occupation.

Case

Three-year-old Stacia asked her mother to fly kites in the park behind their home that early spring morning. Together they prepared the kite with Stacia holding the string while her mother tied the kite and fitted the cross rods. They ran together to the park in to the gusty wind, perfect for kite flying. With Mom running the kite and Stacia holding the string dowel, the kite flew high into the sky. Stacia screamed with joy. A few tugs on the string from Mom brought the kite well over the nearby trees and rooftops. They laughed together as they followed the kite in the sky. The kite danced to an altitude at which it simply floated in the sky. Mom sat on the soggy park grass and Stacia, holding the dowel and giving an occasional tug on the string, sat in her mother's lap. Stacia turned at looked at her mother with complete joy on her face, smiling, so proud and content. They looked at each other—holding that moment. Stacia tucked herself further in to her mother's body and continued to tug the kite, not saying a word, but smiling up at the kite.

The case demonstrates the fluid nature of co-occupation. In the shared experience of flying the kite, there was mutual joy and elation in the outcome and the experience of being together. The eye gaze, the smiles, the nestling into each other—these are observable acts that to an outsider would show tenderness and shared emotionality. A three-year-old might have a difficult time articulating her emotions, but her behavior demonstrates her complete engagement in the experience. In this vignette, the co-occupation was more than flying a kite; it was the full experience of being together. It was the sense of meaning and shared experience that created the co-occupation. Co-occupations involve at least one or more of the following aspects across a spectrum: shared physicality, shared emotionality, and shared intentionality

Aspects of Co-occupation

To illustrate the aspects of co-occupation, reflect on the kite-flying vignette. Flying a kite may be performed independently, but when two individuals share in the kite flying, the occupational experience may become a co-occupation. The individuals may share **physicality** by jointly tugging at the kite string to ensure the kite stays in flight. Shared physicality is when two or more individuals engage in reciprocal motor behavior. For another example of shared physicality, consider breast feeding. When a mother and infant are engaged in breast feeding, the mother and baby are sharing physicality. Throughout the feeding/eating process, the mother and infant are actively involved and responding to each other during the process. The co-occupational process of feeding and eating can be characterized by the observed reciprocal motor behaviors or shared physicality that indicate or depict this process

Shared **emotionality** is when one individual is reciprocally responsive to the other individual's emotional tone. It may be reflected by an individual's smile in response to another individual's laughter. Shared emotionality and physicality may be linked. For example, research describing breast feeding depicts the close link between shared physicality and the emergence of shared emotionality (Simpson, 1999). This motoric act of latching onto the mother's breast (physicality) creates a release of oxytocin in the mother. Oxytocin is a hormone that fosters attachment and bonding in the mother, or emergence of shared emotionality, and this initial bonding leads to the shared physicality of continued nursing.

Finally, individuals may share **intentionality**. Shared intentionality occurs when there is an understanding of each other's role and purpose during engagement of the co-occupation. Intentionality is created in the brain by anticipating what will occur from goal-directed actions. Shared intentionality is characterized by (1) joint goal setting, (2) understanding and knowing each other's intentions, (3) interdependent goal acquisition, and (4) regulation of each other's actions. It is motivated by cooperation, and there is a coordination of task and attention to each other (Warneken, Chen, & Tomasello, 2006). Shared intentionality requires that two individuals have mutually established goals and that the individuals understand the other person's behavior as goal directed (Tomasello & Rakoczy, 2003).

Shared intentionality requires developed cognitive skills of simple expression to highly linguistic skills. Thus, shared intentionality develops over time and is embedded in experience (Bruner, 1995). For example, research has shown that infants begin to develop precursors to shared intentionality by about 9 months of age. The first step in the development of shared intention is joint attention or showing objects to another individual. Joint attention develops between 9 and 12 months of age. Then, shortly after the infant's first birthday (12–15 months), infants will direct attention to distant targets. Finally, between 12 and 18 months, infants appear to understand a shared goal, reciprocal roles, collaboration, and intended actions (Tomasello & Carpenter, 2005).

Shared intentionality may contribute to the creation of meaning (Lazzarini, 2004). Shared meaning requires that both participants have a sense of the outcomes of the actions, both what is expected and what is not expected or is unanticipated.

A spectrum of co-occupations, ranging from foundational to complex, exists depending on the number and degree of aspects (high or low). Using the word *spectrum* is deliberate in that co-occupations may be nested in complexity. It is important to note that all co-occupations, regardless of where they fall within the range of foundational to complex, are equally important. Co-occupations do not require all three aspects of shared physicality, emotionality, and intentionality.

For instance, co-occupations that occur during infancy, such as feeding/eating, provide sustenance for life. Feeding and eating in the neonatal period may be characterized by shared physicality with the beginning of shared emotionality. Shared intentionality will develop as the child matures. Both foundational and complex co-occupations are essential for sustaining life and critical for development and growth. Individual participants such as infants or those individuals with cognitive impairment may not have the ability to understand the other's intentions; however, they may have the ability to reciprocate, and this may become evident through observation of motor processes.

The degree with which a co-occupation is characterized by shared physicality, shared emotionality, and shared intentionality may vary and is dependent on the co-occupation, the age and ability of the individuals engaging in the co-occupation, and sociocultural expectations. For example, when a caregiver is teaching a child to fly a kite for the first time, shared physicality may be high. As the child learns to fly the kite, shared physicality may decrease; however, shared emotionality and shared intentionality may increase.

Engagement in Co-occupation

Engagement in co-occupation may occur with less frequency when an individual has a mental illness. Often, individuals with mental illness experience social isolation, which exacerbates symptoms associated with their illness. For example, social isolation experienced by individuals with serious mental illness is related to increasing symptoms of alcoholism, schizophrenia, and suicide. Reclusive behaviors and social withdrawal are hallmark symptoms of schizophrenia, substance abuse, and major depressive disorder (Ward, 2003). A lack of co-occupational performance may impede participation in activities of daily living and other significant occupations in adult populations.

Conversely, in pediatric populations, co-occupations are essential to survival. That is, infants would die if there was no engagement in reciprocal meaningful activities with significant caregivers. Again, think of the co-occupation of feeding and eating. Without this meaningful co-occupation, infants would not receive the necessary nutrition for survival. Not only are co-occupations essential for survival, the quality or emotional tone of the co-occupational experience, particularly with significant others, impacts bonding and attachment relationships (Kraemer, 1992; Olson, 2004). The quality of an attachment relationship provides the foundation for psychosocial, cognitive, and behavioral development (Kraemer, 1992).

In pediatric populations, psychosocial and emotional development is significantly related to the co-occupations between primary caregiver and child. Co-occupations such as feeding/eating, comforting/self-comforting, and getting to and settling to sleep have been identified in the research literature as significant in early childhood (Olson, 2004). Co-occupational routines that occur between primary caregiver and child have the potential to influence the child's self-regulation, motivation, emotion, and cognition (Barnekow & Kraemer, 2005). If co-occupational routines influence psychosocial and physical development, then occupational therapists need to be adept at understanding the caregivers' concerns and capacities, the child's strengths and needs, and the quality of the co-occupational experience (Barnekow & Kraemer, 2005).

Occupational therapists are instrumental in identifying co-occupation and in thinking about co-occupational performance in children and adults with mental health issues. The key to assessment when evaluating co-occupation is including "the other." That is, observation should always include assessment of the client in relation to the other individual involved in the co-occupation.

Co-occupation in Practice

Extending Gray's (1998) work on occupation as means and ends, we suggest considering co-occupation as both means of therapy and ends of therapy. *Co-occupation as means* occurs when an occupational therapist facilitates co-occupation to address a goal. For example, the occupational therapist may implement cooking as a treatment with a small group of clients diagnosed with depression. The clients are required to plan a meal, decide who is responsible for purchasing items on the menu, work together to prepare the various aspects of the meal, and cleanup. Each activity within the meal planning and preparation facilitates aspects of co-occupational performance. Clients may share physicality while at the grocery store. One client might be pushing the cart as the other client places the grocery items into the cart. They may share emotionality during final preparation of the meal and while eating the meal. Throughout the process, there is shared intentionality as the goal of meal preparation is understood and roles are established and understood within the process. Meal planning, preparation, and cleanup within a group constitute co-occupation as means. Again, meal preparation, eating, and cleanup become a co-occupational process through the sense of meaning and shared experience that the individuals have when involved in the group.

The Lived Experience

Bonnie

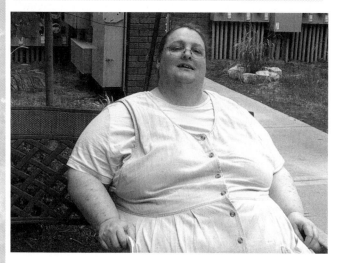

Bonnie describes her struggles with her mood disorder and binge eating. The narrative describes a life that is relatively solitary and passive, but glimmers of hope are associated with making others smile, music, and the support of her occupational therapist.

Today, I can say, "I am alright, I guess." There are days or hours when I can't. When I have to say I have the blues, I'm in my turtle shell, or just in the dumps. I don't really get suicidal anymore. I will just binge on anything chocolate or ice cream. For me, this is practically suicidal behavior anyway.

I have been living on my own for 4½ years now. I have ups and downs with my physical and mental health. Sometimes, I think that the two have a lot to do with each other. I have been asked what it is like to be Bipolar. For me it is a rollercoaster ride that comes on me unexpectedly. I can go months feeling good about life in general and then suddenly hit bottom and feel like I am worthless, friendless and alone. Sometimes, I can talk myself out of it with changing what I am doing. But there are nights when it hits me hard and I feel like things will never change.

I almost never want to get out of bed in the morning, but I do. I hit the pity pool, to the point that I climb into my "turtle shell" and don't want to have much to do with anyone. I don't go to appointments or leave my home much. I just exist. I also am more likely to have bad migraine clusters. My blood sugar is bad because I don't have much control over my eating. I stay up until my eyes hurt and I have a raging migraine. Sometimes I will sleep for hours at a time and miss my meds. Other times I can't sleep for days at a time. Late at night, like now, I am alone and there is nothing to interest me but the games on the Internet.

I used to cope with my stressors by burying myself in book after book. I would read 2 or more books per day. Now it takes me 3 or more days to read one. I don't care about personal hygiene and will only take a bath once a week or so. I feel worthless and don't see how I can get out of it. I don't even try. I am trying my hardest to eat right. When I grocery shop with my case worker or occupational therapist, I may get a little of something unhealthy, but most of the time I just go right on by with a sigh and a wishful glance.

I feel hopeful, most of the time. In fact I see that I can accomplish things. I have learned to cope with making lots of jokes and it makes people smile. It's funny that I can make people smile while I am falling apart inside. Even if it's just making someone smile and laugh. Maybe, that is my legacy. A little bit of sunshine. I will suddenly get an idea to turn some music on or watch something on Ovation channel that catches my eye. I will suddenly care again and even start feeling better. I don't know why it is but music plays a big part in how I feel. The days I listen to the oldies channel, hearing music from the 50s and 60s makes me happy and safe again.

Ways that occupational therapy helps me, is to reverse the mind set I get into. We talk about healthy ways to eat and substitute things like yogurt—the fancy flavors for the thing that they taste like. Going shopping with me and helping me choose fruits and reminding me why I don't want to really eat the Zingers that are right in front of me. She helps me find things that I am good at and encourages me to start on them.

I went through a cognitive therapy class and that helped some, but there is always backsliding and you have to start up again. Hopefully, not sliding back too far down, you have to keep trying every day, because eating disorders are like any other addiction. The only problem is that you can't live without food, so you have to learn control

It doesn't happen all at once, since there is no magic pill to change people, it takes one day at a time, and sometimes one nanosecond at a time to stop where you are and start up and change your habits.

Co-occupation as ends is when the desired outcome is to have an individual engage in co-occupation. The occupational therapists may work with the client individually on tasks and activities with the final goal being planning, preparing, and sharing a meal for the client's family or friends. Under these circumstances, the treatment outcome is co-occupation but the treatment intervention may incorporate a variety of tasks and activities that support the final outcome.

Co-occupation is a construct that is relatively new in the field of occupational therapy and occupational science. However, therapists need to recognize the significance of co-occupation in clients with mental health issues. Engagement in co-occupations facilitates attachment or relational bonds. This in turn has a neurobiological impact on the health of the client (Barnekow & Kraemer, 2005). Engagement in occupation and co-occupation have the potential to transform the lives of people with mental health issues. Our unique focus as *occupational* therapists is to enable these opportunities for enriched, meaning-filled lives.

As you continue in your own occupational journey, recognize that you will best serve your clients by understanding your occupational and co-occupational self.

Summary

The challenge of occupational therapy is how to create opportunities for occupational engagement for our clients. Meyer argued, "Our role consists in giving *opportunities* rather than prescriptions. There must be opportunities to work, opportunities to do and to plan and create, and to learn to use material" (1922, p. 7). Occupational engagement is the human expression of self, both individually and with others. Early on, Wilcock argued for a biological need for occupation (1993). Our world also requires that we engage in occupations for sustenance.

Active Learning Strategies

1. Record of Occupational Engagement

Create a week-long table with each day divided in to half-hour segments. For a week, write down *everything* you do. After the week:

a. Categorize the time into ADLs, school, work, leisure, and rest/sleep.
b. Identify the amounts of time spent in each category (the time should add up to 168 hours for the week).
c. Divide the time for each category by 168 to determine a percentage and create a pie chart that illustrates your week's occupational engagements.

Reflective Questions

- What does this say about your occupational balance?
- Where are you spending most of your time?
- How much control do you have over your choice of occupation? Is this where you want to be spending your time.
- How do your occupations support (or not support) your wellbeing?
- Categorize your time in terms of co-occupation. How much time did you spend alone and how much time with others?

 Record this information and your reflections in your **Reflective Journal**.

2. Activities Box for Co-occupation

a. List all of the co-occupations you have engaged in within the last week. Identify with whom you were interacting.
b. Identify or categorize the aspects (shared physicality, shared emotionality, shared intentionality) of the co-occupational experience.
c. Create a wheel identifying whether the co-occupational experiences were characterized more by shared physicality, shared emotionality, or shared intentionality.
d. Observe an individual diagnosed with a mental health condition during a co-occupation. Answer the reflective questions.

Reflective Questions

- How do occupation and co-occupation give meaning to life (occupation and co-occupation as ends)?
- How do we use occupation and co-occupation as a therapeutic medium (occupation and co-occupation as means)?

 Capture these thoughts in your **Reflective Journal**.

References

American Occupational Therapy Association (AOTA). (1995). Position paper: Occupation. *American Journal of Occupational Therapy, 49,* 1015–1018.

———. (2002). Occupational therapy practice framework: Domain and process. *American Journal of Occupational Therapy, 56,* 609–639.

———. (2008). Occupational therapy practice framework: Domain and process. 2nd ed. *American Journal of Occupational Therapy, 62,* 625–283.

American Psychiatric Association (APA). (2000). *Diagnostic and Statistical Manual of Mental Disorders* (4th ed., text revision). Arlington, VA: Author.

Aubin, G., Hackey, R., & Mercier, C. (1999). Meaning of daily activities and subjective quality of life in people with severe mental illness. *Scandinavian Journal of Occupational Therapy, 6,* 53–62.

Barnekow, K. A., & Kraemer, G. W. (2005). The psychobiological theory of attachment: A viable frame of reference for early intervention providers. *Physical and Occupational Therapy in Pediatrics, 25,* 3–15.

Bruner, J. (1995). From joint attention to meeting of minds: An introduction. In C. Moore & P. J. Dunham (Eds.), *Joint Attention: Its Origins and Role in Development.* Hillsdale, NJ: Erlbaum.

Canadian Association of Occupational Therapy (CAOT). (1994). Position statement on everyday occupations and health. *Canadian Journal of Occupational Therapy, 61,* 294–295.

———. (1997). *Enabling Occupation: An Occupational Therapy Perspective.* Ottawa: CAOT Publications ACE.

———. (2002). *Enabling Occupation: An Occupational Therapy Perspective* (rev. ed.). Ottawa: CAOT Publications ACE.

Christiansen, C., & Baum, C. (1997). Understanding occupation: Definitions and concepts. In C. Christiansen & C. Baum (Eds.), *Occupational Therapy: Enabling Function and Well-being* (pp. 3–25). Thorofare, NJ: Slack.

Clark, F., Azen, S., Zemke, R., Jackson, J., Carlson, M., Mandel, D., Hay, J., Josephson, K., Cherry, B., Hessel, C., Palmer, J., & Lipson, L. (1997). Occupational therapy for independent-living older adults: A randomized controlled trial. *Journal of the American Medical Association, 278,* 1321–1326.

Cottle, T. J., & Klineberg, S. L. (1974). *The Present of Things Future: Explorations of Time in Human Experience.* New York: The Free Press.

Csikszentmihalyi, M. (1990). *Flow: The Psychology of Optimal Experience.* New York: Harper Perennial.

DoRozario, L. (1998). From ageing to sageing: Eldering and the art of being as occupation. *Journal of Occupational Science, 5*(3), 119–126.

Dunlop, D. D., Manheim, L. M., Song, J., Lyons, J. S., & Chang, R. W. (2005). Incidence of disability among preretirement adults: The impact of depression. *American Journal of Public Health, 95,* 2003–2008.

Egan, M., & DeLaat, M. D. (1997). The implicit spirituality of occupational therapy practice. *Canadian Journal of Occupational Therapy, 64*(1), 115–121.

Farnworth, L. (2000). Time use and leisure occupations of young offenders. *American Journal of Occupational Therapy, 54,* 315–325.

Fidler, G. S., & Fidler, J. W. (1983). Doing and becoming: The occupational therapy experience. In G. Kielhofner (Ed.), *Health Through Occupation: Theory and Practice in Occupational Therapy* (pp. 267–280). Philadelphia: FA Davis.

Flaherty, M. G. (1993). Conceptualizing variation in the experience of time. *Sociological Inquiry, 63,* 394–405.

———. (1994). How time flies: Age, memory and temporal compression. *Sociological Quarterly, 35,* 705–721.

———. (1999). *A Watched Pot: How We Experience Time.* New York: New University Press.

Golledge, J. (1998). Distinguishing between occupation, purposeful activity, part 1: review and explanation. *British Journal of Occupational Therapy, 61,* 100–105.

Gray, J. M. (1998). Putting occupation into practice: Occupation as ends, occupation as means. *American Journal of Occupational Therapy, 52,* 354–364.

Hammel, K.W.. (2004). Dimensions of meaning in the occupations of daily life. *Canadian Journal of Occupational Therapy, 71,* 296–305.

Hasselkus, B. R. (1998). Occupation and well-being in dementia: The experience of day-care staff. *American Journal of Occupational Therapy, 52,* 423–434.

———. (2000). From the editor's desk: Reaching consensus. *American Journal of Occupational Therapy, 54,* 127–128.

———. (2002). *The Meaning of Everyday Occupation.* Thorofare, NJ: Slack.

Heinrichs, R. W., Goldberg, J. O., Miles, A. A., & McDermid, V. S. (2008). Predictors of medication compliance in schizophrenia patients. *Psychiatry Research, 15,* 47–52.

Kraemer, G. W. (1992). A psychobiological theory of attachment. *Behavioral and Brain Sciences, 15,* 493–541.

Laliberte-Rudman, D., Yu, B., Scott, E., & Pajouhandeh, P. (2000). Exploration of the perspectives of person with schizophrenia regarding quality of life. *American Journal of Occupational Therapy, 54,* 137–147.

Larson, E. A. (2004). The time of our lives: The experience of temporality in occupation. *Canadian Journal of Occupational Therapy, 71,* 24–35.

Law, M., Steinwender, S., & Leclair, L. (1998). Occupation, health and well-being. *Canadian Journal of Occupational Therapy, 65,* 81–91.

Lazzarini, I. (2004). Neuro-occupation: The non-linear dynamics of intention, meaning and perception. *British Journal of Occupational Therapy, 67,* 342–352.

Lloyd, C., King, R., & Moore, L. (in press). Subjective and objective indicators of recovery in mental illness: A cross-sectional study. *International Journal of Social Psychiatry.*

McColl, M.A. (2003). *Spirituality and Occupational Therapy.* Ottawa, ON: CAOT Publication.

Mechanic, D., Bilder, S., & McAlpine, D. D. (2002). Employing persons with serious mental illness. *Health Affairs, 21,* 242–253.

Meyer, A. (1922). The philosophy of occupational therapy. *Archives of Occupational Therapy, 1,* 1–10.

Minato, M., & Zemke, R. (2004). Time use of persons with schizophrenia living in the community. *Occupational Therapy International, 11,* 177–191.

Mocellin, G. (1995). Occupational therapy: A critical overview, part 1. *British Journal of Occupational Therapy, 58,* 502–506.

Nelson, D. L. (1996). Therapeutic occupation: A definition. *American Journal of Occupational Therapy, 50,* 775–782.

Nuechterlein, K. H., Subotnik, K. L., Turner, L. R., Bentura, J., Becker, D. R., & Drake, R. E. (2009). Individual placement and support for individuals with recent onset schizophrenia: Integrated supported education and supported employment. *Psychiatric Rehabilitation Journal, 31,* 340–349.

Olson, J. A. (2004). Mothering co-occupations in caring for infants and young children. In S. Esdaile & J. Olson (Eds.). *Mothering Occupations: Challenge, Agency, and Participation.* Philadelphia: FA Davis.

Passmore, A. (2003). The occupation of leisure: Three typologies and their influence on mental health in adolescence. *OTJR: Occupation, Participation and Health, 23,* 76–83.

Pierce, D. E. (2001). Untangling occupation and activity. *American Journal of Occupational Therapy, 55,* 138–146.

———. (2003). *Occupation by Design: Building Therapeutic Power.* Philadelphia, PA: FA Davis.

Preston, A. S., Heaton, S. C., McCann, S. J., Watson, W. D., & Selke, G. (2009). The role of multidimensional attentional abilities in academic skills in children with ADHD. *Journal of Learning Disabilities, 42,* 240–249.

Rebeiro, K. L., Day, D., Semeniuk, B., O'Brien, M., & Wilson, B. (2001). Northern initiative for social action: An occupation-based mental health program. *American Journal of Occupational Therapy, 55,* 493–500.

Rowles, G. D. (1991). Beyond performance: Being in place as a component of occupational therapy. *American Journal of Occupational Therapy, 45,* 265–271.

Russinova, Z., & Cash, D. (2007). Personal perspectives about the meaning of religion and spirituality among person with serious mental illness. *Psychiatric Rehabilitation Journal, 30,* 271–284.

Ryff, C. D., & Singer, B. (1996). Psychological well-being: Meaning, measurement, and implications for psychotherapy research. *Psychotherapy and Psychosomatics, 65,* 14–23.

Seamon, D. (2002). Physical comminglings: Body, habit, and space transformed into place. *Occupational Therapy Journal of Research, 22,* 42S–51S.

Simpson, J. A. (1999). Attachment theory in modern evolutionary perspective. In J. Cassidy & P. R. Shaver (Eds.), *Handbook of Attachment: Theory, Research and Clinical Applications* (pp. 115–140). New York: Guildford.

Stedman, T. L. (2005). *Stedman's Medical Dictionary.* Philadelphia: Lippincott, Williams & Wilkins.

Sylvia, L. G., Alloy, L. B., Hafner, J. A., Gauger, M. C., Verdon, K., & Abramson, L. Y. (2009). Life events and social rhythms in bipolar disorder: A prospective study. *Behavior Therapy, 40,* 131–141.

Taylor, B. A, Hoch, H., Potter, B., Rodriguez, A., & Kalaigian, M. (2005). Manipulating establishing operations to promote initiations toward peers with autism. *Research in Developmental Disabilities, 26,* 385–392.

Tomasello, M., & Carpenter, M. (2005). The emergence of social cognition in three young chimpanzees. *Monographs of the Society for Research in Child Development, 70* (1, Serial no. 279).

Tomasello, M., & Rakoczy, H. (2003). What makes human cognition unique? From individual to shared to collective intentionality. *Mind and Language, 18,* 121–147.

Townsend, E. (1993). The 1993 Muriel Driver Lecture: Occupational therapy's social vision. *Canadian Journal of Occupational Therapy, 60,* 174–184.

———. (1997). Occupation: Potential for personal and social transformation. *Journal of Occupational Science: Australia, 4,* 18–26.

————. (2003). Reflections on power and justice in enabling occupation. *Canadian Journal of Occupational Therapy, 70,* 74–87.

Townsend, E., DeLaat, D., Egan, M., Thibeault, R., & Wright, W. A. (1999). *Spirituality in Enabling Occupation: A Learner-Centered Workbook.* Ottawa: CAOT Publications ACE.

Townsend, E., & Wilcock, A. A. (2004). Occupational justice and client-centered practice: A dialogue in progress. *Canadian Journal of Occupational Therapy, 71,* 75–87.

Tuan, Y. (1977). *Space and Place: The Perspective of Experience.* Minneapolis: University of Minnesota Press.

Unruh, A. M., Versnel, J., & Kerr, N. (2002). Spirituality unplugged: A review of commonalities and contentions, and a resolution. *Canadian Journal of Occupational Therapy, 69,* 5–19.

Van Niekerk, L. (2009). Participation in work: A source of wellness for people with psychiatric disabilities. *Work, 32,* 455–465.

Ward, J. D. (2003). Adults with mental illness: Psychiatric diagnoses and related intervention issues. In E. B. Crepeau, E. S. Cohn, & B. A. B. Schell (Eds.), *Willard & Spackman's Occupational Therapy* (10th ed.) (pp. 835–860). Philadelphia: Lippincott Williams & Wilkins.

Warneken, F., Chen, F., & Tomasello, J. (2006). Cooperative activities in young children and chimpanzees. *Child Development, 77,* 640–663.

Warner, R. (2009). Recovery from schizophrenia and the recovery model. *Current Opinion in Psychiatry, 22,* 374–380.

Whiteford, G. E. (2001). The occupational agenda of the future. *Journal of Occupational Science, 8,* 13–16.

————. (2005). Understanding the occupational deprivation of refugees: A case study from Kosovo. *Canadian Journal of Occupational Therapy, 72,* 78–88.

Whiteford, G., Townsend, E., & Hocking, C. (2000). Reflections on a renaissance of occupation. *Canadian Journal of Occupational Therapy, 67,* 61–69.

Wilcock, A. A. (1993). A theory of the human need for occupation. *Occupational Science: Australia, 1,* 17–24.

————. (1998a). *An Occupational Perspective of Health.* Thorofare, NJ: Slack.

————. (1998b). Reflections on doing, being and becoming. *Canadian Journal of Occupational Therapy, 65,* 248–256.

————. (1999). The Doris Sym Memorial lecture: Developing a philosophy of occupation for health. *British Journal of Occupational Therapy, 62,* 192–198.

Wood, W. (1996). Legitimizing occupational therapy's knowledge. *American Journal of Occupational Therapy, 50,* 626–634.

————. (1997). An open letter to new (and not so new) practitioners: What's Robert Frost got to do with it? Flow, passion, and social justice in occupational therapy. *OT Practice, 2,* 42–45.

World Health Organization. (2006). WHO definition of health. Available at: http://www.who.int/about/en (accessed July 12, 2006).

Yerxa, E. J. (1998). Health and the human spirit for occupation. *American Journal of Occupational Therapy, 52,* 412–422.

Yerxa, E. J., Clark, F., Frank, G., Jackson, J., Parham, D., Pierce, D., Stein, C., & Zemke, R. (1990). An introduction to occupational science, a foundation for occupational therapy in the 21st. century. *Occupational Therapy in Health Care, 6,* 1–17.

Zemke, R., & Clark, F. (1996). Co-occupations of mothers and children. In R. Zemke & F. Clark (Eds.), *Occupational Science: The Evolving Discipline* (pp. 213–215). Philadelphia: FA Davis.

Occupation and Wellness

Mona Eklund

> "*Coming here has helped me a lot. The psychotherapy helped me too, but that was in theory. Occupational therapy gave me the practice; getting new habits, daring to do new things, learning what worked, and realizing that what I did was OK.*
>
> —*Karin, 25, after having participated in outpatient psychosocial occupational therapy*

Introduction

Does occupation promote wellness? This is one of the most important questions for occupational therapists, and during almost a century, scholars have argued that this is the case (Law, 2002; Law, Steinwender, & Leclair, 1998; Meyer, 1922/1977; Wilcock, 1998, 2005). It is only recently, however, that researchers have started to present evidence, and initial findings to indicate a relationship between occupation and health among those with a mental illness (Aubin, Hachey, & Mercier, 1999; Eklund, Hansson, & Ahlqvist, 2004; Eklund, Hansson, & Bejerholm, 2001; Goldberg, Britnell, & Goldberg, 2002). Also, recovery and empowerment-oriented frameworks argue that increased participation in meaningful occupations endorses health and wellbeing, mainly through the development of a personal and social identity (Krupa, McLean, Eastabrook, Bonham, & Baksh, 2003). Occupation is a multifaceted phenomenon (Eklund & Leufstadius, 2007) which complicates the discussion of how occupation is related to wellness. The example of a single man living in an apartment of his own illustrates this complexity: he gets up at 7.30 a.m., washes, dresses, and prepares and eats his breakfast. Then he takes the bus to the day-care center for people with mental illness, arrives at about 9.00 a.m., and goes to his workshop, which is a cafeteria. He takes care of the dishes and other cleaning. He works in the cafeteria, with a few breaks for coffee and lunch, until 2.00 p.m. He takes the bus home, and for the rest of the afternoon he watches television. At about 6.00 p.m. he goes to a nearby restaurant and eats dinner. There he sits for a while and just watches people. When he returns home, he again watches television until it is time for bed. A day like this can be described from several angles. We could time the occupations he performed and describe his day in terms of how he uses his time. We could assess his occupational performance according to how well he performed his tasks, both at home and at the day-care center cafeteria. We could also assess the flow of activities over the day, any occurrence of more active periods, and initiatives taken, in order to get a picture of his occupational engagement and general activity level. We could interview him and find out how he perceives the meaning, satisfaction, and value his occupations bring.

Heath and wellness are equally complex concepts. The definition of health stated by the World Health Organization (World Health Organization, 1946) indicates that the individual's own perception, in terms of wellbeing, is the main criterion. According to Medin and Alexandersson (2000), wellbeing may be regarded as a humanistic perspective on health. They proposed two main directions among health definitions, the humanistic and the biological. The humanistic recognizes subjective and sociocultural aspects of health. Ryff (1989) proposed that the humanistic direction of wellness is composed of six dimensions: autonomy, personal growth, environmental mastery, purpose in life, positive relations, and self-acceptance. The biological direction

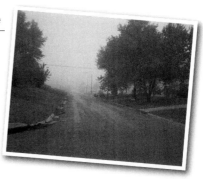

PhotoVoice

I get exercise as I walk around this block. The trees make me feel at peace. Walking gives me more strength. It makes me feel better about myself.

—Glen

considers an individual healthy when his or her body and mind work according to the scientifically identified norm (Medin & Alexandersson, 2000). The biological direction is enacted when a professional such as a doctor or nurse conducts a general physical examination and produces a history and physical document describing the overall health of the individual from the professional's perspective.

Occupation as Actual Doing

What people do in everyday contexts is related to perceptions of health and wellness. Some ways that actual performance of everyday occupations may be framed include time use, general activity level, and grouping into doers and nondoers. The type of daily occupation most investigated for its relationship to wellness is work in terms of open-market employment or sheltered work. Research indicates work is important for people with severe mental illness in alleviating symptoms, strengthening perceived abilities, and increasing a sense of belonging (Arns & Linney, 1993; Bell & Lysaker, 1997; Kennedy-Jones, Cooper, & Fossey, 2005), and those who work rate their quality of life, health, and wellbeing better than those who do not (Eklund et al, 2001). However, contradictory evidence exists. A study focusing on the importance of competitive work compared to other forms of daily occupation failed to demonstrate any differences in self-perceived health-related variables between groups representing different types of daily occupation (Eklund et al, 2004). Participants were described in terms of the following three groups: open-market work or schooling, participation at community-based activity centers, and no regular daily occupation. Although there were no self-perceived differences, the interviewer-rated aspects of health indicated better ratings in the group with open-market work or schooling.

Other occupational categories are less studied in people with mental illness with a few exceptions. Krupa et al (2003) showed that people with mental illness spend more time than a general population sample in passive leisure occupations. Another study found leisure occupations were highly valued for their contribution to meaning in life and considered important for health and wellbeing among people with mental illness (Craik & Pieris, 2006; Pieris & Craik, 2004). The number of studies in this area is limited, but those that exist indicate that leisure becomes even more important in the absence of work.

Time Use

Time use is an aspect of actual doing, and people with a severe mental illness like schizophrenia tend to spend most of their time sleeping, eating, caring for themselves, and performing quiet activities such as sitting or lying and watching other people or objects (Bejerholm & Eklund, 2004; Crist, Davis, & Coffin, 2000; Farnworth, 2003; Krupa et al, 2003; Shimitras, Fossey, & Harvey, 2003; Weeder, 1986). A study focusing on different perspectives of health, self-rated health and wellbeing as well as interviewer ratings of health and functioning found that time spent on work was related to both self-ratings and interviewer ratings of health with a stronger relationship in the interviewer ratings (Eklund & Leufstadius, 2007). The more time spent on work, the

better ratings of health, wellness, and functioning. Thus, work was related to both humanistic and biological aspects of health, as defined by Medin and Alexandersson (2000). Except for work, the only other area of occupation related to health was sleep, with more time spent on sleep related to poorer ratings (interview and self) of health. Similar results were shown in a related study (Leufstadius, Erlandsson, & Eklund, 2006).

Time use is the temporal aspect of occupational balance. People with psychiatric disabilities tend to have distorted and unbalanced temporal occupational patterns (Bejerholm & Eklund, 2004; Leufstadius et al, 2006). A study examining relationships between time use and daily rhythm on the one hand and different aspects of psychiatric symptoms, wellness, social interaction, and sociodemographic characteristics on the other (Leufstadius & Eklund, 2008; Leufstadius et al, 2006) found high time use in work/education was associated with better health, mastery, and quality of life, while a high amount of sleep was associated with lower levels of mastery and social interaction. Individuals belonging to a low-activity group had lower perceived social interaction and mastery than those belonging to two other daily rhythm groups, one characterized by balance and one by a high level of activity (Leufstadius et al, 2006). General psychiatric symptoms explained most of the risk of spending little time in work/education as well as the risk of spending long periods asleep and having an adverse daily rhythm (Leufstadius & Eklund, 2008).

The way people with a mental illness use their time is related to their health and wellbeing, indicating that knowing how people use their time is important when assessing their occupational performance and planning occupational therapy interventions. Time use can also be a variable in occupational therapy assessments and interventions.

Activity Level

A study that included activity level as one of the operationalizations of occupation showed a consistent relationship between general activity level and all measured aspects of an interviewer perspective on health, which included psychosocial functioning, psychiatric symptoms, and general mental health (Eklund & Leufstadius, 2007). No such relationship was found between activity level and self-ratings of health and wellbeing. In terms of the health definition of Medin and Alexandersson (2000), general activity level was related to a biological rather than humanistic view of health.

The previously mentioned studies showing that participation in work and leisure was of importance for wellness may also be regarded as reflecting activity level. Furthermore, the studies by Leufstadius et al (2006) and Leufstadius and Eklund (2008) included a time-use estimate of activity level, or total time in activity. Individuals with a diagnosis of psychosis spent less total time in daily activities than individuals with nonpsychosis. A diagnosis of psychosis and high levels of general symptoms together explained most of the risk of having low total time use in activity. This means that especially people with a severe mental illness are at risk of an inactive and temporally unbalanced daily occupational pattern and need the attention of occupational therapists.

The Lived Experience

Carl

Carl, 35 years old and with Asperger's syndrome, has written a narrative in which he tells about his daily occupations. The focus is not on the occupational therapy but on the daily life he leads after several years in outpatient occupational therapy. Following is part of his story:

Sometimes before breakfast you take a walk. Not too early, but at 8 or 9. It feels nice; you get a kick out of it, in a way. It comes in periods, but it's important to keep up routines and get up. It makes me feel good. I think a lot about weight and such things. You have to see that you have food and order at home. I'm rather picky about that, almost too pedantic at times. But that's something you have to do.

I have a few buddies, we do sports and things. I like to be with people, or talk to people. And do something. Try to find out something to do. That's rather important, I think. I'm quite interested in sports. I grew up with three older brothers, and we played a lot of hockey and tennis in the street. And I've been following a soccer team. Sometimes I think of a soccer match, or I watch TV. And I know some people who have dogs, and I use to take them for a walk. I feel my days go fine, so to say, and that makes me feel good.

Then you go and see your parents. My father has bad lungs so I help them a bit more now, grocery shopping and lifting heavy things. I also feel good about baby-sitting my nieces and nephews. I think it's fun to be with kids and I feel good about being able to help. It's a responsibility, but it's fun too.

Then I have a film interest. I go through what's on TV during the week. That's also something you grew up with, having brothers older than you and starting too early to watch movies for adults. I think it's great fun. Actually, I've always had a soft spot for theatre. I took a few classes on improvisation, and I applied for a theatre school, but the competition was very tough. But I think it's interesting. Acting is fun, and it's fun to follow how movies are built up. How the actors prepare and so on. So I think.

If you feel irritated with someone it's good to do something that diverts you from all that. Sometimes I actually play a game on my cell phone. I take those old games from past times, Game Watch. It's both relaxing and challenging. Music can also be diverting. Or you can play music as a background. Or it can make you more alert. Often when I go to see Katherine [his occupational therapist] I play music to become more wakeful.

What I miss is a job. I would want a job that I like to 100%! But it's difficult. There's always such a competition about everything. I wanted to become a sports journalist, but I've put that on the shelf. I guess I've accepted my situation as it is. I have a certain handicap. I can't change that, but of course I hope for something. They say it's never too late. I studied at the university for several years, but never finished my education. I want a job, job, job!

That's about what I use to do. Then, getting up on time: if you don't get up until 12:30 then the whole day is ruined, more or less. One or two days a week get lost like that. You have to find a way to get up. Then you get done with want you want to do. That's what it's all about, I think.

Occupation as a Subjective Experience

Subjective experiences of occupational performance have drawn a great deal of attention from occupational therapy researchers. The meaning of occupations was emphasized as therapeutic by Meyer in some of the first writings related to occupational therapy (1922/1977). Besides meaning, other subjective experiences include the satisfaction occupational performance may bring and the value attached to occupations. An occupation must be valued before an individual can attribute meaning to that occupation (Persson, Erlandsson, Eklund, & Iwarsson, 2001); therefore, the two are discussed together here.

Satisfaction

Satisfaction with daily occupations has also been measured in relation to health among people with mental illness (Eklund et al, 2001; Eklund et al, 2004). When modeling quality of life, Eklund and Bäckström (2005) found that satisfaction with occupations was second only to positive aspects of the self when determining quality of life. Activity level was another important contributor to the quality-of-life model. Other studies indicate estimates of health and wellness are related to satisfaction with daily occupations, (Eklund et al,

2001, Eklund et al, 2004). Satisfaction with daily occupations is a clear indicator of health and wellbeing, and especially quality of life, in people with mental illness.

Meaning and Value

Researchers and theorists in occupational therapy agree that meaning is an important prerequisite for an occupation to be health promoting (Canadian Association of Occupational Therapists, 2002; Crabtree, 1998; Fisher, 1998; Hammell, 2004; Ivarsson, Söderback, & Ternestedt, 2002; Kielhofner, 2002; Meyer, 1922/1977; Nelson, 1997; Strong, 1998). Bruner (1990) proposed that meaning making has a central place in human action and that meaning is organized in a narrative form (Clark, 1993; Clark, Carlsson, & Polkinghorne, 1997; Helfrich & Kielhofner, 1994; Kirsh, 1996; Mallinson, Kielhofner, & Mattingly, 1996). Other theorists who have emphasized meaning in a way that is compatible with occupational therapy are Antonovsky (1987) and Korotkov (1998), declaring that meaningful occupation fosters the ability to make sense out of chaos. In other words, finding everyday life tasks meaningful, comprehensible, and manageable is the core mechanism that shapes a sense of coherence, which in turn impacts favorably on health and wellbeing.

Goldberg et al (2002), Aubin et al (1999), and Strong (1998) found that the meaning people with mental illness perceive when they occupy themselves is of importance for their health. Goldberg et al (2002) found a relationship between engagement in meaningful occupations and satisfaction with life as a whole. On the other hand, depression accounted for more variance in quality of life than meaningful occupation did. Aubin et al (1999) explored how different operationalizations of the meaning of daily activities were associated with subjective quality of life of adults with serious mental illness. The meaning of activities was defined by three elements: perceived competence, value, and pleasure. They found that perceived competence in daily tasks and rest and pleasure in work and rest activities were positively correlated with subjective quality of life. Findings from Strong (1998) suggested that participation in meaningful occupations could lead to changes in clients' sense of self-efficacy and self-concept. Strong concluded that by helping clients make connections with meaningful occupations and to experience challenges and successes in the context of meaningful work, occupational therapists could facilitate improvements in self-efficacy and self-concept.

Persson et al (2001) presented the values and meaning in occupations model (ValMO) suggesting that in order to generate meaning, an occupation must possess some kind of value. The model distinguishes three types of occupational values: concrete value, symbolic value, and self-reward value. **Concrete value** is about the concrete and visible features of value inherent in occupations. When an occupation attributed with concrete value is performed and finished, the outcome may be a product that brings satisfaction to the doer, such as a meal prepared for the family, improved or newly acquired capacities and skills like learning to drive, or the avoidance of negative consequences. **Symbolic value** is characterized by what an occupation signifies for a person, for example, strengthening his or her gender identity or the bonds to a certain group or culture. **Self-reward value** focuses on immediate rewards that are inherent in the experience of performing a certain occupation. In a self-reward occupation, the person chooses to perform an occupation because he or she simply enjoys doing it. Along with the enjoyment comes an experience of forgetting oneself and time, and a state of flow may occur. A study of how occupational value was linked to health and wellness among people with mental illness found significant associations to all aspects measured (Eklund, Erlandsson, & Persson, 2003), reflecting humanistic as well as biological views of health (Medin & Alexandersson, 2000). Subsequent studies have supported this finding by showing that occupational value is an important factor for other aspects of human life, such as social interaction (Eklund, 2006) and perceived control (Eklund, 2007).

Whereas value can be described in relation to single occupations, meaning is linked to an individual's life story (Persson et al, 2001). For example, when a Swedish woman is cooking meatballs, a very common and traditional dish in Sweden, it brings some value for her in terms of a tasty dish (concrete value), it strengthens her sense of belonging (symbolic value), or it is a fun thing to do (self-reward value). The meaning it brings depends on the role this occupation has play in her life thus far. The meaning is activated by all the times she cooked, served, ate, or tasted this type of meal and all the social and environmental contexts in which this occurred. Thus, the meaning is complex and mostly individual, while the value may be more easily shared by others. This may be one reason

the link between occupational meaning and wellness is less conclusive than those found between satisfaction with daily occupations and occupational value and wellness.

Being and Doing, or Doing and Being?

The psychoanalyst and object relations theorist Winnicott (1971) proposed. that from a developmental perspective, **being** is something that precedes **doing.** "Going-on-being," a quiescent state of being, is vital for an individual to form an identity, and without the feeling of being someone, doing becomes mechanical and meaningless. If a child is deprived of a sense of being, his or her identity and true self will not grow forth. The same is true of adult individuals in crises, including people with mental illness. It is only when a sense of being someone is present that doing can be the foundation for development and health promotion. With their focus on occupation, occupational therapists may focus on doing and neglect the being. The state of being should be considered and incorporated in the clinical reasoning process of occupational therapists; otherwise there is a risk of providing nontherapeutic interventions (Eklund, 2000).

Rowles (1991) emphasized the importance of "being-in-place," understood as people's perceptions of being in a culturally defined spatiotemporal setting that forms the horizon of their everyday lives. For example, the place where an individual feels "at home" often has an influence on his or her sense of identity. Rowles also suggested that this perception could become a component of the self, and in that respect, being-in-place resembles being, as termed by Winnicott (1971). Rowles (1991) and Eklund (2000) proposed a state of being as something that occupational therapists should consider simultaneously with, or even before, doing. Otherwise, occupational therapists tend to emphasize doing as a prerequisite for the feeling of being someone. This is in line with another early object relations theorist, Sullivan (1947), who said that a person is what he does. Among the psychiatrists who largely influenced the young Sullivan during the 1920s was Meyer, one of the founders of occupational therapy.

More recently, occupational therapists have refined the discussion about doing and being. Wilcock (1998) added the term *becoming,* putting emphasis on the developmental potentials lying in the process of doing, being, and becoming and the envisioning of a future self. Gewurtz and Kirsh (2007) corroborated the relevance of doing and becoming when investigating how consumers of mental health services gained insight into their capacity for work. Through doing work, the consumers came to understand their capacity for future work participation and becoming persons with possible work futures. Moreover, Hammell (2004), drawing on Rebeiro, Day, Semeniuk, O'Brien, and Wilson (2001), incorporated the term *belonging,* acknowledging the necessary contribution of social interaction and the sense of being included. Hammell's focus was on how meaning is shaped, and she suggested that it occurs through the dimensions of doing, being, belonging, and becoming.

It is interesting to note that there is an almost century-long concern regarding how being and doing are related, and although the theorists are not unanimous regarding which aspect affects the other, there is agreement that they play an important part in the relationship between occupation and wellness. When it comes to people with mental illness, their sense of identity and of being someone is frequently weakened (Jackson, Tudway, Giles, & Smith, 2009; Van Den Tillart, Kurtz, & Cash, 2009). Therefore, doing must not be focused on in isolation, but the patient's sense of being and belonging should be carefully addressed.

Assessments

The assessments presented in this section provide an overview of an individual's occupational engagement. They are not evaluations of competence but instead focus on patterns, satisfaction, and meaning of occupation.

Time-Use Diary

A yesterday time-use diary asks the person to record what he or she did during the previous 24 hours, complemented with an interview to fill any gaps and sort out any unclear information (Bejerholm & Eklund, 2004). The diary has five columns: time, what I was doing, location, social context, and optional (Figure 46-1). The content of the optional column can be negotiated between the therapist and client. After the time use of a client is mapped, desired changes in time use can be set as treatment goals. The treatment goals may be translated into practical tasks, such as increasing the time spent outside home or diminishing the time spent asleep.

Satisfaction With Daily Occupations

The *Satisfaction with Daily Occupations (SDO)* assessment renders two subscales: activity and satisfaction. The SDO was found to have good psychometric properties (Eklund, 2004; Eklund & Gunnarsson, 2007). This nine-item measure is divided into the areas of work, leisure, domestic tasks, and self-care. Each item is rated in terms of whether or not the person has recently engaged and the occupation (activity) and satisfaction. Satisfaction is rated on a 7-point scale from worst to best possible.

Engagement in Meaningful Activities Survey

Goldberg et al (2002) developed the *Engagement in Meaningful Activities Survey (EMAS)*. Initially, an interview with open-ended questions identifies those activities that are meaningful to the individual, then the individual selects the three most important activities. The survey measures

Time	What I was doing	Geographical location	Social context	Comments (Optional)

Time Use Diary

FIGURE 46-1. Sample time-use diary format.

12 facets of the meaningfulness of activities using a 5-point Likert scale from never to always. Sample items include "the activities I do give me pleasure" and "the activities I do express my creativity." The test–retest reliability was somewhat low for the measure, but the internal consistency was good.

Interventions

This chapter has focused broadly on the relationship of occupational engagement and health. However, there are specific health concerns that are common among people with psychiatric disabilities. According to the Surgeon General's Report on Mental Health (U.S. Department of Health and Human Services, 1999), mental illness ranks second in burden of disease and receives inadequate attention from health-care providers. Health-care providers are often involved in providing services to support healthy lifestyle practices among the general population. Unfortunately, provision of similar services for people with serious mental illness is less common, although the needs for this population are greater and more complex. According to one study, individuals with serious mental illness have a life expectancy that is 25 years shorter than that of the U.S. population, and the major cause of death is cardiovascular disease and not suicide (Colton & Manderscheid, 2006). One contributing cause to this alarming statistic is the increased prevalence of obesity among people with severe mental illness (Allison & Casey, 2001) with a fourfold risk factor for metabolic syndrome (Saari et al, 2005), which is associated with high rates of diabetes. High rates of smoking present another health risk. It is estimated that rates of cigarette smoking among people with schizophrenia are at least two times and possibly more than three times greater than rates among the general population (deLeon & Diaz, 2005). The recovery model has helped shepherd the movement toward interventions directed at promoting health and wellness with an appreciation for the link between psychiatric and physical illness. This section of the chapter discusses interventions that target health and wellness for people with serious mental illness.

Wellness Recovery Action Plans

Mary Ellen Copeland (2000, 2001) developed an individualized system for the development of a wellness plan. The Wellness Recovery Action Plan (WRAP) emerged from a workshop attended by people with mental illness who identified specific wellness tools they used to help manage their symptoms and live a healthier life.

Individuals create a three-ring binder divided into five sections: (1) daily maintenance list, (2) triggers, (3) early warning signs, (4) when things are breaking down, and (5) crisis plan. For each section, the individual developing the WRAP identifies specific indicators and/or behaviors that are relevant to that particular section. For example, in the first section, the person makes a list of words that describe what it is like when he or she is feeling well. Next, a list is made of things the person should do every day to maintain wellness, such as eating a healthy breakfast, spending time outdoors, talking to a friend, and/or journaling. Most importantly, the WRAP is specific and unique to the individual who makes it.

Although WRAP training is commonly used in mental health settings and is compatible with occupational therapy intervention approaches, there is limited research investigating its efficacy. One study examining a WRAP workshop found that it changed consumer and mental health professionals' attitudes and knowledge about recovery (Doughty, Tse, Duncan, & McIntyre, 2008). Another study found very promising results indicating that the WRAP was effective in improving psychiatric symptoms, physical health, and recovery parameters such as hopefulness and empowerment (Cook et al, 2009).

Illness Management and Recovery

Illness Management and Recovery (IMR) is a self-management program that incorporates several approaches including psychoeducation, cognitive behavioral, relapse prevention, and social skills and coping skills training to teach people with severe mental illness how to better manage their health and wellness (Mueser et al, 2006). IMR is a comprehensive and structured program covering 10 topics (recovery strategies,

---

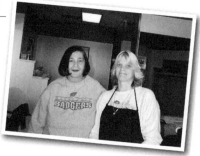

PhotoVoice

This is a picture of me standing with my beautician. I had just had my hair done that day. I really enjoy having my brunette hair done every week. This is significant to me because the money I save from stopping cigarette smoking is the money I now have to pay for getting my hair done. It was hard to quit! I did it "cold turkey," and it's been more than three years.

Evidence-Based Practice

A study of the WRAP program found positive outcomes for a wide range of variables, including symptoms, recovery, hopefulness, self advocacy, physical health, and empowerment (Cook et al, 2009).

➤ Occupational therapists can implement WRAP programming as either a separate intervention or incorporated with other programming.

➤ Individual plans developed using the WRAP model can either focus on general health and lifestyle issues or be directed toward a particular health and wellness concern (e.g., smoking cessation, weight loss).

Cook, J. A., Copeland, M. E., Hamilton, M. M., Jonikas, J. A., Razzano, L. A., Floyd, C. B., Hudson, W. B., MacFarlane, R. T., & Grey, D. D. (2009). Initial outcomes of a mental illness self-management program based on Wellness Recovery Action Plans. *Psychiatric Services, 60,* 246–249.

facts about schizophrenia, stress vulnerability model, social support, using medications effectively, reducing relapses, drug and alcohol use, coping with stress, coping with problems and symptoms, and getting your needs met in the mental health system). Occupational therapists can utilize the existing resources to implement IMR programs in their setting.

IMR is taught in weekly individual or group sessions and requires approximately 9 months to complete the full program. Each session includes time for socialization, individual goal setting and review, teaching new material and practice, and assigning homework. Easy access to the materials has supported the adoption of this model, and several studies are currently underway examining its efficacy. Initial studies indicate the program is well received by participants and that it results in increased knowledge and self-reported improvements in coping (Mueser et al, 2006).

Smoking Cessation

Although tobacco use rates are extremely high in people with serious mental illness, few health professionals provide smoking cessation treatment to this population (Montoya, Herbeck, Svikis, & Pincus, 2005). Nevertheless, the few intervention studies that do exist suggest that people with serious mental illness can benefit from smoking cessation programs. In two separate studies, a statistically significant number of participants remained abstinent, with one group's cessation rates equal to those of individuals without a psychiatric illness in a similar program (Addington, el Guebaly, Campbell, Hodgins & Addington, 1998; George et al, 2000).

The University of Medicine and Dentistry of New Jersey has implemented a fairly large-scale tobacco dependence program for people with mental illness (Foulds et al, 2006). These specialized services do not require that individuals set a quit date, and the duration and frequency of services are open ended. Participants receive both pharmacotherapy and counseling. Results from the program indicate smokers receiving these specialty services have abstinence rates equal to those without a history of mental illness. Figure 46-2 shows a collage created in an occupational therapy group.

Weight Loss

The high rates of obesity in people with serious mental illness has recently raised significant concerns regarding its affect on overall health, mortality, and quality of life (Allison et al, 2009). As a result, lifestyle-modification programs have been developed to specifically target the needs of people with mental illness. A review found that most programs focus on modification of food intake; fewer programs address physical activity (Faulkner, Cohn, & Remington, 2007). Results from these programs indicate modest weight loss is possible for people with serious mental illness.

An occupational therapist working with an interdisciplinary team including a nurse, dietician, and exercise physiologist developed a weight-loss program targeting lifestyle in both nutrition and physical activity (Brown, Goetz, Van Sciver, & Sullivan, 2006). Recovering Energy through Nutrition and Exercise for Weight Loss (RENEW) combines psychiatric rehabilitation principles with evidence-based weight-loss strategies. The year-long program is divided into three phases: intensive, maintenance, and intermittent supports. During the 12-week intensive phase, the group meets weekly for 3 hours, and the focus is on education and the implementation of individualized lifestyle changes at home (e.g., increasing fruit and vegetable intake, decreasing sodas, starting a walking routine). During the 12-week maintenance phase, the meetings are reduced to monthly, but all participants are matched with an intervention leader who serves as a phone buddy and provides weekly phone calls to monitor progress, problem-solve barriers, and provide support. Participants also receive a weekly newsletter. During the final 6-month intermittent support phase, there are no face-to-face meetings, but participants continue to receive weekly phone calls and newsletters. An initial study of the intensive phase found that participants lost an average of approximately 5 pounds. Currently, a randomized controlled trial is underway to examine the effects of RENEW. Figure 46-3 shows a participant in the RENEW weight-loss program who started exercising on a regular basis and lost 12 pounds during the intensive phase of the program.

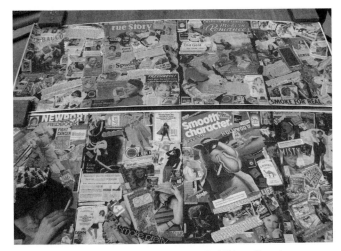

FIGURE 46-2. Jerry, a consumer, created this collage in an occupational therapy group to illustrate the allure of cigarette advertising and the challenges of nicotine addiction for people with mental illness.

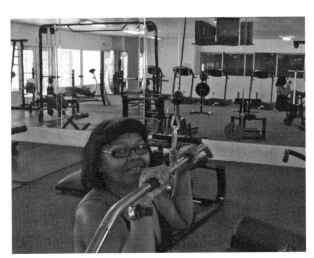

FIGURE 46-3. Claudia, a participant in the RENEW weight-loss program, started exercising on a regular basis and lost 12 pounds during the intensive phase of the program.

Summary

The recovery model speaks to the importance of health and wellness as a key component to successful mental health recovery. Emerging evidence shows that occupational engagement is important for the maintenance of health in people with mental illness. Furthermore, occupational therapists can play a role in addressing major health concerns such as obesity and smoking in this population.

Active Learning Strategies

1. Time-Use Diary

Construct a time-use diary with five columns (see Figure 46-1), and ask a friend or relative to fill in what he or she did during the previous 24 hours. The first column should be a time schedule, the next should leave room for what the person did, the third is for where he or she was, the fourth is for with whom he or she was, and the fifth is optional. You decide what kind of information should be added in the fifth column, but it should be about the personal aspect of occupational performance in terms of the person-environment-occupation model (Law et al, 1996). It could be feelings, perceived meaning, reflections, or any other aspect you would like to add to the diary. Make the diary long enough so that 24 hours can fit in, but fixed intervals are not necessary.

When you get the completed diary back, review and reflect.

Reflective Questions

- Are there any obvious gaps in the information?
- Do you suspect the person who filled in the diary forgot minor doings?
- Do you think he or she left out things of a private character?

Discuss together the pros and cons of a time-use diary, in clinical occupational therapy and in research, and what can be done to make the data collection as trustworthy as possible.

2. The Lived Experience

Reread Carl's narrative and reflect on it.

Reflective Questions

- What types of occupational value and meaning can be traced in Carl's narrative?
- Do they seem to be important for his wellness?

Resources

Assessments

- Engagement in Meaningful Activities Survey: Goldberg, B., Britnell, E. S., & Goldberg, J. (2002). The relationship between engagement in meaningful activities and quality of life in persons disabled by mental illness. *Occupational Therapy in Mental Health, 19*(2), 17–44.
- Satisfaction with Daily Occupations Instrument: Eklund, M. (2004). Satisfaction with daily occupations: A tool for client evaluation in mental health care. *Scandinavian Journal of Occupational Therapy, 11*, 136–142.

Interventions

- Illness Management and Recovery: The Substance Abuse and Mental Health Services Administration (SAMHSA) provides all the materials necessary to implement the program: http://www .mentalhealth.samhsa.gov/cmhs/communitysupport/toolkits
- Wellness Recovery Action Plan: Copeland, M. E. (2000). *Wellness Recovery Action Plan.* West Dummerston, VT: Peach Press. Also see http://www.mentalhealthrecovery.com

References

Addington, J., el Guebaly, N., Campbell, W., Hodgins, D. C. & Addington, D. (1998). Smoking cessation treatment for patients with schizophrenia. *American Journal of Psychiatry, 155*, 974–975.

Allison, D. B., & Casey, D. E. (2001). Antipsychotic-induced weight gain: A review of the literature. *Journal of Clinical Psychiatry, 62*(suppl 7), 22–31.

Allison, D. B., Newcomer, J. W., Dunn, A. L., Blumenthal, J. A., Fabricatore, A. N., Daumit, G. L., Cope, M. B., Riley, W. T., Vreeland, B., Hibbein, J. R., & Alpert, J. E. (2009). Obesity among those with mental disorders: A National Institute of Mental Health report. *American Journal of Preventive Medicine, 36*, 341–350.

Antonovsky, A. (1987). *Unraveling the Mystery of Health.* San Francisco: Jossey-Bass.

Arns, P. G., Linney, J. A. (1993). Work, self, and life satisfaction for persons with severe and persistent mental disorders. *Psychosocial Rehabilitation Journal, 17*, 63–79.

Aubin, G., Hachey, R., & Mercier, C. (1999). Meaning of daily activities and subjective quality of life in people with severe mental illness. *Scandinavian Journal of Occupational Therapy, 6*, 53–62.

Bejerholm, U., & Eklund, M. (2004). Time-use and occupational performance among persons with schizophrenia. *Occupational Therapy in Mental Health, 20*(1), 27–47.

Bell, M. D., & Lysaker, P. H. (1997). Clinical benefits of paid work in schizophrenia: 1-year follow-up. *Schizophrenia Bulletin, 23*, 317–328.

Brown, C., Goetz, J., Van Sciver, A., & Sullivan, D. (2006). A psychiatric rehabilitation approach to weight loss. *Psychiatric Rehabilitation Journal, 29*, 267–273.

Bruner, J. (1990). *Acts of Meaning.* London: Harvard University Press.

Canadian Association of Occupational Therapists. (2002). *Enabling Occupation: An Occupational Therapy Perspective.* Ottawa: CAOT Publications.

Clark, F. (1993). Occupation embedded in real life: Interweaving occupational science and occupational therapy. *American Journal of Occupational Therapy, 47*, 1067–1078.

Clark, F., Carlson, M., & Polkinghorne, D. (1997). The legitimacy of life history and narrative approaches in the study of occupation. *American Journal of Occupational Therapy, 51*, 313–317.

Colton, C. W., & Manderscheid, R. W. (2006). Congruencies in increased mortality rates, years of potential life lost, and causes of death among public mental health clients in eight states. *Preventing Chronic Diseases, 3*(2), 1–14.

Cook, J. A., Copeland, M. E., Hamilton, M. M., Jonikas, J. A., Razzano, L. A., Floyd, C. B., Hudson, W. B., MacFarlane, R. T., & Grey, D. D. (2009). Initial outcomes of a mental illness self-management program based on Wellness Recovery Action Plans. *Psychiatric Services, 60,* 246–249.

Copeland, M. E. (2000). *Wellness Recovery Action Plan.* West Dummerston, VT: Peach Press.

———. (2001). Wellness recovery action plan: A system for monitoring, reducing and eliminating uncomfortable or dangerous physical symptoms and emotional feelings. In C. Brown (Ed.), *Recovery and Wellness: Models of Hope and Empowerment for People with Mental Illness* (pp. 127–150). New York: Haworth Press.

Crabtree, J. L. (1998). The end of occupational therapy. *American Journal of Occupational Therapy, 52,* 205–214.

Craik, C., & Pieris, Y. (2006). Without leisure . . . "it wouldn't be much of a life": The meaning of leisure for people with mental health problems. *British Journal of Occupational Therapy, 69,* 209–216.

Crist, P. H., Davis, C. G., & Coffin, P. S. (2000). The effects of employment and mental health status on the balance of work, play/leisure, self-care, and rest. *Occupational Therapy in Mental Health 15*(1), 27–42.

deLeon, J., & Diaz, F. J. (2005). A meta-analysis of world-wide studies demonstrate and association between schizophrenia and tobacco smoking behavior. *Schizophrenia Research, 76,* 135–157.

Doughty, C., Tse, S., Duncan, N., & McIntyre, L. (2008). The Wellness Recovery Action Plan (WRAP): Workshop evaluation. *Australian Psychiatry, 16,* 450–456.

Eklund, M. (2000). Applying object relations theory to psychosocial occupational therapy: Empirical and theoretical considerations. *Occupational Therapy in Mental Health, 15*(1), 1–26.

———. (2004). Satisfaction with Daily Occupations: A tool for client evaluation in mental health care. *Scandinavian Journal of Occupational Therapy, 11,* 136–142.

———. (2006). Occupational factors and characteristics of the social network in people with persistent mental illness. *American Journal of Occupational Therapy, 60,* 587–594.

———. (2007). Perceived control: How is it related to daily occupation in patients with mental illness living in the community? *American Journal of Occupational Therapy, 61,* 535–542.

Eklund, M., & Bäckström, M. (2005). A model of subjective quality of life for outpatients with schizophrenia and other psychoses. *Quality of Life Research, 14,* 1157–1168.

Eklund, M., Erlandsson, L.-K., & Persson, D. (2003). Occupational value among individuals with long-term mental illness. *Canadian Journal of Occupational Therapy, 70,* 276–284.

Eklund, M., & Gunnarsson, A. B. (2007). Satisfaction with Daily Occupations (SDO): Construct validity and test-retest reliability of a screening tool for people with mental disorders. *Australian Occupational Therapy Journal, 54,* 59–65.

Eklund, M., Hansson, L., & Ahlqvist, C. (2004). The importance of work as compared to other forms of daily occupations for well-being and functioning among persons with long-term mental illness. *Community Mental Health Journal, 40,* 465–477.

Eklund, M., Hansson, L., & Bejerholm, U. (2001). Relationships between satisfaction with occupational factors and health-related variables in schizophrenia outpatients. *Social Psychiatry and Psychiatric Epidemiology, 36,* 79–85.

Eklund, M., & Leufstadius, C. (2007). Occupational factors and aspects of health and wellbeing in individuals with persistent mental illness living in the community. *Canadian Journal of Occupational Therapy, 74,* 303–313.

Farnworth, L. (2003). Time-use, tempo and temporality: Occupational therapy's core business or someone else's business. *Australian Occupational Therapy Journal, 50,* 16–26.

Faulkner G, Cohn T, & Remington G. (2007). Interventions to reduce weight gain in schizophrenia. *Schizophrenia Bulletin, 2007, 33*(3), 654–656.

Fisher, A. G. (1998). Uniting practice and theory in an occupational framework: 1998 Eleanor Clark Slagle Lecture. *American Journal of Occupational Therapy, 52,* 509–522.

Foulds, J. G. K., Steinberg, M. B., Richardson, D., Williams, J. M., Burke, M., & Rhoads, G. G. (2006). Factors associated with quitting smoking at a tobacco dependence treatment clinic. *American Journal of Health Behavior, 30,* 400–412.

George, T. P., Ziedonis, D. M., Feingold, A., Pepper, W. T., Satterburg, C. A., Winkel, J., Rounsaville, B. J., & Koston, R. R. (2000). Nicotine transdermal patch and atypical antipsychotic medication for smoking cessation in schizophrenia. *American Journal of Psychiatry, 157,* 1835–1842.

Gewurtz, R., & Kirsh, B. (2007). How consumers of mental health services come to understand their potential for work: doing and becoming revisited. *Canadian Journal of Occupational Therapy, 74,* 195–207.

Goldberg, B., Britnell, E. S., & Goldberg, J. (2002). The relationship between engagement in meaningful activities and quality of life in persons disabled by mental illness. *Occupational Therapy in Mental Health, 19*(2), 17–44.

Hammell, K. W. (2004). Dimensions of meaning in the occupations of daily life. *Canadian Journal of Occupational Therapy, 5,* 296–305.

Helfrich, C., & Kielhofner, G. (1994). Volitional narratives and the meaning of therapy. *American Journal of Occupational Therapy, 48,* 319–326.

Ivarsson, A.-B., Söderback, I., & Ternestedt, B. M. (2002). The meaning and form of occupational therapy as experienced by women with psychoses. *Scandinavian Journal of Caring Sciences, 16,* 103–110.

Jackson, L., Tudway, J. A., Giles, D., & Smith, J. (2009). An exploration of the social identity of mental health inpatient service users. *Journal of Psychiatric Mental Health Nursing, 16,* 167–176.

Kennedy-Jones, M., Cooper, J., & Fossey, E. (2005). Developing a worker role: Stories of four people with mental illness. *Australian Occupational Therapy Journal, 54,* 116–126.

Kielhofner, G. (Ed.). (2002). *A Model of Human Occupation. Theory and Application* (3rd ed.). Philadelphia: Lippincott Williams & Wilkins.

Kirsh, B. (1996). A narrative approach to addressing spirituality in occupational therapy: Exploring personal meaning and purpose. *Canadian Journal of Occupational Therapy, 63,* 55–61.

Korotkov, D. (1998). The sense of coherence: Making sense out of chaos. In P. T. P. Wong & P. S. Fry (Eds.), *The Human Quest of Meaning. A Handbook of Psychological Research and Clinical Applications* (pp. 51–70). London: Erlbaum.

Krupa, T., McLean, H., Eastabrook, S., Bonham, A., & Baksh, L. (2003). Daily time use as a measure of community adjustment for persons served by assertive community treatments teams. *American Journal of Occupational Therapy, 57,* 558–565.

Law, M. (2002). Participation in the occupations of everyday life. *American Journal of Occupational Therapy, 56,* 640–649.

Law, M., Cooper, B. A., Strong, S., Stewart, D., Rigby, P., & Letts, L. (1996). The person-environment-occupation model: A transactive approach to occupational performance. *Canadian Journal of Occupational Therapy, 63,* 9–23.

Law, M., Steinwender, S., & Leclair, L. (1998). Occupation, health and wellbeing. *Canadian Journal of Occupational Therapy, 65,* 81–91.

Leufstadius, C., & Eklund, M. (2008). Time use among individuals with persistent mental illness: Identifying risk factors for imbalance in daily activities. *Scandinavian Journal of Occupational Therapy, 15,* 23–33.

Leufstadius, C., Erlandsson, L.-K., & Eklund, M. (2006). Time use and daily rhythm in people with persistent mental illness. Relationships to health-related variables and social interaction. *Occupational Therapy International, 13,* 123–141.

Mallinson, T., Kielhofner, G., & Mattingly, C. (1996). Metaphor and meaning in a clinical interview. *American Journal of Occupational Therapy, 50,* 338–346.

Medin, J., & Alexandersson, K. (2000). *Begreppen hälsa och hälsofrämjande: en litteraturstudie* [The concepts of health and health promotion: A literature review]. Lund, Sweden: Studentlitteratur.

Meyer, A. (1922/1977). The philosophy of occupation therapy. Reprinted from *Archives of Occupational Therapy, 1*(1), 1–10, 1922. *American Journal of Occupational Therapy, 31,* 639–642.

Montoya, I. D., Herbeck, D. M., Svikis, D. S., & Pincus, H. A. (2005). Identification and treatment of patients with nicotine problems in routine clinical psychiatry practice. *American Journal of Addictions, 14,* 441–454.

Mueser, K. T., Meyer, P. S., Penn, D. L., Clancy, R., Clancy, D. M., & Salyers, M. P. (2006). The Illness Management and Recovery program: Rationale, development and preliminary findings. *Schizophrenia Bulletin, 32*(S1), S32–S43.

Nelson, D. (1997). Why the profession of occupational therapy will flourish in the 21st century: 1997 Eleanor Clark Slagle Lecture. *American Journal of Occupational Therapy, 51,* 11–24.

Peiris, Y., & Craik, C. (2004). Factors enabling and hindering participation in leisure for people with mental health problems. *British Journal of Occupational Therapy, 67,* 240–247.

Persson, D., Erlandsson, L.-K, Eklund, M., & Iwarsson, S. (2001). Value dimensions, meaning, and complexity in human occupation: A tentative structure for analysis. *Scandinavian Journal of Occupational Therapy, 8,* 7–18.

Rebeiro, K. L., Day, D., Semeniuk, B., O'Brien, M., & Wilson, B. (2001). Northern initiative for social action: An occupation-based mental health program. *American Journal of Occupational Therapy, 55,* 493–500.

Rowles, G. D. (1991). Beyond performance: Being in place as a component of occupational therapy. *American Journal of Occupational Therapy, 45,* 265–271.

Ryff, C. D. (1989). Happiness is everything, or is it? Explorations on the meaning of psychological well-being. *Journal of Personality and Social Psychology, 6,* 1069–1081.

Saari, K. M., Lindeman, S. M., Viilo, K. M., Isohanni, M. K., Jarvelin, M. R., Lauren, L. H., Savolainen, M. J., & Koponen, H. J. (2005). A 4-fold risk of metabolic syndrome in patients with schizophrenia: The Northern Finland 1966 Birth Cohort study. *Journal of Clinical Psychiatry, 66,* 559–563.

Shimitras, L., Fossey, E., & Harvey, C. (2003). Time use of people living with schizophrenia in a north London catchment area. *British Journal of Occupational Therapy, 66,* 46–54.

Strong, S. (1998). Meaningful work in supportive environments: Experiences with the recovery process. *American Journal of Occupational Therapy, 52,* 31–38.

Sullivan, H. S. (1947). *Conceptions of Modern Psychiatry.* New York: Norton.

U.S. Department of Health and Human Services. (1999). *Mental Health: A Report of the Surgeon General.* Rockville, MD: U.S. Department of Health and Human Services, Substance Abuse and Mental Health Services Administration, Center for Mental Health Services, National Institutes of Health, National Institute of Mental Health.

Van Den Tillart, S., Kurtz, M., & Cash, P. (2009). Powerlessness, marginalized identity, and silencing of health concerns: Voiced realities of women living with a mental health diagnosis. *International Journal of Mental Health Nursing, 18,* 153–163.

Weeder, T. C. (1986). Comparison of temporal patterns and meaningfulness of the daily activities of schizophrenic and normal adults. *Occupational Therapy in Mental Health, 6*(4), 27–48.

Wilcock, A. A. (1998). *An Occupational Perspective of Health.* Thorofare, NJ: Slack.

———. (2005). Relationship of occupations to health and well-being. In C. H. Christiansen, C. M. Baum, & J. Bass-Haugen (Eds.), *Occupational Therapy: Performance, Participation, and Well-being* (3rd ed.) (pp. 135–157). Thorofare, NJ: Slack.

Winnicott, D. W. (1971). *Playing and Reality.* London: Tavistock.

World Health Organization. (1946). *Constitution of the World Health Organization.* Adopted by the International Health Conference, New York, June 19–22, 1946; signed on July 22, 1946, by the representatives of 61 states (Official Records of the World Health Organization, no. 2, p. 100) and entered into force on April 7, 1948.

Activities of Daily Living and Instrumental Activities of Daily Living

Catana Brown

> "As for myself, I cannot remember a specific moment when I turned that corner from surviving to becoming an active participant in my own recovery process. My efforts to protect my breaking heart by becoming hard of heart and not caring about anything lasted for a long time. One thing I can recall is that the people around me did not give up on me. They kept inviting me to do things. I remember one day, for no particular reason, saying "yes" to food shopping. All I would do was push the cart. But it was a beginning. And truly, it was through small steps like these that I slowly began to discover that I could take a stand toward what was distressing me.
>
> —Deegan, 1996, p. 96

Introduction

Grocery shopping is an essential living skill that most people perform without giving it much thought. We may get frustrated if we cannot find an item or impatient if the checkout line is moving slowly, but what is grocery shopping like for a person with a mental illness? The grocery store is a busy environment with much information to sort through, social demands from other shoppers and workers, a large and complex space to navigate, intense sensory stimuli, and many, many decisions to be made. What if, in addition to the sensory overload of the grocery store, you also hear voices? What if you experience social anxiety? What if problem-solving and decision-making are an everyday challenge? What if you do not have a car to get to the store? What if you have to face the stigma of using food stamps to purchase your groceries? An everyday task like grocery shopping might be a real hardship for someone dealing with these encumbrances. Occupational therapists can help individuals with mental illness perform basic activities of daily living (ADLs) and more complex instrumental activities of daily living (IADLs) by addressing both client and environmental factors that interfere with a successful and satisfying daily life.

Activities of Daily Living

Activities of daily living are the most basic skills of everyday life. Also called self-care skills, ADLs are tasks that are typically performed in a habitual manner, every day, and across all age groups, genders, and cultures. The Occupational Therapy Practice Framework (AOTA, 2002) identifies 11 ADLs: bathing/showering, bowel and bladder management, dressing, eating, feeding, functional mobility, personal device care (e.g., eyeglass care), personal hygiene and grooming, sexual activity, sleep/rest, and toilet hygiene. In mental health practice, ADL concerns are likely to be related to cognitive, psychological, or sensory issues and less frequently due to motor impairments. The kinds of problems can range from minor, such as poor nail care, to total dependence across all ADLs during the later stages of dementia.

Problems with ADLs can occur at any age, but prevalence rates are higher for the elderly and are a core problem associated with late-stage dementia. Although memory loss is a key feature of dementia, executive dysfunction (i.e., higher-level cognitive processes such as planning, problem-solving, and initiating activity) is most predictive of functional impairment in dementia (Boyle, 2004; Royall, Palmer, Chiodo, & Polk, 2005). Increased attention has been given to the physical impairments associated with Alzheimer's dementia. In a study using the Assessment of Motor and Process Skills, individuals with Alzheimer's dementia had lower motor ability when performing ADL tasks as compared with similar aged adults (Oakley, Duran, Fisher, & Merritt, 2003). The study indicated that people with Alzheimer's disease were slower and had more difficulty with fluid arm and hand movement.

In dementia, typically there is a predictable progression of functional impairment that begins with more complex instrumental ADLs, such as money management, and evolves into a decline in ADLs (Paul et al, 2002). In a 10-year longitudinal study of individuals with mild cognitive impairment, there was limited progression in memory problems and ADL impairment except for those individuals who initially presented with IADL limitations (Purser, Fillenbaum, Pieper, & Wallace, 2005). This suggests that IADL impairment is a good predictor of future dementia and ADL disability in the elderly.

Depression can also have an impact on ADL performance. A large study of 6,871 participants ages 54 to 65 examined risk factors for the development of ADL disability (Dunlop, Manheim, Song, Lyons, & Chang, 2005). Depressed adults were 4.3 times more likely than nondepressed adults to have an ADL disability. ADL disability was defined as the inability to independently perform at least one ADL task (dress, toilet, bathe, eat, walk across a room, and transfer in and out of bed) for a time period of at least 3 months. In a study of severely depressed adults, cognition was associated with IADLs, whereas severity of depression was closely related to basic ADLs (McCall & Dunn, 2003). In depression, typically the barrier is not lack of knowledge or ability to perform the ADL but a lack of volition, interest, or drive for engagement in self-care.

Instrumental Activities of Daily Living

Instrumental activities of daily living are skills that are important for independent living. They are more complex than ADLs and involve the use of objects or materials such as cooking utensils or a checkbook. Although there is no consensus as to the exact tasks that comprise IADLs, Lawton and Brody (1969) were the first to use the term instrumental activities of daily living, and they included the following activities: money management, using the telephone, taking medication, traveling, shopping, preparing meals, doing laundry, and housekeeping.

Different mental disorders can affect IADL performance in distinct ways. For example, because schizophrenia often begins in the late teens or early 20s (Walker, Kestler, Bollini, & Hochman, 2004), many individuals with schizophrenia do not have the opportunity to experience and learn IADLs as part of the typical adult development process. Conversely, individuals with dementia may have developed competence in IADLS as adults but lost their skills due to declining cognitive abilities. For individuals with dementia, it is important to provide interventions that can maintain engagement for as long as possible. In still another situation, individuals with developmental disabilities or attention deficit disorder may need assistance with IADLs as they transition from adolescent to adulthood. This may mean moving from living with family or in supervised settings to more independent living or assuming more responsibilities in a supervised situation.

PhotoVoice

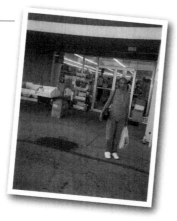

I got my stuff, and I'm outside and I'm leaving. The things I like to buy are eye shadows. I went shopping Wednesday and I like shopping on Sundays too. I always go places and get out. It make me feel happy and think better.

—Barbara

Successful IADL performance is based on a complex interaction of skill knowledge and experience, underlying abilities (cognitive, emotional, social), and environmental resources. First, the individual must have the opportunity to learn the skill. Some individuals with mental illness who have lived in institutional or sheltered settings may not have had the naturally occurring opportunities to, for example, learn how to write a check, use a microwave, or take the bus.

Because of their complexity, IADLs place high demands on cognitive and social skills; therefore, individuals with underlying cognitive and social impairments often have problems with IADLs. For example, memory or attentional impairments can cause safety issues when cooking. Emotional factors such as anxiety and depression can also interfere with performance of IADLS. Depression makes it challenging to engage in IADLs, even when the person has the skills to successfully perform the task. Anxiety can create difficulties in IADLs with social demands such as riding on a crowded city bus.

For many individuals, IADLs are highly ritualized and take place in the same environment. Consequently, recognizing the barriers and facilitators in the particular environment where an IADL is performed is essential to understanding IADL performance. For example, it is important to know if the laundry facilities are located in the home or at a Laundromat. Furthermore, environmental factors such as poverty may mean that individuals with mental illness lack important resources for taking care of IADLs. For example, does the individual have the necessary tools and materials (e.g., a vacuum cleaner) to keep his or her apartment clean?

IADL interventions incorporate both remedial and compensatory strategies. Skills training is used to teach specific IADL tasks. Adaptive devices, cues, and organizational strategies can be useful for simplifying IADL performance and creating a supportive environment. However, intervention approaches discussed in Part II, "The Person," Section 3, "Client Factors," of this textbook are often applied to IADL concerns. For example, if cognitive impairments are an issue, errorless learning or self-talking strategies can be applied to IADL training. A cognitive-behavioral approach may be helpful for individuals whose depression or anxiety is interfering with IADL performance. Motivational interviewing can be used to change behaviors to promote engagement in important IADLs.

Alternatively, interventions that address the environment are also essential. For example, an individual is more likely to be concerned about housekeeping if friends come by to visit. Individuals with limited incomes who are overwhelmed by busy environments can benefit from locating a discount grocery store and shopping at nonpeak times.

In the following sections, four key IADLs are described: home management, money management, medication management, and driving and public transportation. For each, specific suggestions are made for creating a supportive environment, teaching a skill, or simplifying the task. Specific practice models addressing IADLs are discussed in the section "Intervention" in this chapter.

Home Management

Home management is a broad category that includes activities such as house cleaning, meal planning and preparation, shopping, laundry, and small repairs. Effective home management contributes to a better quality of life. A person's home can provide a place of refuge. For many, the home creates opportunities for self-expression and is a reflection of the resident's identity (Marcus, 1997). Deinstitutionalization and supported housing programs have made it possible for more people with serious mental illness to live in their own apartments and homes (Rog, 2004). Unfortunately, successful community living can be tenuous for many, as evidenced by the high numbers of people with mental illness who are homeless (Salkow & Filcher, 2003). Problems with home management can make a person more vulnerable to homelessness because it can lead to eviction (Black, Rabins, German, McGuire, & Roca, 1997).

Consequently, occupational therapists can focus on many different areas to address home management concerns. The therapist may work with the client to create a "home." This can include identifying favorite colors and objects for decorating that reflect the individual's personality. The client may need training in a specific area of home management, such as meal preparation or vacuuming. This training can include teaching and practice as well as environmental adaptations to simplify the task. The various jobs involved in home management can be overwhelming. The therapist may help the client by organizing cabinets and closets, removing unnecessary clutter, creating checklists with cleaning tasks divided throughout the week, and/or teaching work simplification strategies.

Sometimes it is helpful to create an incentive to increase motivation toward home management, such as setting a date for friends to visit the home. Repeated practice with feedback and support is useful for establishing habits that maintain consistent home management patterns. Taking "before and after" pictures can provide both feedback and an incentive to maintain the living space.

Effective home management includes attention to safety issues such as food storage, locking doors, and turning off appliances when not being used. The occupational therapist should be involved in assessing home safety and providing interventions to address any concerns. In some cases, regular monitoring may be needed to ensure the safety of the client.

Money Management

For many individuals with psychiatric disabilities, money management is a significant occupational concern. Individuals with development disabilities may need assistance with very basic money management skills, such as identifying and counting coins and bills (Bochner, Outhred, Pieterse, & Bashash, 2002). Individuals with schizophrenia and severe mood disorders often have third-party payees who assist with money management (Elbogen, Swanson, Swartz, & Wagner, 2003). For individuals with dementia, money management problems are highly associated with memory loss and one of the first areas where significant IADL dysfunction is noted (Tuokko, Morris, & Ebert, 2005).

The availability of money is often a cue for alcohol or drug use among individuals with substance abuse disorders (Rosen, Bailey, & Rosenheck, 2003). In a study of independent living skills and posttraumatic stress disorder in women, money management was the area of greatest deficit and may

be associated with an increased risk of homelessness (Davis & Kutter, 1998).

Perhaps the greatest barrier toward money management that most people with serious mental illness face is not related to skill level but to a lack of financial resources. Most people with serious mental illness lack paid employment and instead live on Social Security Disability Insurance (SSDI) or Supplemental Security Income (SSI) benefits (Kochhar & Scott, 1995). Individuals with serious mental illness who are working are still at a substantial risk for poverty (Rüesch, Graf, Meyer, Rössler, & Hell, 2004). Consequently, strategies to help individuals increase their income (see Chapter 50) or take advantage of existing resources are crucial. Access to food pantries, subsidized housing, thrift shops, and low-cost leisure pursuits are necessary for individuals with serious financial limitations to meet basic needs. Occupational therapists should become aware of local resources and assist clients with accessing these resources.

Close to half of individuals with serious mental illness receiving SSDI or SSI benefits have their money managed by a third-party payee (Elbogen et al, 2003). Individuals with third-party payees are more likely to have substance abuse problems and a primary diagnosis of a psychotic disorder. Studies of payeeship suggest that individuals with serious mental illness who receive this service are generally satisfied and report having sufficient funds to meet basic needs (Dixon, Turner, Krauss, Scott, & McNary, 1999; Elbogen et al, 2003; Rosen, Desai, Bailey, Davidson, & Rosenheck, 2001); however, they do not have sufficient money to participate in enjoyable activities (Elbogen et al, 2003). Occupational therapists can collaborate with clients and payees to develop strategies that allow individuals to have more funds for leisure pursuits.

Occupational therapists can assist individuals without payees and individuals who want to move from payeeship to independent money management to develop strategies and skills for successful money management. One reason that individuals with psychiatric disabilities may have trouble with money management is that they have a restricted sense of future time perspective (Suto & Gelya, 1994). Therefore, saving or imagining the future consequences of spending can be challenging. A spending diary can be used to increase awareness of how much money is spent and on what items

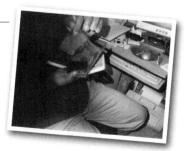

PhotoVoice

This is my wallet. It is empty of money and dreams. Dreams of what I would do if I had money to do the things I did when I had a job to have a full wallet. A full wallet for housing, a car, paying bills, clothes and more. Soon my empty wallet will be no more. As part of my recovery, my wallet will become full again because I will have money to fill it up.

—Sterling

(Figure 47-1). This information may then be used to help individuals create a realistic budget. It is helpful to regularly review income and expenses at the end of each month to determine if the budget is working.

Many other strategies can be used to assist individuals with money management. It may be helpful for the therapist to go with the client the day he or she receives a check to deposit it in the bank or to cash it and pay essential expenses first. Direct deposit and automatic bill payment systems may also help ensure that essential expenses are paid. An envelope system can be created so that money is preassigned for specific monthly expenses. Money management training can also include information on how to make wise purchases, including use of coupons, generic brands, discount and secondhand stores, and so on.

Some individuals may need more basic training, such as counting change, coin identification, or check writing. Compensatory strategies may also be used for these basic skills. For example, computer software was used to help individuals with developmental disabilities use a checkbook (Davies, Stock, & Wehmeyer, 2003). Calculators are another simple compensatory device that may be helpful when shopping.

Spending Diary		
Date	Item	Cost
11/1	Rent	$325.00
11/2	Soda from machine	$1.25
11/2	Cigarettes	$5.33
11/3	Groceries	$27.84
11/4	Cigarettes	$5.33
11/5	Cigarettes	$5.33
11/5	Soda from machine	$1.25
11/6	Dinner at McDonalds	$5.67
11/7	Laundry	$4.50
11/7	Cigarettes	$5.33

FIGURE 47-1. Sample page from spending diary.

Medication Management

There are many reasons why people with psychiatric disabilities do not take medications. Some people may not take medications because of the associated stigma. In a study of individuals with depression, perceived stigma was a more important predictor of medication adherence than symptom severity, duration of the episode, previous hospitalizations, or bothersome side effects (Sirey et al, 2001). Stigma was also the most frequently cited barrier to medication adherence for individuals with schizophrenia (Hudson et al, 2004).

Another major barrier to medication management is negative side effects (Fleck, Keck, Corey, & Strakowski, 2005; Hudson et al, 2004). In this case, individuals weigh the benefits of taking the medication versus the side effects associated with the medication. This is important because psychiatric medications have numerous side effects that range from unpleasant to dreadful. Degree of social support is also associated with medication management. Individuals with psychiatric disabilities are more likely to take their medication when they receive adequate social support from both family and nonfamily members (Voils, Steffens, Flint, & Bosworth, 2005). Finally, forgetfulness can play a major role in adherence to medications. Ordinary forgetfulness, along with the cognitive deficits associated with schizophrenia and dementia, is directly related to medication management (Jeste et al, 2003; Maddigan, Farris, Keating, Wiens, & Johnson, 2003).

Medication management is not just the responsibility of the individual taking the medication but also a concern for the health-care provider. A multisite study revealed that most individuals prescribed antipsychotic or antidepressant medications received dosages either above or below the established guidelines and that most individuals did not received adequate management of their medication side effects (Weinmann, Janssen, & Gaebel, 2005). When side effects are ignored or medications are ineffective, individuals with psychiatric disabilities are less likely to take their medication.

Medication management is a challenging target for IADL intervention. One approach, psychoeducation, teaches individuals with psychiatric disabilities about their illness and the medications they take. Studies of psychoeducation suggest participants increase their knowledge about their illness and medication, but they do not change their behavior toward taking medication (Mueser et al, 2002; Zygmunt, Olfson, Boyer, & Mechanic, 2002). However, psychoeducation is important as a component of a comprehensive program. Effective interventions combine psychoeducation with other strategies, such as reminder systems, self-monitoring, reinforcement, counseling, social support, cognitive-behavioral approaches that target attitudes, and improving quality of care of providers (McDonald, Garg, & Haynes, 2002; Miklowitz, George, Richards, Simoneau, & Suddath, 2003; Vergouwen, Bakker, Katon, Verheij, & Koerselman, 2003). It is interesting to note that although stigma is a primary barrier to medication adherence, stigma is not typically addressed in medication management interventions.

Occupational therapists can take a primary role in designing environments that support medication management. The occupational therapist can create cues and reminder systems or use commercially available products like pill boxes that help the person keep track of medications taken or that beep when it is time to take a medication (see Resources). The social environment can also be a target of intervention. It is important to create social supports and to work to change stigmatizing attitudes among those close to the client.

Driving and Public Transportation

Transportation is a major barrier that prevents individuals with psychiatric disabilities from engaging in daily life activities. Lack of easy access to transportation makes it difficult for individuals with psychiatric disabilities to get to appointments, work, social activities, and leisure pursuits. Many individuals are unable to afford a car and/or the expenses associated with owning a car. The effects of psychiatric illness, particularly dementia, along with medication use, may make it unsafe for some individuals to drive. On the other hand, a diagnosis of mental illness should not automatically exclude someone from driving. Even some individuals with mild dementia are safe to drive (Brown et al, 2005); therefore, a comprehensive evaluation should be conducted to determine driving ability. In dementia, driving safety is associated with scores on the Mini-Mental State Examination; the Clinical Dementia Rating; and specific tests of visuospatial ability, praxis, and executive function (Ott et al, 2005). However, an on-road assessment provides the best evaluation of driving ability (Brown et al, 2005; Lovell & Russell, 2005).

Some individuals with psychiatric disabilities may have limited driving experience or have gone for long periods of time without driving. Occupational therapists can provide interventions to teach driving skills. For driver training, it is important that the therapist have a dual-controlled vehicle and experience in driving instruction. Most certified driver rehabilitation specialists are occupational therapists.

Public transportation is an alternative for those clients who cannot drive, but it presents its own problems. Individuals living in rural, suburban, and even some urban environments may not have access to adequate public transportation systems. Determining the schedule, which bus or train to take, and the correct stop at which to get off are very complicated cognitive tasks. In addition, the social demands of using public transportation may be difficult for people with paranoia or anxiety.

Occupational therapists can assist clients in learning the bus system. The therapist may accompany the client to learn regular routes and practice the experience until the client develops confidence in carrying out the task independently. The therapist may also teach relaxation strategies for individuals with anxiety and provide reassurance and social support until the individual feels comfortable on the bus, subway, or train.

Creative alternatives to transportation may need to be identified when public transportation is limited. In some instances, personal assistant services can be used for transportation (Pita, Ellison, Farkas, & Bleecker, 2001). In other cases, family members, friends, or volunteer agencies may be the only source of transportation.

ADL and IADL Assessments

Different standardized methods of ADL and IADL assessment are available and can be categorized as self-reports or informant reports, simulated performance measures, and real-world performance measures. However, existing standardized measures are limited, and in many cases, the occupational therapist will need to use skilled observation to assess ADL and IADL functioning.

Whenever possible, it is most relevant to conduct the assessment in the environment in which the person will actually perform the skill. The assessment should include observations of the environment and resources available for successful skill performance as well as observation of the skill ability of the individual.

Self-report is widely used for the assessment of ADLs and IADLs; however, problems with insight and cognitive impairment among people with serious mental illness make self-report methods less valid (McKibbin, Brekke, Sires, Jeste, & Patterson, 2004; Patterson, Goldman, McKibbin, Hughs, & Jeste, 2001). Other surveys of functioning are designed to be completed by informants, such as case managers, clinicians, and family members. Ratings by informants are limited by the amount of knowledge the rater has about the individual and the demands created by the physical and social environment where the person lives. Furthermore, in studies comparing different methods, the results of different assessments tend to yield different outcomes. In most cases, self-reports tend to overestimate abilities and informant reports sometimes result in underestimations (Dickerson, Ringel, & Parente, 1997; Rogers, et al, 2003).

The limitations of self-ratings and informant ratings have led to interest in more objective measures that directly assess performance in simulated and real-world settings (McKibbin et al, 2004; Patterson et al, 2001; Rempfer, Hamera, Brown, & Cromwell, 2003). Described next are four observational measures of self-care, followed by a description of several IADL performance measures that use standardized instructions for performance of targeted skills and a standardized rating system for scoring.

Evidence-Based Practice

Different methods of ADL and IADL assessment (self-report, informant report, simulated performance, natural-environment performance) can result in different outcomes.

➤ Occupational therapists should consider biases that might exist in self-reporting or informant reporting.

➤ Performance-based assessments, especially those administered in natural environments, may assess real-world ability more accurately; however, they can also be more time consuming to administer.

McKibbin, C. L., Brekke, J. S., Sires, D., Jeste, D. V., & Patterson, T. L. (2004). Direct assessment of functional abilities: relevance to persons with schizophrenia. *Schizophrenia Research, 72*, 53–67.

The Lived Experience

Willeta Rae Rickey

She was there through the contracted services of an allied health provider, and I sat among my coworkers on a not especially comfortable chair, listening to her presentation. I can recall little of what she had to say all of those years ago, but one thing I do remember: poor hygiene can be a symptom of depression. May she be blessed a thousandfold for her gift of information. As I struggled to keep my life from disappearing into the ever-deepening darkness of depression's abyss, losing function in one area after another, it was to become a silent litany of protest against the onslaught of hopelessness and self-recrimination. "It's a symptom!" cried my aching, angry heart, "a symptom." And then, "Doesn't anybody care?" Receiving counsel from my supervisor on the inadequacies of my personal presentation in the workplace generated a turmoil of negative emotions unlike anything I had experienced before. In time, I became so deeply depressed that I could no longer perform the duties of my position—or any position, and by God's grace, I qualified for a disability retirement. It was to be the saving of me.

Personal hygiene has remained a frequently recurring source of pain. I have experienced uncertainty in how to proceed, not that I never learned how to care for my body, but at times, I have somehow seemed unable to access that information and I have had no confidence that my unclear memories are adequate to society's expectations. I have never recovered my former standards, and when my stress level rises, my self-care efforts are the first to suffer. Even the most basic elements of grooming can feel so overwhelming that it has brought tears to my eyes. I have been through periods of claustrophobia in the small enclosed space of a shower stall. There have been times when my nerves were so fraught that the shower spray has felt like a hail storm. Sometimes, simply being wet has been upsetting. And then there are the times when the problem has not been the distress of the process at all; it has simply seemed to be an eminently pointless exercise.

Even so, I have never ceased to be aware of my hygienic short-comings, whether alone or in the company of others. When I feel especially insecure and vulnerable, I pray that my presence will not offend anyone, and choose a place to sit or stand as far away from other people as I can manage without drawing undue notice. Alternatively, I simply withdraw into the shelter of my four walls until I can manage a more comfortable level of hygiene. Dysfunction in this area is, frankly, miserable.

Why, then, am I embarrassing myself further by writing about it? It is my hope that by sharing my experience, it may serve to illustrate how difficulty in this sensitive area—so very basic to successful functioning in our society—can undercut every effort to assist a person with mental illness to progress toward recovery.

I found the courage to seek assistance from a student of occupational therapy who was assigned to my case as part of her student practicum at the mental health center where I receive services. Although I'm sure she was not expecting such a request when she asked me for suggestions on ways that she might be of help, she proved to be creative, tactful, and very supportive in her efforts. As it transpired, I was unable to consistently perform the steps of the hygienic routine we had developed together. Still, I appreciated her help and encouragement, and her sensitive handling of a difficult issue, which so closely touched upon my very vulnerable self-esteem. Unfortunately, I have witnessed some less praiseworthy instances in which, by all rights, the speaker should have, at the very least, experienced the acrid taste and chewy texture of cheap shoe leather. It is the second reason for offering my thoughts in this way. To wit, a cautionary tale.

Most of us strangers to one another, we sat in the common room of a psychiatric ward—alike only in that not one of us wanted to be there. Some of us were more restive than others. I suppose that's why all of the exits were kept locked. I had never experienced such a situation before, and the loss of freedom was nearly more than I could bear, let alone the mental condition that had caused me to seek help in this place. The sky was dark outside the windows where the drapes had not been pulled. The air was thick with unhappiness, weariness, impatience, and resentment. Some sat trembling, a distressing side effect from the medication they had received. The day had been long, and we endured the tedious wait as the late-comers straggled in—attendance was mandatory.

At last the day's final session was underway. We listened to an inspirational reading, and then the nurse who was facilitating the session asked each of us, in turn, about our success or failure in meeting the day's personal goal which [we] had been required to set during the morning's group session. The woman in the chair next to mine shared her success in having showered and worn clean clothing that day, and in having done so for a period of several days. Sadly, the nurse's face took on a pained look as she tossed off the comment, "Well, if that's where you are . . ." and pointedly moved on to someone else.

Her response made me furious. It seemed to me a cruel humiliation and a betrayal of the trust that had allowed the woman to reveal her wounded psyche—the trust so necessary to those who were seeking to help her. She was released a few days later. I keep wondering how tragically different the outcome might have been if she had been feeling a tad more vulnerable when the ugly incident occurred, a bit more desperate.

As I consider it in hindsight, I realize that the nurse's response was probably an example of those regrettable occasions in which we open our mouths to speak before our brains are fully engaged. Our society is, after all, pretty intolerant of the natural odor of the human body. The question is, "how do we help the mentally ill person who struggles with personal hygiene without causing additional pain in the process?" The issue is complex, and I wish I had a reliable solution. As a step toward that end, I hope to write a booklet that addresses the basic steps of personal hygiene and offers suggestions for overcoming problems such as those I have encountered. Most of all, I would like to reassure those who are struggling that the problem is a symptom of their illness, and not a personal failure. It just may give them enough hope to keep trying.

Observational Measures

Observational measures of self-care described here include the Katz Index of Independence, the Barthel Index, the Functional Independence Measure, the WeeFIM, the Pediatric Evaluation of Disability Inventory, and the Independent Living Skills Survey.

Katz Index of Independence in Activities of Daily Living Scale

The Katz Index of Independence in Activities of Daily Living (Katz ADL) is a very brief assessment of self-care (Katz, 1983). Six items (bathing, dressing, toileting, transferring, continence and feeding) are rated yes or no for independence. The tool is typically completed by a health-care provider. Although the instrument is quick and easy to use, it does not provide information about what aspects of the particular ADL are impaired. In addition, the Katz ADL may not be very sensitive; one study found that 50% of individuals with severe dementia had a perfect score on the measure (Dencker & Gottfries, 1995).

Barthel Index

The Barthel Index was first published by Mahoney and Barthel in 1965 as a quick and easy scale for measuring ADLs. The measure has 10 items: feeding, grooming, bathing, dressing, bowel care, bladder care, toilet use, ambulation, transfers, and stair climbing. The measure is typically completed by the occupational therapist or other health-care worker on the basis of observation of the client. Studies of the Barthel Index indicate that it is a good measure of disability change (Wallace, Duncan, & Lai, 2002) but that it may be less sensitive at higher levels of functioning (O'Connor, Cano, Thompson, & Hobart, 2004)

Functional Independence Measure

The Functional Independence Measure (FIM) was developed for use with the Uniform National Data System for Medical Rehabilitation, making it a widely used instrument in rehabilitation settings (Hamilton, Granger, Sherwin, Zielezny, & Tashman, 1987). The FIM consists of 18 items divided into two domains: physical and sociocognitive. The FIM was developed to expand upon the Barthel Index and make it more comprehensive. The physical domain includes eating, grooming, bathing, dressing upper body, dressing lower body, toileting, bladder management, bowel management, transfer bed–chair–wheelchair, transfer toilet, transfer tub–shower, walk–wheelchair, and stairs. The sociocognitive domain includes comprehension, expression, social interaction, problem-solving, and memory. Each item on the FIM is scored on a 7-point scale, with 7 being the highest level of independence and 1 indicating total assistance. Several studies indicate a high rate of concordance between the Barthel ADL Index and the FIMs (Gosman-Hedstrom & Svensson, 2000; Houldon, Edwards, McNeil, & Greenwood, 2006; Hsueh, Lin, Jeng, & Hsieh, 2006), suggesting that these measures may be comparable.

WeeFIM

The WeeFIM is the corresponding FIM measure for children ages 6 months to 7 years. It includes 18 items measuring self-care, bowel and bladder control, mobility, locomotion, communication, and social cognition using a 7-point scale. The measure can be completed on the basis of observation or parental report. The WeeFIM can distinguish between different groups of children (Msall et al, 1993; Ottenbacher et al, 1996) and is sensitive to change in children with chronic disabilities, particularly in the self-care and social realms (Ottenbacher et al, 2000).

Pediatric Evaluation of Disability Inventory

The Pediatric Evaluation of Disability Inventory (PEDI) is another self-care evaluation for children ages 6 months to 7 years (Haley, Coster, Ludlow, Haltiwanger, & Andrellos, 1992). It can be used with older children with significant developmental delays. The PEDI is more comprehensive than the WeeFIM with 63 self-care items, 59 mobility items, and 65 social function items. Items are rated on a 6-point scale from total assistance to independence. It can be completed on the basis of observation or parental report. There is a comprehensive manual and a computer program available for scoring the PEDI. The PEDI is a norm-referenced test with raw scores, normative standard scores, and scaled scores. It has strong reliability (Haley et al, 1992; Nichols & Case-Smith, 1996) and evidence to support its validity (Nichols & Case-Smith, 1996; Wright & Boschen, 1993).

Independent Living Skills Survey

The Independent Living Skills Survey (ILSS) is a comprehensive questionnaire designed for individuals with serious mental illness (Wallace, Liberman, Tauber, & Wallace, 2000). It includes both an informant and a self-report version. The areas of independent living that are covered include personal hygiene, appearance and care of clothing, care of personal possessions and living space, food preparation, health and safety, money management, transportation, leisure and recreation, work, eating behaviors, and social interaction. Both versions take approximately 20 to 30 minutes to administer. The informant version rates individuals on a 5-point Likert scale of frequency (always to never). The self-report version is answered yes or no.

Studies of reliability and validity indicate the ILSS has adequate internal consistency and interrater reliability. The measure is also sensitive to changes associated with skills training. A study of older adults found the ILSS distinguished individuals with and without schizophrenia (Perivoliotis, Granholm, & Patterson, 2004). Individuals with schizophrenia performed more poorly in most areas, with the largest differences being in appearance/clothing, personal hygiene, food preparation, transportation, leisure and recreation, and job seeking.

Performance-Based Assessments

Performance-based assessments of ADL and IADL include the Kohlman Evaluation of Living Skills, Milwaukee Evaluation of Daily Living Skills, UCSD Performance-based Skills Assessment, Performance Assessment of Self-Care Skills, Test of Grocery Shopping Skills, Cooking Assessments, and Assessment of Motor and Process Skills.

Kohlman Evaluation of Living Skills

The Kohlman Evaluation of Living Skills (KELS) combines interview items with simulated performance (Thomson, 1992). It is practical to administer in a clinical setting because it requires limited equipment and can be administered in 30 to 45 minutes. Seventeen living skills are addressed in the areas of self-care, safety and health, money management, transportation and telephone, and work and leisure. The measure was designed so that the results can be used by occupational therapists to make recommendations regarding the client's living situation. Items are scored as Independent or Needs Assistance. Each item marked Needs Assistance is scored as 1 point, except for the work/leisure items, which are counted as 0.5 points. A score of 5.5 or less indicates that the individual is capable of living independently. Needs Assistance ratings should be considered within the context of the individual's living situation. For example, an individual who scores Needs Assistance may not need to alter his or her living situation or receive training in this area if he or she has a spouse or case manager who can assist with this IADL.

Interrater reliability of the measure ranges from 74% to 94% (Ilika & Hoffman, 1981). In a concurrent validity study, scores on the KELS were associated with living situation (Tateichi, 1984). Individuals who were living independently had better scores on the KELS when compared with people living in a sheltered setting. In another concurrent validity study with older adults in Israel, the KELS was strongly associated with the Routine Task Inventory and the Functional Independent Measure (Zimnavoda, Weinblatt, & Katz, 2002). Two predictive validity studies using the cutoff score to determine ability to live independently for older adults and individuals with psychiatric disabilities were inconclusive (as reported in Thomson, 1992). Brown, Moore, Hemman, and Yunek (1996) found that simulated items on the KELS were not necessarily predictive of performance of the same tasks in the natural environment.

Milwaukee Evaluation of Daily Living Skills

The Milwaukee Evaluation of Daily Living Skills (MEDLS) was designed for individuals with serious mental illness (Leonardelli, 1988). It is similar to the KELS but is more comprehensive and therefore takes longer to administer. However, of the 20 items on the MEDLS, a subset of items can be selected for use based on the concerns of a particular client. The items cover basic communication, bathing, tooth brushing, denture care, dressing, eating, eyeglass care, hair care, maintenance of clothing, makeup use, medication management, nail care, personal health care, safety in the community, safety in the home, shaving, time awareness, use of money, use of telephone, and use of transportation. Most items utilize simulated performance, and items are scored on the basis of established criteria. The total points per item range from 3 to 6. The MEDLS was designed to determine a client's baseline performance prior to treatment, assess treatment effectiveness, and assist in planning related to living situation.

Studies of reliability and validity of the MEDLS are described in the MEDLS manual (Leonardelli, 1988). Interrater reliability coefficients ranged from 0.40 to 1.00, with most items at 0.80 or above. Subtests with the least stability are dressing, hair care, and makeup use. An expert panel supported the face validity of the items. Schretlen et al (2000) studied predictors of functional outcome using the MEDLS in a sample of individuals with serious mental illness. A diagnosis of schizophrenia was predictive of worse scores on the MEDLS. An even stronger predictor of MEDLS outcomes was cognition, particularly auditory divided attention and verbal learning. Another study found a strong correlation between competency assessment using the Hopkins Competency Assessment Test (HCAT) and the MEDLS for individuals with serious mental illness (Jones, Jayaram, Samuels, & Robinson, 1998).

UCSD Performance-Based Skills Assessment

The UCSD Performance-Based Skills Assessment (UPSA) is a measure of capacity to perform IADLs in five areas: household chores, communication, finance, transportation, and planning recreational activities (Patterson et al, 2001). The tasks are simulated so that they can be carried out in a clinic setting. For example, one of the tasks in the household chores category asks the individual to create a shopping list from a recipe for rice pudding. A finance task asks the individual to count out certain amounts of money using coins and bills. It takes about 30 minutes to administer the entire assessment, and scores are based on established criteria.

The UPSA was able to distinguish between individuals with schizophrenia and no mental illness and was correlated with the Direct Assessment of Functional Status (Patterson et al, 2001). Test–retest reliability was 0.94. The developers acknowledge that the UPSA assesses abilities in a simulated setting, which may differ from real-world performance. A study of older individuals with psychosis found all areas of cognition (attention, memory, learning, and executive function) were significantly related to the ability to perform everyday tasks as measured by the UPSA (Twamley et al, 2002). The UPSA was predictive of community living situation and useful in detecting improvement after functional adaptation skills training (Patterson et al, 2003).

Performance Assessment of Self-Care Skills

The Performance Assessment of Self-Care Skills (PASS; Holm & Rogers, 1999) includes 26 tasks in the following categories: functional mobility (e.g., toilet transfers), personal care (e.g., cleaning teeth), IADL with a cognitive emphasis (e.g., setting out medications according to prescription); and IADL with a physical emphasis (e.g., bed making). There are home and clinic versions of the measure. The scoring system for the PASS is more comprehensive than most. Like most performance-based measures, each task is divided into subtasks. For example, the subtasks for medication management are:

1. Reports next time first medication is to be taken correctly.
2. Opens first pill bottle with ease.
3. Distributes pills from the first pill bottle into correct time slots for the next 2 days.
4. Reports next time second medication is to be taken correctly.
5. Opens second pill bottle with ease.
6. Distributes pills from second pill bottle into correct time slots for the next 2 days.

Each subtask is scored on a 9-point scale of "level of independence." The following hierarchically ordered descriptions are used to determine level of independence: verbal supportive, verbal nondirective, verbal directive, gestures, task or environment rearrangement, demonstration, physical guidance, physical support, and total assist. If an individual has difficulty completing a task, support is provided using the hierarchy until the individual is able to complete the subtask. There is also scoring for safety, quality, and process of carrying out the task.

For trained observers, the PASS has high interrater reliability (Holm & Rogers, 1999). Cognitive impairment assessed using the Luria-Nebraska Neuropsychological Battery was a good predictor of performance on the cognitive emphasis IADL subscale for elderly individuals in an acute psychiatric facility (McCue, Rogers, & Goldstein, 1990). Another study found memory was predictive of PASS performance for elderly individuals with dementia, major depression, or no illness (Goldstein, McCue, Rogers, & Nussbaum, 1992). A study comparing perceived skills, perceived habits, and demonstrated skills found that older women with depression perceived themselves as more independent than was demonstrated by performance on the PASS (Rogers & Holm, 2000).

Test of Grocery Shopping Skills

The Test of Grocery Shopping Skills (TOGSS) is a performance-based assessment that is administered in an actual grocery store (Hamera, Brown, Rempfer, & Davis, 2002). It takes approximately 30 to 45 minutes to administer. The measure assesses a person's ability to efficiently and accurately locate 10 items on a grocery shopping list. The TOGGS has three subscale scores:

1. Accuracy (based on finding the correct item, at the correct size and lowest price).
2. Time (to locate the items).
3. Redundancy (the number of aisles entered and number of times the person returns to the same aisle).

In addition, observation of performance in an actual grocery store provides the therapist with information regarding strategy use. For example, does the individual use overhead signs or other available cues to find items, ask for help when needed, or scan the shelf efficiently to locate the correct items? There are two forms of grocery lists so that the measure can be used as a pretest and posttest.

A reliability study of the two forms of the TOGSS indicates combined stability and equivalence reliability coefficients ranging from 0.69 to 0.83 and interrater reliability for trained administrators at 99% to 100% (Hamera et al, 2002). In addition, validity evidence for the TOGSS indicates it is sensitive to differences between individuals with and without psychiatric disabilities (Hamera et al, 2002) and is related to neurocognitive performance in people with schizophrenia (Rempfer et al, 2003).

Cooking Assessments

There are two standardized measures of cooking, both of which were developed by occupational therapists: the Kitchen Task Assessment (KTA; Baum & Edwards, 1993) and the Rabideau Kitchen Evaluation–Revised (RKE-R; Neistadt, 1992). In the KTA, the individual is instructed to make a box of pudding using the instructions on the box. The KTA was designed to evaluate the cognitive processes that underlie successful task completion; initiation, organization, performance of all steps, sequencing, judgment and safety, and completion are rated on a 4-point scale from 0, *independent,* to 3, *not capable.*

In a study of individuals with Alzheimer's disease, the KTA was correlated with neuropsychological measures (Baum & Edwards, 1993). In addition, individuals in later stages of dementia (determined by the Clinical Dementia Rating Scale) performed worse on the KTA than individuals in earlier stages.

Duncombe (2004) used a modified version of the KTA to determine if learning in the clinic was different from learning in the home for individuals with schizophrenia. The modification involved the scoring of the measure. Instead of scoring cognitive abilities, the Duncombe scoring system is based on 40 individuals steps of the task that are scored from 0 to 5 (adapted from the RKE-R system). The modified KTA was able to detect differences in learning after a cooking skills training intervention was provided; however, there was no difference in the amount of improvement for the home and clinic training.

The RKE-R (Neistadt, 1992) is based on a modification of the Rabideau Kitchen Evaluation (Rabideau, 1986). It involves simple meal preparation of a sandwich and hot drink. The task is broken down into 40 steps, and each step is scored on a scale from 0, *independent,* to 3, *unable to perform.* Cues are provided to the individual if (1) assistance is requested, (2) significant frustration is experienced, (3) safety is a concern, or (4) a behavior would interfere with completing the next component step or the task as a whole. The provision of cues is incorporated into the scoring system.

The RKE-R was correlated with the Wechsler Adult Intelligence Scale–Third Edition (WAIS-R) block design scores for people with brain injury (Neistadt, 1992). It detected improvement in cooking performance for individuals with brain injury trained with a meal preparation protocol (Neistadt, 1994).

Assessment of Motor and Process Skills

The Assessment of Motor and Process Skills (AMPS) uses a different approach than the previously described performance measures. Instead of directly assessing the ability to carry out an ADL or IADL skill, the AMPS evaluates particular motor and process skills while the person is carrying out a task of his

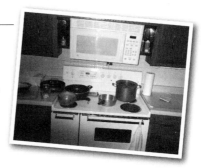

PhotoVoice

I used to do all of the family cooking, but since I got sick I've been unable to do the cooking. The one thing that brought me joy in my life was doing the family cooking, and now it is just a source of pain. I long to get well by medication and by my therapist because nothing would bring me more joy than to be able to cook again.

—Glen

or her choosing. There are 83 possible tasks that are carefully calibrated in terms of difficulty (Fisher 2001). Some tasks fall within the ADL category, such as putting on shoes and socks, although most of the tasks are more complex IADLS tasks.

The therapist observes the client performing two tasks and rates the client in terms of 16 motor skills and 20 process skills. Motor skills include behaviors such as reaching or gripping, whereas performance skills include behaviors such as selecting and organizing. A study of the AMPS for people with developmental disabilities provided valid results, with the exception of some individuals with more severe impairments (Kottorp, Bernspang, & Fisher, 2003). It may be that the overlearning of some tasks by individuals with severe developmental disabilities affects the results.

A study in which the AMPS was used to assess individuals with Alzheimer's disease indicated that poor motor skills was associated with more problems in ADLs (Oakley et al, 2003). A study using the AMPS for individuals with psychiatric conditions suggested that assessment in the home may provide a better indicator of home safety than estimates based on assessment in the clinic (McNulty & Fisher, 2001).

Administration of the AMPS requires specialized training (see Resources). In addition, raters are individually calibrated to enhance the reliability of the measure.

Intervention

There are several different approaches to ADL/IADL intervention with research to support their efficacy. Skills training and applied behavioral analysis have a primary emphasis on teaching the specific ADL and/or IADL skill. Skills training has most often been used for people with serious mental illness such as schizophrenia, bipolar disorder, and major depression. Applied behavioral analysis is an approach that is more frequently applied to individuals with developmental disabilities. Interpersonal and social rhythm therapy was designed for people with bipolar disorder and focuses on creating a routine around the performance of ADLs and IADLs. Finally, the Home Environmental Skills Building Program teaches the caregiver how to create an environment that supports the individual with dementia.

Skills Training

In 1995, the Schizophrenia Patient Outcomes Research Team recommended that skills training be included in the American Psychiatric Association's practice guidelines (Scott & Dixon, 1995). Skills training research indicates that individuals with serious mental illness can learn new skills; less clear evidence exists regarding maintenance and generalizability of skills learned (Bellack, 2004, Heinssen, Liberman, & Kopelowicz, 2000). Skills training interventions for individuals with serious mental illness are founded on learning theory. The skill to be taught is first broken down into its component parts. Target behaviors are taught using a variety of teaching methods designed to compensate for cognitive impairments. The skills are presented through demonstration, didactic instruction, or videotape. Individuals then practice these skills repeatedly, receiving regular feedback based on performance. Social reinforcement and other contingencies are used for motivation. Homework assignments

are utilized to encourage more practice of the skills in the person's natural environment.

The UCLA Social and Independent Living Skills Program is the most studied skills training approach (Eckman et al, 1992; Liberman, Mueser, Wallace, Jacobs, & Eckman, 1986; Liberman et al, 1998; Wallace, Liberman, MacKain, Blackwell, & Eckman, 1992). The modules are intended to be delivered in a small-group format, and it is recommended that training be provided at least twice a week in 1-hour sessions. Most of the modules take 4 months to complete, which stresses the importance of repeated practice. The modules included in the program are:

- Medication Management
- Symptom Management
- Recreation for Leisure
- Basic Conversation
- Community Re-entry
- Job Seeking
- Workplace Fundamentals Training
- Demonstration of Modules Learning Activities

In addition to other learning strategies, problem-solving is a core component of the UCLA modules. In an effort to promote generalization, participants learn a problem-solving strategy that can be applied to novel situations. Each module includes the same learning activities:

1. Introduction to the skill area: defining terms and goal setting.
2. Videotape questions and answers: participants watch actors model the target behaviors.
3. Role-play: participants practice the skills they have learned and receive feedback from trainers and group members.
4. Resource management: participants learn about resources they can use to support skill performance.
5. Problem-solving: participants learn a problem-solving strategy.
6. In vivo exercises: participants practice skills outside the classroom with trainer support.
7. Homework: participants perform skill in real-world situations without trainer support.

One of the studies of the UCLA modules compared skills training to an occupational therapy intervention and found more favorable results for skills training (Liberman et al, 1998). This study greatly concerned occupational therapists. Legitimately, occupational therapists were concerned that the particular craft-based intervention used in the study was presented as generally representing psychosocial occupational therapy. On the other hand, the study did provide important evidence to occupational therapists that craft-based interventions cannot be expected to result in improved living skills.

A criticism of skills training has been the lack of evidence that skills acquired through training will generalize to real-world community situations. In response, Liberman et al (2001) developed In Vivo Amplified Skills Training (IVAST) in which skills training is combined with intensive case management. The case manager works to support skills training by helping with homework assignments, creating opportunities for using skills in the community, and establishing support systems. In an efficacy study of the IVAST program,

IVAST resulted in superior and more rapid improvement in skills when compared with traditional skills training (Glynn et al, 2002).

Reviews of skills training for the most part indicate that skills training results in acquisition of new skills and has a positive effect on role functioning and self-efficacy (Bellack, 2004); however, it should be noted that a meta-analysis (Pilling et al, 2002) was significantly more pessimistic, concluding that skills training was ineffective and not recommended for clinical practice. Mueser (2004) and Bellack (2004) criticize this meta-analysis and argue that only a small sample of the relevant studies was included, and the conclusions are misleading.

The skills training review by Heinssen et al (2000) concludes with recommendations for practitioners. This review addresses client-centered practice concerns and considerations for the environmental context in which IADLs take place. Application of skills training should include the following components:

■ A determination of the particular environments and skills that are problematic and the individual's own personal goals and aspirations.
■ Direct observation in natural environments providing information about both strengths and deficits.
■ Naturally occurring reinforcers to strengthen the skill development process.

Enhancing IADLS through skills training can potentially improve quality of life and promote sustained and successful community living.

Grocery Shopping Skills Training

The interdisciplinary team of Catana Brown (occupational therapist), Edna Hamera (nurse practitioner), and Melisa Rempfer (clinical psychologist) developed a skills training program to teach grocery shopping. The intervention pays particular attention to the environment and uses strategies that teach the participant about the context of the store. The nine-session intervention is administered in a group, and each session includes classroom teaching, practice in an actual grocery store, and homework exercises. The training is built around a script of three questions that help teach the sequencing of grocery shopping; each question includes three strategies (Table 47-1).

An entire session is spent on each question, and then the whole sequence is practiced in only a segment of the store. Finally, the whole process is put together in the whole store and integrated into the larger activity of shopping for and preparing an actual meal. Each skill is taught using a variety of activities so that participants receive repeated practice and regular feedback about performance. A study of individuals with schizophrenia comparing the grocery shopping intervention with a treatment-as-usual control found that individuals in the intervention improved their grocery shopping accuracy and efficiency (Brown et al, 2002)

Designing a Skills Training Intervention

Holmes, Corrigan, Knight, and Flaxman (1995) describe the process of developing a skills training program targeting sleep management. The process they describe incorporates consumer input and can be applied to other skill areas. It is a useful framework for occupational therapists who are developing new skills training modules. The process is broken down into three components, as shown in Table 47-2.

In addition to the process, occupational therapists should integrate a set of strategies that promote engagement and facilitate acquisition and generalization of life skills. Strategies that enhance motivation, facilitate application to real life, match the individual's unique environment, and ensure that skills are learned through repetition and evaluation are outlined in Box 47-1.

Interpersonal and Social Rhythm Therapy

IADLs and the more basic ADLs provide a sense of order and familiarity to daily life. The disruption of routines, such as the timing of sleeping, eating, and exercising, can lead to the onset of bipolar episodes (Malkoff-Schwartz et al, 1998). When sleep–wake cycles are disturbed in individuals who are vulnerable to mood disorders, this can lead to an exacerbation

---

Table 47-1 ● **Grocery Shopping Training**

Question	Strategies
Where is it?	• Use overhead signs • Know the store layout or use a map • Ask for help
Is this what I'm looking for?	• Is it the right size? • Is it the right packaging? • Is it the right flavor, scent, type, etc?
Is this the lowest price?	• Generic items • No frills items: no special packaging or convenience items • Scan the entire shelf from top to bottom to locate lowest priced items

Source: Brown, C., Rempfer, M., & Hamera, E. (2002). Teaching grocery shopping skills to people with schizophrenia. Occupational Therapy Journal of Research, 22(Suppl1), 90S–91S.

Table 47-2 ● **Developing Skills-Training Modules**

Component	Steps
Problem Identification	1. Interview consumers to identify the particular problem using open-ended questions. 2. Create a checklist based on all of the problems generated by the open-ended questions. 3. Administer the checklist to a consumer group. 4. Prioritize the most important problems.
Solution Identification	1. Interview consumers to identify solutions to the problems using open-ended questions. 2. Create a checklist based on all of the solutions generated by the open-ended questions. 3. Administer the checklist to a consumer group. 4. Identify the solutions that the consumers would be most likely to use.
Module Development	1. Create skills-training curriculum about the problem based on the literature and consumer input. 2. Create skills-training curriculum about solutions based on the literature and consumer input.

Source: Holmes, E. P., Corrigan, P. W., Knight, S., & Flaxman, J. (1995). Development of a sleep management program for people with severe mental illness. Psychiatric Rehabilitation Journal, 19, 9–15.

BOX 47-1 ■ Strategies for Skills Training

I. Motivational strategies
- Incorporate both internal and external rewards/motivators
- Match the motivators with the content of a program
- Create an environment that conveys your expectations that participants will learn from the experience
- Use certificates, graduation ceremonies, and so on, to reinforce accomplishments

II. Application to real life
- Make sure that you know what real life is for your group members
- Practice in real-life environments whenever possible
- Facilitate generalization by practicing in multiple real-life environments
- Use homework so individuals can practice skills at home
- Include staff, families, peers, and others in the training

III. Repeated practice
- Teach a topic over multiple sessions
- Incorporate several ways of teaching and practicing the same content
- Use homework for more opportunities to practice
- Encourage families, staff, peers, and others to promote opportunities for practice

IV. Provide feedback about performance
- Make expectations clear
- Use worksheets/quizzes and provide written feedback
- Provide regular verbal feedback for performance
- Have group members work with partners and encourage feedback among peers

V. Evaluate knowledge and/or skill acquisition
- Use quizzes or worksheets that you can review
- Observe performance
- Incorporate question-and-answer sessions or contests
- Have homework that group members turn in

VI. Match environmental and individual needs
- Allow lots of opportunities for choice
- Encourage group members to come up with their own examples
- Use the environments that the group members use
- Adapt the intervention for environmental or individual differences
- Provide multiple suggestions or techniques and help participants determine which strategy works best for them

Evidence-Based Practice

Individuals with serious mental illness can learn new self-care and IADLs; however, training needs to occur over multiple sessions, and the skills are not readily generalizable.

➤ Occupational therapists can use existing manualized ADL and IADL modules or create skill-training interventions using strategies successfully applied in existing skills-training models (simplifying the task, repeated practice, feedback, reinforcements).

➤ Occupational therapists can support generalization by training in multiple real-life environments and encouraging other providers, family members, friends, and so on, to support the individual in using newly learned skills.

Bellack, A. S. (2004). Skills training for people with severe mental illness. *Psychiatric Rehabilitation Journal, 27*, 375–391.

Heinssen, R. K., Liberman, R. P., & Kopelowicz, A. (2000). Psychosocial skills training for schizophrenia: Lessons from the laboratory. *Schizophrenia Bulletin, 26*, 21–46.

An integral part of IPSRT involves keeping a daily record of activities using the Social Rhythm Metric (Monk, Flaherty, Frank, & Hoskinson, 1990). With the Social Rhythm Metric, individuals learn to monitor their routines and strive for regularity in the timing of their daily activities. Individuals with bipolar disorder in IPSRT identify the most unstable rhythms in their lives, set goals for change, and identify triggers that lead to disruptions. They also work to find the right balance of rest and activity. In addition to intervention targeting daily routines, IPSRT includes education about bipolar disorder and medications and family education sessions to gain social support.

Home Environmental Skill-Building Program

The Home Environmental Skill-Building Program (ESP) is an intervention designed for people with dementia in which occupational therapists teach caregivers how to modify the environment (Gitlin, Corcoran, Winter, Boyce, & Marcus, 1999). The intervention occurs over five 90-minute sessions. Three types of strategies are taught: (1) simplification of the physical environment, (2) modification of the caregiver's approach to assisting with ADL and IADL tasks, and (3) involvement of others in the caregiving process. For example, to modify the physical environment, caregivers are encouraged to eliminate clutter and use relevant assistive devices. In terms of the caregiver's approach, recommendations are made to establish daily routines and limit commands to one or two steps. Finally, caregivers are encouraged to utilize social supports, such as involving other family members in caregiving or joining a support group.

In a randomized, controlled trial of the short-term effects of ESP, there was slightly less decline in IADL performance in the treatment group when compared with the control participants (Gitlin et al, 2001). In another study examining the six-month outcomes of ESP, caregiver improvements were detected (Gitlin, Corcoran, Winter, Boyce, & Hauck, 2003). The program was effective in reducing objective and subjective stress, and there was an improvement in overall wellbeing for caregivers.

of the disorder. Therefore, it is hypothesized that "social rhythm disruption" interferes with normal circadian rhythms, which leads to manic symptoms. Interpersonal and social rhythm therapy (IPSRT) was developed as a psychosocial intervention for people with bipolar disorder.

IPSRT uses principles of interpersonal therapy and combines these techniques with an intervention to address daily routines (Frank et al, 2005) like traditional interpersonal therapy (Klerman, Weissman, Rounsaville, & Chevron, 1984), IPSRT targets one of four problem areas: grief, interpersonal role transition, role dispute, and interpersonal deficits. In addition, IPSRT examines how interpersonal problems affect daily routines.

Applied Behavioral Analysis

Applied behavioral analysis (ABA) is often used in teaching new skills to individuals with developmental disabilities. This approach relies heavily on measurement of observable behaviors throughout the process. ABA has a long history with an important publication of the approach going back to Snell in 1974. Snell describes five specific steps to ABA:

1. Direct measurement and task analysis of the positive behavior.
2. Daily measurement of targeted responses before intervention.
3. Development and implementation of a systematic and replicable approach to teaching the behavior.
4. Graphing of the individual's behavior or response to treatment.
5. Controlled single-subject approaches to show that the intervention was responsible for the behavior change.

ABA is criticized for its level of intensity and intrusiveness and limited generalizability (Schoen, 2003). Instruction in natural environments is encouraged to support real-world application.

ABA has evolved over time and often incorporates additional approaches to support the maintenance and generalization of skills. One such approach is correspondence training (Guevremont, Osnes, & Stokes, 1986). In this self-talk approach, a "say, do, report" strategy is used. The individual is instructed to (1) say what he or she is going to do, (2) perform the task, and (3) report that the

task is completed. Using a single-subject design, Stokes, Cameron, Dorsey, and Fleming (2004) found that a multi-component approach incorporating ABA techniques and correspondence training was effective in teaching bowel hygiene to three individuals with developmental disabilities.

Evidence-Based Practice

Disruptions in daily routines can lead to exacerbations of symptoms in people with depression and bipolar disorder.

➤ Interventions for people with mood disorders should include strategies that promote the establishment of regularity in the timing of everyday activities.

Grandin, L. D., Alloy, L. B., & Abramson, L. Y. (2006). The social zeitgeber theory, circadian rhythms, and mood disorders: Review and evaluation. *Clinical Psychology Review, 26,* 679–694.

Summary

ADLs and IADLs are the basic occupations that comprise everyday life. There are many reasons why performance of ADLs and IADLs may be difficult for people with mental illness. Consequently, it requires skilled assessment and intervention on the part of the occupational therapist to best address the individual and specific ADL and IADL needs of the client.

Active Learning Strategies

1. ADL and IADL Performance Interview

Interview a person with a mental illness. Find out which ADLs and IADLs the person performs in a successful and satisfying way and which ones are challenging. From the person's perspective, see if you can learn what is different about one activity he or she is able to do well and one that is difficult. The following questions may be helpful:

- How important is this activity to you?
- What do you like and dislike most about doing it?
- Is it easy or difficult? What makes it easy or difficult?
- Do you do it alone or with others? Do you have any help?
- Where do you do it? What do you like and dislike about the place?
- When do you do it?
- Do you have the money, supplies, and so on, to do it the way you want to?
- How do you feel when you're doing it?

Summarize what you've learned from the interview and formulate ideas for what facilitates and interferes with IADL performance for this individual. What additional information would you like to have to create an intervention plan? What observations or standardized assessments would you want to conduct?

2. ADL and IADL Self-Assessment

Go through this same activity for yourself. Which aspects of IADL performance do you share with the person you interviewed, and which aspects are different?

Reflective Questions
- Many of us take for granted the performance of ADLs and IADLs. For example, we may not put much thought into brushing our teeth; we tend to perform the task almost automatically. Can you recall times when basic ADLs or IADLs were challenging for you? What made it difficult, and why?
- What aspects of mental illness might make an ADL or IADL require more mental or physical effort?
- In terms of barriers to performance, are there differences in the types of barriers you experience versus the barriers for the person you interviewed?
- Are most of the barriers related to person factors or the environment?

 Use your **Reflective Journal** to document your experience and thoughts.

Resources

Assessments
• Asher, I. E. (2007). *Occupational Therapy Assessment Tools: An Annotated Index* (3rd ed.). Bethesda, MD: American Occupational Therapy Association.

Assessment of Motor and Process Skills
• AMPS Project International: http://ampsintl.com

Functional Independence Measure and WeeFim
• Uniform Data System for Medical Rehabilitation
270 Northpointe Parkway, Suite 300
Amherst, New York 14228
(716) 817-7800; Fax: (716) 568-0037
E-mail: info@udsmr.org
Web site: http://www.udsmr.org

Kohlman Evaluation of Living Skills (KELS)
• Thompson, L. K. (1992). *Kohlman Evaluation of Living Skills (KELS)* (3rd ed.). Bethesda, MD: American Occupational Therapy Association.

Independent Living Skills Survey
• Wallace, C. J., Liberman, R. P., Tauber, R., & Wallace, J. (2000). The Independent Living Skills Survey: A comprehensive measure of the community functioning of severely and persistently mentally ill individuals. *Schizophrenia Bulletin, 26,* 631–658. The actual instrument is appended to the article.

Pediatric Evaluation of Disability Inventory (PEDI)
• Health and Disability Research Institute:
http://www.bu.edu/hdr/products/pedi/index.html
PEDI Research Group
Department of Rehabilitation Medicine
New England Medical Center Hospital
#75K/R
750 Washington Street
Boston, MA 02111-1901

Test of Grocery Shopping Skills
• Brown, C., Rempfer, M. & Hamera, E. (2009) *The Test of Grocery Shopping Skills.* Bethesda, MD: AOTA Press.

Intervention
• Interpersonal and Social Rhythm Therapy
• Frank, E. (2005). *Treating Bipolar Disorder: A Clinician's Guide to Interpersonal and Social Rhythm Therapy.* New York, NY: Guilford.

UCLA Social and Independent Living Skills Modules
• Psychiatric Rehabilitation Consultants:
http://www.psychrehab.com/

Medication Management
• E-Pill Medication Reminders: http://www.epill.com Multiple systems for medication management

Transportation
• Association of Driving Rehabilitation Specialists
109 West Street
Edgerton, WI 53534
(608) 884-8833
http://www.driver-ed.org
• Finn, J., Gross, M., Hunt, L., McCarthy, D., Pierce, S., Redepenning, S., Stav, W., Wheatley, C., & Davis, E. S. (2004). Driving evaluation and retraining programs: A report of good practices. Bethesda, MD: AOTA. (This collaborative report from AOTA and the National Highway Traffic Safety Administration is in the public domain and available for free download at http://www.aota.org.)

References

Baum, C., & Edwards, D. F. (1993). Cognitive performance in senile dementia of the Alzheimer's type: The Kitchen Task Assessment. *American Journal of Occupational Therapy, 47,* 431–436.

Bellack, A. S. (2004). Skills training for people with severe mental illness. *Psychiatric Rehabilitation Journal, 27,* 375–391.

Black, B. S., Rabins, P. V., German, P., McGuire, M., & Roca, R. (1997). Need and unmet need for mental health care among elderly public housing residents. *Gerontologist. 37*(6), 717–728.

Bochner, S., Outhred, L., Pieterse, M., & Bashash, L. (2002). Numeracy and money management skills in young adults with Down syndrome. In M. Cuskelly, A. Jobling, & S. Buckley (Eds.), *Down Syndrome Across the Life Span* (pp. 93–106). Philadelphia: Whurr.

Boyle, P. A. (2004). Assessing and predicting functional impairment in Alzheimer's disease: The emerging role of frontal system dysfunction. *Current Psychiatry Report, 6,* 20–24.

Brown C., Dasler P., Munoz J. P., & Cox B. (1999). Lessons learned the hard way . . . Skills training versus psychosocial occupational therapy for persons with persistent schizophrenia. *Mental Health Special Interest Section Quarterly, 22*(2), 3–4.

Brown, C., Moore, W. P., Hemman, C., & Yunek, A. (1996). Influence of instrumental activities of daily living assessment method on judgments of independence. *American Journal of Occupational Therapy, 50,* 202–206.

Brown, C., Rempfer, M., & Hamera, E. (2002). Teaching grocery shopping skills to people with schizophrenia. *Occupational Therapy Journal of Research, 22*(Suppl1), 90S–91S.

Brown, L. B., Ott, B. R., Papandonatos, G. D., Sui, Y., Ready, R. E., & Morris, J. C. (2005). Prediction of on-road driving performance in patients with early Alzheimer's disease. *Journal of the American Geriatric Society, 53,* 94–98.

Davies, D. K., Stock, S. E., & Wehmeyer, M. L. (2003). Utilization of computer technology to facilitate money management by individuals with mental retardation. *Education and Training in Developmental Disabilities, 38,* 106–112.

Davis, J., & Kutter, C. J. (1998). Independent living skills and posttraumatic stress disorder in women who are homeless: Implications for future practice. *American Journal of Occupational Therapy, 52,* 39–44.

Deegan, P. (1996). Recovery as a journey of the heart. *Psychiatric Rehabilitation Journal, 19*(3), 91–97.

Dencker, K., & Gottfries, C. G. (1995) Activities of daily living ratings of elderly people using Katz's ADL Index and the GBS-M scale. *Scandinavian Journal of Caring Sciences, 9,* 35–40.

Dickerson, F. B. (1997). Assessing clinical outcomes: The community functioning of persons with serious mental illness. *Psychiatric Services, 48*(7), 897–902.

Dixon, L., Turner, J., Krauss, N., Scott, J., & McNary, S. (1999). Case managers' and clients' perspectives on a representative payee program. *Psychiatric Services, 50,* 781–786.

Duncombe, L. W. (2004). Comparing learning of cooking in home and clinic for people with schizophrenia. *American Journal of Occupational Therapy, 58,* 272–278.

Dunlop, D. D., Manheim, L. M., Song, J., Lyons, J. S., & Chang, R. W. (2005). Incidence of disability among preretirement adults: The impact of depression. *American Journal of Public Health, 95,* 2003–2008.

Eckman, T. A., Wirshing, W. C., Marder, S. R., Liberman, R. P., Johnston-Cronk, K., Zimmerman, K., & Mintz, J. (1992). Technique for training schizophrenic patients in illness self-management: A controlled trial. *American Journal of Psychiatry, 149,* 1549–1555.

Elbogen, E. B., Swanson, J. W., Swartz, M. S., & Wagner, H. R. (2003). Characteristics of third-party money management for persons with psychiatric disabilities. *Psychiatric Services, 54,* 1136–1141.

Fisher, A. G. (2001). *Assessment of Motor and Process Skills, Vol. 2: User Manual* (4th ed.). Fort Collins, CO: Three Star Press.

Fleck, D. E., Keck, P. E., Corey, K. B., & Strakowski, S. M. (2005). Factors associated with medication adherence in African American and white patients with bipolar disorder. *Journal of Clinical Psychiatry, 66,* 646–652.

Frank, E., Kupfer, D. J., Thase, M. E., Mallinger, A. G., Swartz, H. A., Fagiolini, A. M., Grochocinski, V., Houck, P., Scott, J., Thompson, W., & Monk, T. (2005). Two-year outcomes for interpersonal and social rhythm therapy in individuals with bipolar I disorder. *Archives of General Psychiatry, 62,* 996–1004.

Gitlin, L. N., Corcoran, M., Winter, L., Boyce, A., & Hauck, W. W. (2001). A randomized, controlled trial of a home environmental intervention: Effect on efficacy and upset in caregivers and on daily function of persons with dementia. *Gerontologist, 41,* 4–14.

Gitlin, L. N., Corcoran, M., Winter, L., Boyce, A., & Marcus, S. (1999). Predicting participation and adherence to a home environmental intervention among family caregivers of persons with dementia. *Family Relations, 48,* 363–372.

Gitlin, L. N., Winter, L., Corcoran, M., Dennis, M. P., Schinfeld, S., & Hauck, W. W. (2003). Effects of the Home Environmental Skill-Building Program on the caregiver-care recipient dyad: 6-month outcomes from the Philadelphia REACH initiative. *Gerontologist, 43,* 532–546.

Glynn, S. M., Marder, S. R., Liberman, R. P., Blair, K., Wirshing, W. D., Wirshing, D. A., Ross, D., & Mintz, J. (2002). Supplementing clinic-based skills training with manual-based community support sessions: Effects on social adjustment of patients with schizophrenia. *American Journal of Psychiatry, 159,* 829–837.

Goldstein, G., McCue, M., Rogers, J., & Nussbaum, P. D. (1994). Diagnostic differences in memory test based predictions of functional capacity in the elderly. *Neuropsychological Rehabilitation, 2,* 307–317.

Gosman-Hedstrom, G., & Svensson, E. (2000). Parallel reliability of the Functional Independence Measure and the Barthel ADL index. *Disability and Rehabilitation, 22,* 702–715.

Grandin, L. D., Alloy, L. B., & Abramson, L. Y. (2006). The social zeitgeber theory, circadian rhythms, and mood disorders: review and evaluation. *Clinical Psychology Review, 26,* 679–694.

Guevremont, D. C., Osnes, P. G., & Stokes, T. F. (1986). Programming maintenance after correspondence training interventions with children. *Journal of Applied Behavior Analysis, 19,* 215–219.

Haley, S. M., Coster, W. J., Ludlow, L. H., Haltiwanger, J. T., & Andrellos, P. J. (1992). *Pediatric Evaluation of Disability Inventory (PEDI) 1.0: Development, Standardization and Administration Manual.* Boston: New England Medical Center Hospitals.

Hamera, E., Brown, C., Rempfer, M., & Davis, N. (2002). Test of grocery shopping skills: discrimination of people with and without mental illness. *Psychiatric Rehabilitation Skills, 6,* 296–311.

Hamilton, B. B., Granger, C. V., Sherwin, F. S., Zielezny, M., & Tashman, J. S. (1987). A uniform national data system for medical rehabilitation. In M. J. Fuhrer (Ed.), *Rehabilitation Outcomes: Analysis and Measurements* (pp. 137–147). Baltimore: Brookes.

Heinssen, R. K., Liberman, R. P., & Kopelowicz, A. (2000). Psychosocial skills training for schizophrenia: Lessons from the laboratory. *Schizophrenia Bulletin, 26,* 21–46.

Holm, M. B., & Rogers, J. C. (1999). Performance assessment of self care skills. In B. J. Hemphill-Pearson (Ed.), *Assessments in Occupational Therapy Mental Health* (pp. 117–124). Thorofare, NJ: Slack.

Holmes, E. P., Corrigan, P. W., Knight, S., & Flaxman, J. (1995). Development of a sleep management program for people with severe mental illness. *Psychiatric Rehabilitation Journal, 19,* 9–15.

Houlden, H., Edwards, M., McNeil, J., & Greenwood, R. (2006). Use of the Barthel Index and the Functional Independence measure during early inpatient rehabilitation after single incident brain injury. *Clinical Rehabilitation, 20,* 153–159.

Hsueh, I. P., Lin, J. H., Jeng, J. S., & Hsieh, C. L. (2006). Comparison of the psychometric characteristics of the functional independence measure, 5-item Barthel index and 10-item Barthel index in patients with stroke. *Journal of Neurological and Neurosurgical Psychiatry, 73,* 188–190.

Hudson, T. J., Owen, R. R., Thrush, C. R., Han, X., Pyne, J. M., Thapa, P., & Sullivan, G. (2004). A pilot study of barriers to medication adherence in schizophrenia. *Journal of Clinical Psychiatry, 65,* 211–216.

Ilika, J., & Hoffman, N. G. (1981). Reliability study on the Kohlman Evaluation of Living Skills. Unpublished manuscript.

Jeste, S. D., Patterson, T. L., Palmer, B. W., Dolder, C. R., Goldman, R., & Jeste, D. V. (2003). Cognitive predictors of medication adherence among middle-aged and older outpatients with schizophrenia. *Schizophrenia Research, 63,* 49–58.

Jones, B. N., Jayaram, G., Samuels, J., & Robinson, H. (1998). Relating competency status to functional status at discharge in patients with chronic mental illness. *Journal of the American Academy of Psychiatry & the Law, 26,* 49–55.

Katz, S. (1983). Assessing self-maintenance: Activities of daily living, mobility, instrumental activities of daily living. *Journal of the American Geriatrics Society, 31,* 721–726.

Klerman, G. L., Weissman, M. M., Rounsaville, B. J., & Chevron, E. S. (1984). *Interpersonal Therapy of Depression: A Brief, Focused Specific Strategy.* New York: Basic Books.

Kochhar, S. M., & Scott, C. G. (1995). Disability patterns among SSI recipients. *Social Security Bulletin, 58,* 3–14.

Kottorp, A, Bernspang, G., & Fisher, A. G. (2003). Validity of a performance assessment of activities of daily living for people with developmental disabilities. *Journal of Intellectual Disability Research, 47,* 597–605.

Lawton, M. P., & Brody, E. (1969). Assessment of older people: Self-maintaining and instrumental activities of daily living. *Gerontologist, 9,* 179–186.

Leonardelli, C. A. (1988). *The Milwaukee Evaluation of Daily Living Skills: Evaluation in Long-Term Psychiatric Care.* Thorofare, NJ: Slack.

Liberman, R. P., Blair, K. E., Glynn, S. M., Marder, S. R., Wirshing, W., & Wirshing, D. A. (2001). Generalization of skills training to the natural environment. In H. D. Brenner, W. Boker, & R. Genner (Eds.), *The Treatment of Schizophrenia: Status and Emerging Trends* (pp. 104–120). Seattle: Hogrefe & Huber.

Liberman, R. P., Mueser, K. T., Wallace, C. J., Jacobs, H. E., & Eckman, T. A. (1986). Training skills in the severely psychiatrically disabled: Learning coping and competence. *Schizophrenia Bulletin, 12,* 631–647.

Liberman, R. P., Wallace, C. J., Blackwell, G., Kopelowicz, A., Vaccaro, J. V., & Mintz, J. (1998). Skills training versus psychosocial occupational therapy for persons with persistent schizophrenia. *American Journal of Psychiatry, 155,* 1087–1091.

Lovell, R. K., & Russell, K. J. (2005). Developing referral and reassessment criteria for drivers with dementia. *Australian Occupational Therapy Journal, 52,* 26–33.

Maddigan, S. L., Farris, K. B., Keating, N., Wiens, C. A., & Johnson, J. A. (2003). Predictors of older adults' capacity for medication management in a self-medication program: A retrospective chart review. *Journal of Aging and Health, 15,* 332–352.

Mahoney, F. I., & Barthel, D. W. (1965). Functional evaluation: The Barthel index. *Maryland State Medical Journal, 14,* 61–65.

Marcus, C. C. (1997). *House as a Mirror of Self: Exploring the Deeper Meaning of Home.* Berkeley, CA: Conari Press.

Malkoff-Schwartz, S., Frank, E., Anderson, B., Sherrill, J. T., Siegel, L., Patterson, D., & Kupfer, D. J. (1998). Stressful life events and social rhythm disruption in the onset of manic and depressive bipolar episodes: A preliminary investigation. *Archives of General Psychiatry, 55,* 702–707.

McCall, W. V., & Dunn, A. G. (2003). Cognitive deficits are associated with functional impairment in severely depressed patients. *Psychiatry Research, 121,* 179–184.

McCue, M., Rogers, J. C., & Goldstein, G. (1990). Relationships between neuropsychological and functional assessment in elderly neuropsychiatric patients. *Rehabilitation Psychology, 35,* 91–99.

McDonald, H. P., Garg, A. X., & Haynes, R. B. (2002). Interventions to enhance patient adherence to medication prescriptions. *JAMA, 288,* 2868–2879.

McKibbin, C. L., Brekke, J. S., Sires, D., Jeste, D. V., & Patterson, T. L. (2004). Direct assessment of functional abilities: Relevance to persons with schizophrenia. *Schizophrenia Research, 72,* 53–67.

McNulty, M. C., & Fisher, A. G. (2001). Validity of using the assessment of motor and process skills to estimate overall home safety in persons with psychiatric conditions. *American Journal of Occupational Therapy, 55,* 649–655.

Miklowitz, D. J., George, E. L., Richards, J. A., Simoneau, T. L., & Suddath, R. L. (2003). A randomized study of family-focused psychoeducation and pharmacotherapy in the outpatient management of bipolar disorder. *Archives of General Psychiatry, 60,* 904–912.

Monk, T. K, Flaherty, J. F, Frank, E., & Hoskinson, K. (1990). The Social Rhythm Metric: An instrument to quantify the daily rhythms of life. *Journal of Nervous and Mental Disease, 178,* 120–126.

Msall, M. E., DiGuadio, K., Duffy, L. C., LaForest, S., Braun, S., & Granger, C. V. (1994). WeeFIM: Normative sample on an instrument for tracking functional independence in children. *Clinical Pediatrics, 33,* 431–438.

Mueser, K. T. (2004). To the editor. *Psychological Medicine, 34,* 1365–1367.

Mueser, K. T., Corrigan, P. W., Hilton, D. W., Tanzman, B., Schaub, A., Gingerich, S., Essock, S. M., Tarrier, N., Morey, B., Vogel-Scibilia, S., & Herz, M. I. (2002). Illness management and recovery: A review of the research. *Psychiatric Services, 53,* 1272–1284.

Neistadt, M. E. (1994). A meal preparation treatment protocol for adults with brain injury. *American Journal of Occupational Therapy, 48,* 431–438.

———. (1992). The Rabideau Kitchen Evaluation–Revised: An assessment of meal preparation skill. *Occupational Therapy Journal of Research, 12,* 242–255.

Nichols, D. S., & Case-Smith, J. (1996). Reliability and validity of the Pediatric Evaluation of Disability Inventory. *Pediatric Physical Therapy, 8,* 15–24.

Oakley, F., Duran, L., Fisher, A., & Merritt, B. (2003). Differences in activities of daily living motor skills of persons with and without Alzheimer's disease. *Australian Occupational Therapy Journal, 50,* 72–78.

O'Connor, R. J., Cano, S. J., Thompson, A. J., & Hobart, J. C. (2004). Exploring rating scale responsiveness: Does the total score reflect the sum of its parts? *Neurology, 62,* 1842–1844.

Ott, B. R., Anthony, D., Papandonatos, G. D., D'Abreu, A., Burock, J., Curtin, A., Wu, C. K., & Morris, J. C. (2005). Clinician assessment of the driving competence of patients with dementia. *Journal of the American Geriatric Society, 53,* 829–833.

Ottenbacher, K. J., Msall, M. E., Lyon, N., Duffy, L. C., Ziviani, J., Granger, C. V., Braun, S., & Feidler, R. C. (2000). The WeeFIM instrument: its utility in detecting change in children with developmental disabilities. *Archives of Physical Medicine and Rehabilitation, 81,* 1317–1326.

Ottenbacher, K. J., Taylor, E. T., Msall, M. E., Braun, S., Lane, S. J., Granger, C. V., Lyons, N., & Duffy, L. C. (1996). The stability and equivalence reliability of the functional independence measure for children (WeeFIM). *Developmental Medicine and Child Neurology, 38,* 907–916.

Patterson, T. L., Goldman, S., McKibbin, C. L., Hughs, T., & Jeste, D. V. (2001). UCSD Performance Based Skills Assessment: Development of a new measure of everyday functioning for severely mentally ill adults. *Schizophrenia Bulletin, 27,* 235–245.

Patterson, T. L., McKibben, C., Taylor, M., Goldman, S., Davila-Fraga, W., Bucardo, J., & Jeste, D. (2003). Functional Adaptation Skills Training: A pilot psychosocial intervention study in middle-aged and older patients with chronic psychotic disorders. *American Journal of Geriatric Psychiatry, 11,* 17–23.

Paul, R. H., Cohen, R. A., Moser, D. J., Zawacki, T., Ott, B. R., Gordon, N., & Stone, W. (2002). The Global Deterioration Scale: Relationships to neuropsychological performance and activities of daily living in patients with vascular dementia. *Journal of Geriatric Psychiatry and Neurology, 15,* 50–54.

Perivoliotis, D., Granholm, E., & Patterson, T. L. (2004). Psychosocial functioning on the Independent Living Skills Survey in older outpatients with schizophrenia. *Schizophrenia Research, 69,* 307–316.

Pilling, S., Bebbington, P., Kuipers, E., Garety, P., Geddes, J., Martindale, B., Orbach, G., & Morgan, C. (2002). Psychological treatment in schizophrenia: II. Meta-analyses of randomized controlled trials of social skills training and cognitive remediation. *Psychological Medicine, 32,* 783–791.

Pita, D. D., Ellison, M. L., Farkas, F., & Bleecker, T. (2001). Exploring personal assistance services for people with psychiatric disabilities: Need policy and practice. *Journal of Disability Policy Studies, 12*(1), 2–9.

Purser, J. L., Fillenbaum, G. G., Pieper, C. F., & Wallace, R. B. (2005) Mild cognitive impairment and 10-year trajectories of disability in the Iowa established populations for epidemiologic studies of the elderly cohort. *Journal of the American Geriatrics Society, 53,* 1966–1972.

Rabideau, G. M. (1986). Two approaches to improving the functional performance of a cognitively impaired head injured adult. Masters' thesis. Tufts University: Medford, MA.

Rempfer, M., Hamera, E., Brown, C., & Cromwell, R. L. (2003). Cognition and performance of an independent living skill in people with schizophrenia. *Psychiatry Research, 117,* 103–112.

Rog, D. J. (2004). The evidence on supported housing. *Psychiatric Rehabilitation Journal, 27,* 334–344.

Rogers, J. C., & Holm, M. B. (2000). Daily-living skills and habits of older women with depression. *Occupational Therapy Journal of Research, 20,* S68–S85.

Rogers, J. C., Holm, M. B., Beach, S., Schulz, R., Cipriani, J., Fox, A., & Starx, T. W. (2003). Concordance of four methods of disability assessment using performance in the home as the criterion method. *Arthritis & Rheumatism (Arthritis Care and Research), 49,* 640–647.

Rosen, M. I., Bailey, M., & Rosenheck, R. R. (2003). Principles of money management as a therapy for addiction. *Psychiatric Services, 54,* 171–173.

Rosen, M. I., Desai, R., Bailey, M., Davidson, L., & Rosenheck, R. (2001). Consumer experience with payeeship provided by a community mental health center. *Psychiatric Rehabilitation Journal, 24,* 190–195.

Royall, D. R., Palmer, R., Chiodo, L. K., & Polk, M. J. (2005). Executive control mediates memory's association with change in instrumental activities of daily living: The Freedom House Study. *Journal of the American Geriatrics Society, 53,* 11–17.

Rüesch, P., Graf, J., Meyer, P. C., Rössler, W., & Hell, D. (2004). Occupation, social support and quality of life in persons with schizophrenic or affective disorders. *Social Psychiatry and Psychiatric Epidemiology, 39,* 686–694.

Salkow, K., & Fichter, M. (2003). Homelessness and mental illness. *Current Opinion in Psychiatry, 16,* 467–471.

Schoen, A. A. (2003). What potential does the applied behavior analysis approach have for the treatment of children and youth with autism. *Journal of Instructional Psychology, 30,* 125–130.

Schretlen, D., Jayaram, G., Maki, P., Parke, K., Abebe, S., & DiCarlo, M. (2000). Demographic, clinical and neurocognitive correlates of everyday functional impairment in severe mental illness. *Journal of Abnormal Psychology, 109,* 134–138.

Scott, J. E., & Dixon, L. B. (1995). Psychological interventions for schizophrenia. *Schizophrenia Bulletin, 21,* 621–630.

Sirey, J. A., Bruce, M. L., Alexopoulos, G. S., Perlick, D. A., Friedman, S. J., & Meyers, B. S. (2001). Perceived stigma and patient-rated severity of illness as predictors of antidepressant drug adherence. *Psychiatric Services, 52,* 1615–1620.

Snell, M. E. (1974). *Systematic Instruction of the Moderately and Severely Handicapped.* Columbus: Charles E Merrill.

Stokes, J. R., Cameron, M. J., Dorsey, M. F., & Fleming, E. (2004). Task analysis, correspondence training, and general case instruction for teaching personal hygiene skills. *Behavioral Interventions, 19,* 121–135.

Suto, M., & Gelya, F. (1994). Future time perspective and daily occupations of persons with chronic schizophrenia in a board and care home. *American Journal of Occupational Therapy, 48,* 7–18.

Tateichi, S. A. (1984). Concurrent validity study of the Kohlman Evaluation of Living Skills. Master's thesis. Seattle: University of Washington.

Thomson, L. K. (1992). *The Kohlman Evaluation of Living Skills* (3rd ed.). Bethesda, MD: American Occupational Therapy Association.

Tuokko, H., Morris, C., & Ebert, P. (2005). Mild cognitive impairment and everyday functioning in older adults. *Neurocase, 11*(1), 40–47.

Twamley, E. W., Doshi, R. R., Nayak, G. V., Palmer, B. W., Golshan, S., Heaton, R. K., Patterson, T. L., & Jeste, D. V. (2002). Generalized cognitive impairments, ability to perform everyday tasks and level of independence in community living situations of older patients with psychosis. *American Journal of Psychiatry, 159,* 2013–2020.

Vergouwen, A. C. M., Bakker, A., Katon, W. J., Verheij, T. J., & Koerselman, F. (2003). Improving adherence to antidepressants: A systematic review of interventions. *Journal of Clinical Psychiatry, 26,* 1415–1420.

Voils, C. I., Steffens, D. C., Flint, E. P., & Bosworth, H. B. (2005). Social support and locus of control as predictors of adherence to antidepressant medication in an elderly population. *American Journal of Geriatric Psychiatry, 13,* 157–165.

Walker, E., Kestler, L., Bollini, A., & Hochman, K. M. (2004). Schizophrenia: Etiology and course. *Annual Review of Psychology, 55,* 401–430.

Wallace, C. J., Liberman, R. P., MacKain, S. J., Blackwell, G., & Eckman, T. E. (1992). Effectiveness and replicability of modules for teaching social and instrumental skills to the severely mentally ill. *American Journal of Psychiatry, 149,* 654–658.

Wallace, C. J., Liberman, R. P., Tauber, R., & Wallace, J. (2000). The Independent Living Skills Survey: A comprehensive measure of the community functioning of severely and persistently mentally ill individuals. *Schizophrenia Bulletin, 26,* 631–658.

Wallace, D., Duncan, P. W., & Lai, S. M. (2002). Comparison of the responsiveness of the Barthel Index and the motor component of the Functional Independence Measure in stroke: The impact of using different methods for measuring responsiveness. *Journal of Clinical Epidemiology, 55,* 922–928.

Weinmann, S., Janssen, B., & Gaebel, W. (2005). Guideline adherence in medication management of psychotic disorders: An observational multisite hospital study. *Acta Psychiatrica Scandinavica, 112,* 18–25.

Wright, F. V., & Boschen, K. A. (1993). The Pediatric Evaluation of Disability Inventory: Validation of a new functional assessment outcome instrument. *Canadian Journal of Rehabilitation, 7,* 41–42.

Zimnavoda, T., Weinblatt, N., & Katz, N. (2002). Validity of the Kohlman Evaluation of Living Skills (KELS) with Israeli elderly individuals living in the community. *Occupational Therapy International, 9,* 312–325.

Zygmunt, A., Olfson, M., Boyer, C. A., & Mechanic, D. (2002). Interventions to improve medication adherence in schizophrenia. *American Journal of Psychiatry, 159,* 1653–1664.

Student: K Through 12

Judith S. Gonyea

> "*Education is not to reform students or amuse them or make them expert technicians. It is to unsettle their minds, widen their horizons, inflame their intellects, teach them to think straight, if possible.*
>
> —Robert M. Hutchins

Introduction

John Fitzgerald and his family successfully navigated the world of K–12 (kindergarten through high school) education despite the challenges of occasional tormentors and a system that had not yet fully embraced the concept of inclusion. John was not a typical learner. Equipped with a sensory system that provided inconsistent information—sometimes too much and sometimes too little—John found the classroom was a place of undetermined joys and perils. His primary occupations as learner and classmate were constantly being reframed by the demands of his environment. Despite these challenges, John successfully completed high school, became an Eagle Scout, registered to vote, earned his driver license, and is successfully employed in the community. Finding the *just right* situation for John's learning required collaboration across a broad range of services, providers, and advocates.

Research suggests that more than half of the lifetime cases of mental illness begin before age 14 (Kessler, Chiu, Demler, Merikangas, & Walters, 2005). It is estimated that in the course of one year, more than one in five children and adolescents has a diagnosable emotional disturbance that can interfere with school performance (Koppelman, 2004; U.S. Department of Health and Human Services, 1999). In addition to autism, common disorders include anxiety and mood disorders, behavioral and conduct disorders, learning disorders, and attention deficit hyperactivity disorder (Koppelman, 2004).

Unfortunately, the vast majority of students in need of mental health services do not receive these services (Kutash, Duchnowski, & Lynn, 2006). Unmet mental health needs not only impact academic performance, but also social and occupational functioning (American Occupational Therapy Association [AOTA], 2008). Surveys of school-based practitioners collectively report that therapists are most likely to address fine and gross motor skills, handwriting, perceptual skills, and sensory awareness (Barnes, Beck, Vogel, Grice, & Murphy, 2003; Clark, 2001; Powell, 1994). Practitioners in many of these surveys often report that they feel their level of training has been inadequate, and/or they express confusion about the professional role of occupational therapy

when addressing the complex academic, developmental, personal, social, and emotional needs of children with emotional and behavioral disorders.

Occupational therapists have a disciplinary knowledge base and specialized skill set to address children's mental health needs in school settings. This chapter examines some avenues for practitioners to use occupation-based interventions to address mental health needs in school-aged children. Many of the chapters in Part II of this text explore specific issues and interventions from a diagnostic perspective, and Chapter 36 specifically examines after-school programs. The focus here is to identify some of the learning and social participation challenges faced by children and adolescents with mental illnesses in school settings, to briefly highlight some useful assessments, and to provide an overview of interventions that can be considered with these populations.

Challenges in the K–12 Setting

School mental health is generally defined as mental health service that occurs in a school setting (Kutash et al, 2006). Mental health services in K–12 settings are often challenged by the conventions of the institution. Children with atypical behaviors or perceptions can be overwhelmed by the expectations of the school routine. The meaning or context of school activities may not be evident to them, and the learning may not come easy. Students are routinely asked to make adjustments to new settings, new teachers, new classmates, and expectations that may change with little notice.

Older students may face even more complex adaptation challenges. The onset of psychosis and other serious mental health conditions often occurs during adolescence. Because there are increasing demands for academic production, decisions about future life plans, and socialization demands from peers, students facing the additional challenge of altered perception and thought disorganization may feel too overwhelmed to continue participating in even the most basic routines (Downing, 2006). Eating disorders may also present during this life stage, often accompanied by mood disorders and creating complex psychosocial and health

The Lived Experience

Will

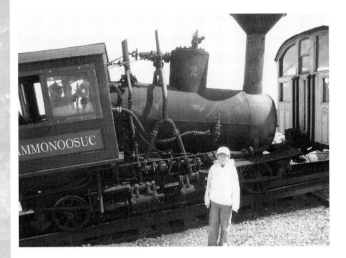

Will was diagnosed at age 3½ with Asperger syndrome. At that age, Will was struggling with many activities of daily living. He could zipper but not button. He could dress himself but only with considerable help. He could not color or draw at all, although he could fingerpaint and make collages. He could not play well with other children, had serious sensitivity to noise, and had anywhere from up to 10 meltdowns a week.

He started receiving speech-language therapy as soon as he was diagnosed and occupational therapy and social skills classes a few months later. Occupational therapy and social skills continued weekly for 3 years (ages 3–5).

Will went to a small, independent school for kindergarten through grade 3, and just this year, he transferred to public school. Will is now in grade 4, mainstreamed, with ongoing speech-language therapy and some help from a reading specialist. He is a good student and has no behavior problems. He has lots of special interests—steam trains, Star Wars, clocks, the presidents—that keep him busy. He is socially and emotionally about a year or two behind his peers, and he struggles to keep up with the flow of conversation and activity of his classmates. He is very sensitive, and he works hard at controlling his emotions.

When I was little, I remember that I didn't like to write with pencils. I liked fingerpainting, 'cause it was fun. It was easy to hold a pencil, but I didn't want to. My brain told me—don't hold a pencil—use fingerpaint. My OT was Miss Dunn. She was nice. And she had a lot of fun with me. She was easy on me, since I was small. She told me to snap my fingers, and I couldn't do it. So she taught me how to snap my fingers. And now, I'm pretty creative, and I'm pretty good at drawing. I draw mostly trains. I prefer drawing with pens because it's easier to get the ink on the paper, and they don't get dull. When pencils get dull, it's hard to get the marks on the paper and it hurts my hand. When my hand hurts, I ask my teacher if I can sharpen it. If I'm home, Mom has me shake out my hands, and we either play Push or Hand Slap to give my hands a rest.

At Country Day school, I liked gym and all the fun stuff. I didn't like anger. I'm always kind to kids and everyone, and I don't like it when they are angry with me.

I was nervous when I started my new school, but it was easy because I know what to say to make new friends. I know how to do that because my mom, and my daycare teachers, and Ms. Marcia, Miss Sue, and Miss Karen from social skills class, and Ms. Bergdoll and Mrs. Schmuck taught me what to say.

I like my new school. My teacher has a schedule for the day and for the week. That way we're organized instead of unorganized. I like to be organized because it's neat. You need to keep your desk neat and tidy. And I like to always know what's happening next. It makes me feel better. At school, math quizzes are easy for me—I can usually answer them quickly. The hard part for me is thinking about words I don't know and figuring out how to spell words.

Having Asperger syndrome mostly makes things easier for me. Some things are harder, but it doesn't happen often. The things that are easy for me are that I like numbers and I have a very good memory. I could tell time when I was 2 years old. It was really easy for me to memorize the multiplication table last year in 3rd grade. When I was in 2nd grade, I memorized all of the presidents of the United States, when they were born, when they served in office, and when they died. And I've read a little bit about each one. And it's easy for me to learn all about steam trains from videos and books and from visiting tourist railroads with my Mom and Dad.

---

problems (Arnow, Sanders, & Steiner, 1999; Santos, Richards, & Bleckley, 2007). The introduction of medications and/or new therapeutic interventions will further challenge students' learning and their participation with peers. Beliefs about competency and personal causation that may be challenging for any adolescent will further erode when an individual must deal with the additional challenges of a serious mental health condition (Henry & Coster, 1997).

John Dewey (1897) was a noted educational psychologist who championed educational reform that could have provided the framework for much of occupational therapy's beliefs regarding motivation and context in the primary and secondary school.

I believe that this educational process has two sides—one psychological and one sociological; and that neither can be subordinated to the other or neglected without evil results following. Of these two sides, the psychological is the basis. The child's own instincts and powers furnish the material and give the starting point for all education. Save as the efforts of the educator connect with some activity which the child is carrying on of his own initiative independent of the educator, education becomes reduced to a pressure from without. It may, indeed, give certain external results, but cannot truly be called educative. Without insight into the psychological structure and activities of the individual, the educative process will, therefore, be haphazard and arbitrary. If it chances to coincide with the child's activity it will get leverage; if it does not, it will result in friction, or disintegration, or arrest of the child's nature." (p. 77)

Meeting children "where they are" and leading them into discovery and participation provides a much less intimidating scenario for different learners and their classmates. This approach to facilitating participation in learning is consistent with occupational therapy's belief in individualizing interventions that recognize each person's attributes and strengths. Nonetheless, practitioners' ability to implement occupation-based interventions can be enhanced by their own research into teaching and learning theories and learning styles. There are several models of learning styles (Jackson, 2005; Kolb, 1984; Sprenger, 2003) that may help practitioners consider a student's approach to learning and design occupation-based methods to support student mastery. Table 48-1 lists some learning styles and occupation-based instructional strategies that may be considered.

Social Participation

For the student with mental health needs, the role of peer may be extremely demanding. Interactions during recess and other free times are far less predictable than those in the classroom. Children who are particularly sensitive to emotional or physical interaction may respond to these demands with self-protective or primal response, failing to demonstrate or even losing essential self-care and interpersonal skills. Kjorstad, O'Hare, Soseman, Spellman, and Thomas (2005) noted these significant skill deficits in children with posttraumatic stress disorder. Socialization skills, such as appropriate expression of emotions, controlling temper, and frustration tolerance, were particularly challenging for many. Others were noted to have tendencies toward withdrawal or nonparticipation.

Javaherian (2006) noted that children from homes in which there is a history of domestic violence may be uniquely challenged by the further influence of a parent's disability or inability to provide safety and support. Knowledge of

appropriate peer interaction may be limited or altogether missing. Similarly, older children with a history of violence, substance abuse, and/or other social conduct disorders may lack the confidence or trust to engage in meaningful peer relationships without support (Javaherian & Hewitt, 2007).

Children with pervasive developmental disorder, autism, and other developmental challenges have also been noted to face particular challenges in control of behavior and adjustment to socially demanding environments (Walz & Baranek, 2006; Watling, 2005). Lack of understanding or an inability to process social expectations can result in restricted participation and/or rejection by their peers. Nonverbal learning disability, for instance, restricts the executive thinking required for more demanding social engagement. McCarthy (2002) noted how these students develop more significant gaps with their peers as social and performance expectations increase in later elementary grades.

High school and teen culture brings on a whole new set of interpersonal challenges, and the occupational therapist should be ready to assess the student's readiness for this increasing social challenge and evaluate social participation with peers during a variety of school activities (e.g., classroom, lunch, recess, assemblies). Working with groups of students struggling with peer interaction, using role-playing, games, or discussion to elicit concerns and practice effective interpersonal techniques, may help support meaningful participation in school activities.

Education

The other major area of school participation concerns education or the learning process itself. This is frequently the source of referral for occupational therapy services as cognitive, perceptual, or neuromusculoskeletal functions restrict participation in school tasks. The ability to complete tasks in the expected amount of time or to effectively communicate verbally or through writing may place the child in academic jeopardy. The No Child Left Behind Act of 2001 (U.S. Department of Education, 2007) has increased the pressure on schools to include students with special needs in typical educational experiences.

For students with mental health challenges, the design of the environment and specific tasks may be particularly challenging. The occupational therapist can help the education team to select opportunities that maximize the student's ability to demonstrate requisite skills in a manner that is least disruptive to the academic environment and that fosters the most acceptance of the student by peers and others. Specifically, the occupational therapist's analysis of the cognitive demands for learning as well as the social and sensory demands for classroom learning may help to identify accommodations that support the student's participation. In individual consultation with the teacher, recommendations for modifications to learning demands or classroom routines that can support both academic learning and socioemotional skill development can be explored. For example, a student who needs to fidget or move about while learning can be encouraged to participate when more active learning opportunities are offered in the classroom; the student can also be accommodated with a separate and movement-enabled testing location for evaluation.

Table 48-1 ● **Matching Learning Styles and Intervention Strategies**

Learning Style	Occupation-Based Strategies
Auditory	Activities that encourage learning through listening: verbal instructions and discussion, structured debates and paired problem-solving, use of YouTube stories
Concrete	Activities that emphasize facts and sequential learning processes: competition, activities requiring attention to detail and practical applications
Kinesthetic	Activities that emphasize movement and experience: gross motor activities; gesture, pantomime, and expressive movement; experiments
Reflective	Activities that include guided reflection: estimating performance, processing results, comparing experiences
Visual	Activities that encourage thinking with pictures: creating movies, art, diagrams, handouts, PowerPoint slideshows; use of imagination in activities

Performance-Based Assessments

The *Occupational Therapy Framework* emphasizes an understanding of clients within their various contexts (AOTA, 2002). This person-first view supports the clinician's understanding of each student as a unique learner with qualities that will influence his or her ability to meaningfully engage in desired and necessary occupations. It is important to note that each person has both chosen roles and roles prescribed by their society, community, family, school, and so on.

Within the context of the K–12 environment are performance demands as peer, learner, and student. Assessment should include an appreciation for the interplay of these roles and how the skills and needs of the student enable or restrict participation. The occupational profile of the child will reflect the various players in his or her life as well as the information available regarding his or her past and future expectations. Younger children and those with more complex disorders or family situations may present a particularly challenging profile to obtain. This should not restrict the initiation of the occupational therapy process, but the therapist should continue to pursue additional information, as available, in order to develop the most meaningful and effective intervention and transition plans.

As a baseline, using a tool such as the Canadian Occupational Performance Measure (Law et al. 1998) or the Social Profile (Donohue, 2007) may provide some insight into the student's ability to identify strengths and needs and interact with others. Affective measures of the student's mood and safety and of family dynamics may also be components of evaluations by psychologists or counselors. Results of these evaluations are important to factor into the overall picture of the student's strengths, needs, and goals.

When appropriate, a child who has an Individualized Education Program (IEP) should be involved in setting education goals. Federal law requires that older students be involved in their own transition planning (Individuals with Disabilities Education Act, 2004). Unfortunately, students' participation in these processes is often quite limited (Cameto, 2005). The Child Occupational Self-Assessment (Keller, Kafkes, Basu, Federico, & Keilhofner, 2005) is a child-centered assessment process that may facilitate a student's participation in educational and transition planning (Harney & Kramer, 2007). This tool is based on the model of human occupation and is designed to encourage the student to self-evaluate his or her competence in the occupations of childhood, including being a student, and to prioritize the relative importance of these various occupations (e.g., doing homework, participating in school activities, meeting role expectations).

Based on an assessment of school performance skills (e.g., ability to write effectively, complete assignments, and interact with peers), a variety of motor, cognitive processing, and visuoperceptual skills tests may be considered, as they would with any school-based referral. Underlying challenges, such as sensory processing deficits, may prevent a student from accurately interpreting the environment and should be a subject of investigation when unexplained emotional challenges emerge. The Sensory Profile (Dunn, 1999) for younger children and the Adolescent/Adult Sensory Profile (Brown & Dunn, 2002) each provide a view of the student's relationship with the sensory environment. For the younger child, parent or teacher report provides the foundation for the assessment. For adolescents, the format is designed for self-reporting, but these students may also need support from other individuals who are most familiar with their reactions to specific types of stimuli. Regarding children with traumatic histories or those with complex developmental disorders, these tests differentiate typically processing children from those who may overly seek sensory stimulation, those who avoid sensory stimulation, those who are overresponsive, and those who are underresponsive, including combinations and variations in response.

These assessments may provide additional information regarding a child's selection or avoidance of particular activities and ways in which the environment can be adapted or the child may acquire adapted skills or coping mechanisms to further his or her participation. A critical interplay takes place among performance skills, performance patterns, and client factors. Altered perceptions of the physical and social environment or difficulty managing responses to the environment will ultimately create a complex scenario that requires attention to all elements, not just the academic performance deficits. Academic performance may reflect more underlying affective deficits than actual neuromotor or processing deficits. Therapists should carefully consider the environment in which these evaluations occur, the student's familiarity and/or comfort with the evaluating therapist, and existing samples of work produced within various academic contexts (e.g., different subject, different teacher). Nonacademic work may also provide further insight into the student's performance potential.

Intervention

It is important for occupational therapists to understand the academic environment before initiating any interventions. Like any home or workplace, each academic environment has its own unique qualities and expectations. Philosophies of learning, teachers' backgrounds and understanding of specific populations, and the community within which the school is located all influence academic demands and expectations. The therapist who rushes in and out may fail to appreciate these unique environmental factors, setting the student up for a much more challenging academic or social experience (Ikiugu, 2007).

Young Children

Cara and MacRae (2005) noted the importance of structure and consistency in programming for younger children. This is true in academic as well as home environments. Therapists need to consider this when selecting both treatment environments and recommendations for ongoing approaches between therapy sessions. While pull-out sessions may be effective when developing a rapport with an otherwise mistrustful student or when working on skills that require specific equipment or a quieter or more private setting, many skills can be demonstrated within more inclusive contexts, such as the classroom, lunchroom, or on the playground (Skog, Vrnig, Castaneda, & Deitz, 2006). Involving peers in activities that promote skills development can increase the potential that these skills will be reinforced on a routine basis and within a more naturalistic context.

Evidence-Based Practice

Kutash (2007) reports on a subset of evidence-based programs (*N* = 20) addressing disruptive and aggressive behavior that can be implemented in schools. These programs use a variety of strategies. Universal intervention strategies are systematic schoolwide and community-oriented approaches designed to address risk factors for all youth in the school. Selective or targeted intervention strategies specifically target at-risk youth to provide supports intended to prevent more serious problem behaviors. Indicated intervention strategies directly focus on youth with significant, demonstrated emotionally and/or behaviorally disordered behaviors (Weisz, Sandler, Durlak, & Anton, 2005).

➤ Occupational therapists can benefit from educating themselves about the multiple evidence-based programs designed to develop emotional and behavioral competencies in school settings.

➤ Occupational therapists should examine programs employing each of these types of intervention strategies to explore methods for integrating occupation-based interventions that complement each of these approaches.

Universal Interventions: Promoting Alternative Thinking Strategies. Kusche, C., & Greenberg, M. (1994). *PATHS: Promoting Alternative Thinking Strategies.* South Deerfield, MA: Developmental Research Programs.

Selective Interventions: First Step to Success. Walker, H. M., Kavanagh, K., Golly, A. M., Stiller, B., Severson, H. H., & Feil, E. G. (1997). *First Step to Success.* Longmont, CO: Sopris West.

Indicated Interventions: Incredible Years. Webster-Stratton, C. (1992). The incredible years: A trouble-shooting guide for parents of children ages 3–8 years. Toronto: Umbrella Press.

Kutash, K. (2007). "Understanding school-based mental health services for students who are disruptive and aggressive: What works for whom?" Proceedings of Persistently Safe Schools: 2007 National Conference on Safe Schools and Communities. Available at: http://gwired.gwu.edu/hamfish/merlin-cgi/p/downloadFile/d/19150/n/off/other/1/name/019pdf (accessed September, 21, 2009).

Weisz, J., Sandler, I., Durlak, J., & Anton, B. (2005). Promoting and protecting youth mental health through evidence-based prevention and treatment. *American Psychologist 60*(6), 628–648.

Sensory integration or sensory processing therapies (Kranowitz, 2003) can promote a sense of control and increased tolerance for varying sensory environments for children identified with specific sensory modulation disorders or those who demonstrate significant hypersensitivity that may be linked to trauma or other life experiences. The ALERT Program and its How Does Your Engine Run? program provides an organized system for introduction of sensory strategies to the primary school population (Shellenberger & Williams, 2002). These programs are designed for group intervention and can form the backdrop for an inclusive occupational therapy program that benefits all students through increased body awareness and self-monitoring skills development.

Adolescents and Teens

Adolescents and older primary students may benefit from interventions that promote teamwork or sports team participation. Feelings of isolation and exclusion from typical peer activities can enhance psychosocial problems in students with and without primary mental health conditions, as noted in a study of boys with developmental coordination disorder by Poulsen, Ziviani, Cuskelly, and Smith (2007). Sensory processing may continue to be a particular challenge for the adolescent and may present in the form of excessive acting out, aggression, and/or withdrawal. Because of their "almost adult" appearance, this can create even more challenges and conflicts within the school setting. Tools for Teens (Henry, 2004) provides a variation on the themes from How Does Your Engine Run? (Shellenberger & Williams, 2002). This type of programming may enable students who often remain in restricted academic environments to develop skills for participating in more mainstream academic activities, which may be particularly relevant for students returning to regular academic environments from residential or other restrictive school or treatment settings.

Using certified therapy dogs, occupational therapists in Albuquerque teamed with teachers and other therapists to promote skills acquisition in students with a variety of disabilities (Scott, Haseman, & Hammeter, 2005). This approach is supported by the Delta Society, a human services organization that works to promote the use of therapy, service and companion animals. The use of therapy dogs may especially be considered when children are struggling despite other forms of intervention. Equine therapy is also used for children's mental health as well as to promote skills development in other areas (Macauley & Gurierrez, 2004; Rollandelli & Dunst, 2003). Integration of this form of therapy can be seen in a variety of mental health and community programs for children, including residential and day school programs.

Schultz (2003) proposes role shifting as a primary intervention to "repeatedly involve the students in those very student role experiences that they were denied because of their bad behavior" (p. CE4). Shultz argues that many students with emotional and behavioral disorders are often routinely denied opportunities to engage in routine school-based occupations (walking in the hall independently, using the school library, having their work displayed in school common areas, etc) because of past behaviors. Role shifting involved engaging students in routine school occupations that encouraged them to participate in meaningful school roles. An example of role shifting that Shultz provides is supporting the students to appropriately use the school library, a space they were routinely denied access to, for self-initiated learning. In her example, Shultz uses routine library activities as her intervention activity but explains the process of convincing both the librarian and the students that they can function effectively in the student role within this environment. Shultz's approach is the epitome of occupation-based intervention. She argues that occupation is the interface between the person and the environment but that the student is the primary agent of change. Our challenge as practitioners is to facilitate the student's discovery of meaning in occupations that support meaningful engagement in the student role.

Also of primary concern when working with adolescents with mental health needs is what comes after high school. Transition to higher education, work, and/or community living presents a new set of contexts and challenges for any students and most especially for students already experiencing emotional challenges (Brollier, Shepherd, & Markley, 1994). Vocational testing and/or prevocational coursework may be provided for some, whereas other students in a more traditional academic track may not be considering the more comprehensive lifestyle choices that lie ahead. Specific life skills, such as knowledge of domestic skills and nutrition, may need to be addressed within the transitional program period.

Fidler (1996) describes the lifestyle performance model that may also provide a viable framework for addressing adolescent concerns, especially when considering transitional skill development toward future community living and roles:

- Taking care of one's self and maintaining one's self in as self-dependent a manner as personal needs and capabilities determine.
- Pursuing personally referenced pleasure, enjoyment, and intrinsic gratification.
- Contributing to the need fulfillment and welfare of others.
- Developing and sustaining reciprocal interpersonal relationships. (p. 144)

The ability for the emotionally challenged teenager to find value in himself or herself is often a daunting prospect, as life experiences have frequently included examples of worthlessness or rejection. Pleasure and enjoyment may have been compromised by physical and/or emotional challenges or may be framed in a socially unacceptable context due to histories of trauma or extreme challenge. Feeling a sense of contribution will mean discovering something of value to share or create, which may also be a foreign experience for many emotionally challenged teens, and development of interpersonal relationship is often fraught with fear of rejection.

Occupational therapy goals that consider these domains create a template for interpersonal relatedness and purpose. Occupational therapy provides a unique perspective for students with emotional challenges within the academic environment. It is important for the occupational therapy practitioner to communicate this role, including the provision of evidence in support of psychosocial and self-management interventions, because faculty, clinicians, and staff may be more familiar with occupational therapy interventions to address motor, cognitive, and/or perceptual deficits.

Summary

The mental health knowledge base and skills set of occupational therapists enable practitioners to make important contributions to address mental health needs in school-aged

Evidence-Based Practice

Occupational therapists can develop interventions that focus on preventing social and emotional difficulties. Bazyk and Bazyk (2009) described an occupation-based, after-school program designed to meet the socioemotional needs of at-risk urban youth ages 7 to 12. The Bazyks' OT HOPE Groups included an introductory conversation period, a structured leisure occupation period, and a discussion period with a focused conversation having a socioemotional theme. Although this program occurred in a faith-based after-school setting and not a school, the elements of the program could be replicated in school-based settings.

➤ Occupational therapists can develop occupation-based programs that help children develop basic socioemotional competencies such as understanding the relationship between feelings and thoughts.

➤ Designing programs that consider safety in both the social and physical environments can address the occupational and socioemotional needs of children at risk for emotional and behavioral problems.

Bazyk, S., & Bazyk, J. (2009). The meaning of occupation-based groups for low income urban youths attending after-school care. *American Journal of Occupational Therapy, 63*(1), 69–80.

children. Several leaders in the field have clarified the school-based mental health practitioner's role, and the profession has begun to develop and disseminate resources that can help practitioners address emotional and behavioral issues that interfere with school functioning and participation in school roles. This chapter identified some of the learning and social participation challenges faced by children and adolescents with mental illnesses in school settings and described the range of assessments and intervention strategies that occupational therapists can employ to address mental health in K–12 populations. To be effective, occupational therapists must collaborate with professionals from multiple disciplines, families, and community organizations, all of whom share a common goal of supporting practices that facilitate social and emotional health of students. Occupational therapy's unique contribution is its use of meaningful occupation to promote students' participation in productive routines and roles in school settings.

Active Learning Strategies

1. Experiential Learning and Journaling

Visit three different public classroom settings (with classroom teachers' permission), one elementary, one middle school or junior high, and one high school. You may want to be part of the group for a while, and then sit in a location where you can be a "fly on the wall." In each setting, complete and compare the following observations:

- Make a list of all of the senses, including proprioception and kinesthesia.
- Keep a record of how each sense is stimulated during your observation (e.g., smells from the cafeteria, sounds from the parking lot, voice of the teacher, things in students' mouths, sunlight in the window). Listen and look for background stimulation.

- Keep a record of how the classroom works, such as how directions are given (steps, complexity of information), where materials are located, how still or active must students be, and how the social culture seems to work. What cues are available to let you know what is acceptable?
- Interview the teachers to determine what skills they were expecting from the students during your observation.
- Identify where the students go during transitions (e.g., cafeteria, gym, playground, buses). With permission, observe the range of opportunities for peer interactions in each of these settings.

Discuss or write about your observations and the skills a student would need for successful participation. Consider how you would adapt for special needs. Include social, physical, and academic (cognitive, etc.) skills.

 Use your **Reflective Journal** to document your personal experiences in these settings.

Resources

Delta Society
- 875 124th Ave NE
  Suite 101
  Bellevue, WA 98005
  Phone: (425) 679-5500
  Website: http://www.deltasociety.org/Page.aspx?pid=183

National Education Association
- 1201 16th Street, NW
  Washington, DC 20036-3290
  Monday–Friday 8:30 a.m.–4:30 p.m. ET
  Phone: (202) 833-4000; Fax: (202) 822-7974
  Website: http://www.nea.org/index.html

United States Department of Education
- U.S. Department of Education
  400 Maryland Avenue, SW
  Washington, DC 20202
  Phone: 1-800-USA-LEARN (1-800-872-5327);
  TTY: 1-800-437-0833; Fax: (202) 401-0689
  Website: http://www.ed.gov/index.jhtml?src=a

Center for School Mental Health (CSMH)
- http://csmh.umaryland.edu
  The CSMH is based at the University of Maryland and directs its efforts to supporting policies and programs that result in effective school mental health promotion. This website provides overviews of CSMH's analysis of programs and research on school mental health, includes concise policy briefs on issues that impact student learning, and is a repository of documents practitioners can use to inform themselves on recent research, policies, and practices related to mental health in schools. Similar sites can be found at UCLA (http://smhp.psych .ucla.edu/) and the University of Miami in Ohio (http://www.units.muohio.edu/csbmhp/ aboutus/index .html).

Collaborative for Academic, Social, and Emotional Learning (CASEL)
- http://www.casel.org
  Social and emotional learning (SEL) focuses on five core competencies: (1)self-awareness, (2) self-management, (3) social awareness, (4) relationships skills, and (5) responsible decision-making. CASEL is a nonprofit organization that seeks to support research and the development of evidence-based practice of SEL. This website describes SEL approaches that can be used by occupational therapists to create opportunities for occupation-based interventions with individual students, classrooms, and school systems.

Positive Behavioral Interventions and Supports (PBS)
- http://www.pbis.org
  This center is supported by the U.S. Department of Education's Office of Special Education. PBS recognizes the considerable impact that the environment has on student behavior and is a clearinghouse of information and resources that can be used to support schoolwide interventions that impact the mental health of all students and especially those with mental illnesses or who are at risk for emotional or behavioral disorders.

National Early Childhood Technical Assistance Center (NECTAC)
- http://www.nectac.org
  This center is supported by the U.S. Department of Education's Office of Special Education Programs and provides resources to ensure that young children with disabilities (0–5 years) and their families receive family-centered, evidence-based services. Using the search term "emotional and behavioral disorders" within the NECTAC website will point you to a number of grant-supported programs, research articles, and practice guidelines specifically relative to young children with mental illnesses.

References

American Occupational Therapy Association (AOTA). (2002). Occupational therapy practice framework: Domain and process. *American Journal of Occupational Therapy, 56,* 609–639.

———. (2008). Frequently asked questions on school mental health for school-based occupational therapy practitioners. Available at: http://www.aota.org/Practitioners/PracticeAreas/Pediatrics/ Browse/School/FAQSchoolMH.aspx. (Accessed September 22, 2009).

Arnow, B., Sanders, M., & Steiner, H. (1999). Premenarcheal verses postmenarcheal anorexia nervosa: comparative study. *Clinical Child Psychology and Psychiatry, 4,* 403–414.

Barnes, K. J., Beck, A. J., Vogel, K. A., Grice, K. O., & Murphy, D. (2003). Perceptions regarding school-based occupational therapy for children with emotional disturbances. *American Journal of Occupational Therapy, 57,* 337–341.

Bazyk, S., & Bazyk, J. (2009). The meaning of occupation-based groups for low income urban youths attending after-school care. *American Journal of Occupational Therapy, 63*(1), 69–80.

Brollier, C., Shepherd, J., & Markley, K. (1994). Transition from school to community living. *American Journal of Occupational Therapy, 48,* 346–349.

Brown, C., & Dunn, W. (2002). *Adolescent/Adult Sensory Profile.* San Antonio, TX: Psychological Corporation.

Cameto, R. (2005). The transition planning process. *NLTS2 Data Brief: Results from the National Longitudinal Transition Study, 4*(1). Available at: http://www.ncset.org/publications/viewdesc .asp?id=2130 (accessed September 26, 2009).

Cara, E., & MacRae, A. (2005). *Psychosocial Occupational Therapy.* Clifton Park, NY: Delmar Learning.

Clark, G. (2001). Children often overlooked for occupational therapy services in educational settings. *School System Special Interest Section Quarterly, 8*(3), 1–3.

Dewey, J. (1897). My pedagogical creed: What education is. *School Journal, 14*(3), 77–80.

Donohue, M. (2007). Interrater reliability of the Social Profile: Assessment of community and psychiatric group participation. *Australian Journal of Occupational Therapy, 54,* 49–58.

Downing, D. (2006). The impact of early psychosis on learning. *OT Practice, 11*(12), 7–14.

Dunn, W. (1999). *Sensory Profile.* San Antonio: Psychological Corporation.

Fidler, G. S. (1996). Lifestyle performance: From profile to conceptual model. *American Journal of Occupational Therapy, 50,* 139–147.

Harney, S., & Kramer, J. M. (2007). Using the Child Occupational Self Assessment to generate student-centered IEP goals. *OT Practice, 12*(20), 10–15.

Henry, D. (2004). *Sensory Integration Tools for Teens.* Dayton, OH: Southpaw Enterprises.

Henry, A., & Coster, W. (1997). Competency beliefs and occupational role behavior among adolescents: Explication of the personal causation construct. *American Journal of Occupational Therapy, 51,* 267–276.

Ikiugu, M. (2007). *Psychosocial Conceptual Practice Models in Occupational Therapy.* St. Louis, MO: Elsevier.

Individuals with Disabilities Act. (2004). Regulations. Part 300: Assistance to States for the Education of Children with Disabilities. 34 C.F.R. 300.321(a)(7).

Jackson, C. J. (2005). *An Applied Neuropsychological Model of Functional and Dysfunctional Learning: Applications for Business, Education, Training and Clinical Psychology.* Sydney, Australia: Cymeon

Javaherian, H. (2006). Helping survivors of domestic violence. *OT Practice, 11*(10), 12–16.

Javaherian, H., & Hewitt, L. (2007). At risk youth: An opportunity to grow. *Occupational Therapy Practice, 12*(14), 7–9.

Keller, J., Kafkes, A., Basu, S., Federico, J., & Keilhofner, G. (2005). *The Child Occupational Self-Assessment* (version 2.1). Chicago: Model of Human Occupation Clearinghouse, Department of Occupational Therapy, College of Applied Health Sciences, University of Illinois.

Kessler, R. C., Chiu, W. T., Demler, O., Merikangas, K. R., & Walters, E. E. (2005). Prevalence, severity, and comorbidity of 12-month DSM-IV disorders in the National Comorbidity Survey Replication. *Archives of General Psychiatry, 62*(6), 617–627.

Kjorstad, M., O'Hare, S., Soseman, K., Spellman, C., & Thomas, P. (2005). The effects of post-traumatic stress disorder on children's social skills and occupation of play. *Occupational Therapy in Mental Health, 21*(1), 39–56.

Kolb, D. (1984). *Experiential Learning: Experience as the Source of Learning and Development.* Englewood Cliffs, NJ: Prentice-Hall.

Koppelman, J. (2004). Children with mental disorders: Making sense of their needs and systems that will help them. *NHPF Issue Brief, No. 799,* National Health Policy Forum. George Washington University, Washington, DC.

Kranowitz, C. (2003). *The Out-of-Sync Child Has Fun.* New York: Penguin Putnam.

Kutash, K. (2007). "Understanding school-based mental health services for students who are disruptive and aggressive: What works for whom?" *Proceedings of Persistently Safe Schools: 2007 National Conference on Safe Schools and Communities.* Available at: http://gwired.gwu.edu/hamfish/merlin-cgi/p/downloadFile/d/19150/n/off/other/1/name/019pdf (accessed September, 21, 2009).

Kutash, K., Duchnowski, A. J., & Lynn, N, (2006). *School-based Mental Health: An Empirical Guide for Decision-Makers.* Tampa: University of South Florida, Louis de la Parte Florida Mental Health Institute, Department of Child & Family Studies, Research and Training Center for Children's Mental Health.

Law, M., Babtiste, S., Carswell, A., McColl, M., Platajko, H., & Pollock, N. (2005). *Canadian Occupational Performance Measure* (4th ed). Toronto: CAOT Publications.

McCarthy, K. (2002). Outside looking in. *OT Practice,* 8–12.

Macauley, B., & Gurierrez K. (2004) The effectiveness of hippotherapy for children with language-learning disabilities. *Communications Disorders Quarterly, 25,* 205–217.

Poulsen A., Ziviani, J., Cuskelly, M., & Smith, R. (2007). Boys with developmental coordination disorder: Loneliness and team sports participation. *American Journal of Occupational Therapy, 61,* 451–462.

Powell, N. (1994). Content for educational programs in school-based occupational therapy from a practice perspective. *American Journal of Occupational Therapy, 48,* 130–137.

Rollandelli, P., & Dunst C. (2003) Influences of hippotherapy on the motor and social-emotional behavior of young children with disabilities. *Bridges. Practice-Based Research Syntheses. Research and Training Center on Early Childhood Development. Puckett Institute,* 2(1), 1–14.

Santos, M., Richards, C. S., & Bleckley, M. (2007). Comorbidity between depression and disordered eating in adolescents. *Eating Behaviors, 8,* 440–449.

Schultz, S. (2003). Psychosocial occupational therapy in schools: Identify challenges and clarify role of occupational therapy in promoting adaptive functioning. *OT Practice, 8,* CE1–CE8.

Scott, K., Haseman, J., & Hammeter, R. (2005). Kids, dogs, and the occupation of literacy. *OT Practice, 10*(3), 16–20.

Shellenberger, S., & Williams, M. (2002) "How does your engine run?": The ALERT program for self-regulation. In A. G. Fisher, E. A. Murray, & A. C. Bundy (Eds.), *Sensory Integration: Theory and Practice* (pp. 342–345). Philadelphia: FA Davis.

Skog, K., Vrnig, E., Castaneda, C., & Deitz, J. (2006). Promoting participation and success on the playground. *OT Practice, 11*(21),11–16.

Sprenger, M. (2003). *Differentiation through Learning Styles and Memory.* Thousand Oaks, CA: Corwin Press.

U.S. Department of Education. (2007). *No Child Left Behind.* Available at: http://www.ed.gov/nclb/landing.jhtml?src=pb (accessed November 2007).

U.S. Department of Health and Human Services. (1999). *Mental Health: A Report of the Surgeon General—Executive Summary.* Rockville, MD: U.S. Department of Health and Human Services, Substance Abuse and Mental Health Services Administration, Center for Mental Health Services, National Institutes of Health, National Institute of Mental Health.

Walz, N., & Branek, G. (2006). Sensory processing patterns in persons with Angelman syndrome. *American Journal of Occupational Therapy, 60,* 472–479.

Watling, R. (2005). Interventions for common behavior problems in children with disabilities. *OT Practice, 10*(15), 12–15.

Weisz, J., Sandler, I., Durlak, J., & Anton, B. (2005). Promoting and protecting youth mental health through evidence-based prevention and treatment. *American Psychologist 60*(6), 628–648.

Student: Adult Education

Sharon A. Gutman and Victoria P. Schindler

> "There was a time when living independently in a middle class lifestyle was not even something I could dream about, but supported education helped me set, and then go about achieving, goals that have altered the downward spiral that was my life.
>
> —Jasper, 1997, p. 52

Introduction

This chapter describes how **supported education** services for adults with psychiatric disabilities can help people reenter the student role and pursue personal educational goals. Supported education services can help adults with psychiatric disabilities to complete a general equivalency diploma (GED), enroll in community-based adult education classes, begin technical training certification, or pursue college-level coursework (Mowbray, Megivern, & Holter, 2003). The onset of many psychiatric illnesses commonly occurs between late adolescence and early adulthood (Megivern, Pellerito, & Mowbray, 2003). It is in this developmental period that people traditionally complete high school and begin employment and/or postsecondary education. The onset of a psychiatric illness within this developmental period frequently disrupts the completion of secondary education and entrance into paid employment and/or postsecondary education. Consequently, many people with psychiatric disabilities are unable to earn a diploma or degree necessary to attain economic and social independence. Instead, many experience gaps in their foundational academic knowledge and social skills. Such gaps negatively impact employment options and restrict people to low-wage, entry-level positions that do not offer access to adequate health care.

This chapter describes supported education services for adults with psychiatric disabilities and illustrates how such programs have helped adults to participate more fully in educational forums in the larger community. Evaluation and intervention methods are discussed, and a summary of research studies offering empirical support for the effectiveness and client satisfaction of supported education services is provided.

Role of Occupational Therapy in Supported Education

Several public laws have been created in an effort to preserve the right of people with psychiatric disabilities to receive access to and accommodations supporting educational pursuit.

The Americans with Disabilities Act (ADA; U.S. Department of Justice, 2006), Individuals with Disabilities Education Act (IDEA; U.S. Department of Education, 2006), and the Rehabilitation Act (Special Education and Rehabilitation Services, 2004) all mandate the full inclusion of people with disabilities—including psychiatric disabilities—in educational settings. However, while such legislation ensures access and reasonable accommodations that support the full participation of people with psychiatric disabilities in educational settings, many colleges and universities have not developed supported education services for this population. More commonly, institutions of higher education have developed services for people with physical and learning disabilities (Dowrick, Anderson, Heyer, & Acosta, 2005). Stigmatization and misperception may account for this disparity in supported education service provision. Despite advances in pharmacology that have helped people with psychiatric disabilities to attain greater daily life function and stability, many still inaccurately believe that people with psychiatric disabilities cannot endure the rigors of academic requirements (Mowbray et al, 2005). Yet research has demonstrated that when people with psychiatric disabilities are provided with reasonable accommodations, supportive services, and ongoing counseling, they are able to successfully pursue personal educational goals (Mowbray et al, 2003).

Occupational therapists are uniquely qualified to develop and provide supported education services for adults with psychiatric illness. Because they are trained to help people resume functional life roles after the onset of disability, occupational therapists can assist adults with psychiatric disabilities to regain the adult student role in the larger community (Gutman, Kerner, Zombek, Dulek, & Ramsey, 2009). The occupational therapy techniques of activity analysis and synthesis can be used to break down educational skills into component parts. Specific educational material can be broken down into smaller cognitive tasks that initially match the client's skill level. Therapists can then progressively increase the challenge level of such tasks until the larger educational skill as a whole is mastered. The same is true for learning and memory strategies, social interaction skills with peers and instructors, and illness management techniques. Occupational therapists can also uniquely contribute to supported education services by helping to make environmental modifications to the educational setting. Classrooms can be adapted to decrease sensory overload and facilitate concentration. Therapists can also help students to learn compensatory strategies to increase organization, classroom participation, and school performance.

The student role is highly valued in our society, and the ability to succeed in the student role is critical to one's future life conditions and the availability of resources. Because of the relationship between success in the student role and adult life conditions, the development of supported education services cannot be understated. The unique expertise that occupational therapists possess is critically needed by clients who desire to succeed in an academic environment and to become contributing members of society, able to independently meet housing, health care, and social participation needs.

Occupations of the Adult Student with a Psychiatric Disability

Adults with psychiatric disabilities commonly have a history of past failure experiences in the educational system (Megivern et al, 2003). As children or adolescents, such students may have been labeled with behavioral problems. In adolescence, when the onset of symptoms commonly becomes pronounced, students frequently do not receive appropriate support to complete high school and often drop out without developing the skills needed to obtain and maintain employment (Mowbray et al, 2003). A spiral of low-wage employment or unemployment ensues. People frequently cannot pay for needed health care and consequently are unable to access the resources necessary to manage psychiatric symptoms. Without appropriate intervention, both physical and mental status suffer over time.

In adulthood, people with psychiatric disabilities commonly identify educational pursuit as a desired occupational goal (Dowrick et al, 2005). If people are able to step back into the student role in adulthood, the occupations needed to succeed in that role are much more complex than they are for a younger student with less responsibility. In addition to

managing their psychiatric disability, most adult students must simultaneously work to pay for housing, food, child care, transportation, health care, and/or school. Time-management skills are critical in order to organize and prioritize the various responsibilities associated with each of these occupations. Juggling these responsibilities can induce stress that, if not addressed appropriately, can exacerbate an illness. Participation in therapy or counseling to receive assistance with stress management associated with the new role of student can be helpful for adult learners with psychiatric disabilities.

Adult learners with psychiatric disabilities must often become advocates for themselves to access and receive appropriate accommodations that can help them succeed in school. Such skills are often difficult for people with low self-esteem and confidence resulting from past failure experiences. Advocacy requires that instructors and administrators, who may be perceived as unapproachable school authority figures, be notified of a student's disability and the specific accommodations that would help that student succeed in the educational setting.

Adult students with psychiatric disabilities have the additional burden of managing their illness. Illness management involves an array of occupations, including maintaining a medication schedule, regularly attending therapy, and refilling prescriptions when needed. Illness management also involves the ability to identify one's symptoms and seek help when symptoms appear in order to prevent illness exacerbation.

Assuming the responsibilities of new roles and occupations can be both exciting and anxiety provoking. While the prospect of becoming a student and pursuing desired educational goals is often stimulating, it can also arouse long-standing fears and insecurities. Many adult learners with psychiatric disabilities report experiencing a series of unsuccessful trials before they feel sufficiently comfortable to actually enroll in a class and attend it through its entirety (Jasper, 1997; Orrin, 1997; Weiner, 1996). Instead, their educational path is often marked by a series of beginnings and withdrawals—classes are begun with enthusiasm but then ended as students experience anxiety, fear, or illness. Supported education can help to break this cycle.

In addition to the anxiety experienced when new roles are assumed, adult learners with psychiatric disabilities may also experience disruption in their familiar relationships as a result of the assumption of the student role. Others who have previously served as a stable support for the student may react negatively to the student's new educational occupations. Pursuing one's goals may cause others to reevaluate and feel inadequate about their own accomplishments. Relationships may change as the adult learner grows and attains new skills. Spouses, children, and friends may resent the time and financial commitments that the adult learner has made in order to participate in educational occupations. When significant others do not support the adult learner's educational activities, he or she is less likely to maintain perseverance to complete desired occupational goals.

All of these stressors become compounded when adult learners have comorbid physical health problems, have comorbid substance abuse disorders, or may be homeless or in danger of becoming homeless. Physical health problems, substance abuse disorders, and homelessness are commonly

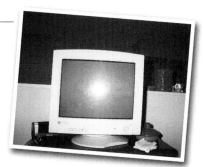

PhotoVoice

Omen-Amen
Photovoice
Psychokenesis
The PK Zone
$E = M \times C^2$
Flux Capacitor
Void
    For a
successful life
I aim to go back to college and
to achieve a very good grade there.

—Grady

seen in the lives of adults with psychiatric disorders who failed to receive adequate treatment early in the course of their illness (Jones et al, 2004; McQuistion, Finnerty, & Hirschowitz, 2003). Supported education services must often work collaboratively with the social service agencies that specifically address these problems.

The occupational skills necessary to successfully assume the student role as an adult learner with a psychiatric disability fall into three categories: specific academic occupations, specific social occupations, and balancing requirements for academic success and health-care management. These occupations are detailed in Tables 49-1, 49-2, 49-3, and 49-4.

Assessments

The process of assessment can be challenging and stigmatizing for adult students with psychiatric disabilities. Participation in the formal assessment process may remind students of periods when they were patients in treatment and may elicit anxiety and feelings of inadequacy. If students experienced

poor academic and test performance in the past, present evaluations may remind them of that time period and arouse further performance anxiety. Consequently, formal evaluations must be selected with sensitivity and with full consent of the adult student.

Adult education assessment can be divided into four categories: evaluations that assess (1) career interests, (2) academic skills, (3) psychosocial adjustment, and (4) overall function in the student role.

Assessment of Career Interests and Academic Skills

Evaluations that assess career interests and academic skills have largely been developed by professionals other than occupational therapists but are still relevant to use in the occupational therapy assessment process. The Harrington-O'Shea Career Decision-Making System (Harrington, 1993) is an evaluation designed to help students determine career goals. This scale helps students to clarify career interests, identify educational requirements for specific employment

Table 49-1 ● **Specific Academic Occupations**

Occupation	Abilities Required
Classroom attendance	• Arrange transportation to and from class • Notify instructors of absences • Obtain notes and class material when absent
Participation	• Maintain concentration during class activities • Take notes while aurally processing class material • Ask questions when further clarification is needed • Appropriately contribute to class discussions
Time management	• Schedule all educational assignments and activities in a realistic way that supports their completion in accordance with due dates • Schedule sufficient time for both educational and noneducational activities (e.g., work, child care, elder care, leisure activities)
Prioritization	• Prioritize several educational activities and schedule them accordingly • Compare the importance of educational and noneducational responsibilities and schedule them according to need
Note-taking	• Record essential information during class or reading while simultaneously processing information received aurally and visually • Study
Study skills	• Learn and apply new material • Include such activities as outlining, highlighting, and self-testing
Test-taking	• Demonstrate learning of new material in a formal evaluation situation, such as completing a multiple-choice test administered in a classroom setting
Completion of homework assignments (paper, writing, reading, etc)	• Carry out assigned work independently and outside of the classroom environment • Demonstrate self-initiative, the ability to impose self-structure, and the ability to set goals and carry them out in accordance with due dates • Break down academic tasks into smaller, manageable components; understand the order in which each component should be implemented; and perform each component until the whole activity is completed
Stress management	• Identify when feeling overwhelmed by academic activities • Implement appropriate actions to alleviate such feelings • Understand which educational activities can trigger stress • Schedule stress-relieving activities to prevent illness exacerbation
Sensory overload reduction	• Identify when feeling overwhelmed by the amount of sensory stimulation entering central nervous system (e.g., sitting too long in class, reading textbook material without scheduling breaks) • Modify study setting and use compensatory strategies to avoid sensory overload before it occurs
Filing and updating formal documents (e.g., financial aid, admission, registration)	• Identify forms required for education • Take initiative to complete such forms, or seek assistance with their completion by due dates • Maintain a calendar indicating which forms need to be renewed or updated

Table 49-2 ● Specific Social Occupations

Occupation	Abilities Required
Social norms of classroom behavior	• Raise hand to answer or ask a question • Speak when called on by the instructor rather than randomly shouting out loud • Allow the instructor and fellow students to speak without interruption • Remain seated quietly during classroom activities without creating disruption • Refrain from speaking to fellow students during classroom instruction (unless such interaction is required by specific classroom exercises) • Refrain from monopolizing classroom and small group discussions • Refrain from answering questions in a tangential manner that strays from the class topic
Interaction with fellow students	• Appropriately greet fellow students and introduce self upon initial meeting • Maintain appropriate personal space of fellow students • Maintain appropriate eye contact • Understand the norms of turn-taking in conversation • Understand topics of appropriate conversation • Understand the norms of initiating and terminating a conversation • Understand the meaning of nonverbal cues in social interaction and refine behavior in response to such cues • Understand and respect boundaries regarding personal space and personal information
Interaction with instructors	Interaction with instructors consists of all of the above social interaction norms with fellow students as well as • Feel sufficiently comfortable to advocate for reasonable accommodations to support academic success • Feel sufficiently comfortable to ask for assistance or feedback regarding academic performance if needed • Feel sufficiently comfortable to ask and answer questions during class • Refrain from interrupting the instructor during class • Refrain from challenging the instructor in a hostile manner during or after class
Appropriate self-care and attire	• Maintain grooming habits • Wear appropriate clothing in the academic environment
Advocacy for rights and reasonable accommodations	• Feel sufficiently comfortable to speak to administrators and instructors regarding psychiatric disability and the specific accommodations that would support educational participation • Seek assistance from a clinical or legislative advocate if not sufficiently comfortable or able to independently speak to administrators and instructors

Table 49-3 ● Balancing Requirements for Academic Success and Health-Care Management

Occupation	Abilities Required
Identify symptoms indicating illness exacerbation	• Understand own unique constellation of symptoms • Understand when symptoms appear • Understand connection between symptoms and illness exacerbation rather than attributing symptoms to external factors • Understand that the appearance of symptoms necessitates help from designated health-care providers and family members
Maintain contact information and procedures to follow in case of illness exacerbation	• Identify appropriate people who can provide help in the event of illness exacerbation • Provide copies of the list to critical people (health-care professionals, case managers, school advisors, and family members) who can help to contact designated individuals in the event of illness exacerbation • Carry out the indicated procedures to seek help
Manage medications	• Understand at which times during the day or evening medications should be taken • Understand the correct dosage of each medication • Consistently adhere to a medication schedule • Follow the correct steps to refill medications (so that gaps in medication administration do not occur) • Understand the possible side effects of each medication • Distinguish between medication side effects and illness symptoms (so that needed medications are not discontinued based on a false belief that medications cause illness)
Participate in supportive therapy	• Understand the need to receive therapeutic assistance to manage stresses associated with being an adult learner who has a psychiatric disability • Make a commitment to consistently attend therapy

Table 49-4 ● **Assessments of Psychosocial Adjustment**

Area of Assessment	Name of Assessment	Brief Description
Self-esteem (Rosenberg, 1965)	Rosenberg Self-Esteem Scale	Ten-item scale to measure the self-acceptance aspect of self-esteem
Coping (Pearlin & Schooler, 1978)	Coping Mastery Scale	Assesses psychological ability. Self-administered paper and pencil assessment of how individual manages everyday stress.
Anxiety (Zung, 1971)	Zung Anxiety Scale	Self-report measure to assess changes in expressed anxiety
Interpersonal self-efficacy (Vitkux & Horowitz, 1987)	Interpersonal Self-Efficacy Index (ISE)	Fifteen-item questionnaire used to rate various aspects of self-efficacy with respect to solving interpersonal problems
Social attitudes (Beiser et al, 1987)	Social Response Questionnaire (SRQ)	Seventeen-item measure of informal labeling of persons with psychiatric disabilities. Asks respondent to rate the degree to which each adjective describes a person with mental illness
Quality of life (Lehman, 1991)	Lehman's Quality of Life Inventory	Two items that ask how individuals feel about their life as a whole
Self-image (Offer, Ostrov, & Howard, 1981)	Offer Self-Image Questionnaire (OSIQ)	Measures 10 aspects of adolescent functioning
Empowerment (Pearlin & Schooler, 1978)	Empowerment Scale	Thirteen-item measure
Symptoms (Derogatis & Melisaratos, 1983)	Brief Symptom Inventory	Ten-item measure

positions, and determine appropriate types of postsecondary training. The Wide Range Achievement Test–Revision 3 (Wilkinson, 1993) evaluates basic reading and math skills and can identify students needing remedial education and tutoring. The ASSET Test (Barrett, Vachman, & Huisingh, 1991) is another academic measure that assesses language, math, and reading skills.

Assessment of Psychosocial Adjustment

A large body of evaluations has been created for the purpose of assessing psychosocial adjustment. Many of these scales have been developed by professionals in psychology and address factors such as self-esteem, coping, anxiety, self-efficacy, social attitudes, quality of life, self-image, empowerment, and symptom identification. Such evaluations can be used at baseline and postintervention to determine if students are able to increase their psychosocial adjustment as a result of participation in supported education services.

Assessment of Functional Performance in the Student Role

Three standardized occupational therapy evaluations have been developed to assess functional performance in the student role. These scales—the Tasks Skills, Interpersonal Skills, and School Behavioral Scales—are standardized evaluations intended to be used conjointly to provide collective information about an adult learner's ability to function in the student role despite psychiatric disability (Schindler, 2004). The Task Skills and Interpersonal Skills Scales are 5-point rating scales with high levels of reliability, internal consistency, and convergent validity. The School Behavior Scale is a 5-point rating scale with high internal consistency. These scales are observational measures intended to be completed by an occupational therapist. Each scale requires approximately 10 minutes to complete. The scales can be used as baseline and postintervention measures to determine if client progress has been made.

Additionally, therapists can use the Occupational Therapy Practice Framework (American Occupational Therapy Association, 2002) and the International Classification of Function, Disability, and Health (ICF; World Health Organization, 2006) to further assess functional performance in the student role. For example, the following information is important to assess: (1) past educational participation and achievement; (2) current educational goals; (3) cognitive, sensoriperceptual, neuromusculoskeletal, and psychosocial skills; and (4) learning styles, routines, and habits related to educational participation. The Adolescent/Adult Sensory Profile (Brown & Dunn, 2002) can also help occupational therapists to gain a greater understanding of how sensory processing problems—related to psychiatric disability—can affect school performance. The Allen Cognitive Level Screen (Allen, 1996) can provide a quick assessment of a student's cognitive functioning.

Intervention

Three supported education program models are documented in the literature: (1) onsite services, (2) mobile support services, and (3) self-contained classrooms (Collins, Bybee, & Mowbray, 1998; Collins, Mowbray, & Bybee, 2000; Mowbray et al, 2005). The goal of these services is to provide support to adults with psychiatric disabilities to reenter the student role in some type of academic forum—for example, GED preparation courses, community-based adult education classes, technical training certification programs, or college-level coursework.

Onsite Model

In the **onsite model**, students attend college courses while simultaneously receiving supported education services in the form of individual counseling or a support group (Collins et al, 1998, Mowbray et al, 2003). This model is specifically intended for students with psychiatric disabilities who already have developed the academic and social skills needed to begin coursework. Supported education services may focus on advocacy skills, tutoring in specific academic areas, and the creation of classroom accommodations. This is the most common type of supported education service model and is routinely provided by mental health departments already existing at institutions of higher learning (Collins et al, 1998; Collins et al, 2000; Unger, 1992). Students who have previously enrolled in college and then experienced psychiatric symptoms commonly self-identify the need for such services.

At Wayne County College in Detroit, Michigan, both individual and group support are provided for students enrolled in college courses (Mowbray, Collins, & Bybee, 1999). Group support meetings are held twice weekly and focus on the group's specified needs. The group cofacilitators include a staff person and a self-identified consumer who has firsthand knowledge of the experience of attending college with a psychiatric disability. This program also provides individual counseling through which students are consistently assigned to one staff person. The assigned counselor meets with each student on a regular and as-needed basis.

Mobile Support Model

The **mobile support model** addresses the needs of students as they attend integrated college courses or technical training programs. In this model, staff members travel to students to provide assistance at the institution at which the student is attending courses. Staff members are routinely housed in a community-based mental health center and commonly provide services at several postsecondary educational sites (Collins et al, 1998; Collins et al, 2000; Unger, 1992). The mobile support model frequently provides several different types of service. Ongoing support and monitoring is offered through regular meetings with students on the academic campus. Academic tutoring, case management, and crisis intervention are also offered as needed. Staff members meet with students in settings that students identify as the most comfortable for them (e.g., the college student center, library, coffee shop). Staff members also provide a link between the student and college personnel by providing advocacy services to students needing fair treatment in the areas of financial aid and reasonable accommodations (Collins et al, 1998; Collins et al, 2000; Cook & Jonikas, 1992).

An example of a mobile support program is offered at Laurel House in Stamford, Connecticut (Dougherty & Campana, 1996). This mobile support program is based on a **clubhouse model** in which clients of Laurel House are provided with support to reenter the student role at a nearby college or technical school. Support staff members have flexibility in the provision of a wide range of services both on and off campus. Staff members visit students on campus to provide assistance with administrative needs (i.e., help with admissions, registration, and financial aid) as well as ancillary needs (e.g., housing and employment). Psychosocial services are provided at Laurel House to help students adjust to and deal with the stresses of being a student. Laurel House provides a familiar environment for students to obtain tutoring, complete assignments, or study after class.

Self-Contained Classroom Model

The **self-contained classroom model** provides the opportunity for students to attend a specialized curriculum designed to help them obtain the foundational academic skills and confidence needed to enter college or technical training courses in the larger community (Collins et al, 1998; Collins et al, 2000; Hoffman & Mastrianni, 1992; Unger, Anthony, Sciarappa, & Rogers, 1991). The self-contained classroom model is intended for people who have been out of school for a lengthy period of time and require skills building before fully entering postsecondary settings. Self-contained classrooms customarily provide specialized instruction in study skills, basic writing and reading, basic math, vocational exploration, and navigating the administrative aspects of an educational institution. This type of supported education model provides a venue for networking among students facing similar challenges and sharing parallel goals (Housel & Hickey, 1993). The self-contained classroom is intended to help people reintegrate into mainstream educational classes in the future semesters.

A self-contained classroom model is described by Collins et al (2000). This supported education curriculum has three objectives: to help students (1) manage the campus environment, (2) explore career options, and (3) manage stress associated with the student role. The curriculum is developed and implemented by two instructors in a classroom setting. The curriculum includes activities designed to enhance basic academic skills, teach students about library resources, and offer assistance in the completion of financial aid and registration forms. The philosophy underlying this model is the assumption that students can use the self-contained classroom as a bridge to gain the confidence and skills needed to succeed in a mainstream classroom in the future.

Programs With Combined Models

Most supported education programs integrate features of each of the previously described models. In the Houston model (Housel & Hickey, 1993), specialized case managers travel to students in the educational setting, familiar mental health professionals are physically present on campus to provide support, and specialized educational training is offered through self-contained classrooms.

The Chicago-based community scholar program Thresholds is another well-known supported education program that combines self-contained classrooms, onsite support, and mobile-support services (Cook & Jonikas, 1992; Cook & Solomon, 1993). A structured curriculum addresses career decision-making, study skills, time management, relaxation techniques, test-taking strategies, memory-enhancement techniques, library research skills, and writing skills. Once participants complete the structured curriculum, they are encouraged to enroll in regular college or technical training programs. Onsite and mobile support services are also provided as students complete coursework in academic institutions.

Supported Education Programs Developed by Occupational Therapists

While supported education services for adult students with psychiatric disabilities have increased in number throughout the country, such services are still uncommon and infrequently found in most institutions of higher learning (Dowrick et al, 2005). Despite federal acts (U.S. Department of Education, 2006; U.S. Department of Justice, 2006) that mandate the right to educational access and accommodations

Evidence-Based Practice

In 1998, Collins et al conducted the Michigan Supported Education Research Program to determine if one of three supported education models—the self-contained classroom, onsite service, or a control group—was more effective than the others. Approximately 400 participants were assigned to three types of supported education groups: (1) an onsite support group in which participants explored career and educational options, (2) a self-contained classroom that addressed basic academic skills; and (3) a control group in which the participants independently pursued their education but were given the option of contacting a counselor if needed. It was found that the self-contained classroom model was more effective at developing academic competency, while the onsite support group model was more effective at motivating the participants to pursue educational goals. The control group was found to be the least effective at developing academic competency and motivating one's pursuit of educational goals.

A study of three postsecondary supported education programs for students with psychiatric disabilities was conducted to determine education and employment outcomes and predictors of school completion and employment fit. Approximately 124 students were surveyed over five semesters. The study demonstrated that students were able to complete 90% of their college courses with a grade point average of 3.14. The school retention rate was found to be comparable to that of the general population of part-time students (Unger, Pardee, & Shafer, 2000).

➤ When providing supported education interventions, occupational therapists should insure that both mental health professionals in the community and educators in the academic setting collaborate to provide students with a range of needed support.

➤ Supported education programs are most effective when they integrate the use of (1) preparatory classes to build academic and social skills, (2) ongoing support provided through individual and/or group counseling, and (3) professional mental health services through which students can receive needed medical intervention.

Collins, M. E., Bybee, D., & Mowbray, C. T. (1998). Effectiveness of supported education for individuals with psychiatric disabilities: Results from an experimental study. *Community Mental Health Journal, 34,* 595–613.

Unger, K. V., Pardee, R., & Shafer, M. S. (2000). Outcomes of postsecondary supported education programs for people with psychiatric disabilities. *Journal of Vocational Rehabilitation, 14,* 195–199.

in the postsecondary setting, supported education services for adults with psychiatric disabilities continue to be rare rather than routine (services for people with physical and learning disabilities are much more common). Most supported education programs in the country have been developed largely by professionals in social work and psychology. Yet occupational therapists can make distinct contributions to this service area through our understanding of occupational role adaptation and participation.

In response to the need for supported education services, the occupational therapy departments at Richard Stockton College of New Jersey (Pomona, New Jersey) and Columbia University (New York City) have collaboratively developed the Bridge Program (Gutman et al, 2009). This supported education service is specifically designed for adults with chronic psychiatric disabilities who have fallen into the cycle of unemployment/low-wage employment and inability to access appropriate health care. The Bridge Program is a self-contained classroom with group learning activities and individual mentoring. It provides a one-semester course for adults with psychiatric disabilities that helps students to (1) obtain the basic academic skills needed to succeed in an educational environment, (2) enhance the social and behavioral skills needed to interact with professors and fellow students, and (3) identify resources specifically for the adult learner. One-to-one mentoring is also provided to help students (1) maintain their motivation to remain in and complete the Bridge Program, (2) identify available educational opportunities beyond the program, (3) complete admission and financial aid applications, (4) study for the GED and college entrance examinations, (5) locate community resources needed to support educational pursuits (e.g., child care, computer skills workshops), and (6) apply material learned in each module to the participants' personal educational goals.

The Bridge Program's 12 sessions include time management and prioritization, stress management, study and test-taking skills, effective reading skills, basic writing skills, basic computer skills, introduction to the Internet, basic algebra, use of library resources, social skills in the academic environment, public speaking techniques, and exploration of educational/vocational interests (Gutman et al, 2009). After completion of the program, students are invited to attend an ongoing support group to provide assistance as they begin to reenter the student role in the larger community.

In its pilot year, 12 of the 16 participants who successfully completed the Bridge Program went on to complete a GED or enrolled in some form of further education, such as adult education classes, GED preparation classes, technical training certification programs, and community college classes (Gutman et al, 2009). Two Bridge Program sites are now offered: one at Richard Stockton College and one at Columbia University. The program uses the same model at each school and is sponsored by the occupational therapy programs at both institutions. Referrals for each site come from local mental health agencies. Occupational therapy students participate in the program as instructors and mentors.

In a similar supported education program conducted by the occupational therapy program at Kean University (Union, New Jersey), called Pathways to Success, students and faculty conduct six separate educational courses for clients referred from local mental health agencies (Stern, 2006). Each course runs for 6 weeks, once per week. In past years, course topics have included computer skills, stress management, public speaking, and study skills. Clients from local mental health agencies are invited to select the course or courses in which they wish to participate. Courses provide the opportunity for clients to gain confidence and explore their desire to reenter the student role (Knis-Matthews, Bokara, DeMeo, Lepore, & Mavus, 2007).

The supported education program at the University of Southern California (USC; Los Angeles) is implemented through USC's Occupational Therapy Faculty Practice. Therapists provide support to USC students who self-identify the need for supported education services. Students are typically seen once a week; continued contact may be

The Lived Experience

The following narrative is based on an interview with a 56-year-old man who has dealt with chronic depression for most of his life. In the last year, he has participated in a supported education program, the Bridge Program, to pursue desired educational goals. The narrative illustrates that recovery processes are normally characterized by a series of gains and setbacks; few are linear, progressive courses.

After high school I tried college because my parents wanted me to go and I guess I was trying to please them. But that was a disaster. I flunked out. I guess I wasn't prepared for that level of work and self-discipline and I never thought I was entitled to ask for help. I always thought that I was just bothering the instructors who must have more important things to do than bother with me. Maybe it was also my self-esteem; it wasn't very good. And in college the level of social interaction seemed even more complex and beyond my ability to understand. I guess I flunked out of college for all of these reasons.

The college I went to was a small liberal arts college in Staten Island. That was one thing my parents stressed, "You're going to college." They were working-class people and they didn't want to see me struggle the way they did. Certainly, there is nothing wrong with being working class but they wanted a better life for me. But when I graduated from high school and went away to school I wasn't ready academically or socially. I hadn't developed the social skills that other people had developed all throughout elementary, junior high, and high school. When I got to college it was a real shock because the other students had social knowledge from normal development that I had never acquired. Even though I lived in the dorm I was still isolated there. Things hadn't changed for me. And when I failed it was a disaster. I felt so low about myself. It was devastating for me because I had failed at the one thing my parents wanted me to do. That was *really* devastating.

I attended college for one year as a biology major. I think I wanted to work in a lab but I wasn't very clear about my own desires and my future goals. I came home after one year—after I flunked out. I was just so defeated over this incident that I had zero confidence in myself because I had failed at the very thing that I thought I wanted to do and that my parents wanted me to do. My parents were very angry and disappointed—they took it personally. They felt that they had failed. So, that didn't help either. I just felt like a screw-up and I didn't do anything for a very long time. I didn't attempt education again until last year when I started the Bridge Program.

In 2005 I had reached a point where I felt that my therapy had helped me to make important strides in my recovery. I had heard about the Bridge Program and wanted to try it. I wanted to try to accomplish what I had failed at before. Maybe it was about pleasing my parents again. I am a bit ashamed of that. That's a bad reason to do anything. My dad died 17 years ago. My mom is now in a nursing home and unaware of what's going on. So I'm carrying them around in my pocket. It's kind of scary to acknowledge that kind of thing. I also felt that I was becoming too dependent on my own treatment; it's becoming real safe to go to therapy even though it's helping me. So, I wanted to take the risk of getting out in the community and doing things myself. I wanted to set a goal to return to school and see if I could achieve this. I wanted to move away from the safety of therapy and use the support systems and skills I learned through counseling. I wanted to challenge my own self-destructive behaviors and transition back into the community. The problem is, when I try new things I tend to go back to the old familiar self-destructive behaviors and negative thinking. So the Bridge Program is a little scary for me; not as scary as classroom work though.

In the Bridge Program all of the instructors and mentors have helped me to have greater confidence in myself. They have conveyed to me their belief in my abilities. My own belief in my abilities is coming less easily. Last year my mentors in the program helped me to enroll in a certification program for medical reception at the local community college. I began to take a computer skills course as a trial run. I was doing fine. In fact I had received Bs on both exams. But I started doubting myself again and soon I started falling back into the same old self-destructive behaviors and I stopped going to class. I guess as much as I want to make changes I'm still afraid. I'm scared to rely on myself. It's not easy for me to face this. This past semester my mentor helped me to sign up for the same course again. I was doing well and thinking that I could finish this time. But then I had to have a cardiac catheterization procedure and right after my mother had a stroke. I couldn't handle the stress of these two events happening so closely and I withdrew from the class again. But next semester I want to try again. I can't look at what happened harshly. I have to think, "There is a lot of good about me and it is up to me to discover that stuff and use it to change my life in positive ways."

maintained through e-mail or phone communication. Examples of specific accommodations include helping students to modify their schedules so that they can (1) reduce the length of the school day, (2) receive additional tutoring, (3) register for a reduced class load, (4) take tests in a quiet environment without distractions, (5) have more time in testing situations, and (6) make modifications to their study habits and setting to increase alertness and organization (M. K. Wolfe, personal communication, November 27, 2006).

The college setting is a nonstigmatizing environment in which adults with mental health concerns can begin to participate more fully in desired social and community member roles. Because the student role is highly esteemed in the larger society, adults with psychiatric disabilities who assume the student role through supported education report increased confidence and self-esteem (Gutman et al, 2009; Mowbray et al, 2003). Students report that they begin to view themselves as functioning, productive members of society rather than as psychiatric patients. The pursuit of postsecondary education is also an age-appropriate occupation for young adults and adults in midlife who desire a career change. Students in supported education services in the postsecondary educational setting commonly state that they prefer such services precisely because they are provided in the natural environment. Students state that receiving services in the natural environment encourages them to feel like contributing members of the larger community (Gutman et al, 2007; Lawrence, 2004). For these reasons, supported education programs in the postsecondary setting can uniquely facilitate community participation by providing age-appropriate services in a normalized setting that is highly esteemed by both mental health consumers and the larger society.

Summary

Supported education is a service-delivery model with evidence to support its efficacy. Because occupational therapists receive distinct training in functional adaptation and activity analysis, they can uniquely contribute to the development of supported education services. By ensuring that supported education services for people with psychiatric disabilities become routine and customary—as it has become for other groups with disabilities—occupational therapists can make a valuable contribution to this population as well as help to regain the profession's footing in mental health practice.

Active Learning Strategies

1. Simulation of Auditory Hallucinations

Turn on a television and a radio talk show (in the same room). Adjust the volume level of each to high. Then begin either reading a textbook chapter or writing an essay. Maintain this activity for at least 5 minutes and then answer the following questions.

Reflective Questions
- How difficult was it for you to concentrate on the reading or paper assignment? How much of the assignment were you able to complete?
- Did you feel frustrated or agitated? What other feelings did you experience?
- Were you able to tune out the voices in order to attend to your reading or writing?

  This activity is intended to simulate the experience of auditory hallucinations, or hearing voices while one is attempting to concentrate on educational activities. This activity simulates the inability to control the presence, volume, and statements of such auditory hallucinations.

Record your observations in your
Reflective Journal.

2. Simulation of Obsessions and Compulsions

Read the following paragraph. Each time you read the words *wash, washes,* or *washed,* get up, wash your hands, sit back down, and continue reading where you left off.

  A ten-year-old boy named Peter awakes one morning to the sound of school children as they play kickball on their way to school. Peter hurries to get out of bed and wash before breakfast. He takes the large bar of soap from the sink and places it between both hands. He rubs his hands together rigorously and creates a stream of suds and bubbles that fall to the floor. Peter begins his wash routine with his palms, soaps each finger, scrubs under each nail, and then rinses thoroughly. He dresses, too, choosing only clothing that seems clean and freshly washed. Soon Peter is dressed and joins his younger brother in the kitchen. Peter's younger brother, Seth, is messy and doesn't wash behind his ears. This

bothers Peter and he refuses to let Seth touch him. One day Peter counted every time he washed his hands. He counted up to 19 but then lost count. He wanted to start over and begin counting again, but his parents wouldn't let him because it was time for him to go to bed. But Peter couldn't sleep. He lay awake wishing he could wash his hands one more time. Ever since that day, Peter feels that he must wash his hands at least 20 times to remain clean. Peter feels compelled to keep his clothes clean, too. If Seth touches him before they go to school, Peter insists that he must change his clothing. He once made his mother wash all of his clothes because Seth had hidden in his closet to surprise him.

Reflective Questions
- What was it like for you to repeatedly stop reading and wash your hands? Were you able to concentrate on the story?
- Did you begin to resent having to wash your hands? Did you feel frustrated?

  This activity is intended to simulate the symptoms of obsession and compulsion. It is designed to help readers better understand how obsessions and compulsions—which commonly accompany various psychiatric illnesses—can disrupt simple daily activities and turn them into long, drawn-out rituals. Although many people with such symptoms feel compelled to perform specific activities, they can also feel resentment, frustration, and a loss of control over their actions. Imagine what this reading activity would be like if you were a student who felt compelled to wash your hands at least once every two paragraphs. What would such a compulsion do to your ability to be a student?

3. Simulation of Tangential and Fragmented Thoughts

Set up the following four activities: (1) read a chapter in a textbook, (2) develop an outline for an essay about climatic changes, (3) heat a pot of soup on a stove, and (4) develop a monthly budget based on needed expenses. Set a timer to go off at 3-minute intervals. Then begin the first activity. When the timer goes off, switch to the second activity. Continue to switch activities each time the alarm rings. Stop this activity in 15 minutes and answer the following questions:

Reflective Questions

- How well were you able to switch attention and focus on the tasks of a different activity? Were you able to concentrate sufficiently on any of the four tasks?
- Were you able to satisfactorily complete any of the four activities? Which activities were the most difficult to concentrate on? Were you able to focus completely on the next activity, or did you continue to think about the demands of the other activities?
- What happened to the soup? Were you able to cook it without incident, or did it accidentally boil?

This activity is intended to simulate the symptoms of psychiatric illnesses involving flight of ideas, uncontrolled rumination, and tangential and fragmented thought processes, symptoms commonly present in schizophrenia and bipolar illness. It offers an opportunity to understand what it might be like to participate in educational activities while experiencing such symptoms.

 Record the experience in your **Reflective Journal**.

Acknowledgment

This chapter is dedicated in memory of Dr. Karen Stern, who was one of the first occupational therapists to develop supported education services for adults with chronic psychiatric disabilities. Dr. Stern staunchly advocated for access and accommodations that could help students with psychiatric disabilities to participate fully in postsecondary educational environments. Her work helped many people transform potential capabilities into valued skills that positively changed their quality of life. Dr. Stern's work will undoubtedly continue to serve as an important model for the profession's involvement in supported education for many years to come.

Resources

Accommodations for People With Psychiatric Disabilities in Educational Settings
- From Boston University's Center for Psychiatric Rehabilitation: http://www.bu.edu/cpr/reasaccom/educa-accom.html

Review of Supported Education Programs and Recommendations
- http://www.psychosocial.com/IJPR_11/Supported_Ed_Strategies_Leonard.html

Substance Abuse and Mental Health Services Administration
- Toolkit for implementing the supported education model: http://mentalhealth.samhsa.gov/cmhs/CommunitySupport/employment_education/evidence.asp

References

Allen, C. K. (1996). *Allen Cognitive Level Screen (ACLS) Test Manual.* Colchester, CT: S & S Worldwide.

American Occupational Therapy Association. (2002). Occupational therapy practice framework: Domain and process. *American Journal of Occupational Therapy, 56,* 609–639.

Barrett, M., Vachman, L., & Huisingh, R. (1991). *Assessing Semantic Skills Through Everyday Scenes.* Moline, IL: Linguisystems.

Beiser, M., Waxler-Morrison, N., Iacono, W. G., Lin, T., Fleming, A. E., & Husted, J. (1987). A measure of "sick" label in psychiatric disorder with physical illness. *Social Science Medicine, 25,* 251–261.

Brown, C., & Dunn, W. (2002). *Adolescent/Adult Sensory Profile: User's Manual.* San Antonio, TX: Psychological Corporation.

Collins, M. E., Bybee, D., & Mowbray, C. T. (1998). Effectiveness of supported education for individuals with psychiatric disabilities: Results from an experimental study. *Community Mental Health Journal, 34,* 595–613.

Collins, M. E., Mowbray, C. T., & Bybee, D. (2000). Characteristics predicting successful outcomes of participants with severe mental illness in supported education. *Psychiatric Services, 51,* 774–780.

Cook, J. A., & Jonikas, J. A. (1992). Models of vocational rehabilitation for youths and adults with severe mental illness. *American Rehabilitation, 18*(3), 6–12.

Cook, J. A., & Solomon, M. L. (1993). The Community Scholar Program: An outcome study of supported education for students with severe mental illness. *Psychosocial Rehabilitation Journal, 17,* 83–87.

Derogatis, L., & Melisaratos, N. (1983). The Brief Symptom Inventory: An introductory report. *Psychological Medicine, 13,* 595–605.

Dougherty, S. J., & Campana, K. A. (1996). Supported education: A qualitative study of the student experience. *Psychiatric Rehabilitation Journal, 19*(3), 59–69.

Dowrick, P. W., Anderson, J., Heyer, K., & Acosta, J. (2005). Postsecondary education across the USA: Experiences of adults with disabilities. *Journal of Vocational Rehabilitation, 22*(1), 41–47.

Gutman, S. A., Kerner, R., Zombek, I., Dulek, J., & Ramsey, A. (2009). Supported education for adults with psychiatric disabilities: Effectiveness of an occupational therapy program. *American Journal of Occupational Therapy, 63,* 245–254.

Gutman, S. A., Schindler, V. P., Furphy, K. A., Klein, K., Lisak, J. M., & Durham, D. P. (2007). The effectiveness of a supported education program for adults with psychiatric disabilities: The Bridge Program. *Occupational Therapy in Mental Health, 23*(1), 21–38.

Harrington, T. (1993). *Harrington-O'Shea Career Decision-Making System Revised Manual.* Circle Pines, MN: Planning Associates.

Hoffman, F. L., & Mastrianni, X. (1992). The hospitalized young adult: New directions for psychiatric treatment. *American Journal of Orthopsychiatry, 62,* 297–302.

Housel, D. P., & Hickey, J. S. (1993). Supported education in a community college for students with psychiatric disabilities: The Houston Community College Model. *Psychosocial Rehabilitation Journal, 17,* 41–50.

Jasper, C. A. (1997). Life before supported education: The long journey. *Journal of the California Alliance for the Mentally Ill, 8*(2), 51–53.

Jones, D. R., Macias, C., Barreira, P. J., Fisher, W. H., Hargreaves, W. A., & Harding, C. M. (2004). Prevalence, severity, and co-occurrence of chronic physical health problems of persons with serious mental illness. *Psychiatric Services, 55,* 1250–1257.

Knis-Matthews, L., Bokara, J., DeMeo, L., Lepore, N., & Mavus, L. (2007). The meaning of higher education for people diagnosed with a mental illness: Four students share their experiences. *Psychiatric Rehabilitation Journal, 31*(2), 107–114.

Lawrence, J. (2004). Mental health survivors: Your colleagues. *International Journal of Mental Health Nursing, 13,* 185–190.

Lehman, A. F. (1991). *Quality of Life Core Version.* Baltimore: University of Maryland, School of Medicine, Center for Mental Health Services Research.

McQuistion, H. L., Finnerty, M., & Hirshowitz, E. S. (2003). Challenges for psychiatry in serving people with psychiatric disorders. *Psychiatric Services, 54,* 669–676.

Megivern, D., Pellerito, S., & Mowbray, C. (2003). Barriers to higher education for individuals with psychiatric disabilities. *Psychiatric Rehabilitation Journal, 26,* 217–231.

Mowbray, C. T., Collins, M. E., Bellamy, C. D., Megivern, D. A., Bybee, D., & Szilvagyi, S. (2005). Supported education for adults with psychiatric disabilities: An innovation for social work and psychosocial rehabilitation practice. *Social Work, 50*(1), 7–20.

Mowbray, C. T., Collins, M., & Bybee, D. (1999). Supported education for individuals with psychiatric disabilities: Long-term outcomes from an experimental study. *Social Work Research, 23,* 89–100.

Mowbray, C. T., Megivern, D., & Holter, M. C. (2003). Supported education programming for adults with psychiatric disabilities: Results from a national survey. *Psychiatric Rehabilitation Journal, 27,* 159–167.

Offer, D., Ostrov, E., & Howard, K. L. (1981). *The Adolescent: A Psychological Self-Portrait.* New York: Basic Books.

Orrin, D. (1997). How I earned my MSW despite my mental illness. *Journal of the California Alliance for the Mentally Ill, 8*(2), 61–63.

Pearlin, L. I,. & Schooler, M. (1978). The structure of coping. *Journal of Health and Social Behavior, 19,* 2–21.

Rosenberg, M. (1965). *Society and the Adolescent Self-Image.* Princeton, NJ: Princeton University Press.

Schindler, V. P. (2004). Occupational therapy in forensic psychiatry: Role development and schizophrenia. *Occupational Therapy in Mental Health, 20*(3/4).

Special Education and Rehabilitation Services. (2004). *The Rehabilitation Act.* Available at: http://www.ed.gov/policy/speced/leg/rehabact.doc (accessed October 31, 2006).

Stern, K. (2006). "Pathways to Success: A Supported Education Program for Adults with Psychiatric Disabilities." Paper presented at Mental Health Partnerships of New Jersey, Kean University, Union, New Jersey.

Unger, K. V. (1992). *Adults with Psychiatric Disabilities on Campus.* Health Resource Center, American Council for Education (Rep. No. H030C00001-91). Washington, DC: Department of Education.

Unger, K. V., Anthony, W. A., Sciarappa, K., & Rogers, E. S. (1991). A supported education program for young adults with long-term mental illness. *Hospital and Community Psychiatry, 42,* 838–842.

Unger, K., V., Pardee, R., & Shafer, M. S. (2000). Outcomes of postsecondary supported education programs for people with psychiatric disabilities. *Journal of Vocational Rehabilitation, 14,* 195–199.

U.S. Department of Education. (2006). *Individuals with Disabilities Education Improvement Act of 2004 (IDEA).* Available at: http://www.ed.gov/policy/speced/guid/idea/idea2004.html (accessed December 12, 2006).

U.S. Department of Justice. (2006). *Americans with Disabilities Act.* Available at: http://www.ada.gov (accessed December 12, 2006).

Vitkux, J., & Horowitz, L. M. (1987). Poor social performance of lonely people: Lacking a skill or adopting a role? *Journal of Personality and Social Psychology, 52,* 1266–1273.

Weiner, E. (1996). An exploratory qualitative study of three university students with mental illness and the perceived role their families play in their university education. *Psychiatric Rehabilitation Journal, 19*(3), 77–80.

Wilkinson, G. S. (1993). *Wide Range Achievement Test–Revised 3.* Wilmington, DE: Jastak Association.

World Health Organization. (2006). *International Classification of Functioning, Disability, and Health.* Available at: http://www.who.int/classifications/icf/en (accessed December 9, 2006).

Zung, W. W. K. (1971). A self-rating anxiety scale. *Archives of General Psychiatry, 26,* 112–118.

Work as Occupation

Deborah B. Pitts

> "Work, especially the opportunity to aspire to and achieve gainful employment, is a deeply generative and re-integrative force in the life of every human being."
>
> —Beard, Propst, and Malamud, 1982, p. 47

Introduction

The human occupation of work has had a central place in the philosophy and practice of occupational therapy since the founding of the profession (Hall & Buck, 1919; Meyer, 1922/1977; Reilly, 1966). This centrality results from the necessity of work, in its broadest definition, in the daily lives of most humans, both ancient and modern. In modern life, lack of opportunity to work not only has profound financial implications, but the psychological and social impact of not working can be equally devastating (Dewey, 1902; Jakobsen, 2004; Wilcock, 1993). Studies show that persons with psychiatric disabilities consistently identify the desire and preference to work (Uttaro & Mechanic, 1994; Van Dongen, 1996). In addition, work and opportunities for meaningful occupation are central to recovery for persons with psychiatric disabilities (Davidson, 2003; Kennedy-Jones, Cooper, & Fossey, 2005; Krupa, 2004; Scheid & Anderson, 1995; Strong, 1998; Van Dongen, 1996). However, despite the importance of work and the desire to work, persons with psychiatric disabilities are much less likely than any other disability group to be working, with unemployment rates ranging from 32% to 62% (Cook, 2006) and as high as 85% to 92% in some studies (Anthony, Cohen, Farkas, & Gagne, 2002).

A significant barrier keeping those who want to work unemployed is the belief held by many mental health professionals that people with psychiatric disabilities cannot and perhaps should not work given their vulnerability (Cook, 2006; Henry & Lucca, 2004). Occupational therapists can facilitate work and work reentry by first believing that work is possible—that is, by "[believing] in the potential productivity of the most severely disabled psychiatric client" (Beard, Propst, & Malamud, 1982, p. 47). With stigma being such a critical barrier to participation for persons with psychiatric disabilities (Corrigan, 2005; Link, Struening, Neese-Todd, Asmussen, & Phelan, 2001) and hope being so critical to recovery (Deegan, 1996; Klyma, Juvakka, Nikkonen, Korhonen, & Isohanni, 2006; Woodside, Landeen, Kirkpatrick, & Byrne, 1994), occupational therapists must take up this perspective, which is fully consistent with our perspective on human occupational potential (Wicks, 2001). With these beliefs in our hearts and minds, we can use our knowledge about occupation, disability, and recovery to collaborate with persons with psychiatric disabilities to plan interventions that address the person and environmental factors that may act as barriers to their work participation.

Importance of the Worker Role

Work is most typically distinguished from other areas of occupation, particularly activities of daily living/instrumental activities of daily living and play/leisure, because of its role in facilitating identity development and social participation. Yerxa (1998) draws on Jahoda's (1981) research regarding the importance of work to assert a link between engaging in occupation and health, particularly mental health (Box 50-1). In occupational therapy, we acknowledge that work or productive occupations are not restricted to paid employment and can include household work, care giving, education, or volunteer experiences (American Occupational Therapy Association [AOTA], 2002; Reberio & Allen, 1998).

Developing a Worker Role

The childhood occupation of play has a formative or developmental influence on work choices and work behaviors that occur in adolescence and adulthood. Although not always seen as a direct causal influence, these early occupational experiences are believed to mediate the development

---

BOX 50-1 ■ Latent Consequences of Work

- Employment imposes a time structure on the individual's day.
- Employment implies regularly shared experiences.
- Employment links individuals to goals and purposes transcending their own.
- Employment defines important aspects of personal status and identity.
- Employment enforces activity, providing a predictable demand for action.

The Lived Experience

Quiet Please . . . I'm concentrating!

Joe Crespo

Work has been an important aspect in my continued quest to recover from schizophrenia. Although my work history has been both intermittent and turbulent, just knowing that I haven't crashed signifies that there will be smoother rides in the future with fewer landings.

One of my favorite movies has a quote saying, "What one man can do another can do." Anthony Hopkins says it again, "What one man can do another can do." He says it again screaming at his partner to yell it with him, "WHAT ONE MAN CAN DO ANOTHER CAN DO!" The movie was *The Edge*. The quote is in reference to killing a bear. They are lost in the woods and this bear is stalking them already having eaten their other friend. They end up killing the bear with a makeshift spear, a wild beast five hundred pounds their size. This five-hundred-pound bear is SCHIZOPHRENIA.

My mind was so disconnected to anything a person of sound body and mind could expect to experience. I saw my mother and father go to work everyday and no matter how disconnected I was I knew that their going to work meant a roof over "our" shoulders and food to eat. No matter how bad I felt about myself I saw, knew and hoped that one day I could go back to work and get on with my life. A few years went by after the diagnosis and onset of my illness. I was suicidal and in a state nobody in their wildest dreams could imagine. I was aware of my mental state and wanted out. This was my first thought. But how was I to get out of this state of torment? I started thinking about what had happened to me. I had had a good life, played sports, had friends and had all the makings of a great life ahead of me, And then this blockbuster.

One day my father asked me if I wanted to type the names and addresses of business cards into his computer. I accepted the offer. No matter how messed up my head was, I was still able to type. I had taken typing in high school and still remembered how to do it. I got a job with a call center down the street and ended up staying there for two years. I loved going to work and I loved knowing how to type. The first day was agonizing worrying I was not going to be able to learn the job and worrying I was not going to be able to connect with other people. But smiles and laughter helped me see that I was just as capable to learn as everybody else, and oh yes, I had some money in my pocket as my dad used to emphasize. I was around others who believed in the work I did. They kept me and let others go, and I was proud of my accomplishments. About a year into my employment a supervisor told me that I should do data entry. They gave me more and more responsibilities doing data entry. It hit me that I was good at data entry and I wanted to see where it would lead me. Being around supportive people made a world of difference, my supervisor made me believe in myself with her data entry epiphany.

Along with a severe mental illness, I had a crushing dependence on alcohol. So even during this time of employment I began drinking again. It got me through each day along with my normal regime of medications that helped drown out the demons enough to let me sleep. So I drank alone in the garage, went to bed at a reasonable time and went to work in the morning. I did this for quite awhile, and while the drinking allowed me to sleep and get up in the morning, it also gave me a horrible feeling of being dependent on something that would mask my thought disorder. Now my internal thought disorder had now been externalized in my speech. As time went on, I started stuttering on the phone. It got so bad that I could barely pronounce any words at all. I was humiliated for the longest time knowing that others could hear me talk that way, but management was still on my side. They told me it was not that bad, but still I was embarrassed. I knew I did not stutter like that and it had to be the alcohol that was numbing my brain from the night before. It made me believe that I was so calm inside, when I was an utter wreck both inside and out, but I stayed on until I could no longer take it. I walked out one day and left my job. Schizophrenia had won again. Now all I had was alcohol, and a life that had gone nowhere in two years.

Feeling self-defeated and alone I still remembered the supervisor's words and I was revitalized. It wasn't defeat or schizophrenia that had won, it was the dark shadows that pervaded my spirit. The five-hundred-pound bear that nobody could figure out how to kill was now mine to figure out. Freely accepting this formula to be put on my shoulders was the worst mistake I have ever made, for I was not the same as I was when I was young. I was not in high school any more playing basketball, hitting shot after shot. I was not in my prime with friends having a blast and being the life of the party. I was not Mr. Baseball Card collector, blackjack dealer, I was Joe and I was lost. I had been through a tremendous amount of both physical and mental pain and was dealing with schizophrenia, which no single word could capture. I simply was not the same person anymore. The question now was how I was going to sustain myself while consuming alcohol and having shattered self-esteem and trying to kill a bear as ANOTHER MAN CAN DO! The job hadn't paid me much. I was free to get back on track and look for a data entry position that paid more money, to start thinking about having a life of which I knew nothing about.

Around this time I started thinking of going back to school. I had never been a really good student before, but I had always tried my hardest. I always harped to other people that it took me five times the amount of time to learn something new than a "normie." All I needed to transfer to a four-year university was one course in mathematics. I was horrible at math. It had been three or four years of thinking about how math was keeping me from transferring. Then one day it hit me. I told myself I was going to do it. I was going to pass math. I was going to study six or seven hours a day or more and I was going to pass. I was going to kill that five-hundred-pound bear. So I signed up to kill that bear. I knew it was going to be tough, but from the first day I studied six hours a day. As I was doing the problems I was figuring out questions I had about life. I was not just doing the problems. I think this is what was different and the reason why it took me so long. Doing the problems was kind of like therapy. It was still tough, but I was learning. I showed up every day to class and when the first test came around I ended up with a "C." I realized when I got the test back that I had not answered five questions that were on the back of the test. The teacher would write the distribution of grades on the chalkboard and I was amazed that half of the class had failed and I had gotten a C. I was mad at

The Lived Experience — cont'd

myself for not answering those questions, but I kept on studying six or seven hours a day. There is no question that I was progressing. The medications must have been working because as I said before there was no way I could have even thought about math unless I was in a semistable place. Work had also helped. I do not think without the work experience at the call center

I would have been able to pass math, and I did. I passed with a "B" grade. I was officially a university student. I probably cracked a real smile for the first time in my life. Something that was so deeply engraved in my brain had vanished through hard work. They say that hard work cures all. I prefer to say there is no cure, only hope of one!

of the occupational skills and person factors necessary for future work success and satisfaction (Bundy, 1991; Florey, 1981; Parham & Fazio, 1997; Reilly, 1974). Larson (2004) introduced a perspective on the developmental influences of childhood work to occupational science and occupational therapy. She draws on educational research which notes that children are more likely to experience activities as work when the activity is required rather than optional, chosen by caregivers (e.g., teachers) rather than by themselves, is effortful, useful and involves others.

In Western societies, our earliest formal work experiences usually begin in early adolescence. Typical early work experiences for adolescents in the United States include working within the family business, child care, nonskilled odd jobs around one's neighborhood, and volunteer experience often associated with membership in school-based service clubs or national service organizations. In developing countries, participation in formal work may begin much earlier in childhood and impact/limit engagement in play. In recent years, occupational therapists internationally have become more involved in global efforts at promoting occupational justice (Wilcock & Townsend, 2000). This includes efforts to counter child labor and to promote the development of work experiences through which individuals and their families can sustain a meaningful existence (Kronenberg, Algado, & Pollard, 2005).

Through early work experiences, young people continue the development of what are considered critical vocational behaviors. Reilly (1974) drew on the vocational psychology and career development literature in her early theorizing regarding play and proposed the developmental stages of exploration, competence, and achievement in occupational behavior. Vocational and rehabilitation literature defines critical vocational behaviors as occupational choice, job acquisition, and job retention, or simply to **choose, get, and keep** work (Anthony, Cohen, Farkas, & Gagne, 2002; Farley, Little, Bolton, & Chunn, 1993). Major task demands and work-related competencies consistent with the choose, get, and keep model are summarized in Table 50-1. In addition to the development of critical vocational behaviors, Erikson's (1959) psychosocial model of development emphasizes the critical challenge of identity versus role confusion during this period of vocational development.

During early adolescence, it is not only early work experiences but engagement in leisure occupations that influence later work participation. This perspective is partially informed by the work of Stebbins (1992), who described **serious leisure** as particularly engaging and time/skill-intensive. Serious leisure influences identity development and therefore

may influence future career choices (Lobo, 1999; Passmore, 1998). Passmore (1998) studied adolescent leisure experiences and was able to distinguish particular categories of leisure activity that may support the development of worker role skills. Specifically, achievement-oriented leisure activities demanded self-control, collaboration with others, and time-management for successful participation; and social leisure activities afforded the development of the social negotiation skills associated with successful interpersonal relationships.

Work and career decisions are typically made in late adolescence and early adulthood, although it is now understood that given the influence of technology and globalization on the nature of work, workers may go through multiple work transitions that require renewed decision-making at later points in life. Decisions, no matter when they are made, are most typically informed by the interaction among our **occupational self-knowledge** (e.g., personal causation, interests, values), our actual **occupational skills and capacities**, and our access to resources and supports needed to obtain a particular type of work (Kielhofner, 2002). Specific work competencies are obtained in a variety of ways, including education, training, and on-the-job experience. Although self-knowledge and actual work capacities are important, occupational therapy, as well as other rehabilitation professions, has been criticized for

Table 50-1 ● **Major Task Demands and Examples of Work-Related Competencies in the Choose, Get, Keep Model**

Choose	Get	Keep
Major Task Demands		
Select an appropriate and suitable occupational goal	Find employment opportunities	Adapt to the workplace
Plan to achieve the goal	Acquire a job	Retain employment
Examples of Work-Related Competencies		
Self-knowledge Work knowledge Job decision-making skills	Work orientation/motivation Job-finding skills Self-presentation (e.g., resumes, applications, interviews) Job performance skills	Basic work habits and behaviors Personal and environmental coping skills Interpersonal relationship skills Work attitudes and values

Farley, R. C., Little, N. D., Bolton, B., & Chunn, J. (1991). Employability Assessment and Planning in Rehabilitation and Educational Settings. Fayetteville, AK: Arkansas Research & Training Center in Vocational Rehabilitation.

its overreliance on person factors as predictors of success at work. The occupational justice and disability studies have turned our profession's attention to the structural barriers, including poverty and discrimination, that impact access to preparation for certain types of work (Townsend, 2003).

In developed countries, retirement is understood to be that time when workers transition out of full-time paid employment, with a significant reduction in demands related to productive occupations. Although generally understood as a desired time, studies show that transition from work to retirement can be difficult for some people and may result in significant risks for physical and mental health (Jonsson, Borell, & Sadlo, 2000). In addition, as cost of living has increased in the United States, retirement is often being extended beyond the well-accepted retirement ages of 65 to 67. Many older persons therefore do not have the choice to transition out of work life and must remain engaged in some type of work, even if only part time. In addition, grandparents have increasingly assumed care responsibilities for grandchildren when parents cannot afford child care. In developing countries with subsistence economies, ritualized end-of-work life is less common, and the elderly may remain engaged in work routines as long as their physical capacities support their participation.

Work and Psychiatric Disabilities

Work is a lifelong process that may be affected by the development of psychiatric disorders. In childhood, when developmental delay, sensory modulation difficulties, physical or sexual trauma, or the diagnosis of serious emotional disorders

occurs, play and chore experiences may be disrupted and impact the development of occupational skills, competence, and identity (Reilly, 1974; Parham & Fazio, 1997; Kielhofner, 2002). Due to the emergence of a psychiatric disorder during adolescence, vocational developmental opportunities may be disrupted, and as a result, the person may miss opportunities for work maturity (Fabian, 2000; Gioia, 2005). Schizophrenia in particular is understood as emerging in adolescence or young adulthood (American Psychiatric Association, 2000). Gioia (2005) proposes a model for understanding the interruption in career development that results from the emergence of psychiatric disorders. The model is based on her research into the experience of persons with schizophrenia that focused on their personal perspectives regarding their beliefs and experiences with work as well as the impact of their illness on their sensibilities about future work. Like other models regarding the recovery experience in schizophrenia (Davidson & Strauss, 1992), she argues that individuals must integrate their illness experience into their ongoing career development. They must bring together internal and external resources, as well as illness management and work strategies, to confront the internal and external barriers that may impede work participation. Emphasizing the individuality of each person's experience, she proposes three phases of vocational recovery: work as restoration, reformulation of vocational identity, and future work direction. Figure 50-1 depicts the individual work and illness trajectory for an individual with schizophrenia.

Persons with psychiatric disorders, particularly schizophrenia, are known to experience neurocognitive impairments that significantly impact their functioning (see Chapter 14). These

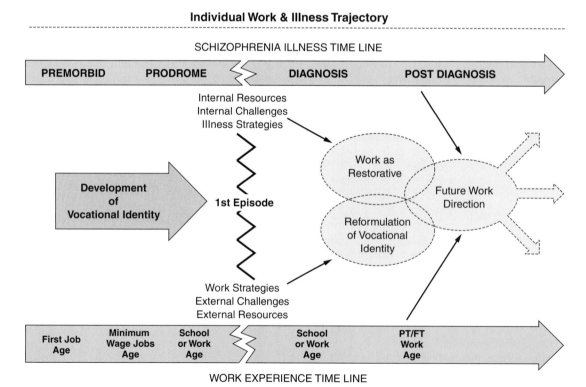

FIGURE 50-1. The impact of schizophrenia on the development of the worker role. *Adapted with permission from Gioia, D. (2005). Career development in schizophrenia: A heuristic framework. Community Mental Health Journal, 41(3), 315.*

impairments are understood to be distinct phenomenon from the psychiatric symptoms; include impairments of attention, memory, and executive function; and impact occupational performance (Goia, 2005; Green, 1996), including work (McGurk & Meltzer, 2000). McGurk and Mueser (2004) found persons with psychiatric disabilities who were working were more likely to have fewer cognitive impairments and less severe symptoms. Although there is some debate regarding the impact of psychiatric symptoms on work performance, recent studies have clearly demonstrated that although negative symptoms do have some impact, positive symptoms are not predictive of work functioning (Anthony, Rogers, Cohen, & Davies, 1995; Bell & Lysaker, 1995). Given the importance of cognition on human performance and the studies demonstrating its relationship to work functioning, cognition has become a major focus of research regarding work, work interventions, and work outcomes across the life span and an individual's employment career.

Given the nature of many psychiatric disorders, symptom exacerbations may occur during an individual's working life. Depending on his or her coping response to the symptom exacerbation, the person may be disengaged from the workforce for some time or may decide to change his or her type of work to mediate the stress. For many persons with psychiatric disabilities, an additional strategy for managing stress is to work part time rather than full time. In addition, transition to retirement may come earlier because it offers a viable and socially valued alternative to work.

As noted in the introduction, persons with psychiatric disabilities consistently state that working and having access to work opportunities is significant to their recovery. Qualitative studies find that persons with psychiatric disabilities identify several benefits to working, including access to meaningful social roles, regular daily activity and social connectedness, and enhanced mental health and self-efficacy (Honey, 2003; Kirsh, 2000; Provencher, Greg, Mead, & Mueser, 2002; Strong, 1998;). Research also shows that when persons with psychiatric disabilities choose to work, they must balance these positive benefits with the challenges and risks of working. A major risk is the loss of or reduction in benefits (e.g., Social Security disability, Medicaid/Medicare health coverage, food stamps, housing subsidies) typically associated with earning an income. Individuals with psychiatric disabilities, even if they are making a reasonable salary and receiving health benefits, often worry about the consequences of losing their job and then having to engage in the lengthy and challenging process of reapplying for benefits. Persons with psychiatric disabilities must go through a process of "weighing up" (Honey, 2003, p. 388) and may determine that to work is too risky to their financial and mental and physical health status (Honey, 2003; Nagle, Cook, & Polatajko, 2002).

Many factors can present barriers to work for people with psychiatric disabilities. An important review (Cook, 2006) identified the following list:

- Low educational attainment
- Lowered productivity
- Unfavorable labor market dynamics
- Lack of effective vocational services
- Lack of effective clinical services
- Labor force discrimination

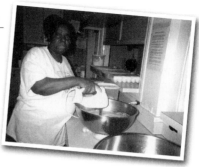

PhotoVoice

In my job I've learned to bake a cake from scratch. I can enjoy the pleasure of cooking and smiling and being myself.
Having a job makes me feel like I am somebody.
Working is part of recovering from my mental illness.

—Janet

- Failure of protective legislation
- Poverty-level income
- Linkage of health care to disability beneficiary status
- Disadvantages upon labor force reentry
- Employment disincentives
- Ineffective work incentive legislation

It is important that occupational therapists identify the specific barriers faced by a particular individual so that interventions can target the issue. In many cases, interventions must address environmental or policy-level concerns.

Federal Policy Designed to Support Work Participation

Federal policy has been implemented in the United States to increase the access that persons with disabilities, including those with psychiatric disabilities, have to gainful work. These include Section 504 of the Rehabilitation Act of 1973 as amended in 1992 and 1998, the Americans with Disabilities Act of 1990, the Ticket to Work and Work Incentives Improvement Act of 1999, and Medicaid funding for personal assistance services (PAS). Each policy addresses specific barriers that persons with disabilities experience as they attempt to enter or reenter the work world.

Section 504 of the Rehabilitation Act of 1973 protects the civil rights of persons with disabilities. It prohibits discrimination on the basis of disability by the federal government, federal contractors, and recipients of federal financial assistance. Organizations that receive federal funds are required to make their programs accessible to individuals with disabilities. This policy promotes access of persons with psychiatric disabilities to employment services as well as to work opportunities in the federal government.

The *American with Disabilities Act (ADA) of 1990* prohibits employers (in both government and private sectors) from discriminating against a **qualified individual with a disability** who can perform the **essential functions** (i.e., the fundamental or critical duties) of the job with or without **reasonable accommodations**. In addition, the ADA requires employers to provide reasonable accommodations if requested by the employee with a disability as long as they do not impose an undue hardship on the viability of the business. It is the employee's decision to request accommodations; the employer may not ask questions that are likely to elicit information about a disability before making an offer of employment. Assisting persons with disabilities to determine their need and preference for reasonable accommodations is an important function for employment service providers. Employment service providers can assist the person in identifying the specific types of accommodations needed for a particular job and work environment. Occupational therapists are particularly skilled in this area given our understanding of the functional effects of medical and psychiatric disorders and activity analysis, which can be used to evaluate the task and contextual dimensions of work environments.

The ADA protects all persons with a disability, including persons with psychiatric disabilities. MacDonald-Wilson, Rogers, Massaro, Lyass, and Crean (2002) explored the nature of the functional limitations that might create the need for reasonable accommodations by persons with psychiatric disabilities. They found that functional limitations were most commonly experienced by the study participants in their efforts to interact with others, learn the job task, maintain work stamina/pace, manage symptoms and tolerate stress, work independently, modify work performance, and follow schedule/attend work. With regard to the types of reasonable accommodations, they found that job coach involvement on the job, job coach assistance in hiring, flexible scheduling, changes in training and supervision, and modified job duties were most frequently provided.

Requesting reasonable accommodations can be problematic for persons with psychiatric disabilities because it requires disclosure of aspects of their disability in the face of profound stigma and negative stereotypes associated with mental illness (Dalgin & Gilbride, 2003; Ralph, 2002). In addition, the **direct-threat** exemption of the ADA further complicates decisions to disclose given the widely held perception that persons with psychiatric disabilities are dangerous (Campbell & Kaufmann, 1997). The direct-threat standard of the ADA supports the efforts of employers to provide a safe working environment for all employees and allows them to lawfully exclude an employee who poses a direct threat in the workplace. The Equal Employment Opportunity Commission provides enforcement guidance on the implementation of the ADA and psychiatric disabilities. Disclosure, then, becomes a complex decision process that requires the person with a psychiatric disability to consider issues of confidentiality (Mechanic, 1998), shame (Ralph, 2002), and concern about negative responses from employers and coworkers (Dalgin & Gilbride, 2003). Although persons with psychiatric disabilities disagree on whether or not to disclose, it does appear that having access to social support is necessary to "survive" the disclosure experience (Ralph, 2002). Occupational therapists promoting work participation for persons with psychiatric disabilities can offer that social and emotional support along with technical expertise regarding the nature and type of reasonable accommodations to request.

The *Ticket to Work and Work Incentives Improvement Act* implemented by the Social Security Administration introduced new incentives and expanded on existing incentives to promote return to work for persons with disabilities who received Social Security benefits. Beneficiaries of both Social Security Disability Insurance (SSDI) and Supplemental Security Income (SSI) are eligible for specific incentives, including federal financial resources to obtain return to work assistance (i.e., Ticket to Work). This limits the adjustments in SSDI/SSI payment as a result of work earnings and allows individuals to extended medical coverage with Medicare/Medicaid once employed. SSDI/SSI beneficiaries receive a ticket, or voucher, that allows them to use Social Security funds to pay for employment services. In addition, when SSDI beneficiaries choose to work, their Social Security payments are not affected unless they earn over the substantial gainful activity (SGA) amount (SGA amount in 2010: $1,000). For SSI beneficiaries, the impact of earnings on their Social Security is graduated so that after the first $85.00 of earnings, their Social Security payment is reduced $1 for every $2 of earnings. Another important incentive specifically designed for SSI beneficiaries is the Plan for Achieving Self-Support (PASS), which supports individuals in achieving a work goal.

O'Day and Killeen (2002) found that these incentives, as currently implemented, may benefit only a small number of individuals with psychiatric disabilities. Nevertheless, given that fear of losing benefits is identified as a barrier for work participation of SSDI/SSI beneficiaries, educating and facilitating access to these work incentives is an important responsibility of any employment services provider, including occupational therapists. In addition, MacDonald-Wilson, Rogers, Ellison, and Lyass (2003) found that mental health consumers, their families, and in many instances their service providers were uninformed regarding the work incentives. Tremblay, Smith, Xie, & Drake (2004) found that specialized benefits counseling resulted in significantly greater improvements in earnings in comparison to employment service recipients who did not receive the counseling. Occupational therapists working with persons with psychiatric disabilities on work entry or reentry must be fully informed of the work incentive programs and must educate the individuals they serve regarding work incentives as they apply to their personal situation.

Medicaid-funded personal assistance services (PAS), also called in-home support services (IHSS) for persons with disabilities, have been implemented in most states and until recently were limited to persons with physical disabilities. PAS "refers to a range of human and mechanical assistance provided to persons with disabilities of any age who require help with routine activities of daily living (ADLs) and health maintenance activities" (Doty, Kasper, & Litvak, 1996, p. 377). Consumer-directed personal assistance services (CD-PAS) represent an innovation in the provision of PAS and are consistent with the overall direction in self-determination in social, rehabilitation, health, and mental health services. In CD-PAS, rather than the medical/social professional prescribing and managing the services, the person with the disability assumes responsibility for all aspects of the PAS he or she receives. When accessing the PAS option through Medicaid for persons with psychiatric disabilities to support work participation, it is critical to distinguish PAS from the employment- provided support services. Pita, Ellison, Farkas, and Bleecker (2001) studied persons with psychiatric disabilities who had accessed PAS through their state Medicaid programs and found the service "helped them 'a lot' with daily life" (p. 7). In particular, they found the program useful for assistance with transportation, household routines, and organizing daily tasks. Workplace-based PAS are increasingly being accessed by persons with physical disabilities, and persons with psychiatric disabilities may also find PAS on the job to facilitate their work retention. In addition, serving as a PAS worker may provide an employment choice for persons with psychiatric disabilities.

Work Assessments

Occupational therapy assessment of work readiness, preferences, and performance for persons with psychiatric disabilities is informed by our understanding of human occupational development, the functional impairments associated with psychiatric disorders, and the demands of workplace settings. Assessment of work is an ongoing process that focuses on the critical vocational behaviors of occupational choice, job acquisition, and job retention (i.e., choose, get, keep). The assessment of a person's occupational choice has recently been expanded in the field of psychiatric rehabilitation to include readiness assessment. **Readiness assessment** is an important first step in any rehabilitation assessment process, and it is argued that it must come before conducting functional and resource assessments (Cohen & Mynks, 1993; Rogers et al, 2001; Smith et al, 1998). Readiness assessment is based on theoretical models that propose stages of behavioral change. Such models offer explanations for our successful—and failed—attempts to eliminate problems or develop helpful habits and daily routines. These models also argue that interventions designed to facilitate behavioral changes must be matched with each specific stage of change in order to result in positive outcomes (i.e., success in changing) (Prochaska & Norcross, 2001; Rogers et al, 2001). When conducting a readiness assessment, the occupational therapist must engage the person in thoughtful discussions and/or values clarification activities (i.e., individual or group exercises) focused on the person's satisfactions/dissatisfactions with his or her current situation, commitment to change, environmental awareness, personal preferences, and sources of personal support (Cohen & Mynks, 1993). Through the readiness assessment process, individuals can identify the lifestyle and environmental changes they want to make in their worker role.

As in other areas of occupation, assessment approaches for facilitating work participation include interview, self-report, and behavioral observation. Along with readiness, occupational development and choice are most effectively assessed through interview and/or self-report approaches. Although interview and self-report approaches are also important for eliciting individuals' perceptions of their job search and job retention experiences, observational approaches are likely to be more useful in fully understanding their behavioral success. Psychometric measures of task performance developed for use with nondisabled populations have been found to be less effective in assessing the work functioning of persons with psychiatric disabilities. As a result, **situational assessments** have become the preferred approach for assessing work function of persons with psychiatric disabilities (Bolton, 1988; MacDonald-Wilson, Rogers, & Anthony, 2001).

The Occupational Therapy Practice Framework (AOTA, 2002) provides guidance for the assessment process in occupational therapy that includes first the development of an occupational profile and then an analysis of occupational performance. Given recent understandings of the impact of sensory and cognitive disruptions on occupational performance, particularly work, these areas in particular should be targeted in an occupational therapy evaluation.

The Occupational Profile

In the context of work assessment, the **occupational profile** focuses particularly on the person's engagement in childhood occupations as preparatory experiences for work and engagement in adolescent occupational experiences, especially work and school, as sources for the development of self-knowledge around potential work interests, values, self-efficacy, and competencies. In addition, the occupational therapist elicits the person's perceptions regarding person factors and contextual barriers to work participation. The occupational profile is most often completed using interviews, particularly those with a narrative perspective, and/or self-report assessments.

Interviews

Occupational Performance History Interview–II (OPHI-II) uses a semistructured and narrative interview approach to help the occupational therapist understand the individual as an occupational being. Informed by the model of human occupation (MOHO), the suggested interview questions are organized in five thematic areas, including occupational roles, daily routine, occupational behavior settings, activity/occupational choices, and critical life events (Kielhofner et al, 2004). This assessment can be used with adolescents (at least 12 years of age) through seniors.

Familiarity with the MOHO is important to interpret the findings from the interview. The clinician uses the information to complete a set of rating scales and key forms, specifically the Occupational Identity, Occupational Competence, and Occupational Behavior Settings. Each item is rated using a 4-point adaptive scale (4, most adaptive response; 1, least adaptive response) (Kielhofner et al, 2004).

Reliability and validity of the OPHI-II including interrater reliability, concurrent validity, and predictive validity, has been demonstrated in several studies. Further, a study investigating the nature of the interview questions found that the narrative approach to questions effectively generated rich occupational stories and more meaningful information for intervention planning. Cross-cultural validity has also been demonstrated (Kielhofner 2002).

Worker Role Interview (WRI) is a work-based assessment developed by proponents of the MOHO (Braveman et al, 2005). The WRI is a semistructured interview that elicits information consistent with the MOHO components of volition, habituation, and environment. The information derived from the WRI is expected to be integrated with findings from observational assessments of a person's specific work competencies. Although originally developed for use with injured workers who are expecting to return to a particular type of work, recent updates of the tool have been developed for use with persons who may have been out of the workforce for some time due to extended illness or disability (Braveman et al, 2005). Interview findings are utilized to complete a general rating scale that includes 16 items specifically related to the MOHO components, including personal causation, values, interests, roles, habits, and the environment. Each item on the 4-point rating scale is operationally defined (Braveman et al, 2005). Dependability of the WRI, including internal, test–retest, and interrater validity, has been established. Cross-cultural validity has also been demonstrated (Kielhofner, 2002).

Work Environment Impact Scale (WEIS) is another work-based assessment developed by proponents of the MOHO. The WEIS uses a semistructured interview format to elicit the person's perception of their work environment, including the physical, social, and temporal aspects. It was developed for use with persons with physical and/or psychiatric disabilities. The nature of the questions limit its use with persons who have been out of work for some time; they focus on a current work environment or a work environment to which the person expects to return (Moore-Corner, Kielhofner, & Olson, 1998). After completion of the interview, the practitioner completes a 17-item rating scale that focuses on the physical space, social contacts and supports, temporal demands, objects utilized, and daily job functions. Each item is rated on a 4-point scale that indicates the degree to which the person perceives that aspect of the environment to support or interfere with his or her success and satisfaction at work (Moore-Corner et al, 1998). Dependability of the WEIS, including overall construct validity and interrater agreement, has been established. In addition, these studies indicate it can be used cross-culturally (Kielhofner, 2002).

Self-Report Assessments

Adult/Adolescent Sensory Profile (Brown & Dunn, 2002; Brown, Tollefson, Dunn, Cromwell, & Filion, 2001) is a self-report measure designed to identify sensory-processing patterns and effects on occupational performance. It is informed by Dunn's model of sensory processing (Dunn, 1997). The instrument can also be used to develop individuals' awareness of their sensory-processing needs and strategies to optimize the desired sensory environment. Respondents answers questions regarding how they generally respond to sensations as opposed to how they respond to a particular event or situation at one point in time. Based on the intersection of two continua (neurological threshold and behavioral response/self-regulation), Dunn's model describes quadrants identified as Low Registration, Sensation Seeking, Sensory Sensitivity, and Sensation Avoiding. Each quadrant has its own score. There are 60 items with 15 items for each quadrant. These quadrants cover the sensory processing categories of taste/smell, movement, visual, touch, activity level, and auditory; these categories are distributed throughout the quadrants. Psychometric evidence supports the claim that scores from the profile can provide reliable and valid inferences about an individual's sensory-processing patterns (Brown & Dunn, 2002).

Occupational Self-Assessment (Baron, Kielhofner, Iyenger, Goldhammer & Wolenski, 2002) is informed by the MOHO and is designed to facilitate an understanding of individuals' perceptions of their occupational competence and the impact of aspects of the environment on their occupational performance. This instrument serves as both an intervention

planning tool and an outcome measure, so it can be administered multiple times to identify change in response to the occupational therapy intervention. Studies have examined the validity and reliability of the Occupational Self-Assessment and found that it works well across cultural, language, and diagnostic differences (Kielhofner & Forsyth, 2001).

The recently updated *Self-Directed Search (SDS)* was developed by John Holland and has been used in career counseling for over 30 years (Spokane & Holland, 1995). Although not originally developed for use with persons with psychiatric disabilities, it has been used by vocational and psychiatric rehabilitation practitioners because of its low cost, ease of use, and exploratory design. It requires a certain level of self-knowledge and knowledge of the world of work, so it has some limitations depending on the person's development in these areas.

The SDS is based on Holland's theory of persons in vocational environments (Holland, 1997) and includes an Assessment Booklet, which matches the person to Holland's six interest or personality types, and the Occupations Finder, which the individual uses to find compatible job titles (Spokane & Holland, 1995). The psychometric properties of the instrument have been validated (Holland, 1997), as have the realistic, investigative, artistic, social, enterprising, and conventional (RIASEC) types (Spokane & Holland, 1995) originally identified by Holland. By completing the Assessment Booklet, which includes questions related to activity preferences and competencies, interest in particular job titles, and estimates of work ability and skill, the individual obtains a three-letter code (e.g., SIE) that is used to identify job titles in the Occupations Finder. The SDS also includes a Leisure Activities Finder that can be used as part of a work/leisure intervention (Spokane & Holland, 1995).

Work Environment Scale (WES) uses a person–environment fit perspective consistent with occupational therapy practice and provides a method for facilitating the match between individuals' and the social environment of their work settings (Moos, 1994). The WES facilitates occupational decision-making prior to work entry and evaluates individuals' experience in their current work contexts. The 90-item self-report instrument elicits information about the person's perception of social relationships at work, the degree of social support for personal growth in the workplace, and maintenance and change characteristics of the social environment.

Analysis of Occupational Performance

During the **analysis of occupational performance**, the occupational therapist elicits more targeted information regarding the performance skills/patterns, person factors, activity demands, and contextual barriers that may need intervention to facilitate successful work participation. Assessment approaches most commonly used during the analysis of occupational performance are observational or proxy measures of work-related functioning.

Situational Assessments

Work Behavior Inventory (WBI) was developed to meet the need for a situational assessment to measure the onsite work performance of persons with psychiatric disabilities. It is quick to administer and measures changes in work behavior over time, so it can serve as an outcomes measure for work rehabilitation interventions (Bryson, Bell, Lysaker, & Zito, 1997). The WBI consists of five behavioral scales (Work Habits, Work Quality, Personal Presentation, Social Skills, and Cooperativeness) and provides a global rating of the individual's work behavior. Each scale consists of behavioral descriptors developed and tested to represent critical work behaviors. Each behavioral descriptor is rated on a 5-point scale measuring the consistency of the quality of the individual's work performance, from *needs improvement to superior performance*. Administration of the WBI requires the practitioner to have access to the individual's worksite and involves a combination of a 10- to 15-minute observation of the individual performing work duties and a semistructured interview with the worksite supervisor. The practitioner administering the measure should be knowledgeable of work behaviors and the impact that psychiatric disabilities may have on an individual's social and task performance in work environments (Bryson et al, 1997). Dependability of this tool, including concurrent validity, interrater reliability for individual behavioral descriptors, and overall inventory total and discriminant validity comparing schizophrenia substance abuse samples, has been demonstrated in several studies (Bryson et al, 1997; Bryson, Bell, Greig, & Kaplan, 1999).

Vocational Cognitive Rating Scale (VCRS) was developed by Greig, Nicholls, Bryson, and Bell (2004) to provide a contextualized measure of the impact of common neurocognitive impairments experienced by persons with psychiatric disabilities in the workplace. The VCRS has 16 behavior-based items rated on a 1 to 5 severity scale (the lower the number, the greater severity). The ratings for each item are determined by a rehabilitation practitioner following a brief observation of the person at work and an interview with the worker's supervisor. The tool has been used in a variety of workplace settings to monitor and communicate to clients about their work performance. Dependability, including interrater reliability, internal consistency, concurrent and predictive validity, and good discriminate validity to distinguish between workers and nonworkers, was demonstrated in the initial study of the tool (Greig et al, 2004).

Volitional Questionnaire (VQ) (de las Heras, Geist, Kielhofner, & Li, 2003), informed by the MOHO, is an observational assessment of volition and is useful when self-report assessments are not feasible. Some clients have difficulty verbally articulating their goals, interests, and values but can communicate them through their active engagement in their environments. Although not specifically designed as a work assessment, given its observational approach, it could be used with persons who have had little work experience and who are also less able to articulate their activity preferences. It may have particular usefulness in psychosocial clubhouses (see Chapter 39), which are specifically designed to engage individuals with psychiatric disabilities in work experiences through the work-ordered day and transitional employment placements. The VQ contains 14 items that describe behaviors reflecting values, interests, and personal causation. The rating focuses on individuals' volitional behaviors in their environments rather than on the environmental support needed to engage. The VQ is supported by a detailed manual (de las Heras et al, 2003). Content validity and interrater reliability studies (de las Heras, 1993a, 1993b) have been completed.

Interventions to Promote Work Participation

Facilitating entry or reentry into employment has been a focus of occupational therapy intervention in the United States since the founding of the profession. The founding meeting of the National Society for the Promotion of Occupational Therapy (NSPOT) was held in 1917 at Consolation House, a curative workshop founded by George E. Barton in Clifton Springs, New York. Barton, an architect, experienced his own recovery from tuberculosis through engagement in occupation. Herbert J. Hall countered the prevailing wisdom of his time regarding the "rest cure" as the proper intervention for neurasthenia and promoted the "work cure" (Anthony, 2005a, 2005b). Barton and Hall, along with other founders, believed that occupational therapy had a moral obligation to assist persons with disabilities to regain their capacity to be self-supporting (Peloquin, 1994; Quiroga, 1995).

As a result of early jurisdictional claim disputes between the civilian and military governmental departments over the rehabilitative care of the war-wounded, occupational therapy's focus became prevocational. A prevocational perspective meant that occupational therapy interventions, as medical interventions, would target functional recovery, or restoration. It would be the role of the civilian Federal Board for Vocational Education, what we now know as the Rehabilitation Services Administration, to address vocational rehabilitation, or the specific preparation of persons with disabilities to enter work (Gritzer & Arluke, 1985). The term *prevocational* has fallen out of favor largely because of consumer and professional critics who argued that rehabilitation's focus on preparatory processes for work entry acted as a barrier to real work entry or reentry for persons with psychiatric disabilities. This critique is most well understood as vocational rehabilitation has moved from a train–place perspective to a place–train perspective (Becker & Drake, 2003; Corrigan, 2001).

Occupational therapy's focus on the development of prevocational interventions and theoretical models to support those interventions may also have served as a barrier to our contributing to more recent innovations in employment services that emerged during the 1980s and 1990s, particularly for persons with psychiatric disabilities. However, occupational therapy's participation in these community- and evidenced-based employment interventions has increased, and occupational therapy researchers are contributing to the body of knowledge regarding the meaning of work as occupation as well as its critical role in recovery, and they are also providing guidance for facilitating work reentry and retention (Eastabrook, Krupa, & Horgan, 2004; Kirsh, Cockburn, & Gewurtz, 2005; Krupa, 2004; Krupa, Lagarde, & Carmichael, 2003; Strong, 1998). Occupational therapists' increased participation in community-based employment services for persons with psychiatric disabilities has likely been influenced by several factors, including (1) our profession's vigorous effort to promote occupational participation for all persons, including those at risk for disability; (2) clear evidence from recovery research that work matters; (3) growth of community- based interventions as alternatives to psychiatric hospitalization for persons with psychiatric disabilities; (4) regulatory and financial mechanisms designed to support community-based services; and, (5) individual efforts of particular occupational therapists who have advocated for occupational therapy representation in these community mental health settings. Kirsh, Cockburn, and Gewurtz (2005) completed a comprehensive review of the literature regarding vocational outcomes for persons with psychiatric disabilities and summarized the implications of these findings for occupational therapists (Box 50-2). Their arguments regarding the fit between occupational therapy practice and the key characteristics of interventions that facilitate work outcomes include our commitment to self-direction for persons with psychiatric disabilities; our fundamental belief in the value of occupational engagement for individuals' overall health and wellbeing; and our understanding of the interaction between person, occupation, and environment.

Informed by innovations in practice technologies, better understandings of the nature of psychiatric disability, and most importantly by social and political movements that have foregrounded the civil rights and occupational needs of persons with psychiatric disabilities, interventions to promote work entry and reentry for persons with psychiatric disabilities have been developed. In the main, these work participation approaches emphasize integrating people with psychiatric disabilities into real-work contexts of their choice. Employment program approaches identified in the literature and public policy include transitional employment, supported employment, social enterprises/affirmative business, and self-employment.

Transitional Employment

Transitional employment (TE) represents one of the oldest of the employment models and is usually described in relationship to the psychosocial clubhouse (see Chapter 39). A transitional employment placement (TEP) is a time-limited placement (e.g., 3–6 months) in a competitive job at a prevailing wage in a real-work context. Psychosocial rehabilitation clubhouses innovated this approach and offer it as part of their continuum of work opportunities along with the clubhouse-based work-ordered day, community-based independent employment (Beard, Propst, & Malamud, 1982), and more recently supported employment (Bond & Jones, 2005). For clubhouses, the TEP represents a work opportunity particularly designed to address common employment barriers experienced by persons with a psychiatric disability, including limited or no work history, lack of self-efficacy regarding potential for work, and/or lack of clarity around preferred work/career goals. By participating in one or more TEPs, clubhouse members are given the opportunity to develop their sense of efficacy as a worker, to build a work history, and to try out different kinds of work experiences to further clarify their career/work preferences. Clubhouses work with local business to develop TEPs, and every effort is made to include a variety of job types, generally entry level and unskilled. In addition to meeting the needs of the clubhouse members, a key element in the development of TEPs is meeting the employer's needs for qualified workers.

Although the clubhouse-based transitional employment approach has received criticism as being outdated and no longer needed in light of the evidence regarding supported employment (Bilby, 1992), efforts to document its benefits have been made, particularly by the International Center for Clubhouse Development (ICCD; http://www.iccd.org). McKay, Johnsen, and Stein (2005) investigated the employment outcomes of an ICCD-certified clubhouses in Massachusetts and found that job tenure and higher earnings were positively related to the length of time a person had been a member of the clubhouse. An earlier study by Henry, Barreira, Banks, Brown, and McKay (2001) also found that clubhouse members who had worked a TEP were more likely than members who had not worked a TEP to obtain competitive employment.

Supported Employment

Supported employment (SE), as an evidence-based practice, is the most replicated employment services model for persons with psychiatric disabilities (Bond & Jones, 2005). Introduced in the early 1980s, this model of vocational rehabilitation was initially designed to meet the needs of persons with developmental disabilities who had spent their work careers in preparatory contexts called sheltered workshops. Supported employment eliminated prevocational training and promoted a **place–train approach** to work entry. The approach was quickly adopted for other disability groups, including persons with psychiatric disabilities, for whom the traditional approach of train–place had been common. The Rehabilitation Act Amendments of 1998, Title IV of the Workforce Investment Act of 1998, defined supported employment as "competitive work in integrated work settings, or employment in integrated work settings in which individuals are working toward competitive work, consistent with the strengths, resources, priorities, concerns, abilities, capabilities, interests, and informed choice of the individuals, for individuals with the most significant disabilities for whom competitive employment has not traditionally occurred; or for whom competitive employment has been interrupted or

---

BOX 50-2 ■ Program Characteristics That Influence Work Outcomes for Persons With Psychiatric Disabilities

- Specific focus on work
- Inclusion of a vocational or employment specialist on the mental health team
- Job matching, attention to client preferences and choices
- Ongoing, available supports
- Rapid placement and on-the-job training
- Problem-solving approach to work and daily living
- Pay for work
- Attention to the work environment
- Team approach
- Support and education for employers and coworkers
- A range of services that are available and accessible

intermittent as a result of a significant disability; and who, because of the nature and severity of their disability, need intensive supported employment services . . . to perform such work" (p. 20).

The individual placement and support model of supported employment was developed by Becker and Drake (1993, 2003) and has provided guidance for the development of supported employment services for persons with psychiatric disabilities within the United States and internationally (Bond, 2004). The key characteristic of supported employment programs for persons with psychiatric disabilities include the following:

- Integration and coordination of employment assistance services with the mental health services that the person is receiving.
- Service eligibility based on the person's expressed desire to work; individuals are not screened out based on illness or employment history.
- Competitive employment in a job consistent with the person's preferences is the goal.
- There is no extended assessment or preparatory phase: job-search begins immediately upon program entry.
- Individualized support is provided on a time-unlimited basis as needed by the person.
- Social Security benefits counseling is provided to assist the person in effectively managing Social Security, health insurance, and other government benefits to support his or her successful entry into and retention of work. (Bond & Jones, 2005, p. 378–379).

Effectiveness studies of supported employment for persons with psychiatric disabilities consistently show that those with psychiatric disabilities receiving supported employment services provided in a manner consistent with the key characteristics described here are more likely than controls to gain and sustain employment (Bond, 2004; Bond et al, 2001; Bond & Jones, 2005; Cook et al, 2005). In addition, these studies indicate that nonvocational outcomes such as better control of symptoms, higher self-esteem, and improved quality of life are experienced by recipients of supported employment services over other vocational rehabilitation approaches (Bond, 2004). As a result of these studies, supported employment is identified as an evidence-based mental health practice by the Center for Mental Health Services (CMHS). In the United States, most state mental health authorities have adopted supported employment as part of their recovery-oriented mental health service system (National Association of State Mental Health Program Directors, 2002). Figure 50-2 illustrates a model of cognition, symptoms, and work in supported employment.

Affirmative Businesses/Social Firms

Beginning in the 1970s in Italy, affirmative businesses/social enterprises have been developed internationally to provide employment opportunities for persons with psychiatric disabilities (Warner & Mandiberg, 2006). Affirmative businesses/social firms are designed to increase the economic self-sufficiency of persons with psychiatric disabilities (Shaheen, Williams & Dennis, 2003). Social enterprises are intended to both operate as a financially viable business and

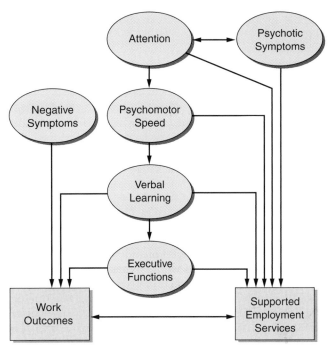

FIGURE 50-2. A model of cognition, symptoms, and work in supported employment. *Adapted with permission from McGurk, S. R., & Mueser, K. T. (2004). Cognitive functioning, symptoms, and work in supported employment: A review and heuristic model. Schizophrenia Research, 70, 162.*

meet the needs of disenfranchised workers. Also referred to as worker cooperatives, these businesses typically offer services, such as cleaning or repair, or sell handmade products. An asset of this model is the supportive atmosphere that is developed among workers in the agency. All workers are guaranteed a fair-market wage, and the business does not accept governmental subsidies to support revenues. Although not as popular in the United States, affirmative businesses

---

Evidence-Based Practice

Employment assistance services for persons with psychiatric disabilities are more likely to result in positive work outcomes when they are integrated with mental health services and focus on immediate work entry in real-world employment settings rather than prevocational training (Bond, 2004; Cook et al, 2005).

➤ Occupational therapists can advocate direct access to work participation for persons with psychiatric disabilities and promote the development of supported employment, transitional employment, or affirmative businesses/social forms.

➤ Occupational therapists working to promote work participation should insure that any employment assistance they provide is integrated and coordinated with the person's mental health services.

Bond, G. R. (2004). Supported employment: Evidence for an evidence-based practice. *Psychiatric Rehabilitation Journal, 27*(4), 345–356.

Cook, J. A., Leff, H. S., Blyler, C. R., Gold, P. B., Goldberg, R. W., Mueser, K. T., et al. (2005). Results of a multisite randomized trial of supported employment interventions for individuals with severe mental illness. *Archives of General Psychiatry, 62*, 505–512.

may be developed as part of the supported employment approach described earlier (Warner & Mandiberg, 2006).

Cognitive and Neurocognitive Enhancement Strategies

Given that neurocognitive deficits impact successful work functioning of persons with psychiatric disorders (McGurk & Meltzer, 2000), interventions have been developed that pair cognitive and neurocognitive enhancement strategies to facilitate work participation. Computer-assisted cognitive rehabilitation (CCAR) focuses on remediating common cognitive deficits, including attention and concentration, psychomotor speed, learning and memory, and executive functions, as well as cognitive behavioral strategies focused on social problem-solving.

Bell, Bryson, Breig, Corcoran, and Wexler (2001) found that study participants in a work therapy program plus neurocognitive enhancement therapy (NET) improved significantly in comparison to controls on executive functioning, working memory, and affect recognition. McGurk, Mueser, and Pascaris (2005) found that study participants in a supported employment program who participated in the Thinking Skills for Work program were more likely to work, worked more jobs, worked more hours, and earned more wages than controls. The Thinking Skills for Work program consists of thorough cognitive assessment, participation in 24 hours of computer-based cognitive exercises, and consultation between the cognitive specialist and employment specialist to insure that cognitive strengths and challenges are considered in the job development process.

Cognitive-behavioral approaches targeting social perception can also facilitate successful work participation when integrated into an employment services intervention. The Indianapolis Vocational Intervention Program (IVIP) uses a cognitive-behavioral perspective and specifically targets social perceptions within work contexts. Participants in the IVIP attend weekly group sessions that include didactic content and skills training (i.e., Thinking About Work, Barriers to Work, Workplace Relationships, and Realistic Self-Appraisal) while participating in a work placement. Lysaker, Bond, Davis, Bryson, and Bell (2005) found that participants in the IVIP worked more and performed better at work tasks than controls. The intervention was also effective in sustaining hope and self-esteem across the work placement period.

In addition to cognitive rehabilitation approaches, "errorless learning" has been investigated for its efficacy in facilitating the learning of work tasks by persons with psychiatric

disorders (Kern, Liberman, Kopelowicz, Mintz, & Green, 2002). Errorless learning was developed as an education approach for children with learning disabilities and targets the impact of neurocognitive deficits on learning. The components of errorless learning include (1) a thorough task analysis; (2) teaching that begins with simple tasks at which success is likely, then trains on hierarchically ordered exercises; and (3) overlearning (e.g. continued practice of a skill even after it is learned). The researchers found errorless learning superior to conventional training approaches on two work tasks for persons with psychiatric disabilities.

Summary

For many individuals, work is central to defining identity. People with psychiatric disabilities are often deprived of the worker role, and this occupational deprivation can contribute to a negative sense of self. From its beginnings, the occupational therapy founders were concerned with the importance of work and health for people with psychiatric disabilities. Although occupational therapy, particularly in the United States, lost some of its footing in this practice arena, it has regained a position here. Occupational therapists are beginning to contribute significantly to both the research and clinical practice related to promoting employment for people with psychiatric disabilities.

Evidence-Based Practice

People with psychiatric disabilities can work even when experiencing persistent symptoms and may be able to sustain that work longer when exposed to training and environmental supports that specifically target neurocognitive deficits (McGurk, Mueser, & Pascaris, 2005).

➤ Occupational therapists can actively encourage and explicitly support the expressed desires and efforts of persons with psychiatric disabilities to work.

➤ Occupational therapists can use existing cognitive enhancement strategies or create cognitive enhancement interventions that successfully apply understandings from existing cognitive training models.

McGurk, S. R., Mueser, K. T., & Pascaris, A. (2005). Cognitive training and supported employment for persons with severe mental illness: One-year results from a randomized controlled trial. *Schizophrenia Bulletin, 31*(3), 898–909.

Active Learning Strategies

1. Childhood Occupations

Reflect on engagement in your childhood occupations—play and chores.

Reflective Questions
• How are these activities related to your choice of occupational therapy as a profession?

• Did you have chores?
• How did your family's rules and reinforcements prepare you for work behaviors?

 Capture your thoughts in your **Reflective Journal**.

2. Personal Work Experiences

Reflect on your early work experiences.

Reflective Questions
- How did you get that work?
- What work behaviors did you learn/practice?
- How did this work influence your future career decisions?
- How did work impact other areas of your life?
- What environmental constraints limited your access to occupational experiences?
- What environmental affordances promoted your access to occupational experiences?
- What critical life events influenced your occupational development?

 Document your reflection about your personal work experience in your **Reflective Journal**.

3. Career Choice and Satisfaction

Reflect on your decision to become an occupational therapist.

Reflective Questions
- Did you consider other careers?
- What were they, how old were you, and what influenced your thoughts about those careers?
- To what degree did the social aspects of your work environment influence your satisfaction and tenure with that job?
- What effects, positive and negative, did work have on your overall health and mental health?

4. Interview

Interview a person with a psychiatric disability who is working. Explore what influenced his or her decision to work. Has this individual experienced stigma in the workplace? Has he or she requested reasonable accommodations? What was his or her experience with that process? What is this person's perception about the relationship between working and his or her overall health, mental health, and recovery?

Resources

Accommodations in the Workplace for People with Psychiatric Disabilities
- Center for Psychiatric Rehabilitation at Boston University: http://www.bu.edu/cpr/jobschool/potentialjob.html

Incentives to Work for People on SSI/SSDI
- The Work Site of the Social Security Administration: http://www.ssa.gov/work

Supported Employment Toolkit
- Provides specific information on implementing supported employment services: http://mentalhealth.samhsa.gov/cmhs/communitysupport/toolkits

References

American Occupational Therapy Association (AOTA). (2002). Occupational therapy practice framework: Domain and process. *American Journal of Occupational Therapy, 56,* 609–639.

American Psychiatric Association. (2000). *Diagnostic and Statistical Manual of Mental Disorders: DSM-IV-TR* (4th ed., text rev.). Washington, DC: American Psychiatric Association.

Anthony, S. H. (2005a). Dr. Herbert J. Hall originator of honest work for occupational therapy (1904–1923): Part I. *Occupational Therapy in Health Care, 19*(3), 3–19.

———. (2005b) Dr. Herbert J. Hall originator of honest work for occupational therapy (1904–1923): Part II. *Occupational Therapy in Health Care, 19*(3), 21–32.

Anthony, W. A., Cohen, M. R., Farkas, M. D., & Gagne, C. (2002). *Psychiatric Rehabilitation* (2nd ed.). Boston: Center for Psychiatric Rehabilitation.

Anthony, W. A., Rogers, E. S., Cohen, M., & Davies, R. R. (1995). Relationships between psychiatric symptomatology, work skills and future vocational performance. *Psychiatric Services, 46*(4), 353–358.

Baron, K., Kielhofner, G., Iyenger, A., Goldhammer, V., & Wolenski, J. (2002). *The Occupational Self-Assessment (OSA) (Version 1.2).* Chicago: University of Illinois, College of Applied Health Sciences, Department of Occupational Therapy, Model of Human Occupation Clearinghouse.

Beard, J. H., Propst, R. N., & Malamud, T. J. (1982). The Fountain House model of psychiatric rehabilitation. *Psychosocial Rehabilitation Journal, 5*(1), 47–53.

Becker, D. R., & Drake, R. E. (1993). *A Working Life: The Individual Placement and Support (IPS) Program.* Concord, NH: New Hampshire-Dartmouth Psychiatric Research Center.

———. (2003). *A Working Life for People With Severe Mental Illness.* New York: Oxford University Press.

Bell, M. D., Bryson, G., Greig, T., Corcoran, C., & Wexler, B. E. (2001). Neurocognitive enhancement therapy with work therapy: Effects on neuropsychological test performance. *Archives of General Psychiatry, 58*(8), 763–768.

Bell, M. D., & Lysaker, P. H. (1995). Psychiatric symptoms and work performance among persons with mental illness. *Psychiatric Services, 46*(5), 508–510.

Bilby, R. (1992). A response to the criticisms of transitional employment. *Psychosocial Rehabilitation Journal, 16,* 69–82.

Bolton, B. (1988). Vocational assessment of person with psychiatric disorders. In J. A. Ciardiello & M. D. Bell (Eds.). *Vocational Rehabilitation of Persons with Prolonged Psychiatric Disorders.* Baltimore, MD: Johns Hopkins University Press, 165–180.

Bond, G. R. (2004). Supported employment: Evidence for an evidence-based practice. *Psychiatric Rehabilitation Journal, 27*(4), 345–356.

Bond, G. R., Becker, D. R., Drake, R. E., Rapp, C. A., Meisler, N., Lehman, A. F., et al. (2001). Implementing supported employment as an evidence-based practice. *Psychiatric Services, 52*(3), 313–322.

Bond, G. R., & Jones, A. (2005). Supported employment. In R. E. Drake, M. R. Merrens, & D. W. Lynde (Eds.), *Evidence-Based Mental Health Practice: A Textbook* (pp. 367–394). New York: W.W. Norton. & Company.

Braveman, B., Robson, M, Velozo, C. Kielhoner, G., Fisher, G., Forsyth, K., & Kerschbaum, J. (2005). *A User's Guide to Worker Role Interview, Version 1.0.,* Chicago: Model of Human Occupation Clearinghouse, University of Illinois at Chicago.

Brown, C. & Dunn, W. (2002) *Adolescent/Adult Sensory Profile.* Psychological Corporation, San Antonio, TX.

Brown, C., Tollefson, N., Dunn, W., Cromwell, R., & Filion, D. (2001). The Adult Sensory Profile: Measuring patterns of sensory processing. *American Journal of Occupational Therapy, 55*(1), 75–82.

Bryson, B., Bell, M. D., Greig, T., & Kaplan, E. (1999). The Work Behavior Inventory: Prediction of future work success of people with schizophrenia. *Psychiatric Rehabilitation Journal, 23*(2), 113–118.

Bryson, G. Bell, M. D., Lysaker, P., & Zito, W. (1997). The Work Behavior Inventory: A scale for the assessment of work behavior for people with severe mental illness. *Psychiatric Rehabilitation Journal, 20*(4), 47–55.

Bundy, A. C. (1991). Play theory and sensory integration. In A. G. Fisher, E. A. Murray & A. C. Bundy (Eds.) *Sensory Integration Theory and Practice* (pp. 46–68). Philadelphia: FA Davis.

Campbell, J. & Kaufmann, C. L. (1997). Equality and differences in the ADA: Unintended consequences for employment of people with mental health disabilities. In R. J. Bonnie and J. Monahan (Eds.) *Mental Disorders: Work, Disability and the Law* (pp. 221–240). Chicago: University of Chicago Press.

Cohen, M., & Mynks, D. (1993). *Compendium of Activities for Assessing & Developing Readiness for Rehabilitation Services.* Boston: Center for Psychiatric Rehabilitation.

Cook, J. A. (2006). Employment barriers for persons with psychiatric disabilities: Update of a report for the President's Commission. *Psychiatric Services, 57*(10), 1391–1405.

Cook, J. A., Leff, H. S., Blyler, C. R., Gold, P. B., Goldberg, R. W., Mueser, K. T., et al. (2005). Results of a multisite randomized trial of supported employment interventions for individuals with severe mental illness. *Archives of General Psychiatry, 62,* 505–512.

Corrigan, P. W. (2001). Place-then-train: An alternative paradigm for psychiatric disabilities. *Clinical Psychology: Science and Practice, 8,* 334–349.

———— (Ed). (2005). *On the Stigma of Mental Illness: Practical Strategies for Research and Social Change.* Washington, DC: American Psychological Association.

Dalgin, R. S., & Gilbride, D. (2003). Perspectives of people with psychiatric disabilities on employment disclosure. *Psychiatric Rehabilitation Journal, 26*(3), 306–310.

Davidson, L. (2003). *Living Outside Mental Illness: Qualitative Studies of Recovery in Schizophrenia.* New York: New York University Press.

Davidson, L., & Strauss, J. S. (1992). Sense of self in recovery from severe mental illness. *British Journal of Medical Psychology, 65,* 131–145.

Deegan, P. (1996). Recovery as a journey of the heart. *Psychiatric Rehabilitation Journal, 19*(3), 91–97.

de las Heras, C. G. (1993a). *Validity and Reliability of the Volitional Questionnaire.* Unpublished master's thesis, Tufts University, Boston, MA.

————. (1993b). *The Volitional Questionnaire.* Unpublished manual, Santiago, Chile.

de las Heras, C. G., Geist, R., Kielhofner, G., & Li, Y. (2003). *The Volitional Questionnaire (VQ) (version 4.0).* Chicago: Model of Human Occupation Clearinghouse, Department of Occupational Therapy, College of Applied Health Sciences, University of Illinois at Chicago.

Dewey, J. (1902). Interpretation of Savage Mind. *Psychological Review, 9,* 217–230. Available at: (http://www.brocku.ca/MeadProject/Dewey/Dewey_1902c.html) accessed April 5, 2010.

Doty, P., Kasper, J., and Litvak, S. 1996. Consumer-directed models of personal care: Lessons from Medicaid. *Milbank Quarterly* 74(3): 377–409.

Dunn, W. (1997). The impact of sensory processing abilities on the daily lives of young children and their families: A conceptual model. *Infants and Young Children, 9(4),* 23-35.

Eastabrook, S., Krupa, T., & Horgan, S. (2004). Creating inclusive workplaces: Employing people with psychiatric disabilities in evaluation and research in community mental health. *Canadian Journal of Program Evaluation, 19*(3), 71–88.

Erikson, E. H. (1959). *Identity and the Life Cycle.* New York: International Universities Press.

Fabian, E. S. (2000). Social cognitive theory of careers and Individuals with serious mental health disorders: Implications for psychiatric rehabilitation programs. *Psychiatric Rehabilitation Journal, 23*(3), 262–269.

Farley, R. C., Little, N. D., Bolton, B., & Chunn, J. (1993). Employability assessment and planning in rehabilitation and educational settings. Fayetteville: Research and Training Center in Vocational Rehabilitation; University of Arkansas.

Florey, L. L. (1981). Studies of play: Implications for growth, development, and for clinical practice. *American Journal of Occupational Therapy, 35,* 519–524.

Gioia, D. (2005). Career development in schizophrenia: A heuristic framework. *Community Mental Health Journal, 41*(3), 307–325.

Green, M. F. (1996). What are the functional consequences of neurocognitive deficits in schizophrenia. *American Journal of Psychiatry, 153,* 321–330.

Greig, T. C., Nicholls, S. S., Bryson, G. J., & Bell, M. D. (2004). The Vocational Cognitive Rating Scale: A scale for the assessment of cognitive functioning at work for clients with severe mental illness. *Journal of Vocational Rehabilitation, 21,* 71–81.

Gritzer, G., & Arluke, A. (1985). *The Making of Rehabilitation: A Political Economy of Medical Specialization, 1890–1980.* Berkley: University of California Press.

Hall, H. J., & Buck, M. M. C. (1919). *The Work of Our Hands.* New York: Moffat, Yard & Company.

Henry, A. D., Barreira, P., Banks, S., Brown, J., & McKay, C. (2001). A retrospective study of clubhouse-based transitional employment. *Psychiatric Rehabilitation Journal, 24*(4), 344–354.

Henry, A. D., & Lucca, A. M. (2004). Facilitators and barriers to employment: The perspectives of people with psychiatric disabilities and employment service providers. *Work 22*(3), 169–182.

Holland, J. L. (1997). *Making Vocational Choices: A Theory of Vocational Personalities and Work Environments* (3rd ed.). Odessa, FL: Psychological Assessment Resources.

Honey, A. (2003). The impact of mental illness on employment: Consumers' perspectives. *Work 20*(3), 267–276.

Jahoda, M. (1981). Work, employment, and unemployment values, theories, and approaches in social research. *American Psychologist, 36*(2) 184–191.

Jakobsen, K. (2004). If work doesn't work: How to enable occupational justice. *Journal of Occupational Science, 11*(3), 125–134.

Jonsson, H., Borell, L., & Sadlo, G. (2000). Retirement: An occupational transition with consequences for temporality, balance and meaning of occupation. *Journal of Occupational Science, 7*(1), 29–37.

Kennedy-Jones, M., Joanne Cooper, J., & Fossey, E. (2005) Developing a worker role: Stories of four people with mental illness. *Australian Occupational Therapy Journal 52,* 116–126.

Kern, R. S., Liberman, R. P., Kopelowicz, A., Mintz, J., & Green, M. F. (2002). Applications of errorless learning on improving work performance in persons with schizophrenia. *American Journal of Psychiatry, 159,* 1921–1926.

Kielhofner, G. (2002). *A Model of Human Occupation. Theory and application* (3rd Edition). Baltimore: William and Wilkins.

Kielhofner, G., & Forsyth, K. (2001). Measurement properties of a client self-report for treatment planning and documenting therapy outcomes. *Scandinavian Journal of Occupational Therapy, 8,* 131–139.

Kielhofner, G., Mallinson, T., Crawford, C., Nowak, M., Rigby, M., Henry, A., & Walens, A. (2004). *A User's Manual for the Occupational Performance History Interview (Version 2.1) OPHI-II.* Chicago: Model of Human Occupation (MOHO) Clearinghouse, Department of Occupational Therapy, College of Applied Health Sciences, University of Illinois.

Kirsh, B. (2000). Work, workers, and workplaces: A qualitative analysis of narratives of mental health consumers. *Journal of Rehabilitation 66*(4), 24–30.

Kirsh, B., Cockburn, L., & Gewurtz, R. (2005). Best practice in occupational therapy: Program characteristics that influence vocational outcomes for persons with serious mental illnesses. *Canadian Journal of Occupational Therapy, 72,* 265–279.

Klyma, J., Juvakka, T., Nikkonen, M., Korhonen, T., & Isohanni, M. (2006). Hope and schizophrenia: An integrative review. *Journal of Psychiatric and Mental Health Nursing, 13,* 651–664.

Kronenberg, F., Algado, S. S., & Pollard, N. (Eds.). (2005). *Occupational Therapy without Borders: Learning from the Spirit of Survivors.* New York: Elsevier Churchill Livingstone.

Krupa, T. (2004). Employment, recovery and schizophrenia: Integrating health and disorder at work. *Psychiatric Rehabilitation Journal, 28*(1), 8–15.

Krupa, T., Lagarde, M., & Carmichael, K. (2003). Transforming sheltered workshops into affirmative. *Psychiatric Rehabilitation Journal , 26*(4), 359–367.

Larson, E. A. (2004). Children's work: The less considered childhood occupation. *American Journal of Occupational Therapy, 58,* 369–379.

Link, B. G., Struening, E. L., Neese-Todd, S., Asmussen, S., & Phelan, J. C. (2001). Stigma as a barrier to recovery: The consequences of stigma for the self-esteem of people with mental illnesses. *Psychiatric Services 52*(12), 162–166.

Lobo, F. (1999). The leisure and work occupations of young people: A review. *Journal of Occupational Science, 6*(1), 27–33.

Lysaker, P. H., Bond, G., Davis, L. W., Bryson, G. J., & Bell, M. D. (2005). Enhanced cognitive-behavioral therapy for vocational rehabilitation in schizophrenia: Effects on hope and work. *Journal of Rehabilitation Research & Development, 42*(5), 673–682.

MacDonald-Wilson, K. L., Rogers, E. S., & Anthony, W. A. (2001). Unique issues in assessing work function among individuals with psychiatric disabilities. *Journal of Occupational Rehabilitation 11*(3), 217–232

MacDonald-Wilson, K., Rogers, E., Ellison, M., & Lyass, A. (2003). A study of the social security work incentives and their relation to perceived barriers to work among persons with psychiatric disability. *Rehabilitation Psychology, 48*(4), 301–309.

MacDonald-Wilson, K. L., Rogers, E. S., Massaro, J. M., Lyass, A., & Crean, T. (2002). An investigation of reasonable workplace accommodations for people with psychiatric disabilities: Quantitative findings from a multi-site study. *Community Mental Health Journal, 38*(1), 35–50.

McGurk, S. R., & Meltzer, H. Y. (2000). The role of cognition in vocational functioning in schizophrenia. *Schizophrenia Research, 45*(3), 175–184.

McGurk, S. R., & Mueser, K. T. (2004). Cognitive functioning, symptoms, and work in supported employment: A review and heuristic model. *Schizophrenia Research, 70,* 147–173.

McGurk, S. R., Mueser, K. T., & Pascaris, A. (2005). Cognitive training and supported employment for persons with severe mental illness: One-year results from a randomized controlled trial. *Schizophrenia Bulletin, 31*(3), 898–909.

McKay, C., Johnsen, M., & Stein, R. (2005). Employment outcomes in Massachusetts clubhouses. Psychiatric. *Rehabilitation Journal, 29*(1), 25–33.

Mechanic, D. (1998). Cultural and organizational aspects of application of the American with Disabilities Act to persons with psychiatric disabilities. *Milbank Quarterly, 76*(1), 5–23.

Meyer, A. (1922/1977). Philosophy of occupation therapy. Reprinted from the Archives of Occupational Therapy, vol. 1, pp. 1–10, 1922. *American Journal of Occupational Therapy, 31*(10).

Moore-Corner, R. A., Kielhofner, G., & Olson, L. (1998). *A User's Manual for Work Environment Impact Scale, Version 2.0.* Chicago: Model of Human Occupation Clearing house, University of Illinois.

Moos, R. (1994). *Work Environment Scale Manual: Development, Applications, Research* (3rd ed.). Palo Alto, CA: Consulting Psychologists Press.

Nagle, S., Cook, J. V., & Polatajko, H. J. (2002). I'm doing as much as I can: Occupational choices of person with severe and persistent mental illness. *Journal of Occupational Science, 9*(2), 72–81.

National Association of State Mental Health Program Directors. (2002). *Performance Measures for Mental Health Systems.* Alexandria, VA: National Association of State Mental Health Program Directors Research Institute.

O'Day, B., & Killeen, M. (2002). Does U.S. federal policy support employment and recovery for people with psychiatric disabilities? *Behavioral Sciences and the Law, 20,* 559–583.

Parham, L. D., & Fazio, L. S. (Eds.). (1997). *Play in Occupational Therapy for Children.* St. Louis, MO: Mosby.

Passmore, A. (1998). Does leisure support and underpin adolescents' developing worker role? *Journal of Occupational Science, 5*(3), 161–165.

Peloquin, S. M. (1994). Moral treatment: How a caring practice lost its rationale. *American Journal of Occupational Therapy, 48,* 167–173.

Pita, D. D., Ellison, M. L., Farkas, M., & Bleecker, T. (2001). Exploring personal assistance services for people with psychiatric disabilities: Need, policy, and practice. *Journal of Disability Policy, 12*(1), 2–9.

Prochaska, J. O. & Norcross, J. C. (2001). Stages of change. *Psychotherapy, 38,* 443–448.

Provencher, H. L., Gregg, R., Mead, S., & Mueser, K. T. (2002). The role of work in the recovery of persons with psychiatric disabilities. *Psychiatric Rehabilitation Journal, 26*(2), 132–144.

Quiroga, V. (1995). *Occupational Therapy: The First Thirty Years, 1900 to 1930.* Bethesda, MD: American Occupational Therapy Association.

Ralph, R. O. (2002). The dynamics of disclosure: Its impact on recovery and rehabilitation. *Psychiatric Rehabilitation Journal, 26*(2), 165–172.

Reberio, K. L., & Allen, J. (1998). Voluntarism as occupation. *Canadian Journal of Occupational Therapy, 65,* 279–285.

Rehabilitation Act Amendments. (1998). Title IV of the Workforce Investment Act of 998, Pub Law 105–220, 112 Stat 936.

Reilly, M. (1966). A psychiatric occupational therapy program as a teaching model. *American Journal of Occupational Therapy, 20*(2): 61–67.

———. (1974). *Play as Exploratory Learning.* Beverly Hills: Sage Publications.

Rogers, E. S., Martin, R., Anthony, W., Massaro, J., Danley, K., Crean, T., & Penk, W. (2001). Assessing readiness for change among persons with severe mental illness. *Community Mental Health Journal, 37*(2), 97–112.

Scheid, T. L., & Anderson, C. (1995). Living with chronic mental illness: Understanding the role of work. *Community Mental Health Journal, 31*(2), 163–176.

Shaheen, G., Williams, F., & Dennis, D. (2003). *Work as Priority a Resource for Employing People Who Have a Serious Mental Illness and Who Are Homeless.* DHHS Pub. No. SMA 03-3834. Rockville, MD: Center for Mental Health Services, Substance Abuse and Mental Health Services Administration.

Smith, T. E., Rio, J., Hull, J. W., Hedayat-Harris, A., Goodman, M., & Anthony, D. T. (1998). The rehabilitation readiness determination profile: A needs assessment for adults with severe mental illness. *Psychiatric Rehabilitation Journal, 21*(4), 380–387.

Spokane, A. R., & Holland, J. L. (1995). The self-directed search: A family of self-guided career interventions. *Journal of Career Assessment, 3*(4), 373–390.

Stebbins, R. (1992). *Amateurs, Professionals and Serious Leisure.* Toronto: McGill-Queens University Press.

Strong, S. (1998). Meaningful work in supportive environments: Experiences with the recovery process. *American Journal of Occupational Therapy, 52*(1), 31–38.

Townsend, E. A. (2003). Reflections on power and justice in enabling occupation. *Canadian Journal of Occupational Therapy, 70,* 74–87.

Tremblay, T., Smith, J., Xie, H., & Drake, R. E. (2004). The impact of specialized benefits counseling services on Social Security Administration disability beneficiaries in Vermont. *Journal of Rehabilitation, 70*(2), 5–11.

Uttaro, T., & Mechanic, D. (1994). The NAMI consumer survey analysis of unmet needs. *Hospital and Community Psychiatry, 45,* 372–274.

Van Dongen, D. J. (1996). Quality of life and self-esteem in working and nonworking persons with mental illness. *Community Mental Health Journal, 32*(6), 535–548.

Warner, R., & Mandiberg, J. M. (2006). An update on affirmative businesses or social firms for people with mental illness. *Psychiatric Services 57,* 1488–1492.

Wicks, A. (2001). Occupational potential: A topic worthy of exploration. *Journal of Occupational Science, 8*(3), 32–35.

Wilcock, A. A. (1993). A theory of the human need for occupation. *Journal of Occupational Science, 1*(1), 17–23.

Wilcock, A. A., & Townsend, E. A. (2000). Occupational terminology interactive dialogue: Occupational justice. *Journal of Occupational Science, 7,* 84–86.

Woodside, H., Landeen, J., Kirkpatrick, H., & Byrne, C. (1994). Hope and schizophrenia: exploring attitudes of clinicians. *Psychosocial Rehabilitation Journal 18,* 140–144.

Yerxa, E. J. (1998). Health and the human spirit for occupation. *American Journal of Occupational Therapy, 52*(6), 412–418.

Social Participation

Chris Lloyd and Frank P. Deane

> A healthy social life is found only when in the mirror of each soul the whole community finds its reflection, and when in the whole community the virtue of each one is living.
>
> —Rudolf Steiner

Introduction

People with psychiatric disabilities face many social and economic barriers that impact their quality of life and ability to fully engage in occupations involving social participation with community, family, peers, and friends. They find themselves excluded from many aspects of daily life, such as education, employment, housing, social networks, health care, and community life, including leisure participation. Stigma and discrimination prevent many of their basic human needs from being met, and their recovery is compromised by social disadvantage. The recovery movement is supported by government policy and aims to transform the mental health service system to one based on recovery rather than disability.

A number of chapters in this text address social participation issues, such as the chapters on recovery, stigma, public policy, and culture, as well as those specific to environments in which social participation takes place, such as family, work, school, and leisure. This chapter explores ways in which occupational therapy practitioners can play an important role in delivering recovery-focused interventions that support the development of relationships and companionship with peers, friends, partners, and pets, which are vitally important to social participation occupations.

Social Exclusion

In the United Kingdom, the Social Exclusion Unit identified five main reasons why psychiatric disability leads to and reinforces **social exclusion** (Office of the Deputy Prime Minister [ODPM], 2004):

1. Stigma and discrimination against people with psychiatric disability is pervasive throughout society.
2. Low expectations are often shown by professionals of what people with psychiatric disability are able to achieve.
3. Lack of responsibility for promoting vocational and social outcomes is often shown by service providers who do not always work effectively.
4. Lack of ongoing support to enable people with psychiatric disability to work.
5. Barriers to engaging in the community

Psychiatric disability can lead to a vicious cycle of social exclusion. Even a short episode of mental health problems can have long-term impact on a person's life, relationships, housing, and employment opportunities. This occurrence can lead to unemployment, homelessness, debt, and social isolation. Unfortunately, these situations can lead to a worsening of a person's mental health, and a cycle of exclusion kicks in. Preventing the cycle of social exclusion from occurring and breaking this cycle when it does occur is important. Early intervention plays a key role in keeping people at work and maintaining their social supports (ODPM, 2004)

Stigma and discrimination can contribute to a person's preferring to stay in the safety of mental health services rather than engage in mainstream society. There is a lack of clear responsibility for improving the vocational and social outcomes for people with psychiatric disability; therefore, different services do not always work effectively to meet the identified needs of individuals and do not maximize available resources (Davidson, O'Connell, Tondora, Styron, & Kangas, 2006). Traditionally, there has been a focus on the diagnosis of the psychiatric disability and medical symptoms rather than on vocational and social roles. Professionals often do not have the time, training, or local contacts to deliver recovery-focused interventions designed to assist people to work or participate in their local community. People require support to enable them to seek, obtain, and maintain work (ODPM, 2004).

Stigma

The *Macquarie Dictionary* (Delbridge et al, 1998) defines stigma as "a mark of disgrace; a stain, as on one's reputation" and "a characteristic mark or sign of defect, degeneration, disease, etc." (p. 2080). It is this "mark" that produces negative reactions from others. The signs or symptoms that mark a person are behaviors identified by others as deviant in some way, such as talking out loud to someone who is not present or an unkempt appearance.

Labels, specifically diagnostic labels, become signals in the same way as symptoms. The ways in which signals such as symptoms and labels lead to stereotypes and subsequent discrimination have been described as a social-cognitive process (Corrigan & Kleinlein). Chapter 28 provides a deeper understanding of this phenomenon. Because stigma is a main factor in influencing how a person living with a mental illness experiences and seeks social participation, it is briefly discussed here.

Labeling theory proposes that social and contextual factors are critical in determining who gets labeled, and often these factors are not specifically related to deviant behavior. For example, an individual is less likely to be labeled with a psychiatric disability by laypersons if he or she is in a closer personal relationship with them; labeling depends on the relational distance between the observer and the person (Phelan & Link, 1999). Thus, when a person is fully socially engaged and has multiple relationships, it is less likely that he or she will experience stigma associated with labeling.

Although it has been argued that labeling theory overemphasizes the social influence of others and does not sufficiently account for self-labeling, it has been countered that self-labeling is also a highly socially dependent process (Phelan & Link, 1999). Self-labeling is associated with what is more commonly called **self-stigma**. Self-stigma is thought to occur because people with psychiatric disability live in societies that widely reinforce stigmatizing ideas (e.g., media portrayals) to the extent that persons with the psychiatric disability themselves come to accept and internalize these views and consequently experience negative reactions such as poor self-esteem, which may be more damaging than perceived stigma from others (Barney, Griffiths, Jorm, & Christensen, 2006; Corrigan & Kleinlein, 2005; Corrigan & Calabrese, 2005; Kelly & Jorm, 2007; Link, Struening, Neese-Todd, Asmussen, & Phelan, 2001).

Effects of Stigma on Social Participation

Public discrimination can reduce the willingness of individuals to interact with others who have psychiatric disabilities in social activities, sport, church, employment, or educational contexts. This may be manifest in direct refusal to allow access to such opportunities (e.g., housing). In a comparison of individuals with schizophrenia and individuals with diabetes, it was found that work-related stigma was significantly greater for those with schizophrenia. Specifically, 47% of those with schizophrenia reported they

had not been offered a job after their illness was revealed, compared with only 25% of those with diabetes (Lee, Lee, Chiu, & Kleinman, 2005). Forty-five percent of those with schizophrenia said they had been laid off after disclosing their illness.

There is increasing evidence that patients' concerns about stigma lead to more impaired social functioning in interactions with people outside of their family (e.g., Perlick et al, 2001). However, it is also clear that many people with psychiatric disabilities also feel stigmatized by their own family members, with 54% of a sample of people with schizophrenia reporting they felt disliked or disposed by family members because of their illness (Lee et al, 2005).

Self-stigma also impacts social participation because persons with psychiatric disability may fear that they will be rejected by other people. Many individuals avoid social interaction and withdraw due to anxiety and fear of rejection. A study of 510 outpatients with schizophrenia revealed that "40.6% deliberately avoided most social contacts" as a result of stigmatization (Lee et al, 2005, p. 155). This avoidance and withdrawal has the effect of reducing opportunity for meaningful community participation.

Recovery

What is recovery? Recovery is a journey toward a new and valued sense of identity, role, and purpose outside of the constraints of having a psychiatric disability. It is about living well despite limitations resulting from the illness, its treatment, and personal and environmental conditions (Queensland Health, 2005). Recovery is a unique and deeply personal journey. Recovery is fully addressed in Chapter 1, and it is briefly addressed here because of its link to social participation. Social participation can be understood as one of the processes by which recovery is pursued.

Mental health consumers have shaped our understanding of recovery. The results of a study conducted by Andresen, Oades, and Caputi (2003) found the component processes of recovery include hope, self-identity, meaning in life, and responsibility. These processes are all important in terms of supporting a person with a psychiatric disability to pursue friendships, seek or carry out employment or school roles, and take on volunteer opportunities—all activities associated with social participation.

Key facets of recovery involve hope and finding meaning, purpose, and direction for one's own life experiences. It is promoted when people with psychiatric disability are treated with equality and respect. Recovery occurs when people are empowered to take ownership and to play an active role in their own recovery process (Mezzina et al, 2006). Recovery involves establishing social roles and making social connections, which may be accomplished through activities, relationships or occupations (Marrone, Foley, & Selleck, 2005).

Social Networks

People with psychiatric disability are frequently described as being withdrawn and isolated (Topor et al, 2006). This isolation is a consequence of the social conditions under

The Lived Experience

Danni

The following are brief excerpts from an interview with Danni, a 53-year-old woman with schizophrenia who currently lives alone with six cats (and is a previous owner of dogs and goats).

Interviewer: *Danni, I know you have six cats; what do you see as the benefits of pet ownership?*

Danni: *They are friendly, loving, and don't answer you back! [laughs]. They give me much enjoyment. With my cats, if I am feeling down or sick they will come up to me and sit in my lap. They seem to have a sixth sense. They purr and follow me around. They are very therapeutic.*

I: *How do they contribute to social interactions with others?*

Danni: *Neighbors interact with me because of the cats. We talk about them. One of my cats has now gone to the neighbors. The neighbor has never had a cat before, she finds it very rewarding and wants to keep her. Even when I had dogs, when walking the dogs, people would often stop and talk. We would take the dogs on the RSPCA Paws walk where everyone takes their pets.*

I: *What's that about?*

Danni: *The RSPCA raises money. It is a 5 kilometre walk that you take your dogs on and other people sponsor you. It's a good day out, very rewarding and quite funny. Different people dress their dogs up. If you want to talk about goats, that's another kettle of fish! If you were ever stressed out—you'd be more stressed out!*

I: *What was the problem?*

Danni: *They eat anything! They would get off their tethers when ever they could. They ate all the roses. They ate everything in the vegetable garden. They were naughty but quite funny.*

I: *So, what are the hassles or downsides to pet ownership?*

Danni: *When they go missing or they get sick. You have the worry of the vet bills. The downside is if you have neighbors that don't like pets that cause hassles, but I'm lucky that way. The downside with dogs was we were working and we could not walk them enough, we could not get them enough exercise, but that was about it.*

I: *What contact do you have with your family?*

Danni: *I have no family. . . . I left home when I was 16 and I then came out to Australia and did not stay in contact with my sister and mother. My father died when I was 18.*

I: *Do you have anyone that you consider "like" family now?*

Danni: *My ex-partner's mother.*

I: *What kinds of relationship do you have with her?*

Danni: *I'm like a daughter really. I take her shopping. Depending when she wants to go, sometimes once a week, sometimes once a fortnight, depending what she wants. I take her to the doctors. I take her to the theatre sometimes. If something goes wrong at her house, I go over to see if I can help or get someone who can.*

I: *Do you have contact with other people through your relationship with her?*

Danni: *She's got family and I've met all of them . . . they keep in touch with me. If there is someone's special birthday, I'm invited. If there is a wedding, I'm sometimes invited. It's Mum's birthday coming up in August and we are organizing a surprise party.*

I: *Who is "we"?*

Danni: *Me at the moment [laughs]. Everyone is getting in touch with me. They will help me organize everything.*

---

which many people with psychiatric disability live, namely, stigmatized and impoverished. Unfortunately, after the diagnosis, there is often a disruption in the person's life; he or she has fewer life experiences, and the number of people surrounding the individual tends to diminish.

The study conducted by Topor et al (2006) found that people with psychiatric disability identified the importance of relationships as playing a major role in the course of their illness. They identified three aspects of the contributions that family members and long-term friends made to the recovery process: standing alongside the person, being there for the person in recovery, and moving on with recovery. The unequal relationships that developed during the illness begin to change.

Practitioners have an important role in the work of recovery. Topor et al (2006) identified the position of the practitioner in serving as an intermediary for various interventions that involved money, activities, groups, housing, and opportunities for socializing as important. They also did more than their formal role required, and they did something different from what the person had come to expect from professionals, such as choosing to remain with the person and giving the person special treatment. Social interaction is of importance to the recovery process. Strong social networks can promote a sense of wellbeing, help develop confidence, and allow greater access to employment, education, and volunteerism.

Social networks can also influence engagement in leisure and exercise occupations, thereby benefiting the participants in varied ways, physically, socially, emotionally, and spiritually. Therapists can emphasize the capacity for ongoing support through organized exercise groups (e.g., sporting clubs, walking groups, consumer-supported groups) and naturally occurring social networks or opportunities (e.g., friends who exercise together, walking to get coffee, walking pets).

Family and Social Participation

Although the rates at which individuals with severe mental illness maintain contact with their family is likely to vary among studies, some level of contact with family appears relatively high. A U.K. study involved the review of case

PhotoVoice

Friendships make life successful. You rejoice, celebrate, console, cajole, reminisce, laugh, and cry with friends. Friends encourage you to do things out of your comfort zone. Friends keep pace with your recovery as you keep pace with theirs. Friends have the uncanny ability to finish your sentence. Friendships make life successful for everyone.'

—Mary

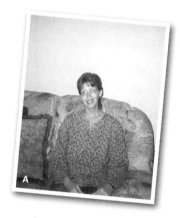 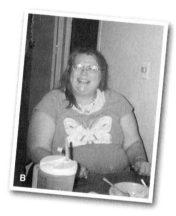 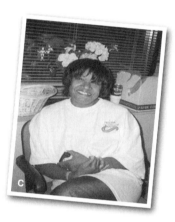

files of 257 clients receiving treatment from Community Mental Health Teams in London (Krupnik, Pilling, Killaspy, & Dalton, 2005). Evidence of contact between the client and family over the preceding year was found in 81% of the case files. However, only 55% of these contacts were clearly face to face. This raises concerns that although clients are still connected with their families, the quality of this contact and of the relationships is likely to also be highly variable.

Similar levels of perceived social support from relatives were found in a longitudinal study of 183 people with schizophrenia and affective disorders in Switzerland (Muller, Nordt, Lauber, & Rossler, 2007). At baseline, 82% of participants felt they had a social role with close relatives, and about 3 years later this percentage remained essentially the same. Further, the perceived social support received from close relatives remained stable at the 3-year period.

Finally, in the United States, the reanalysis of data from 902 individuals with schizophrenia from the Schizophrenia Patient Outcomes Research Team (PORT) client survey and a Veterans Affairs extension found that 87% had social contact with their family in the year prior to the interview (Resnick, Rosenheck, Dixon, & Lehman, 2005). The intensity of family contact was measured as the number of in-person or telephone interactions between the person with schizophrenia and the most frequently contacted family members. This was rated on a 5-point scale ranging from 1, representing no contact in the prior year, to 5, representing at least daily contact. An average for the total sample of 4.07 (standard deviation = 1.00) was obtained, suggesting relatively intensive contact (Resnick et al, 2005).

Contact with family appears to affect other aspects of social participation for people with psychiatric disabilities. A longitudinal study of 114 individuals with schizophrenia followed up over 5 years, using a global outcome measure derived from 10 different measures, suggested that after 5 years, 33% of the sample was worse, 5% unchanged, and 62% better overall (Harvey, Jeffreys, McNaught, Blizard, & King, 2007). However, social isolation, living apart from relatives, longer illness, and being an inpatient when assessed 5 years earlier were related to overall outcomes. Those who were socially isolated or did not have relationships with family tended to have poorer social and clinical outcomes.

In another study of people with schizophrenia, the degree of residential independence was related to their frequency

Evidence-Based Practice

Generally, both consumers and their families tend to be more socially isolated and to have smaller social networks.

➤ Occupational therapists can provide families with education about mental illness, communication skills, and problem-solving to promote social connections.

➤ Occupational therapists need to consider that general involvement with the family is associated with a number of positive outcomes for the consumer.

Pekkala, E., & Merinder, L. (2001). Psychoeducation for schizophrenia. *Cochrane Database of Systematic Reviews, 2,* CD002831.

of family contact, performance of activities of daily living, and social presentation and participation (Dickerson, Ringel, & Parente, 1999). A Dutch study of 73 young people (mean age 21 years) with psychosis who were followed up over 5 years (Lenior, Dingmans, Linszen, De Haan, & Schene, 2001) highlighted the role of family in activities of daily living. Sixty-nine percent of the sample received help with daily activities from their parents (mostly house keeping). Forty-four percent were accompanied by parents to outpatient appointments, with 34% of parents checking medication compliance or helping to make decisions about treatment (37%).

Measures of Functioning and Disability

Improvement in functioning is an important part of recovery for people with severe mental illness. Mental health professionals and services often gauge recovery and service outcomes by focusing on different domains of functioning and not necessarily on the functional issues of most concern to consumers (Fossey & Harvey, 2001). A number of tools measure aspects of social participation and can be used by occupational therapists to measure changes over time and inform intervention and life planning. The Life Skills Profile, the Health of the Nation Outcome Scales, the Multidimensional Scale of Independent Functioning, the St. Louis Inventory of Community Living Skills, the Satisfaction with Daily Occupations, the Camberwell Assessment of Need Short Appraisal Schedule, the Multnomah Community Ability Scale, and the Socially-valued Role Classification Scale can be used to measure aspects of social participation. It is not necessary to use the whole scale; the subscales that measure the aspects you are interested in can be administered.

Life Skills Profile

The Life Skills Profile (LSP) was developed to measure function and disability in people with schizophrenia (Parker, Rosen, Emdur, & Hadzi-Pavlovic, 1991; Rosen, Hadzi-Pavlovic, & Parker, 1989) but can be used with a wide range of mental disorders. The LSP has since been widely used to assess social disability in severe, prolonged or relapsing mental illness (Rosen, Trauer, Hadzi-Pavlovic, & Parker, 2001). Consistent with contemporary rehabilitation and recovery approaches, the scoring emphasizes functional strengths rather than weaknesses (Rosen et al, 2001).

The LSP is a 39-item measure with items assessing levels of psychosocial functioning and disability with five subscales: self-care, nonturbulence, social contact, communication, and responsibility. Higher scores represent more positive functioning.

Examples of items include *Does this person generally show warmth to others? Is the person generally well groomed (e.g., neatly dressed, hair combed)? Is this person willing to take psychiatric medications when prescribed by a doctor? Is this person violent to others?* The LSP is widely used in mental health settings, both inpatient and outpatient, to assess outcome over time. The psychometric properties of this scale have been reported by Parker et al (1991) and Trauer, Duckmanton, and Chui (1995).

Health of the Nation Outcome Scales

The Health of the Nation Outcome Scales (HoNOS) was developed for use as a routine measure of consumer outcomes in U.K. mental health services (Wing, Curtis, & Beevor, 1996). The HoNOS addresses problems resulting from overactive, aggressive, disruptive, or agitated behavior; suicidal thoughts or behavior; nonaccidental self-injury; problem drinking or drug taking (substance use); cognitive problems involving memory, orientation, understanding; problems associated with physical illness or disability; problems associated with hallucinations and delusions; depressed mood; other mental and behavioral problems; problems with making supportive social relationships; problems with activities of daily living (overall disability); problems with living conditions; and problems with occupations and activities. Subscale scores are computed for behavior (items 1–3), impairment (items 4–5), symptoms (items 6–8), and social skills (items 9–12). A total score is derived by adding the 12 item scores. Ratings are made on a 5-point scale ranging from 0 (no problems with the period rated) to 4 (severe to very severe). The HoNOS has been validated in Canada (Kisely, Campbell, Crossman, Gleich, & Campbell, 2007), the United Kingdom (Bebbington, Brugha, Hill, Marsden, & Window, 1999), and Australia (Trauer et al, 1999).

Multidimensional Scale of Independent Functioning

The Multidimensional Scale of Independent Functioning (MSIF) is a relatively new instrument for rating functional disability over a 1-month time period in psychiatric outpatients (Jaeger, Berns, & Czobor, 2003). The MSIF uses a semistructured interview to obtain information and is scored using anchors on a 7-point scale for rating independent functioning in work, education, and residential domains. Independent functioning is further broken down into three dimensions: role position (RP, the actual role that the individual is expected to perform), support (SU, the amount of assistance an individual receives in the specified role position or task), and performance (PE, the quality of the productive activities compared to normal expectations within the role environment as well as their timeliness and the reliability with which they are performed). Global MSIF ratings within each environment (work, education, residential) are then made to reflect the overall level of independent functioning (Jaeger et al, 2003).

St. Louis Inventory of Community Living Skills

The St. Louis Inventory of Community Living Skills (SLICLS) was developed as a relatively brief level of functioning measure, with a focus on discrete community living skills (Evenson & Boyd, 1993). The scale was designed to be useful in measuring the level of specific skills needed for community or group home residence. Skills are assessed in the following areas: (1) personal hygiene, (2) grooming, (3) dress skills, (4) self-care (basic homemaking such as bed making, cleaning area, organizing possessions), (5) communication, (6) safety, (7) handling time, (8) handling money, (9) leisure activities, (10) clothing maintenance, (11) meal preparation,

(12) sexuality, (13) use of resources, (14) problem solving, and (15) health practices.

Each item is rated on a 7-point scale from few or no skills to self-sufficient, very adequate. This measure can be completed in 2 or 3 minutes by someone familiar with the client. The SLICLS has been validated in the United States (Fitz & Evenson, 1995) and Hong Kong (Au, Tam, Tam, & Ungavri, 2005).

Satisfaction with Daily Occupations

The Satisfaction with Daily Occupations (SDO) consists of nine items regarding the occupational areas of work, leisure activities, domestic tasks, and self-care (Eklund, 2004). Each item consists of a two-part question. The first part queries whether or not the client presently performs the targeted kind of activity. The second asks the client to rate his or her satisfaction with the activity on a 7-point scale from 1, worst possible, to 7, best possible. This means, for example, that a person in employment rates his or her satisfaction with having a job, and a client without work rates that situation.

Camberwell Assessment of Need Short Appraisal Schedule

The Camberwell Assessment of Need Short Appraisal Schedule (CANSAS) is a structured interview in which staff, client, and carer views of need can be recorded separately (Andresen, Caputi, & Oades, 2000). It was designed specifically to inform clinical practice and to serve as a service evaluation tool. The 22 items of need include accommodation, food, household skills, self-care, daytime activities, physical health, psychotic symptoms, information on condition, psychological distress, safety to self, safety to other, alcohol, drugs, company, intimate relationships, sexual expression, child care, basic education, telephone, transport, money, and benefits.

Multnomah Community Ability Scale

The Multnomah Community Ability Scale (MCAS) is a 17-item instrument that measures the functioning level of people with a mental illness who live in the community, and the scale is designed to be completed by case managers (Barker, Barron, McFarland, & Bigelow, 1994). This instrument provides a measure of the client's severity of disability. The scale is scored from 1 (extreme problem) to 5 (no impairment), with a "don't know" category. The MCAS consists of the following items: physical health, intellectual functioning, thought processes, mood abnormality, response to stress and anxiety, ability to manage money, independence in daily life, acceptance of illness, social acceptability, social interest, social effectiveness, social network, meaningful activity, medication compliance, cooperation with treatment, alcohol/drug abuse, and impulse control. Section 1 addresses interference with functioning, which covers physical and psychiatric symptoms that make life more difficult for the client (5 questions); section 2 addresses adjustment to living and how the client functions in his or her daily life and has adapted to the disability of mental illness (3 questions);

section 3 addresses social acceptability (5 questions); and section 4 addresses behavioral problems that make it more difficult for the client to integrate successfully in the community or comply with prescribed treatment (4 questions). Studies have addressed the reliability and validity of the MCAS (Barker et al, 1994; Hendrys, Dyck, McBride, & Whitbeck, 2001; Zani, McFarland, Wachal, Barker, & Baron, 1999).

Socially Valued Role Classification Scale

The Socially Valued Role Classification Scale (SRCS) focuses on role categories that are either socially responsible or economically valued by the wider community (Waghorn, 2005). The role categories are ranked in order of increasing similarity to competitive employment while also considering the extent of external demands and responsibility outside the home. These roles include (1) home duties and self-care; (2) caring for others; (3) personal development, rehabilitation, and voluntary work; (4) formal study or approved training; and (5) competitive employment. Role status is classified by systematically combining information related to (1) hours of participation, (2) whether support from others was provided, (3) standard of performance, and (4) whether multiple roles were present. The aim is to establish whether role performance is above average, about average, definitely below average, could not assess, or not applicable. Support needs are assessed dichotomously as to either support received/required or not received/required (Waghorn, Chant, & King, 2007).

Interventions for Social Participation

This section addresses interventions that promote social participation for people with psychiatric disabilities. It begins with a more general discussion of recovery-oriented services, and then addresses interventions targeting occupations that might stimulate social connectedness to others through community arts, peer support, and pets therapy.

Evidence-Based Practice

There are a variety of assessment measures that focus on functioning and can be used to inform planning and interventions.

► Occupational therapists can use measures that focus on functioning to determine what problems the consumer has.

► Occupational therapists can use the same measures of functioning to measure whether or not their intervention has been successful.

Fossey, E. M., & Harvey, C. A. (2001). A conceptual review of functioning: Implications for the development of consumer outcome measures. *Australian and New Zealand Journal of Psychiatry, 35,* 91–98

Recovery-Oriented Service Provision

Although the recovery philosophy has been widely accepted in mental health policy in many Western nations around the world (e.g., Australian Health Ministers, 2003; Turner-Crowson & Wallcraft, 2002), the capacity to successfully implement recovery-oriented services has thus far met with mixed success. Fischer and Chamberlin (2005) state that piecemeal approaches that offer only selected programs without systemwide uptake of the recovery paradigm have had limited effects at improving recovery for consumers.

The American Association of Community Psychiatrists (AACP) provided guidelines for recovery-oriented services in part because "the majority of services in the country continue to practice more traditional models of service delivery, and many of the consumers of behavioral health services remain unaware of the promise of recovery and its potential for improving the quality of their lives" (Sowers, 2005, p. 760). Occupational therapists who work in behavioral health services can help link outcomes to recovery and quality of life indicators through promoting full participation in everyday life in the community.

One of the initial stages in developing recovery-oriented services is attempting to change the attitudes of administrators, managers, and mental health workers. Rickwood (2004, p. 3) suggested that "implementing a recovery orientation requires an attitude shift for many service providers in order to support consumer rights and provide the types of services that maximize wellbeing for people with mental illness." Modification of attitudes of mental health professionals and individuals with psychiatric disability is a key component of most general mental health competencies as well as specific recovery-oriented competencies (Coursey et al, 2000; New Zealand Mental Health Commission, 2001). Attitude shift also means being prepared to work collaboratively with consumers and viewing them as partners in their own care. This is consistent with an emphasis in occupational therapy supporting client-centered practice (Law & Mills, 1998).

The American Association of Community Psychiatrists (AACP) Guidelines for Recovery Oriented Services (2009) include a number of domains that have direct relevance to community participation activities. They specify the need for a mission, vision, and strategic plan that reflects a commitment to fostering recovery with a focus on "developing and strengthening the community of recovery persons." These should be supported by organizational structures such as participation of consumers in administrative and governing bodies (Sowers, 2005, pp. 761–762). Occupational therapists can support and promote the people they serve to take board positions in a variety of mental health community agencies.

With regard to the guideline concerning training and continuing education, it is recommended that professionals have exposure to consumers in nonclinical settings. Interactions with consumers in a range of community activities outside of treatment settings (e.g., sport, art, education) ensure such opportunities. Occupational therapists who provide continuing education should consider inviting their consumers to co-present with them as colleagues, including finding ways to offer scholarships or financial assistance to facilitate such participation. Potential barriers needing accommodation include transportation, financial, and social supports.

A wide range of "success-facilitating processes" is specified, with many of the resources being directly related to community participation, such as child care and transportation. A recovery-oriented system should also support opportunities for a "full array of training, education and employment opportunities" (p. 769) and "independent living and supporting housing" (Sowers, 2005, p. 770).

From such descriptions, it is clear that recovery-oriented services encompass a broad set of services and service outcomes. In addition to attitude change, successful revisions to existing services will require rethinking the way professionals have traditionally seen their roles. In many cases, it will require greater flexibility and expansion of roles or improved coordination between providers to meet the needs of consumers.

Community Arts

Community arts practices can benefit the health and wellbeing of participants and the wider community (VicHealth, 2002a). The arts assist people by increasing self-esteem, confidence, and social networks (ODPM, 2004). One major area of evidence for the health impacts of community arts is individual personal development. These areas have been identified as self-confidence and self-esteem, education and skills acquisition, employability and learning about health (VicHealth, 2002a). By being involved in community arts, social connections are facilitated across individuals, groups, families, and communities. Diverse people are brought together around a common project and a sense of purpose. These projects connect socially isolated participants to the mainstream and connect the mainstream to socially isolated participants. The process of public acknowledgment through the presentation of quality work is an important aspect of connecting individuals to the wider community (VicHealth, 2002b). For example, Figure 51-1 shows Cindy Dilegame and her mosaic-tiled bowling ball, which was created in the

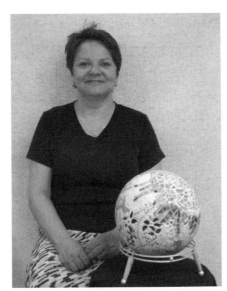

FIGURE 51-1. Cindy Dilegame and her mosaic-tiled bowling ball, which was created in the Occupational Therapy Clinic at the Northern Arizona VA Health Care System.

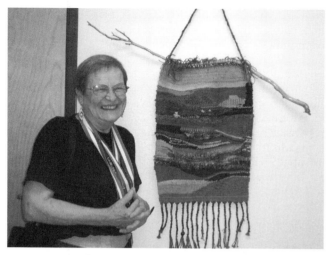

FIGURE 51-2. Betty Long and her weaving, created in the Occupational Therapy Clinic at the Northern Arizona VA Health Care System.

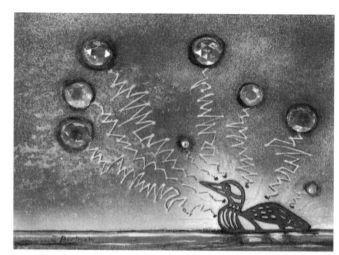

FIGURE 51-4. Artwork titled "Electric Loon" by Jessica Bortnak, a participating artist at the Northern Initiative for Social Action.

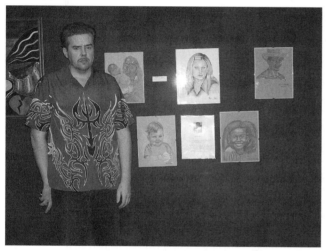

FIGURE 51-3. Ray LaPorte, participating artist at the Northern Initiative for Social Action at a community art exhibit.

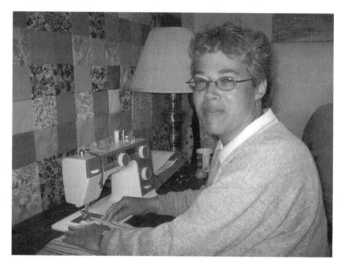

FIGURE 51-5. Quilter Odette St. Gelais participates in Warm Hearts/Warm Bodies, a program of the Northern Initiative for Social Action.

Occupational Therapy Clinic at the Northern Arizona VA Health Care System. Figure 51-2 shows Betty Long and her weaving project, which was created at the same clinic.

Participation in community arts projects is a powerful tool for advocacy because it creates and enlarges understanding of unfamiliar people and issues. Participating in community arts projects provides people with a valued identity. They move from being classified according to diagnosis or deficits to active description of what they can do. For example, a "person with psychiatric disability" becomes an "actor, singer, or artist." Being publicly recognized through presentation of work brings a sense of pride to the participants and allows the public to appreciate the talents of people about whom they may have held misconceptions (VicHealth, 2002b). Community arts grants and sponsored art fairs may also stimulate economic benefits for the artists as well as for the sponsoring agencies.

The Northern Initiative for Social Action (NISA) is a consumer-driven occupational initiative that provides a variety of opportunities for participation (Figures 51-3, 51-4, and 51-5). The mission of the program includes the following: "We believe in an accepting social environment in which

all persons are considered equal and capable." NISA has an active community arts program.

Peer Support

According to Mead, Hilton, and Curtis (2001), peer support is a system of giving and receiving help founded on key principles of respect, shared responsibility, and mutual agreement on what is helpful. The primary goal is to responsibly challenge the assumptions about mental illness and at the same time validate for individuals who they really are and where they have come from. Peer support becomes a natural extension and expansion of community, a simultaneous movement toward autonomy and community building. Peer support may be either financially compensated or voluntary (Solomon, 2004).

Peer support has been delineated into six categories: self-help groups, Internet support groups, peer-delivered services, peer-run or peer-operated services, peer partnerships, and peer employees (Solomon, 2004).

- *Self-help groups:* These are voluntary, small group structures for mutual aid in the accomplishment of a specific purpose, such as GROW, a mutual support group for people with psychiatric disorders.
- *Internet online support groups:* Communication in Internet support groups is frequently conducted through e-mail or bulletin boards. These types of groups offer a high degree of anonymity.
- *Peer delivered services:* This type of service is provided by individuals who identify themselves as having a mental illness and who have received/are receiving treatment and who deliver services for the primary purpose of helping others with a mental illness.
- *Peer-run or peer-operated services:* These are services that are planned, operated, administered, and evaluated by people with psychiatric disabilities. They have some paid staff and a significant number of volunteers. Examples include drop-in centers, clubhouses, crisis services, vocational and employment services, and psychosocial educational services (review Chapter 35 and Chapter 39).
- *Peer partnerships:* These services are not freestanding legal entities and share the control of the operation of the program with others without psychiatric disability. For example, a peer-run drop-in center may operate within a mental health system.
- *Peer employees:* This includes both individuals who fill designated unique peer positions and peers who are hired into traditional mental health positions. Examples of specifically designed peer positions include peer companion, peer advocate, consumer case manager, peer specialist, and peer counselor.

Consumer-delivered services are becoming more common in mental health service delivery, such as case management teams, crisis services, and vocational and employment coaches, as well as programs such as mutual help/self-help groups, peer support programs, and drop-in centers (Salzer & Shear, 2002). The involvement of consumers as mental health service providers has been influenced by a growing consumer movement, expansion of disability rights, and the legitimization of self-help and peer support. A number of reasons given for consumer employment include (Mowbray et al, 1996) the following:

- Meaningful work contributes to increased self-esteem, acquisition of specific work skills, and career choices.
- Including consumers as mental health workers can increase the sensitivity of programs and services about recipients.
- Consumers can serve as effective role models for clients.
- Including consumers is an expression of affirmative action and consistent with contemporary civil and disability rights policies.

Being involved in peer support can increase an individual's social networks and may offer acceptance, support, understanding, empathy, and a sense of community, leading to an increase in hope and autonomy and an assumption of personal responsibility, Importantly, a structured process of social interaction may allow people to adopt socially valued roles in which they no longer are restricted to the passive role of patient (Davidson et al, 1999).

Peer Education and Advocacy through Recreation and Leadership (PEARL) is an intervention based on principles of peer helping and psychosocial rehabilitation (Gammonley & Luken, 2001). People with a mental illness are trained and supported to serve as advocates for improving peer socialization, recreation involvement, and community inclusion among participants in psychosocial rehabilitation settings. Peer-initiated recreation experiences can promote recovery by providing opportunities to learn and practice skills in the natural environment with natural supports. According to Gammonley and Luken, promoting recovery requires that providers offer individualized supports and services that emphasize community membership, self-determination, meaningful relationships, hope, and collaboration among stakeholders.

Occupational therapists can be involved by either providing referrals to peer support services or acting as a consultant within a peer support program.

Family Psychoeducation

Family psychoeducation is an evidence-based intervention provided in a group format for family members of an individual with a psychiatric disability (Jewel, Downing, & McFarlane, 2009). The goals of family psychoeducation include (1) developing supportive relationships among families with similar experiences, (2) improving relationships within the family, and (3) improving outcomes for the family member with mental illness. Family psychoeducation includes education about mental illness as well as the teaching of strategies to problem-solve difficult family situations. In addition, social connectedness is an important part of family psychoeducation. Typically, families spend time in each session socializing informally with other families. Multifamily contact is encouraged both within and outside of the intervention session. Evidence indicates that family psychoeducation is effective in reducing relapse rates and improving symptoms in the individual with mental illness and enhancing family outcomes (Murray-Swank & Dixon, 2004). This approach is discussed in more detail in Chapter 29.

Pets

Pets have the capacity to provide company, get people with psychiatric disability out into the community when exercising an animal, and facilitate interaction through organized

---

Evidence-Based Practice

Peer support is a way in which consumers may experience an increase in social networks and gain acceptance, support, and understanding.

➤ Occupational therapists may need to consider opportunities to promote opportunities for peer support.

➤ Occupational therapists may need to consider creating opportunities for consumers to be included, such as co-presenting at conferences and co-writing an article.

Davidson, L., Chinman, M., Kloos, B., Weingarten, R., Stayner, D., & Tebes, J.K. (1999). Peer support among individuals with severe mental illness: A review of the evidence. *Clinical Psychology: Science and Practice, 6,* 165–187.

activities such as animal obedience, agility, or shows. **Animal-assisted therapy (AAT)** usually refers to "interactions between patients and a trained animal, along with its human owner or handler, with the aim of facilitating patients' progress toward therapeutic goals" (Barker & Dawson, 1998, p. 797). Research on the therapeutic potential of pets is as diverse as the animals and contexts in which they have been used. For example, there is equine-facilitated psychotherapy for children (Rothe, Vega, Torres, Soler & Pazos, 2005) and adults (Bizub, Joy, & Davidson, 2003); dogs used with both children (Kogan, Granger, Fitchett, Helmer & Young, 1999; Reichert, 1998) and adults (Barker & Dawson, 1998; Kovacs, Kis, Rozsa, & Rozsa, 2004); cats and dogs used with elderly people with schizophrenia (Barak, Savorai, Mavashev, & Beni, 2001); and dolphins used to treat adults with depression (Antonioli & Reveley, 2005).

Increasing evidence shows that pet owners have some health advantages over non–pet owners (Friedman & Thomas, 1995). In particular, those who own pets appear to have lower blood pressure compared with non–pet owners (e.g., Anderson, Reid, & Jennings, 1992), and reduced blood pressure seems particularly related to touching (petting) an animal (Vormbrock & Grossberg, 1988). It has been theorized that one of the reasons people with mental or physical illnesses appear to benefit from AAT is that their marginalized status places them in a position of needing additional attention (Odendaal, 2000). Companion animals provide attention in a reciprocal way. Further, Odendaal theorizes that a range of physiological effects (such as lowered blood pressure, neurochemical changes) accompany such individualized feelings of attachment ("affiliation behavior"). Although reliable changes in some of these physiological measures have been attained in human–animal interactions, much more research is needed to clarify the mechanisms and role they play during positive interaction (Odendaal, 2000).

Velde, Cipriani, and Fisher (2005) provide three case studies and summarize the views of pets as an intervention by occupational and other therapists. Pet ownership can provide a meaningful life role, particularly that of caretaker. Pet care provides a valued occupation, leisure activities, and companionship. Interactions with pets can potentially enhance range of motion, strength, balance, and mobility. Pets provide topics of conversation in interactions with others and have been used to facilitate both verbal and nonverbal social responses (Velde et al, 2005).

Three recent studies assessed the role of AAT in the treatment of people with schizophrenia (Barak et al, 2001; Kovacs et al, 2004; Nathans-Barel, Feldman, Berger, Modai, & Silver, 2005). The length of the AAT varied from 10 weekly 1-hour sessions with a therapy dog (Nathans-Basrel et al, 2005) to once weekly 3-hour group sessions with dogs or cats for 12 months (Barak et al, 2001). All three studies had relatively small samples of between seven and 20 inpatients with schizophrenia. One small study was an uncontrolled prepost intervention over 9 months that found improvements in domestic and health-related activities (Kovacs et al, 2004).

The other two studies both allocated patients to the AAT group or a control group based on some degree of matching. One control group involved reading and discussion of current news (Barak et al, 2001), and the second involved activities similar to the AAT activities but without the presence of the dog (Nathans-Barel et al, 2005). AAT treatments encouraged mobility through walking the dogs, interpersonal contact, communication, and reinforced activities of daily living such as hygiene and self-care (through feeding and grooming the dogs). There were significantly greater reductions in anhedonia (i.e., improved ability to experience pleasure) and improvements in motivation, utilization of leisure (Nathans-Barel et al, 2005), and social functioning (Barak et al, 2001) in the AAT group compared to controls. However, no significant differences were noted between groups for negative symptoms, positive symptoms, general psychopathology, (Nathans-Barel et al, 2005), impulse control, or self-care (Barak et al, 2001).

In a study using a larger sample of 230 hospitalized psychiatric patients, a single 30-minute group interaction with a therapy dog and the dog's owner was compared with a single therapeutic recreation session (Barker & Dawson, 1998). A pretreatment and posttreatment crossover study design was used, and it was found that for those receiving the AAT session there were significant pre–post reductions in state anxiety among people with psychotic disorders, mood disorders, and other psychiatric disorders. For those receiving the therapeutic recreation session, there were reductions only in state anxiety for the mood disorders group. However, overall there were no significant differences in anxiety change after AAT and after participation in therapeutic activity. Both

PhotoVoice

This picture is of "Tippy" my 9-year-old mixed terrier companion dog. He was sick in this picture as he had a serious back strain. He hurt his back while in the backyard as he frightened off the neighbor dog. He could barely walk and yelped in pain whenever he moved. I ran him to the emergency vet clinic and he was given a shot to ease the pain. He is so important to me and I love him so much that the thought of losing him was devastating. Today he is back to normal yet I have feelings of sadness that he is 9 years old and is aging. He is my therapy and knows more about my moods than anyone I know.

I even read a book on aging companion animals and have learned how to massage his aging bones and muscles. I hope for many, many more good years with this beautiful little beast. My companion dog "Tippy."

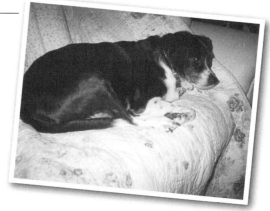

—Jan

appeared to produce similar levels of change overall (Barker & Dawson, 1998).

In summary, AAT of between 9 and 12 months appears to offer some benefits over control groups for long-term hospitalized patients with schizophrenia. However, the effect of shorter doses of AAT compared with other active interventions has not been established.

Summary

This chapter examined the impact that having a psychiatric disability has on individuals and their ability to socially participate, and it discussed the importance of providing recovery-oriented care. Occupational therapists are able to play an important role in providing interventions that promote recovery and social inclusion within the community. The occupations that engage people with others (family, friends, peers, and at the community level), such as employment, education, leisure and exercise, arts, pets, and active social networks, are areas in which occupational therapists can be involved.

> ### Evidence-Based Practice
>
> Pets have the capacity to provide company and create opportunities for people with psychiatric disability to exercise, facilitate interaction, and to have lowered blood pressure. However, while studies of animal-assisted therapy of between 9 and 12 months' duration appear to offer some benefits over control groups for long-term hospitalized patients with schizophrenia, the effects of shorter doses of AAT compared to other active interventions is not established.
>
> ➤ Occupational therapists can use AAT to help consumers gain meaningful life roles.
>
> ➤ Occupational therapists can use pets in therapy to reduce anhedonia, improve motivation, utilization of leisure, and social functioning.
>
> Barak, Y., Savorai, O., Mavashev, S., & Beni, A. (2001). Animal-assisted therapy for elderly schizophrenia patients: A one-year controlled trial. *American Journal of Geriatric Psychiatry, 9,* 439–442.

Active Learning Strategies

1. Peer Support Groups

Gather information about the peer-support groups that are available in the local community. What is the purpose of the group? Who are the attendees of the group? How often do they meet?

2. Pets and Social Interactions

Talk to someone you know who owns a dog or cat. Ask them what positive experiences pet ownership gives them. Ask specifically about examples in which having a pet dog or cat has contributed to social interactions with others. What do they see as the hassles or downside of pet ownership? Think about how these experiences might inform your recommendations about pet ownership for people with mental illness.

3. Family Contact

Reflect on the frequency and types of contacts you have with your family. Consider both your immediate and extended family.

Reflective Questions

- Consider the labels associated with our relationships with particular members of our family (e.g., daughter, brother, mother, nephew). Beyond the labels, what are the roles you have in your family (e.g., emotional support, practical support person, advisor, role model, sympathetic listener etc)?
- Which roles do you most value?
- How have these relationships helped to expand your social networks and engagement with other people?
- How can you assess, reestablish, or expand the family roles of individuals with mental illness?

 Capture your thoughts in your **Reflective Journal.**

References

American Association of Community Psychiatrists (AACP). (2009). AACP Guidelines for Recovery Oriented Services. Available at: http://www.communitypsychiatry.org/publications/clinical_and_administrative_tools_guidelines/ROSGuidelines .aspx (accessed February 2010).

Anderson, W. P., Reid C. M., & Jennings G. L. (1992). Pet ownership and risk factors for cardiovascular disease. *Medical Journal of Australia, 157,* 298–301.

Andresen, R., Oades, L., & Caputi, P. (2003). The experience of recovery from schizophrenia: Towards an empirically validated stage model. *Australian and New Zealand Journal of Psychiatry, 37,* 586–594.

Andresen, R., Caputi, P., & Oades, L. G. (2000). Interrater reliability of the Camberwell Assessment of Need Short Appraisal Schedule. *Australian and New Zealand Journal of Psychiatry, 34,* 856–861.

Antonioli, C., & Reveley, M. A. (2005). Randomised controlled trial of animal facilitated therapy with dolphins in the treatment of depression. *British Medical Journal, 331,* 1–4.

Au, R. W. C., Tam, P. W. C., Tam, G. W. C., & Ungavri, G. S. (2005). Cross-cultural validation of the St. Louis Inventory of Community Living Skills for Chinese patients with schizophrenia in Hong Kong. *Psychiatric Rehabilitation Journal, 29*, 34–40.

Australian Health Ministers. (2003). *National Mental Health Plan 2003–2008.* Canberra: Australian Government Publishing Service.

Barak, Y., Savorai, O., Mavashev, S., & Beni, A. (2001). Animal-assisted therapy for elderly schizophrenic patients: A one-year controlled trial. *American Journal of Geriatric Psychiatry, 9*, 439–442.

Barker, S., Barron, N., McFarland, B. H., & Bigelow, D. A. (1994). A community ability scale for chronically mentally ill consumers: Part I. Reliability and validity. *Community Mental Health Journal, 30*, 363–383.

Barker, S. B., & Dawson, K. S. (1998). The effects of animal-assisted therapy on anxiety ratings of hospitalized psychiatric patients. *Psychiatric Services, 49*, 797–801.

Barney, L. J., Griffiths, K. M., Jorm, A. F., & Christensen, H. (2006). Stigma about depression and its impact on help seeking intentions. *Australian and New Zealand Journal of Psychiatry, 40*, 51–54.

Bebbington, P., Brugha, T., Hill, T., Marsden, L., & Window, S. (1999). Validation of the Health of the Nation Outcome Scale. *British Journal of Psychiatry, 174*, 389–394.

Bizub, A. L., Joy, A., & Davidson, L. (2003). "It's like being in another world": Demonstrating the benefits of therapeutic horseback riding for individuals with psychiatric disability. *Psychiatric Rehabilitation Journal, 26*, 377–384.

Carless, D., & Douglas, K. (2007). Narrative, identity and mental health: How men with serious mental illness re-story their lives through sport and exercise. *Psychology of Sport and Exercise, 9*(5), 575–594.

Corrigan, P. W., & Clabrese, J. D. (2005). Strategies for assessing and diminishing self-stigma. In P. W. Corrigan (Ed.). *On the Stigma of Mental Illness: Practical Strategies for Research and Social Change* (pp. 239–256). Washington DC: American Psychological Association.

Corrigan, P. W., & Kleinlein, P. (2005). The impact of mental illness stigma. In P. W. Corrigan (Ed.), *On the Stigma of Mental Illness: Practical Strategies for Research and Social Change* (pp. 11–44). Washington DC: American Psychological Association.

Coursey, R. D., Curtis, L., Marsh, D. T., et al. (2000). Competencies for direct service staff members who work with adults with severe mental illnesses in outpatient public mental health/managed care systems. *Psychiatric Rehabilitation Journal, 23*, 370–377.

Davidson, L., Chinman, M., Kloos, B., Weingarten, R., Stayner, D., & Tebes, J. K. (1999). Peer support among individuals with severe mental illness: A review of the evidence. *Clinical Psychology: Science and Practice, 6*, 165–187.

Davidson, L., O'Connell, M., Tondora, J., Styron, T., & Kangas, K. (2006). The top ten concerns about recovery encountered in mental health system transformation. *Psychiatric Services, 57*, 640–645.

Delbridge, A., Bernard, J. R. L., Blair, D., Butler, S., Peters, P., & Yallop, C. (Eds.). (1998). *The Macquarie Dictionary* (3rd ed.). Sydney: Macquarie University Library.

Dickerson, F. B., Ringel, N., & Parente, F. (1999). Predictors of residential independence among outpatients with schizophrenia. *Psychiatric Services, 50*, 515–519.

Eklund, M. (2004). Satisfaction with Daily Occupations: A tool for client evaluation in mental health care. *Scandinavian Journal of Occupational Therapy, 11*, 136–142.

Evenson, R. C., & Boyd, M. A. (1993). The St. Louis Inventory of Community Living Skills. *Psychosocial Rehabilitation Journal, 17*, 93–97.

Firtz, D., & Evenson, R. C. (1995). A validity study of the St. Louis Inventory of Community Living Skills. *Community Mental Health Journal, 31*, 369–377.

Fisher, D. B., & Chamberlin, J. (2005). The role of mental health consumers in leading the recovery transformation of the mental health system. In N. A. Cummings, W. O'Donohue, T. William, & M. A. Cucciare (Eds.), *Universal Healthcare: Readings for Mental Health Professionals* (pp. 219–242). Reno, NV: Context Press.

Fossey, E. M., & Harvey, C. A. (2001). A conceptual review of functioning: Implications for the development of consumer outcome measures. *Australian and New Zealand Journal of Psychiatry, 35*, 91–98.

Friedman, E., & Thomas, S. A. (1995). Pet ownership, social support and one-year survival rates after acute myocardial infarction in the cardiac arrhythmia suppression trial (CAST). *American Journal of Cardiology, 72*, 1213–1217.

Gammonley, D., & Luken, K. (2001). Peer education and advocacy through recreation and leadership. *Psychiatric Rehabilitation Journal, 25*, 170–178.

Harvey, C. A., Jeffreys, S. E., McNaught, A. S., Blizard, R. A. & King, M. B. (2007). The Camden Schizophrenia Surveys III: Five-year outcome of a sample of individuals from a prevalence survey and the importance of social relationships. *International Journal of Social Psychiatry, 53*, 340–356.

Hendrys, M., Dyck, McBride, D., & Whitbeck, J. (2001). A test of the reliability and validity of the Multnomah Community Ability Scale. *Community Mental Health Journal, 37*, 157–168.

Jaeger, J., Berns, S., & Czobor, P. (2003). The Multidimensional Scale of Independent Functioning: A new instrument for measuring functional disability in psychiatric populations. *Schizophrenia Bulletin, 29*, 153–167.

Jewell, T. C., Downing, D., & McFarlane, W. R. (2009). Partnering with families: Multiple family group psychoeducation for schizophrenia. *Journal of Clinical Psychology, 65*, 868–878.

Kelly, C. M., & Jorm, A. F. (2007). Stigma and mood disorders. *Current Opinion in Psychiatry, 20*, 13–16.

Kisely, S., Campbell, L. A., Crossman, D., Gleich, S. & Campbell, J. (2007). Are the Health of the Nations Outcome Scales a valid and practical instrument to measure outcomes in North America? A three-site evaluation across Nova Scotia. *Community Mental Health Journal, 43*, 91–107.

Kogan, L. R., Granger, B. P., Fitchett, J. A., Helmer, K. A., & Young, K. J. (1999). The human-animal team approach for children with emotional disorders: 2 case studies. *Children and Youth Care Forum, 28*, 121.

Kovacs, Z., Kis, R., Rozsa, S., & Rozsa, L. (2003). Animal-assisted therapy for middle-aged schizophrenic patients living in a social institution. A pilot study. *Clinical Rehabilitation, 18*, 484–486.

Krupnik, Y., Pilling, S., Killaspy, H., & Dalton, J. (2005). A study of family contact with clients and staff of community mental health teams. *Psychiatric Bulletin, 29*, 174–176.

Law, M., & Mills, J. (1998). Client-cent red occupational therapy. In M. Law (Ed.), *Client-Centered Occupational Therapy* (pp. 1–18). Thorofare, NJ: Slack.

Lee, S., Lee, M. T. Y., Chiu, M. Y. L., & Kleinman, A. (2005). Experience of social stigma by people with schizophrenia in Hong Kong. *British Journal of Psychiatry, 186*, 153–157.

Lenior, M. E., Dingmans, P. M. J., Linszen, D. H., De Haan, L., & Schene, A. H. (2001). Social functioning and the course of early onset schizophrenia: Five-year follow-up of a psychosocial intervention. *British Journal of Psychiatry, 179*, 53–58.

Link, B. G., Struening, E. L., Neese-Todd, S., Asmussen, S., & Phelan, J. C. (2001). The consequences of stigma for the self-esteem of people with mental illnesses. *Psychiatric Services, 52*, 1621–1626.

Marrone, J., Foley, S., & Selleck, V. (2005). How mental health and welfare to work interact: The role of hope, sanctions, engagement, and support. *American Journal of Psychiatric Rehabilitation, 8*, 81–101.

Mead, S., Hilton, D., & Curtis L. (2001). Peer support: A theoretical perspective. *Psychiatric Rehabilitation Journal, 5*(2), 134–141.

Mezzina, R., Borg, M., Marin, I., Sells, D., Topor, A., & Davidson, L. (2006). From participation to citizenship: How to regain a role, status, and a life in the process of recovery. *American Journal of Psychiatric Rehabilitation, 9, I39–61.*

Mowbray, C. T., Moxley, D. P., Thrasher, S., et al. (1996). Consumers as community support providers: Issues created by role innovation. *Community Mental Health Journal, 51,* 47–67.

Muller, B., Nordt, C., Lauber, C., & Rossler, W. (2007). Changes in social network diversity and perceived social support after psychiatric hospitalization: Results from a longitudinal study. *International Journal of Social Psychiatry, 53,* 564–575.

Murray-Swank, A. B., & Dixon, L. (2004). Family psychoeducation as an evidence-based practice. *CSN Spectrums, 9,* 905–912.

Nathans-Barel, I., Feldman, P., Berger, B., Modai, I., & Silver, H. (2005). Animal-assisted therapy ameliorates anhedonia in schizophrenia patients: A controlled pilot study. *Psychotherapy and Psychosomatics, 74,* 31–35.

New Zealand Mental Health Commission. (2001). *Recovery Competencies for New Zealand Mental Health Workers.* Wellington, NZ: New Zealand Mental Health Commission.

Odendaal, J. S. J. (2000). Animal-assisted therapy: Magic or medicine? *Journal of Psychosomatic Medicine, 49,* 275–280.

Office of the Deputy Prime Minister (ODPM). (2004). *Mental Health and social Exclusion.* Wetherby, UK: ODPM Publications.

Parker, G., Rosen, A., Emdur, N., & Hadzi-Pavlovic, D. (1991). The Life Skills Profile: Psychometric properties of a measure assessing function and disability in schizophrenia. *Acta Psychiatrica Scandinavica, 83,* 145–152.

Pekkala, E., & Merinder, L. (2001). Psychoeducation for schizophrenia. *Cochrane Database of Systematic Reviews, 2,* CD002831.

Perlick, D. A., Rosenheck, R. A., Clarkin, J. F., et al. (2001). Adverse effects of perceived stigma on social adaptation of persons diagnosed with bipolar affective disorder. *Psychiatric Services, 52,* 1627–1651.

Phelan, J. C., & Link B. G. (1999). The labeling theory of mental disorder (I): The role of social contingencies in the application of psychiatric labels. In A. V. Horwitz & T. L. Scheid (Eds.), *A Handbook for the Study of Mental Health: Social Contexts, Theories & Systems* (pp. 139–149).Cambridge: Cambridge University Press.

Queensland Health. (2005). *Sharing Responsibility for Recovery: Creating and Sustaining Recovery Oriented Systems of Care for Mental Health.* Brisbane, Australia: Queensland Health.

Reichert, E. (1998). Individual counseling for sexually abused children: A role for animals and storytelling. *Child and Adolescent Social Work Journal, 15,* 177–185.

Resnick, S. G., Rosenheck, R. A., Dixon, L., & Lehman, A. F. (2005). Correlates of family contact with the mental health system: Allocation of a scarce resource. *Mental Health Services Research, 7,* 113–121.

Rickwood, D. (2004). Recovery in Australia: Slowly but surely. *Australian e-Journal for the Advancement of Mental Health, 3,* 1–3.

Rosen, A., Hadzi-Pavlovic, D., & Parker, G. (1989). The Life Skills Profile: A measure assessing function and disability. *Schizophrenia Bulletin, 15,* 515–337.

Rosen, A., Trauer, T., Hadzi-Pavlovic, D., & Parker, G. (2001). Development of a brief form of the Life Skills Profile: The LSP-20. *Australian and New Zealand Journal of Psychiatry, 35*(5), 677–683.

Rothe, E. Q., Vega, B. J., Torres, R. M., Soler, S. M.C., & Pazos, R. M. M. (2005). From kids and horses: Equine facilitated psychotherapy for children. *International Journal of Clinical and Health Psychology, 5,* 373–383.

Salzer, M. S., & Shear, S. L. (2002). Identifying consumer-provider benefits in evaluation of consumer-delivered services. *Psychiatric Rehabilitation Journal, 25,* 281–288.

Solomon, P. (2004). Peer support/peer provider services underlying processes, benefits, and critical ingredients. *Psychiatric Rehabilitation Journal, 27,* 392–401.

Sowers, W. (2005). Transforming systems of care: The American Association of Community Psychiatrists Guidelines for Recovery Oriented Services. *Community Mental Health Services, 41,* 757–774.

Topor, A., Borg, M., Mezzina, R., Sells, D., Marin, I., & Davidson, L. (2006). Others: The role of family, friends, and professionals in the recovery process. *American Journal of Psychiatric Rehabilitation, 9,* 17–37.

Trauer, T., Callaly, T., Hantz, P., et al. (1999). Health of the Nation Outcome Scales. *British Journal of Psychiatry, 174,* 380–388.

Trauer, T., Duckmanton, R. A., & Chui, E. (1995). The Life Skills Profile: A study of its psychometric properties. *Australian and New Zealand Journal of Psychiatry, 29,* 492–499.

Turner-Crowson, J., & Wallcraft, J. (2002). The recovery vision for mental health services and research: A British perspective. *Psychiatric Rehabilitation Journal, 25,* 245–254.

Velde, B. P., Cipriani, J., & Fisher, G. (2005). Resident and therapist views of animal-assisted therapy: Implications for occupational therapy practice. *Australian Occupational Therapy Journal, 52,* 43–50.

VicHealth. (2002a). *Promoting Mental Health and Wellbeing Through Community and Cultural Development.* Melbourne, Australia: Globalism Institute, School of International and Community Studies, RMIT University.

————. (2002b). *Creative Connections: Promoting Mental Health and Wellbeing Through Community Arts Participation.* Melbourne, Australia: VicHealth.

Vormbrock, J. K., & Grossberg, J. M. (1988). Cardiovascular effects of human-pet dog interactions. *Journal of Behavioral Medicine, 11,* 509–517.

Waghorn, G. (2005). Work-related subjective experiences, work-related self-efficacy and vocational status among community residents with schizophrenia or schizoaffective disorder. Doctoral thesis. University of Queensland, Brisbane.

Waghorn, G., Chant, D., & King, R. (2007). Classifying socially valued role functioning among community residents with psychiatric disorders. *American Journal of Psychiatric Rehabilitation, 10*(3), 185–221.

Wing, J., Curtis, R., & Beevor, A. (1996). *Health of the Nation Outcome Scalesx: Report on Research.* London: Royal College of Psychiatrists.

Zani, B., McFarland, B., Wachal, M., Barker, S., & Barron, N. (1999). Statewide replication of predictive validation for the Multnomah Community Ability Scale. *Community Mental Health Journal, 35,* 223–229.

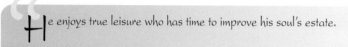

Leisure and Play

Valerie Howells

> "He enjoys true leisure who has time to improve his soul's estate.
>
> —Henry David Thoreau

Introduction

Persons with mental illness may face numerous complexities when attempting to engage in meaningful activity that can be called "leisure." These complexities might involve cost, location, other people, challenges of skill level, and the symptoms of mental illness that might get in the way of engagement in meaningful leisure activity. For a person coping with depression, interests might be less compelling and avoided if they involve too much energy. Having to leave one's home and go into the community might be barriers to full participation for a person living with schizophrenia and poverty. Overcoming homelessness and lack of space for the equipment that supports one's leisure interests might also serve as a barrier to engaging in valued leisure interests. All of these factors will either help or hinder the individual's occupational engagement, and each must be considered in order to effectively support his or her performance.

This chapter uses findings from an ethnographic study that took place at an inclusive arts studio for people with and people without mental illness as a backdrop for examining the concept of leisure (Howells & Zelnik, 2005). The voices of participants at the studio are used throughout the chapter to highlight the experience of individuals with mental illness in pursuing a meaningful leisure interest—in this case, art.

Throughout the chapter, the terms *individuals with mental illness, people with mental illness,* and *individuals with psychiatric disabilities* are used to describe a large group of people. However, these individuals must not be lumped into a group, even though they are described as such. Each person and his or her leisure interests are distinctive; therefore, we must conceptualize each client as a unique being and tailor our interventions to the individual. It is not simple, and ultimately it is about one person.

Leisure and Play Defined

What exactly is leisure? Leisure has been studied in social science fields as diverse as psychology, therapeutic recreation, sociology, gerontology, and political science, to name a few. Writers in these fields note that multiple definitions exist for leisure but agree that leisure is multidimensional (Coleman & Iso-Ahola, 1993; Gunter, 1987; Lee, Dattillo, & Howard, 1994). In the field of occupational therapy, Primeau (1996) articulated that the dimensions of time, activity, and experience distinguish leisure from work.

The Occupational Therapy Practice Framework (AOTA, 2008) identifies leisure and play as areas of occupation. **Leisure** is defined as "a nonobligatory activity that is intrinsically motivated and engaged in during discretionary time, that is, time not committed to obligatory occupations such as work, self-care, or sleep" (Parham & Fazio, 1997, p. 250). This definition of leisure focuses on the time and activity dimensions of leisure but does not directly address the experience dimension, that is, the subjective aspects of leisure. Writers both within and outside the field of occupational therapy concern themselves with the meaning of the experience to the individual engaged in the activity, framing this dimension of leisure as a state of mind. Their premise is that it is essential to explore what the activity means to the individual and to understand the *quality* of the activity as viewed by the person who is doing it. Suto (1998) notes that it is this subjective experience of leisure that is most compatible with the person-environment-occupation model. She suggests that occupational therapists adopt Reid's (1995) definition of leisure to direct their practice and aid in the development of theory related to leisure. Reid's definition states:

> Leisure will be defined as those activities which produce intrinsic rewards and provide the participant with life enhancing meaning and a sense of pleasure. It should be understood that many such activities can often appear to be work-like in form and may occur in one's vocation. What often separates work from leisure is the attitude with which it is undertaken and the reward which is gained from experience. With work, the reward is often only monetary; leisure usually involves intrinsic value. Leisure, then, is as much an attitude or state of mind as it is a type of activity. (p. 14)

This definition speaks to the subjective dimension and reminds us that whether the activity is categorized and experienced as work or leisure is dependent on the experience and meaning it engenders in the individual who is engaged in the doing.

While the literature that addresses the theoretical aspects of leisure in occupational therapy is quite limited (Lobo, 1998; Primeau, 1996; Suto, 1998), many authors have explored the concept of play. However, just as with leisure, there is no consensual definition of play or agreement on the precise dimensions that comprise it (Bundy, 2005). The Occupational Therapy Practice Framework (AOTA, 2008) defines **play** as "any spontaneous or organized activity that provides enjoyment, entertainment, amusement, or diversion" (Parham & Fazio, 1997, p. 252), but in the early years of occupational therapy, play was used primarily as a diversion, for skill development or remediation. Allesandrini (1949) identified play as "a serious undertaking . . . [of] purposeful activity". Reilly (1974) described play as a biosocial phenomenon that was the primary vehicle in childhood for the development of skills, abilities, interests, and habits. Reilly's view promoted the idea of play as mastery, an antecedent to work on the developmental continuum.

More recently, both Bundy (1993) and Florey & Greene (1997) addressed the importance of intrinsic motivation in play. Florey and Greene describe play as activity that is done for its own sake without reliance on external rewards. Bundy's playfulness model focuses on three characteristics of play: intrinsic motivation, internal control, and freedom to suspend reality. She suggests that playfulness as a characteristic is not specific to play but rather can be seen in individuals doing any activity.

Both play and leisure are considered areas of occupation; therefore, occupational therapists address performance concerns related to exploration and participation in these areas. **Exploration** refers to an individual's ability to identify play or leisure activities, interests, skills, or opportunities. **Participation** is the act of doing the occupation, planning for the occupation, maintaining a balance with other areas of occupation, and obtaining and appropriately using related tools and supplies (AOTA, 2008). In her editorial on participation's relationship to occupation and health, Baum (2003) writes that in order to enable participation, one cannot focus solely on an individual's function but rather must direct attention to eliminating physical, social, societal, or attitudinal barriers.

Participation in play and leisure has many benefits for people across the life span regardless of the conditions they may experience. Play affords children the opportunity to develop skills, to learn about and master their environments and their bodies, and to experience competence. Bundy (1993) notes that children who are more playful are more successful: they have a greater degree of internal control, are more internally motivated, have more freedom from the constraints of reality, and can respond to interactional cues.

Leisure is believed to positively influence health, enhance wellbeing, improve coping skills, buffer stress, and provide a means to augment self-identity and development (Coleman & Iso-Ahola, 1993; Kleiber, Hutchinson, & Williams, 2002; Nagle, Cook, & Polatajko, 2002; Reid, 1995; Samdahl & Kleiber, 1989; Tinsley, Hinson, Tinsley, & Holt,1993). These outcomes were identified in two studies of adolescents (Passmore, 2003; Passmore & French, 2003). Based on their findings, the authors created three categories of leisure: achievement (sports, music, any form of competition), social (doing with others), and time-out leisure ("vegging out"). The adolescents in the studies stated that their involvement in leisure occupations led to personal growth, better health, and competence, where they gained skills used in the activities. However, an analysis of findings in Passmore's study (2003) demonstrated that while participation in achievement and social leisure had a significant positive relationship with mental health, this relationship was not true for time-out leisure. The author notes that this finding may be because young people who perceive themselves to be less able chose more isolative activities. This may be particularly true for adolescents with disabilities, because they may not have access to the same opportunities for leisure or may struggle with feelings of incompetence due to self- or social stigma.

Having leisure occupations available and accessible enhances quality of life. These are critical issues for persons with mental illness. How can involvement in play or leisure affect individuals with mental illness? A participant in the art studio describes how making art affects her:

Usually when I do something like [art], it affects other parts of my life in one way or another. It might be a change in my own cognitive thinking . . . better self-esteem about my accomplishments, a little bit of comparison, a little bit of seeing. Or it might be feeling a little more of where I really am—as a person who could be an artist, who could maybe have things in galleries or things around town.

The experience of doing art creates possibilities and allows this individual to see a different vision of the future for herself. Exemplifying Bundy's description of the characteristic of suspension of reality in play, this individual is able to imagine herself as an artist in the future and to consider her talents, perhaps more realistically, in the context of the art studio and in comparison to other artists and class participants. The same sense of mastery can occur for an athlete who completes a challenging cross-country run and achieves his record time, for a pianist performing for others at a community event, and so forth.

Factors That Affect Leisure and Play

Engagement in leisure occupations is thought to have many benefits for all members of society. Examining leisure and mental illness requires that we also consider other variables that could impact exploration and participation. Occupational therapists are developing and investigating concepts related to occupational engagement that must be examined in conjunction with the occupations of play and leisure in order to more fully comprehend how participation is affected in persons with mental illness. These concepts include occupational balance, flow, occupational deprivation, and occupational alienation.

Leisure and Occupational Balance

The idea of maintaining **occupational balance** is referred to in the Occupational Therapy Practice Framework's (AOTA, 2008) definition of participation. Occupational therapists

The Lived Experience

Susan (a pseudonym)

Art as an activity is expensive. I enjoy it very much . . . it takes space, it takes people, it takes new skills, learning new skills. . . . There is no space in my [present] apartment to even have a sewing machine. My apartment is so small that if I put my sewing machine up it would take half of the apartment. At home in [former city of residence], I had the ironing board up. In fact, I had two ironing boards. I had two sewing machines, one on this side of the table, the serger on the other side of the table. . . . Here if I even just unfold the sewing machine, I'll feel like it's taking up half the space in the place. I had a loom. There is no place in my apartment to even put the loom—a small loom, table top. My loom, in fact, is now corroding on the balcony. I think my sewing project for last year was I sewed a button on a pair of shorts. Yeah, I did keep a needle and a spool of thread out. . . . So, I feel like it was a combination of environment and restrictions and the depression itself which just made me feel like, "Well, you don't deserve to enjoy anything anyway so just forget it," you know?

After participating in the art group, Susan spent more time in the community, took art classes, created meaningful relationships, and pursued her art. Making art in the context of the studio did not change her illness, but it certainly changed the quality of her life.

So anyway, after two things now, two times of kind of coming to the brink [depression and suicidal thoughts leading to hospitalization] and trying to figure out, "Okay, well what do you need to, you know, feel good?" I think that art is it. I still am not convinced that I am kitchy enough to really make money, okay? I just want you to know that I think that, yes, its satisfying and I enjoy the people and the place and this group thing is really powerful for me."

have long been proponents of balance in one's daily routines, appreciating that balance is influenced by cultural beliefs and context. Adolph Meyer, a psychiatrist and one of the founding fathers of occupational therapy in the United States, promoted the idea of balance in work, rest, play, and sleep. Occupational balance, like leisure, is defined and interpreted by the individual. As such, there are very different views of what constitutes leisure and balance, depending on the individual's experience. This is confirmed in a study by Craik and Pieris (2006) who reported that individuals with mental illness had difficulty assigning occupations to categories and that context often determined whether the occupation was considered leisure or not. It is the pattern of our occupations, then, in conjunction with our subjective experience, that may lead to wellbeing (Backman, 2004).

In their article about the importance of work in the lives of individuals with psychiatric disabilities, Marrone and Golowka (1999) describe the effect that one area of occupation can have on another. They report that the ability to engage in leisure is often lost in the early stages of mental illness and that participation in work activities can enhance self-esteem and serve as "a prompt" for involvement in new activities, such as leisure. Although they do not name it as such, they are clearly describing occupational balance when they state that when leisure is performed "in tandem with working, leisure then has more meaning" (p. 190). Considering the work–leisure balance in this way may be helpful to occupational therapists who often think of leisure as a precursor to work or a means of developing the skills necessary to be successful in work occupations.

Leisure and Flow

Numerous studies have explored the relationship between flow and leisure activities (Havitz & Mannell, 2005; Hull, Michael, Walker, & Roggenbuck, 1996; Mannell, Zuzanek, & Larson, 1988). Csikszentmihalyi (1993) described **flow** as a state of consciousness that occurs when someone is involved in an activity with high but manageable challenges that requires the full use of his or her skills. During this flow state, the individual is completely absorbed in the activity and loses all track of time. The person may undergo a "sense of transcendence" during these periods and experience greater happiness and satisfaction in these states. Flow can have long-term effects, including an enhanced sense of self, and can lead to greater enjoyment in activities.

Many participants in the art studio described experiences similar to Csikszentmihalyi's description of flow when they engaged in making art. As one participant said:

[Art] gets my mind off of really worrying a lot, worrying more than I think I need to. It really does take me to a place where sometimes I almost feel totally absorbed in it. I've done potters wheel type of work and I can be really lost in that. Time can go by—five hours, well, not that long but three or four hours . . . it's sort of a rest. It's a sort of meditation. It quiets my mind down.

Emerson, Cook, Polatajko, and Segal (1998) interviewed individuals with schizophrenia in order to determine if this group of people could experience enjoyment. Results of their study demonstrated that people with schizophrenia recounted experiences of enjoyment and that these experiences also included connecting socially with others. The individuals in the study reported feeling excited when engaged in challenging activities with heightened concentration and experiences of losing track of time. These findings challenged Csikszentmihalyi's (1990) assertion that flow states are not experienced in this population of people.

Another study conducted by McCormack, Funderburk, Lee, and Hale-Fought (2005) examined the day-to-day experience of clients served by community mental health centers to determine if the frequently reported mood states of boredom and anxiety in individuals with severe mental illness were related to the degree of challenges offered by the activities in which they participated. The results of their study showed that most activities in which people participated offered little challenge or stimulation. The authors of the study suggest the preponderance of these types of activities might be due to avoidance of challenging situations as a means of coping. When participants engaged in activities that provided high challenge matched to their skills (flow), there was not a significant association with anxiety or boredom.

Leisure and Occupational Deprivation

Occupational deprivation is defined as a "state of prolonged preclusion from engagement in occupations of necessity and/or meaning due to factors which stand outside of the control of the individual" (Whiteford, 2004, p. 222). The lack of choice that accompanies occupational deprivation can occur as a result of external forces such as poverty, cultural beliefs, or public policies. Individuals with mental illness identify significant contextual barriers that affect their participation in social and leisure activities. The most commonly reported external barriers include limited finances (often due to unemployment and poverty); both social/institutional stigma and self-stigma; lack of social support; and lack of transportation (Davidson, Haglund, et al, 2001; Deegan, 1993; Hodgson, Lloyd, & Schmid, 2001; Nagle et al, 2002; Pieris & Craik, 2004). In addition, being incarcerated or homeless also contribute to these barriers, where simply surviving may be the focus, rather than pursuit of meaningful leisure interests.

Participants at the art studio often referred to the challenge of engaging in art in the face of poverty. When asked about her thoughts on attending classes at the art studio as a way to resume her artwork, one participant said:

Well, I hope I can get reconnected to my sense of color, which I feel is gone, and my sense of order, which I feel I've lost. [Where I'm living now] is a very hostile environment to me so I really feel like I've been roughing it. . . . [When asked about doing art she replies] Do art compared to survival? I'm still going towards the survival side and the challenge of survival keeps getting higher and higher, so, to me, the thing of art, it just keeps going down. So, I'm hoping to at least get some increase [in doing art] there [at the art studio] so I can at least feel connected to a quality of life that I'm accustomed to or at least that I've known before.

As can be seen in this narrative, the harsh realities of poverty and living on the edge make pursuit of leisure interests a challenge. Yet at the same time, engaging in meaningful pursuits provides an avenue toward an enhanced quality of life.

Stigma profoundly affects individuals in their everyday life. Society holds strong negative stereotypes about mental illness, and individuals often seek social distance from those they perceive as mentally ill. This labeling frequently results in people with mental illness living segregated lives and experiencing isolation, self-stigma, and the loss of opportunity to be members of the community in which they live (Corrigan, 2005; Link & Phelan, 2001). All of the participants at the art studio spoke of stigmatizing experiences—either those they had experienced personally (if they had a mental illness) or stereotypical beliefs they held (if they did not have a mental illness). However, over time, art created a common ground, providing participants with a means of connecting with each other and changing their views. The shared experience of art allowed people to deconstruct their beliefs about mental illness and incited a change in the studio on both an individual and a cultural level. During the exit interviews, participants referred to art as an equalizer and a means of breaking down barriers (Zelnik & Howells, 2006). You will hear these ideas in the words that follow.

I know in the very beginning everybody was kind of in their own little area 'cause there wasn't . . . there was still that feeling that everything was very new. . . . But by the second set of courses you could see that the comfort level was there and so people felt more like moving around, intermixing, and talking.

Stigma presents a formidable challenge to people's desire to engage in their communities. It can severely affect participation and can be more difficult to manage than the symptoms of the illness itself (Corrigan, 2005).

Individuals with mental illness also frequently experience disruptions in their occupational functioning as a result of their condition. **Negative symptoms** such as **avolition, anhedonia,** and **anergia** can impair their ability to participate in everyday activities. Consider the person who runs daily as a means to overcoming depression, who sings in a choir to cope with anxiety, or who watches a football game with family and friends in an alcohol- and drug-free place to overcome substance abuse and social isolation. Before attending the art studio, one participant shared the following comment in her initial interview:

I was kind of glad when you called me because I've been sort of on a downer for a few months. . . . I need something. I need something to get me out, and something I like. I think the struggle to get going has more to do with my depression.

Although the constellation of symptoms that an individual experiences are unique to that person (Zelnik & Howells, 2007), deficits in social and cognitive functioning that affect performance may include a reduced ability to concentrate and pay attention, thought disorders, hypersensitivity, deficits in social skills and judgment, disorganized thoughts, disorganized speech, and disheveled appearance. In addition to coping with the symptoms of mental illness, people must also manage medication side effects such as dry mouth and sensitivity to sunlight, which can be very disruptive and limit the location of leisure pursuits.

Avolition and related symptoms are often identified in the literature as the reasons for the social isolation experienced by people with mental illness (Link & Phelan, 2001).

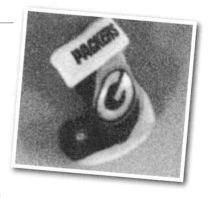

PhotoVoice

This is a picture of Green Bay Packer stocking. I've been a fan of the Green Bay Packers for a lot of years. When they win I feel fulfillment which is good for my mental health.

However, Davidson, Staynor, et al (2001) challenges this view, stating, "This literature has gone so far as to characterize people with negative symptoms as 'empty shells' who can no longer 'think, feel, or act' having 'lost the capacity both to suffer and to hope'" (Andreasen, 1984, pp. 62–63). In this view, the lack of social support experienced by people with psychiatric disabilities is seen as having been brought about primarily by "the ravages of the disorder itself, leaving the person isolated, apathetic, and no longer even desiring companionship or love" (p. 276). Davidson, Staynor, et al are addressing issues of social functioning from the perspective of a recovery model that seeks to support individuals to resume role functioning and activities through skills development and environmental supports. Andreason's description is an example of how social stigma can be reinforced by diagnostic nosology. Occupational therapists working in community mental health programs need to be strengths-based and offer encouragement, support, and opportunities to engage in meaningful and challenging leisure occupations of interest to the person.

Leisure and Occupational Alienation

Occupational alienation is "a sense of isolation, powerlessness, frustration, loss of control, and estrangement from society or self that results from engagement in occupation that does not satisfy inner needs" (Wilcock, 2006). Individuals with mental illness often experience occupational alienation because they more commonly engage in passive pursuits such as watching TV or listening to a radio rather than active or social leisure (Krupa, McLean, Eastabrook, Bonham, & Baksh, 2003; Shimitras, Fossey, & Harvey, 2003). Passive pursuits appear to more readily lead to feelings of boredom and do not encourage social interaction or recovery. This often results from lack of access to active leisure, lack of friends or partners to do things with, and the external barriers identified earlier in this chapter, such as lack of finances to pursue certain occupations and transportation limitations. Also, people with mental illness may not be employed and therefore do not have the social network that work can potentially create (Davidson, Haglund, et al, 2001; Shimitras et al, 2003).

Social isolation has long been a problem for people with mental illness. They frequently report being lonely, lacking opportunities for social interaction, and experiencing the loss of friends and family. It is believed that participation in leisure activities can create a sort of scaffolding or social support to act as a buffer during stressful periods (Iso-Aloha & Park, 1996). Leisure occupations can be highly social in nature. The social quality of leisure was referred to by informants in Nagle et al's (2002) study who remarked that it was important not only to do things but to do things with others. Social connections were viewed as supporting health and doing. The people in this study also embraced the opportunity to be around people who were not mentally ill, and they expressed a desire to be included in the broader community.

In a qualitative study examining factors related to quality of life for individuals with schizophrenia, participants reported that social interaction was a major factor that affected the quality of their lives. One theme that emerged in the study was that of connecting and belonging. Participants viewed connecting and belonging as essential, and activity was often used as a vehicle for interacting (Laliberte-Rudman,

Yu, Scott, & Pajouhandeh, 1999). As Davidson (2001) notes, personal narratives suggest that people with mental illness long to engage with others and experience a sense of belonging. The qualitative studies mentioned throughout this chapter consistently report participants' views about the importance of being socially connected. In these studies, people with psychiatric disabilities comment on their desire to be with others and indicate that leisure activity often provides this opportunity (Deegan, 1993; Krupa et al, 2003; Shimitras et al, 2003).

Leisure and Play Assessments

Using an occupation-based, client-centered, top-down approach, therapists often begin the assessment process by using an interview or self-report measure to identify areas of occupation in which there may be an issue. Interview tools such as the Canadian Occupational Performance Measure (COPM) or the Occupational Performance History Interview II (OPHI-II) and self-report measures such as the Occupational Self-Assessment (OSA) are valuable tools with which to begin this process. If leisure exploration or participation are identified as a problem, then the therapist may select a specific assessment to address that area. However, valid and reliable tools with which to assess the occupations of both play and leisure are lacking. Numerous authors have called for the development of measurement tools in this area (Bundy, 2005; Havitz & Dimanche, 1997; Nilsson & Fisher, 2006; Ragheb, 1996).

In a study of occupational therapists' evaluation of leisure, Turner, Chapman, McSherry, Krishnagiri, & Watts (2000) found that leisure was primarily addressed through informal interviews despite the availability of standardized assessments. Leisure was used principally as a means, rather than as an end, to develop skills to engage the person in meaningful leisure pursuits. Therapists practicing in the psychosocial area appeared to value leisure more than those practicing in other areas.

If therapists use measures that assess only time use or categories of interest, then they may discount the subjective dimension of leisure that can affect engagement. Primeau (1996) cautions therapists to consider the meaning of the experience to the client as well as to observe the affective expression of the person engaged in various activities. Given the subjective character of leisure, qualitative approaches that seek to fully understand the experience and meaning of the leisure activity to the individual may be the most effective method of gathering a complete picture of the occupation of leisure for an individual. The therapist will want to gather data about the past and present interests of a client and the uniqueness of those interests, as well as what makes particular activities important to the client. This information can be applied to interventions designed to help the client to explore and create new or alternative activities with comparable qualities and lead the client to have similar, positive experience or to avoid negative experiences.

Therapists may also work with individuals who are either unable or are hesitant to give voice to their leisure interests. During the Craik and Pieris study (2006), participants with serious mental illness demonstrated difficulty verbalizing their experiences and the value of their leisure occupations when initially questioned, needing prompts. The authors cautioned that it may not be adequate to base findings on verbalizations alone. In these cases, it is imperative that the occupational therapist use observation to determine the leisure interests and patterns of the client. Assessments such as the Volitional Questionnaire (de las Heras, Geist, Kielhofner, & Li, 2002), although not specific to leisure occupations, address behaviors that reflect the personal causation, values, and interests of the individual engaged in an activity. Assessments such as this may help the therapist to think about the volitional traits of the person, thereby coming to some understanding of what is meaningful and important to that individual.

Although there are only a limited number of assessments designed specifically to assess the play and leisure occupations of persons with mental illness, they can be classified into those that are used with children and adolescents and those that are used with adults.

Assessments for Children and Adolescents

Bundy (2005) states that there are five factors that can be evaluated in children's play: the activity, the child's motivation, the way in which the child approaches play, the child's capacity to play, and the environmental factors affecting play. Assessment of play should ideally address all five factors; however, no single instrument does this, nor does a test battery exist. Bundy's (2005) work in *Measuring Occupational Performance* offers a review of recommended play assessments.

Play and social behavior can be evaluated in children with psychosocial problems using both structured and unstructured play approaches. Unstructured approaches, in combination with a play history taken from parents, are used with children under the developmental age of three. With preschool-aged children, both structured and unstructured approaches can be used. The child's developmental age determines the task/play and objects the child is given, the degree of structure provided, and the people present (i.e., only the individual, one peer, or a group of peers). Interviewing school-aged children about their play and validating the information with parents is a valuable tool for finding out about play/leisure preferences, interests, and social interactions. Observing the child in natural settings with peers allows the therapist to gain insight into the social interaction, task performance and behavior.

The Pediatric Interest Profiles, developed by Henry (2000), are standardized assessments that can be used with children and adolescents to assess their interests and involvement in play and leisure occupations. They include a Kid Play Profile for ages 6 to 9, a Preteen Play Profile for ages 9 to 12, and an Adolescent Leisure Interest Profile for ages 12 to 21.

The Kid Play Profile consists of 50 items or activities. Children who respond affirmatively to doing an activity are then asked if they like the activity and with whom they do it. The questions and responses on the form are represented by both drawings and words. Respondents can circle or color their responses to each item.

The Preteen Play Profile consists of 59 items grouped into eight activity categories: sports, outside, summer, winter, indoor, creative, lessons-classes, and social. An affirmative response to the initial question is followed by four other questions, including how often the activity is done, how much the respondent likes the activity, how good they feel they are at the activity, and with whom they do the activity. As with the Kid Play Profile, both drawings and words are used to describe the activities. Both the Kid Play Profile and the Preteen Play Profile can be easily administered and serve as a mechanism for children to express their feelings and thoughts about their play experiences.

The Adolescent Leisure Interest Profile (ALIP) consists of 83 items grouped into eight categories. For each item, the respondent is asked, "How interested are you in this activity?" and "How often are you in this activity?" Affirmative answers are followed by three more questions related to how well they feel they perform the activity, how much they enjoy it, and with whom they do it. Unlike the Kid and Preteen Profiles, no drawings are used—adolescents use a check mark to indicate their answer (Henry, 1998).

Studies of the Kid Play and Preteen Play profiles demonstrate that children between the ages of 6 and 12 can understand and respond to the format. Test–retest reliability and internal consistency of total scores for both profiles were acceptable (Kielhofner et al, 2002). Studies of the ALIP have demonstrated good test–retest reliability and good internal consistency, with Henry (1998) reporting test–retest scores ranging from 0.53 to 0.85 and Trottier, Brown, Hobson, and Miller (2002) reconfirming test–retest reliability. It is interesting to note that adolescents in the Trottier et al study complained about the length of time needed to complete the test and needed clarification about the meaning of some of the activities. Henry (1998) acknowledged that there may be cultural, ethnic, and geographical bias in the ALIP.

Assessments for Adults

There are several assessments that may be used with adults, including the Leisure Satisfaction Scale, the NPI Interest Checklist, the Occupational Questionnaire, Soederback and Hammarlund's 14 Dimensions of Leisure, and others.

The Leisure Satisfaction Scale (LSS), developed by Beard and Ragheb (1980), is a standardized self-report measure that includes six subscales: psychological, educational, social, relaxational, physiological, and aesthetic. These subscales address 51 needs thought to be satisfied through engagement in leisure. Respondents rate the items using a 5-point Likert scale from *Never true for you* to *Always true for you*. There is also a short form of the LSS consisting of four statements in each of the six areas. Administration of the short form can be completed in 10 minutes.

The LSS has been used by occupational therapists in studies of individuals with mental illness (Lloyd, King, Lampe, & McDougall, 2001), adolescents (Trottier et al, 2002), and a group of nurses (DiBona, 2000). The Trottier et al study (2002) reaffirmed the findings of the authors of the LSS. Internal consistency of both studies was comparable, with Trottier et al reporting an alpha coefficient of 0.87 compared to Beard and Ragheb's score of 0.93. Lloyd et al (2001) administered the LSS with 100 clients of a community mental health rehabilitation service in Australia. The authors of this study reported that respondents' leisure satisfaction was similar to that of the general population. This finding differs from that of other studies, which typically report that individuals with mental illness lack both leisure interests and satisfaction. The authors also reported a strong correlation between the total score on the LSS and the social contact subscale, indicating concurrent validity. That is, clients who were less satisfied with their leisure had less social contact, and clients who were highly satisfied with their leisure were most likely to have high ratings of social contact when externally rated.

The NPI Interest Checklist was developed by Matsutsuyu (1969) as a means of gathering data about a client's interests. Matsutsuyu developed the instrument for use with adults in an inpatient psychiatric unit. As originally designed, the interest checklist sought to classify both the intensity and the type of interest. Part I included 80 items that comprised manual skills, physical sports, social recreation, activities of daily living, and cultural/educational. Respondents were to identify whether they had a strong interest, casual interest, or no interest in the item. Part II offered the client the chance to add items not included in the list, and Part III asked the client to give a historical account of his or her interests and hobbies in narrative form. In 1978, factor analytic studies by Rogers, Weinstein, and Figone failed to establish the validity of the categories of interest that comprised the instrument; this could reinforce the earlier mentioned concept that people classify their leisure interests on the basis of their attitude about the activity, not on the activity itself. However, the instrument has been shown to discriminate between populations—individuals who are disabled identify fewer interests and participate less in their interests (Kielhofner et al, 2002). The checklist was modified by Kielhofner and Neville in 1983. The Modified Interest Checklist, which can be used with adolescents or adults, contains 68 items scored by level of interest (i.e., strong interest, some interest, or no interest) during the past 10 years and the last year. Respondents are asked to identify if they currently participate in the activity or if they hope to participate in the activity in the future. After completing the checklist, it is recommended that the therapist discuss the answers with the client (Kielhofner et al, 2002).

Although it does not solely address leisure, the Occupational Questionnaire (Smith, Kielhofner, & Watts, 1986) is an example of a tool that occupational therapists can use to understand an individual's time use. Persons are asked to identify how they spend their time during a weekday and a weekend day. The form can be used as a semistructured interview if this method is preferable and can also be used individually or in a group (Kielhofner et al, 2002). Participants record their activities in half-hour increments and respond to four questions about each half hour. They first indicate if they consider the activity to be work, a daily living task, recreation, or rest, then describe their feelings of competence with, importance of, and enjoyment in the activity. This form is much like a time diary, and the therapist can have the individual fill out the form for a specific day or for a "typical" day. The questions speak to the subjective experience of the individual and allow the therapist to know the meaning of the activity to the person.

Soederback and Hammarlund (1993) created a leisure-time frame of reference with an assessment for use in clinical decision-making. They conducted an analysis of the literature and, from this analysis, identified 16 dimensions of leisure: time, intrinsic motivation, free choice of activity, capability, structure of social and culture environment, leisure-time activity engaged in, goals, pleasure for pleasure's sake, diversion, recreation, relaxation, self-fulfillment,

influence on individual, leisure role, leisure behavior, and satisfied harmonious person. Their assessment consists of questions related to these dimensions. The authors suggest beginning the assessment process with an interview and then proceeding to specific assessments that address the problem areas identified in the interview.

When assessing the leisure pursuits or interests of older adults, Bundy (2001) recommends that, rather than ask the typical question "What do you do for leisure?" the therapist should ask what activities they do that lead them to forget about the world around them and become totally focused on the activity. This is a logical adaptation if one recalls that leisure as a category is deceptive and that activities can have multiple and different meanings to each individual. The suggestion is one that therapists working with adolescents and adults should also consider incorporating. Bundy developed a model of leisure that addresses the concepts of control, motivation, and disengagement, all of which affect the person's degree of absorption in the leisure pursuit. In the model, the first three concepts occur on a continuum from external to internal (control), low to high (motivation), and none to complete (disengagement). When assessing and planning intervention strategies with older adults, therapists can employ these continua by asking the client to rate his or her leisure involvement or using them to think about and assess the experience (Bundy, 2001).

Leisure Intervention

Meyer adeptly summarizes the goal of occupational therapy intervention when he states: "Our role consists in giving *opportunities* rather than prescriptions. . . . It takes, above all, resourcefulness and ability to respect at the same time the native *capacities and interests* of the patient" (Meyer, 1977, p. 641).

Indeed, there is no precise prescription for how to incorporate play and leisure into interventions with individuals with mental illness. In fact, there often may not be a need for "treatment," per se, but rather for opportunities to explore and access interests. Many of the participants at the art studio

---

Evidence-Based Practice

Few valid and reliable tools exist for assessing leisure. It is essential to understand the meaning of the activity to the individual as well as the time and activity dimensions of leisure.

➤ Occupational therapists need to use qualitative measures or existing interview tools, along with time diaries and checklists, to examine the meaning of leisure experiences for clients.

➤ Occupational therapy researchers can aid in the practitioner's understanding of their client's leisure by developing valid assessments.

Nilsson, I., & Fisher, A. G. (2006). Evaluating leisure activities in the oldest old. *Scandinavian Journal of Occupational Therapy, 13*, 31–37.

Primeau, L. A. (1996). Work and leisure: Transcending the dichotomy. *American Journal of Occupational Therapy, 50*(7), 569–577.

Suto, M. (1998). Leisure in occupational therapy. *Canadian Journal of Occupational Therapy, 65*(5), 271–278.

spoke of making art as "therapeutic" but not as "therapy." This is an important distinction. Intervention strategies must take into account the person, the occupations that are meaningful to them, and the environmental factors surrounding their exploration and participation in play and leisure.

Interventions with Children and Adolescents

Play interventions are typically used more as a means that target multiple skills and behaviors than as an end or outcome. However, the goal of intervention can be play itself or helping the child to develop playfulness. Just as when working with adults, the therapist needs to know the child's favored activities and incorporate these activities into the treatment.

Small-group activities with a focus on learning how to share, interact in a respectful manner, and cooperate with other group members are valuable tools to use with children who exhibit behavioral problems in middle childhood and adolescence. Florey and Greene (1997) note that it is difficult for beginning therapists to work with children and adolescents with behavioral disorders during middle childhood because their behaviors are often not predictable, are inconsistent, or may be difficult to distinguish from behaviors considered typical or normal. No matter the age of the child with psychosocial problems, play and leisure create ideal ways to intervene, with the goal of either enhancing skills (means) or exploring and participating in play or leisure interests (ends). Fazio (2001) describes the use of community-based clubs that provide occupation-centered activities for children who are in the middle childhood/adolescent stage. These clubs occur in the context of larger community organizations such as the YMCA and 4-H and provide the child/adolescent with a natural setting in which to develop social behaviors and roles through engagement in play and leisure.

Regardless of the child's age, certain skills are valuable for the occupational therapist to employ. Keen observational skills are essential. It is also critical that the therapist be self-aware and be able to recall his or her own playful self in order to create, imagine, and use symbolic play with the child (G. D. Reeves, personal communication, January, 2007). Activity analysis skills will assist in determining the physical, cognitive, and social demands of each activity. Because many children with psychosocial problems have experienced failures with task or social performance, it is important to carefully select play and leisure activities that will create a challenge–skill match and to design varied opportunities that offer choice.

The environment in which the play takes place should be carefully considered. It must contain ample objects that are interesting, encourage exploration, and provide new experiences, and it should offer an opportunity to interact with people and even animals. The space needs to be large enough to allow freedom of movement.

Interventions with Adults

Leisure interventions with adults are also used as both a means and an end. Often, leisure is used to help people regain skills that have diminished as a result of their illness or the context in which they live. Common goals related to intervention as a means include improving social skills, enhancing self-esteem or self-confidence, regaining or

developing roles, regaining physical abilities, and developing relationships.

Just-Right Challenges

Because some individuals with psychiatric disabilities have experienced repeated failures, social stigma, or both, it is important to carefully plan leisure activities so that they are just-right challenges. Understanding the challenge–skill ratio is an important consideration when developing programs. Therapists need to provide activities that are meaningful, challenging, and match the skill level of the person in order to achieve the possibility of experiencing flow.

Contextual Considerations

The immediate context in which the intervention occurs as well as the broader community context must be carefully considered. It should provide emotional safety (Rebeiro & Cook, 1999; Suto & Frank, 1994); opportunities for choice and control, mastery, and autonomy; and the chance to develop skills in an environment that provides reasonable challenges. Bejerholm and Eklund (2004) comment on the importance of environment in their study of time use and occupational performance in persons with schizophrenia. For the people in their study, the environment did not provide stimulus for seeking out activity or interacting. The authors state, "Arranging and reshaping the environment would most likely shape opportunities for promoting occupational performance . . . diminishing the gap between the clients adaptive capacity and the environmental demands" (p. 41). Occupational therapists can partner with clients to alter, modify, and adapt environments so that they are more conducive to successful leisure performance. This might include finding a bowling alley that is not collocated with a bar for the person who is establishing new routines that support abstinence from alcohol or sending an e-mail reminder on the morning of a community event that was planned the previous week.

Social Considerations

Rebeiro and Cook (1999) discuss the impact that participation in a group can have in the lives of individuals with severe mental illness. They conducted an exploratory study

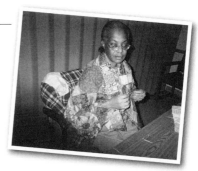

PhotoVoice

I have a quilt, and I sew on it every other Monday. I think I might make another one, oo. I sew it together, and Lisa is my teacher. I feel happy and peaceful. Brown color, blue, and purple. Lisa gave me quilt pieces. I hand cut every piece of it, and sew across the line. It is kind of hard to do. It is beautiful. It shows a brilliant color and shape. I showed it to my art teacher. My art teacher was glad to see it too.

—Barb

with eight women who regularly attended an occupation-based women's group. Results of the study demonstrated that the group created a place of safety, a sense of belonging, and opportunities to risk attempting new skills, ultimately leading to an enhanced sense of self through engaging in occupation. The authors make the point that because the group was homogeneous, it provided a safe social context, offered acceptance, and was free from stigma. Depending on the individual, homogenous groups of this kind that involve leisure activities can be very valuable treatment strategies. However, other individuals may prefer to seek out social and leisure opportunities that exist in the broader community (Figure 52-1).

Model Programs

Intervention strategies in psychiatric rehabilitation are directed toward enhancing the skills of individuals and developing environmental supports. The assumption of this model is that by intervening and creating change in these two areas, the individual will be able to engage in valued roles and occupations (Anthony, Cohen, Farkas, & Gagne, 2002). While these principles have been applied more broadly, they can also be applied to facilitating engagement in leisure interests. **Supported socialization** is one method in this tradition that can assist individuals with mental illness to engage in social and recreational activities in their natural environment (Davidson, Staynor, et al, 2001). The Partnership Project is a supported socialization program designed to reduce loneliness and improve community integration for people with psychiatric disabilities (Davidson, Staynor, et al, 2001; Stayner, Davidson, & Tebes, 1996). Participants in the project were randomly assigned to one of three groups. One group paired individuals with psychiatric disabilities who resided in the community with volunteers who also had personal histories of psychiatric illness. Another group paired people with psychiatric disabilities with volunteers who did not share this personal history. The final group was a stipend-only group; participants received money but were not paired with partners. All the participants in the study were given a stipend of

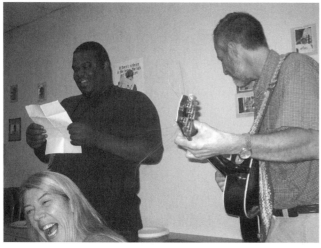

FIGURE 52-1. Tramell sings with Dan Orlett, a nurse, and enjoys a newfound activity, singing with a group of people.

$28 a month to help with the costs of participating in social and recreational activities, and all agreed to engage in activities of their choosing for a few hours a week over a 9-month period. Prior to involvement in the program, participants reported feeling lonely and isolated, indicating that this was not how they preferred to spend their time. The people with whom they did have contact were primarily other consumers or mental health professionals. This is a common experience in the social worlds of many individuals with psychiatric disabilities. Participants also reported they longed to be more involved in social activities with a greater variety of people in their community. All of the participants in the study reported that relationships were important to them. Lastly, participants acknowledged that stigma and financial limitations significantly affected their participation in social and recreational interests.

Davidson, Staynor, et al (2001) reported two outcomes for the individuals in the stipend-only group. Some individuals in this group reported that they did not experience significant change in their social lives, continued to feel stigmatized, and often used their stipend to help pay their bills. Other individuals in this group used their stipend to engage in activities that were normally not available to them due to cost. This group found that having some extra cash helped their social lives because they could do things with friends and not rely on them financially. Many people in the stipend-only group did not feel that involvement in the program affected their daily lives, yet all those who did engage in activity in the community, even though they had no partner, felt some benefit from being able to participate in new activities.

People in the groups with partners/volunteers reported many common themes and stated that the program increased their socialization and participation. Participants acknowledged that making a commitment (contract) to spend time with their partner helped them to overcome social and self stigma, anxiety and awkwardness, and lack of motivation. The authors of the study reported that the aspects of the "contract" that helped people to overcome the internal and external obstacles to social and recreational participation with their new partners included feelings of unconditional acceptance from their partner and having consistent and regular interaction with their partner. Social support and a small amount of money helped these participants create a place for themselves in their communities and experience a sense of belonging and a sense of efficacy.

Participants in the art studio shared similar experiences, discussing the importance of connecting and belonging within the context of meaningful occupation. Occupational therapists may want to look carefully at these kinds of programs as models for intervention. Clearly, these models are therapeutic and enhance feelings of wellbeing even though they are not "therapy."

The Active Advice Pilot Project (Heasman & Atwal, 2004) was a leisure education program for individuals with psychiatric disabilities. The program, which involved unemployed people diagnosed with mental illness over the course of 6 months, was designed to help clients resume involvement in meaningful leisure as a means of improving their quality of life and increasing their involvement in their communities. The evaluation process included the administration of the Occupational Case Analysis Interview and Rating Scale (OCAIRS) and the interest checklist. One activity from the checklist was chosen, and a plan was developed to aid the individual in participation. Authors of the project reported that the plan could include any of the following interventions: education; social support by volunteers, peers, or staff; or graded interventions. The results indicated that 47% of the participants were successful in achieving their plans. Many participants in this study were hesitant to engage in leisure without a partner, were anxious about meeting strangers, and struggled to follow through on their plans. A number of networking strategies were used, including a database of individuals with similar interests, volunteers, and a newsletter that provided information about community events. The authors note that for some participants, involvement in the project was the end (outcome), and for others, it provided a means for engagement in the broader community.

Adjusting to Changing Interests and Abilities

As individuals age, some of their leisure activities may change or cease. However, certain familiar or favorite activities may continue to be meaningful to them. It is therefore crucial not to assume that older adults are no longer interested in learning new activities or are unable to participate in active leisure or recreational activities (Iso-Ahola, Jackson, & Dunn, 1994). Depending on the specific diagnosis, older adults with mental illness may experience cognitive changes that impair their ability to perform. In this case, the therapist will need to adapt the activity, if possible, or identify characteristics of the activity that made it meaningful and attempt potential substitutions. These individuals may also experience physiological changes that must be taken into consideration.

> ## Evidence-Based Practice
>
> Stigma can profoundly affect the lives of people with mental illness, including their involvement in social and leisure pursuits in their communities.
>
> ➤ Occupational therapists can partner with their clients to address issues related to occupational deprivation and alienation to enhance leisure and social participation.
>
> ➤ Occupational therapists should consider developing programs based on the supported socialization model.
>
> Corrigan, P. (2005). *On the Stigma of Mental Illness: Practical Strategies for Research and Social Change.* Washington, DC: American Psychological Association.
>
> Davidson, L., Haglund, K. E., Stayner, D. A., Rakfeldt, J., Chinman, M. J., & Tebes, J. K. (2001). "It was just realizing . . . that life isn't one big horror": A qualitative study of supported socialization. *Psychiatric Rehabilitation Journal, 24*(3), 275–292.

Summary

People benefit from participation in leisure activities that are safe, conducive to active "play," meaningful, and associated with successful performance. This is perhaps especially critical to those with mental illness. It is essential that as occupational therapists we partner with our clients to help them achieve this goal. We must listen carefully to their stories and only after careful listening proceed in ways that make our interventions relevant. Relevant interventions can profoundly shift people's lives. This chapter has provided tools for assessing and intervening in the lives of children, adolescents, and adults with mental illness around leisure and play. Full participation and engagement in occupations that hold meaning and value is the intended outcome of successful occupational therapy intervention.

Active Learning Strategies

1. Leisure Exploration and Participation

Select a new leisure occupation to learn. Spend 2 months engaged in the occupation, devoting time each week to performing this occupation. Record your experience in a journal—the dates you participate, the amount of time you spend, what you do, and the meaning of the experience to you. Respond to the following focused questions at the end of each week. At the conclusion of the learning activity, reflect on how you could employ your new knowledge when you approach leisure occupations with clients.

- *Week 1:* How did you decide which occupation you would do? In what ways does your culture affect your options? What facilitates your options? What limits your options? How did you begin doing your selected occupation? What does it feel like to do something new and unfamiliar?

- *Week 2:* Have you experienced problems with occupational participation as a result of occupational deprivation, alienation, or for any other reason? If so, how has this affected your experience? If not, what are potential problems that could be experienced by someone who desired to pursue this occupation? How does what you do shape society, and how does society shape what you do?

- *Week 3:* Consider the other people who are doing this occupation. In what ways are you connected to them? If you are engaged in an occupation that takes place in a group, how has the group affected your participation and experience? If you are involved in an occupation that is individual, how has engaging in a singular pursuit affected your participation and experience?

- *Week 4:* Where does your occupation fit in your own development? What experiences in your past affect your present experience? How does your experience compare to cultural expectations for a person of your age and situation? What do you feel/think about this? How does your occupational choice reflect your family history? What potential does this occupation have to affect your future?

- *Week 5:* Consider your entire routine of occupations. In what ways does your selected occupation affect you (your health, wellbeing, feelings of competency, self esteem, etc)? How do you presently use time in your life? How has adding this occupation affected your occupational balance?
- *Week 6:* Have you had any moments when you experienced flow in this occupation? If so, think about all the factors that led to this experience. If not, try to determine what prevents this.

- *Week 7:* Describe the "therapeutic" aspects of the occupation for you. Are there "limitations"? How might it be modified/graded? For whom would this occupation be appropriate?
- *Week 8:* What have you learned about yourself while doing this occupation? How can you apply this knowledge to practice?

 Record your responses to these questions in your **Reflective Journal**.

Source: Adapted from an assignment originally developed by Virginia A. Dickie.

References

Alessandrini, N. A. (1949). Play: A child's world. *American Journal of Occupational Therapy, 3,* 9–12.

American Occupational Therapy Association (AOTA). (2008). Occupational therapy practice framework: Domain and process (2nd ed.). *American Journal of Occupational Therapy, 62,* 625–683.

Andreasen, N. C. (1984). *The Broken Brain: The Biological Rrevolution in Psychiatry.* New York: Harper & Row.

Anthony, W., Cohen, M., Farkas, M., & Gagne, C. (2002). *Psychiatric Rehabilitation* (2nd ed.). Boston: Center for Psychiatric Rehabilitation.

Backman, C. L. (2004). Occupational balance: Exploring the relationships among occupations and their influence on well being. *Canadian Journal of Occupational Therapy, 71*(4), 202–209.

Baum, M. C. (2003). Participation: Its relationship to occupation and health. *OTJR: Occupation, Participation and Health, 23*(2), 46–47.

Beard, J. G., & Ragheb, M. G. (1980). The leisure satisfaction measure. *Journal of Leisure Research, 12*(1), 20–33.

Bejerholm, U., & Eklund, M. (2004). Time use and occupational performance among persons with schizophrenia. *Occupational Therapy in Mental Health, 20*(1), 27–47.

Bundy, A. C. (1993). Assessment of play and leisure: Delineation of the problem. *American Journal of Occupational Therapy, 47,* 217–222.

———. (2001). Leisure. In B. R. Bonder & M. B. Wagner (Eds.), *Functional Performance in Older Adults* (2nd ed.) (pp. 196–217). Philadelphia: F.A. Davis.

———. (2005). Measuring play performance. In M. Law, C. Baum, & W. Dunn (Eds.), *Measuring Occupational Performance: Supporting Best Practice in Occupational Therapy* (2nd ed.) (pp. 129–149). Thoroughfare, NJ: Slack.

Coleman, D., & Iso-Ahola, S. E. (1993). Leisure and health: The role of social support and self-determination. *Journal of Leisure Research, 25*(2), 111–128.

Corrigan, P. (2005). *On the Stigma of Mental Illness: Practical Strategies for Research and Social Change.* Washington, DC: American Psychological Association.

Craik, C., & Pieris, Y. (2006). Without leisure . . . "it wouldn't be much of a life": The meaning of leisure for people with mental health problems. *British Journal of Occupational Therapy, 69*(5), 209–216.

Csikszentmihalyi, M. (1990). *Flow: The Psychology of Optimal Experience.* New York: Harper & Row.

———. (1993). Activity and happiness: Towards a science of occupation. *Occupational Science: Australia, 1*(1), 38–42.

Davidson, L., Haglund, K. E., Stayner, D. A., Rakfeldt, J., Chinman, M. J., & Tebes, J. K. (2001). "It was just realizing . . . that life isn't one big horror": A qualitative study of supported socialization. *Psychiatric Rehabilitation Journal, 24*(3), 275–292.

Davidson, L., Stayner, D. A., Nickou, C., Styron, T. H., Rowe, M., & Chinman, M. L. (2001). "Simply to be let in": Inclusion as a basis for recovery. *Psychiatric Rehabilitation Journal, 24*(4), 375–388.

Deegan, P. (1993). Recovering our sense of value after being labeled mentally ill. *Journal of Psychosocial Nursing, 31,* 157–164.

de las Heras, C. G., Geist, R., Kielhofner, G., & Li, Y. (2002). *The Volitional Questionnaire (VQ) (Version 4.0).* Chicago: Model of Human Occupation Clearinghouse, Department of Occupational Therapy, College of Applied Health Sciences, University of Illinois at Chicago.

DiBona, L. (2000). What are the benefits of leisure? An exploration using the leisure satisfaction scale. *British Journal of Occupational Therapy, 63*(2), 50–58.

Emerson, H., Cook, J., Polatajko, H., & Segal, R. (1998). Enjoyment experiences as described by persons with schizophrenia: A qualitative study. *Canadian Journal of Occupational Therapy, 65*(4), 183–192.

Fazio, L. S. (2001). *Developing Occupation-Centered Programs for the Community: A Workbook for Students and Professionals.* Upper Saddle River, NJ: Prentice Hall.

Florey, L. L., & Greene, S. (1997). Play in middle childhood: A focus on children with behavior and emotional disorders. In L. D. Parham & L. S. Fazio (Eds.), *Play in Occupational Therapy for Children* (pp 126–143). St Louis, MO: Mosby.

Gunter, B. G. (1987). The leisure experience: Selected properties. *Journal of Leisure Research, 19,* 115–130.

Havitz, M. E., & Dimanche, F. (1997). Leisure involvement revisited: Conceptual conundrums and measurement advances. *Journal of Leisure Research, 29*(3), 245–278.

Havitz, M. E., & Mannell, R. C. (2005). Enduring involvement, situational involvement, and flow in leisure and non-leisure activities. *Journal of Leisure Research, 37*(2), 152–177.

Heasman, D., & Atwal, A. (2004). The active advice pilot project: Leisure enhancement and social inclusion for people with severe mental health problems. *British Journal of Occupational Therapy, 67*(11), 511–514.

Henry, A. D. (1998). Development of a measure of adolescent leisure interests. *American Journal of Occupational Therapy, 52*(7), 531–539.

———. (2000). *The Pediatric Interest Profiles: Surveys of Play for Children and Adolescents.* San Antonio, TX: Therapy Skill Builders.

Hodgsen, S., Lloyd, C., & Schmid, T. (2001). The leisure participation of clients with a dual diagnosis. *British Journal of Occupational Therapy, 64*(10), 487–492.

Howells, V., & Zelnik, T. (2005). [*The Effectiveness of a Community Arts Studio: Assessing Change in the Lives of Participants with and without Mental Illness.*] Unpublished raw data.

Hull, R. B., Michael, S. E., Walker, G. J., & Roggenbuck, J.W. (1996). Ebb and flow of brief leisure experiences. *Leisure Sciences, 18,* 299–314.

Iso-Ahola, S. E., Jackson, E., & Dunn, E. (1994). Starting, ceasing, and replacing leisure activities over the life-span. *Journal of Leisure Research, 26*(3), 227–240.

Iso-Ahola, S. E., & Park, C. J. (1996). Leisure-related social support and self-determination as buffers of stress-illness relationship. *Journal of Leisure Research, 28*(3), 169–187.

Kielhofner, G., Forsyth, K., Federico, J., Henry, A., Keponen, R, Oakley, F., & Pan, A. W. (2002). Self-report assessments. In G. Kielhofner (Ed.), *Model of Human Occupation* (3rd ed.) (pp. 213–236). Baltimore: Lippincott, Williams & Wilkins.

Kielhofner, G., & Neville, A. (1983). *The Modified Interest Checklist.* Chicago: Model of Human Occupation Clearinghouse, University of Illinois – Chicago.

Kleiber, D. A., Hutchinson, S. L., & Williams, R. (2002). Leisure as a resource in transcending negative life events: Self-protection, self-restoration, and personal transformation. *Leisure Sciences, 24,* 219–235.

Krupa, T., McLean, H., Eastabrook, S., Bonham, A., & Baksh, L. (2003). Daily time use as a measure of community adjustment for persons served by assertive community treatment teams. *American Journal of Occupational Therapy, 57*(5), 558–565.

Laliberte-Rudman, D., Yu, B., Scott, E., & Pajouhandeh, P. (1999). Exploration of the perspectives of persons with schizophrenia regarding quality of life. *American Journal of Occupational Therapy, 54*(2), 137–147.

Lee, Y., Datillo, J., & Howard, D. (1994). The complex and dynamic nature of leisure experience. *Journal of Leisure Research, 26*(3), 195–211.

Link, B. G., & Phelan, J. C. (2001). Conceptualizing stigma. *Annual Review Sociology, 27,* 363–385.

Lloyd, C., King, R., Lampe, J., & McDougall, S. (2001). The leisure satisfaction of people with psychiatric disabilities. *Psychiatric Rehabilitation Journal, 25*(2), 107–113.

Lobo, F. (1998). Social transformation and the changing work–leisure relationship in the late 1990s. *Journal of Occupational Science, 5*(3), 147–154.

Mannell, R. C., Zuzanek, J., & Larson, R. (1988). Leisure states and "flow" experiences: Testing perceived freedom and intrinsic motivation hypothesis. *Journal of Leisure Research, 20,* 289–304.

Marrone, J., & Golowka, E. (1999). If work makes people with mental illness sick, what do unemployment, poverty, and social isolation cause? *Psychiatric Rehabilitation Journal, 23*(2), 187–193.

Matsutsuyu, J. (1969). The interest check list. *American Journal of Occupational Therapy, 23,* 323–328.

McCormack, B. P, Funderburk, J. A., Lee, Y., & Hale-Fought, M. (2005). Activity characteristics and emotional experience: Predicting boredom and anxiety in the daily life of community mental health clients. *Journal of Leisure Research, 37*(2), 236–253.

Meyer, A. (1977). The philosophy of occupational therapy. *American Journal of Occupational Therapy, 31*(10), 639–644.

Nagle, S., Cook, J. V., & Polatajko, H. J. (2002). I'm doing as much as I can: Occupational choices of persons with a severe and persistent mental illness. *Journal of Occupational Science, 9*(2), 72–81.

Nilsson, I., & Fisher, A. G. (2006). Evaluating leisure activities in the oldest old. *Scandinavian Journal of Occupational Therapy, 13,* 31–37.

Parham, L. D., & Fazio, L. S. (Eds.). (1997). *Play in Occupational Therapy for Children.* St Louis, MO: Mosby.

Passmore, A. (2003). The occupation of leisure: Three typologies and their influence on mental health in adolescence. *OTJR: Occupation, Participation and Health, 23*(2), 76–83.

Passmore, A., & French, D. (2003). The nature of leisure in adolescence: A focus group study. *British Journal of Occupational Therapy, 66*(9), 419–426.

Pieris, Y., & Craik, C. (2004). Factors enabling and hindering participation in leisure for people with mental health problems. *British Journal of Occupational Therapy, 67*(6), 240–247.

Primeau, L. A. (1996) Work and leisure: Transcending the dichotomy. *American Journal of Occupational Therapy, 50*(7), 569–577.

Ragheb, M. G. (1996). The search for meaning in leisure pursuits: Review, conceptualization and a need for a psychometric development. *Leisure Studies, 15,* 245–258.

Rebeiro, K. L., & Cook, J. V. (1999). Opportunity, not prescription: An exploratory study of the experience of occupational engagement. *Canadian Journal of Occupational Therapy, 66*(4), 176–187.

Reid, D. G. (1995). *Work and Leisure in the 21st Century: From Production to Citizenship.* Toronto: Wall & Emerson.

Reilly, M. (1974). *Play as Exploratory Learning.* Beverly Hills, CA: Sage Publications.

Rogers, J., Weinstein, J., & Figone, J. (1978). The interest checklist: An empirical assessment. *American Journal of Occupational Therapy, 32,* 628–630.

Samdahl, D. M., & Kleiber, D. A. (1989). Self-awareness and leisure experience. *Leisure Sciences, 11,* 1–10.

Shimitras, L., Fossey, E., & Harvey, C. (2003). Time use of people living with schizophrenia in a north London catchment area. *British Journal of Occupational Therapy, 66*(2), 46–54.

Smith, N. R., Kielhofner, G., & Watts, J. (1986). The relationship between volition, activity pattern, and life satisfaction in the elderly. *American Journal of Occupational Therapy, 40,* 278–283.

Soederback, I., & Hammarlund, C. (1993). A leisure-time frame of reference based on literature analysis. *Occupational Therapy in Health Care, 8*(4), 105–133.

Stayner, D. A., Davidson, L., & Tebes, J. K. (1996). Supported partnerships: A pathway into community life for persons with serious psychiatric disabilities. *Community Psychologist, 29*(3), 14–17.

Suto, M. (1998). Leisure in occupational therapy. *Canadian Journal of Occupational Therapy, 65*(5), 271–278.

Suto, M., & Frank, G. (1994). Future time perspective and daily occupations of persons with chronic schizophrenia in a board and care home. *American Journal of Occupational Therapy, 48,* 7–18.

Tinsley, H. E. A., Hinson, J. A., Tinsley, D. J., & Holt, M. S. (1993). Attributes of leisure and work experiences. *Journal of Counseling Psychology, 40,* 447–455.

Trottier, A. N., Brown, G. T., Hobson, S. J. G., & Miller, W. (2002). Reliability and validity of the Leisure Satisfaction Scale (LSS short form) and the Adolescent Leisure Interest Profile (ALIP). *Occupational Therapy International, 9*(2), 131–144.

Turner, H., Chapman, S., McSherry, A., Krishnagiri, S., & Watts, J. (2000). Leisure assessment in occupational therapy: An exploratory study. *Occupational Therapy in Health Care, 12*(2/3), 73–85.

Whiteford, G. (2004). When people cannot participate: Occupational deprivation. In C. H. Christiansen & E. A. Townsend (Eds.), *Introduction to Occupation* (pp. 221–242). Upper Saddle River, NJ: Prentice Hall.

Wilcock, A. A. (2006). *An Occupational Perspective of Health* (2nd ed.). Thorofare, NJ: Slack.

Zelnik, T., & Howells, V. (2006). "The Impact of an Integrated Community Arts Studio on Stigmatizing Beliefs and Experiences." Paper presented at the annual meeting of the American Psychiatric Association, Toronto.

———. (2007). Mood disorders. In B. J. Atchison & D. K. Dirette (Eds.), *Conditions in Occupational Therapy* (pp. 91–112). Baltimore: Lippincott, Williams & Wilkins.

Rest and Sleep

Doris Pierce and Karen Summers

> "The whole of human organization has its shape in a kind of rhythm. It is not enough that our hearts should beat in a useful rhythm, always kept up to a standard at which it can meet rest as well as wholesome strain without upset. There are many other rhythms which we must be attuned to: the larger rhythms of night and day, of sleep and waking hours, of hunger and its gratification, and finally the big four—work and play and rest and sleep.
>
> —Adolf Meyer, 1922/1977

Introduction

Sleep is the occupation that takes up approximately one-third of our lives. It is the occupation without which we would soonest die. Sleep is also the foundation of all our waking occupations. The quality of our sleep impacts the quality of everything we do each day. Although sleep was once regarded as a form of unconsciousness, it is now described as an active state, with structured neurological phases, and important for renewing our mental and physical health each day (American Academy of Sleep Medicine, 2004). Disruptions to sleep are the focus of sleep medicine and negatively affect health, immunity, cognition, mood, development, and life quality. Yet, because our culture strongly values productivity, life-threatening sleep problems are routinely ignored (Walsh, Dement, & Dinges, 2005). As the father of sleep medicine, William C. Dement, said, "We live in a sleep-sick society" (Dement & Vaughan, 1999).

Of course, paralleling the larger culture, some occupational therapists may question whether sleep really is an occupation. According to Pierce (2001), "An occupation is a specific individual's personally constructed, non-repeatable experience . . . a subjective event in perceived temporal, spatial and socio-cultural conditions that are unique to that one-time occurrence (p. 139)." Sleep meets these criteria. It is personally constructed and nonrepeatable: only you can know your sleep experience last night, each of your nights is different, and their meaning is best known by you. Its temporal conditions include a beginning, a duration, phases, and an ending. It occurs in a specific physical space with associated objects. It may occur within a shared or solitary experience, but it certainly has social and culture meaning to you. Sleep is definitely an occupation.

Sleep disorders are disruptions to the largest and most health-impacting occupational pattern in human life. Understanding the occupation of sleep and the manifestations of its disorders offers occupational therapy an opportunity to help our current clients as well as to strategically contribute our expertise on occupations to the young specialty of sleep medicine. Many occupational therapy clients with

specific diseases or lifestyles are at risk for sleep disorders that threaten their health and life quality. Sleep issues may also underlie the disruptions of important occupational patterns treated by occupational therapists, such as learning in classroom settings or safely completing industrial work tasks.

This chapter provides an overview of sleep: its basic neurophysiology, contextual features, and life-span variations. Sleep debt, disorders, and populations especially at risk for sleep problems, as well as the sleep interventions currently available through sleep medicine clinics, are described here. Most important, we describe how and why the occupation of sleep offers an exciting new area of practice for occupational therapists, whereby they can contribute to the field by adding interventions with our current clients and in providing new opportunities for our profession to serve the occupational needs of our "sleep-sick society" in partnership with sleep medicine.

The Physiology of Sleep

Sleep is a biological process that is highly influenced by our behavior and interactions with the social and physical environment.

Circadian Rhythms

Sleep is an occupation that occurs on a daily basis and in a predictable way, nested within the **circadian rhythm**. The circadian rhythm is the physiological 24-hour time pattern of human life (Czeisler, Buxton, Khalsa, 2005; Scheer, Cajochen, Turek, & Czeisler, 2005; Turek, Dugovic, & Laposky, 2005; Van Dongen & Dinges, 2005). It includes usual periods of being alert and awake, an energy dip, and sleep. The average adult who works during the day experiences highest energy in the morning, an energy dip in the early afternoon, a revival of energy for the rest of the day, and then sleeps through the night. The pattern of the circadian rhythm is set in childhood within the family pattern of a usual awakening and sleep time. Older people in Western culture tend to get up and go to bed earlier than do younger adults, perhaps due to lifestyle changes since they acquired their circadian patterns in childhood.

The circadian rhythm is the physiological, temporal structure around which everyday routines are built. Because we anticipate waking, sleeping, and different levels of energy at different times of the day, we develop patterns of typical activities in which we engage at certain times of the day: morning self-care and grooming routines upon waking, meals evenly spaced over the day and evening, high-energy tasks such as work or school in the morning and afternoon, more leisurely and restorative activities in the later afternoons and evenings, end of day self-care and transition to sleep, and sleep through the night.

Persons who have atypical circadian rhythms are more vulnerable to disrupted routines as well as poor quality sleep. Some of the many people susceptible to desynchronized circadian rhythms and disorganized daily routines include shift workers, new mothers, people with chronic or acute illnesses including mental illness, and persons who are blind or have head injuries. Because many of our occupational therapy clients experience threats to their sleep quality and circadian rhythms, it is important for occupational therapists to understand sleep and circadian rhythms in order to recognize challenges to their clients' routines and health.

Zeitgebers

The word **zeitgeber** is German for time giver. A zeitgeber is a cue in nature that keeps the human body well organized with a recurring and physiologically varying 24-hour cycle. Zeitgebers entrain the body to nature's rhythms, telling it when to sleep, wake, be highly active, or relax. Zeitgebers also shape physiological cycles of hunger, thirst, and elimination. These physiological rhythms are the template within which most humans enact their everyday routines and activities of getting up and dressed, eating, working most of the day, a midday break to eat, slightly lowered energy in the afternoon, a meal again in the evening, and less energetic activities prior to bedtime. Of course, not everyone's day fits perfectly into the pattern provided the body by the zeitgeber's of nature. Some individuals—night-shift workers, for example—create daily patterns that are contradictory to the cues of nature. This leads to health and sleep challenges.

The most powerful zeitgeber that nature provides is light. Sunrise and sunset set our body clocks. Not only the light but the length of the day affects us, as do the variation of temperature between day and night. Before electricity was discovered, all humans actively coordinated their activities to the daylight because those were usually the best hours for outside work, travel, or any activities that required good light. Eating and levels of activity that occurred on a daily basis further reinforced a stable body rhythm entrained to nature. Now, because of the availability of electric light, it is possible to go through life with only minimal awareness of and synchronization with such cues. This "unnatural" pattern confuses the body and can cause desynchronization and health problems.

Sleep Neurotransmitters

Zeitgebers cue the body clock through the actions of a series of neurotransmitters throughout the nervous system. Decreases in light are perceived through histamine receptors in the eyes and communicated through the optic nerves to the suprachiasmatic nuclei (SCN). The SCN are located just above the intersection of the optic nerves. The SCN communicate to the pineal gland to either secrete or cease secreting melatonin. Melatonin is commonly known as the sleep hormone (Scheer et al, 2005; Van Dongen & Dinges, 2005). It is manufactured by the body from the protein tryptophan. Tryptophan is found in turkey, among other foods, and has been credited for many Thanksgiving after-dinner naps. Melatonin can also be purchased in vitamin and health food stores as a sleep aid. Melatonin triggers the hypothalamus to slow body activities and brain functions, begin lowering body temperature, and initiate sleep. In the morning, the eyes sense the increasing light of dawn and sunrise even through closed lids, the histamine receptors communicate this to the SCN, and the body begins to stir and wake for the day's activities.

The Role of Sleep in Health and Growth

Sleep is the activity that uses the largest portion of our lives—approximately one third. Without sufficient sleep, our health gradually declines. The impacts of inadequate sleep on health in today's society are so common and so misunderstood in Western culture that we accept them as usual variations in our health. For example, students and professors often get sick right during and after exam week. This pattern is due to increasing sleep debt over the semester. Since the immune system reconstitutes the body's supply of interleukins during deep sleep, failure to get enough deep sleep for extended periods results in a compromised immune system. Without immune sufficiency, everyday viruses and infections against which we are usually defended result in very real illnesses. Although we may try to figure out who is to blame for "giving" us a cold or the flu, it may be that we caused our own illness by degrading our immune system defenses through poor rest (Krueger & Majde, 2005; Siegel, 2005). Sleep deprivation has been used as an effective form of torture throughout history and across cultures. Beyond the illnesses that result from sleep debt's effect on our immune systems, extended sleep deprivation will cause a loss of thermoregulation, or cooling, of the body that will lead to death, usually within a couple of weeks of complete lack of sleep (Coren, 1996).

Sleep also plays an important role in recovery from illness. That is why, if you imagine a person who is ill, you envision him or her in bed and drowsy. The body defends itself by increasing temperature to fever levels in order to create a more hostile environment for pathogens. It also forces the individual into extended deep sleep in order to pump out emergency supplies of immune defenses.

Sleep and Cognition

It is common knowledge that a good night's sleep is the best preparation for any important cognitive challenge, such as taking a test. Studies have shown that decreased sleep results in slower reaction times, lowered performance on intelligence tests, irritability, and poorer problem-solving (Curcio, Ferrara, & DeGennaro, 2006; Haimov, Hanuka, & Horowitz, 2008). Mood is related to sleep. Learning is affected by sleep. This is especially a concern in children, who are often in sleep debt as they try to match schedules with busy two-career parents, staying awake into the evening for important family time. The next day at school, the child is fidgety and tired, trying hard to stay focused through a grueling day of school.

Napping

Naps are those brief sleep periods that typically occur in the afternoon within the physiological dip in energy that is a natural part of the everyday circadian rhythm (Bliwise, 2005). Having an afternoon nap is a healthy way to regain energy for the rest of the day and maintain health. Many cultures highly value the nap. In Europe and South America, it is called a siesta. In China, it is called the *hsiuhsi*. In the past, during this afternoon time, much business would stop as everyone caught a short, restorative nap. In the modern economies of today, however, this nap break is not as popular as it was in the past.

Unfortunately, in the United States and other Western countries, the nap is not respected. In a culture where productivity is valued above all else, "time is money" and time spent napping is lost productivity. Ironically, the cost to national economies of the lowered productivity of tired workers who are not allowed to break for a nap is so great that it is probably immeasurable (Bolge, Doan, Kannan, & Baran, 2009). Tiredness can also result in deaths, accidents, and mistakes that entail far more serious costs to us than just lowered productivity. A well-timed nap could prevent many of these unfortunate results of our culture's unhealthy attitude toward the human need for sleep. Many great men of history are well known for their tendency to nap: Thomas Alva Edison, Henry Ford, and Albert Einstein (Anthony, 1997). It is time we learned from their examples the power of the nap for keeping the mind sharp and creative!

Sleep Architecture, Types, and Phases

Sleep occurs in a pattern that is phased and rhythmic. This pattern is often called **sleep architecture**, so named because a hypnogram produced by a sleep lab looks like a city skyline (Bliwise, 2005; Thomas & Chokroverty, 2005). During sleep, brain activity can be tracked by electroencephalograph, or EEG. Typically, a hypnogram shows the brain waves during a full night's sleep. The brain activity changes from one type to another as the sleep type changes.

The Stages of NREM Sleep

Non–rapid eye movement, or NREM, sleep is the largest portion of adult human sleep and has four phases. During NREM sleep, the body is fully active. You can turn and adjust your body and covers for comfort without fully waking. The four stages of NREM sleep are like a ladder descending from very light sleep to deepest dreamless sleep. Healthy sleep begins with Stage 1, when you begin to doze off, yet you would notice if something happened in the room.

Stage 2 is a transitional stage, where brain waves are slowing and the body is moving toward deep sleep. Stages 3 and 4 are the deep sleep phases in which the body gets its best rest and the immune system produces its protective metabolic components. On EEG, deep sleep shows slow synchronous waves.

REM Sleep

REM, or rapid eye movement, sleep displays high brain activity levels (Krueger & Majde, 2005, Siegel, 2005). REM is known as paradoxical sleep because its neurophysiological readings look more like a waking state than like deep sleep. REM occurs five or six times during the night and accounts for 30% of sleep in a healthy adult. Dreams occur during REM. There are many theories regarding why humans dream, but the consensus at this point is that dreams help the brain to purge, reconstitute, and reorganize (Cartwright, 2005; Domhoff, 2005; Pace-Schott, 2005; Stickgold, 2005). REM sleep is also different in other ways. Memory becomes inactive during REM, and there is no body movement below the neck. The cessation of body temperature regulation also makes REM sleep susceptible to disruption in too cold or too warm sleep environments. You will pop out of REM if you get too cold or too warm, but when you adjust your covers and fall back to sleep, you enter the phases of NREM sleep. Repeatedly sleeping in spaces that are not at a comfortable temperature produces REM deprivation, resulting in cognitive and mood impairments, even if the recommended hours of sleep per night are being maintained.

Typical Sleep Patterns

For healthy adults, the typical sleep pattern includes several cycles that begin with stage 1 NREM sleep, progress to stage 4, and then move into nREM sleep. These NREM–REM cycles are shorter in the beginning of the night and longer at the end but are about 90 minutes in length. You may awaken for brief periods between cycles, look around, and doze off again. Generally, in the earlier part of the night, the portion of REM sleep is less than a third of the cycle, and toward the end of the night, the portion of REM sleep is more than a third. Therefore, the deepest and best quality of REM sleep occurs for most of us around 6:00 am.

Interruptions to these typical sleep cycles are at the root of most sleep problems. When sleep is disrupted, whether by environmental or physiological causes, the brain returns to the beginning of the cycle. For example, persons with severe sleep apnea, who wake repeatedly throughout the night due to breathing difficulties, have fragmented sleep that includes lots of stage 1 and 2 NREM light sleep, little stage 3 and 4 sleep, and almost no REM sleep at all.

The Context of Sleep

The degree to which sleep is grounded in physiological mechanisms has resulted in a largely decontextualized view of this occupation. Yet all occupations have context, just as all blankets have texture. Looking closely at sleep uncovers interesting aspects of its social, spatial, and temporal contexts. Occupational therapists well understand such subtleties because they must work to assist their clients within the contextual features of their everyday lives.

The Social Context of Sleep

The social context of sleep seems, at first glance, nonexistent. Are we not alone in peaceful sleep, unaware of our surroundings? Actually, many are not. A recent study of bed sharing in couples describes their development of bed-sharing skills, negotiation of a shared bed routine, important activities that occur in bed before sleep, valuing of shared sleep, and impacts of illness and sleep disorders on both persons in a bed-sharing couple (Rosenblatt, 2006). Bed partners of persons with sleep apnea, restless legs syndrome, and snoring suffer a level of sleep debt that nearly matches that of the person with the symptoms. This study describes an occupational pattern of Western culture that is large and obvious once we turn our attention to it, yet it has remained unnoticed in research. Similarly, the social context of children's sleep has remained mostly out of awareness. Although not as well accepted in Western cultures, newborns, nursing infants, and toddlers often sleep with their parents. Children who are ill, disabled, anxious, or toilet-training are constantly in interaction with their parents during the night. Some people even sleep with their pets.

The Temporal Context of Sleep

The temporal context of sleep is shaped by its physiological timing within the 24-hour cycle. Personal and family routines for sleep support the maintenance of this daily rhythm. Mothers make efforts to develop sleep routines in their children (Pierce, 2001). Adults with sleep disorders usually have poor sleep routines and have difficulty supporting a regular sleep rhythm. Without synchrony with the temporal patterns of environmental zeitgebers, sleep will be disordered. Persons who work evening and night shifts require especially strong and regular sleep routines to support the adequacy of their sleep. **Sleep hygiene** is the use of effective lifestyle choices to support good sleep, such as monitoring caffeine, nicotine, and alcohol intake; not exercising too close to bedtime; keeping a regular sleep schedule; using a bedtime routine; and maintaining an effective sleep environment.

The Spatial Context of Sleep

The spatial context of sleep may be the most concrete. Since the invention of the electric light, humans sleep an average of two hours less each night than previously (Coren, 1996). Dement and Vaughan (1999) call our modern world an "electric cave," referring to famous experiments in which sleep–wake cycles were studied in persons living for 32 days in Mammoth Cave (Kentucky) without zeitgebers to keep them to a 24-hour rhythm. The characteristics of the sleep space that are critical to the quality of sleep include light, temperature, sound, and air quality (Hirshkowitz & Smith, 2004). If your bedroom is too light, too noisy, too warm, too cold, or too dry, your sleep will be disrupted. For persons with allergies or asthma, it is important that the sleep space be as allergen-free as possible. Also, the sleep furnishings contribute to sleep: the bed, the pillows, and the bedding. Sleepwear must be comfortable. For persons with sleep disorders, such as apnea, the bedroom may include special equipment, such as a continuous positive airway pressure machine and mask to support adequate oxygenation during sleep. It is also important to keep the bedroom peaceful and uncluttered.

Sleep Across the Lifespan

Just as the body changes with age, so does sleep. The amount of sleep time and the amount of time spent in different sleep stages also changes throughout the life span. As shown in Table 53-1, people require the highest amount of sleep at birth, and then the amount of sleep diminishes until they reach adulthood (Carskadon & Dement, 2005). The guidelines in Table 53-1 are a recommendation only. Some individuals need more sleep than is suggested to function at their best. However, some individuals may still function with less than the recommended dozing time.

Infancy and Childhood Sleep

Newborns tend to sleep 16 to 18 hours a day. Fifty percent of their sleep is REM, which is the largest percentage of REM sleep humans experience throughout their lifetime. Newborns have the shortest healthy sleep cycles in humans, lasting about 55 minutes. Newborns spend a lot of their day asleep but wake frequently even at night. Melatonin, a neurotransmitter that gives the body the message to sleep, has to be synchronized in newborns. The infant begins to stabilize its hormone level during his or her first 3 months. Thereafter, a more stable sleep pattern may emerge (Dileo, Reiter, & Taliaferro, 2002).

As the child grows, the total amount of sleep decreases. At 3 to 5 years old, 11 to 13 hours of sleep are needed in each 24-hour cycle. The naps have shortened in length and usually occur only once instead of twice a day. The amount of sleep spent in REM decreases, and the length of the sleep cycle increases.

Sleep is important to human functioning across the life span. However, sleep plays an important role in children. This is when the body grows and the brain develops. Lack of sleep can impair the child's ability to develop (Tikotzky et al, 2010). Sleep also plays a role in the child's health. The body's immune system works to fight off disease while the child is asleep (World Health Organization, 2004). For a child who has special needs or a chronic illness, sleep is even more crucial.

Table 53-1 ● **Sleep Requirements Over the Life Span**

Age	Hours Suggested	Source
1–2 months	10.5–18	Sleep foundation.org
3–11 months	9–12	Sleep foundation.org
1–3 years	12–14	Sleep foundation.org
3–5 years	11–13	Sleep foundation.org
5–12	10–11	Sleep foundation.org
Teenagers	8.5–9	Kidshealth.org
Adults	8–8.5	National Heart, Lung and Blood Institute

Despite the importance of sleep in childhood, many children do not get the amount of sleep that is suggested for them. Lack of sleep can be attributed to the overscheduling of today's child and the 24-hour world we live in today. As a result, the child will have sleep debt and have difficulty functioning appropriately. Frequently, instead of appearing drowsy, the child may demonstrate the opposite behavior of "hyperness": they move and fidget to stay awake, which can be problematic especially in school when they need to attend to a task. Other symptoms of sleep deprivation in children are emotional lability, impulsiveness, aggression, and trouble awakening. No one wants to see these behaviors in children. However, few parents or educators realize that if the child would get the appropriate amount of sleep, his or her functioning and behavior would improve. In addition, children who have sleep disturbances are at more risk to develop mental illness later in life.

Teen Sleep

As the child becomes a teenager, the amount of sleep continues to decrease and melatonin levels begin to fall. Ironically, despite the need for less sleep as they grow older, this population is chronically sleep deprived (Curcio et al, 2006). Teenagers have busy schedules, including academics, extracurricular activities, recreation, and jobs. In addition, teenagers typically prefer to stay up late and sleep later in the morning. This pattern does not match well with school hours and contributes to their sleep debt. However, some school systems are beginning to recognize that teenagers are often not good learners in early mornings and are starting the high school day later.

While changes in sleep patterns do typically occur in teenagers, it is important that caregivers note any abrupt changes in sleep patterns or suddenly increased sleep debt. This can be a sign of depression and increased risk of suicide. Sleep causes impulsivity, impairs judgment, and can lead to exacerbation of a preexisting psychopathology (Carskadon, 2002; Xianchen, 2006).

Adult Sleep

Adults should be getting an average of at least 8 hours of sleep a night. With very busy schedules, however, most adults do not reach this threshold. Adult sleep is also impacted by those with whom we share a bed (Rosenblatt, 2006). A partner who snores can significantly reduce the sleep quality of his or her partner. Also, partners have to compromise on the temperature of the room, type of mattress, and covers. Children, pets, and caregiving for aging parents can also disrupt sleep.

Sleep in the Elderly

When an adult reaches the senior years, sleep patterns continue to change. There is more light stage 1 sleep and less deep stage 4 sleep (Bliwise, 1997, 2005; Collier & Skitt, 2003). As a result, elders are often too easily aroused from sleep. This profound effect is exacerbated by the elderly typically having more pathophysiologic conditions that further compound their sleep issues. These conditions include periodic leg movements, nocturia, diabetes, cardiovascular disease, gastrointestinal issues, chronic pain, nocturnal cough, and disordered breathing. In addition, Alzheimer's disease and Parkinson's disease occur more frequently in the older population and are both linked to sleep disturbances. Thus, it is no surprise that maintaining healthy sleep through the night, a form of insomnia, is prevalent in the elderly.

Changes in occupational routine and life conditions can also impact the sleep routine of older people. For example, senior citizens can have depression and anxiety secondary to retirement, death of a spouse, relocation, and financial stress that can impair their sleep. In long-term care environments, sleep can be impaired by nighttime noise from other residents and staff. Despite the many challenges to sleep in the elderly, their sleep issues commonly go undiagnosed.

Sleep Debt

Because sleep is undervalued in Western cultures, **sleep debt** is common. Sleep debt is a physical condition of tiredness due to inadequate sleep. The easy acceptance of the need for people to have their morning caffeine before they should even be required to communicate is indicative of the degree to which many of us consider sleep debt to be a normal state. Many people live such tired lives that they do not even know they are in sleep debt. Yet sleep debt can impair health, mood, endurance, coordination, reaction times, cognition, and memory (Dinges, Rogers, & Baynard, 2005). Extreme sleep debt will result in lack of coordination, depression, disorganized thinking, and hallucinations. Sleep debt can cause deadly accidents. Though sleep debt may be tolerable in a grumpy fellow office worker, it does not seem as acceptable in the driver of the tractor-trailer barreling toward us, in our emergency room physician, or in the pilot of our next cross-country flight.

Even an hour of lost sleep can make a tremendous difference in our reaction times and safety. In a large study of 2 years of traffic fatalities and accidents in Canada, the week following the spring change to daylight savings (in which 1 hour of sleep is lost by everyone), traffic accidents increased by 7% (Coren, 1996). In the fall of the same year, when clocks were set back (1 hour of extra sleep for all), accidents were reduced by 7%.

A lack of REM sleep can occur despite an appropriate number of hours of sleep because repeated disruptions of the sleep cycle cause the cycle restart in light sleep, so the person rarely reaches the REM phase that follows deep sleep. REM sleep can be disrupted by sleep apnea, some antidepressants and monoamine oxidase inhibitors, or by sleeping in noisy or lighted environments. A symptom of REM sleep debt is hypnic myoclonia, a sudden muscle movement and visual image as you fall asleep. Sometimes hypnic myoclonia feels like you are falling and wakes you up. It results from entering directly into REM sleep rather than reaching REM though the other phases and is caused by REM sleep debt. Extreme REM sleep debt will cause "waking dreams," or hypnagogic hallucinations.

Sleep debt is an increasing problem in children. With more women in the workforce, children often stretch the length of their waking day into the evening in order to get the amount of time with their parents that they need

(Komada et al, 2009). By the time the whole family arrives home and gets dinner ready, it is already late. Instead of being in bed by eight o'clock, a preschooler or school-aged child may stay up until nine or ten at night. Sleep debt affects children's coordination, mood, and ability to resist illnesses, just as it does in adults. It looks different in children, however. Instead of appearing more slow-moving than usual or compensating for their tiredness with careful doses of caffeine, children get even more energetic when sleep deprived. So, although that child in the classroom who is disruptive and overly active may be suffering from attention deficits, those deficits are not necessarily caused by an attention disorder (Chervin, 2005a). Sleep debt causes very similar symptoms in children.

Sleep Disorders

While most people have experienced sleep disturbances for a night or two at some point in their lives, a more serious sleep disorder may exist if this pattern persists over a period of time. In order to confirm the condition, a physician must make the diagnosis. The American Academy of Sleep Medicine developed the *International Classification of Sleep Disorders, Version 2* (ICSD-2) in 2004 to assist physicians in diagnosing sleep disturbances (Kryger, 2005; Thorpy, 2005). The disorders are divided into eight categories with different types of sleep disorders contained within the categories:

1. The insomnias (primary, secondary)
2. The sleep-related breathing disorders (central and obstructive sleep apnea)
3. The hypersomnias (not caused by a breathing disorder)
4. The circadian rhythm sleep disorders
5. The parasomnias
6. The sleep-related movement disorders
7. Isolated symptoms, apparently normal variants and resolved issues
8. Other sleep disorders

Insomnias

Insomnia is a major category of sleep disorders (Buysee, 2005). It is the most common sleep disorder, occurring in 10% to 50% of the population (Jindal, Buysee, & Thase, 2004). Insomnia occurs when an individual has difficulty initiating sleep, maintaining sleep, getting enough sleep, or has impaired sleep quality. Depending on the type of symptoms, different types of insomnia may be diagnosed. In addition to having difficulty sleeping at night, individuals frequently have symptoms during the day such as drowsiness. As a result, the individual's ability to perform waking occupations is impaired. When working with a client who has insomnia, it is important to understand the type they are experiencing. For example, does the individual wake up in the night several times to urinate and then go back to sleep? Or is he or she unable to fall back to sleep? In order to help clients with sleep disorders, the occupational therapist must understand the pattern of their sleep.

While sleep disturbances such as insomnia are frequently listed as symptoms of mental illnesses and treated as a secondary condition, a trend in the literature is beginning to question which comes first. Some authors suggest that the insomnia may precede a mental illness instead of resulting from it (Collier & Skitt, 2003; Ford & Kamerow, 1989; Gupta, 2006; Weissman et al, 1997). In other words, the disruption of sleep may be causing the disorder. This "the chicken or the egg" debate will continue. No matter how this question is resolved, the fact remains that sleep is important to wellbeing, and poor sleep will result in poor health and impaired function. The irony may be that an occupation, sleep, rather than a medical condition, may be impairing the ability to perform all other waking occupations. In fact, directly improving the occupation of sleep may be the most effective strategy to increasing the function of our clients.

Sleep-Related Breathing Disorders

Sleep-related breathing disorders include diagnoses in which respiration is impaired while sleeping. For example, sleep apnea is classified as a sleep-related breathing disorder (Schwab, Kuna, & Remmers, 2005). Central sleep apnea results from central nervous system dysfunction impairing breathing. Obstructive sleep apnea in adults is characterized by frequent breathing stops (apneas) due to an obstruction in the breathing passages. Excessive weight, allergies, and any conditions affecting airway size can also contribute to apnea. Individuals frequently present with snoring with this condition. Apneas cause frequent brief awakenings during the night and reduction in the amount of REM sleep. In addition to impairing the individual's sleep, these conditions can impair the ability of their bed partner's ability to maintain peaceful sleep. These conditions must be diagnosed through a sleep study and are treatable through the use of a breathing machine, surgery, weight loss, and improved sleep hygiene. It is interesting that in a culture that does not value sleep, we are experiencing an epidemic of obesity that may be tied to reduced amounts of sleep.

Hypersomnias Not Due to a Breathing Disorder

Hypersomnias not due to a breathing disorder occur when an individual demonstrates excessive daytime sleepiness and difficulty staying awake during the day. As a result, the individual may fall asleep unintentionally and at inappropriate times, as in narcolepsy. In some individuals, however, hypersomnias may result in the opposite problem: hyperactivity. Such individuals need to keep moving in order to avoid falling asleep (Kryger, 2005). Narcolepsy is the most commonly known hypersomnia, but it can be hard to accurately diagnose. In some cases, narcolepsy has been misdiagnosed as schizophrenia (Douglas, Hays, Pazderka, & Russell, 1991). Clearly, an understanding of sleep disorders is especially important for therapists working in mental health settings.

Circadian Rhythm Sleep Disorders

Circadian rhythm sleep disorders present as individual sleep patterns that are out of sync with society's expectations of the time for sleep. Delayed sleep phase is a type of circadian rhythm sleep disorder that happens when sleep occurs later than the desired society norms. In these cases,

The Lived Experience

Gregory

I've had sleep problems for at least 15 years. The first time I was really aware of it was when I had a kind of panic attack. I think I was actually near to death because when I woke up I was gasping for breath and I felt trapped. It was a real fight-or-flight response. I was worried about work, I needed to make some changes in my career, so I thought it was anxiety and I went to a psychiatrist. He never asked me about my sleep or even suggested a physical, and we did talking therapy. He gave me Xanax. And with Xanax, you can sleep no matter what.

After that, Doris was so concerned about my snoring and my stopping breathing that I went to a head, neck, and throat surgeon and had an uvulectomy, some soft palate tissue removal, and removal of scar tissue and polyps from my nose from a lifetime of allergies. It took a couple of months for all that tissue to heal. After that I felt different, I could breathe through my nose. My wife says I was a much happier person after that, the dark rings under my eyes disappeared and I was not so grumpy, but I don't remember that.

Years later, I went for allergy testing. I found out I was allergic to every grass that grows, most trees, cats, dogs, corn, wheat, mushrooms, tomatoes, bananas, melons, and oranges. I started taking allergy medications, and later added allergy shots. I avoid the foods I am allergic to, but it's difficult. None of my allergists ever asked me how my breathing affected my sleep. Sleep was not a consideration. They did do an MRI and found that my nasal passages are distorted by years of swelling from hay fever, which I have had since childhood.

My wife kept saying to ask my doctor about a sleep study because she really thought I needed one. I stopped breathing at night and she knew that was wrong. Plus, it was hard for her to sleep with all my loud snoring and stopping breathing and kicking my legs to wake up and breath. I guess I didn't care if I died. I was asleep. You don't know you are stopping breathing when you are asleep. Sometimes, I was so loud, she was forced to sleep somewhere else.

After about two years of allergy treatment, I asked my general practitioner if she could recommend a sleep study doctor. I told her about my stopping breathing and how loud my wife said I snored. She just noted this in my chart. Doris kept insisting I needed a sleep study. It was a sore point for us. I really did not want to go through that horrible surgery again. The second time I asked my general practitioner for a referral, she sent me for a sleep study. I was concerned about the sleep study because at that point in time I was waking up to urinate every hour and I thought it would be difficult for them to come in and

unplug me so I could go to the bathroom. When I woke up, I had to go like right now. I got there at 9:30 at night. By 11:30, they had me all hooked up and I was ready to sleep. There were at least 30 electrodes on me. They were everywhere. They wired me up, I went to sleep for one hour, and then I woke up. At that time, the technician came in and I told her I had to go. She said, "I'm glad you are up because we want to try the continuous positive airway pressure (CPAP) machine because we can tell you are stopping breathing and we need to monitor you." They put a mask on me and I went back to sleep and I slept for four hours. That was the first time I had slept four hours without waking up since . . . well, since I can remember.

When I met with my sleep doctor, we went over the chart and he said I was "state fair material" because I stopped breathing 177 times within 2 hours. He said I had obstructive apnea and my oxygen level was in the extreme danger zone. The doctor says, to help with the apnea, "I want you to work on losing weight." My general practitioner said, "Try Weight Watchers." But, I'm an American male and I'll do it my own way. I will try to increase my physical activity and watch my portions.

The first thing I noticed when I started sleeping with the CPAP machine was I was sleeping for six hours without getting up to pee. Then my dreams started changing, they were not anxiety-based dreams. They were happy dreams, just dreams. I didn't wake up laughing, but I didn't wake up going, "Oh, shit!" any more. I wasn't remembering dreams before the CPAP machine. If I remembered anything it was because it was upsetting. Another thing I remember about sleeping for a block of hours was the depth of field of my vision changed. I have two sets of glasses, one for computer and one for driving, they are both for myopia. After sleeping a block of hours for several days, I could read the dashboard of my car in my driving glasses. I could switch back and forth, which I couldn't do before.

My mental acuity, I'm bouncing back. Instead of just being in survival mode, I'm more active in my self-directed endeavors at work. I can think of what I need to do and enjoy doing it, instead of just going through the motions and just being there. I play guitar, and I am able to analyze and recall melodies and chord structures much more clearly. My wife says I'm happier, I crack jokes, and "my dark cloud seems to be disappearing." She is so glad I don't fall asleep now when she is talking to me, or when we watch a movie. I feel fortunate that my wife insisted that I have a sleep study. If she had not insisted, I would not have done it. I would probably have heart and brain damage without medical intervention. It really was headed that way. And marriage damage.

---

the individual's body is not entrained to the rising and setting of the sun. Chrono-physiological changes are the underlying cause of circadian rhythm disorders (Monk, 2005). Night-shift workers are especially prone to circadian rhythm sleep disorders. Also, when a traveler moves across several time zones quickly, this same condition may occur for a short time and is officially termed "circadian rhythm sleep disorder not due to a substance or known physiological condition, jet lag" (Arendt, Stone, & Skene, 2005).

Parasomnias

The sixth type of sleep disorder is **parasomnia**. Parasomnias are actions that accompany sleep that are either experienced or physical in nature (Mahowald, 2005; Mahowald & Schenck, 2005). They are undesired, and the individual may be unaware of them. Examples of parasomnias include bruxism (teeth grinding), sleep terrors, and sleep walking. Because the individual is unaware of his or her actions, the results could be dangerous. For example, people with parasomnias may eat during their sleep and not remember it the next day or may leave their home in the middle of the night (Hirshkowitz & Smith, 2004).

Parasomnias can occur in adults as well as children. Sleep terrors, a form of parasomnia that usually occurs in children, is especially frightening because children have difficulty separating dreams from real life. This can be confusing for them and their caregivers. Another parasomnia that frequently occurs in children is sleep-related enuresis, or frequent urination during sleep (Sheldon, 2005).

Sleep-Related Movement Disorders

Sleep-related movement disorders occur when the body moves involuntarily during sleep (Bliwise, 2005). Restless leg syndrome (RLS) is a common example of this condition. The symptoms can include sensations of something crawling inside your legs or arms, restlessness, and daytime sleepiness, and RLS occurs more often in women than in men. (Hirshkowitz & Smith, 2004; Kantrowitz, 2006). Periodic leg movement disorder (PLMD) is another type of sleep-related movement disorder. This involuntary movement of the legs and sometimes arms usually occurs in a regular pattern of movements. Unlike RLS movements, which can occur while awake, the movements related to PLMD occur only during sleep.

Other Sleep Disorders

The last category, other sleep disorders, encompasses conditions that are hard to classify in the other categories. Environmental sleep disorder is one example. This condition occurs when a factor in the environment results in impaired sleep and insomnia. The factors could include noises, light, or temperatures that are too hot or too cold. As a result, the individual has difficulty sleeping. Noise is a frequent disturbance for individuals who live and sleep in a group setting, such as a long-term care facility or a dormitory (Thorpy, 2005).

Populations at Special Risk for Sleep Problems

While sleep disorders can take place in isolation, they frequently co-occur with another condition. Sleep disturbances commonly occur in conjunction with many diagnoses that occupational therapists regularly treat in their practice. Because the occupation of sleep plays a major role in supporting individuals' participation in their daily lives, sleep issues need to be addressed in occupational therapy. To better serve their clients, occupational therapists need to be aware of these comorbid conditions.

Psychiatric Disorders

Individuals with mental illness are at high risk for sleep disorders (Becker, 2006). Insomnia occurs in 50% of serious psychiatric disorders (Lichstein, Nau, McCrae, & Stone, 2005). Disturbed sleep is a recognized symptom of many types of mental illness, including depression and anxiety (American Psychiatric Association, 2000; Stein & Mellman,

2005). In fact, 40% to 50% of all individuals with chronic insomnia have anxiety or depressive disorders. Sleep disorders are definitely linked with mental illness. Depression can cause sleep disturbances, and sleep disturbances can be a precursor to depression and exacerbate symptoms. Clients with insomnia should be screened for mental illness, and conversely, individuals with depression should be screened for sleep issues. Since sleep disorders frequently are comorbid with mental illness, clients who are hospitalized in a psychiatric inpatient unit should have their sleep issues addressed (Collier, Skitt, & Cutts, 2003).

Different types of sleep disorders can be seen in different types of mental illness. For example, individuals who have trouble falling asleep may have depression, while those who wake early and cannot fall back to sleep may be showing a symptom of anxiety. Further complicating diagnoses of sleep disorders, sleep patterns may change. For example, an individual with bipolar disorder may be getting too little sleep in a manic phase and too much sleep during a depressive phase. Changes in sleep patterns may signal the oncoming of a new phase of the condition and be a key to treatment. Clients with bipolar disorder should learn to monitor their sleep patterns so that when they recognize a change in sleep patterns, they can seek assistance before their status changes (Benson & Zarcone, 2005).

Sleep is a state of calmness. As a result, sleep can be especially beneficial and restorative for a person with an anxiety disorder. It is important for individuals with anxiety disorders to have the appropriate amount of sleep along with good quality sleep as part of a healthy lifestyle. If the individual does not get enough restorative sleep, the lack of sleep can increase the arousal level of an already anxious person. The increased anxiety further inhibits sleep, leading to a self-perpetuating cycle of lack of sleep and anxiety (Stein & Mellman, 2005).

To be diagnosed with generalized anxiety disorder, the individual may present with sleep disturbances including initiating sleep, staying asleep, or unsatisfying sleep. In particular, individuals with posttraumatic stress disorder (PTSD) frequently have nightmares and insomnia. Although, they often have sleep disturbances, sleep issues are not their main complaint when they consult with a physician. Therefore, individuals with PTSD should be screened for sleep disorders. While individuals with obsessive disorder do not present with sleep disorders specifically, they may demonstrate obsessions around their sleep routines. For example, they may repeatedly check to see if their alarm clock is set for the morning. Anxiety disorders are frequently comorbid with other mental illness, which may lead to other sleep disturbances.

Also, sleep disturbances are noted as part of the diagnostic criteria for mood disorders. Individuals with depression report insomnia most frequently and have an increased incidence of sleep disturbances (Benca, 2005). According to Livingston, Blizard, and Mann (1993), impaired sleep increases the risk of depression in the elderly population. In addition to sleep patterns being disrupted due to depression, some of the medications used in the treatment of depression can cause sleep disturbances (Schweueitzer, 2005). Antidepressants, particularly serotonin reuptake inhibitors (SSRIs), can disturb the sleep pattern. Because individuals with depression frequently have sleep disturbances, the medication's effect on sleep may not always be evident. When individuals with Parkinson's disease present with symptoms of depression and anxiety, they often have sleep disturbances (Trenkwalder, 2005). With treatment to improve sleep, the individual's quality of life can improve. In individuals with Parkinson's disease, sleep should be assessed along with depression and anxiety symptoms (Borek, Kohn, &, Friedman, 2006).

Individuals with schizophrenia frequently deal with insomnia. Hofstetter, Lysaker, and Mayeda (2005) demonstrated that poor sleep quality may impact quality of life and ability to demonstrate coping skills in individuals with schizophrenia. Sleep studies demonstrate that these individuals have reduced slow-wave sleep and reduced REM sleep latency (Monti & Monti, 2005). Since the definition of insomnia is that the person does not sleep at night, these individuals may not be responding to their body clock (Foster, 2006). People with schizophrenia may have trouble sleeping at socially acceptable times and thus have erratic sleep patterns. As a result, they feel stress that can lead to psychosis. Helping these individuals reset their body clock through light therapy may help (Foster, 2006).

Insomnia and eating disorders are not frequently linked, but individuals with anorexia nervosa often have insomnia. Bulimia nervosa, another eating disorder, is not consistently linked with sleep disturbances, incidences of hypersomnolence after eating binges may occur with this condition. A sleep-related eating disorder occurs when food is consumed during a partial arousal from sleep of which the person is unaware (Benca & Schenck, 2005). All individuals with eating disorders should have their sleep addressed.

Individuals with medication or substance abuse may have sleep issues caused by the abuse, by withdrawal from the substance, or by self-medication for sleep issues. Many people think alcohol will help them sleep, but the opposite is true. Total sleep time, sleep efficiency, and slow-wave sleep are decreased by alcohol (Gillin, Drummond, Clark, & Morre, 2005).

Neurological Disabilities

Several neurological conditions commonly co-occur with sleep disorders and often can be seen in childhood. Some of these conditions include sensory processing disorder, autism, attention deficit hyperactivity disorder (ADHD), and attention deficit disorder (ADD). As children and adults, these individuals often have difficulty regulating themselves during waking occupations. They also have difficulty with initiating sleep and maintaining a healthy sleep state. They have difficulty interpreting cues from their bodies and their environments that indicate it is time to sleep. The social cues needed to develop typical circadian rhythms are missed. They do not recognize the "norm" of sleeping at night and being awake during the day (Richdale & Prior, 1995).

People with brain injuries, blindness, and low vision also have difficulties perceiving the zeitgebers of light and dark to establish sleep patterns. These individuals need to maintain good sleep hygiene to help ensure regular sleep patterns.

It is not uncommon for individuals with complex clinical syndromes to have their sleep disorder go completely unaddressed. Examples include Asperger's syndrome (hypersomnia

and sleep breathing disorders), autism (insomnia), and Down syndrome (sleep breathing disorders). Treating their sleep disorders could improve their function (Kryger, 2005).

Occasionally, individuals with excessive daytime sleepiness (EDS), which involves the hypothalamic areas of the nervous system, also have weight gain. This can complicate matters by increasing sleepiness, which can also contribute to weight gain. This vicious cycle between gaining weight and sleep deprivation requires recognition and interruption by health care providers if it is not to become a life pattern of poor sleep, ill heath, and limited quality of life (Kryger, 2005).

Alzheimer's and Dementia

The elderly (see "Sleep in the Elderly" earlier in this chapter) are at risk for sleep disturbances that occur frequently with aging (WHO, 2004). Individuals with Alzheimer's and other forms of dementia often become confused about day and night (Petit, Montplaisir, & Boeve, 2005). This condition is called sundown syndrome. Also, individuals with traumatic brain injury may have disruption of the hypochiasmatic nuclei, which interferes with sleep patterns. Both of these conditions can interfere with sleep of patients in medical institutions.

Movement and Breathing Limitations

Typically, the body moves during sleep to maintain comfort. Individuals with conditions that impair their movements may have difficulty maintaining comfort during sleep. Such conditions include cardiovascular accident, spinal cord injury, and cerebral palsy. Others may be able to move but only with associated pain that disrupts sleep. Chronic pain conditions such as arthritis often impair sleep (Lavigne, McMillan, & Zucconi, 2005).

The body and the brain continue to need oxygen throughout the night. When the amount of oxygen is restricted, sleep disturbances can occur. In addition to the category of sleep disorders related to breathing disorders, other more common conditions can impair breathing, such as allergies, the common cold, and chronic obstructive pulmonary disease. Anyone can have their sleep impaired from time to time due to common ailments. Since some of the conditions can cause snoring, this also has an impact on the person's bed partner. When you share a bed, you are at risk for a sleep disturbance.

Factory Workers, Truckers, Pilots, Parents, and Caregivers

Shift workers often have disturbed sleep patterns due to the unusual time patterns of their daily occupations and the misfit of those patterns with the rest of the culture. They negotiate between their shift work schedule and the more typical schedules of their families, friends, and community services, resulting in a flexing and disrupted sleep schedule. As a result, they have excessive sleepiness during both work and daytime hours, which can cause serious driving and workplace accidents. Disrupted sleep also puts them at greater risk for gastrointestinal and cardiovascular diseases (WHO, 2004).

Another neglected population at risk for disturbed sleep patterns is parents, especially single parents. Newborns, who sleep in short cycles, and children with teething, toilet-training, illnesses, and other nighttime needs, can disrupt their parents' sleep. In fact, all caregivers are at risk for sleep disturbances, especially caregivers of persons with special needs. Caregiving can be physically and emotionally demanding. It is important for all caregivers to get as much sleep as possible so they can carry out their responsibilities safely, effectively, and without negative impacts on their own health.

Lastly, women encounter more sleep issues than men, have different sleep architecture (Armitage, Baker, & Parry, 2005; Wolfson & Lee, 2005), and report insomnia more often than adult men (Phillips et al, 2008). Women's risk for insomnia also increases during female hormone conditions, including menstruation, pregnancy, and menopause. Sleep disorders also interrupt the production of hormones that modulate hunger and satiety. Since women have more fragmented sleep, this impacts them more, resulting in weight gain. Restless legs syndrome is another condition that has more prevalence in women than in men (Kantrowitz, 2006). Cultural factors also impair women's sleep. Women are typically the primary caregivers for children and parents who can require assistant during the night. Females should be aware of their increased risks for sleep disturbances.

Sleep Medicine Professionals

Sleep medicine is a relatively young specialty (Dement, 2005). Medicine has been in existence for hundreds of years. Its early years were focused on generalist interventions. Advances in surgery, pharmaceuticals, and psychiatry pulled medicine from its generalist focus toward the emergence of specialties. Viewed within the long history of medicine, the emergence in the 1980s of the specialty of sleep medicine is a recent development. As sleep medicine and its interventions evolve, an awareness of the importance of sleep seeps increasingly into the consciousness of the public. Research is demonstrating the relationships that exist between sleep debt and a variety of health issues: workplace injuries, dangers to others from inadequate sleep in pilots and truck drivers, and the contribution of disturbed sleep to obesity, depression, and compromised immune function. Many common health conditions treated by physicians are associated with sleep disturbances: bipolar disorders, schizophrenia, depression, respiratory conditions, and others. Instead of being overlooked as a suspended, unconscious part of life, sleep is beginning to be regarded as a critical base of everyday functioning. Like being unable to eat, work, or communicate, the disruption of the activity of sleep strikes at the very core of enacting a satisfying, peaceful, and meaningful human life.

The Sleep Team

Several types of professionals are involved in sleep medicine teams (Chervin, 2005b). The sleep medicine physician is a specialist who has completed additional residencies in order to focus his or her practice on sleep disorders. There is board certification for sleep specialists, who may come from the fields of neurology, psychiatry, psychology, or osteopathy. A pulmonologist or internist may also be involved in sleep disorders treatment, especially in addressing the effects of sleep apnea on the heart and lungs. Otolaryngologists, often called ENTs, perform surgeries to reduce snoring. Some dentists specialize in creating custom-made oral appliances to reduce snoring and aid nighttime breathing. The sleep somnographer manages a sleep study laboratory, usually accredited by the Academy of Sleep Medicine. They record patterns of sleep, brain activity, blood oxygenation, respiration, and body movements during sleep and return the results of the sleep study to the referring sleep specialist.

Emerging Role for Occupational Therapists

The relatively recent emergence of sleep medicine and the present rapid development of its interventions offers opportunities for occupational therapists to form partnerships with sleep medicine professionals in order to better serve individuals with sleep disorders. Such innovative practice not only provides a new arena for the profession but also gives occupational therapy a strategic stage upon which to display the important tie of occupation to health. Addressing disruptions to sleep, an activity that occupies the largest portion of our lives and without which we would soonest die, can highlight the unique contribution of occupational therapists and their knowledge base.

Within this intervention picture, several potentially useful strategies for sleep assessment and intervention remain unaddressed: sleep environment assessment and modification and sleep routine assessment and establishment within the individual's and family's lifestyle. These aspects of sleep medicine are uniquely suited to the knowledge base and skills of occupational therapists. However, they require program development and research in order to offer occupational therapists some guidance as to what they may offer to sleep medicine teams. Many occupational therapists are already treating clients with sleep disturbances and can begin by more effectively addressing sleep issues within their own interventions. For example, many children with sensory-processing disorders have sleep problems that are highly disruptive to their own and their families' lives. Initial and ongoing assessment, monitoring, home programming and modifications, and consultation with the family can be seamlessly integrated into existing occupational therapy practice. Individuals with more severe sleep issues should be referred to a reputable sleep physician, complete with a brief report from the occupational therapist. Over time, the physician will increasingly value this partnership and perspective.

Approaching a sleep medicine team or physician to offer to develop occupational therapy services to support their current interventions should be done in the same way that any new service is developed: with adequate background preparation, with a collegial attitude, seeking to learn, providing carefully tailored information, and initiating exploratory discussions. Early services may be offered at no cost in order to develop programming that is responsive to clients, the needs of the team, and the constraints of the system. It is not necessary to start with a large number of clients. Most importantly, such innovative services must continually evolve on the basis of feedback from all stakeholders to better meet the needs of the clients. Reflecting deeply on each intervention, an occupational therapist seeking to develop services to support the sleep medicine team is likely to find that assessing and modifying sleep environments and habits, both accustomed areas of interventions with other populations, should prove quite successful. Collecting data as the interventions progress, such as case studies, simple outcome measures, and client satisfaction scores and statements, is also a useful way to contribute. This information will serve not only to improve interventions but also to support their effectiveness in the eyes of the team and reimbursers. In regard to reimbursement, the physician's referral should go a long way toward assuring the necessity of the occupational therapy assessments and interventions provided. The therapist must be prepared, however, to provide logical, informed, and data-based responses to questions of reimbursers, given the innovative nature of these services.

Screening, Evaluation, and Interventions to Improve Sleep

Occupational therapists are well situated to recognize and assist with sleep problems. Many of our clients are specifically at risk for sleep disorders, as stated in a previous section. Understanding and supporting healthy patterns of daily occupation is our forte, and sleep is certainly the biggest occupation of all. Sleep problems can also affect our clients' abilities to accomplish their desired occupational outcomes, such as functioning well in the classroom or returning to full-time work.

Screening for Sleep Issues

The American Occupational Therapy Association's Practice Framework: Domain and Process (AOTA, 2002) includes sleep under client factors. Not only is sleep a primary occupation in our lives and health, but it also impacts our ability to perform all of our waking occupations. Sleep can be considered the base or foundation occupation upon which other occupations rest. Because sleep plays such a major role in everyone's lives, occupational therapists should inquire about their clients' sleep in every initial evaluation. The therapist should assess the client's entire 24-hour day, not just his or her awake time. If occupational therapists do not query about their clients' sleep, they could overlook major impacts on client function and undermine the effectiveness of their own interventions.

The therapist should inquire about basic sleep amounts and whether the client is satisfied with his or her sleep. If your client is in a special population at risk for sleep disorders, his or her sleep pattern should receive extra attention. If the client reports concerns about sleep or the therapist suspects that the client has a sleep disorder or significant sleep debt, further investigation may need to be conducted. Resist the tendency to dismiss sleep problems as normal for at-risk populations, as so often happens.

Do some background research about sleep medicine in your community. Seek recommendations from colleagues in regard to reputable sleep laboratories and specialists. If you are treating a population at risk for sleep issues, it may be useful to prepare an information page on sleep problems and resources that you can provide to clients. If you recommend a formal sleep study, the client will probably need to go first to his or her general practitioner in order to receive insurance coverage for the sleep assessment. Providing a brief written overview of what you have noted about your client's sleep report and why it may warrant an assessment will be very helpful to your client in bringing the sleep issue to the attention of the general practitioner. Often, general practitioners dismiss sleep concerns and are hesitant to refer patients to this relatively new specialty. Sometimes their knowledge of sleep medicine and disorders is not up to date. Make efforts to support your clients if they choose to seek a formal sleep evaluation.

For more data to support your understanding of your client or his or her need for a sleep study, a 2-week sleep diary is an excellent method. The sleep diary combines the temporal aspects of sleep with the client's opinion of his or her sleep quality. The diary should log the time the individual goes to bed and wakes up in the morning. The client should record as accurately possible upon waking how long it took to fall asleep. He or she should also note any awakenings and how long they lasted. In addition, the quality of sleep should be rated on a scale of 1 to 10. The sleep diary should note any significant events during the day that may affect nighttime sleep, such as naps, excessive daytime sleepiness, or consuming large amounts of alcohol or caffeine. The diary should also list any medications the client may be taking so that the occupational therapist can check on their potential impacts on sleep. It is worth noting here that although individuals with insomnia frequently perceive they are getting less sleep than they actually are, this does not mean they do not have sleep issues. Their concerns about their sleep disturbances should be respected.

The Multiple Sleep Latency Test is a formalized method used in sleep clinics to assess sleep debt. The procedure is to put the client in a dark room and then time how long it takes him or her to fall asleep. Typically, a person falls asleep within 10 to 20 minutes. Falling asleep in 5 or 6 minutes indicates the need to increase the usual amount of sleep. If a person falls asleep after 6 minutes but in less than 10, then the test is inconclusive and the client requires further assessment (Milter, Carskadon, & Hirshkowitz, 2005). Sleep debt can also be assessed by self-report or by the occupational therapist in a nonstandardized method. Ask how long it takes the client to fall asleep when he or she goes to bed at night. If your client is consistently falling asleep as soon as his or her head hits the pillow, that person probably has sleep debt. Also inquire whether the client falls asleep consistently when in a darkened room, watching television, or at a movie. If the individual consistently falls asleep under these conditions, he or she may have a sleep debt. If this is the case, a formalized sleep assessment would be beneficial.

Occupational Profile of Sleep

In addition to a formal assessment performed at a sleep clinic, or for those who choose not to seek formal assessment, many clients would benefit from an occupational sleep profile, such as the one shown in Figure 53-1. The purpose of the profile is to investigate your client's sleep routines. As with any assessment, your role as an occupational therapist is to gather input from your client and then analyze it. Then you can make recommendations to improve the client's sleep. While some aspects of sleep, such as snoring or the amount of sleep, can be observed directly by a sleep clinician or a bed partner, only the individual can report how he or she feels while asleep. For example, does the person feel rested after waking up? Does he or she feel anxious about getting enough sleep?

In order to get the best information from your client, ask open-ended questions and make the client comfortable. Explain the question further if the client has difficulty answering it. Suggest possible answers only as a last resort. For example, only if the client has difficulty identifying the reason for his night awakenings might you provide suggestions to consider, such as pain, urination, or stress. Have the client provide as much information as possible. For instance, during one interview with a parent, a mother stated that her child slept fine. With further discussion, it was discovered that the child slept under the bed. If you ask only yes-or-no questions, you may not get the answers you need.

OCCUPATIONAL PROFILE OF SLEEP

Client: _____ Date: _____

Client Record #: _____ DOB: _____

Diagnosis/Respiratory conditions: _____

Precautions/Allergies: _____

List medications (including herbal supplements)   Time   Amount

_____

_____

SLEEP ROUTINE

What are your concerns about your sleep? _____

How long has this occurred? _____

How long does it take to fall asleep? _____ Time you typically fall asleep: _____

What time do you wake up in the a.m.? _____ Amount of a typical night's sleep _____

Do you sleep through the night? _____ How often do you wake? _____

What is the cause of awakenings if known? _____

How long does it take to fall back asleep? _____

Describe how you feel when you wake up (restful, tired): _____

Do you take naps—frequency, length and time of the day? _____

Describe sleep pattern on the weekend: _____

Do you have increased stress in your life—describe: _____

Is sleep a priority in your life? _____

AWAKE ROUTINE

Do you participate in other occupations in your bedroom? (work, computer, read, television):

_____

Exercise regularly: Yes No   Type: _____ Time of day? _____

What time do you eat your meals? _____

Drink caffeinated beverages? Yes No How much? _____ Time of day? _____

continued on next page

FIGURE 53-1. Occupational Profile of Sleep.

OCCUPATIONAL PROFILE OF SLEEP (continued)

Drink alcoholic beverages? Yes No   How much? _____ Time of day? _____

Smoke? Yes No How much? _____   Are you around smoke on a regular basis? Yes No

Describe your nightly routine from dinner to bedtime: _____

_____

SLEEP ENVIRONMENT

Bed size: king, queen, full or twin   Mattress type and condition: _____

Linens type and texture: _____

Type of Pajamas: _____

Temperature: _____ Light level: _____ Noise level: _____

Bed sharers: partner, children, pets, other: _____

Describe your sleep environment: _____

Additional information: _____

SLEEP PATTERNS

Do you snore? _____ Do you move around in your sleep? _____

Do you move your legs, have the urge to move them, or pain? _____

Do you breathe through your mouth? _____

Any changes in sleep due to menstruating, pregnancy, or menopause: _____

FIGURE 53-1. Occupational Profile of Sleep **cont'd**

The Occupational Profile of Sleep collects information on the client's medical history, sleep routines, sleep patterns, awake routines, and sleep environment. All these factors have important impacts on sleep. The questions in each section will help you determine possible causes of sleep issues. Once you gather the information and analyze the data, you will be able to provide intervention suggestions to improve sleep. (The next section, "Sleep Interventions," will help you consider intervention strategies you might use.)

A basic medical history can provide clues to sleep issues. Some diagnoses can put clients at risk for sleep issues. (Refer to the previous section on populations at risk for sleep problems to identify these conditions.) In addition to examining their primary diagnosis, you will need to get information on supplementary conditions. Respiratory conditions are especially important to sleep quality. If a person has difficulty breathing because of allergies, asthma, or even a cold, they may awake frequently in order to breathe, which prevents reaching deep sleep and feeling rested the following day.

In addition to medical conditions, the medications a client takes can impact sleep (Schweitzer, 2005). Some medications cause drowsiness, while others can make it difficult to sleep. Even over-the-counter medications such as antihistamines can cause drowsiness. As an occupational therapist, it is important to be aware of the medications your client

is taking and their impact on occupational performance. If you are not familiar with the client's medication and its side effects, check the *Physician's Desk Reference* (2009). In addition to the medication type, the dose and timing of the medications can impact the individual's ability to actively engage in waking occupations. Sometimes medication dose and timing changes can improve client function. Clients with depression are often prescribed antidepressants, which have sedative side effects and are also used to treat insomnia: trazodone, mirtazapine, fluoxetine, sertraline, paroxetine, venlafaxine, bupropion, and nefazodone (Becker, 2006). While occupational therapists cannot prescribe medications, they can discuss the impact of the medications on their clients with the physician. Also, they should educate their clients on the side effects of drugs and support them in self-advocating their needs to their physicians.

The sleep routine section of the profile gathers information about the quantity and quality of your client's sleep. The first question allows the client to state concerns about sleep and how long they have been occurring. This information helps to guide you in your investigation. The amount of sleep is important to determine if the person is getting enough sleep. However, quality is as important as quantity. Sleep fragmentation can impair sleep. If the person is waking up during the night, try to determine what may be causing the awakening. Is it due to physiological reasons (breathing issues, urination, hunger, or pain)? Is there an environmental cause, such as noise or light? Do they have nightmares, or are they stressed? The individual may have no idea of the cause. Once you determine awakenings exist, also explore how long the client stays awake before falling back to sleep. Is he or she able to return to slumber?

Although you may not have the opportunity to view your client sleeping, you still need to understand his or her sleep patterns. This next section of the profile investigates how the body functions during sleep. For example, if the client breathes through the mouth, he or she may have respiratory issues such as allergies or enlarged tonsils. If a client has any of these conditions listed in this section of the profile, then a referral to a sleep specialist or a physician is recommended. In addition, females should be aware that hormonal changes can impact their sleep.

The awake routine section assesses the client's occupations during the day. Most people understand that activities during the night can impact their sleep. Many do not understand how actions during the day can impair sleep. This section enables you to investigate the client's daily routine.

The sleep environment can also impact sleep. The last section of the profile provides questions to help you understand the client's sleep environment. If possible, an on-site assessment of the natural sleep environment is even better. This will provide you with a more accurate picture and additional clues to possible improvements that may enhance your client's sleep quality.

The last question on the profile is open ended to allow the client to express any issues that were not addressed. This also allows you the opportunity to gather more information about your clients' individual preferences, including their sensory processing. There is no one answer to everyone's sleep issues, so it is important to know clients as individuals and as an occupational beings and to use that information to help them improve their sleep.

Evidence-Based Practice

A qualitative study of individuals with psychiatric disabilities and insomnia found that most people avoid telling health professionals about their sleep problems (Collier, Skitt, & Cutts 2003). In addition, the sleep problems that most affected their quality of life did not always fit the criteria for a sleep disorder diagnosis.

➤ This study supports the importance of collaborating with the client to identify their own definition of insomnia and personal goals for sleep

➤ After conducting a sleep profile, occupational therapists can then identify the barriers to sleep and consider what might be the best intervention (e.g. creating a more conducive environment for sleep; establishing sleep routines; changing negative thinking about sleep)

Collier, E., Skitt, G., & Cutts, H. (2003). A study on the experience of insomnia in a psychiatric inpatient population. Journal of Psychiatric and Mental Health Health Nursing, 10, 697–704.

Sleep Interventions

Once the client's sleep profile is completed, the occupational therapist can make recommendations to improve sleep. Since sleep is a complex occupation, there is no single, easy fix. Because an individual's sleep issues do not develop overnight, they cannot be fixed quickly. If a contributing factor to the sleep disorder is a disruptive routine, it takes time to change a person's routines and habits. Also, some interventions may need to be tried before the most effective approach can be discovered. Each trial of an intervention must last several nights in order to determine what will work. Researchers recommend trying the approach for 3 days to 3 weeks before deciding if a technique is or is not effective (Hoch & Reynolds, 1986).

Often, people turn to the easy answer of taking medications to resolve their sleep issues. However, medication tends to mask the cause of the sleep disorder and treats only the symptoms. In fact, lifestyle redesign and nonpharmacological interventions are preferable for the treatment of most sleep disorders (Collier & Skitt, 2003). Also, chronic insomnias respond better to non-pharmacological interventions (Morin et al, 1999). Medications should be used in the short term, no more than 3 weeks at a time for acute situations, and not for long-term situations (Collier & Skitt, 2003). Although sleep medications may treat the symptoms of sleep deprivation, they do not resolve the underlying cause. As a result, the condition causing the sleep disturbance remains. For example, the person may be suffering from lack of sleep due to stress. Taking sleep medications does not remove the stress (Kantrowitz, 2006).

Melatonin is a hormone produced in the brain and regulates circadian rhythms. When the eyes sense darkness, melatonin is released, triggering the body to fall asleep. Natural melatonin is available over the counter but is not regulated by Food and Drug Administration. Always consult with your physician before taking any medications or supplements. While melatonin is easily available and many use it to treat jet lag, minimal evidence exists in regard to its effectiveness. According to review of current research by Buscemi et al (2005), melatonin is not effective for treating primary sleep disorders but may be useful in the treatment for individuals with difficulty falling asleep, such as in delayed sleep phase. Individuals with visual impairments may benefit from melatonin to help set their circadian rhythms. If they are having sleep issues, they should consult their physician (Hirshkowitz & Smith, 2004).

Because the evidence demonstrates the benefits of nonpharmacological interventions for sleep disorders, lifestyle redesign and behavioral techniques should be implemented. Despite the evidence of its effectiveness, this is not the chosen method in most sleep medicine approaches (Morin, 2005). Occupational therapists have the expertise to implement changes in lifestyle and can offer clients additional supports to improve their sleep (Clark et al, 1997).

One of the most effective methods to improve sleep is education (Collier & Skitt, 2003). Once clients understand the importance of sleep and sleep hygiene, they may be more invested in making choices and lifestyle changes to improve sleep. In today's Western culture, the focus is very much on productivity. For many, it is almost a game they play every day of the week, taking pride in how much they can get done each day. By educating clients on the role that sleep plays in their daily lives, occupational therapists can assist them in changing their daily routines and making sleep a higher priority.

The best treatment for disturbed sleep is to develop good sleep hygiene. This is particularly true in treating insomnia. Sleep hygiene includes having a relatively unvarying sleep schedule, an effective routine for falling asleep, an adequate amount of sleep, and living habits throughout the day that do not negatively impact sleep. For example, foods you eat or drink and when you exercise during the day can impact your ability to fall asleep at night. Good sleep hygiene helps to set your body clock, helping the body know when it is time to shift into sleep. If not already in place, use of a standard bedtime and waking time will have a positive impact on sleep quality. You should go to bed and wake up at the same time each day, including on the weekend. Though nothing may sound better to a tired person than sleeping in on the weekend, this pattern is disruptive to the establishment of the circadian rhythm that underlies sleep hygiene. Instruction in sleep hygiene may be beneficial for individuals who have bipolar disorder (Benca, 2005) and schizophrenia. Frequently, individuals with schizophrenia do not have a daily routine, much less a sleep routine. As a result, they may develop habits not conducive to good sleep. Individuals with schizophrenia would benefit from instruction in sleep hygiene to help increase their ability to function (Benson & Zarcone, 2005).

If a person is waking during the night, information on sleep routine from the sleep profile should help guide the therapist to an intervention. If a physiological reason is causing the awakenings, a medical examination may be required. If the person is having insomnia or difficulty falling back to sleep, behavioral techniques may be helpful.

Clients who are unable to fall asleep within 15 to 35 minutes should get up out of bed and do a quiet activity until they feel sleepy enough to go back to bed (Hayter, 1983; Wade, 2006). Staying in bed while awake is counterproductive to establishing a good sleep pattern. The bed should be used only for sleeping and intimacy with a partner. For those who are trying to establish improved sleep patterns, watching television or even reading in bed should be avoided. This sends a clear message to the body that the bed is for sleeping. The bedroom should be free of any clutter or furnishings associated with other occupations such as work. This is referred to as stimulus control therapy (Morin, 2005).

Another behavioral technique to help induce sleep is sleep restriction. The amount of time spent in bed is initially reduced in order to establish a pattern of several nights of sound sleep. Once healthy sleep is occurring on a regular basis, increases in the amount of sleep are made very gradually until the individual maintains the amount of sleep recommended for his or her age (Morin, 2005). In addition to behavioral techniques to help encourage sleep, cognitive therapy techniques can also be beneficial. Clients with sleep disorders need to change their beliefs about sleep. If they learn to view sleep as a positive activity, the sleep pattern can be changed. Having stressful thoughts about not falling asleep can make falling asleep even harder. When you combine these interventions with techniques to decrease stress, a person can become less stressed and thus sleep better (Morin, 2005). This treatment is recommended for individuals with anxiety disorders and posttraumatic stress disorder (Stein & Mellman, 2005).

Here is an example from occupational therapy of an intervention that demonstrated the benefit of changing thought patterns about sleep (Scott, 1999). A group of occupational therapy students had children who were hospitalized for serious medical conditions make a Native American dream catcher to stop nightmares. Although the dream catcher may not have literally prevented the nightmares, the children participated in a project that gave them a sense of increased control and that did prevent the nightmares. Being in the hospital can be scary for children, and the dream catcher gave them an action they could take on their own behalves. The belief that the dream catcher would only let in the nice dreams worked for them. The children expressed that the nightmares stopped after they had made their dream catchers.

The bedtime routine is a critical component of healthy sleep. Everyone has a different sleep routine, but it might include putting on pajamas, face washing, tooth brushing, and settling into a quiet activity. The bedtime routine is best done before feeling sleepy rather than after. Also, taking a bath is a traditional part of the nightly routine for many. A warm bath can help induce sleep. After the bath, body temperature drops and may continue to drop to help induce sleep. Some individuals find bath time alerting, however, and should avoid bathing close to bedtime. Everyone should include a quiet activity in the bedtime routine to help them settle down, such as reading a book or listening to relaxing music. Watching television or surfing the Internet should be avoided because they are highly stimulating in content and include light-emitting screens that are alerting. Quiet bedtime activities should include dim lighting to indicate to the body that it is time to sleep. It is best that the client collaborate in examining and redesigning his or her own routine so that it results in a routine that really fits.

In order to fall asleep, a person should be relaxed. This means not thinking or participating in stressful activities before bedtime. If your client goes to bed with things on his or her mind that disrupt the ability to sleep, recommend writing them down before going to bed and visualizing addressing them the next day. Relaxation training includes thinking relaxing thoughts, meditation, muscle relaxation techniques, and massage. These can be calming and enjoyable activities that encourage sleep (Morin, 2005).

Regular mealtimes are another way to help set the body's clock. Individuals with sleep disorders should avoid caffeine in the afternoons and evenings. Caffeine is a stimulant and can stay in the body for hours. A popular myth is that alcohol can help you sleep. Although a hot toddy may initially create relaxation and sleepiness, it will result later in the night in waking and difficulty falling back to sleep. Alcohol is a carbohydrate and impacts blood sugar levels. After the alcohol is metabolized, sugar levels drop and cause awakening. This is the body's way of communicating hunger and the need for more food in order to stabilize sugar levels. On the other hand, some foods can help with sleep. For example, the protein tryptophan, found in turkey and milk, can help stimulate sleep. A light snack before bedtime, with protein or decaffeinated tea, may help with sleep, but heavy food should be avoided near bedtime.

Exercise is a healthy activity, and a fit body sleeps better than an unfit body. Exercise, however, should be done earlier in the day or evening. It is alerting and should be avoided during the 2 to 3 hours just before bedtime. Everyone needs time to wind down before sleep. Running a 5-minute mile will not accomplish this task. Even though the activity may cause tiredness, it will not encourage immediate sleep.

Rhythmical vestibular input can be quite calming. Babies tend to fall asleep when they are cradled or rocked. A hammock slowly moving back and forth also encourages restful sleep. Still, a note of caution must be included here. If an intervention works for falling asleep and a person becomes dependent on that strategy, then he or she will need it every night to fall asleep. This is especially true for children. If falling asleep to the hum and gentle breeze of a ceiling fan is what works to improve sleep, keep in mind that it might be hard to take that ceiling fan on family vacations. If children can learn to fall asleep without any special equipment, they will sleep easier in the long run. Sleep is critically important, however, so if the ceiling fan helps, then go ahead and turn it on.

Adapting the Sleep Environment

In addition to good sleep hygiene, a person must have a comfortable environment that is conducive to sleep. If the environment is not inviting and calming, consistent high-quality sleep will be hard to achieve. This section provides suggestions to decrease environmental problems that may be impairing the ability to sleep, addressing sleep furnishings, temperature, light, sound, and bed partners. The best method for an occupational therapist to assess the client's sleep environment is to make a home visit. If this is not possible, have the client describe his or her sleep environment.

The bed is the most important furnishing of the sleep environment. The comfort of the mattress greatly impacts sleep. Therefore, your clients should have a mattress that is comfortable to them. This is an area where personal preference plays a large role. If the current mattress is comfortable, then this is not a problem area. If the mattress is uncomfortable enough to cause soreness upon waking, or is too hard or saggy, it may be time for the client to purchase a new mattress. Encourage your clients to lie down on the mattress before buying it to make sure it is comfortable (Hirshkowitz & Smith, 2004). Although a mattress can be a large purchase, if it improves sleep, health, and mood, then the investment is worth it.

The pillow is also important to a good night's sleep. The type selected also depends on personal preference. There is no one correct pillow for everyone. Waking up with neck pain is a sign that a new pillow may help. Just like a mattress, pillows should be tried out in the store in order to find one that fits (Hirshkowitz & Smith, 2004). Lying on your side or back, the pillow should support the neck in a way that keeps the spine straight. For clients with allergies or respiratory issues, pillows and mattresses should be covered with a zippered plastic covering to prevent them from being exposed to dust mites.

Although the mattress and pillow are the biggest factors in making the bed comfortable, linens also play a role. Once again, personal preference is the key. The texture of the sheets should be comfortable. Also, the weight of the blanket or comforter is an important factor to consider. Some people prefer a heavy blanket, providing calming proprioceptive input, while others may want the lightest cover possible. This is also true of pajamas for those who wear them. Lycra material in sheets or pajamas can help provide proprioceptive input.

The temperature of the sleep environment needs to be just right for sleeping. In order to fall asleep, the body temperature must drop. However, if the room is too cold, a person will have trouble staying asleep. Be aware that people perceive temperature differently. Elderly people tend to be colder than most adults and will want more warmth in the bedrooms. Bigger people tend to be warmer and will want a cooler sleeping space. Men tend to like a cooler environment than do women. Once again, there are individual preferences. In order for the room to be comfortable, it should also be free of clutter. As mentioned earlier, the bedroom should be a place only for sleep.

The visual system cues the body to recognize day and night by responding to environmental light. In our modern society, lights can be on for 24 hours, which is not conducive to sleep. For sleep, a room should be completely dark. No television or computer screens should be on. The light triggers the brain to believe it is daytime and this interferes with sleep. Dark out curtains may be needed to block light from the outside. An eye mask could also be worn to help block out light. A nightlight is appropriate for children if they feel they need it. Individuals who have difficulty waking up in the morning may also benefit from morning light. The sunrise can help the body awake, or alarm clocks that bring light up slowly when it is time to wake can also be used. Light therapy may help people with depression, dementia, and sundown syndrome. Being exposed to natural and full-spectrum light during the day can help to set the body's clock for sleep at night. With better sleep, agitation and negative effects on mood may decrease.

In order to sleep, the room should be as quiet as possible. A white noise machine or fan may be needed to drown out unavoidable noises in the household, institution, or neighborhood where a client sleeps. Also, earplugs could be used to help block out more proximal noises, such as a bed partner's snoring. There should be no noise from televisions, computers, or radios. Relaxing music that is used to help with falling asleep should be on a timer or automatically stop when the CD is over in order to avoid noise throughout the evening.

Bed partners can also impact sleep. Frequently, the snoring of a bed partner is a serious threat to sleep. If the above suggestions for decreasing noise do not work, the partner may need to seek medical help, or bed-sharing for sleep may have to be discontinued to protect sleep quality. Although co-sleeping with nursing infants and toddlers is a choice made by many families, family pets and older children should have their own sleep spaces and should respect the needs of the adults of the family for healthy sleep.

While most people have some control over their own sleep environment, individuals who live in institutional settings, such as long-term care facilities, have little control. As a result, people have trouble sleeping with all the noise and lights common to those settings. The Sh-h-h-h Project was developed to help patients sleep better in the hospital through nonpharmacological procedures (Dreher, 1996). "Sleep baskets" containing materials for the sleep interventions, including lotion for back rubs, lavender oil for aromatherapy, decaffeinated tea, and ear plugs, were distributed. Calming music was available through the in-room television sets, and warmed blankets were available to the elderly.

In addition to the nonpharmacological interventions and environmental modifications, staff in these settings can make changes to their routines to help clients sleep better. Staff should consider whether waking a patient to perform a task such as taking their vitals is more beneficial than the quality of uninterrupted sleep. Sometimes such monitoring is necessary. A reduction in unnecessary waking will improve sleep, help clients heal faster, and make them feel more relaxed the next day. Noise can interfere with patients' sleep also, especially at shift change. Reducing talk between staff and work procedure noises that occur just outside of people's rooms during sleep hours can go a long way toward improving institutional sleep environments (Dreher, 1996).

Summary

In this chapter, we shared our vision of the role that occupational therapy can play in addressing an epidemic of sleep problems that especially affect client populations to whom we provide service. Sleep is easily the largest occupation in life, is required of all persons on a daily basis, and has the strongest tie to health. Yet the strong focus in Western culture on productivity has created a blind spot in regard to the occupation of sleep. Sleep is fascinating: its neurophysiology, its daily rhythms, its contextual shaping, and its developmental differences. Sleep debt and disorders can be addressed through education, improved sleep routines, and changes to the sleep environment. These are areas of expertise for occupational therapists. The logic is clear, but program development is required if occupational therapists are to conquer this exciting new frontier of sleep interventions.

Active Learning Strategies

1. Sleep Diary

Keep a sleep diary for 2 weeks. Include sleep schedule, quality of sleep, and any unusual conditions. Analyze the patterns you find in your sleep diary and describe them. Describe your own sleep routine.

2. Occupational Profile of Sleep

Analyze your own sleep routine, environment, and patterns using the using the Occupational Profile of Sleep. What did you find out about your sleep that you did not already realize? What changes might improve your sleep?

Or, with a partner, practice your professional interviewing skills by administering to each other the Occupational

Profile of Sleep. If you were an occupational therapist collecting this profile, what would your initial plan be for addressing any sleep issues that were identified? Do you recognize any sleep debt in your friends or family members? What might be the causes of their sleep debts?

3. Two in a Bed

If you regularly share a bed, read *Two in a Bed* by Paul Rosenblatt, a study of the social context of sleep. Describe or discuss how the points made in this study are congruent or incongruent with your own experiences of bedsharing.

References

American Academy of Sleep Medicine. (2004). *International Classification of Sleep Disorders: Diagnostic and Coding Manual* (2nd ed.). Westchester, IL: American Academy of Sleep Medicine.

American Occupational Therapy Association (AOTA). (2002). Occupational therapy practice framework: Domain and process. *American Journal of Occupational Therapy, 56,* 609–639.

American Psychiatric Association. (2000). *Diagnostic and Statistical Manual of Mental Disorders: DSM-IV-TR* (4th ed., text rev.). Washington, DC: American Psychiatric Association.

Anthony, W. A. (1997). *The Art of Napping.* New York: Larson.

Arendt, J., Stone, B., & Skene, D. (2005). Sleep disruption in jet lag and other circadian rhythm–related disorders. In Kryger, Roth, & Dement (Eds.). *Principles and Practice of Sleep Medicine* (4th ed.) (659–672). Philadelphia: Elsevier Saunders.

Armitage, R., Baker, F., & Parry, B. (2005). The menstrual cycle and circadian rhythms. In Kryger, Roth, & Dement (Eds.). *Principles and Practice of Sleep Medicine* (4th ed.) (pp. 1266–1277). Philadelphia: Elsevier Saunders.

Becker, P. (2006). Treatment of sleep dysfunction and psychiatric disorders. *Current Treatment Options in Neurology, 8,* 367–375.

Benca, R. (2005). Mood disorders. In Kryger, Roth, & Dement (Eds.). *Principles and Practice of Sleep Medicine* (4th ed.) (pp. 1311–1326). Philadelphia: Elsevier Saunders.

Benca, R., & Schenck, C. (2005). Sleep and eating disorders. In Kryger, Roth, & Dement (Eds.). *Principles and Practice of Sleep Medicine* (4th ed.) (pp. 1337–1344). Philadelphia: Elsevier Saunders.

Benson, K., & Zarcone, V. (2005). Schizophrenia. In Kryger, Roth, & Dement (Eds.). *Principles and Practice of Sleep Medicine* (4th ed.) (pp. 1327–1336). Philadelphia: Elsevier Saunders.

Bliwise, D. (1997). Sleep and aging. In W. Orr & M. Pressman (Eds.), *Understanding Sleep: The Evaluation and Treatment of Sleep Disorders* (pp. 441–464). Washington, DC: American Psychological Association.

———. (2005). Normal aging. In Kryger, Roth, & Dement (Eds.). *Principles and Practice of Sleep Medicine* (4th ed.), (pp. 24–38). Philadelphia: Elsevier Saunders.

Bolge, S. C., Doan, J. F., Kannan, H., & Baran, R. W. (2009). Association of insomnia with quality of life, work productivity, and activity impairment. *Quality of Life Research, 18,* 415–422.

Borek, L., Kohn, R., & Friedman, J. (2006). Mood and sleep in Parkinson's disease. *Journal of Clinical Psychiatry, 67,* 958–1005.

Buscemi, N., Vandermeer, B., Friesen, C., et al. (2005). Manifestations and management of chronic insomnia in adults. *Evidence Report/Technology Assessment, 125,* 1–10.

Buysee, D. (2005). Overview of insomnia: Definitions epidemiology, differential diagnosis, and assessment. In Kryger, Roth, &

Dement (Eds.). *Principles and Practice of Sleep Medicine* (4th ed.) (pp. 702–713). Philadelphia: Elsevier Saunders.

Carskadon, M. (2002). Regulation of sleepiness in adolescents: Update, insights, and speculation. *Sleep, 25,* 606–614.

Carskadon, M., & Dement, W. (2005). Normal human sleep: An overview. In Kryger, Roth, & Dement (Eds.). *Principles and Practice of Sleep Medicine* (4th ed.) (pp. 13–23). Philadelphia: Elsevier Saunders.

Cartwright, R. (2005). Dreaming as a mood regulation system. In Kryger, Roth, & Dement (Eds.). *Principles and Practice of Sleep Medicine* (4th ed.) (pp. 565–572). Philadelphia: Elsevier Saunders.

Chervin, R. (2005a). Attention deficit, hyperactivity and sleep disorders. In S. Sheldon, R. Ferber, & M. Kryger (Eds.). *Principles and Practice of Pediatric Sleep Medicine* (4th ed.). Philadelphia: Elsevier Saunders.

———. (2005b). Use of clinical tools and tests in sleep medicine. In Kryger, Roth, & Dement (Eds.). *Principles and Practice of Sleep Medicine* (4th ed.) (pp. 602–614). Philadelphia: Elsevier Saunders.

Clark, F., Azen, S., Zemke, R., et al. (1997). Occupational therapy for independent-living older adults: A randomized controlled trial. *Journal of the American Medical Association, 50,* 1321–1326.

Collier, E., & Skitt, G. (2003). Non-pharmacological interventions for insomnia. *Mental Health Practice, 6,* 29–32.

Collier, E., Skitt, G., & Cutts, H. (2003). A study on the experience of insomnia in a psychiatric inpatient population. *Journal of Psychiatric and Mental Health Health Nursing, 10,* 697–704.

Coren, S. (1996). *Sleep Thieves.* New York: Free Press.

Curcio, G., Ferrara, M., & DeGennaro, L. (2006). Sleep loss, learning capacity and academic performance. *Sleep Medicine Review, 10,* 323–337.

Czeisler, C., Buxton, O., & Khalsa, S. (2005). The human circadian timing system and sleep–wake regulation. In Kryger, Roth, & Dement (Eds.). *Principles and Practice of Sleep Medicine* (4th ed.) (pp. 375–394). Philadelphia: Elsevier Saunders.

Dement, W. (2005). History of sleep physiology and medicine. In Kryger, Roth, & Dement (Eds.). *Principles and Practice of Sleep Medicine* (4th ed.) (pp. 1–12). Philadelphia: Elsevier Saunders.

Dement, W., & Vaughan, C. (1999). *The Promise of Sleep.* New York: Random House.

Dileo, H., Reiter, R., & Taliaferro, D. (2002). Chronobiology, melatonin, and sleep in infants and children. *Pediatric Nursing, 28,* 35–39.

Dinges, D., Rogers, N., & Baynard, M. (2005). Chronic sleep deprivation. In Kryger, Roth, & Dement (Eds.). *Principles and Practice of Sleep Medicine* (4th ed.) (pp. 67–76). Philadelphia: Elsevier Saunders.

Domhoff, G. (2005). The content of dreams: Methodologic and theoretical implications. In Kryger, Roth, & Dement (Eds.). *Principles and Practice of Sleep Medicine* (4th ed.) (pp. 522–554). Philadelphia: Elsevier Saunders.

Douglas, A., Hays, P., Pazderka, F., & Russell, J. (1991). Florid refractory schizophrenias that turn out to be treatable variants of HLA-associated narcolepsy. *Journal of Nervous and Mental Disease, 179,* 12–17.

Dreher, H. (1996). Beyond the stages of sleep: An emerging nursing model of sleep phases. *Holistic Nursing Practice, 10,* 1–11.

Ford, D., & Kamerow, D. (1989). Epidemiologic study of sleep disturbances and psychiatric disorders: An opportunity for prevention? *Journal of American Medical Association, 262,* 1479–1484.

Foster, R. (2006). Poor sleep can accompany schizophrenia. *Science News, 170,* 109.

Gillin, J., Drummond, S., Clark, C., & Moore, P. (2005). Mediation and substance abuse. In Kryger, Roth, & Dement (Eds.). *Principles and Practice of Sleep Medicine* (4th ed.) (pp. 1345–1358). Philadelphia: Elsevier Saunders.

Gupta, S. (2006). Sleeping, snoring and the blues. *Time, 168,* 88.

Haimov, I., Hanuka, E., & Horowitz, Y. (2008). Chronic insomnia and cognitive functioning among older adults. *Behavioral Sleep Medicine, 6,* 32–54.

Hayter, J. (1983). Sleep behaviors of older persons. *Nursing Research, 32,* 242–246.

Hirshkowitz, M., & Smith, P. B. 2004. *Sleep Disorders for Dummies.* New York: Wiley.

Hoch, C. C., & Reynolds, C. F. (1986). Sleep disorders in the elderly and what to do about them. *Geriatric Nursing, 7,* 24–27.

Hofstetter, J., Lysaker, P., & Mayeda, A. (2005). Quality of sleep in patients with schizophrenia in association with quality of life and coping. *BMC Psychiatry, 5,* 13–24.

Jindal, R., Buysee, D., & Thase, M. (2004). Maintenance treatment of insomnia: What can we learn from the depression literature? *American Journal of Psychiatry, 161,* 19–24.

Kantrowitz, B. (2006). The quest for rest. *Newsweek, 147,* 50–56.

Komada, Y., Adachi, N., Matsuura, N., et al. (2009). Irregular sleep habits of parents are associated with increased sleep problems and daytime sleepiness of children. *Tohoku Journal of Experimental Medicine, 219,* 85–89.

Krueger, J., & Majde, J. (2005). Host defense. In Kryger, Roth, & Dement (Eds.). *Principles and Practice of Sleep Medicine* (4th ed.) (pp. 256–265). Philadelphia: Elsevier Saunders.

Kryger, M. (2005). Differential diagnosis of pediatric sleep disorders. In S. Sheldon, R. Ferber, & M. Kryger (Eds.), *Principles and Practice of Pediatric Sleep Medicine* (4th ed.) (pp. 17–25). Philadelphia: Elsevier Saunders.

Kryger, M., Roth, T., & Dement, W. (Eds.). (2005). *Principles and Practice of Sleep Medicine* (4th ed.). Philadelphia: Elsevier Saunders.

Lavigne, G., McMillan, D., & Zucconi, M. (2005). Pain and sleep. In Kryger, Roth, & Dement (Eds.). *Principles and Practice of Sleep Medicine* (4th ed.) (pp. 1246–1255). Philadelphia: Elsevier Saunders.

Lichstein, K., Nau, S., McCrae, C., & Stone, K. (2005). Psychological and behavioral treatments for secondary insomnias. In Kryger, Roth, & Dement (Eds.). *Principles and Practice of Sleep Medicine* (4th ed.) (pp. 738–748). Philadelphia: Elsevier Saunders.

Livingston, G., Blizard, B., & Mann, A. (1993). Does sleep disturbance predict depression in elderly people? A study in inner London. *British Journal of General Practice, 43,* 445–448.

Mahowald, M. (2005). Other parasomnias. In Kryger, Roth, & Dement (Eds.). *Principles and Practice of Sleep Medicine* (4th ed.) (pp. 917–925). Philadelphia: Elsevier Saunders.

Mahowald, M., & Schenck, C. (2005). REM sleep parasomnias. In Kryger, Roth, & Dement (Eds.). *Principles and Practice of Sleep Medicine* (4th ed.) (pp. 897–916). Philadelphia: Elsevier Saunders.

Meyer, A. (1922). The philosophy of occupational therapy. *Archives of Occupational Therapy, 1,* 1–10.

Milter, M., Carskadon, M., & Hirshkowitz, M. (2005). Evaluating sleepiness. In Kryger, Roth, & Dement (Eds.). *Principles and Practice of Sleep Medicine* (4th ed.) (pp. 1417–1423). Philadelphia: Elsevier Saunders.

Monk, T. (2005). Shift work: Basic principles. In Kryger, Roth, & Dement (Eds.). *Principles and Practice of Sleep Medicine* (4th ed.) (pp. 673–679). Philadelphia: Elsevier Saunders.

Monti, J., & Monti, D. (2005). Sleep disturbance in schizophrenia. *International Review of Psychiatry, 17,* 247–253.

Morin, C. (2005). Psychological and behavioral treatments for primary insomnia. In Kryger, Roth, & Dement (Eds.). *Principles and Practice of Sleep Medicine* (4th ed.) (pp. 726–737).

Morin, C. M., Hauri, P. J., Espie, C. A., Spielman, A. J., Buysee. D. J., & Bootzinn, R. R. (1999). Nonpharmacological treatment of chronic insomnia: An Academy of Sleep Medicine Review. *Sleep, 22,* 1134–1356.

Pace-Schott, E. (2005). The neurobiology of dreaming. In Kryger, Roth, & Dement (Eds.). *Principles and Practice of Sleep Medicine* (4th ed.) (pp. 551–564). Philadelphia: Elsevier Saunders.

Petit, D., Montplaisir, J., & Boeve, B. (2005). Alzheimer's disease and other dementias. In Kryger, Roth, & Dement (Eds.). *Principles and*

Practice of Sleep Medicine (4th ed.) (pp. 853–862). Philadelphia: Elsevier Saunders.

Phillips, B. A., Collop, N. A., Drake, C., et al. (2008). Sleep disorders and medical conditions in women. *Journal of Women's Health, 17,* 1191–1199.

Physician's Desk Reference. (2009). PDR (63rd ed.). New York: Thomson Reuters.

Pierce, D. (2001). Occupation by design: Dimensions, therapeutic power and creative process. *American Journal of Occupational Therapy, 55,* 249–249.

Richdale, A., & Prior, M.(1995). The sleep/wake rhythm in children with autism. *European Child and Adolescent Psychiatry, 4,* 175–186.

Rosenblatt, P. (2006). *Two in a Bed: The Social System of Couple Bed Sharing.* Albany, NY: State University of New York Press.

Scheer, F., Cajochen, C., Turek, F., & Czeisler, C. (2005). Melatonin in the regulation of sleep and circadian rhythms. In Kryger, Roth, & Dement (Eds.). *Principles and Practice of Sleep Medicine* (4th ed.) (pp. 395–404). Philadelphia: Elsevier Saunders.

Schwab, R., Kuna, K., & Remmers, J. (2005). Anatomy and physiology of upper airway obstruction. In Kryger, Roth, & Dement, 2005 (Eds.). *Principles and Practice of Sleep Medicine* (4th ed.) (pp. 983–1000). Philadelphia: Elsevier Saunders.

Schweitzer, P. (2005). Drugs that disturb sleep and wakefulness. In Kryger, Roth, & Dement (Eds.). *Principles and Practice of Sleep Medicine* (4th ed.) (pp. 499–518). Philadelphia: Elsevier Saunders.

Scott, A. H. (1999). Wellness works: Community service health promotion groups led by occupational therapy students. *American Journal of Occupational Therapy, 53,* 566–574.

Sheldon, S. (2005). Sleep-related enuresis. In S. Sheldon, R. Ferber, & M. Kryger (Eds.). *Principles and Practice of Pediatric Sleep Medicine* (4th ed.) (pp. 293–304). Philadelphia: Elsevier Saunders.

Siegel, J. (2005). REM sleep. In Kryger, Roth, & Dement (Eds.). *Principles and Practice of Sleep Medicine* (4th ed.) (pp. 120–135). Philadelphia: Elsevier Saunders.

Stein, M., & Mellman, T. (2005). Anxiety disorders. In Kryger, Roth, & Dement (Eds.). *Principles and Practice of Sleep Medicine* (4th ed.), (pp. 1297–1310). Philadelphia: Elsevier Saunders.

Stickgold, R. (2005). Why we dream. In Kryger, Roth, & Dement (Eds.). *Principles and Practice of Sleep Medicine* (4th ed.) (pp. 579–587). Philadelphia: Elsevier Saunders.

Thorpy, M. (2005). Classification of sleep disorders. In Kryger, Roth, & Dement (Eds.). *Principles and Practice of Sleep Medicine* (4th ed.) (pp. 615–625). Philadelphia: Elsevier Saunders.

Tikotzky, L., De Marcas, G., Har-Toov, J., Dollberg, S., Bar-Haim, Y., & Sadeh, A. (2010). Sleep and physical growth in infants during the first 6 months. *Sleep Research, 19*(1), 103–110.

Trenkwalder, C. (2005). Parkinsonism. In Kryger, Roth, & Dement (Eds.). *Principles and Practice of Sleep Medicine* (4th ed.) (pp. 801–810).

Turek, F., Dugovic, C., & Laposky, A. (2005). Master circadian clock, master circadian rhythm. In Kryger, Roth, & Dement (Eds.). *Principles and Practice of Sleep Medicine* (4th ed.) (pp. 318–320). Philadelphia: Elsevier Saunders.

Van Dongen, H., & Dinges, D. (2005). Circadian rhythms in sleepiness, alertness, and performance. In Kryger, Roth, & Dement (Eds.). *Principles and Practice of Sleep Medicine* (4th ed.) (pp. 435–443). Philadelphia: Elsevier Saunders.

Wade, A. (2006). Sleep problems in depression: How do they impact treatment and recovery? *International Journal of Psychiatry in Clinical Practice, 10,* 38–44.

Walsh, J., Dement, W., & Dinges, D. (2005). Sleep medicine, public policy and public health. In Kryger, Roth, & Dement (Eds.). *Principles and Practice of Sleep Medicine* (4th ed.) (pp. 648–656). Philadelphia: Elsevier Saunders.

Weissman, M. M., Greenwald, S., Nino-Murcia, G., & Dement, M. D. (1997). The morbidity of insomnia uncomplicated by psychiatric disorders. *General Hospital Psychiatry, 19,* 247–250.

Wolfson, A., & Lee, K. (2005). Pregnancy and the postpartum period. In Kryger, Roth, & Dement (Eds.). *Principles and Practice of Sleep Medicine* (4th ed.) (pp. 1278–1286). Philadelphia: Elsevier Saunders.

World Health Organization. (2004). WHO technical meeting on sleep and health. Presented in Bonn, Germany January 22–24.

Xianchen, L. (2006). Sleep and youth suicidal behavior; a neglected field. *Current Opinion in Psychiatry, 19,* 288–293.

Spiritual Occupation

Emily Schulz

> "You will find as you look back upon your life that the moments when you have truly lived are the moments when you have done things in the spirit of love.
> —Henry Drummond, Scottish Evangelist and Scientist, 1851–1897

Introduction

This chapter explores the nature and clinical use of spiritual occupation, especially as experienced by persons who live with serious mental illness. First, spiritual occupation is described and defined, followed by an examination of how people engage in spiritual occupation across the life span. Several assessments that touch upon spiritual aspects are briefly presented, followed by a discussion of intervention models and techniques relative to application of the spiritual in mental health practice. To appreciate the full person-environment-occupation perspective, refer to Chapter 31, which contains content related to the spiritual dimension of the person (both therapist and client) and the environment within which therapy is provided. Those occupations that provide meaning and purpose in one's life that likely have an impact on the experience of mental health recovery are highlighted in this chapter.

Description of Spiritual Occupation

Many readers may be wondering what is meant by the term *spiritual* and whether or not spiritual is synonymous with religion. Although for some people, religion may mean the same thing as spirituality, other individuals may not be religious but may still consider themselves to be spiritual. From that perspective, therefore, spirituality is a broader term that can include the concept of religion (Thoresen, 1998).

A definition of **spirituality** for occupational therapy has been developed on the basis of a literature review from helping professions, including occupational therapy: "Experiencing a meaningful connection to our core self, others, the world, and/or a Greater Power, as expressed through our reflections, narratives, and actions" (Schulz, 2002, p. 4). **Connectedness** in spirituality can be conceptualized as having a vertical element (a greater power, such as the Divine, values, and/or beliefs) and a horizontal element (self, others, and the world) (Ross, 1995; Schulz, 2008), as is seen in Figure 54.1. Spirituality involves that which uplifts the spirit, affirms life, and generates positive and loving connections (Hawkins, 2002).

This concept of connectedness and uplifting spirit may, for some individuals, play a role in mental health and wellbeing.

Occupational therapists promoting recovery-oriented programs in mental health and substance abuse should consider spiritual occupations as a potential source of healing. They should also consider that for persons struggling with past harmful relationships, finding a meaningful way to disconnect with sources of distress and abuse may be helpful to their spiritual wellbeing. **Spiritual occupation** encompasses the expressive aspect of spirituality, which is brought forth and made outwardly apparent through a being's reflections, narratives, and actions (Schulz, 2008). Reflections may include such spiritual occupations as introspection, contemplation, intuition, logical thinking, prayer, and meditation—any process that occurs within the individual relative to meaningful connections (positive, loving, life affirming) to a greater power, self, others, and the world.

Narratives involve storytelling through the read, written, or spoken word and depict the inner spiritual workings of a being when shared by others. Spiritual occupation in the form of narratives can be inspiring, healing, and uplifting in nature. The sacred texts and scriptures from different religions are one example; witnessing about a religious, spiritual, or positive life experience is another; and the use of prose or poetry to inspire and uplift or bring clarity to a situation is still another. This text incorporates first-person narratives in The Lived Experience feature as a means of conveying the lived experience of persons with psychiatric disability and mental health recovery. The variety of narratives in this text and in the mental health literature overall promotes an appreciation for narrative writing and journaling as a spiritual occupation.

The manner in which individuals tell stories about their lives and about others is very powerful and shows others what kind of spiritual connectedness those individuals are experiencing at that moment. Do the individuals who are sharing stories tell them with integrity? Do their words match their actions, or do they say one thing and do another? Do they use words as a weapon or as a healing balm? Again, the level to which the spiritual occupation of narratives is used to uplift, affirm, and generate positive loving connections to a greater power, self, others, and the world indicates where the speaker or writer is in his or her spirituality. Occupational therapists who focus on understanding the

Three Dimensional Spirituality Model

The Mystery that is Spirituality

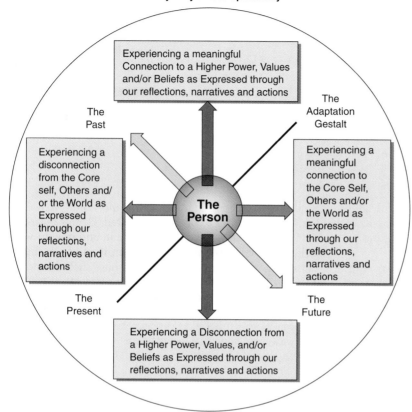

Experiencing a meaningful Connection to a Higher Power, Values and/or Beliefs as Expressed through our reflections, narratives and actions

The Past

The Adaptation Gestalt

Experiencing a disconnection from the Core self, Others and/or the World as Expressed through our reflections, narratives and actions

The Person

Experiencing a meaningful connection to the Core Self, Others and/or the World as Expressed through our reflections, narratives and actions

The Present

The Future

Experiencing a Disconnection from a Higher Power, Values, and/or Beliefs as Expressed through our reflections, narratives and actions

FIGURE 54-1. Three-dimensional spirituality model. Connectedness in spirituality can be conceptualized as having a vertical element (a greater power such as the Divine, values, and/or beliefs) and a horizontal element (self, others, and the world). *Adapted with permission from Schulz, E. (2008). OT-Quest assessment. In B. J. Hemphill-Pearson (Ed.), Assessments in Occupational Therapy Mental Health: An Integrative Approach (pp. 263–289). Thorofare, NJ: Slack.*

spiritual nature of the persons they serve and the occupations that reflect their spiritual values and beliefs can provide guidance as to how these practices might be incorporated into everyday routines that enhance their state of mental and spiritual wellbeing.

Spiritual occupation in the form of actions is the most outward and visible sign of the spiritual process of experiencing meaningful connectedness to self, others, the world and greater power, occurring within the individual. There are several examples of spiritual occupations in the form of actions described in this chapter; however, the ones mentioned are only a minute portion of the infinite possible spiritual occupations in which one can engage.

The Occupational Therapy Practice Framework (AOTA, 2008) recognizes that people engage in **religious observances** ("an organized system of beliefs, practices, rituals, and symbols designed to facilitate closeness to the sacred or transcendent"; Moreira-Almeida & Koenig, 2006, p. 844) as well as in occupations that give their lives meaning, more broadly reflected in values, beliefs, and spirituality. Simply put, **spiritual occupations** are those reflections, narratives, and actions that are meaningful, uplifting to the spirit, that affirm life, and that generate positive and loving connections to a greater power, self, others, and/or the world. When spiritual occupations are part of a person's daily routines, they can be understood as important to his or her sense of wellbeing and can contribute to a person's recovery process.

Spiritual Occupation Across the Life Span

Spiritual occupations that occur across the life span, from an individual perspective, are as varied as the individuals who engage in them. For individuals, spiritual occupations may

PhotoVoice

The Bedtime Prayer Cross
This is how I get through each day and night to have and maintain a successful life. It gives me balance in my life that makes me feel comfortable and under control. When I look at the cross I am hopeful I will get through the tough times too.

—Grady

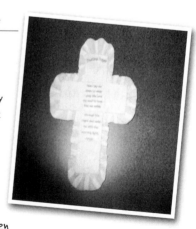

or may not involve religious content. Depending on the level of meaning of the activity for the person, examples of developmentally appropriate spiritual occupations not related to religion could include a child playing, an adolescent raking leaves for a neighbor who needs assistance, an adult cooking a meal for a loved one, and an elderly person volunteering at a homeless shelter.

From a group or community-level perspective, most cultures and religions typically have rituals that mark certain milestones in life. An exhaustive description of each and every religious and cultural ritual and tradition is beyond the scope of this chapter. However, generally speaking, many cultural and religious traditions have some kind of ceremony or ritual that involves welcoming a child or newcomer into the family/community, a coming-of-age ceremony, a marriage ceremony, and burial traditions. These ceremonies mark the natural flow of human life and are imbued with meaning for the groups involved. They are spiritual occupations that take place at a group or community level rather than at an individual level.

Holidays are also spiritual occupations that occur at the community level (Luboshitzky & Gaber, 2001). It has been suggested that spiritual occupations that occur in groups are considered to be highly therapeutic (Wilding, 2007). For persons who live with serious mental illness and their families, their ability to engage in these significant spiritual occupations may also have been affected by the course of their condition. In facilitating the recovery process, restoring spiritual occupations may also expand potential sources of support through a spiritual community.

Assessments

The most well-known occupational therapy assessment that includes a spiritual component to it is the Canadian Occupational Performance Measure (COPM) (Law et al, 2005). This assessment has been well researched with a variety of populations. It includes spirituality as part of the major life areas in which people engage. As such, the COPM helps to ameliorate the potential awkwardness that some therapists may feel about broaching the topic of spirituality with clients (Engquist, Short-DeGraff, Gliner, & Oltenbruns, 1997). The COPM is designed to identify those areas of life that the person is interested in changing and measures aspects of performance and satisfaction in one's life at varied time intervals appropriate to the goals and setting.

Another assessment tool designed specifically to address the issue of spirituality in occupational therapy practice is the OT-Quest (Occupational Therapy Quality of Experience and Spirituality Assessment Tool). This assessment, developed by the author of this chapter, obtains both qualitative and quantitative information regarding the spirituality of the person completing it. To date, only one research study has been conducted of this tool (Schulz, 2008); therefore, more research regarding its reliability and validity as well as its effectiveness in the clinic is warranted. Details regarding the OT-Quest, how to use it and score it, and how to write goals with the information gained from it and from the research are published elsewhere (Schulz, 2008). The lived experience narratives in this chapter use a number of the questions asked in the OT-Quest as a means of eliciting information shared in the narratives. In addition, the exercises at the end of this chapter provide reflective activities to gain awareness of personal spiritual experiences.

Intervention Models and Techniques

A three-dimensional model of spirituality for use in guiding clinical reasoning in occupational therapy practice has been developed and is described in detail elsewhere (Schulz, 2008). The model is based on the definition of spirituality described earlier in this chapter. According to the model, spirituality includes three dimensions: a vertical element related to connectedness to a greater power, values, and beliefs; a horizontal element related to connectedness to self, others, and the world (Ross, 1995); and a third element of time (Smith, 1992). Figure 54-1 provides a visual representation of this model.

The spirituality of a being appears to evolve, change, and grow over time, influenced by life experiences and the individual's adaptive responses to challenges that are experienced across the life span (Schulz, 2002). The concept of time includes the notion of past, present, and future (linear time) as well as the historical and cultural context in which the person lives.

When addressing spirituality and using spiritual occupation in occupational therapy practice, the therapist begins by gaining clarity about his or her own spiritual process. Once clear about his or her spirituality, the therapist is freed up to be in a state of unconditional positive regard with his or her clients' spirituality.

A necessary therapeutic skill needed in any intervention, but especially when addressing the highly personal area of spirituality and using spiritual occupation with a client, is the ability to view the client with unconditional positive regard (Rogers, 1951). Unconditional positive regard for the client is required of the therapist regardless of whether or

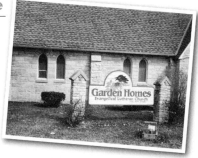

PhotoVoice

This picture is that of a church I attended. The church reminds me of the days when I sort of liked going to church. Now that I'm 53 years old I really don't like to go to church. The reason church was ok with me as a child is I felt better when I was young. I guess I fear God and he is a mystery to me. This is something I'm still working on.

The Lived Experience

Two narratives follow to provide a gender-balanced perspective regarding spiritual occupation and to demonstrate that everyone's spiritual path and thus the spiritual occupations in which they engage are entirely unique to each individual. Each person is at a different place with his or her spirituality, and each person has a completely personal and distinctive spiritual journey. Thus, some of what is shared in these two narratives may resonate with the reader, and some may not. It does not matter whether or not the therapist holds the same view as a client; what matters is whether or not the therapist can be unconditionally accepting of a perspective different from his or her own.

The questions that were used to elicit these narratives are based on Schulz's (2008) three-dimensional model of spirituality. After The Seeker and The Knower answered the questions, they devised some spiritual goals based on their responses, in collaboration with the author, and those goals follow each narrative.

The Seeker

The writer of this narrative is a female in her early 50s. She is a wife, mother of three children, and a professor. In this narrative, she describes how a profoundly tragic personal loss spurred her on to begin seeking spiritual answers—thus, she is referred to as "The Seeker."

Q: What are the most important underlying beliefs or values which guide your life?
A: That life is no accident. I was placed (or chose) to be on this earth for a purpose. Everything that happens is part of a divine plan.

Q: How, if at all, do you establish and maintain a relationship with the Divine in your life?
A: Constant dialog. I do a lot of activities that require little thinking, so during these times, I am constantly reflecting, questioning, and communicating with the divine.

Q: How do your beliefs/values influence the way in which you connect to yourself?
A: God don't make 'em better than me! Really, I believe that I was given what I needed to do what I was put here to do. By doing, the meaning helps me in the direction I am supposed to go. Meaning comes from the divine.

Q: What activities do you do to maintain a positive relationship with yourself?
A: Anything creative. I find out about myself, accept myself, and love myself through creative activities.

Q: How do your beliefs/values influence the way in which you connect to other beings?
A: I don't judge as harshly. I listen and accept. Walk away if they bring me pain. Embrace them if they are struggling also.

Q: What activities do you do to maintain a positive relationship with other beings?
A: Creative stuff and interaction with plants and animals. I find acceptance and love in these activities and therefore have the ability to give it.

Q: How do your beliefs/values influence the way in which you connect to the world (society, nature, the planet, the universe)?
A: Don't sweat the small stuff: it's all small stuff. From a universal perspective, the only thing that will count in the long run is how we treat others and deal with the challenges of life. Everything else will pass away.

Q: What activities do you do to maintain a positive relationship with the world (society, nature, planet, and universe)?
A: Actually, I am finding that energy work does this for me. I am trying to evolve to the level of "seeing" energy. The more I do this or energy therapy, the more connected I feel to the world around me.

Q: Describe a challenge that you have recently experienced in your life.
A: My son took his own life. He died in my arms. None of us saw this coming. He was the image of my beloved father. He was a source of great pride. Living with this and all of the facets of this loss is a daily exercise.

Q: How, if at all, did a creative process help you to get through that challenge?
A: At first, the creative process was lost along with so much else. That was real scary. I did not realize one could lose that. Ever so slowly, it began to reemerge as I found myself surrounded by physical ugliness (90-year-old house). First, I was driven to carve a mantle with a Dremel. Quite a mess, but a good outlet for anger and demanding concrete creativity. Next, a dark, dirty hall was made lighter. A sky was painted on the ceiling. Symbolic maybe? The toughest was a trump l'oeil on built-in cabinets. I cried as I struggled with this. It used to be so easy. But persistence paid off and each cabinet door was a little easier. By this time, I was well enough to start searching for answers. Reading was interspersed with fabric art. (My spouse sensed a need and surprised me with a new sewing machine.) I now have a room (totally remodeled) for my creative area.

Q: How, if at all, did a spiritual process help you to get through that challenge?
A: I don't feel it did as such. My spirituality underwent a phase transition. It became different as I struggled to survive.

Q: In what ways, if at all, were the creative process and the spiritual process linked for you?
A: The creative process opened me up to connect with the divine. During the periods of high creativity, I felt peace. My soul could rest. Seeking a connection with the divine has become a necessary part of my life balance.

Q: In what ways, if at all, did you use inner reflection to get through that challenge? (Examples are introspection, contemplation, logical thinking, intuition, meditation, prayer.)
A: Inner reflection was a double-edged sword. Trying to answer why. At the same time, some of the answers were very painful. Again, I would logically go through all of the facts as I knew them over his lifetime and try to make sense. Then I would scream out at God for allowing this to happen. Then I would tell myself that there had to be a reason and I would find it. Prayer is useless when the pain is so great and you are mad as hell at the divine. Meditation just made you dwell on it more. Logical pursuit of the question gave me a focus and direction.

The Lived Experience—cont'd

Q: *In what ways, if at all, did you use narratives (storytelling through the read, written, or spoken word) to get through that challenge?*

A: *In the beginning, when you are still too numb to think, the written word provided basic information. I used this information as a reference point until I was able to function at a higher level.*

Q: *In what ways, if at all, did you take action to get through that challenge?*

A: *I realized when I was at my best and worst and made the decision to position myself where the less pain was. This was pure survival. I did it without regard to family. They were still paralyzed and could not make any changes. I was going under for the third time. Fortunately, they trusted and loved me enough they followed my lead.*

Q: *Given where you have come from and where you are now in your life, where would you like to be in the future relative to your relationship to the Divine, yourself, other beings, and the world?*

A: *I want to support others. Way too much pain in this world to handle it ourselves. We need each other. I want to be more in sync with the divine. Be more sensitive to this universal energy that makes us all one. More evolved spiritually.*

Goals

1. Life balance: Activities in all areas of life will make room for a creativity element. On a frequent basis (at least once a week), infuse creativity to a part of the day.
2. Connectivity: Spiritual connectivity to others will be a focus of interaction. Consciously setting the ego aside in interactions (at least once a week) will be a key factor in this. Consciously saying "I am not going to judge this person during this interaction, I am going to try to meet them where they are."
3. Energy sensitivity: Evolution of the ability to "see" the energy around me in all living things. Practice doing so by quieting the mind, quieting the soul, softening the eyes, and looking in the negative spaces or between forms at least 10–15 minutes a week.
4. Responsibility to the next generation: Mentoring and teaching those on the same path as opportunities present, such as giving a class, offering a presentation or workshop, offering energy work as needed.

The Knower

The narrative writer is a male in his early 60s. He is a husband, father of 3 children, and a social activist. In this narrative, he describes his spiritual beliefs and how those beliefs—which stem from a deep place of knowing for him—permeate and guide every aspect of his life. Thus, he is referred to as "The Knower."

Q: *What are the most important underlying beliefs or values which guide your life?*

A: *Simply put, the guiding principle which guides my life is "what goes around comes around." I believe that karma*

is at work both in our individual and collective experiences and that we create our reality based on how we think, and feel and breathe life into our thoughts and feelings (if that makes any sense). I also believe that values must be lived, and the extent to which I am able to align my lifestyle with my ideals (that which I value) will I achieve a sense of satisfaction, fulfillment, and peace and produce karmic patterns that are in support of my intentions and goals in life. I feel that I am somehow "hard wired" to act on my beliefs, and it is through this "breathing life in to them" that they become real to me. Action is the heart and soul of my belief system. I am guided by the belief that everyone's beliefs matter, but those that matter most are those which are acted upon, so it is incumbent that we take seriously the challenge to make our beliefs living realities. And I am also driven by the desire to make my life speak a certain truth that is ever evolving and focused on the advancement of my understanding of how things work in the universe.

Q: *How, if at all, do you establish and maintain a relationship with the Divine in your life?*

A: *The Divine becomes present in my life when an ideal is acted upon through life choices, particularly those that require sacrifice and risk. When I find myself giving form to an idea, concept, or vision, I am filled with a sense of divine purpose. "Give it form" the divine whispers in my ear. Don't just believe in something . . . live it, dance with it, sacrifice for it, experiment with it, turn it on its ear, then listen to it. There are countless ways of experiencing the Divine that are available to me, but actualizing a vision is how I am accustomed to sensing the Divine in my life. Dream it, then create it. Then watch it evolve.*

Q: *How do your beliefs/values influence the way in which you connect to yourself?*

A: *My sense of self is connected primarily to actualizing beliefs I hold, thus the chief connection I have with myself is value-based. When I have a notion about something that makes sense to me, I have to make it real by giving it form. And because I'm at the Peace Abbey 7 days a week, I find like any good gardener, a desire to keep planting those crops that best take root in the soil, climate, and general conditions of the plot of earth I'm given. The Peace Abbey is a garden for goodness and that which grows best is that which is rooted in altruism. No question about that.*

Q: *What activities do you do to maintain a positive relationship with yourself?*

A: *Meditation, recitation of the prayers for peace of the world's religions and poetry, and rearranging objects, pictures, assembling symbols in a room to produce a certain feeling that generate a particular mood or message that conveys a certain truth I am feeling gives me enormous positive feelings and feedback. My surroundings are easels that I imbue meaning on and through the re-creating of a space, room, building, memorial, I establish a positive relationship with self, and by extension, others. The saying "what is within surrounds us" is so true . . . and*

Continued

The Lived Experience—cont'd

I must, if I'm to be happy, well-adjusted, and fulfilled, continually create environments that reflect my beliefs and values, dreams and aspirations for a better world.

Q: How do your beliefs/values influence the way in which you connect to other beings?

A: Because who I am is so visible and public through the environments (programs, projects, organizations) I create, it both encourages and hinders my social life. While most people hold certain beliefs that may or may not be endorsed by those around them, they are nevertheless, by comparison, somewhat hidden.

Q: What activities do you do to maintain a positive relationship with other beings?

A: Working on issues of peace, social justice, animal rights, and veganism are among the most important shared activities with others.

Q: How do your beliefs/values influence the way in which you connect to the world (society, nature, the planet, the universe)?

A: I believe in democratic socialism because I hold that there is enough for everyone so long as the system doesn't overly reward a few at the expense of others. The vegan life style is my chosen path because it leaves a smaller "foot print" on the planet, is more nurturing and thoughtful, compassionate and loving.

Q: What activities do you do to maintain a positive relationship with the world (society, nature, planet, and universe)?

A: Everything listed on the Peace Abbey Web page (www.peaceabbey.org) is how I go about maintaining a positive relationship with the world around me. The most fulfilling is participating in Stonewalk. [Author's note: Some of the Peace Abbey programs include the Peace Seeds, City Care program, Solidarity Bread, Morning Meeting, and Stonewalk; since they are clear examples of spiritual occupations involving connecting to others or connecting to the world.]

Q: Describe a challenge that you have recently experienced in your life.

A: Dealing with the ongoing financial difficulties of the Peace Abbey is the biggest test of my beliefs and values.

Q: How, if at all, did a creative process help you to get through that challenge?

A: The creative process is the most essential aspect of my journey because I am most comfortable experimenting with my life. I like to imagine ways for peace to be furthered, and then creatively implement them through a program or project. Since the life blood of all such undertaking is funding, validating a more authentic response to the funding requirements of an organization like the Peace Abbey is the most creative thing I can do with my life. It is as important as the very programs that seek funding.

Q: How, if at all, did a spiritual process help you to get through that challenge?

A: The notion of "experimentation," which by its very nature is spiritual (doing something that either doesn't make complete sense by conventional thinking, hasn't been done before, or is deemed too improbable), helps me meet the challenge of the Abbey's financial difficulties. I resonate with the poem "The Road Not Taken" by Robert Frost, as well as the saying from George Bernard Shaw that Bobby Kennedy recited in his stump speeches: "Some men see things as they are and say 'why?' I dream of things that never were and say 'why not?'" I am drawn to approaches to problem solving that are more dependent on serendipity, chance, synchronicity than focus-grouped, scientifically proven ways of meeting a particular challenge.

Q: In what ways, if at all, were the creative process and the spiritual process linked for you?

A: I have found that there is nothing as creative as that which is spiritual for it draws on elements of the human psyche that are endlessly connected to everything that has existed, does exist, and will exist. Sensing this on a deep intuitive level enables me to remain secure and steadfast. I think that this understanding, while spiritual in nature, is the biggest source of my creativity. Through meditation, prayer, visualization, and activist pacifism, a steady flow of spiritual creativity surfaces that keeps me energized and focused.

Q: In what ways, if at all, did you use inner reflection to get through that challenge? (Examples are introspection, contemplation, logical thinking, intuition, meditation, prayer.)

A: As much as anything, my vision is furthered by meditation and seeking to live my life as a form of prayer. I like seeing my life as a prayer because it requires an intuitive understanding of praxis. Putting belief into action.

Q: In what ways, if at all, did you use narratives (storytelling through the read, written or spoken word) to get through that challenge?

A: As I tell people who visit the Abbey about our struggle to "attract" funding rather than "asking for support," I am encouraged by the sheer logic and nobility of trusting in human nature versus fine-tuning a fundraising appeal. I find that storytelling, sharing example after example of people stepping forward to "offer" rather than having to be "asked," provides an opportunity for me to better understand the dynamics at work when people come from that deep place of personal giving. The more I tell of people like the two anonymous contributors, the more I believe in human goodness and the worthiness of my path in life.

Q: In what ways, if at all, did you take action to get through that challenge?

A: Interestingly, the path of action that I took appeared to be non-action, though it was putting my beliefs in action by not acting or not fundraising. Sort of the Zen of fundraising . . . allowing people to rise to the occasion versus making them feel obligated in some way.

Q: Given where you have come from and where you are now in your life, where would you like to be in the future relative to your relationship to the Divine, yourself, other beings, and the world?

A: The future that matters most is one that has me staying on track with my vision wherever that leads. And my

The Lived Experience—cont'd

vision, such as it is, requires a willingness to sacrifice and risk because what I believe in is out of synch with the way the world is at present. My world, however, is totally a reflection of my vision of how the world could be, should be.

Goals

1. Life balance: Be involved with people whom you admire but are not doing the same kind of work and see how they refresh their energy (i.e., what books they read, movies/plays they see, food they eat, recreation they enjoy). On a frequent basis (at least once a week) break from the routine that has defined your life and see how the quality of life might be enhanced by doing activities that you are in sync with but might not have engaged in for a period of time or have never done before. (Example for The Knower: Go to a country western concert, since you avoid that genre of music.)
2. Connectivity: Volunteer to serve, in an acceptable capacity, in an organization that you may be in disagreement with (Examples for The Knower: Republican State Committee, Beef Growers Association, National Rifle Association) and seek to better understand those dynamics within the lives of their members that provide insight into their humanity and explore the commonality that exists between you and them. Without compromising the integrity of your life, step into the shoes of others and see why the shoe fits for others without judging them (at least once a month).

3. Energy sensitivity: Be aware of how attitudes and perceptions change the energy field around you and others, and as a result, hinder your ability to be sensitive to what you and others really need. Strive to take an extra moment to "read" the nuances of body language, facial expressions, mannerisms, et cetera, as they can be more useful than the spoken word when it comes to appreciating the energy they are personally experiencing within their bodies and imagine what the typical response might be in return from those around them. Do this intentionally as often as you can (at least once a week) without being judgmental but sensitive to the life experiences they're creating energetically. Come to appreciate the "feeling tone" around relationships, both positive and negative.
4. Responsibility to one's ideals: Like the flow of the Tao, allow the passion of your life to sweeten with rest and activity. "Staying on track" presumes I'm staying on the same train, which may or may not be the case. Explore other ways of living your ideals besides your current approach. While staying true to your dream, allow your dream to be reinvented from time to time in ways you're not accustomed to or necessarily comfortable with. Expand your comfort zone (at least once a week). (Example for The Knower: Visit a Harley Davidson store and engage people in nonpolitical conversation and learn from those you rarely get to meet.)

---

not the client's spiritual perspective is in accordance with the therapist's own viewpoint. **Unconditional positive regard** involves having a sincere, nonjudgmental acceptance of another being and his or her viewpoint while still maintaining the integrity of one's own perspective. for example, a Jewish occupational therapist is tasked with developing a creative solution to the problem of a Catholic nun who wants to hold her rosary in her painful arthritic hands while she prays. The Jewish occupational therapist does not suddenly become Catholic, nor does the Catholic nun suddenly become Jewish, merely because they are in a therapy session together. Neither tries to convert the other to his or her own belief system. Nor does the Jewish therapist express, verbally or nonverbally, any irritation or judgment regarding the Catholic nun's religious beliefs simply because they differ from his own. Rather, the Jewish therapist, while still maintaining his own beliefs, respectfully facilitates the Catholic nun's desired spiritual occupation of using the rosary.

Another important point for therapists to remember is that clients may be in a state of distress when receiving therapy; that is, something traumatic and challenging may have occurred in their lives that prompted therapy. Therefore, as a therapist, it is important to be in a strong mental, emotional, and spiritual state before engaging others in therapy. One of the strengths of using spirituality and spiritual occupations therapeutically is that positive mental and emotional states are fostered by them. The combination of one's own skillful therapeutic use of self, use of unconditional positive regard, peaceful and steady mental/emotional state, and

spiritual occupations will go a long way toward helping clients in distress be able to engage in therapy and begin the process of recovery.

After addressing the therapist's own spiritual process, what spiritual occupations might be pursued with the client? The therapist should always take the client's lead on this. For example, if the client's religious or spiritual background is different from that of the therapist, the therapist can ask the client to share some information about spiritual occupations or religious rituals that are meaningful to the client. The therapist can also research the client's religion or spiritual path to become informed about it and better serve the client. The client is the expert in his or her own spirituality and spiritual occupations. However, most people will not openly share this type of information unless they are asked. The COPM is a good assessment tool to use to elicit such information (Law et al, 2005).

Once the therapist has a clear understanding of the spiritual occupations, religious and/or secular rituals that hold meaning for the client, the next step is to assist the client to incorporate them into his or her routines in an effort to enhance mental health recovery and life. Depending on the client's state and circumstances, doing so may involve scheduling time for the client to be able to engage in the chosen spiritual occupations as well as modifying the environment and/or the occupational form for them to do so. For example, helping a woman coping with depression reengage in daily mass attendance might begin by determining if a close friend who is a member of that

Evidence-Based Practice

Koenig (2008) reports that religious involvement is often used to cope with stress as well as mental and physical health problems. It is associated with a reduction in psychological distress, lessens depression, and enhances mental health recovery. Positive emotions, including hope, happiness, optimism, and higher quality of life are all associated with religious involvement. Koenig advocates for physicians and other health professionals to identify the religious or spiritual practices of their clients so that their health-promoting activities can be incorporated into their overall plan for health.

➤ Occupational therapy practitioners should identify the spiritual occupations the person reports as effective coping strategies that are important to him or her.

➤ Asking about what provides meaning and purpose in the individual's life will give clues as to daily occupations that can be incorporated into a plan for healthy living.

Koenig, H. G. (2008). *How Religious Beliefs and Practices Are Related to Stress, Health and Medical Services.* Paper presented at a Heritage Foundation Symposium, December 3, 2008. Available at: http://www.hoje.org.br/site/arq/artigos/How_Religious_Beliefs_and_Practices_Are_Related.pdf (accessed October 24, 2009).

person's spiritual community could pick up and accompany her to mass. Helping a man with bipolar disorder return to his status as an elder in his church once he has overcome a manic episode might be an important resumption of role performance and community connectedness. Incorporating time and place for quiet reflection and meditation in the early morning and prior to going to bed at nighttime might facilitate a sense of stability and serve as a calming occupation for a person overcoming an anxiety disorder.

Summary

This chapter provides a framework for understanding the spiritual nature of persons and several tools to determine the ways engagement in spiritual occupation might bring about a sense of purpose and meaning. Based on an unconditional positive regard for the individual and his or her spiritual beliefs and practices, the therapist works with the person with mental illness to promote a positive state of spirituality through engagement in chosen spiritual occupations.

Active Learning Strategies

1. Connectedness to the Self

Whenever a therapist plans to apply spirituality in practice or use spiritual occupation as an intervention, it is useful to first know his or her own spiritual path and level of comprehension regarding the nature of spiritual occupation. In essence, the therapist must connect with and understand his or her personal spirituality before attempting to use it clinically. Respond in writing to the following questions (based on the three-dimensional model of spirituality).

Reflective Questions

- What are the most important underlying beliefs or values that guide your life?
- How, if at all, do you establish and maintain a relationship with the Divine in your life?
- How do your beliefs/values influence the way you connect to yourself?
- What activities do you do to maintain a positive relationship with yourself?
- How do your beliefs/values influence the way you connect to other beings?
- What activities do you do to maintain a positive relationship with other beings?
- How do your beliefs/values influence the way you connect to the world (society, nature, the planet, the universe)?
- What activities do you do to maintain a positive relationship with the world?
- Describe a challenge that you have recently experienced in your life.

- How, if at all, did a creative process help you to get through that challenge?
- How, if at all, did a spiritual process help you to get through that challenge?
- In what ways, if at all, were the creative process and the spiritual process linked for you?
- In what ways, if at all, did you use inner reflection (introspection, contemplation, logical thinking, intuition, meditation, prayer) to get through that challenge?
- In what ways, if at all, did you use narratives (storytelling through the read, written, or spoken word) to get through that challenge?
- In what ways, if at all, did you take action to get through that challenge?
- Given where you have come from and where you are now in your life, where would you like to be in the future relative to your relationship to the Divine, yourself, other beings, and the world?

 Use your **Reflective Journal** to document your thoughts about your spiritual self.

2. Creating Goals

After completing exercise 1, write four goals for yourself based on your responses to the 16 questions. You may include the categories brought forth by "The Seeker" and "The Knower" in the chapter narratives (life balance, connectivity, energy sensitivity, responsibility to the next generation, and responsibility to one's ideals) or create your own personally relevant categories, or use a combination thereof.

Document your goals in your
Reflective Journal.

3. Applying Spiritual Occupation
in Practice

a. Imagine you are the occupational therapist for The Seeker, as she has been admitted to the inpatient psychiatric hospital where you work for severe depression after her son's death. (Although this did not actually happen to the narrative writer, it is certainly a possible scenario for other parents experiencing the loss of a child.) Examine the perspective of the The Seeker and compare it with your own. Identify the ways in which your perspectives coincide and the ways in which they clash. What will you do to prepare yourself to be in a state of unconditional positive regard with her during therapy? Give examples and be specific.

b. Look again at The Seeker's spiritual occupations mentioned in her narrative and goals. Make a list of the ones that are unfamiliar to you. Choose one to explore further, and write down your findings. Give examples and be specific.

c. Based on The Seeker's narrative, identify which spiritual occupations you would employ with her in therapy, and explain why. Give examples and be specific.

d. Imagine that you are the occupational therapist for The Knower. He also has been admitted to the inpatient psychiatric hospital where you work for severe depression after losing his Peace Abbey due to financial insolvency. (Although this did not happen to the narrative writer, it is a potential scenario for someone who loses his or her life's work for any reason.) Examine the perspective of the The Knower and compare it with your own. Identify the ways in which your perspectives coincide and the ways in which they clash. What will you do to prepare yourself to be in a state of unconditional positive regard with him during therapy? Give examples and be specific.

e. Look again at The Knower's spiritual occupations mentioned in his narrative and goals. Make a list of the ones that are unfamiliar to you. Choose one to explore further, and write down your findings. Give examples and be specific.

f. Based on The Knower's narrative, identify which spiritual occupations you would use with him as an intervention, and explain why. Give examples and be specific.

g. Imagine that you are an occupational therapist running a support group for persons with severe depression in an outpatient mental health clinic. The Seeker and The Knower are two of the people in your group of six clients. Knowing what you do about them, what kinds of spiritual occupations could you address in a group setting that would be therapeutic for them and the rest of the group? Give examples and be specific.

Resources

- Peace Abbey, a multifaith retreat center. http://www.peaceabbey.org
- A set of 12 prayers for peace representing 12 religious traditions. http://www.peaceabbey.org/abbey/peace_seeds_prayers.pdf
- National Center for Complementary and Alternative Medicine. http://nccam.nih.gov/health/providers
- Spiritual practices recommended for influencing health and wellbeing of cancer patients. http://www.cancer.gov/cancertopics/pdq/supportivecare/spirituality/patient
- Located at Duke University, the Center for Spirituality, Theology and Health was founded in 2007 to promote scholarship and research on the influence that spirituality, beliefs, and practices of caring have on individual and community health. http://www.spiritualityandhealth.duke.edu

References

American Occupational Therapy Association (AOTA). (2002). Occupational therapy practice framework: Domain and process. *American Journal of Occupational Therapy, 56,* 609–639.

Engquist, D. E., Short-DeGraff, M., Gliner, J., & Oltenbruns, K. (1997). Occupational therapists' beliefs and practices with regard to spirituality and therapy. *American Journal of Occupational Therapy, 51*(3), 173–180.

Hawkins, D. A. (2002). *Power vs. Force: The Hidden Determinants of Human Behavior.* Carlsbad, CA: Hay House.

Koenig, H.. (2008). "How Religious Beliefs and Practices Are Related to Stress, Health and Medical Services." Paper presented at a Heritage Foundation Symposium, December 3. Available at: http://www.hoje.org.br/site/arq/artigos/How_Religious_Beliefs_and_Practices_Are_Related.pdf (accessed October 24, 2009).

Law, M., Baptiste, S., Carswell, A., McColl, M. A., Polatajko, H., & Pollock, N. (2005). *Canadian Occupational Performance Measure.* Ottawa: Canadian Association of Occupational Therapists.

Luboshitzky, D., & Gaber, L. B. (2001). Holidays and celebrations as a spiritual occupation. *Australian Occupational Therapy Journal, 48*(2), 66–74.

Moreira-Almeida, A., & Koenig, H. G. (2006). Retaining the meaning of the words religiousness and spirituality: A commentary on the WHOQOL SRPB group's "A cross-cultural study of spirituality, religion, and personal beliefs as components of quality of life" (62[6], 2005, pp. 1486–1497). *Social Science and Medicine, 63,* 843–845.

Rogers, C. (1951). *Client-Centered Therapy: Its Current Practice, Implications and Theory.* London: Constable.

Ross, L. (1995). The spiritual dimension: Its importance to patient's health, well-being and quality of life and its implications for nursing practice. *International Journal of Nursing Studies, 32*(5), 457–468.

Schulz, E. (2002). *The meaning of spirituality in the lives and adaptation processes of individuals with disabilities.* Unpublished doctoral dissertation, Texas Woman's University, Denton, Texas.

———. (2008). OT-Quest assessment. In B. J. Hemphill-Pearson (Ed.), *Assessments in Occupational Therapy Mental Health: An Integrative Approach* (pp. 263–289). Thorofare, NJ: Slack.

Smith, H. (1992). *Forgotten Truth: The Common Vision of the World's Religions.* San Francisco: Harper.

Thoresen, C. E. (1998). Spirituality, health, and science: The coming revival? In S. Roth-Roemer, & S. R. Kurpius (Eds.), *The Emerging Role of Counseling Psychology in Health Care* (pp. 409–431). New York: W.W. Norton;.

Wilding, C. (2007). Spirituality as sustenance for mental health and meaningful doing: A case illustration. *Medical Journal of Australia. 186*(10), S67–S69.

Grief and Bereavement

Noralyn Davel Pickens

> "The pain—it came up from my chest and engulfed me—I was weak and overwhelmed. People told me to do things to take my mind off of it. It didn't help. I needed just to sit, be still and feel my pain. I knew I had to really feel it to heal."
>
> —Mimi, age 30, after death of her husband

Introduction

Grief is experienced by all persons at some point in life. Grief is the cognitive, emotional, physical, social, behavioral, and spiritual reactions to personal loss (DeSpelder & Strickland, 2005). Understanding the complexities of grief is important for occupational therapists, because prolonged or complicated grief can either lead to or exacerbate mental health problems, which in turn affect a person's occupational patterns. Bereavement, a closely related term, "takes us out of the normal patterns of our daily lives and disrupts the smooth unfolding of our life stories" (Attig, 2002, p. 8). Bereavement can take a person on a new life trajectory with changed roles and responsibilities.

This chapter describes three dimensions of the grief and bereavement experience that are of concern to occupational therapy: typical and complicated grief, the challenges and concerns for clients with serious mental illness as they grieve, and the losses and grief families experience as a result of a loved one's mental illness.

Case: Gloria: A Tale of Three Deaths

Gloria is in good physical health, has a good marriage and a small but close group of friends. Gloria experienced the deaths of three significant people in two years. The first year, her father died after a long struggle with amyotrophic lateral sclerosis (ALS). His death was expected and seen almost as a relief to her father and family. The length of dying time allowed for funeral planning, sharing of history and stories, and good-byes. Once it came, it was a rather peaceful death. Gloria felt she and her siblings became closer as a result of the time together with their father. She had forced herself to reflect on death, the afterlife, and her own life's trajectory. As a result, her religious faith and community became a greater part of her life.

One year later, Gloria's younger brother was brutally murdered. His death was completely unexpected and lacked closure as the case went unsolved. Her brother had been the "family clown" and, after struggling with a difficult divorce and drug addiction, was getting his life "back together." Later that same year, Gloria's daughter gave birth to a child who died six days later. Although they were aware the child had health problems, they seemed manageable, and the death was unexpected.

In contrast to her father's death, the deaths of her brother and grandchild cut short their lives and truncated plans for continued lives together. There was a loss of potential and of current and future relationships. Adding to Gloria's pain was her family's struggle coming to terms with the death of her brother, as well as her desire to lessen her daughter's grief. Gloria began to have difficulty sleeping, and she would frequently wake from a dream about her brother. She sometimes felt his death was a dream and that he would be over for Sunday dinner, as he often was. She no longer looked forward to preparing that or any other meal.

Gloria tried to spend time with her daughter, who had simply closed the nursery room with all the new furniture, toys and gifts, and who invariably slept the day away or went for long walks alone. Friends encouraged her daughter to "move on" and "try again" (i.e., to have another child). It seemed her daughter needed more time to grieve than what her social group felt necessary.

As time went on, Gloria accepted support from her friends, sought spiritual help from her pastor, and regrounded herself in her daily occupations, including her Sunday meals. Reflecting on the experiences, she notes that nothing could have prepared her for the range of emotions she felt, from overwhelming loss and sorrow to intense anger and frustration. She is comforted by the memories of the family's time together with their father. The sense that his death was "acceptable" gave her a context to make sense of the other deaths. Gloria often imagines her father, brother, and grandchild being together, which gives her comfort. After a long period, her daughter sought professional help and began to make sense of her own loss. The healing began, but it would be a life-long experience of loss.

The Experience of Grief

Many of us have experienced loss of a significant relationship through death. Factors that contribute to our experience include how the death occurred, our relationship to the person at the time of death, and our personal beliefs and understanding of death. We also grieve over losses of cherished relationships, pets, homes, jobs, and objects. Although this chapter emphasizes the grief and bereavement over loss of loved ones, it is important to recognize the many losses our clients with serious mental illness experience; for them, these losses are often multilayered and complex. The multiple losses of home, family, job, and sense of sanity would be devastating to anyone. This is where occupational therapists can play an important role in fostering healthy life patterns and a sense of normality within the changed reality.

Grief is an emotional reaction to a loss (Corr, Nabe, & Corr, 1997). We experience and express grief emotionally, physically, cognitively, behaviorally, socially, and spiritually (Corr et al, 1997; DeSpelder & Strickland, 2005; Kastenbaum, 1998):

■ Emotionally: sadness, anger, guilt, anxiety, loneliness, fatigue, helplessness, shock, yearning, emancipation, relief, numbness
■ Physically: hollowness in stomach, tightness in chest, oversensitivity to noise, shortness of breath, lack of energy, sense of depersonalization, weakness
■ Cognitively: disbelief, confusion, preoccupation
■ Behaviorally: sleep or appetite disturbances, absent-mindedness, withdrawal, loss of interest in activities, crying, sighing, restlessness, hostility, visiting and cherishing objects, avoiding objects and places
■ Socially: difficulties in interpersonal relationships and groups
■ Spiritually: loss of meaning or hostility toward God

Bereavement is a reaction to loss that encompasses the emotional and physical reactions of grief and mourning. It involves a psychological process of letting go of relationships. For some, it is a sense of being deprived of something cherished (DeSpelder & Strickland, 2005). Bereavement also describes a *state of being* in which people are referred to as "bereaved." This state can persist for a period of months to years.

Mourning is behavioral action and integration of grief and bereavement (DeSpelder & Strickland, 2005; Kastenbaum, 1998). The action or outcome of grief and bereavement provides the opportunities for occupation that foster healing and growth following loss. Mourning is a culturally driven experience that includes rituals and tasks carried out by the bereaved in coping with the death of their loved one. These rituals and tasks of mourning can be part of a healthy response to death.

Review of Grief Theory

Theories abound on the process of grief (Bowlby, 1961; Kübler-Ross, 1969; Lindemann, 1944; Parkes, 1971; Parkes & Weiss, 1983; Rando, 1984; Worden, 1991). In general, all follow a similar pattern of shock and disbelief, then acute mourning, followed by resolution. Although most appear to be "stage" theories, with a closer reading, nearly all theories describe interactive movement among the "stages." Bowlby (1973) describes a fluid process of four phases in grief and "reorganization."

1. Phase I—emotional numbing and disbelief
2. Phase II—yearning and searching
3. Phase III—disorganization and despair
4. Phase IV—reorganization

The first phase, emotional numbing and disbelief, is a cognitive–emotional protective measure. This phase may last only a few hours, but for individuals with difficulty coping with stressors or major life events, the phase can be long lasting and become a barrier to reality. The second phase, yearning and searching, can involve emotional swings accompanied by variable energy-level swings and preoccupation with thoughts of the loved one. In the third phase, the death becomes a reality, and the person may withdraw, isolate, and experience fatigue and depression. Reorganization into new life patterns is phase four. This is a gradual and difficult process of recognizing the deceased's place in one's life. One can make sense of the death in the scope of life and mortality (Freeman, 2005).

Of these theories, the Kübler-Ross theory has risen to public awareness and become a part of popular culture. Although Kübler-Ross's and other stage theories demonstrate order, it has been widely accepted that a person may move in and out of phases in a nonlinear fashion; the stages are not mutually exclusive, and there is overlap among the phases.

Until recently, however, these stage theories went untested, while remaining ubiquitous in pedagogy. Implementing a longitudinal cohort design involving 233 participants who experienced the death of a loved one by natural causes, Maciejewski, Zhang, Block, and Prigerson (2007) studied *how* people experience grief; if grief is experienced in stages, at what magnitude and duration? The proposed stages included a typical sequence of disbelief, yearning, anger, depression, and acceptance.

The findings provides "partial support for the stage theory of grief" (p. 721); however, they suggest that *disbelief* wanes by 1 month postdeath and that the primary negative response is yearning, not depression. Anger peaked at approximately 5 months, with depression peaking around 6 months. Acceptance demonstrated a steady increase from the first month postdeath. The authors call attention to a yearning experience rather than depression. All negative responses were in decline by 6 months. The authors suggest that continuation of negative responses beyond this time indicates a need for further evaluation of an abnormal grieving process.

The stage theories of grief have supporters and detractors. Moules (1998) suggests that the traditional grief theories impede healing by setting expectations of what *should* occur. It is important to allow the natural grieving process to occur, as subjectively experienced, and not set false expectations for our clients.

Complicated Grief

Grief is a natural and expected response to a loss. Most people who are grieving a loss will come to accept their loved one's death within a few months. However, for some people grief becomes an overwhelming experience and consumes much of their lives. **Complicated grief** is a departure from normal grief patterns in the duration or intensity of the emotional, psychological, and physical symptoms of grief (Stroebe, Hansson, Stroebe, & Schut, 2001). People experiencing complicated grief have intrusive thoughts about the deceased that interfere with daily activities, or they may avoid certain people and situations that were formerly connected to and hold memories of the deceased individual.

Horowitz et al (1997) first developed diagnostic criteria for complicated grief that were later expanded upon by Prigerson and Jacobs (2001). Prigerson and Jacobs use the term **traumatic grief** to reflect the traumatic distress experience of the bereaved person. Table 55-1 outlines the diagnostic criteria for traumatic grief.

Complicated grief is closely related to depression and anxiety, but research has demonstrated that each of these conditions present as distinct clinical entities with clusters of symptoms that make them distinguishable from one another (Boelen & Van den Bout, 2005). Depression and anxiety can be comorbid conditions along with complicated (or traumatic) grief and should be treated as such. It is recommended that formal intervention for grief occur only when it becomes complicated grief, or in cases in which the death was traumatic in nature or the grieving person already has compromised coping mechanisms and little social support (Wagner, Knaevelsrud, & Maercker, 2001).

Experience of Grief Over the Life Span

The needs and concerns of individuals who grieve differ across the life span. Older adults often experience multiple losses with age: home, physical health, friends, and family.

Table 6-1 ● **Diagnostic Criteria for Traumatic Grief**

Criterion A: Three of the following four symptoms of separation distress:
1. Intrusive thoughts about the deceased
2. Yearning for the deceased
3. Searching for the deceased
4. Loneliness as a result of the death

Criterion B: Four of the following eight symptoms of traumatic distress:
1. Purposelessness or feelings of futility about the future
2. Subjective sense of numbness, detachment, or absence of emotional responsiveness
3. Difficulty acknowledging the death (e.g., disbelief)
4. Feeling that life is empty and meaningless
5. Feeling that part of oneself has died
6. Shattered worldview (e.g., lost sense of security, trust, and control)
7. Assumes symptoms or harmful behaviors of or related to the deceased person
8. Excessive irritability, bitterness, or anger related to the death

Criterion C: Duration of the disturbance (symptoms listed) is at least 2 months

Criterion D: The disturbance causes clinically significant impairment in social, occupational, or other important areas of functioning.

Source: Prigerson, H. G., & Jacobs, S. C. (2001). Traumatic grief as a distinct disorder: A rationale, consensus criteria and a preliminary empirical test. In M. S. Stroebe, R. O. Hansson, W. Stroebe, & H. Schut (Eds.), Handbook of Bereavement Research: Consequences, Coping and Care (pp. 588–613). Washington, DC: American Psychological Association.

As older adults are living longer, they are experiencing deaths of spouses, siblings, and adult children. Adults with strong self-efficacy demonstrate less grief over time and are better able to make meaning of the death in relation to their lives. From their work with widows and widowers in midlife, Bauer and Bonanno (2001) found that adults who were able to make realistic and pragmatic statements about their abilities and life situations demonstrated the best overall emotional health following the death of their loved one.

Families with children at home cope with grief in complex ways. Symptoms of grieving families include changes in communication patterns, role confusion, acting out, withdrawal and isolation as a family, and overprotection of family members (Kastenbaum, 1998).

Losses are complicated for adolescents. They may be thrust into new roles with the need to develop new meanings and values. They may find themselves in mixed roles (i.e., that of caregiver and bereaved), roles they are not emotionally prepared to take on (Kastenbaum, 1998). Adolescents may act out in school and withdraw from extracurricular activities and peer groups. They may self-medicate through drugs and alcohol.

In grieving their parents or primary caregivers, children experience a loss of security and connection to a person who represented the larger world. Weiss (2001) suggests that the loss of a parental relationship creates an insecure environment and, reflecting on Bowlby's work, suggests that the child can return to typical patterns of childhood occupations only when the child identifies himself or herself as a protected being. Children's egotism affects their grieving. For example, if a child had an argument with the person before the death, he or she may feel guilty, believing that he or she somehow "wished" the person dead. Young children sometimes complain of physical problems similar to those experienced by their family member before they died; for example, stomach pain or headaches. Children may become overprotective of others and may suffer depression and real physical problems. They may have intrusive thoughts about death, act out of fear or anger, and detach from close relationships. They need healthy means with which to express their grief.

Mourning Rituals

A mourning ritual is an act or pattern of acts that express loss through a task or activity. Rituals hold meaning for families and loved ones who take comfort in performing acts at specific times to remember a person who died. Mourning rituals help to reframe relationships through acting on one's memory of the loved one. Rituals can be times of private prayer, personal acts, or group activities focused on the memory of the deceased.

Current Western society provides limited time for formal mourning rituals. In many work environments, mourning is minimized to 3 to 5 work release days. Many religious and ethnic groups continue formal grieving practices, such as the Jewish custom of sitting Shiva for 7 days after the death of a loved one. Their formal mourning period is recognized with a visit to the temple 30 days later for Sheloshim and 1 year later for Yahrzeit. For Muslims, 7 days of prayer and wearing black clothing for 40 days is required of family members of the deceased (Gilanshah, 1993). In the traditional Hmong culture, all normal work ceases at the death until after the burial, at which time only certain work may be resumed; women may not do needlework because it symbolizes a "slippery road" for the deceased (Bliatout, 1993). However, for many mourners, the formal grief time is only a few hours at a memorial service. Long past is the formal social ritual of visiting family graves and lengthy formal mourning.

Perhaps in response to the lack of formal ritual in today's society, families develop private grief rituals. Gudmundsdottir and Chesla (2006) found that, following the death of a child, families created special memorial spaces with photos and items of the deceased child, carried special "tokens" (small cherished items that remind one of the child), or privately visited the cemetery to be "close" to the body. These private rituals helped maintain a sense of closeness to the deceased child and served as a reminder of the family as it once was.

Intervention for Grief

Occupational therapists can assist clients in finding healthy expressions for their grief. Our understanding of the richness of everyday occupation turns even simple actions into acts of meaning (Hasselkus, 2002). Everyday occupations become daily rituals of healing and memory holding. For many, it is important to acknowledge the death in everyday life. Intentional acts to honor the memory of the loved one can include regular "memory walks" during which one walks paths frequented by the deceased, preparing meals or treats that were favored by the deceased, and spending time with other people who were loved by the deceased.

Formal acts of mourning can include creating family heirlooms. Ilott (2006) found that the process of commissioning an artist to create heirloom pieces from family objects and materials was therapeutic in her grief process. Thibeault (1997) collected mementos of her father to pass on to her nieces and nephews, children who were unable to appreciate their grandfather's creative mind before his progressive illness. A newer form of memorializing the dead is through the World Wide Web (de Vries & Rutherford, 2004). "Cyberspace cemeteries" provide a space for tribute through word and images in a medium ever-present among people today.

When clients are not experiencing complicated grief, yet are struggling with the everyday tasks of living, occupational therapists can foster a sense of self-efficacy—the "I can do" attitude and self-perception (Bauer & Bonanno, 2001). Occupational therapists may need to address the new skills needed for success in instrumental daily living skills. For example, a healthy interdependent couple may have divided household responsibilities for decades. Teaching the surviving spouse skills in homemaking, finances, or transportation will increase self-confidence and help ease the transition while promoting confidence for living alone. Where there is a need for support and sharing outside the family, it is important to provide information about grief support groups, which often are affiliated with local hospitals and religious institutions.

Adolescents and young children have special needs in their grieving process. Children need to be allowed open communication of thoughts, feelings, and questions that may come much later. Young children may be given the choice to attend the funeral, an experience that can make the death "real." Following a death in which parents are overwhelmed, finding a trusted relation or friend to provide care allows a sense of freedom and protection for the children. Children need assurances that people are available to love and care for them (Dyergrov & Dyergrov, 2005; Kastenbaum, 1998). Creative expressions of grief are very valuable to adolescents and children. Artwork; written work such as family stories, poetry, or letters to the deceased; music and creative movement can help a young person come to understand the complicated experience of grief. Schools need to be notified of the death in order to provide opportunities for grief support. Schools need to provide "safe" people (e.g., counselors) and places for children to go if they need to express their grief away from their peers (Stevenson, 2002).

The anniversary of the death is an important day of remembrance. Families may have day-long gatherings of friends and loved ones at which photos, films, and cherished objects are shared. Special religious services may be held in honor of the loved one. The anniversary can be created as a healing experience through sharing, memorializing, and honoring the deceased.

Special Challenges and Concerns for Clients with Mental Illness

People who live with serious mental illness have often already coped with significant losses of family, friends, and lifestyle. Yet when a major loss of family occurs, such as a death of a parent or child, the individual's ability to manage his or her grief presents a huge challenge. Macias et al (2004) emphasize the need to support persons with mental illness by assuring them that grief is a normal reaction to loss and "not a reflection of their emotional fragility" (p. 425).

Loss of a Parent

For persons with serious mental illness, the death of a parent can bring about a severe depression and dramatic loss of functioning that can persist for years (Mazure, Bruce, Maciejewski, & Jacob, 2000; Piper, Ogrodniczuk, Azim, & Weideman, 2001). For example, an adult child with mental illness may continue to live in his or her aging parent's homes, which allows for an interdependence in which both the adults (child and parent) function at higher levels than if

---

alone. However, when the remaining parent dies, this person may experience the multiple losses of support systems, companions, housing, and income (Jones et al, 2003). The family home may be sold, his or her daily companion is gone, and the person may have few people whom he or she trusts and can turn to. The person may not have the daily living skills required to find new housing, perform complex homemaking tasks, or make financial decisions.

Persons with serious mental illness can be overlooked or "uninvited" to wakes and funerals due to concern for acting-out behavior. They often do not get the same grief support from friends and family that others do (Jones et al, 2003; Macias et al, 2004). Additionally, they may feel responsible for the death. Depending on the severity of the mental illness, they may have difficulty communicating feelings and thoughts, which can then be expressed in psychotic episodes or delusional experiences of their loved one (Martins, 2002).

Loss of Children

Loss of children is a related issue for people with serious mental illness. Having a child (or children) permanently taken away is as profound an experience as a death. Anywhere from 23% to 68% of mothers with severe mental illness have their children taken away from them permanently (Schen, 2005). Hospitalization and other prolonged periods away from their children increase the likelihood that they will lose custody of their children. The experience of grief over their child(ren) can be reflected in delusional experiences of parenting small children or a profound yearning for motherhood. The symptomatology of the parent with serious mental illness becomes a primary concern for health care providers and other family members, while consideration for the parent's loss of their parent–child relationship is often overlooked by others. Although there may be a strong rationale for removing the child, the parent with serious mental illness still grieves the loss and may do so without support or understanding.

Intervention for Clients with Mental Illness

For clients already struggling with serious mental illness, the death of a significant person justifies evaluation of the client's support systems and overall health. We need to recognize the losses our clients with serious mental illness have already experienced and their sometimes profound skills at adapting to their losses. Yet the fragility of mental health can be shattered by a significant loss of parent, child, or other beloved individual. It is important that we do not attempt to "rescue" the individual, patronize him or her, or diminish the loss. Attempt to understand how the deceased individual impacted the life of your client. Help your client create memory books, memorials, or healthy mourning rituals. Engage the client in the development of practical life planning.

If a midlife client is in a regular treatment program, prepare him or her for life changes. Occupational therapists can assist in preparation for the loss of a parent to lower the risk of complicated grief. For example, if the parent is the consistent personal and housing support, how can the person with serious mental illness look for alternative supports that would assist in the transition and loss and find meaning? Similar to older couples residing together, persons with

mental illness who live with parents often experience an interdependence that can be life affirming and provide a source of esteem (Jones et al, 2003). How can this void be filled or healed? Address needs in instrumental activities of daily living (IADL), such as housing, finances, and homemaking. As noted earlier, for grieving spouses, occupational therapists can help foster a sense of self-efficacy through IADL training. The development of social and practical resources may be more beneficial than introspective therapy (Jones et al, 2003).

Grief and Loss for Families of People with Serious Mental Illness

The personal loss experienced by family members of a person with a serious mental illness is similar to grief experienced when a loved one dies (Stein, Dworsky, Phillips, & Hunt, 2005). It is a loss of a companion, "potential," or an expected future. This grief is frequently not acknowledged or validated by friends and community (Young, Bailey, & Rycroft, 2004). However, the loved one's mental illness can be persistent, without an end in sight. The closure and integration that occurs in typical grieving becomes a moving target without resolution (Davis & Schultz, 1998).

Parental Grief

The first full episodes of many mental illnesses occur between mid-teen and young adult years. Prior to the onset of mental illness, parents expect a "normal" life for their child. Even after a number of depressive or psychotic episodes have occurred, many parents maintain hope for their child's mental health. Adjustment to the loss of the child's "normality" requires parents to "undergo a complex reorganization of lifestyle, self-perception, role, economic security, and belief systems" as they accept their offspring's mental illness (MacGregor, 1994, p. 163.) It is a slow unraveling, understanding, and acceptance of the loss of the expected future and transition to a new reality.

As their child matures, parents worry about the future and experience a lack of control within the health care system. They often have mixed feelings of being upset by the changes yet feeling resentful of the need and demands made by the adult child. Parents may feel trapped, stigmatized and have impaired relationships with others in the family (Rose, Mallinson, & Gerson (2006).

In a recent study, parents reported that having a child with schizophrenia was the most "distressful" life event endured. The level of contact with their child does not correlate to more or less grief, but more contact did intensify "intrusive" thoughts, such as preoccupations with the child's health, whereabouts, and safety. Parents experienced more negative emotions and less wellbeing than did parents of children without mental illness (Godress, Ozgul, Owen, & Foley-Evans, 2005).

Sibling Grief

Siblings also experience grief when a brother or sister has serious mental illness. As serious mental illness often appears in late adolescence and young adulthood, close siblings may be well aware of the changing experience of their brother or sister. They may see themselves at risk and need counseling and education along with the family (Riebschleger, 1991).

Siblings experience differences in the relationship in terms of reciprocity. They lose a peer and become a caregiver (Hatfield & Lefley, 2005). In contrast, some siblings avoid family and siblings responsibilities, become depressed themselves, and may fear for their own children's mental health (Ufner, 2005). Siblings often are forced to review their world perspective and life trajectory in relation to their mentally ill brother or sister.

Children and Partner's Grief

Children and partners experience losses when their parent or spouse has serious mental illness. Children grieve for what they do not have; they may feel different from their peers and awkward when talking about parents with their friends (Young, Bailey, & Rycroft, 2004). They avoid bringing friends home and take on adult caregiving roles early in life.

Spouses and partners are impacted by a change from the initial relationship expectations and struggle with new responsibilities in the relationship. The health of the relationship declines as the relationship loses balance. Partners avoid discussing the mental illness for fear of the impact on themselves and their children. Without support, the family can become isolated and controlled by the stigma of the mental illness.

Traumatic Death

Traumatic deaths present a different set of challenges for the bereaved. Negative emotional responses are longer lasting, and participants have greater difficulty making sense of the loss (Currier, Holland, & Neimeyer, 2006). An abrupt death may be psychologically disruptive; the mind had no preparation for the death and must quickly accommodate the knowledge. Children and adolescents are especially challenged by the confusion surrounding traumatic deaths. They are limited in their ability to understand the sudden change in family structure and may feel overwhelmed and insecure in their familial attachments (Adams, 2002).

Suicide can be viewed as shameful, criminal, and in some communities, sinful. If police and courts are involved, the families often have limited exposure to the details of the death. Families can be stigmatized by guilt and shame. As a result, their grief is challenging for other family and friends to support. Suicide adds a double edge to the sword of pain experienced in grief, as society often finds it unapproachable. In the case of a troubled relationship, the death prevents any future reconciliation, and there is a loss of hope for desired closure. The bereaved may need assistance to reframe the relationship, let go of that hope, and accept the relationship as it was. Families need to understand that mental illness can be a cause of death in the case of suicide (Martins, 2002).

Children and young siblings are affected more deeply by suicide than by a "natural" death (Pfeffer, Jiang, Kakuma, Hwang, & Metsch, 2002). They experience confusion, shock, and fear and often feel very alone as their parents struggle with their own feelings. The risk for posttraumatic stress disorder is very high for siblings who lived in the same home as the deceased, a higher risk than for parents due to the sibling receiving less attention (Dyregrov & Dyregrov, 2005). Children are often "lost" in the family grief, in part due to adults' inability to understand and express the complex emotions surrounding suicide.

Intervention for Families

Beyond the interventions described previously, families with a mentally ill loved one have special needs. Parents and siblings need acknowledgment and validation of the experience of grief and loss. Children of persons with mental illness also need to acknowledge their ongoing losses. Families require education about serious mental illness and may need assistance in changing their assumptions to find new and unexplored roles for the family member with serious mental illness. Provide information on local support groups for families and, in the case of suicide, a group that can address understanding of the suicide and unique expressions of grief.

Assessments

Occupational therapy does not have any assessment tools specific to occupation and grief, but a number of tools from the disciplines of psychology and nursing have utility for practice. The following scales are selected as instruments that target specific issues discussed in this chapter.

Evidence-Based Practice

When a death is sudden and unexpected, grief can be confusing, and the need to make sense of the loss is often a critical aspect of the grieving process (Rando, 1984). Rituals and memorials are created to hold loved ones close. Engagement in everyday occupations are important to grieving and healing and can support an individual's reconstruction of meaning and purpose following loss.

➤ Maintaining occupations can help individuals and families stabilize during periods of stress and loss. For example, one mother described cooking meals represented holding or "cooking my family together" (Gudmundsdottir & Chesla, 2006).

➤ Participation in occupation can support the adaptation process by helping individuals to "rebuild meaning, purpose and understanding" after loss (Hoppes, 2005, p. 85.).

Gudmundsdottir, M., & Chesla, C. A. (2006). Building a new world: Habits and practices of healing following the death of a child. *Journal of Family Nursing, 12,* 143–164.

Hoppes, S. (2005). When a child dies the world should stop spinning: An autoethnography exploring the impact of family loss on occupation. *American Journal of Occupational Therapy, 59*(1), 78–87.

Rando, T. (1984). *Grief, Dying, and Death: Clinical Interventions for Caregivers.* Champaign, IL: Research Press.

The Grief Experience Questionnaire (GEQ) may be helpful for adults with serious mental illness, those at risk for suicide, and those who are grieving a stigmatizing death. The GEQ addresses factors related to suicidal bereavement, such as culpability and disgrace. It is a 55-item self rating instrument utilizing a 5-point Likert scale. It has strong internal consistency and factor structure. Construct validity evaluation suggests its strength in differentiating between normal and suicidal bereavement (Niemeyer & Hogan, 2001).

The Inventory of Complicated Grief-Revised (ICG-R) by Prigerson and Jacobs (2001) was designed to distinguish between normal and complicated grief. The items have a present experience focus rather than reflecting on past emotions. It is a 19-item tool with a 5-point frequency rating scale. The tool demonstrates ability to predict long-term dysfunction. It has strong internal consistency, test–retest reliability, and convergent and criterion validity.

The Hogan Sibling Inventory of Bereavement (HSIB) focuses on the loss of brothers and sisters in childhood and adolescence (Hogan, 1990). Developed from qualitative interviews with bereaved siblings, its 46 items reflect the nature of the sibling experience. For example, question stems begin "since my brother or sister died..." The HSIB uses a five point Likert rating scale ("almost always true" to "hardly ever true"). It has strong internal consistency. Construct validity was established; high scores on the HSIB correlate with poor self-concept. The HSIB is a useful tool to address grief and bereavement in children and adolescents (Niemeyer & Hogan, 2001).

The Mental Illness Version of the Texas Inventory of Grief (MIV-TIG), adapted from the Texas Revised Inventory of Grief, addresses grief-related symptoms, specifically for individuals who have a family member with mental illness. A reliable and valid tool, the MIV-TIG is useful in measuring the current impact of mental illness on the family as it assesses and delimitates between initial and present feelings about the loved one's loss of mental health (Miller, Dworkin, Ward, & Barone, 1990).

Summary

Occupational therapists are beginning to illuminate how engagement in occupation facilitates coping and supports the reconstruction of meaning and purpose in the lives of people who have experienced personal loss. This chapter described various dimensions of the grief and bereavement experiences. Using a life-span perspective, the challenges and concerns for individuals and families and for clients with serious mental illness as they grieve were explored. Occupation is a medium to support the bereavement process and to foster healing and growth following loss. Engagement in occupation can be a powerful mechanism by which people address the challenges associated with grief and restore wellbeing and mental health after loss.

Active Learning Strategies

1. Self-Reflection

Reflect on the person with whom you feel most secure.

Reflective Questions
- What about this person and your relationship shape who you are?
- What would it be like if he or she were to die?
- How would your life change?
- What resources and supports would you need?

 Capture your thoughts in your **Reflective Journal**.

2. Experience with a Death

Reflect on a death you have experienced.

Reflective Questions
- What was your *first* experience of the death?
- How did you initially react?
- What did others say to you that was helpful?
- What did others say to you that was *not* helpful?
- What did you *do* in your grieving?
- What life patterns have changed?

- How do you think of that person now?
- What brings him or her "back" to you?
- How has this experience changed over time?

 Write about your experiences in your **Reflective Journal**.

3. Grief Rituals

Consider what you know about grief rituals of cultures other than your own. Research different traditions by interviewing members or religious leaders of different cultural groups. Interview chaplains who work in interfaith environments (e.g., many hospitals) on their experiences with different grief rituals.

4. Reflections on Occupation and Death

Poetry, as an art form, is a method of communicating a range of responses to experiences in our lives that have filled us with ecstasy, agony, and every emotion in between. Read these two poems. For each poem, identify how the artist's words provide a lens on the impact of grief or loss on a person's pattern of daily occupation.

FUNERAL BLUES
W. H. Auden

Stop all the clocks, cut off the telephone,
Prevent the dog from barking with a juicy bone,
Silence the pianos and with muffled drum
Bring out the coffin, let the mourners come.
Let aeroplanes circle moaning overhead
Scribbling on the sky the message He Is Dead,
Put crêpe bows round the white necks of the public doves,
Let the traffic policemen wear black cotton gloves.

He was my North, my South, my East and West,
My working week and my Sunday rest,
My noon, my midnight, my talk, my song;
I thought that love would last for ever: I was wrong.
The stars are not wanted now: put out every one;
Pack up the moon and dismantle the sun;
Pour away the ocean and sweep up the wood.
For nothing now can ever come to any good.

OTHERWISE
Jane Kenyon

I got out of bed
on two strong legs.
It might have been
otherwise. I ate
cereal, sweet
milk, ripe, flawless
peach. It might

have been otherwise.
I took the dog uphill
to the birch wood.
All morning I did
the work I love.

At noon I lay down
with my mate. It might
have been otherwise.
We ate dinner together
at a table with silver
candlesticks. It might
have been otherwise.
I slept in a bed
in a room with paintings
on the walls, and
planned another day
just like this day.
But one day, I know,
it will be otherwise.

Auden, W. H. (2007). *Selected Poems*. Edited by Edward Mendelsen. New York: Vintage International.
Kenyon, J. (1996). *Otherwise*. St. Paul, MN: Graywolf Press.

 Write down your thoughts about these poems in your **Reflective Journal**.

Resources

- **SAMHSA—Substance Abuse and Mental Health Services Administration:** SAMHSA's information center offers resources for people dealing with grief and loss. The resources here describe the grieving process, differentiate grief from depression, and provide multiple sources that can be used for education, support, and advocacy. http://mentalhealth.samhsa.gov/publications/allpubs/KEN-01-0104/default.asp
- **Growth House, Inc.:** This Web site is a useful source of information and resources covering a broad range of death and dying, life-threatening illness, and end-of-life care issues. The stated mission of this organization is to both educate the public and facilitate global professional collaboration. This site includes a search engine that is specifically linked to a database of full-text materials about end-of-life care. http://www.growthhouse.org
- **Transformations:** This Web site provides self-help and multiple bulletin boards for consumer support and discussion of recovery issues. Registration allows consumers to share resources and participate in bulletin boards for a variety of mental health topics, including anxiety, bipolar disorder, codependency, depression, and addiction. http://www.transformations.com

References

Adams, D. W. (2002). The consequences of sudden traumatic death: The vulnerability of bereaved children and adolescents and ways professionals can help. In G. R. Cox, R. A. Bendiksen, & R. G. Stevenson (Eds.), *Complicated Grieving and Bereavement: Understanding and Treating People Experiencing Loss* (pp. 23–40). Amityville, NY: Baywood Publishing.

Attig, T. (2002). Relearning the world: Always complicated, sometimes more than others. In G. R. Cox, R. A. Bendiksen, & R. G. Stevenson (Eds.), *Complicated Grieving and Bereavement: Understanding and Treating People Experiencing Loss* (pp. 7–19). Amityville, NY: Baywood Publishing.

Bauer, J., & Bonanno, G. A. (2001). I can, I do, I am: The narrative differentiation of self-efficacy and other self-evaluations while adapting to bereavement. *Journal of Research in Personality, 35,* 434–448.

Bliatout, B. T. (1993). Hmong death customs: Traditional and acculturated. In D. P.Irish, K. F. Lundquist, & V. J. Nelson (Eds.), *Ethnic Variations in Dying, Death and Grief: Diversity in Universality* (pp. 79–100). Washington, DC: Taylor & Francis.

Boelen, P. A., & Van den Bout, J. (2005). Complicated grief, depression, and anxiety as distinct post-loss syndromes: A confirmatory factor analysis study. *American Journal of Psychiatry, 162,* 2175–2177.

Bowlby, J. (1961). Processes of mourning. *International Journal of Psychoanalysis, 42,* 317–340.

———. (1973). *Attachment and Loss* (3 vols.). New York: Basic Books [1973–83].

Corr, C. A., Nabe, C. M., & Corr, D. M. (1997). *Death & Dying, Life & Living* (2nd ed.). Boston: Brooks/Cole.

Currier, J. M., Holland, J. M., & Neimeyer, R. A. (2006). Sense-making, grief, and the experience of violent loss: Toward a mediational model. *Death Studies, 30,* 403–428.

Davis, D. J., & Schultz, C. L. (1998). Grief, parenting and schizophrenia. *Social Science and Medicine, 46,* 369–379.

DeSpelder, L. A., & Strickland, A. L. (2005). *The Last Dance: Encountering Death and Dying* (7th ed.). Boston: McGraw Hill.

deVries, B., & Rutherford, J. (2004). Memorializing loved ones on the World Wide Web. *OMEGA, 49*(1), 5–26.

Dyregrov, K., & Dyregrov, A. (2005). Siblings after suicide—"The forgotten bereaved." *Suicide and Life Threatening Behavior, 35*(6), 714–724.

Freeman, S. J. (2005). *Grief and Loss: Understanding the Journey.* Belmont, CA: Thomson Learning.

Gilanshah, F. (1993). Islamic customs regarding death. In D. P. Irish, K. F. Lundquist, & V. J. Nelson (Eds.), *Ethnic Variations in Dying, Death and Grief: Diversity in Universality* (pp. 137–145). Washington, DC: Taylor & Francis.

Godress, J., Ozgul, S., Owen, C., & Foley-Evans, L. (2005). Grief experiences of parents whose children suffer from mental illness. *Australian and New Zealand Journal of Psychiatry, 39*(1–2), 88–95.

Gudmundsdottir, M., & Chesla, C. A. (2006). Building a new world: Habits and practices of healing following the death of a child. *Journal of Family Nursing, 12,* 143–164.

Hasselkus, B. (2002). *The Meaning of Everyday Occupation.* Thorofare, NJ: Slack, Inc.

Hatfield, A. B., & Lefley, H. P., (2005). Future involvement of siblings in the lives of persons with mental illness. *Community Mental Health Journal, 41*(3), 327–338.

Hogan, N. S. (1990). Hogan Sibling Inventory of Bereavement. In J. Touliatos, B. Permutter, & M. Strauss (Eds.), *Handbook of Family Measurement Techniques* (p. 524). Newbury Park, CA: Sage.

Hoppes, S. (2005). When a child dies the world should stop spinning: An autoethnography exploring the impact of family loss on occupation. *American Journal of Occupational Therapy, 59*(1), 78–87.

Horowitz, M. J., Siegel, B., Holen, A., Bonanno, G. A., Milbrath, C., & Stinson, C. H. (1997). Diagnostic criteria for complicated grief. *American Journal of Psychiatry, 154,* 904–910.

Ilott, I. (2006). A special occupation: Commissioning an heirloom. *Journal of Occupational Science, 13,* 145–148.

Irish, D. P., Lundquist, K. F., & Nelson, V. J. (1993). *Ethnic Variations in Dying, Death and Grief: Diversity in Universality.* Washington, DC: Taylor & Francis.

Jacques, N. D., & Hasselkus, B. R. (2004). The nature of occupation surrounding dying and death. *OTJR: Occupation, Participation and Health, 24*(2), 43–55.

Jones, D., Harvey, J., Giza, D., Rodican, C., Barreira, P. J., & Macias, C. (2003). Parental death in the lives of people with serious mental illness. *Journal of Loss and Trauma, 8,* 307–322.

Kastenbaum, Robert. (1998). *Death, Society and Human Experience* (6th ed.). Boston: Allyn & Bacon.

Kübler-Ross, E. (1969). *On Death and Dying.* New York: Macmillan.

Lindemann, W. (1944). Symptomatology and management of acute grief. *American Journal of Psychiatry, 101,* 141–148.

Macias, C., Jones, D., Harvey, J., Barreira, P., Harding, C., & Rodican, C. (2004). Bereavement in the context of serious mental illness. *Psychiatric Services, 55,* 421–426.

MacGregor, P. (1994). The unrecognized response to mental illness in a child. *Social Work, 39,* 160–166.

Maciejewski, P. K., Zhang, B., Block, S. D., & Prigerson, H. G. (2007). An empirical examination of the stage theory of grief. *Journal of the American Medical Association, 297,* 716–723.

Martins, L. (2002). Minding mental illness in the grief process. In G. Cox, R. A. Bendiksen, & Stevenson, R. G. (Eds.), *Complicated Grieving and Bereavement: Understanding and Treating People Experiencing Loss.* Amityville, NY: Baywood Publishing.

Mazure, C., Bruce, M., Maciejewski, P., & Jacobs, S. (2000). Adverse life events and cognitive-personality characteristics in the prediction of major depression and antidepressant response. *American Journal of Psychiatry, 157,* 896–903.

Miller, F., Dworkin, J., Ward, M., & Barone, D. (1990). A preliminary study of unresolved grief in families of seriously mentally ill patients. *Hospital and Community Psychiatry, 41,* 1321–1325.

Moules, N. J. (1998). Legitimizing grief: Challenging beliefs that constrain. *Journal of Family Nursing, 4,* 142–166.

Neimeyer, R. A., & Hogan, N. S. (2001). Quantitative or qualitative? Measurement issues in the study of grief. In M. S. Stroebe, R. O. Hansson, W. Stroebe, & H. Schut (Eds.), *Handbook of Bereavement Research: Consequences, Coping and Care* (pp. 89–116). Washington, DC: American Psychological Association.

Parkes, C. M. (1971). The first year of bereavement: A longitudinal study of the reaction of London widows to the death of their husbands. *Psychiatry, 33,* 444–467.

Parkes, C. M., & Weiss, R. (1983). *Recovery from Bereavement.* New York: Basic Books.

Pfeffer, C., Jiang, H., Kakuma, T., Hwang, J., & Metsch, M. (2002). Group interventions for children bereaved by the suicide of a relative. *Journal of the American Academy of Child and Adolescent Psychiatry, 41,* 505–513.

Piper, W., Ogrodniczuk, J., Azim, H., & Weideman, R. (2001). Prevalence of loss and complicated grief among psychiatric outpatients. *Psychiatric Services, 52,* 1069–1074.

Prigerson, H. G., & Jacobs, S. C. (2001). Traumatic grief as a distinct disorder: A rationale, consensus criteria and a preliminary empirical test. In M. S. Stroebe, R. O. Hansson, W. Stroebe, & H. Schut (Eds.), *Handbook of Bereavement Research: Consequences, Coping and Care* (pp. 588–613). Washington, DC: American Psychological Association.

Rando, T. A. (1984). *Grief, Dying and Death: Clinical Interventions for Caregivers.* Champaign, IL: Research Press.

Riebschleger, J. L. (1991). Families of chronically mentally ill people: Siblings speak to social workers. *Health & Social Work, 16*(2), 94–103

Rose, L. E., Mallinson, R. K., & Gerson, L. D. (2006). Mastery, burden and areas of concern among family caregivers of mentally ill persons. *Archives of Psychiatric Nursing, 20*(1), 41–51.

Schen, C. R. (2005). When mothers leave their children behind. *Harvard Review of Psychiatry, 13,* 233–243.

Stein, C. H., Dworsky, D. O., Phillips, R. E., & Hunt, M. G. (2005). Measuring personal loss among adults with serious mental illness. *Community Mental Health Journal, 41,* 129–139.

Stevenson, R. G. (2002). It's never easy! Children, adolescents and complicated grief. In G. R. Cox, R. A. Bendiksen, & R. G. Stevenson (Eds.), *Complicated Grieving and Bereavement: Understanding and Treating People Experiencing Loss* (pp. 275–287). Amityville, NY: Baywood Publishing.

Stroebe, M. S., Hansson, R. O. , Stroebe, W., & Schut, H. (Eds.). (2001). *Handbook of Bereavement Research.* Washington, DC: American Psychological Association.

Thibeault, R. (1997). A funeral for my father's mind: A therapist's attempt at grieving. *Canadian Journal of Occupational Therapy, 64,* 107–114.

Ufner, M. J. (2005). Lifespan effects of having a sibling with schizophrenia. *Dissertation Abstracts International: Section B: The Sciences and Engineering, 65*(10-B), pp. 50–69. AAT 3149990.

Wagner, B., Knaevelsrud, C., & Maercker, A. (2001). Internet-based treatment for complicated grief: Concepts and case study. In M. S. Stroebe, R. O. Hansson, W. Stroebe, & H. Schut (Eds.), *Handbook of Bereavement Research: Consequences, Coping and Care* (pp. 409–432). Washington, DC: American Psychological Association.

Weiss, R. S. (2001). Grief, bonds and relationships. In In M. S. Stroebe, R. O. Hansson, W. Stroebe, & H. Schut (Eds.), *Handbook of Bereavement Research: Consequences, Coping and Care* (pp. 47–62). Washington, DC: American Psychological Association.

Worden, J. W. (1991). *Grief Counseling and Grief Therapy: A Handbook for the Mental Health Practitioner* (2nd ed.). New York: Springer.

Young, J., Bailey, G., & Rycroft, P. (2004). Family grief and mental health: A systematic, contextual and compassionate analysis. *Australian and New Zealand Journal of Family Therapy, 25*(4), 188–197.

Glossary

acculturation—The processes that occur when people from different cultural groups have continuous contact, which results in changes in the cultural patterns of either or both of the groups

acquire knowledge—The cycle of assessing, processing, and understanding information

action—Actually making a change

action stage—Stage during which the individual is implementing behavioral change

activating events (A)—The cause of behavioral and emotional consequences that individuals experience

activities of daily living (ADLs)—Tasks that are typically performed in a habitual manner, every day, and across all age groups, genders, and cultures

acute dynamic factors—Characteristics that can change extremely quickly, such as the deterioration in mood or thought processing often seen in the exacerbation of mental illness or negative behavioral outcomes as a result of alcohol intoxication

acute pain—Pain that comes on quickly, can be severe, but lasts a relatively short time. Acute pain and its associated physiologic, psychological, and behavioral responses are almost always caused by tissue irritation or damage in relation to injury, disease, disability, or medical procedures

acute stressors—Any short-term event or situation that induces emotional distress in a given client and goes away quickly

adaptation—Adjustment of a person to fluctuating circumstances within or external to the individual

affective dimensions—One dimension of pain referring to fear, tension, and autonomic properties

after-school program (ASP)—An intervention offered to children between ages 5 and 18 during the school year and after normal school hours

agnosia—Loss of comprehension of visual, auditory, or other sensations, although sensory sphere is intact

agoraphobia—Anxiety about or avoidance of open places or situations from which one may feel unable to get away or help may not be available given paniclike symptoms

allostasis—The physiological changes that accompany the body's readiness activities

Alzheimer disease—The most common type of dementia, which is an age-related, neurological, degenerative disorder that predominately affects persons over age 65

Americans with Disabilities Act of 1990 (ADA)—Legislation passed by the U.S. Congress in 1990 to ensure the rights of persons with disabilities and to prohibit discrimination on the basis of disability in employment, public services, transportation, public accommodation, communications, state and local governments, and the U.S. Congress. An individual with a disability is defined by the ADA as one with a physical or mental impairment that limits one or more major life activities, a person with a history or record of an impairment, or a person perceived by others to have such an impairment.

analgesic—Pain-relieving medication

analysis of occupational performance—The process of examining the client's occupational performance with the intention to elicit more targeted information regarding the performance skills/patterns, person factors, activity demands, and contextual barriers that may need intervention to facilitate successful work participation

anchoring and adjustment heuristic—A heuristic used when people start with an anchor and then make adjustments with additional information

anergia—Lack of energy

anger—A feeling of tension and hostility, typically accompanied by anxiety aroused by a perceived threat to self, possessions, personal rights, or core values

anhedonia—Absence of pleasure from those activities that would ordinarily be enjoyable

animal-assisted therapy (AAT)—Interactions between clients and a trained animal, along with its human owner or handler, with the aim of facilitating client's progress toward therapeutic goals

anorexia nervosa—Disorder described as the intense fear of being fat, a disturbance of body image, and an obsession with food and thinness, associated with the refusal to maintain a normal weight for one's age and height. This obsession translates into severe food restriction and extreme weight control behaviors, which lead to major weight loss

antidepressants—Medications used for relieving symptoms of depression

antisocial personality disorder—Disorder characterized by a pervasive pattern of disregard for and violation of the rights of others that begins in childhood or early adolescence and continues into adulthood. Symptoms of conduct disorder will have been present prior to age 15, and for the person being diagnosed, the individual must be 18 years of age

anxiety—Unpleasant emotional state associated with psychophysiological changes in response to an intrapsychic conflict; in contrast to fear, the danger or threat in anxiety is unreal. Potential issues include an uncomfortable feeling of impending danger, an overwhelming awareness of being powerless, inability to perceive the unreality of the threat, prolonged feeling of tension, and exhaustive readiness for the expected danger with physiological conditions including an increased heart rate, disturbed breathing, trembling, sweating, and vasomotor changes

anxiety disorders—A category of conditions involving anxiety reactions in response to stress, including phobic disorder, panic disorder with agoraphobia, agoraphobia without history of panic disorder, social phobia, simple phobia, generalized anxiety disorder, obsessive compulsive disorder, and posttraumatic stress disorder

aphasia—Absence or impairment of the ability to communicate through speech, writing, or signs because of brain dysfunction

apraxia—Inability to perform purposive movements, although there is no sensory or motor impairment

arena-style assessment—An assessment in which one team member is the evaluation facilitator and is primarily responsible for interacting with the child during the actual assessment, and another team member may serve as coach. This person assists the facilitator during the assessment and facilitates discussion after the evaluation. All other team members observe the child's responses during the evaluation

Asperger's disorder—A severe and sustained impairment of social interaction and functioning. Considered to be on the autism spectrum, there are no clinically significant delays in language, cognitive, or developmental age–appropriate skills

assertive community treatment (ACT)—A community-oriented intensive case management developed in response to the deinstitutionalization movement of psychiatric rehabilitation. The key objectives of ACT are to reduce the hospital admission rate among individuals with the most serious disabilities, develop skills for community living, and promote proper utilization of mental health services

assigning homework—Requiring clients, as part of their daily lives outside of therapy sessions, to experiment with, apply, practice, or supplement what is addressed in therapy

associated conditions—Conditions directly related to the etiology of the primary impairment (e.g., early dementia, heart defects, low muscle tone)

asylums—Psychiatric hospitals (intended to protect and treat people with mental illness); a place and space dedicated for the relief of care of the destitute or sick, especially those with mental illness

at risk—The possibility of a child being diagnosed as developmentally delayed; risk is identified among children born with significant biological risks or who are living in a high-risk environment

attention deficit-hyperactivity disorder (ADHD)—Disorder characterized by a persistent pattern of inattention and/or hyperactivity-impulsivity that is more frequent and severe than is typically observed in individuals at a comparable level of development

attention deficit-hyperactivity disorder, combined type—Subtype of ADHD used if six (or more) symptoms of hyperactivity-impulsivity have persisted for at least 6 months. Most children and adolescents with the disorder have the combined type. It is not known whether the same is true of adults with the disorder

attention deficit-hyperactivity disorder, predominantly hyperactive-impulsive type—Subtype of ADHD used if six (or more) symptoms of hyperactivity-impulsivity (but fewer than six symptoms of inattention) have persisted for at least 6 months. Inattention may often still be a significant clinical feature in such cases

attention deficit-hyperactivity disorder, predominantly inattentive type—Subtype of ADHD used if six (or more) symptoms of inattention (but fewer than six symptoms of hyperactivity-impulsivity) have persisted for at least 6 months. Hyperactivity may still be a significant clinical feature in many such cases, whereas other cases are more purely inattentive

attenuation theory—Approach suggesting that unattended information is not totally blocked but is turned down, distinguished from filter theory suggesting that unattended messages are fully blocked and unattended

atypical antipsychotics—A functional category of newer (since the 1990's) antipsychotic drugs thought to exert their action predominantly through serotonergic blockade. They are considered the "second generation" of antipsychotics.

atypical autism—Characterized by either that there were no characteristics of autism before age 3 or the child does not meet the criteria for one of the areas of impairment as identified in the DSM-IV-TR diagnosis of autism

atypical subtype—A subtype of depressive episodes characterized by mood brightening with positive events and neurovegetative functions that are reversed from the melancholic (e.g., appetite is increased, sleep is excessive, and the person may feel leaden paralysis, as if he or she is unable to move). Symptoms are worse at night in atypical depression, and the individual is highly sensitive to rejection by others

autism spectrum disorder (ASD)—A nonspecific diagnosis of any developmental disorder characterized by poor social abilities and impaired communication and commonly includes autism, Asperger's disorder, and pervasive developmental disorder not otherwise specified (PDD-NOS)

autogenic training (AT)—A method of self-induced deep relaxation, derived from hypnosis. It involves the silent repetition of phrases about homeostasis

automatic processing—Processing of information that guides behavior but without conscious awareness and without interfering with other conscious activity that may be going on at the same time

autonomy—Capacity of the client for self-direction and making his or her own choices, as opposed to authority, in which the therapist tells the client what to do

availability heuristic—A heuristic used when people estimate frequency or make decisions based on how easy it is to think of an example

avoidance—Withdrawal, distraction, use of substances, or other methods of staying away from the stressor

avolition—One of five negative symptoms of schizophrenia, including lack of attention to grooming and hygiene, difficulty persisting at work or school activities, and physical inertia

background and personal history—Life experiences within one's family of origin, extended family, neighborhoods, schools, spiritual community, society, and world

basic activities of daily living (BADLs)—Activities that focus on self-care, such as bathing, dressing and toileting

becoming—A person's sense of future or potential transformation and self-actualization

behavioral experiments—The most important behavioral strategy testing the client's thoughts, beliefs, and related behaviors as part of discovering his or her relative utility or validity. The typical behavioral experiment involves creating a hypothesis to test, predicting the outcome, undertaking the test or "experiment," evaluating the result, and then using this feedback to revise or create new perspectives

behavioral strategies—Some type of actions to manage stress, such as confronting a person about a conflict or engaging in physical activity to manage the feelings

behavioral strategies and techniques—Procedures that focus on activating or monitoring overt observable behaviors such as "doing" an action, activity, or behavioral experiment or on covert behaviors such as self-reported thoughts and feelings and may be used to directly or indirectly impact beliefs

being—Existing within the environment

belief system (B)—A shared system of beliefs and values that systematically define a way of perceiving the social, cultural, physical, and psychological world

belonging—Being a member of the environment

bereavement—A reaction to loss that encompasses the emotional and physical reactions of grief and mourning. It involves a psychological process of letting go of relationships

bibliotherapy—Use of specific reading materials as a therapeutic intervention

binge-eating/purging type—Subtype of anorexia nervosa in which most individuals who binge eat also purge through self-induced vomiting or the misuse of laxatives, diuretics, or enemas. Some individuals included in this subtype do not binge eat but do regularly purge after the consumption of small amount of food

biopsychosocial model—A conceptual model that assumes that psychological and social factors must also be included along with the biologic in understanding a person's condition

bipolar disorder—One of mood disorders characterized by recurrent episodes of both ends of an extreme from the low, sad, and unpleasant mood of depression to the elevated, elated, and energized mood of mania

bipolar I disorder—A disorder characterized by one or more manic episodes or mixed episodes (i.e., frequent fluctuations between low and expansive mood)

bipolar II disorder—A disorder characterized by one or more major depressive episodes and at least one hypomanic episode

bizarre delusion—Outside of the realm of possibility

board and care home—Living arrangements that provide shelter, food, and 24-hour supervision or protective oversight and personal care services to residents. Other terms for board and care homes include *homes for the aged, residential care homes, adult foster care, domiciliary care,* and *assisted-living facilities*

body mass index (BMI)—A rough method of assessing weight status calculated by dividing an individual's weight (in kilograms) by the square of his or her height (in meters). Normal BMI ranges between 20 and 25

bradykinesia—A decrease in spontaneity; slowed movement

bradyphrenia—Abnormal slowness of respiration, specifically a low respiratory frequency

capitation—A form of reimbursement for health-care services in which the health insurer assigns a finite number of patients to the care of a subcontracting provider. The health-care provider is paid a predetermined amount for each patient enrolled in his or her care. This arrangement provides incentives to the provider to limit health-care costs by placing the provider at financial risk if the cost of care provided exceeds the payment received

case management—Individualized process or method for ensuring that a consumer is provided with needed services in a coordinated, effective, and efficient manner

catastrophic reactions—Emotional and physical reactions to tasks, such as yelling or hitting due to frustration with a task the person can no longer perform

categorization—The process in which ideas and objects are recognized, differentiated, and understood. Categorization implies that objects are grouped into categories, usually for some specific purpose

central executive—Process that moves information in and out of short-term memory and integrates new information that is coming in with long-term memory stores

Certified Alcohol and Drug Counselors (CADC)—Professionals who assist clients affected by the use of alcohol or other drugs by focusing on gaining and maintaining skills for a substance-free lifestyle

childhood disintegrative disorder (CDD)—A personality disorder of children marked by regression in many areas of functioning after at least 2 years of normal development. Individuals exhibit social, communicative, and behavioral characteristics similar to those of autistic disorder

choose, get, and keep model—A vocational behavior approach that includes selecting an appropriate and suitable occupational goal and planning to achieve the goal, finding employment opportunities and acquiring a job, and adapting to the workplace and retaining employment

chronic, intermittent stressors—An agent, condition, or other stimulus that persistently but irregularly causes stress to an individual

chronic, permanent stressors—An agent, condition, or other stimulus that continuously causes stress to an individual

chronic/persistent pain—Pain that persists beyond its typical course of recovery. Unlike acute pain, persistent pain does not appear to serve a biologic purpose and is often experienced in the presence of minimal or no apparent tissue damage. Persistent pain typically produces significant changes in mood, thoughts, attitudes, lifestyle, and environment

circadian rhythm—The physiological 24-hour time pattern of human life. It includes usual periods of being alert and awake, an energy dip, and sleep

circadian rhythm sleep disorders—Disorders characterized by a persistent or recurrent pattern of sleep disruption that results from a mismatch between the individual's endogenous circadian sleep–wake system and external demands regarding the timing and duration of sleep

classical (or respondent) conditioning—A procedure in which a neutral stimulus is repeatedly paired with a stimulus (unconditioned stimulus) that naturally elicits a response (unconditioned response) until the neutral stimulus (conditioned stimulus) comes to elicit that response (now the conditioned response) by itself. It is also called Pavlovian conditioning and respondent conditioning

classification—A systemic arrangement into classes or groups based on perceived common characteristics; a means of giving order to a group of disconnected facts

client-centered practice—Emphasis on a client's autonomy and right to choose goals and/or interventions based on his or her identified needs for services

clinical depression—A serious medical illness that lasts for weeks, months, and sometimes years. Individuals with clinical depression are unable to function as they used to. Often they have lost interest in activities that were once enjoyable to them, and they feel sad and hopeless for extended periods of time. It may even influence someone to contemplate or attempt suicide

clubhouse model—A comprehensive and dynamic program of support and opportunities for people with severe and persistent mental illnesses. Clubhouse participants are called *members* (as opposed to *patients* or *clients*), and restorative activities focus on their strengths and abilities, not on their illness. The clubhouse is unique in that it is not a clinical program, meaning there are no therapists or psychiatrists on staff. Additionally, all participation in a clubhouse is strictly on a voluntary basis

cognition—Thinking skills, including language use, calculation, perception, memory, awareness, reasoning, judgment, learning, intellect, social skills, and imagination

cognitive behavior modification (CBM)—A remedial approach used in behavior therapy to influence various classes of disorders such as anxiety, fears, phobias, aggression, and disorders of conduct. CBM combines elements of behavior therapy (e.g., modeling, feedback, reinforcement) with cognitive approaches (e.g., cognitive think aloud) to teach individuals to self-regulate for the purpose of changing their own behavior

cognitive behavior therapy (CBT)—An active, problem-oriented treatment task that seeks to identify and change maladaptive beliefs, attitudes, and behaviors that contribute to emotional distress

cognitive interventions—Treatments to identify and modify the consumer's thoughts, feelings, beliefs, and attitudes related to pain, disability, and quality of life. It is assumed that an individual's affect and behaviors are greatly influenced by cognitive appraisal whereby the person interprets events in terms of their perceived significance

cognitive reconstruction—One of the elements for eating disorder treatment, delivered via individual and/or group therapy to improve ego strength, conflict resolution, personal identity, and self-acceptance at normal body weight

cognitive restructuring—Any psychological method used to remove negative thoughts or irrational roadblocks that harm a person's emotional health and replace those thoughts with neutral or more positive perspectives

cognitive skills—Thinking skills, including language use, calculation, perception, memory, awareness, reasoning, judgment, learning, intellect, social skills, and imagination

cognitive strategies—Efforts to analyze the situation to fully understand the nature of the threat or challenge

cognitive-behavioral strategies—Ways to identify and change maladaptive cognitions, beliefs, and attitudes about pain and promote the use of adaptive behavioral coping skills training (e.g., cognitive restructuring), relaxation training (with or without biofeedback), imagery, distraction, and hypnosis

collaboration—1. A prescribed process of integration in which there is planned communication and deliberate sharing of information. The providers of care may enter into a formal contractual relationship, delineating separate responsibilities for each diagnostic category (i.e., one provider addresses the mental health problem and the other addresses the substance use problem). 2. A recursive process whereby the therapist and client work together in an intersection of common goals as partners

collectivism—A frame of reference whereby an individual's behavior and worth are determined by the valued group

community development—A process of building local communities to support the wellbeing of both individual community members and the community as a whole

community integration—The opportunity to live in the community and be valued for one's uniqueness and abilities, like everyone else. Community integration encompasses housing, employment, education, health status, leisure/recreation, spirituality/religion, citizenship and civic engagement, valued social roles (e.g., marriage, parenting), peer support, and self-determination. Community integration should result in community presence and participation of people with psychiatric disabilities similar to that of all others without a disability label

Community Mental Health Centers Act of 1963 (CMHA)—An act to provide federal funding for community mental health centers (also known as the Community Mental Health Centers Construction Act, Public Law 88-164, or the Mental Retardation and Community Mental Health Centers Construction Act of 1963). The purpose of the CMHA was to provide for community-based care as an alternative to institutionalization

comorbid conditions—Diseases that are unrelated to the primary condition but co-occur with the associated condition (e.g., influenza, glaucoma, breast cancer)

compensatory approach—Intervention approach whereby the therapist adapts the environment, task, or teaching method to compensate for the cognitive impairment

competence—Analogous to self-efficacy. A belief in individual's own capability, which motivates him or her to act

complicated grief—An emotional reaction to a loss that is prolonged, persistent, and severe and is sometimes called *abnormal grief*. It interferes with a person's entire life, diminishing his or her interests and desires in life, and often takes the form of severe depression

concept formation—Learning to conceive and respond in terms of abstract ideas based on an action or object

concrete value—The type of occupational value characterized by the concrete and visible features of value inherent in occupations

conduct disorder—Disorder characterized by a repetitive and persistent pattern of behavior in which the basic rights of others or major age-appropriate societal norms or rules are violated. These behaviors fall into four main categories: aggressive conduct that causes or threatens physical harm to other people or animals, nonaggressive conduct that causes property loss or damage, deceitfulness or theft, and serious violations of rules

connectedness—Association with or related to others, especially to influential or important people

consequences (C)—The end result of a behavior, which may be positive, negative, or neutral

consultant—A health-care worker who acts in an advisory capacity

consultation—Meeting of two or more health-care practitioners to evaluate the nature and progress of disease in a particular client and to establish diagnosis, prognosis, and/or therapy. It is a level of integration in which the service provider informally and occasionally communicates information about the person's status to the other providers

consumer-operated services—Peer-run, self-help organizations or groups that are administratively and financially controlled by persons participating in mental health services (consumers). They are not simply mental health services delivered by consumers, but are independent, peer-run programs. In general, they offer mutual support, community-building, and advocacy

consumer-survivor movement—A diverse association of individuals (and organizations representing them) who are either currently consumers (clients) of mental health services or consider themselves survivors of psychiatry or mental health services, or who simply identify as "expatients" of mental health services. The movement campaigns for more choice and improved services and/or empowerment and user-led alternatives. Common themes are "talking back to the power of psychiatry," rights protection and advocacy, and self-determination

contemplation—An action of considering the pros and cons of changing when the person starts thinking about the problem or concern

contemplation stage—Stage during which an individual starts to consider changing

contingency management (CM)—An intervention strategy that, using the principles of operant conditioning, provides reinforcing consequences for substance-abusing individuals who meet treatment goals

controlled processing—Processing of information that is conscious, effortful, and planned

co-occupation—Mutually engaging in occupation

co-occurring disorders (COD)—Two or more disorders (often a substance-related disorder and a mental disorder) occurring at the same time in an individual

coping—Adapting to and managing change, stress, or opportunity (e.g., acute or chronic illness, disability, pain, death, relocation, work, changes in family structure, new relationships, or new ideas)

coping process—Process involving information processing, emotions, and a behavioral response

corticobasal ganglionic degeneration—A neurological disorder in which brain cells atrophy and die in the basal ganglia and the cortex of the brain. While the disease produces symptoms similar to those found in Parkinson's disease it does not respond to parkinsonian medications

cultural competence—Sensitivity to the cultural, philosophical, religious, and social preferences of people of varying ethnicities or nationalities. Professional skill in the use of such sensitivities facilitates optimal care of individuals and families

cultural context—Customs, beliefs, activity patterns, behavior standards, and expectations accepted by the society of which the individual is a member. It includes political aspects, such as laws that affect access to resources and affirm personal rights. Opportunities for education, employment, and economic support are also included

cultural formulation outline—A resource for a systematic review of a person's cultural background and the role of culture in the manifestation of symptoms and dysfunction. It includes the cultural identity of the individual,

cultural explanations of the illness, cultural factors related to the environment and individual functioning, cultural elements of the clinician–patient relationship, and a general discussion of how cultural considerations may influence the diagnosis and treatment of a psychiatric condition

cultural practices—The doing of culture, or the discrete, observable, objective, and behavioral aspects of human activities related to culture in which people engage

cultural safety—The concept extending notions of cultural sensitivity or cultural competency, which often ignore the power dynamics between those providing and those seeking services, particularly marginalized populations. This concept suggests that health care providers must recognize the broader sociopolitical aspects of providing care to marginalized persons

cultural worldview—The way in which a person or group looks at the world and their place in it. It is a belief system grounded in moral and ethical reasoning, magicoreligious beliefs, cosmology, values, social relationships, and the person's connection to nature

culturally and linguistically appropriate services—Services that are respectful and responsive to the cultural and linguistic needs of consumers and their families

culture—Something that is learned and shared among members of a group and that is cumulative and dynamic, including a system of shared meaning through language and nonverbal communication. It is value laden and defines norms for roles, relationships, obligations, beliefs, health practices, and behavior

culture bound syndromes—Recurrent, locality-specific patterns of aberrant behavior and troubling experience that may or may not be linked to a particular DSM-IV-TR diagnostic category. Many of these patterns are indigenously considered to be "illness," or at least afflictions, and most have local names. Cultural-bound syndromes are generally limited to specific societies or culture areas and are localized, folk, diagnostic categories that frame coherent meanings for certain repetitive, patterned, and troubling sets of experiences and observations

culture emergent model—An inquiry-centered approach to developing the knowledge, attitudes, and skills for culturally competent practice. In this process-oriented approach, the specific culture is irrelevant. The model stresses the development of skills for cross-cultural interactions, that is, learning to ask questions

culture-specific expertise—A strong base of cultural information for all groups

cyclothymic disorder—A chronic (at least 2-year period) mood disturbance characterized by fluctuating hypomanic symptoms and depressive symptoms that are not of sufficient number or severity to reach criteria for either manic episodes or major depressive episodes

decisional balance—Identifying the pros and cons of both changing and not changing

declarative memory—Conscious awareness of events and objects, including encoding, storing, and retrieving information

deep processing—An activity of finding meaning in facts in order to result in better remembering

defensive retreat, or denial—Defense mechanism in which the existence of unpleasant realities is disavowed; refers to a keeping out of conscious awareness any aspects of either internal or external reality that, if acknowledged, would result in anxiety

delirium—An acute, reversible state of disorientation and confusion. Delirium is marked by disorientation without drowsiness; hallucinations or delusions; difficulty in focusing attention; inability to rest or sleep; and emotional, physical, and autonomic overactivity

delusions—Distortions in thought or false beliefs

dementia—An acquired syndrome that results from a disease or disorder of the brain that affects cognition, or thinking, and memory. It disrupts perception, information processing, problem-solving, judgment, sequencing of tasks, recognition and naming of objects, mood and affect, writing and calculating, and other functions necessary to carry out daily activities

depression—A temporary mood state or chronic mental disorder characterized by feelings of sadness, loneliness, despair, low self-esteem, and self-reproach; accompanying signs include may include psychomotor retardation or less frequently agitation, withdrawal from social contact, and vegetative states such as loss of appetite and insomnia

depressive episode—The period characterized by a depressed mood and loss of interest or pleasure in life activities for at least 2 weeks

determination stage—Stage during which a person considers change, recognizes the challenges, but also builds a determination to at least start to change some of the behaviors

developmental delay—An impairment in the performance of tasks or the meeting of milestones that a child should achieve by a specific chronological age. The diagnosis of a developmental delay is made with use of standardized tools assessing cognitive, physical, social, and emotional development as well as communication and adaptive skills

developmental regression—The second phase of Rett's disorder beginning from 2 to 4 years of age. Its duration can range from weeks up to 1 year. This stage includes the loss of skills characteristic for the developmental stage

dialectical behavior therapy (DBT)—A comprehensive cognitive-behavioral treatment protocol for complex and difficult-to-treat mental disorders that combines individual psychotherapy with psychosocial skills training

diathesis stress model—A view that abnormal behavior is a function of a series of stressors in predisposed individuals (due to hereditary, temperamental, and sociocultural factors)

direct service provider—Professional who provides for the basic care and training of individuals with disabilities. This involves the areas of daily living skills development, speech and language development, mobility, learning, and vocational development as directed by state and federal regulation

direct source of poverty—Necessary expenses such as for therapy and special equipment that consume a client's financial resources

direct threat—A significant risk to the health or safety of others that cannot be eliminated by reasonable accommodation

disability—A physical or mental impairment that substantially limits one or more of an individual's major life activities, defined by the U.S. government; this includes individuals with a record of an impairment and those regarded as having such an impairment/loss of function at the level of the whole person, which may include inability to communicate or to perform mobility, activities of daily living, or necessary vocational or avocational activities, thereby limiting full participation in everyday life

disability communities—Collectives of individuals and their families who share a disability experience; may join together in advocacy or supporting one another

disability rights movement—Effort to improve the quality of life of people with disabilities. For people with physical disabilities accessibility and safety are primary issues that this movement works to reform

disaffiliation—People whose circumstances have devolved to such a level of disruption that they are viewed as "other" (e.g., street people or the homeless)

diseases of adaptation—Stage of exhaustion that is responsible for the onset of diseases

disruptive behavior disorder, not otherwise specified—Disorder characterized by conduct, or oppositional defiant behaviors that do not meet the criteria for conduct disorder or oppositional defiant disorder

diversion—The routing of patients away from one facility to others. In forensic occupational therapy settings, offenders are sent to a residential or nonresidential setting as an alternative to incarceration

divided attention—Aspect of consciousness carrying out more than one task at a time

doing—Acting on the environment and interacting with other people

domestic violence—Intentionally inflicted injury perpetrated by and on family member(s); varieties include spouse abuse, child abuse, and sexual abuse, including incest. May include any abuse that occurs within one's home by others who share that home

double stigma—A stigma resulting from prejudice and discrimination that occurs when the individual has a mental illness and belongs to an ethnic minority group

drop-in centers—A place for give-and-take exchange of information within a neighborhood or community. An easy-to-find location on home turf makes it convenient and easy for people to get information on a program or plan and to express their concerns and issues. A drop-in center offers informal, continuing contact with the community

drugs and illicit drugs—Any substances that are not sanctioned by custom or law, such as marijuana or cannabis (including hashish), cocaine (including crack), heroin (opioids), hallucinogens (including LSD, PCP, peyote, mescaline, mushrooms, and Ecstasy), inhalants, and psychotherapeutics (including nonmedical use of prescription-type pain relievers, tranquilizers, stimulants [including methamphetamines], and sedatives)

dual diagnosis capable—The term used when admitting a client with a co-occurring disorder to a program that is primarily oriented to one diagnostic classification over the other; the personnel are appropriately trained and services are available to address the integrated assessment and intervention processes

dual diagnosis enhanced program—Program in which a high level of integration exists, with no one orientation to a primary diagnostic category

dynamic risk factors—Variables of risk that can change over time and can include socioeconomic, marital, or employment status, family support, criminal network, and substance abuse

dynamic sizing—The practitioner's capacity to ask himself or herself whether what he or she knows about a person's cultural group fits the particular individual being treated

dynamic systems theory—Concept that all of the components of a system are interrelated; if there is a change in one aspect of the system, the other components are affected

dysfunctional thought record (DTR)—A worksheet widely used in cognitive therapy to help patients respond to automatic thoughts and to change negative mood states

dysthymic disorder, or dysthymia—Disorder characterized by features similar to major depressive disorder, but symptoms are less severe and must be present chronically (a period of at least 2 years) rather than episodically. In children, irritability may be observed more than depressed mood. Feelings of inadequacy, guilt, and excessive anger are commonly experienced in dysthymia, along with periods of social withdrawal and reduced activity or productivity

early intervention—A multidisciplinary, coordinated, natural environment–based system (i.e., least restrictive environment) of service provision to eligible children birth to 3 or 5 years of age and their families (depending on governmental jurisdiction); provided under the U.S. Individuals with Disabilities Education Act, Part C. Services are designed to address identified developmental delays and at risk situations of the child and/or the family

early onset stagnation—The first phase of Rett's disorder beginning at 5 months of age and continuing for weeks to months

eating disorders—A disorder characterized by severe disturbances in eating behavior. It includes two specific diagnoses, anorexia nervosa and bulimia nervosa. Anorexia nervosa is characterized by a refusal to maintain a minimally normal body weight. Bulimia nervosa is characterized by repeated episodes of binge eating followed by inappropriate behaviors such as self-induced vomiting; misuse of laxatives, diuretics, or other medications; fasting; or excessive exercise

education programs—Informal programs including training programs during which consumers learn recovery and advocacy skills. These programs are typically time limited. Using a consumer-led group format, consumers meet to acquire new information or gain new skills

electroconvulsive shock treatment (ECT)—The use of an electric shock to produce convulsions and thereby treat drug-resistant or especially severe psychiatric disorders such as major depression

emergency hospitalization—The practice of hospitalizing a person detained against his or her will for, on average, 3 to 5 days while a hearing is convened to evaluate whether there is probable cause to hold the individual

emotion—An evaluative mental state produced by a neural impulse. Emotions include a combination of physiological arousal, subjective experience, and behavioral or affective expression

emotion dysregulation—Emotional responses that are not adaptive to the particular situation. Dysregulated emotion does not always involve a negative emotion (although most frequently it does), but it involves an emotional experience that interferes with goal-oriented activity

emotion regulation—Efforts to control emotional states

emotion regulation skills—Ability to control emotional states. Emotions can be regulated before or after they occur. One way that emotions are regulated is by reframing the meaning of events or putting perspective on events before they occur

emotional functions—Appropriate range and regulation of emotions; self-control

emotional stress—A sustained, damaging emotional response and the inability to control such responses

emotionality—The observable behavioral and physiological component of emotion; it is a measure of a person's emotional reactivity to a stimulus

employee assistance programs—Confidential resources to assist employees with life issues that impact their ability to focus on or meet employment expectations

empowerment—Increasing the spiritual, political, social, or economic strength of individuals and communities. It often involves developing confidence in one's own capacities

enculturation—The process whereby an individual is taught the norms of the culture

engagement phase—The initial stage of wraparound process that focuses on team development through face-to-face contact with the family and either personal or telephone contact with potential team members

entitlement programs—The kind of government program that provides individuals with personal financial benefits (or sometimes special government-provided goods or services) to which an indefinite (but usually rather large) number of potential beneficiaries have a legal right (enforceable in court, if necessary) whenever they meet eligibility conditions that are specified by the standing law that authorizes the program

environment—The milieu; the aggregate of all of the external conditions and influences affecting the life and development of an individual

environmental press—Occurs when forces in the environment, together with individual need, evoke a response

environment-focused interventions—Environmental solutions that have the potential to indirectly influence a person's thoughts and beliefs. Educating family, friends, caregivers, and health care professionals using the same teaching-learning and cognitive behavior treatment strategies and techniques used with clients is an environmentally focused intervention that can indirectly have a profound impact on modifying a person's dysfunctional beliefs

episodes—Distinct periods and features of mood disturbance

episodic memory—Memory for events that have happened to the person. It is organized temporally, or by when it occurred

essential functions—Tasks and responsibilities that the individual who holds the job would have to perform, with or without reasonable accommodation, in order to be considered qualified for the position

established risk—A child's diagnosed condition that places him or her at risk for delays in social/emotional, cognitive, or physical development

ethnicity—The state or fact of belonging to a particular ethnic group. Ethnic group refers to a social group characterized by a distinctive social and cultural tradition maintained from generation to generation, a common history and origin, and a sense of identification with the group

ethnocentrism—The universal tendency of humans to appraise ways of thinking, acting, and believing according to their own experience and cultural background; that is, to see the world and what passes for normal behavior through one's own cultural lens

evaluative dimensions—One dimension of pain referring to the subjective overall intensity of the pain experience (e.g., annoying, miserable, unbearable)

evidence-based medicine (EBM)—The process of applying relevant information derived from peer-reviewed medical literature to address a specific clinical problem; the application of simple rules of science and common sense to determine the validity of the information; and the application of the information to the clinical issue

evidence-based practice—The conscientious and judicious use of current best evidence in making decisions about the care of clients. Health services are bolstered by a strong scientific base, preferably accumulated through a plethora of randomized clinical trials performed by different research teams in multiple research sites and even in different places of the world

evocation—Drawing on the client to identify his or her own goals and values toward change. This is different from education that focuses on providing knowledge or skills to the client

exclusion—Disconnection from the situation or society overall

executive dysfunction—Inability to think abstractly and to plan, initiate, sequence, monitor, and stop complex behavior

executive function—A theorized cognitive system that controls and manages other cognitive processes. The concept is used to describe a loosely defined collection of brain processes which are responsible for planning, cognitive flexibility, abstract thinking, rule acquisition, initiating appropriate actions and inhibiting inappropriate actions, and selecting relevant sensory information

expectancies—The act, action, or state of looking forward to or awaiting some occurrence or outcome

exploration—An individual's ability to identify play or leisure activities, interests, skills, or opportunities

expressed emotion—A qualitative measure of the "amount" of emotion displayed, typically in the family setting, usually by a family or caretakers. Theoretically, a high level of expressed emotion in the home can worsen the prognosis in clients with mental illness or act as a potential risk factor for the development of psychiatric disease

extrinsic motivation—A tendency to obtain some outcome that is separate from the inherent satisfaction of the activity itself

Fairweather Lodge model—A psychosocial rehabilitation model combining congregate living with collaborative employment. A typical Fairweather Lodge is an affordable dwelling for four to eight people who share in running the home, including domestic chores and purchase and preparation of food. The residents make their own house rules and manage their own activities. In addition, they run a small business chosen by consensus and jointly planned

faith background—One's spiritual or religious experiences and beliefs

family—A social system consisting of a group of individuals whose occupations are interrelated. It is not limited to a specific family structure, the number or gender of the people in the family group, or the biological (genetic) relationships among family members. It is people who voluntarily consider themselves to be family as a result of their interaction, situation, psychological attachment, or capacity to reciprocally satisfy social needs

family intervention (FI)—Intervention of more than one member of a family in the same session; family relationships and processes are explored in order to reduce relapse rates, enhance the social adjustment of people with psychotic disorders, and reduce caregiver stress and burden

family respite—Brief periods of relief for families providing caregiving to persons living in the community

family-centered care—A social model that promotes competencies based on the family life style

feelings—An inner subjective sensation without a physiological response

fetal alcohol spectrum disorder (FASD)—Disorder characterized by problems in infants caused by a woman's alcohol use during pregnancy. It includes fetal alcohol syndrome (FAS), alcohol-related neurodevelopmental disorder, and other alcohol-related birth defects, which manifest themselves in a wide range of behavioral, cognitive, physical, and health-related problems throughout childhood with carryover into adulthood

fidelity measures—Assessment tools examining the extent to which a program's implementation is true to the program model. Fidelity measures rate programs against an agreed-upon list of components within a program model

filter theory—Approach suggesting there is a limit to the amount of information a person can attend to at any one point in time. Therefore, individuals use an "attentional filter" that lets in some information and blocks the rest. Only the information that is allowed in can be utilized later. The filter prevents people from experiencing information overload

flow—A timeless experience in an inherently satisfying activity wherein a person's skill just meets the challenge of the situation

forensic occupational therapy—The application of mental health specialty practice in legal contexts. Forensic mental health occupational therapists work with individuals with mental disorders who have committed a crime and are consigned by law into custody at a correctional setting

forensic setting—A setting pertaining to or connected with the correctional system

formal neighborhood profiles—An accurate representation of a neighborhood community with regard to information about the population, employment rates, business and industry, land use, educational opportunities, housing, recreational resources, and health services

frontotemporal lobe dementia or Pick disease—A degenerative brain disease that particularly affects the frontal and temporal lobes. As in other frontal lobe dementias, Pick disease is characterized clinically by changes in personality early in the course, deterioration of social skills, emotional blunting, behavioral disinhibition, and prominent language abnormalities

full integration—The ideal level of integration as it involves a single intervention plan that addresses both substance abuse and mental health conditions

gatekeeping—Deciding the allocation, limitation, or rationing of services. Decisions are based on a variety of factors including need; cost; the potential for success of the proposed therapy; and the availability of facilities, staff, and equipment in order to control costs

generalized adaptation syndrome—A group of common symptoms during illness characterized as representing the body's ordinary physiological reaction to unfavorable conditions, passing through the alarm reaction, resistance or adaptation, and finally exhaustion stage

generalized anxiety disorder (GAD)—Anxiety disorder characterized by at least 6 months of persistent and excessive anxiety and worry

graded activity programs—Programs implementing a biomechanical approach whereby purposeful activities are graded from low to high in demand with regard to performance components (e.g., range of motion, strength, and endurance)

grief—An emotional reaction to a loss

group—A social microcosm in which members have the opportunity to interact with each other

growth—Development, maturation, or expansion of physical structures or cognitive and psychosocial abilities. Particularly, cognitive growth is evidenced by the progressive maturation of thought, reasoning, and intellect, especially in school-aged children. Psychosocial growth involves the development of personality, judgment, and temperament across one's lifetime, as experience in work, play, and emotional interactions with others broaden

guided discovery—A process therapists use to help clients reflect on how they process information. Through answering questions or reflecting on thinking processes, a range of alternative thinking is opened up for each client. This alternative thinking forms the blueprint for changing perceptions and behaviors

guided imagery—The purposeful use of images to reduce stress and distract attention away from intrusive thoughts. In this technique, the participant focuses on a relaxing environment (e.g., a peaceful garden) of his or her choice

guidelines for best practice—The best indicators about how to promote the client's recovery

gustatory systems—Systems relating to taste

habituation—The process by which occupation is organized into patterns or routines

habituation system—One of the subsystems of the model of human occupation forming structure and routine to daily life

hallucinations—Distortions in perception

health-care literacy—The consumers' ability to read, understand, and use health-care information, including having the social skills and motivation to gain access to this information and the cognitive skills to process and use the information to make appropriate decisions about their health

heritage consistency—The degree to which an individual's lifestyle reflects his or her traditional ethnic, religious, and cultural heritage

heuristics—A simple way to rapidly come to a solution that is hoped to be close to the best possible answer, or "optimal solution"

homeless shelters or transitional housing—Temporary, safe housing that typically provides a place to stay for one night to 30 days

homeostasis—The ability to maintain a favorable balance and adjust when external circumstances create abnormal circumstances

hope—The expectation that something desired will occur. Can be considered an important therapeutic tool in promoting mental health recovery

Housing First—An approach to ending homelessness that centers on providing homeless people with housing quickly and then providing services as needed

human and social services sector—Housing, employment, and income supports primarily for individuals who have serious and persistent mental illness

Human Rights Watch, 2003—An independent, nongovernmental organization supported by contributions from private individuals and foundations worldwide. It accepts no government funds, directly or indirectly. Human Rights Watch conducts regular, systematic investigations of human rights abuses in some 70 countries around the world

Huntington's disease—Inherited progressive degenerative disease of cognition, emotion, and movement. The disease, which affects men and women equally, is transmitted by a single autosomal dominant gene on the short arm of chromosome 4 and usually diagnosed in the late 30s to early 40s

hyperactivity-impulsivity—Manifestations of disturbed behavior in children or adolescents characterized by constant overactivity, distractibility, impulsiveness, inability to concentrate, and aggressiveness

hyperresponsive—Characterized by an abnormal high degree of responsiveness (to a sensory or emotional stimulus)

hypersomnia—Excessive daytime sleepiness lasting more than 1 hour at a time for every day for several months; the inability to feel refreshed after sleeping; excessively long periods of sleep (total sleep time of more than 10 hours a day); with no evidence of cataplexy or narcolepsy

hypomanic episodes—The periods similar to manic episodes, with periods of elevated, expansive, or irritable mood, but symptoms are at a lower intensity and without marked impairment in social or occupational functioning. Hypomania may even include brief periods of high efficiency or creativity

hyporesponsive—Characterized by a diminished degree of responsiveness (as to a physical or emotional stimulus)

hypothalamic-pituitary-adrenal axis (HPA)—A regulatory network that operates in response to stress and consists of chemical messengers that prepare the body for the fight-or-flight response and then a return to homeostasis, or relaxation, when the threat has been removed

identifying ABCs—A method that provides a framework to identify the activating events (A), irrational beliefs (B), and emotional and behavioral consequences (C) related to specific situations, beliefs, and thoughts or emotions that are interfering with a person's wellbeing

imitative behavior—One of the socializing techniques allowing group members to observe the interactions and behaviors of the group leaders and other group members, and then experiment with applying these interactions themselves

implementation phase—The third stage of the wrap-around process in which the team meets regularly to discuss the effectiveness of the interventions and adjust the plan accordingly. This phase continues until the team identifies adequate progress and begins to move ahead with the final phase of transition

inattention—Lack of attention

inclusive programs—Programs in which students, regardless of the severity of their disability, receive appropriate specialized instruction and related services within an age-appropriate general education classroom in the school that they would attend if they did not have a disability

independent employment (IE)—The fact that people with mental illnesses obtain and maintain jobs without support

independent living centers (ILC)—Nonresidential, nonprofit, and community-based organizations that coordinate services including counseling, training, rehabilitation, assistance with devices, and respite care by and for people with all types of disabilities and assist them to achieve their maximum potential within their families and communities

independent living movement (IL)—Effort focusing on personal assistance services and the removal of architectural and transportation barriers to allow individuals with disabilities to manage their daily life activities and fully participate in the life of the community

indirect source of poverty—Burden of care may present as an indirect source of poverty due to the number of hours of care needed which impact employability and income of the parent or caregiver

Individualized Family Service Plan (IFSP)—A plan of care that identifies the family's resources, desired outcomes for their child, activities to achieve the noted outcomes, developmental strengths and needs of their child, and plans for transition if the child is approaching his or her third birthday

infant mental health—An infant's capacities to feel and know about their environment and the people with whom they interact

information processing theory—A system for studying the communication process through the detailed analysis of all aspects of a process, including the encoding, transmission, and decoding of signals; not concerned in any direct sense with the meaning of a message

insomnia—Inability to sleep, in the absence of external impediments (e.g., noise, a bright light) during the period when sleep should normally occur; may range from restlessness or disturbed slumber to a shorter than normal length of sleep or to absolute wakefulness

instrumental activities of daily living (IADLs)—More complex activities than BADLs that require interaction with the environment and/or others such as grocery shopping, using public transportation, and money management

integrated assessment—Evaluation conducted when a person screens positive for the presence or history of mental illness and a substance use history; in general, it focuses on whether there are co-occurring disorders, delineates the specific diagnoses involved, determines the client's readiness for change, identifies the client's strengths and problem areas as they affect the process of recovery, and establishes the service needs of the person

integrated intervention—Treatment process conducted when all aspects of the co-occurring diagnostic conditions are addressed in a comprehensive plan, whether in a single contact or series of contacts over time

integrated screening—Initial patient evaluation conducted in a brief manner at the point of first contact with the individual; determines the likelihood of a co-occurring disorder and does not lead to a diagnosis; however, it determines whether there is a need for an in-depth integrated assessment and referral to a range of experts

integration—The bringing together of various parts so as to function as a harmonious whole

intellectual disability (replacing the term *mental retardation*)—Developmental disability characterized by significantly subaverage general intellectual functioning accompanied by significant limitations in adaptive functioning. Degrees of retardation are commonly measured in terms of I.Q.; for example, mild (50–55 to approximately 70), moderate (35–40 to 50–55), severe (20–25 to 35–40), and profound (below 20–25)

intensive outpatient programs (IOP)—An intermediate level of mental health care. Individuals are seen as a group two to five times a week (depending on the structure of the program) for 2 to 3 hours at a time. The clinical work is primarily done in a group setting, with individual sessions scheduled periodically generally outside group hours

intentionality—The use of a therapist's skilled interaction that elicits the desired response

interdependence—A dynamic of being mutually and physically responsible to and sharing a common set of principles with others. It is the result of an individually chosen balance between personal abilities and aspirations and environmental resources that support occupational functioning

interdisciplinary teaming—Team consisting of members who value each other's work and who communicate routinely and effectively. Interdisciplinary teams set goals collaboratively and through consensus. The child's family may not be considered team members

interests—One of the components of a volitional system, or things that give pleasure and satisfaction

internal working model—A unique, individualized conceptualization of self that is embedded in and influenced by the surrounding sociocultural environment. This model, composed of beliefs, goals, and strategies, provides a framework that defines identity

interpersonal and social rhythm therapy (IPSRT)—A therapeutic approach that has been used successfully for those individuals with bipolar disorder. In IPSRT, additional emphasis is placed on developing stable rhythms for daily routines, such as sleeping and eating, and social roles, such as a parent, spouse, worker

interpersonal learning—Broad and complex therapeutic factor occurring when the therapy group looks at the interpersonal distortions or misperceptions of others that impair social interaction. Through repeated opportunities for members to develop misperceptions of each other and then later correct those misperceptions, skills are gained as to how to correct or check their thoughts about one another

interpersonal psychotherapy (IPT)—A psychotherapeutic approach that focuses on clients' problems in interpersonal and social functioning as a means of symptom relief

intrinsic motivation—An innate tendency to seek novelty and strive for challenge and mastery

involuntarily outpatient commitment—Less restrictive, court-ordered mechanism that requires a consumer to submit to outpatient services if the person has a history of decompensation that has required involuntary commitment to inpatient facilities, has a history of severe and persistent mental illness and lacks insight into the need for treatment, and/or has a demonstrated risk of homelessness or incarceration

involuntary commitment—The practice of using legal means or forms as part of a mental health law to commit a person to a mental hospital, insane asylum, or psychiatric ward against his or her will and/or over his or her protests

labeling theory—The approach concerning how the self-identity and behavior of individuals may be determined or influenced by the terms used to describe or classify them; it is associated with the concept of a self-fulfilling prophecy and stereotyping (also known as social reaction theory). Unwanted descriptors or categorizations (including terms related to deviance, disability, or a diagnosis of mental illness) may be rejected on the basis that they are merely "labels," often with attempts to adopt a more constructive language in its place

late motor deterioration—The last phase of Rett's disorder beginning when the third stage and ambulation ceases; this stage can continue for decades. The fourth stage also has subgroups for individuals who once walked and for those who never walked and is characterized by severe disability, wheelchair dependency, and distortion and wasting of the extremities

legal aid societies—Nonprofit entities that provide civil legal assistance for individuals who cannot afford their own legal counsel

leisure—A nonobligatory activity that is intrinsically motivated and engaged in during discretionary time, that is, time not committed to obligatory occupations such as work, self-care, or sleep

Lewy body dementia—Same as diffuse Lewy body disease. A degenerative cerebral disorder of old people, characterized initially by progressive dementia or psychosis, and subsequently by parkinsonian findings, usually with severe rigidity; additional manifestations may include involuntary movements, myoclonus, dysphagia, and orthostatic hypotension. They present diffusely in the nuclei of the hypothalamus, basal forebrain, and brainstem

limbic-cortical circuit—A body structure that modulates arousal and alerting behaviors in organisms and allows for storage and retrieval of memories to enable approach/avoidance behaviors. This structure interacts in survival activities, such as eating, drinking, and reproduction, as well as during social interaction, emotion regulation, and activities related to pleasure and ego satisfaction

linear continuum paradigm—The paradigm of helping persons with psychiatric disabilities to find housing that can become a home that is safe and offers a base from which they may be fully engaged in their community as citizens

lived experience—The subjective perception of one's experience of health or illness. It is considered consistent with studying human experience from a qualitative, phenomenological perspective.

logos reasoning—The use of logical arguments to persuade an audience

long-term memory—The phase of the memory process considered as the permanent storehouse of information that has been registered, encoded, passed into the short-term memory, coded, rehearsed, and finally transferred and stored for future retrieval; cognitive abilities access material and information retained in long-term memory

low registration—A pattern of sensory processing characterized by high threshold and passive response; when people have low registration, they miss input that others take in. They may be slow to respond or may require repetition and cues

maintenance—Keeping a behavioral change for at least 6 months

maintenance stage—Stage during which an individual is learning to maintain the change he or she has implemented. The person consolidates and builds on the skills he or she has learned

major depressive disorder—Disorder characterized by one or more instances of a major depressive episode but no occurrence of a manic episode

malformation syndromes—Rare syndromes characterized by failure of typical development, including mental and physical retardation, infant death, and various other abnormalities; a localized error of morphogenesis resulting in a primary structural defect

manic episode—The period characterized by an abnormally elevated, expansive, or irritable mood for at least one week, in conjunction with other criteria, such as inflated self-esteem or grandiosity, decreased need for sleep, rapid speech, psychomotor agitation, and involvement in high-risk activities

marginality—Lack of integration with cultural experiences and norms

mastery—Success; possession of consummate skill

melancholic subtype—A subtype of depressive episodes characterized by loss of pleasure in nearly all activities and/or lack of pleasure even when something good happens, along with such symptoms as early morning awakenings, increased depression in the morning, marked weight loss, excessive guilt, and psychomotor retardation or agitation

memory impairment—An inability to learn new information and/or recall past information

Mental Health Parity Act of 1996—Legislation signed into U.S. law on September 26, 1996, requiring that annual or lifetime dollar limits on mental health benefits be no lower than any such dollar limits for medical and surgical benefits offered by a group health plan or health insurance issuer offering coverage in connection with a group health plan

mental hygiene movement—The science and practice of maintaining and restoring mental health; a branch of early 20th-century psychiatry that has become an interdisciplinary field including subspecialties in psychology, nursing, social work, law, occupational therapy and other professions

metacognition—Cognition about your own cognition; an awareness of what you know and what you do not know. It includes anticipating your abilities to cognitively manage situations and recognize errors as they occur

milieu therapy—The process of establishing a planned treatment environment where everyday interactions and therapeutic events are designed and integrated into the institution's daily routine with the goal of providing clients with opportunities for socialization and productivity

Mini Mental Status Examination (MMSE)—A commonly used assessment tool to quantify a person's cognitive ability. It assesses orientation, registration, attention, calculation, and language

minimal coordination of services—The term used when the service provider is aware of the co-occurring disorder (COD) and may be aware that the person is receiving help elsewhere for the other diagnostic category. One provider may have referred the client to another provider, but there is no contact or follow-up among service providers

mixed episodes—The periods characterized by rapid changes in moods occurring nearly daily

mobile support model—A system addressing the needs of students as they attend integrated college courses or technical training programs. In this model, staff members travel to students to provide assistance at the institution the student attends. Staff members are routinely housed in a community-based mental health center and commonly provide services at several postsecondary educational sites

modeling—Acquiring and learning a new skill by observing and imitating behavior being performed by another

modified labeling theory—The approach indicating that expectations of labeling can have a large negative effect, that these expectations often cause clients to withdraw from society, and that those labeled as having a mental disorder are constantly being rejected from society in seemingly minor ways, but when taken as a whole, all of these small slights can drastically alter their self-concepts. For a person who is labeled, he or she anticipates and perceives negative societal reactions, and this potentially damages quality of life

monoamine oxidase inhibitors (MAOIs)—A group of antidepressants that inhibit enzymatic breakdown of monoamine neurotransmitters of the sympathetic/adrenergic system; not used as first-line therapy because of the risk of hypertensive crisis after consumption of foods or beverages containing pressor amines, including cheese, chocolate, beer, and wine

mood disorders—Any mental disorder that has a disturbance of mood as the predominant feature. Mood disorders, including dysthymic disorder, are divided into the depressive disorders (unipolar depression), the bipolar disorders, and two disorders based on cause (i.e., due to a general medical condition or substance-induced mood disorder)

mood disorders with postpartum onset—Mood disorders characterized by more serious symptoms than increased crying, anxiety, and insomnia, including psychotic hallucinations and/or delusions. It can increase the risk of the mother harming herself or her baby. It is diagnosed if onset occurs within 4 weeks after childbirth

moral treatment—An approach to mental disorder based on humane psychosocial care or moral discipline that emerged in the 18th century and came to the fore for much of the 19th century, deriving partly from psychiatry or psychology and partly from religious or moral concerns. The movement is particularly associated with reform and development of the asylum system in Western Europe at that time. It fell into decline as a distinct method by the 20th century, however, due to overcrowding and misuse of asylums and the predominance of biomedical methods. The movement is widely seen as influencing certain areas of psychiatric practice up to the present day

motivational interviewing—A counseling approach that recognizes that consumers who need to make behavior changes approach intervention at different levels of readiness. This nonjudgmental approach attempts to increase consumers' awareness of potential problems faced by the behavior and to engage them in identifying reasons (motivations) for change

motor and praxis skills—Ability of planning of movement or motion in response to an environmental demand or occupational engagement

mourning—Behavioral action and integration of grief and bereavement

multicultural context—A person's family, community, and the effects of stigma associated with mental illness in society that influences their cultural identity

multifamily psychoeducation group (MFPG)—A group of families, other caregivers, and friends who participate in the psychoeducation. They are supportive of persons with mental illnesses working together with mental health professionals as part of an overall clinical treatment plan for people with mental illnesses

mythos reasoning—The use of images and stories rather than facts to persuade an audience

narrative—A short story about individual's life or health from his or her point of view

negative symptoms—Any abnormality indicative of a mental or physical disorder characterized by absence of typical function, such as flat affect, social withdrawal, and difficulty initiating activity

neighborhood profile—A description of important neighborhood characteristics and a visual map locating important resources and activities

neighborhood regeneration—Process of eliminating barriers and creating supports that promote satisfying and productive daily life for people in that community

nociception—The perception of physical pain

nonbizarre delusion—A belief that in actuality is untrue but is in the realm of possibility

non–rapid eye movement (NREM)—Slow oscillation of the eyes during the portion of the sleep cycle when no dreaming occurs

normal sensory function—An ability to effectively process the sensory information and result in an appropriate adaptive response

normalization—Any process that makes something more normal, which typically means conforming to some regularity or rule or returning from some state of abnormality

objective burden—The challenges of addressing a myriad of practical problems associated with mental illness including managing positive (e.g., hallucinations and delusions) and negative (e.g. lack of motivation, poor daily living skills and hygiene) symptoms and adapting to a family member's mood swings and socially inappropriate or self-destructive behaviors

obsessive-compulsive disorder—Anxiety disorder characterized by obsessions (which cause marked anxiety or distress) and/or compulsions (which serve to neutralize anxiety)

occupation—Everything people do to occupy themselves throughout a 24 hour day, including taking care of oneself (self-care), enjoying life (leisure), and contributing to social and economic everyday life in one's community (productivity)

occupational alienation—A sense of isolation, powerlessness, frustration, loss of control, and estrangement from society or self that results from engagement in occupation that does not satisfy inner needs

occupational balance—Balance in one's daily routines, appreciating that balance is influenced by cultural beliefs and context

occupational competence—The personal sense of achievement in one's performance of daily activities

occupational deprivation—State of prolonged preclusion from engagement in occupations of necessity and/or meaning due to factors outside the control of the individual

occupational enrichment—The deliberate manipulation of environments to facilitate and support engagement in a range of occupations congruent with those that the individual might normally perform

occupational justice—The equitable opportunity and resources to enable people's engagement in meaningful occupations

occupational profile—A method of systematically describing a person's occupational history, patterns of daily living, interests, values, and needs often performed at the beginning of a therapeutic relationship with an occupational therapy practitioner

occupational self-knowledge—An individual's insight of his or her occupational performance, which includes personal causation, interests, and values

occupational skills and capacities—An individual's ability to perform his or her occupations, including ADLs, work, and leisure activities that are important, meaningful, and purposeful to the individual

olfactory systems—Systems relating to the sense of smell

Olmstead v. L.C. and E.W.—A public entity shall administer services, programs, and activities in the most integrated setting appropriate to the needs of qualified individuals with disabilities A further prescription, here called the "reasonable-modifications regulation," requires public entities to "make reasonable modifications" to avoid "discrimination on the basis of disability" but does not require measures that would "fundamentally alter" the nature of the entity's programs

ombudsman—An official who is typically appointed by an agency, government, employer, or school and charged to investigate and address complaints reported by individuals

onsite model—A system specifically intended for students with psychiatric disabilities who already have developed the academic and social skills needed to begin coursework. In the onsite model, students attend college courses while simultaneously receiving supported education services in the form of individual counseling or a support group

operant conditioning—A procedure developed by B. F. Skinner in which a spontaneously emitted behavior (operant behavior) is either rewarded (reinforced) or punished and, as a result, then occurs with a frequency that is either increased (in the case of reinforcement) or decreased (in the case of punishment). It may be referred to as instrumental conditioning

opioids, or narcotics—Medications producing insensibility or stupor

oppositional defiant disorder (ODD)—Disorder where a recurrent pattern of negativistic, defiant, disobedient, and hostile behavior is displayed toward authority figures that persists for at least 6 months

pain—An unpleasant sensory and emotional experience associated with actual or potential tissue damage or described in terms of such damage

pain behavior—Actions or reactions that a person says or does (e.g., moaning or taking pain medication) or does not do (e.g., job attendance), which communicates to others the presence of pain. Pain behaviors are observable and readily influenced by spiritual, cultural, familial, and environmental factors

panic attack—Episode of the sudden onset of intense apprehension, fearfulness, or terror in a discrete period, often associated with feelings of impending doom. During these attacks, one experiences symptoms such as shortness of breath, palpitations, chest pain or discomfort, choking or smothering sensations, and fear of "going crazy" or losing control

panic disorder—Anxiety disorder characterized by recurrent unexpected panic attacks about which there is persistent concern, with or without agoraphobia

parasomnia—Any of several abnormal experiences or behaviors associated with sleep (e.g., bruxism, night terrors, or sleepwalking)

Parkinson's disease—A slowly progressive neurological condition usually resulting from deficiency of the neurotransmitter dopamine as the consequence of degenerative, vascular, or inflammatory changes in the basal ganglia; characterized by tremor, rigidity, bradykinesia, and postural instability

partial hospitalization programs (PHP)—A program used to treat mental illness and substance abuse. In partial hospitalization, the client continues to reside at home but commutes to a treatment center up to 7 days a week. Since partial hospitalization focuses on overall treatment of the individual, rather than purely on safety, the program is not used for acutely suicidal people

participation—The act of doing the occupation, planning for the occupation, maintaining a balance with other areas of occupation, and obtaining and appropriately using related tools and supplies

peer support programs—Informal private programs consisting of self-help groups and peer support systems where people in recovery provide services to one another to assist with any issues others may be having difficulty with in their life. These programs help them clarify their concerns and explore their available resources

performance capacity—The mental and physical abilities that underlie skilled performance

performance subsystem—One of the subsystems of the model of human occupation comprising the mental and physical constituents (e.g., bones, muscles, nervous system) that provide the capacity for the person to engage in occupational performance

personal agency—Ways in which people meet goals by being exercised individually

personal assistance services (PAS)—Services providing help to people with disabilities to assist them with tasks essential for daily living

personal causation—One of the components of a volitional system, which is personal assessment of abilities and closely linked to self-efficacy as a contributor to motivation

personal constitution—Physical, psychological, and emotional factors that influence an individual's spiritual context and outlook

personal context—Features of the individual that are not part of a health condition or health status which includes age, gender, socioeconomic and educational status

personal questioning—Occurs when a person continually asks himself or herself questions related to feelings of helplessness, fear, frustration, anxiety, and irritability, such as "Why me? How did I let this happen?"

personal spiritual experience—The individual's own source for spiritual, religious, and mystical experiences, which affects the degree to which the individual participates in spiritual practices and the value he or she places on the spiritual dimension of life

person-environment-occupation (PEO) model—A conceptual model used by occupational therapists to guide clinical reasoning and plan interventions. It emphasizes that occupational performance is influenced by the capacity of the individual, the characteristics of the occupation, and the resources and task demands of the environment

person-first language—A form of politically correct linguistic prescriptivism aiming to avoid perceived and subconscious dehumanization when discussing people suffering from disabilities. The basic idea is to replace, for example, "disabled people" with "people with disabilities," thus emphasizing that they are people first and the disability is second. Further, the concept favors the use of "having" rather than "being" (e.g., "she has a learning disability" instead of "she is learning disabled")

pervasive developmental disorder (PDD)—A class of childhood-onset disorders characterized by severe and pervasive impairment in several areas of development: reciprocal social interaction skills, communication skills, or the presence of stereotyped behavior, interests, and activities

phonological loop—Analogous to inner speech or what you do when you talk yourself through a task

photovoice—A methodology used in the field of health care and education that combines photography with grassroots social action. Participants are asked to represent their community or point of view by taking photographs and writing narratives that convey lived experience. It is often used among marginalized populations and is intended to give insight into how they conceptualize their circumstances. As a form of community consultation, photovoice attempts to bring the perspectives of those "who lead lives that are different from those traditionally in control of the means for imaging the world" into the policymaking process

physical context—The nonhuman aspects of contexts. which includes accessibility to and performance within environments; inclusive of natural terrain, plants, animals, buildings, furniture, objects, tools, or devices

physical harm reduction—One of the elements for eating disorder treatment via weight gain and/or symptom interruption to minimize risk

physicality—The state or quality of being physical

place-train approach/perspective—An approach that emphasizes placing a person in a housing or working situation first and then offering the training and support to facilitate successful everyday living

planning phase—The second stage of a wraparound process in which the team is brought together to review family strengths, develop a collaborative mission statement, identify needs across all life domains, prioritize those needs, and identify strategies and actions to meet those needs

play—Any spontaneous or organized activity that provides enjoyment, entertainment, amusement, or diversion

policy problem—Increased mental health costs and decreased access to mental health care

polygenic—Involving the combined action or effects of multiple genes

polysubstance dependence—Disorder reserved for behavior during the same 12-month period in which the person was repeatedly using at least three groups of substances (not including caffeine and nicotine) where no single substance predominates

positive symptoms—Any abnormality indicative of a mental or physical disorder characterized by aberrations in behavior or behavior that is not typically present in other individuals, such as hallucinations, delusions, disorganized thinking, and disorganized behavior

posterior cortical atrophy—A neurodegenerative disease that leads to a dementing syndrome involving distinct neuropsychological deficits of higher visuospatial functions. Although most patients are seen initially with neurological complaints, in some cases, secondary manifestations, such as affective symptoms, might appear in the foreground

posttraumatic stress disorder (PTSD)—Anxiety disorder characterized by the reexperiencing of an extremely traumatic event accompanied by symptoms of increased arousal and by avoidance of stimuli associated with the trauma, and numbed response to environmental stimuli

precontemplation—No thought or intention of changing in the near future. It is a similar concept of denial but based on little to no awareness of how a behavior might have serious disabling consequences

precontemplation stage—Stage during which a person resists change as he or she cannot see any reason to change the behaviors

preparation—The process of getting something ready for change when the person recognizes that the pros outweigh the cons in terms of changing

primary progressive aphasia—A form of dementia marked by the inability to recall the names of things, to read, or to express oneself with speech and gradually worsens possibly producing other cognitive deficits. Early in the course of the disease, brain functions pertaining to daily living are preserved (e.g., understanding speech, correct social behavior, and practicing hobbies). Associated with nonspecific degeneration of neurons in the left hemisphere of the brain

procedural memory—Memory about how to do something. Procedural memory takes longer to be created and is less susceptible to errors. It is also more implicit, meaning it is less consciously accessible

procovery—Attaining a productive and fulfilling life regardless of the level of health assumed attainable

prodromal period—The time between the emergence of early signs of the illness and the point at which the diagnostic criteria for the disorder are met

program for assertive community treatment (PACT)/assertive community treatment (ACT)—Community-based treatment, rehabilitation, and support services that help people with major mental illness improve to the point at which they can be discharged from the hospital, transfer into community living, and be connected with the services to support successful community integration

progressive—Typically used to describe the course of a disease in an unfavorable direction

progressive dementia—A type of dementia characterized by a gradual to rapid decline in the ability to care for oneself, including Alzheimer disease and vascular dementia, which make up 90% of all dementia-related disease

progressive muscle relaxation (PMR)—A strategy used to relieve excess tension that can result in muscle spasms, pain, and fatigue. PMR involves focusing attention on a muscle group, systematic tensing and relaxing of major musculoskeletal groups for several seconds, passive focusing of attention on how the tensed muscle feels, release of the muscles, and passive focusing on the sensations of relaxation

progressive supranuclear palsy—A disorder clinically seen as postural instability, along with falls and gait disturbances. The inability to gaze downward is an early sign. Oral motor involvement leads to dysarthria or speech disorders

protective factors—Factors that prevent the developmental process of eating, such as assertion skills; independence; autonomy; opportunity to invest in a variety of roles; ability to use stress management techniques; positive self-esteem; family environment that is not overly concerned with appearance, beauty, and thinness; family relationships that allow the person to develop a sense of belonging as well as individuation; and social environment that is not overly concerned with beauty and thinness

protracted duration—The experienced passage of time perceived as too slow

pseudostationary period—The third phase of Rett's disorder beginning once the second phase subsides and continuing for years or decades. It has also been termed the "wake-up" period and marks a time during which regression slows so that it is unapparent, and some communication skills may return

psychiatric rehabilitation (PsyR) or psychosocial rehabilitation—A combination of services incorporating social, educational, occupational, behavioral, and cognitive interventions aimed at long-term recovery and maximization of self-sufficiency

psychoeducation—A means of providing persons with psychiatric illnesses with the skills to comanage their illnesses. Skills taught may include improving adherence to treatment regimens, managing stressful events and symptom relapses, and enhancing social and familial function

psychosocial clubhouses—International community of people who share the lived experience of mental illness and recovery. They offer a physical place where people are afforded respect and varied opportunities to pursue valued and chosen occupations that hold meaning and purpose

psychosocial functional enablement—One of the elements for eating disorder treatment via individual and/or group psycho-educative, creative, and experiential occupation-focused activities to improve occupational performance and perceived self-competence

psychosocial interventions—Modalities designed to help clients attain independence, recovery, employment, meaningful interpersonal relationships, and improved quality of life

psychosocial issues—Concerns that include both psychological and social aspects

public housing agencies (PHAs)—A nonprofit organization that works to preserve and improve public and affordable housing through advocacy, research, policy analysis, and public education. As a multibillion-dollar asset, public housing is the cornerstone of affordable housing and community development

qualified individual with a disability—An individual with a disability who, with or without reasonable modification to rules, policies, or practices, the removal of architectural, communication, or transportation barriers, or the provision of auxiliary aids and services, meets the essential eligibility requirements for the receipt of services or the participation in programs or activities provided by a public entity

quota system—An individualized preset number of exercise or activity repetitions or duration based on a consumer's mean baseline scores

rational emotive behavior therapy (REBT)—A comprehensive, active-directive, philosophically and empirically based psychotherapy that focuses on resolving emotional and behavioral problems and disturbances and enabling people to lead happier and more fulfilling lives

readiness assessment—An assessment to determine whether an individual is ready to perform the worker role. Through this assessment, the person can identify the specific lifestyle and environmental changes he or she wants to make relative to the worker role

reasonable accommodations—Change in the work environment or in the way things are customarily done that enables an individual with a disability to enjoy equal employment opportunities

recidivism—Used to describe the repetition of antisocial acts as well as the relapse of a disease or behavioral pattern

recovery—A journey of healing and transformation enabling a person with a mental health problem to live a meaningful life in a community of his or her choice while striving to achieve his or her full potential

recovery movement—A political process shifting attention to the rights and needs of persons living with mental illness and emphasizing choice and self-determination as an individual pursues a life with personal purpose and meaning

recovery standards—State or federal policies that advocate for mental health recovery being addressed by all public mental health agencies

redefinition—The act of giving a new definition

reeducation—Efforts aimed at instilling new beliefs in people that are different from their previous ones

reentry centers—Structured and supervised residential settings for offenders just prior to or after their release from prison that support in job placement, counseling, and other services

regression—A return of symptoms or a more primitive mode of behavior due to loss of function

relapse—The recurrence of a disease or symptoms after a period of improvement or recovery

relatedness—Being connected; associated

religious observances—An organized system of beliefs, practices, rituals, and symbols designed to facilitate closeness to the sacred or transcendent

REM (rapid eye movement)—Symmetric, quick scanning eye movements occurring often during sleep commonly associated with dreaming

remediation—The correction of something bad or defective

remediation approach—Intervention approach in which cognitive impairment is targeted and intervention is directed at improving a particular skill

remission—Significant improvement or recovery from a condition which may or may not be permanent

representativeness heuristic—A rule of thumb wherein people judge the probability or frequency of a hypothesis by considering how much the hypothesis resembles available data

resident mobility—The movement of residents in and out of a neighborhood over time. High levels of resident mobility are believed to compromise the development and stability of social networks that could support occupation

resilience—A character trait associated with the ability to endure stressful situations without suffering the physiological or psychological consequences, such as illness or disease, typically associated with such adversity

respondent—The behavior elicited by a reflexive or classically conditioned stimulus

responsive social skills training—An intervention that combines problem-solving with social skills training in a group setting. In a responsive social skills training group, clients are invited to report any recent events that have occurred in their lives that they would like to work on with the group. In addition, clients are invited to identify social situations that they anticipate coming up in the future

restricting type—Subtype of anorexia nervosa described as presentations in which weight loss is accomplished primarily through dieting, fasting, or excessive exercise

Rett's disorder (RD)—A developmental disorder marked by mental retardation, impaired language use, breath holding and hyperventilation, seizures, loss of communication skills, tremors of the trunk, difficulty walking, and abnormally small development of the head, occurring almost exclusively in girls (in about one of every 10,000 to 15,000 female children) after the age of 6 to 18 months

salutogenesis—The sense of coherence describing people for whom life is viewed as manageable, meaningful, and comprehensible

schema—Mental representation that creates structure out of related concepts. Schema goes beyond categories in that it includes information about the relationship of a concept

school mental health—Mental health service that occurs in a school setting

scientific-minded—Approaching each new person without assumptions, while at the same time considering cultural hypotheses about that person that can be tested and modified

script—A type of schema that describes the sequence of events expected to occur in a familiar activity

secondary conditions—Diseases that an individual with an intellectual disability experiences at a higher rate than the general population and, in many cases, are preventable (e.g., hypertension, obesity, depression)

secure base—A caregiver who promotes exploration and learning about the environment by providing a safe, comfortable atmosphere

selective attention—Aspect of consciousness sorting out and focusing on the relevant sensory stimuli in the environment

selective norepinephrine reuptake inhibitors (SNRIs)—A group of chemical compounds that selectively inhibit reuptake of norepinephrine by the presynaptic neurons; thought to exert an antidepressant effect

selective serotonin reuptake inhibitors (SSRIs)—A class of drugs that selectively prevent the reuptake of serotonin; used for the treatment of depression, obsessive-compulsive behaviors, eating disorders, and social phobias

self-advocacy—Speaking up for oneself; it means that although a person with a disability may call upon the support of others, the individual is entitled to be in control of his or her own resources and how they are directed. It is about having the right to make life decisions without undue influence or control by others

self-contained classroom model—An approach that helps people reintegrate into mainstream educational classes in the future semesters. The self-contained classroom model is intended for people who have been out of school for a lengthy period of time and require skill building before fully entering postsecondary settings

self-determination—Refers to the freedom with which an individual can choose important life and occupational issues such as where to live, what to do with one's time, who to spend time with, and when, where and how to get help when experiencing a problem

self-monitoring—A self-regulatory or self-management process that involves paying deliberate attention to some aspect of one's behavior

self-regulation—A self-directive process through which learners transform their mental abilities into task-related skills for learning. Includes continuously monitoring progress toward a goal, checking outcomes, and redirecting unsuccessful efforts

self-reward value—The type of occupational value characterized by immediate rewards that are inherent in the experience of performing a certain occupation

self-stigma—The prejudice people with mental illness turn against themselves

semantic memory—Memory for facts

sensation avoiding—A pattern of sensory processing that is characterized by low threshold and active response; people with a processing preference of sensation avoidance create or choose environments that reduce sensory input. They can do well in low-stimulus situations or settings that others find dull

sensation seeking—A pattern of sensory processing characterized by high threshold and active response; sensation-seeking individuals actively engage with the environment to meet sensory needs

sense of self—The anthropological view of the person, which includes the person's understanding of what it means to be human, the components that constitute the self (e.g., body, spirit, soul, feelings, will, mind, and heart), and how the person perceives the self (e.g., lovable/unworthy, good/bad, or capable/incapable)

sensory dimensions—One dimension of pain including temporal, spatial, pressure, and thermal properties

sensory dysfunction—The neurological inability to properly process the sensory information and result in an inappropriate adaptive response

sensory integration—The neurobiological process involved in organizing multiple sensations from the environment and the person's own body. Sensory integration is followed by an adaptive response, which involves a purposeful, goal-directed response to a sensory experience

sensory integrative theory—The framework for understanding how behaviors, coordination, and development are impacted by the integration of sensory input at the neurobiological level

sensory modalities—Part of the nervous system responsible for processing sensory information. Commonly recognized sensory systems are those for vision, hearing, somatic sensation (touch), taste, and olfaction (smell). However, there are two additional senses, the proprioceptive and vestibular senses, that provide information essential to effective movement

sensory processing—The means by which an individual obtains information about the world and his or her own body. Sensory processing is the larger construct that encompasses sensory integration

sensory processing disorder—Characterized by an inability to interpret and organize varied stimuli, including those acquired by the following 7 senses: tactile, proprioceptive, visual, vestibular, auditory, gustatory, and olfactory

sensory sensitivity—A pattern of sensory processing characterized by low sensory thresholds and a passive self-regulation strategy; when people have a sensory sensitivity pattern of sensory processing, they notice things that others do not notice

sensory-perceptual skills—Ability to receive and differentiate varied types of sensory stimuli

serious leisure—The systematic pursuit of an amateur, hobbyist, or volunteer core activity that is highly substantial, interesting, and fulfilling and where, in the typical case, participants find a career in acquiring and expressing a combination of its special skills, knowledge, and experience

service integration—Integration of mental health and substance abuse services

severe emotional disturbance (SED)—A diagnosable mental, behavioral, or emotional disorder that severely disrupts people's ability to function socially, academically, and emotionally at home, in school, or in the community, and has been apparent for more than 6 months

shock—A sudden disturbance, either mental or physical

short-term memory—The phase of the memory process in which stimuli that have been recognized and registered are stored briefly. While decay occurs rapidly, typically within seconds, information may be held indefinitely by using rehearsal as a holding process by which to recycle material repeatedly through short-term memory

simpatico—The ability to empathize with others and remain agreeable, even if it means personal sacrifice

situational assessments—An assessment of work function of people with psychiatric disabilities. This assessment is intended to elicit the person's perceptions of their job search and job-retention experiences and to fully understand the person's behavioral success

sleep architecture—The organization of brain wave activity related to each of the stages of sleep

sleep debt—A physical condition of tiredness due to inadequate sleep

sleep hygiene—The use of effective lifestyles choices to support good sleep, such as monitoring caffeine, nicotine, and alcohol intake; not exercising too close to bedtime; keeping a regular sleep schedule; using bedtime routines; and maintaining an effective sleep environment

sleep-related breathing disorders—Disorders marked by sleep disruption, leading to excessive sleepiness or insomnia judged to be due to abnormalities of ventilation during sleep such as sleep apnea

sleep-related movement disorders—Disorders marked by the involuntary body movement during sleep

social capital—Community assets that engender cooperation among community members: interpersonal networks, bonds, and institutions that support communities, maintain their cohesiveness, and help them cope with crises

social cognition—The processes and functions that allow a person to understand, act on, and benefit from the interpersonal world

social context—The availability and expectations of significant individuals, such as family, friends, and caregivers. Includes larger social groups influential in establishing norms, role expectations, and social routines

social exclusion—A multidimensional process of progressive social change where groups and individuals are detached from social relations and institutions thereby preventing them from full participation in the typical activities of the society in which they live

social justice—The ideal of a just society in which social relations and social conditions are fair and equal, particularly in regard to the poorest and most marginalized members of society

social learning theory or social cognitive theory—The approach by which people learn new behavior through overt reinforcement or punishment or via observational learning of the social factors in their environment. If people observe positive, desired outcomes in the observed behavior, then they are more likely to model, imitate, and adopt the behavior themselves

social persuasion—Verbal encouragement

social phobia—Any of a variety of phobic disorders characterized by clinically significant anxiety provoked by exposure to certain types of social or performance situations, often leading to avoidance of these situations

social skills—An ability to facilitate interaction and communication with others. Social rules and relations are created, communicated, and changed in verbal and nonverbal ways. The process of learning such skills is called socialization

social skills training (SST)—A process of optimizing social functioning of individuals with disabilities and improving their repertoire of skills for community functioning such as identifying and mending problems in social relationships, daily life, work, and leisure

socializing techniques—Learning processes directed towards effective group participation

sociocultural contexts—Milieus shaped by the accepted norms, rules, assumptions, and expectations governing what is understood to be significant within a particular community or social group as well as what is taken to be or not to be appropriate

Socratic questioning—Disciplined, deep, and systematic questioning that can be used to pursue thought in many directions and for many purposes, including to explore complex ideas, to get to the truth of things, to open up issues and problems, to uncover assumptions, to analyze concepts, to distinguish what we know from what we do not know, and to follow logical implications of thought

somatic/emotional states—The physical and emotional response to an activity

specialty care system—The "traditional" mental health continuum of specialty services, such as specialty inpatient units, partial hospitalization programs, and intensive outpatient programs

spiritual context—The primary orientation of a person's life which inspires and motivates that individual; it is the essence of the person giving meaning and substance to the person's life

spiritual environment—The experience of conscious involvement in the project of life integration through self-transcendence toward the ultimate value one perceives

spiritual occupation—Reflections, narratives, and actions that are meaningful, uplifting to the spirit, affirm life, and generate positive and loving connections to a greater power, self, others, and/or the world. When spiritual occupations are a part of a person's daily routines, they can be understood as important to their sense of wellbeing and can contribute to a person's recovery process

spirituality—Experiencing a meaningful connection to our core self, others, the world, and/or a Greater Power, as expressed through our reflections, narratives, and actions

stable dynamic factors—Characteristics that remain unchanged for longer periods of time but are treatable, such as alcoholism, drug abuse, or attitudes toward violence

stages of change model—A model for changing health behaviors including addictions. It is also referred to as the transtheoretical model

state hospitals—Public institutions that provide inpatient services to those with serious mental illness

states—Characteristics associated with a specific point in time and circumstance

static dementia—Dementia characterized by the degree of cognitive impairment that can remain relatively stable for years, by such as that caused by traumatic brain injury or stroke. If the dementia is due to a static condition, there may be some improvement, a stepwise decline, or a plateau in decline, although full recovery is rare

static risk factors—Unchanging characteristics of the individual, such as their age at first offense, gender, or history of prior convictions or violence

stigma—An attribute that is deeply discrediting, resulting in the marginalization of that person in the eyes of others

stress inoculation training—A cognitive-behavioral treatment for posttraumatic stress disorder. The basic goal of stress inoculation training is to help a person gain confidence in his or her ability to cope with anxiety and fear stemming from reminders of the trauma. During stress inoculation training, the therapist helps the client become more aware of reminders (also called "cues") of fear and anxiety. In addition, clients learn a variety of coping skills that are useful in managing anxiety, such as muscle relaxation and deep breathing

stressor sequences—A cascade of adversity, often resulting from a single event, such as loss of a job

structural stigma—A sociopolitical process in which the policies of private or governmental structures restrict the opportunities of stigmatized groups

subjective burden—Emotional responses of dealing with catastrophic events including feelings of grief; symbolic loss of the hopes, dreams, and aspirations that were held for a loved one with mental illness; a sense of chronic sorrow; empathic pain; and the emotional "roller coaster" that individuals may feel they are riding during the relapse and remission their loved one experiences; feelings of anger, guilt, and resentment

substance abuse—A maladaptive pattern of substance use manifested by recurrent and significant adverse consequences related to the repeated use of substances

substance dependence—A substance use disorder characterized by having cognitive, behavioral, and physiological symptoms indicating that the individual continues use of the substance despite significant substance-related problems

substance-induced disorders—Disorders related to drug use but excluding drug dependency. Substance-induced disorders include intoxication, withdrawal, and other substance-induced mental disorders such as delirium and psychosis

substance intoxication—Characterized by the development of a reversible substance-specific syndrome due to recent ingestion of (or exposure to) a substance

substance-related disorders—Disorder related to taking a drug of abuse (including alcohol), to the side effects of a medication, and to toxin exposure. Substance-related disorders are divided into two groups: substance use disorders and substance-induced disorders

substance use disorders—Disorders that include substance dependence and substance abuse. Substance use disorders include both dependence on and abuse of drugs usually taken voluntarily for the purpose of their effect on the central nervous system or to prevent or reduce withdrawal symptoms

substance withdrawal—A substance-induced disorder characterized by the development of a substance-specific maladaptive behavioral change, with physiological and cognitive concomitants, due to the cessation of, or reduction in, heavy and prolonged substance use

suffering—The negative affective response to pain. Suffering is personal and can be manifest as fear, anxiety, or depression

supported education—The process of helping people with a diagnosis of mental illness participate in an education program so they may receive the education and training they need to achieve their learning and recovery goals and become gainfully employed in the job or career of their choice

supported employment (SE)—A competitive employment arrangement for people with disabilities that includes integration within their community

supported socialization—One method that can assist individuals with mental illness to engage in social and recreational activities in their natural environment

supported/supportive housing—The approach to match the needs of the consumer with the appropriate housing type, which is linked to the amount of support necessary. The consumer then moves from one level of care to another as his or her level of support needs changes

supportive social environment—An essential factor in a client's ability to change dysfunctional beliefs and to develop more adaptive beliefs as part of psychosocial recovery

susto—Spanish term described as a folk illness associated with Latino cultures. Similar to posttraumatic stress disorder, susto occurs after an individual experiences a shocking or frightening experience. The belief is that the situation is so frightening that it causes the soul to leave the body

symbolic value—The type of occupational value characterized by what an occupation signifies for a person, for example, strengthening his or her gender identity or the bonds to a certain group or culture

synchronicity—A normal relationship between experience and time passage

syndrome—A group of symptoms, signs, laboratory findings, and physiological disturbances that are linked by a common anatomical, biochemical, or pathological history, usually defining a disease

taijinkyofusho (TKS)—Japanese term similar in meaning to social phobia in the West. The phobia in TKS is manifested as fear of offending others, while in Western cultures, social phobia most often involves a fear of embarrassment or humiliation

temporal compression—The experienced passage of time which seems to have quickened

temporal context—Stage of life, as well as time of day, year, and duration; the location of occupational performance in time. May be both external and internal, including objective and subject perception of time

TIC TOC technique—Procedure that focuses on identifying and reframing thoughts or cognitions that interfere with undertaking and accomplishing desired tasks. First, the client identifies a task that he or she wants or needs to do but is avoiding or resisting. Then the client completes a three-column worksheet that includes identification of TICS (task interfering cognitions), related thought distortions (e.g., emotional reasoning, all-or-nothing thinking, minimization, mind-reading, or overgeneralization), and a reframed TOC (task-oriented cognition) related to the problematic task

tolerance—The point at which an individual stops exercising due to pain or fatigue

traits—Enduring characteristics that exist across situations

transactional model—A framework for evaluating the processes of coping with stressful events. Stressful experiences are construed as person–environment transactions that depend on the impact of an external stressor. The person's appraisal of the stressor and the social and cultural resources at his or her disposal contribute to the framework from which a person learns healthy coping.

transcultural health care—Formal areas of study and practice in the cultural beliefs, values, and lifeways of diverse cultures and in the use of knowledge to provide culture-specific or culture-universal care to individuals, families, and groups of particular cultures

transdisciplinary teams—Teams consisting of members informed by the theories and strategies of the other disciplines involved. Transdisciplinary team members are dedicated to learning and working across disciplinary boundaries. The child's family is considered an integral part of the team and is empowered to participate in assessment, goal planning, and treatment

transition phase—The last stage of the wraparound process in which the initial plan of care has been implemented and modified over time, and the appropriate interventions have been successfully delivered to produce the desired outcomes. This phase occurs in a thoughtful manner that engages the entire team in decision-making, supports rather than abandons, and helps people move to a life free of system interference rather than simply moving people from services

transitional employment (TE)—One of the oldest of the employment models, usually described in relationship to the psychosocial clubhouse. The goal of transitional employment is to give individuals work experience so they are able to transition into other jobs that will enhance their self-sufficiency

traumatic grief—A disorder that reflects the traumatic distress experience of the bereaved person. The symptoms of traumatic grief include intrusive thoughts about the deceased, yearning for the deceased, searching for the deceased, and loneliness as a result of the death

treatment mall approach—Decentralized program with clients coming from different areas of the hospital to attend the program. It is structured around an educational or classroom model, with a large selection of courses available for patients to choose from

tricyclic antidepressants (TCAs)—One of a group of antidepressant drugs so named because of their three-ringed structure; they inhibit the uptake of serotonin and noradrenaline but cause anticholinergic side effects

typical antipsychotics—Dopamine antagonists, which work primarily by blocking D2 receptors in the brain and are used to treat psychosis (in particular, schizophrenia). They may also be used for the treatment of acute mania, agitation, and other conditions

unconditional positive regard—Blanket acceptance and support of a person regardless of what the person says or does

unipolar—Just one side of the affective spectrum

unipolar depression—A mood disorder characterized by recurrent episodes of depression, which is the low, sad, unpleasant mood of an extreme in the continuum of typical moods

unitary disorder—Presence of only one diagnosis, either a mental health diagnosis or a substance use disorder

universalist—A person who sees a disability from a social perspective, recognizing the need to examine the broader contexts beyond personal factors that impact the social participation of individuals with disabilities

validation—A communication technique used for clients with moderate to late dementia in which the caregiver makes statements to the client that demonstrate respect for the client's feelings and beliefs. This method helps prevent argumentative and agitated behavior

values—One of the components of a volitional system, which is a set of beliefs about what is important and worthy for the individual

vascular dementia—A steplike deterioration in intellectual functions with focal neurologic signs, such as the result of multiple infarctions of the cerebral hemispheres

vestibular system—Systems interpreting stimuli from the inner ear receptors regarding head position and movement and is responsible for balance through detection of the position and movement of the head in space

vigilance—Ability to sustain attention over time

virtual environment—An environment in which communication occurs by means of airways or computers and an absence of physical contact; it includes, among a broad variety of electronic methods of communication, e-mail, Internet searches, electronic monitoring of seniors in their homes or institutions, social networking, and telerehabilitation

visuospatial sketchpad—A tool that plays a role in spatial orientation and problem-solving that involves visual input around locating objects and the self. People use it to find their way around a building as well as in smaller spaces such as organizing words and sentences on a page

volition—A person's motivation for action and different occupations. Volition is one of the subsystems of model of human occupation. It influences both the individual's choice of occupation and his or her persistence when engaging in that occupation

voluntary admissions—The process of accepting clients. The concept includes clients accepted for medical and nursing care in a hospital or other health care institution

voluntary sector—The sphere of social activity undertaken by organizations that are for nonprofit and nongovernmental. This sector is also called the third sector, in reference to the public sector and the private sector. Civic sector is another term for the sector, emphasizing the sector's relationship to civil society. It includes support groups, advocacy, and self-help resources

waiver—An exemption from some aspect of a federal/state/local health care statute that gives a facility the right to deliver care in a manner that varies from published standards

wholeness—The concept that the entire family is greater than the sum of each individual family member

Woodley House—A series of nationally recognized programs based on a unique residential care recovery approach. Woodley House provides varying mental health services to over 300 consumers each year. A compassionate continuum of care, Woodley House leads the way in returning people suffering from mental illness to productive and independent lives

working memory—Process for short-term memory storage and active manipulation of new information; that is, the person is "working with" the information temporarily

work-ordered day—A building block of the clubhouse philosophy; each day is structured to mirror the expectations and relationships of a workplace for preparing members for future employment

wraparound—A planning process that brings people together from different parts of the whole family's life. With help from one or more facilitators, people from the family's life work together, coordinate their activities, and blend their perspectives of the family's situation

zeitgeber—A cue in nature that keeps the human body well organized with a recurring and physiologically varying 24-hour cycle. Zeitgebers entrain the body to nature's rhythms, telling it when to sleep, wake, be highly active, or relax

Index of Assessments

Because this textbook is organized according to the person-environment-occupation model rather than assessments, different assessment measures are interspersed throughout the chapters. This index was developed as a reference tool to enable readers to quickly identify the chapters in which a particular assessment is addressed. Entries refer to the chapter(s), and not the page number, where the content on the relevant assessment is found. In some cases, an assessment is discussed in detail, whereas in other cases, it is simply identified as a relevant measure.

Index of Interventions

Because this textbook is organized according to the person-environment-occupation model rather than interventions, different intervention methods are interspersed throughout the chapters. This index was developed as a reference tool to enable readers to quickly identify the chapters in which a particular intervention is addressed. Entries refer to the chapter(s), and not the page number, where the content on the relevant intervention is found. In some cases, an intervention is discussed in detail, whereas in other cases, it is simply identified as a relevant method.

Index